# NCLEX-RN® REVIEW

## Sixth Edition

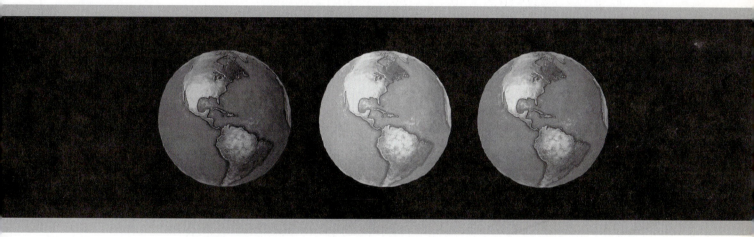

Rebecca Caldwell Oglesby, MSN, RN

Instructor of Nursing, BSN Program
The Presbyterian School of Nursing at Queens University of Charlotte
Charlotte, North Carolina

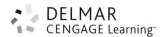

DELMAR
CENGAGE Learning™

Australia • Canada • Mexico • Singapore • Spain • United Kingdom • United States

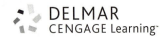
**DELMAR**
CENGAGE Learning™

**NCLEX-RN® Review, Sixth Edition**
Rebecca Caldwell Oglesby

Vice President, Career and Professional Editorial:
Dave Garza

Director of Learning Solutions: Matthew Kane

Senior Acquisitions Editor: Maureen Rosener

Managing Editor: Marah Bellegarde

Senior Product Manager: Patricia Gaworecki

Editorial Assistant: Meaghan O'Brien

Vice President, Career and Professional Marketing:
Jennifer McAvey

Marketing Director: Wendy Mapstone

Senior Marketing Manager: Michele McTighe

Marketing Coordinator: Scott Chrysler

Production Director: Carolyn Miller

Production Manager: Andrew Crouth

Senior Content Project Manager: Stacey Lamodi

Senior Art Director: Jack Pendleton

Technology Project Manager: Erin Zeggert

For product information and technology assistance, contact us at
**Cengage Learning Customer & Sales Support, 1-800-354-9706**
For permission to use material from this text or product, submit all requests online at **www.cengage.com/permissions.**
Further permissions questions can be e-mailed to
**permissionrequest@cengage.com**

Library of Congress Control Number: 2008930400

ISBN-13: 978-1-4180-5315-4

ISBN-10: 1-4180-5315-5

**Delmar**
5 Maxwell Drive
Clifton Park, NY 12065-2919
USA

Cengage Learning is a leading provider of customized learning solutions with office locations around the globe, including Singapore, the United Kingdom, Australia, Mexico, Brazil, and Japan. Locate your local office at: **international.cengage.com/region**

Cengage Learning products are represented in Canada by Nelson Education, Ltd.

To learn more about Delmar, visit **www.cengage.com/delmar**

Purchase any of our products at your local college store or at our preferred online store **www.ichapters.com**

Printed in Canada
1 2 3 4 5 6 7 12 11 10 09

# Dedication

For my husband Mike, who patiently endured this work;
For my colleagues, who never doubted me;
For dear friends, who believed in me;
For Echo Heron, who inspired me;
For nursing students, whose compassion I revere.

# A Message from the National Student Nurses' Association

The National Student Nurses' Association (NSNA) is pleased to bring you the NSNA endorsed *NCLEX-RN® Review*, Sixth Edition. Using this book will better prepare you to meet the challenge of passing the exam the first time around.

NSNA is committed to the professional development of today's nursing student. We recognize the challenges of succeeding in today's complex health care environment. This outstanding book maintains high standards both in content and in presentation. The contributing experience of the clinicians and educators will help you achieve NCLEX success!

# CONTENTS

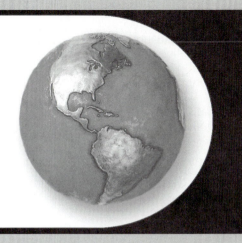

## UNIT 1
## PREPARING FOR THE NCLEX EXAMINATION • 1

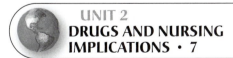

## UNIT 2
## DRUGS AND NURSING IMPLICATIONS • 7

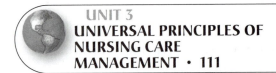

UNIT 3
**UNIVERSAL PRINCIPLES OF NURSING CARE MANAGEMENT · 111**

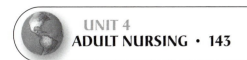

UNIT 4
ADULT NURSING • 143

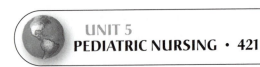

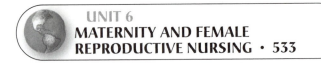

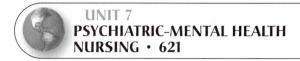

## UNIT 7
## PSYCHIATRIC-MENTAL HEALTH NURSING · 621

## APPENDIX · 685

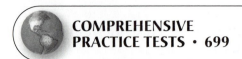

## COMPREHENSIVE PRACTICE TESTS · 699

# CONTRIBUTORS

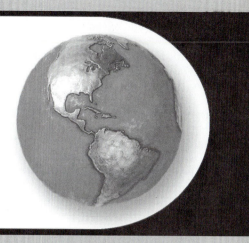

## EDITOR

**Rebecca Caldwell Oglesby, MSN, RN**
Instructor of Nursing, BSN Program
The Presbyterian School of Nursing at Queens University
   of Charlotte
Charlotte, North Carolina

## CONTRIBUTORS

**Margaret Ahearn-Spera, RN, C, MSN**
Director, Medical Patient Care Services
Danbury Hospital
Danbury, Connecticut
Assistant Clinical Professor
Yale University School of Nursing
New Haven, Connecticut

**Cynthia Blank-Reid, RN, MSN, CEN**
Trauma Clinical Nurse Specialist
Temple University Hospital
Philadelphia, Pennsylvania
Clinical Adjunct Associate Professor
Drexel University College of Nursing and Health Professions
Philadelphia, Pennsylvania

**Elizabeth Blunt, PhD (c), MSN**
Assistant Professor and Director, Graduate Nursing
   Programs
Drexel University College of Nursing and Health Professions
Philadelphia, Pennsylvania

**Margaret Brenner, RN, MSN**
Senior Consultant
Pinnacle Healthcare Group, Inc.
Paoli, Pennsylvania

**Nancy Clarkson, MEd, RN, BC**
Professor and Chairperson
Department of Nursing
Finger Lakes Community College
Canandaigua, New York

**Deborah L. Dalrymple, RN, MSN, CRNI**
Associate Professor of Nursing
Montgomery County Community College
Blue Bell, Pennsylvania

**Judy Donlen, DNSc, RN**
Executive Director, Southern New Jersey
Perinatal Cooperative
Pennsauken, New Jersey

**Judith L. Draper, APRN, BC**
Assistant Professor
Drexel University College of Nursing and Health Professions
Philadelphia, Pennsylvania

**Theresa M. Fay-Hillier, MSN, RN, CS**
Adjunct Faculty
Drexel University College of Nursing and Health Professions
Philadelphia, Pennsylvania

**Marcia R. Gardner, MA, RN, CPNP, CPN**
Assistant Professor
Drexel University College of Nursing and Health
   Professions
Philadelphia, Pennsylvania

**Jeanne Gelman, MSN, MA, RN**
Professor Emeritus, Psychiatric-Mental Health Nursing
Widener University
Chester, Pennsylvania

**Theresa M. Giglio, MS, RD**
Instructor, LaSalle University
Philadelphia, Pennsylvania

**Judith M. Hall, RNC, MSN, IBCLC, LCCE, FACCE**
Mary Washington Hospital
Fredericksburg, Virginia

**Marilyn Herbert-Ashton, MS, RN, BC**
Virginia Western Community College
Roanoke, VA

**Marilyn Herbert-Ashton, RN, C, MS**
Director, Wellness Center
F. F. Thompson Health Systems, Inc.
Adjunct Professor of Nursing
Finger Lakes Community College
Canandaigua, New York

**Holly Hillman, RN, MSN**
Assistant Professor
Montgomery County Community College
Blue Bell, Pennsylvania

**Lorraine C. Igo, MSN, EdD, RN**
Assistant Professor
Drexel University College of Nursing and
    Health Professions
Philadelphia, Pennsylvania

**Nancy H, Jacobson, MSN, APRN-BC, CS**
Staff Development Coordinator
Rydal Park
Rydal, Pennsylvania

**Nancy H. Jacobson, RN, CS, MSN**
Senior Manager
The Whitman Group
Huntington Valley, Pennsylvania

**Charlotte D. Kain, EdD, RN, C**
Professor Nursing, Health Care of Women
Montgomery County Community College
Blue Bell, Pennsylvania

**Roseann Tirotta Kaplan, MSN, RN, CS**
Adjunct Faculty
Drexel University College of Nursing and Health Professions
Philadelphia, Pennsylvania

**Constance O. Kolva Taylor, MSN, RN**
Kolva Consulting
Harrisburg, Pennsylvania

**Mary Lou Manning, PhD, CPNP, RN**
Director, Infection Control and Occupational Health
The Children's Hospital of Philadelphia
Adjunct Assistant Professor
University of Pennsylvania School of Nursing
Philadelphia, Pennsylvania

**Judith C. Miller, MSN, RN**
President, Nursing Tutorial and Consulting Services
Clifton, Virginia

**Eileen Moran, MSN, RN, C**
Clinical Educator
Abington Memorial Hospital
Abington, Pennsylvania

**Marie O'Toole, EdD, RN**
Associate Professor, College of Nursing
Rutgers, The State University of New Jersey
Newark. New Jersey

**Faye A. Pearlman, MSN, RN, MBA**
Assistant Professor
Drexel University College of Nursing and Health Professions
Philadelphia, Pennsylvania

**Janice Selekman, DNSc, RN**
Professor and Chair
Department of Nursing
University of Delaware
Newark. Delaware

**Robert Shearer, CRNA, MSN**
Assistant Professor
Drexel University College of Nursing and Health Professions
Philadelphia, Pennsylvania

**Magdeleine Vasso, MSN, RN**
Assistant Professor
Drexel University College of Nursing and Health Professions
Philadelphia, Pennsylvania

**Anne Robin Waldman, MSN, RN, C, AOCN**
Clinical Nurse Specialist
Albert Einstein Medical Center
Philadelphia, Pennsylvania

**Virginia R. Wilson, MSN, RN, CEN**
Assistant Professor, Graduate Nursing Programs
Drexel University College of Nursing and Health Professions
Philadelphia, Pennsylvania

## TEST ITEM WRITERS

**Frances Amorim, MSN, RN**
Clinical Lecturer
University of Pennsylvania, School of Nursing
Philadelphia. Pennsylvania

**Eileen B. Augente, MA, RN, CDE**
Instructor, Long Island University
Brooklyn, New York
Clinical Nurse Specialist, Diabetes
Amityville, New York

**Pamela Bellefeuille, RN, CS, CEN, TRNCCP, MN**
Clinical Nurse Specialist, Manager
Emergency Department, Kaiser
Santa Rosa, California

**Jean E. Berry, MSN, RN**
Assistant Professor
Bloomsburg University
Bloomsburg, Pennsylvania

**Janice Caie-Lawrence, MSN, RN**
Assistant Professor
University of Detroit Mercy
Detroit, Michigan

**Susan Chaney, MSE, RN, C**
Staff Nurse, Harbor View Mercy Hospital
Psychiatric Division of St. Edward Mercy
    Medical Center
Fort Smith, Arkansas

**Jane A. Claffy, MSN, RN, C**
St. Vincent's Hospital School of Nursing
New York City, New York

**H. Allethaire Cullen, RNP, CS, MSN, CEN**
Director of Education
Education Empowerment
Coventry, Rhode Island

**Janet Curley, EdD(C), RN, CEN**
Adjunct Lecturer
Pace University
New York, New York

**Sandra H. Faria, DSN, RN**
Florida State University School of Nursing
Tallahassee, Florida

**Elizabeth A. Fisk, MS, RN**
Associate Professor
Fitchburg State College
Fitchburg, Massachusetts

**Judith M. Hall, RNC, MSN, IBCLC, LCCE, FACCE**
Lactation Consultant and Childbirth Educator
Mary Washington Hospital
Fredericksburg, Virginia

**Shirley Sullivan Hall, MSN, RN**
Assistant Professor
School of Nursing Hampton University
Hampton, Virginia

**Janice L. Hinkle, MSN, RN, CNRN**
Instructor
Thomas Jefferson University
Philadelphia, Pennsylvania

**Susan Jaskowski, MSN, CCRN, CRNP, RN**
Pediatric Neurosurgery Nurse Practitioner
Penn State University Hershey Medical Center
Hershey, Pennsylvania

**Nancy Kirk, MSN, RN**
Lead Instructor, Medical Surgical Nursing and
    Pharmacology
The Health Institute of Tampa Bay
St. Petersburg, Florida

**Kathleen I. Marchiondo, MSN, RN**
Assistant Professor
Research College of Nursing
Kansas City, Missouri

**Cheryl Martin, MSN, RN, C**
Associate Professor of Nursing
Bethel College
Mishawaka, Indiana

**Patricia A. Middlemiss, MSN, RN**
Assistant Professor of Nursing
Gwynedd-Mercy College
Gwynedd Valley, Pennsylvania

**Anna P. Moore, MS, RN**
Assistant Professor
Southside Regional Medical Center
School of Nursing
Petersburg, Virginia

**Patricia A. Mynaugh, PhD, RN**
Associate Professor
Villanova University College of Nursing
Villanova, Pennsylvania

**Lynda C. Opdyke, MSN, RN**
Facilitator, Academic Affairs
Mercy School of Nursing
Charlotte, North Carolina

**Joan Opelia, MSN, RN**
Consultant
Nursing Tutorial and Consulting Services
Clifton, Virginia

**Deborah L. Panning, MSN, RN, C**
Unit Manager
Brandywine Hospital School of Nursing
Coatesville, Pennsylvania

**Carol Park, MSN, RN, CS**
School of Nursing
Sentara Norfolk General Hospital
Norfolk, Virginia

**Mary Reuland, MS, RN**
College of St. Catherine
Minneapolis Campus
Minneapolis, Minnesota

**Kathy Rodgers, MSN, RN, CNS, CCRN, CEN**
Critical Care Clinical Nurse Specialist
St. Elizabeth Hospital
Beaumont, Texas

**Mary Jean Ricci, MSN, RN, C**
Holy Family College
Philadelphia, Pennsylvania

**Nancy G. Runton, MSN, CPNP**
Pediatric Nurse Practitioner
Virginia Pediatric Group, LTD
Fairfax, Virginia

**Linda F. Samson, PhD, RNC, CNAA**
Dean, School of Health Sciences
Clayton State College
Morrow, Georgia

**Fran Schuda, MSN, RN, CCRN**
Director, Training and Development
Episcopal Hospital
Philadelphia, Pennsylvania

**Ruth Schumacher, MSN, RN**
Lecturer, Department of Maternal-Child Nursing
College of Nursing
The University of Illinois at Chicago
Chicago, Illinois

**Cheryl J. Smally, MSN, MSS, RN**
St. Luke's College of Nursing and Health Sciences
Sioux City, Iowa

**Lorry L. Smith, MSN, RN**
Clinical instructor, Baccalaureate Nursing
Eastern Kentucky University
Richmond, Kentucky

**Diane L. Spatz, PhD, RN, C**
University of Pennsylvania
Philadelphia, Pennsylvania

**Martha L. Tanicala, MSN, RN, CPN**
Instructor
St. Vincent Medical Center School of Nursing
Toledo, Ohio

**Susanne M. Tracy, MN, MA, RN**
Associate Professor
Rivier—St. Joseph School of Nursing
Nashua, New Hampshire

**Rosemarie Trouton, MSN, RN**
Clinical Nurse Educator, Pediatrics
Hershey Medical Center
Hershey. Pennsylvania

**Wanda May Webb, MSN, RN, CS**
Level Coordinator
Brandywine School of Nursing
Coatesville, Pennsylvania

**Mary Jo Westien, MS, APRN, CS**
Brigham Young University
Provo, Utah

**Diane Wieland, MSN, RN, CS**
Assistant Professor
Thomas Jefferson University
College of Allied Health Sciences
Department of Nursing
Philadelphia, Pennsylvania

**Judy Winterhalter, DNSc, RN, CS**
Associate Professor
Gwynedd-Mercy College
Gwynedd Valley, Pennsylvania
Psychotherapist
North Penn Counseling Center
Lansdale, Pennsylvania

**Evelyn Wolynies, MSN, RN**
Clinical Nurse Specialist
Neuropsych Huntington's Disease
University of Medicine and Dentistry of New Jersey
Cooper Hospital
Camden, New Jersey

**Catherine Y. Zion, MS, RN**
Clinical Instructor
Macon College School of Nursing
Macon, Georgia

## REVIEWERS

**Judy Bourrand, MSN, RN**
Ida V. Moffett School of Nursing
Samford University
Birmingham, Alabama

**Mary Kathie Doyle, BS, CCRN**
Instructor
Maria College
Troy, New York

**Mary Lashley, PhD, RN, CS**
Associate Professor
Towson University
Towson, Maryland

**Melissa Lickteig, EdD, RN**
Instructor, School of Nursing
Georgia Southern University
Statesboro, Georgia

**Darlene Mathis, MSN, RN APRN, BC, NP-C, CRNP**
Assistant Professor
Ida V. Moffett School of Nursing
Samford University
Birmingham, Alabama

**Barbara McGraw, MSN, RN**
Instructor
Central Community College
Grand Island, Nebraska

**Carol Meadows, MNSc, RNP, APN**
Eleanor Mann School of Nursing
University of Arkansas
Fayetteville, Arkansas

**Maria Smith, DSN, RN, CCRN**
Professor, School of Nursing
Middle Tennessee State University
Murfreesboro, Tennessee

# PREFACE

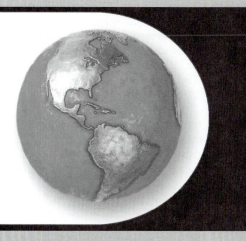

Endorsed by the National Student Nurses' Association (NSNA), the *NCLEX-RN® Review, Sixth Edition* has been developed expressly to meet your needs as you study and prepare for the all-important NCLEX-RN® licensure examination. Taking this exam is always a stressful event in the best of circumstances; it constitutes a major career milestone and NCLEX success is the key to your future ability to practice as a registered nurse.

## NEW TO THIS EDITION

The *NCLEX-RN® Review, Sixth Edition* has been revised to meet the standards set by the National Council's State Boards of Nursing's (NCSBN) most current test plan. More than 3000 unique and challenging NCLEX questions have been included. Additionally, each question is followed by a comprehensive rationale for each answer given as well as the identifying areas of cognitive level, client need, nursing process, and subject area. Additional emphasis on pharmacology and delegation in the form of 500 new questions has been added throughout the practice material since these areas have a greater emphasis on the actual exam.

Alternative format questions are throughout the practices tests and include the newest addition to the exam: the charting question. These new questions have been added to the test-taking software included with the book.

New content currently being tested on the exam is included in the text such as conscious sedation, complementary and alternative medicine (CAM), and herbal medicines.

More user-friendly charts and images have been included throughout the review content, followed by diet and nutrition appendices and eleven 100-question practice tests.

## Test-Taking Software

The CD-ROM included with this text holds a pool of over 3000 questions (2000 new, 1100 from text) in an environment that simulates the test taking experience. Tests are downloaded in varying lengths just like the actual exam. You can test your knowledge and test taking skills in two ways: learning and test modes. In learning mode, the rationale for correct and incorrect responses are immediately given after each question. In test mode, you will receive a score after completing a test. Questions answered incorrectly may be reviewed after completing the exam.

In either mode, once the test is completed, you have the option to view and print the results displayed as bar-graph percentages that represent the areas of the test plan, cognitive levels, subject area, and nursing process. This element gives you a clear and concise visual presentation of the results that further enhance and maximize study time.

## Free PDA Downloads

Practice for the exam on-the-go with PDA portability! Downloads can be accessed from the CD-ROM providing over 500 practice questions with rationales. Practice tests are downloaded in tests of varying lengths just like the actual examination. Test and learning modes are available in both Windows® and Palms® operation systems.

### Organization, Content, and Features

Unit 1, Preparing for the NCLEX Examination is an introductory unit that covers:

- Explanation of the test plan
- Test construction
- How computerized adaptive testing (CAT) works
- Study tips and techniques

Unit 2, Drugs and Nursing Implications groups drugs by classifications and similarities to help you in consolidating this important but sometimes overwhelming information. Unit 2 includes:

- Drug classification prototypes
- Related drug variances from the prototype
- Drug action mechanisms
- Drug uses and adverse effects
- Nursing implications and discharge teaching

Unit 3, Universal Principles of Nursing Care and Management includes:

- Nursing practice standards
- Legal and ethical aspects of nursing
- Delegation
- Prioritization
- Coordinating the health care team and client care

Units 4 through 7 cover adult, pediatric, maternity, and psychiatric-mental health nursing. Each of these units covers a systematic approach to review the subject matter:

- Introductory review of anatomy and physiology along with basic theories and principles

- The Nursing Process integrated with a body systems approach:
  - Assessment: review of both history and physical examination
  - Analysis: includes appropriate NANDA nursing diagnoses
  - Planning: discusses client goals
  - Implementation: identifies the interventions to achieve client goals
  - Evaluation: lists outcome criteria
- Review of the pertinent disorders for each system that includes:
  - General characteristics
  - Pathophysiology
  - Psychopathology
  - Medical/surgical management
  - Assessment data
  - Nursing interventions and client education

The concept, scope, and design of this text represent the commitment of the author and publishing team to help the graduate nurse reach full professional potential.

Good luck on your NCLEX-RN® examination!

# LIST OF ABBREVIATIONS

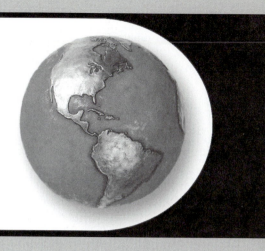

| | |
|---|---|
| AA | Alcoholics Anonymous |
| ABGs | arterial blood gases |
| ABE | acute bacterial endocarditis |
| ac | before meals |
| ACOA | Adult Children of Alcoholics |
| ACE | angiotensin-converting enzyme |
| ACh | acetylcholine |
| ACTH | adrenocorticotropic hormone |
| ADA | American Dietetic Association |
| ADH | antidiuretic hormone |
| ADL | activities of daily living |
| AFB | acid-fast bacillus |
| AIDS | acquired immune deficiency syndrome |
| AKA | above the knee amputation |
| ALG | antilymphocytic globulin |
| ALL | acute lymphocytic leukemia |
| ALT | alanine aminotransferase |
| An | analysis |
| ANA | American Nurses Association or antinuclear antibodies |
| ANLL | acute nonlymphocytic leukemia |
| ANS | autonomic nervous system |
| Ap | application |
| A-P | anterior-posterior |
| APTT | activated partial thromboplastin time |
| ARC | AIDS-related complex |
| ARDS | adult respiratory distress syndrome |
| As | assessment |
| ASA | acetylsalicyclic acid (aspirin) |
| ASD | atrial septal defect |
| ASO | antistreptolysin |
| AST | aspartate aminotransferase |
| ATG | antithymocytic globulin |
| ATN | acute tubular necrosis |
| ATP | adenosine triphosphate |
| AV | atrial-ventricular |
| BCG | Bacillus Calmette-Guérin |
| BID | twice a day |
| BKA | below the knee amputation |
| BMR | basal metabolic rate |
| B&O | suppositories containing belladonna |
| BP | blood pressure |
| BPD | bronchopulmonary dysplasia |
| BPH | benign prostatic hypertrophy |
| BSE | breast self-examination |
| BUN | blood urea nitrogen |
| CABG | coronary artery bypass graft |
| C | Celsius |
| Ca | calcium |
| CAD | coronary artery disease |
| CAT | computerized adaptive testing |
| CBC | complete blood count |
| CCK-PZ | cholecystokinin and pancreozymin |
| CCU | coronary care unit |
| CDC | Centers for Disease Control and Prevention |
| CEA | carcinoembryonic antigen |
| CF | cystic fibrosis |
| CHD | congenital heart disease |
| CHF | congestive heart failure |
| CHO | carbohydrate |
| CI | chloride |
| CL | cognitive level |
| cm | centimeter |
| CN | client need |
| CNM | certified nurse midwife |
| CNS | central nervous system |
| Co | comprehension |
| $CO_2$ | carbon dioxide |
| COPD | chronic obstructive pulmonary disease |
| CP | cerebral palsy |
| CPAP | continuous positive airway pressure |
| CPD | cephalopelvic disproportion |
| CPK | creatine phosphokinase |
| CPR | cardiopulmonary resuscitation |
| C&S | culture and sensitivity |
| CSF | cerebrospinal fluid |
| CST | contraction stress test |
| CT | computed tomography |
| CTZ | chemoreceptor trigger zone |
| CV | cardiovascular |
| CVA | cerebrovascular accident |
| CVP | central venous pressure |
| CVS | chorionic villi sampling |
| D&C | dilatation and currettage |
| DDAVP | desmopressin |
| DDST | Denver Developmental Screening Test |
| DES | diethylstilbestrol |
| DIC | disseminated intravascular coagulation |
| dL | deciliter |
| DMT | a hallucinogen |

**xix**

| | |
|---|---|
| DNA | deoxyribonucleic acid |
| DPT | diphtheria, pertussis, and tetanus toxoid |
| dr | dram |
| DT | diphtheria and tetanus toxoid |
| DTs | delirium tremens |
| DTaP | diphtheria-tetanus-acellular pertussis vaccine |
| DTP | diphtheria, tetanus, and pertussis toxoid |
| DVT | deep venous thrombosis |
| ECG | electrocardiogram |
| ECT | electroconvulsive therapy |
| ED | Emergency department |
| EDC | estimated date of confinement |
| EEG | electroencephalogram |
| EMG | electromyography |
| ENT | ear, nose, throat |
| EP | erythrocyte protoporphyrin |
| ERT | estrogen replacement therapy |
| ESR | erythrocyte sedimentation rate |
| ETOH | ethyl alcohol |
| Ev | evaluation |
| fl dr | fluid dram |
| fl oz | fluid ounce |
| F | Fahrenheit |
| FAD | flavin adenine dinucleotide |
| FDA | Food and Drug Administration |
| FHT | fetal heart ones |
| FHR | fetal heart rate |
| FSH | follicle-stimulating hormone |
| FSP | fibrin split products |
| ft | feet |
| FTT | failure to thrive |
| g | gauge or gram |
| GI | gastrointestinal |
| gr | grain |
| gtt(s) | drop(s) |
| GTT | glucose tolerance test |
| GU | genitourinary |
| GVHD | graft versus host disease |
| h | hour |
| HA | headache |
| $H_2$ | histamine 2 |
| HBIG | hepatitis B immunoglobulin |
| HBV | hepatitis B vaccine |
| HCG | human chorionic gonadotropin |
| HGI | hydrochloric acid or hydrochloride |
| $HCO_3$ | bicarbonate |
| HCS/HPL | human chorionic somatomammotropin/ human placental lactogen |
| He | health promotion/maintenance |
| HELLP | hemolysis, elevated liver enzymes, lowered platelets |
| Hct | hematocrit |
| Hg | mercury |
| Hgb | hemoglobin |
| HbA1c | hemoglobin A1c |
| HgbS | abnormal hemoglobin seen in sickle-cell anemia |
| Hib | *Haemophilus influonzae* type B |
| HIV | human immunodeficiency virus |
| HLA | human leukocyte antigen |
| HMD | hyaline membrane disease |
| HNP | herniated nucleus pulposus |
| $H_2O$ | water |
| $H_2O_2$ | hydrogen peroxide |
| hr(s) | hour(s) |
| $HSV_2$ | herpes simplex virus type 2 |
| I & O | intake and output |
| I & Os | intake and outputs |
| IA | intra-arterial |

| | |
|---|---|
| ICP | intracranial pressure |
| ICU | intensive care unit |
| ID | identification |
| IDDM | insulin-dependent diabetes mellitus |
| IDM | infant of diabetic mother |
| IgG | immunoglobulin G |
| IM | intramuscular |
| Im | implementation |
| IMV | intermittent mandatory ventilation |
| in | inch |
| IPPB | intermittent positive pressure breathing |
| IQ | Intelligence quotient |
| ISG | immune serum globulin |
| ITP | idiopathic thrombocytopenic purpura |
| IUD | intrauterine device |
| IUGR | intrauterine growth retardation |
| IV | intravenous |
| IVP | intravenous pyelogram |
| JRA | juvenile rheumatoid arthritis |
| K | potassium or knowledge (in question code for comprehensive practice tests) |
| kcal | kilocalories |
| KCL | potassium chloride |
| kg | kilogram |
| KUB | kidney, ureter, bladder |
| L | liter |
| lb | pound |
| LDH | lactic dehydrogenase |
| LE | lupus erythematosus |
| LGA | large for gestational age |
| LH | luteinizing hormone |
| LOA | left occiput anterior |
| LOC | level of consciousness |
| LOP | left occiput posterior |
| LP | lumbar puncture |
| LPN | licensed practical nurse |
| L/S | lecithin/sphingomyelin |
| LSD | lysergic acid diethylamide |
| LVN | licensed vocational nurse |
| m | meter or minim |
| min | minim *or* minutes |
| MAO | monamine oxidase |
| MAOI | monamine oxidase inhibitors |
| MAR | medication administration record |
| mcg | microgram |
| MCT | medium chain triglycerides |
| MD | medical doctor |
| mEq | milliequivalent |
| mg | milligram |
| MI | myocardial infarction |
| mL | milliliter |
| MLC | mixed leukocyte culture |
| mm | millimeter |
| MMR | measles, mumps, rubella |
| MRI | magnetic resonance imaging |
| MSH | melanocyte-stimulating hormone |
| mU | milliunit |
| Na | sodium |
| NANDA | North American Nursing Diagnosis Association |
| NEC | necrotizing enterocolitis |
| ng | nanograms |
| NG | nasogastric |
| NIDDM | non-insulin-dependent diabetes mellitus |
| NP | nursing process |
| NPO | nothing by mouth |
| NS | normal saline |
| NSAIDs | nonsteroidal anti-inflammatory drugs |
| NSS | normal saline solution |

| | | | |
|---|---|---|---|
| NST | nonstress test | R | respirations |
| $O_2$ | oxygen | RA | rheumatoid arthritis |
| OB-Gyn | obstetrics-gynecology | RAIU | radioactive iodine uptake |
| OBS | organic brain syndrome | RBC | red blood cell |
| OCD | obsessive-compulsive disorder | RDA | recommended daily allowances |
| OCT | oxytocin challenge test | RDS | respiratory distress syndrome |
| OD | right eye | RF | rheumatic fever |
| OMD | organic mental disorder | RIA | radioimmunoassay |
| OOB | out of bed | RN | registered nurse |
| OPV | oral polio vaccine | RNA | ribonucleic acid |
| OR | operating room | ROA | right occiput anterior |
| OS | left eye | ROM | range of motion |
| OTC | over-the-counter | ROP | right occiput posterior |
| OU | both eyes | $S_3$ | third heart sound |
| oz | ounce | SA | sinoatrial |
| P | pulse | Sa | safe, effective care environment |
| PA | pulmonary artery | SBE | subacute bacterial endocarditis |
| PABA | para-aminobenzoic acid | Sub-Q | subcutaneous |
| PACU | postanesthesia care unit | SGA | small for gestational age |
| PAP | pulmonary artery pressure | SGOT | serum glutamic-oxylacetic transaminase |
| Pap | Papanicolaou | SGPT | serum glutamic-pyruvic transaminase |
| PCA | patient-controlled analgesia | SIDS | sudden infant death syndrome |
| $pCO_2$ | partial pressure of carbon dioxide | SL | sublingual |
| PCP | *Pneumocystis carinii* pneumonia or phencyclidine | SLE | systemic lupus erythematosus |
| | | STD | sexually transmitted disease |
| PCWP | pulmonary capillary wedge pressure | T | temperature or thoracic |
| PDA | patent ductus arteriosus | TB | tuberculosis |
| PEEP | positive-end expiratory pressure | TBI | total body irradiation |
| PG | phosphatidylglycerol | tbsp | tablespoon |
| $PGE_2$ | prostaglandin $E_2$ | TCAs | tricyclic antidepressants |
| Ph | physiological integrity | Td | adult tetanus toxoid and diphtheria toxoid |
| PICCs | peripherally implanted central catheters | TEF | tracheoesophageal fistula |
| PID | pelvic inflammatory disease | TENS | transcutaneous electrical nerve stimulator |
| PIH | pregnancy-induced hypertension | TET | tetralogy |
| PKU | phenylketonuria | THC | tetrahydrocannabinol |
| Pl | planning | TIA | transient ischemic attack |
| PMI | point of maximal impulse | TID | three times a day |
| PND | paroxysmal nocturnal dyspnea | TPN | total parenteral nutrition |
| PNS | parasympathetic nervous system or peripheral nervous system | TPP | thiamin pyrophosphate |
| | | TSE | testicular self-examination |
| PO | by mouth | TSH | thyroid-stimulating hormone |
| $PO_2$ | partial pressure of oxygen | tsp | teaspoon |
| post-op | postoperative (after surgery) | TUR | transurethral resection |
| PPD | purified protein derivative | TURP | transurethral prostatectomy |
| PPN | peripheral parenteral nutrition | ug | microgram |
| pre-op | preoperative | UC | ulcerative colitis |
| prep | preparation | URI | upper respiratory infection |
| PRN | as needed | UTI | urinary tract infection |
| Ps | psychosocial integrity | VBAC | vaginal birth after cesarean |
| PSA | prostate-specific antigen | VDRL | Venereal Disease Reactive Laboratory |
| PT | prothrombin time | VER | visual evoked response |
| PTCA | percutaneous transluminal coronary angioplasty | VF | ventricular fibrillation |
| | | VMA | vanillylmandelic acid |
| PTH | parathormone | VS | vital signs |
| PTSD | post-traumatic stress disorder | VSD | ventricular septal defect |
| PTT | partial thromboplastin time | VT | ventricular tachycardia |
| PTU | propylthiouracil | WBC | white blood count or white blood cell |
| PUBS | percutaneous umbilical blood sampling | WBCs | white blood cells |
| PUC | pediatric urine collector | wk | week |
| PVC | premature ventricular contraction or polyvinyl chloride | WNL | within normal limits |
| | | < | less than |
| PVD | peripheral vascular disease | > | greater than |
| q | every | | |
| QID | four times a day | | |

# UNIT 1

# PREPARING FOR THE NCLEX EXAMINATION

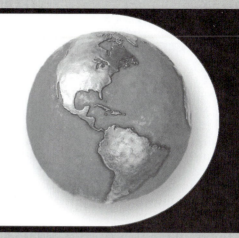

This first unit of the NCLEX-RN® Review will provide you with the important information you need to know about the construction of the National Council Licensure Examination for Registered Nurses (NCLEX-RN®, often referred to as "state boards"), with tips on how to study and with test-taking techniques you can use to improve your success when writing the examination.

## UNIT OUTLINE

# Understanding the NCLEX Examination

## THE TEST PLAN

The NCLEX-RN® examination questions are based on a test plan of client needs with concepts and processes fundamental to the practice of nursing integrated throughout the categories. These categories are nursing process, caring, communication and documentation, and teaching and learning. The latest plan went into effect in April 2007.

## Categories of Client Needs

The health care needs of clients across the life span in a variety of settings are grouped under four broad categories, some with several subcategories. The four main categories are safe, effective care environment; health promotion and maintenance; psychosocial integrity; and physiological integrity.

A. Safe, Effective Care Environment
   This category has two subcategories: management of care and safety and infection control. These two subcategories account for 21–33% of test items, which measure the nurse's ability to provide and direct nursing care that enhances the care delivery setting in order to protect clients and their families/ significant others and other health care personnel.
   1. Management of care comprises 13–19% of test items. This includes, but is not limited to, advocacy, client rights, confidentiality, delegation, ethical practice, legal rights and responsibilities, and supervision.
   2. Safety and infection control comprises 8–14% of test items. This includes, but is not limited to, disaster planning, emergency response plan, and error prevention.

B. Health Promotion and Maintenance
   The second major category comprises 6–12% of test items and measures the nurse's ability to provide and direct nursing care of clients and their families/significant others that incorporates the knowledge of expected growth and development principles, prevention, and/or early detection of health problems and strategies to achieve optimum health. This includes, but is not limited to, the aging process, ante/intra/postpartum and newborn care, developmental stages and transitions, growth and development, health and wellness, self-care, and techniques of physical assessment.

C. Psychosocial Integrity
   The third category comprises 6–12% of test items and measures the nurse's ability to provide and direct care that promotes and supports the emotional, mental, and social well-being of the families/significant others experiencing stressful events as well as clients with acute or chronic mental illness. This includes, but is

not limited to, abuse/neglect, behavioral interventions, cultural diversity, end of life, grief and loss, psychopathology sensory/perceptual alterations, stress management, and therapeutic communications.

D. Physiological Integrity
   The fourth major category has four subcategories: basic care and comfort, pharmacological and parenteral therapies, reduction of risk potential, and physiological adaptation. These subcategories account for 53–67% of test items and measure the nurse's ability to promote physical health and wellness by providing care and comfort, reducing risk potential, and managing health alterations.
   1. Basic care and comfort comprises 6–12% of test items and includes, but is not limited to, alternative and complementary therapies elimination, mobility/immobility, and rest and sleep.
   2. Pharmacological and parenteral therapies comprises 13–19% of test items and includes, but is not limited to, central venous access devices, dosage calculation, intravenous therapy, and medication administration.
   3. Reduction of risk potential comprises 13–19% of test items and includes, but is not limited to, diagnostic tests, laboratory values, monitoring conscious sedation, and therapeutic procedures.
   4. Physiological adaptation comprises 11–17% of test items and includes, but is not limited to, fluid and electrolyte imbalances, hemodynamics, pathophysiology, and radiation therapy.

## Levels of Cognitive Ability

The practice of nursing requires application of knowledge, skills, and abilities. To assess the candidates' ability in these areas, a majority of the test items are written at the application or higher levels of cognitive ability, which requires more complex thought processing. Bloom's taxonomy for the cognitive domain serves as a basis for writing and coding the test items.

## HOW THE TEST IS CONSTRUCTED

A. The National Council of State Boards of Nursing Inc. is the central organization for the independent member boards of nursing, which includes the 50 states, the District of Columbia, Guam, and the Virgin Islands. The member boards are divided into four regional areas, which supervise the selection of test item writers (representing educators and clinicians), whose names are suggested by the individual state boards of nursing. This provides for regional representation in the testing of nursing practice. All test items are validated in at least two approved nursing textbooks or references.

B.  The National Council contracts with a professional testing service to supervise writing and validation of test items by the item writers. This professional service works closely with the Examination Committee of the National Council in the test development process. The National Council and the state boards are responsible for the administration and security of the test.

C.  The exam is a computer exam known as CAT, which stands for Computerized Adaptive Testing. The exam is taken on a computer utilizing state-of-the-art technology.

There are several formats for questions. Multiple-choice questions with four choices, single-answer items or ones that require more than one response. There may be fill-in-the-blank questions or ones that ask the test taker to identify the area on a picture or a graphic, or drag-and-drop. The computer screen displays the question and the answer choices. There may also be questions that require responses to be placed in priority order. Each of these types of questions are integrated throughout the sample tests in this book.

Each candidate is oriented to the computer before the exam starts. Because the exam is geared to the candidate's skill level, each candidate will have a unique exam. Each exam will include approximately 15 experimental questions dispersed throughout the exam, so the candidate will be able to answer all the questions with equal effort. The experimental questions will not be counted for or against the candidate. Some candidates will be finished in a little over an hour; others will use the entire allotted time. The minimum number of questions candidates must answer is 75, and the maximum they may answer is 265. There is not a time limit for each question, but a 6 hour limit for the entire exam, which includes the exam instructions explaining how to use the mouse, the space bar, and the enter key; samples representing each type of question in the exam; and rest breaks.

D.  The exam is given at Pearson Professional Testing Centers across the United States. The candidate submits credentials to the State Board of Nursing in the state in which licensure is desired. Once the credentials are accepted, the candidate calls the testing service for an appointment, which will be scheduled within 30 days.

## HOW THE TEST IS SCORED

A.  The NCLEX-RN® is scored by computer and a pass/fail grade is reported.

B.  A criterion-referenced approach is used to set the passing score. This provides for the candidate's test performance to be compared with a consistent standard of criteria. Passing the exam will determine if the candidate is safe to practice as an entry-level nurse by using critical thinking skills to make nursing judgements.

## HOW CANDIDATES ARE NOTIFIED OF RESULTS

A.  Candidates in the following states may access their unofficial results within two days via the NCLEX Candidate Web site or from the NCLEX-RN®. Quick Results line: Arizona, Colorado, Connecticut, District of Columbia, Florida, Georgia, Illinois, Idaho, Indiana, Iowa, Kansas, Kentucky, Louisiana, Maine, Maryland, Massachusetts, Michigan, Minnesota, Missouri, Montana, Nebraska, Nevada, New Jersey, New Mexico, New York, North Carolina, North Dakota, Ohio, Oklahoma, Oregon, Pennsylvania, South Carolina, South Dakota, Tennessee, Texas, Utah, Vermont, Washington, Wisconsin, Wyoming.
Website: www.pearsonvue.com/nclex
NCLEX Quick Results line: 1-900-776-2539.

B.  Unsuccessful candidates are provided with a diagnostic profile that describes their overall performance on a scale from low to high, and their performance on the questions testing their abilities to meet client needs.

 **Preparation and Test Taking**

## USING THE TEST PLAN TO YOUR BEST ADVANTAGE
### Performing a Self-Needs Analysis

The first step to take when preparing to study for the NCLEX-RN® is to perform a self-needs analysis to identify your knowledge base in relation to the information provided in the test plan.

A.  Look carefully at the elements of the test plan (Categories of Client Needs), which are also reported to those who fail the test.

B. Go through your notes and text references. Select what is important and star, underline, or highlight this information.
C. Categorize this information in terms of material that needs to be learned or material that needs only to be reviewed.

## Planning for Study

A. Look at the period of time available to you for study between now and when you are scheduled to take the NCLEX-RN®. Ideally, plan to study up to four nights before the test, allow three nights for review, and the night before the test for relaxation. If you have limited time for study, plan your time so that you have at least one night for nothing but review.
B. Identify your maximum concentration time for profitable study. It is better to block out short periods of time (45–60 minutes, interspersed with planned breaks) that can be quality study time, rather than setting aside 3 hours of time to study, which may only produce 90 minutes of quality study time.
C. When you decide what your maximum time for profitable study is, then that is the block of time you should set aside on a regular basis for study purposes. Within the confines of your allocated study time, make sure you establish a schedule that permits you to cover completely all the material to be learned.
D. Nursing research has shown that reviewing more than 5,000 questions before sitting for the exam produces greater success rates of passing.

## How to Study

A. To promote maximum concentration, ensure that your study materials are your prime area of focus.
B. Make sure you are mentally alert and in a room where you will be free from outside interruptions. If possible, choose a room with no telephone.
C. Do not smoke, do not nibble on snacks, and do not answer the telephone. This will allow you to direct your energy to the study activity.
D. Proceed with your planned study periods in an organized manner by choosing an approach that will be meaningful to you. Some content lends itself to study using concepts, while other content is best studied using systems.
E. Use methods of memory improvement that will work for you. Mnemonic devices (where a letter represents the first letter of each item in a sequence) are an effective means of retrieving material. Mental imagery is the technique of forming pictures in your mind to help you remember details of the sequence of events, such as the administration of an injection. Try practicing self-recitation to improve your study habits. Reciting to yourself the material being learned will

promote retention of information being studied. Concentrate on the information you identified in your self-needs analysis as needing to be learned.
F. The final step of your study program involves organizing the material so that you will be able to learn all the "need to learn" and review all the "need to review" information within the allotted study time period. Your schedule should have allowed you to complete your review so you can close your books and do something relaxing on the night before the examination.

# FINAL PREPARATION FOR TEST TAKING

In addition to having studied appropriately to assure yourself of a good knowledge base, there are measures you can take to be in prime physiologic and psychologic shape for writing the examination.

## Physiologic Readiness

To prime yourself physiologically, you should meet your own needs for nutrition, sleep, and comfort.
A. You will function best if you are well nourished.
  1. Plan to eat three well-balanced meals a day for at least 3 days prior to the examination.
  2. Be careful when choosing the food you consume within 24 hours of the examination.
    a. Avoid foods that will make you thirsty or cause intestinal distress.
    b. Minimize the potential of a full bladder midway through the examination by limiting the amount of fluids you drink and by allowing sufficient time at the test site to use the bathroom before entering the room.
B. Assess your sleep needs.
  1. Determine the minimal amount of sleep you need in order to function effectively.
  2. Plan to allow sufficient time in your schedule the week before the examination to provide yourself with the minimum sleep you need to function effectively for at least 3 days prior to the examination.
C. Plan your wardrobe ahead of time.
  1. Shoes and clothes that fit you comfortably will not distract your thought processes during the examination.
  2. Include a comfortable sweater.
  3. Your clothes for the test day should be ready to wear by the night before the examination.
D. If you wear glasses or contact lenses, take along an extra pair of glasses.
E. If you are taking medications on a regular basis, continue to do so during this period of time. Introduction of new medications should be avoided until after completion of the examination.

## Reducing Psychologic Stress

While a certain amount of anxiety will stimulate your nervous system to focus keenly on the examination, excess anxiety will interfere with your ability to concentrate on the examination and, indeed, hinder your success. You must approach the examination with a positive attitude. You have graduated from a school of nursing that has prepared you to provide safe and effective nursing care to your clients. Trust that the curriculum in your school of nursing was designed to include all the important concepts and principles necessary for safe nursing practice. Feel confident that you accessed multiple resources to allow you to learn the content. Most of the tests you wrote while in school were developed in the style used for the NCLEX-RN®. Keeping these points in mind will enable you to approach the examination with a positive frame of reference for success.

Minimize the anxiety-producing situations related to writing the examination by carefully planning your pre-examination activities. Make a list of the important things you need to accomplish.

A. Rehearse the route or means of transportation you plan to take to the test location, preferably at the same time of the day on which you actually will be going. Check your local resources for road conditions that might necessitate altering your planned route. In your time assessment, include parking your car, locating where you are to report for registration, and locating the bathrooms. To ensure adequate travel time and to minimize stress related to getting to the test site on time the morning of the test, add an extra 30 minutes to the total time needed for the rehearsal run.
B. Have your admission materials readily available.
C. If you are staying overnight near the test site, be sure you pack everything you will need. Before retiring for the night, make your rehearsal run to the test location in preparation for the next day.
D. Plan to use relaxation exercises to control your anxiety level. If you have been using a specific method of relaxation successfully, then continue using it during this period of time. If you have not, consider trying one of the following.
    1. Yoga or meditation before the exam
    2. Guided imagery: requires using your imagination to create a relaxing sensory scene on which to concentrate.
    3. Breathing exercises.
E. For any of the methods to achieve the desired results, you must be willing to commit the time necessary to implement their prescribed protocols.

## TAKING THE TEST

While having a good knowledge base is important for success in test-taking situations, the following strategies can be used to maximize your skill in choosing the correct answers.

A. Take your seat and give yourself an opportunity to implement the method of relaxation you have been practicing.
B. Read the directions carefully, and then be sure to follow them carefully.
C. Plan to manage your time effectively. While taking the CAT test, work steadily. You do not have to answer a specific number of questions in a given time period. If you take the maximum length of time, your score will reflect the number of questions you have completed.
D. Read the stem of the question carefully. This is the part of the question that describes what is being asked.
E. Read the stem a second time to key in on important words and then reword the question to determine the purpose of the question.
F. Move to the answer choices. In a single multiple-choice item there will be one correct and three incorrect choices. Incorrect answers are called distractors. A multiple-choice item that has more than one correct answer may have fewer distractors.
G. Consider if the question is asking about 1) a needed assessment that should be done first, 2) Maslow's Hierarchy of Needs, or 3) a safety issue. Keep these in mind for each question.
H. Carefully evaluate the answer choices for key words. Be sure to appreciate the universality of words such as *each, all, never,* and *none;* the limitations of words such as *rarely, most,* and *least;* and the latitude offered by words such as *usually, frequently,* and *often.*
I. Read each option twice. Use the space bar on the keyboard to highlight each answer choice.
J. Answer it by saying to yourself
    1. *Yes,* it answers what is being asked.
    2. *No,* it does not answer what is being asked.
    3. *Maybe* it answers what is being asked.
K. Use this procedure for all the answer choices. When you first read the question, if an obvious answer comes to mind, restrain your desire to look for it in the answer choices. For a single multiple-choice item, read all the choices to make sure your thought was indeed the only *yes* answer. For this type of question, if you are fortunate enough to have only one *yes* answer, then you have eliminated the three distractors. For a multiple multiple-choice item, you likely have the correct answers and have eliminated the other distractors.
L. If you identified more than one *yes* option for a single multiple-choice item, then evaluate those other options in terms of which is more *yes* than *maybe.* If you have no *yes* answer, then evaluate the *maybe* choices for one that leans more toward *yes.*
M. Always choose the answer that has the highest likelihood for being *yes* (correct). Look critically at the answer choices for clues. If you see choices that are opposites, frequently one is the correct answer. For example:

During insertion of a central venous catheter, in which position should the client be placed?
1. A supine position.
2. Trendelenburg's position.
3. Reverse Trendelenburg's position.
4. A high-Fowler's position.

Choices 2 and 3 are opposites, and in this case 2 is the correct answer.

N. If you have an answer that contains more than one option, all of the options must be correct for that choice to be correct. If you can eliminate one of the options in an answer, you can automatically eliminate the other answer choices with that option. For example:

What complications can occur from the administration of TPN?
1. Hyperglycemia and hypocalcemia.
2. Hyperglycemia and hyperkalemia.
3. Hypoglycemia and hypercalcemia.
4. Hyperkalemia and hypercalcemia.

Hypercalcemia and hyperkalemia are distractors. Eliminate the choices with these options and there is only one correct choice remaining.

O. Look for options that do not meet the requirements of the stem. For example:

Which medication is used to lyse (break up) already formed clots?
1. Warfarin sodium (Coumadin).
2. Heparin sodium (Lipo-Hepin).
3. Streptokinase (Kabikinase).
4. Vitamin K.

Choices 1, 2, and 3 are all used in the treatment of formed clots. Choice 4 is necessary for clot formation and therefore does not meet the requirements for the stem and must be eliminated as a possibility. Now choose among the remaining options. 3 is correct.

P. If the stem asks for the exception or which choice is not the answer, you are looking for the *no* answer rather than the *yes* answer. For example:

Individuals from which group would be excluded from getting TB?
1. Lower socioeconomic groups.
2. Malnourished and debilitated individuals.
3. Individuals on steroid therapy.
4. White females with a history of alcohol abuse.

Choices 1, 2, and 3 are all at risk and therefore, *yes* responses. Choice 4 is the *no* response and, therefore, the correct answer.

Q. Be careful to avoid reading elements into the question that are not specifically included in the stem and answer choices.

R. Assume you have a doctor's order and all the equipment or supplies you need. Remember, the questions are based on texts and not the "real world."

S. When you have decided on an answer, press the return key. The computer will ask if this is your desired answer choice. If it is, then press the enter key again and your choice will be recorded. If you wish to review the answer choices again, use the space bar to do so and then press the enter key when you have made your decision. The computer will again ask if this is your desired answer choice. If it is, then press the enter key again to record your choice.

T. A calculator will be accessible on the desktop of the computer screen.

# HOW TO USE THIS BOOK

As you go through each unit of this book, use it to perform your self-needs analysis and as a basis for study. You will make the best use of both your time and the book if you use the study skills suggested earlier in this unit.

A. For more detailed information on the particular subjects you feel need extra study, review those subjects in current textbooks, and scan the list of suggested readings at the end of each unit for further resources.

B. The questions interspersed throughout Units 2 through 7 are typical of the board questions, and they will help you to become more familiar with the style of questions found in the NCLEX-RN®.

C. When setting up your study time include time to take the practice tests on the enclosed disk in the back of this book. You may take these tests once, before you start studying, to help you with your needs analysis. When you have completed studying, you may take them again, to evaluate for test performance.

D. While taking the practice tests, apply the test-taking strategies discussed earlier in this unit.

## *REFERENCES AND SUGGESTED READINGS*

Benson, H. RelaxationResponse.org. Retrieved November 8, 2008, from http://relaxationresponse.org.

Bloom, B. S., Engelhart, M. D., Furst, E. G., Hill, W. H., Krathwohl, D. R., et al. (Eds.). (1956). *Taxonomy of educational objectives: The classification of educational goals.* Handbook I, The cognitive domain. New York: David McKay.

Flynn, P. (1980). *Holistic health: The art and science of care.* Bowie, MD: Brady.

Levy, J. (1989). *The fine arts of relaxation and meditation.* New York: Wisdom Publications.

National Counsel of State Boards of Nursing, Inc. (2008). *NCLEX-RN® Examination.* Chicago: Author.

Wilson, L. O. (2006). Beyond Bloom—A new Version of the Cognitive Taxonomy. Retrieved August 14, 2008, from http://www.uwsp.edu/education/lwilson/curric/newtaxonomy.htm.

# UNIT 2
# DRUGS AND NURSING IMPLICATIONS

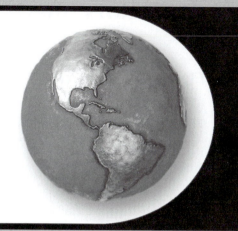

Today's nurse needs to have a firm foundation in pharmacology. Important aspects of current nursing practice deal with effectiveness of medications, detecting adverse effects, drug interactions, and incorporating client teaching concerning drug use. Clients, including pregnant women and nursing mothers, should be taught adverse effects of drugs and not to take OTC drugs or herbals while on prescribed medication without consulting their physician.

This unit, Drugs and Nursing Implications, provides a review of all major drug classifications. The first part of the unit contains a review of pharmacokinetics, drug administration, and calculations. Keep in mind that pediatric drug doses typically are calculated per kilograms of body weight. Following these introductory concepts, multiple choice questions for each drug classification are provided.

Each major drug classification is represented by a prototype drug. A review of action, use, adverse effects, nursing implications, discharge teaching (where applicable), and related drugs is in chart form when appropriate or otherwise listed with pertinent comments. At times, a prototype drug may not be used because one particular drug might not represent a drug group. For example, in the laxative drug group, there is not one single representative or prototype drug. If no prototype drug is used, this is indicated under the drug classification.

**Factors Affecting Drug Action**

## DEFINITION OF A DRUG

A. According to the Food and Drug Administration (FDA), a drug is any substance used to diagnose, cure, mitigate, treat, or prevent a condition or disease.

B. Drugs come from three main sources: plants (e.g., digoxin), animals (e.g., insulin), and synthetic chemicals (e.g., meperidine).

C. Most of the drugs used today are synthetic chemicals and are associated with fewer allergic reactions.

## FACTORS AFFECTING DRUG ACTION

### Absorption

A. Absorption refers to the time the drug enters the body until it enters the bloodstream.

B. Many factors affect the rate and amount of absorption.
1. Dosage form
2. Route of administration
   a. Parenteral: absorption generally rapid
   b. Intravenous (IV) and intra-arterial (IA): most rapid absorption
   c. Intramuscular (IM) and subcutaneous (SC)
      1) Absorption is relatively fast if given in an aqueous base but can be delayed if given in an oil base
      2) Speed of absorption depends on condition of blood flow
      3) Impaired peripheral circulation and shock will delay absorption
   d. Intradermal: absorption is slow and confined to area injected (e.g., purified protein derivative—PPD)
   e. Oral: rate and degree of absorption can vary depending on GI motility, presence of food in stomach, gastric pH, and use of other drugs
3. Lipid solubility: affects absorption as it passes through gastric intestinal mucosa.
4. Gastrointestinal (GI) motility
   a. Stomach empties more slowly with food and will delay oral drug absorption.
   b. Most oral drugs are best absorbed if given before meals or between meals.
      1) Diarrhea can cause drugs not to be absorbed

2) Constipation may delay drug absorption, potentially causing toxicity

### Distribution

A. Once in bloodstream, drugs are distributed within the body. Distribution can take as long as several hours, depending on blood flow (in various areas of the body) and cardiac output.

B. Plasma-protein binding
1. Medications connect with plasma proteins (primarily albumin) in vascular system.
2. Strong attachments have a longer period of drug action.
3. Clients with reduced plasma proteins such as in kidney or liver disease could receive a heightened drug effect.

C. Volume of distribution
1. Client with edema has an enlarged area in which a drug can be distributed and may need an increased dose.
2. Smaller dose may be needed for client with dehydration.

D. Barriers to drug distribution: prevent some medications from entering certain body organs.
1. Blood-brain barrier
   a. Helps preserve homeostasis in brain.
   b. To pass through this barrier, drug must be lipid soluble and loosely attached to plasma protein.
2. Placental barrier
   a. Shields fetus from possibility of adverse drug effects.
   b. Many substances (drugs, nicotine, alcohol) do cross placental barrier.

E. Obesity: body weight plays a role in drug distribution because blood flows through fat slowly, thus increasing time before drug is released.

F. Receptor combination
1. A receptor is an area on a cell where drug attaches and response takes place.
   a. Receptor is usually protein or nucleic acid.
   b. Other substances that can be receptors are enzymes, lipids, and carbohydrate residues.
2. Drugs can have an agonist or antagonist effect.
   a. Agonist will connect itself to the receptor site and cause pharmacological response.

**b.** Antagonist will attempt to attach, but because attachment is uneven, there is no drug response.

**3.** There can be competition at receptor site when more than one drug tries to occupy it.

## Metabolism

**A.** Process of metabolism is a sequence of chemical events that change a drug after it enters the body.

**B.** Liver is principal site of drug metabolism.

**C.** Oral medications
  **1.** Go directly to the liver via the portal circulation before entering systemic circulation.
  **2.** Many medications become entirely inactivated by the liver the first time they go through it.

**D.** Age
  **1.** Age of an individual influences metabolism of drugs.
  **2.** Infants and elderly have reduced ability to metabolize some drugs.

**E.** Nutrition: liver enyzmes involved in metabolism rely on adequate amounts of amino acids, lipids, vitamins, and carbohydrates.

**F.** Insufficient amounts of major body hormones such as insulin or adrenal corticosteroids can reduce metabolism of drugs in liver.

## Excretion

**A.** Process by which drugs are eliminated from body
  **1.** Drugs can be excreted by kidneys, intestines, lungs, mammary, sweat, and salivary glands.
  **2.** Most important route of excretion for most drugs is kidneys.

**B.** Renal excretion
  **1.** Carried out by glomerular filtration and tubular secretion, which increase quantity of drug excreted.
  **2.** Another renal process that results in excretion is tubular reabsorption.
    **a.** Drug metabolites in urine can be reverted back into bloodstream.
    **b.** Decreases quantity of drug excreted.

**C.** Drugs can affect elimination of other drugs
  **1.** Example: probenecid is sometimes administered with penicillin to prevent excretion of penicillin and thus increase effects of penicillin.
  **2.** Example: antacids increase elimination of aspirin, thus decreasing its effects.

**D.** Blood concentration levels
  **1.** Affect drug elimination
  **2.** When peak blood level of drug is reached, excretion becomes greater than absorption and blood levels of drug begin to drop.

**E.** Half-life: time required for total amount of drug to decrease by 50%.

## Accumulation

**A.** Therapeutic levels
  **1.** Important goal is for drug to reach therapeutic levels and maintain therapeutic level.
  **2.** Can be maintained when liver or renal function remain unchanged.

**B.** Loading dose
  **1.** Sometimes given to raise therapeutic level quickly before drug has chance to be eliminated.
  **2.** For client safety, loading doses are given in several smaller doses over short periods of time.
  **3.** Once therapeutic level is achieved, a smaller daily maintenance dose is given to maintain therapeutic levels; digoxin may be given this way.

**C.** Toxicity: occurs when drug is eliminated more slowly than it is absorbed, causing excessive drug concentration.

## Underlying Disease

**A.** Disease can lead to variable drug response.

**B.** Diseases that may affect drug response
  **1.** Cardiovascular disease
  **2.** Gastrointestinal disease
  **3.** Liver disease
  **4.** Kidney disease

## Client's Age

**A.** Pediatric: drug dosages are based on body weight—milligrams per kilogram (mg/kg).

**B.** Geriatric: careful drug history should be obtained, including over-the-counter (OTC) drugs to determine whether there are drug interactions or adverse effects.

### Sample Questions

**1.** What is the result of taking antibiotics with food?
  1. Prevent side effects.
  2. Enhance action of drug.
  3. Delay rate of absorption.
  4. Increase rate of absorption.

**2.** What occurrence may be caused due to the decreased serum albumin levels in the elderly?
  1. Toxic drug effects.

2. Enhanced absorption.
3. Enhanced drug distribution.
4. An increase in the therapeutic effects.

3. If a central nervous system (CNS) depressant is administered to an infant, toxic effects can occur due to what action?
   1. Increased drug absorption.
   2. Increased drug distribution.
   3. Decreased drug half-life.
   4. Decreased drug excretion.

## Answers and Rationales

1. **3.** Taking food will decrease the rate of absorption. Furthermore, taking dairy products with an antibiotic such as tetracycline will cause calcium (Ca+) to bind to the drug and decrease absorption.

2. **1.** Toxic drug effects occur because there is less albumin or protein for the drug to bind to in the elderly.

3. **3.** The blood-brain barrier is not fully developed in infants and CNS depressants can readily penetrate.

# Drug Administration

## ASSESSMENTS APPROPRIATE TO ALL MEDICATION ADMINISTRATION

A. Confirm client diagnosis and appropriateness of medication.
B. Identify all concurrent medications.
C. Identify any potential contraindications or allergies.
D. Identify client's knowledge of medications.

## ANALYSIS

Nursing diagnoses for the client receiving medications may include:
A. Risk for injury related to side effects of medications.
B. Deficient knowledge: drug effects related to lack of previous experience.
C. Noncompliance related to side effects, financial, or other difficulties, limiting ability to take medications.

## PLANNING AND IMPLEMENTATION

A. Identify appropriate goals such as, "Client will explain rationale for medication prior to discharge."
B. Prepare and administer medications according to the following principles.

## TECHNIQUES OF DRUG ADMINISTRATION

### General Principles for All Medications

A. Verify all new or questionable orders on the medication administration record (MAR) against physician orders for completeness.
B. Prepare medications in a quiet environment.
C. Wash your hands. Observe standard precautions, as appropriate.
D. Collect all necessary equipment, including straws, juice or water, stethoscope.
E. Review MAR for each client carefully to ensure safety: note medication, dosage, route, expiration date, and frequency.
F. Research drug compatibilities, action, purpose, contraindications, side effects, and appropriate routes.
G. Find medication for individual client and calculate dosage accurately. Confirm normal range of dose, particularly in pediatrics.
H. Check expiration date on medication and look for any changes that may indicate decomposition (color, odor, and clarity).
I. Compare label three times with the medication to decrease risk of error.
   1. When removing package from drawer
   2. Before preparing medication
   3. After preparing medication
J. Check need for prn medications.
K. Be sure medications are identified for each client.
L. Check for any allergies and perform all special assessments before administration.

M. Confirm client's identity by checking at least two of the three possible mechanisms for identification to ensure safety.
   1. Ask client his name.
   2. Check client's identi-band and ask him to state his date of birth.
   3. Check bed tag (this is least reliable method).
N. Provide privacy, if needed.
O. Inform client of medication, any procedure, technique, purpose, and client teaching as applicable.
P. Stay with client until medication is gone; do *not* leave medication at bedside.
Q. Assist client as needed, and leave in position of comfort.
R. Give medication within 30 minutes of prescribed time.
S. Chart administration immediately in ink.
T. Circle initials and document rationale if drug not administered.
U. Report any errors immediately and complete appropriate institutional documentation.
V. Liquid medications—all routes of administration—must *not* be mixed together unless compatibility is verified.
W. Observe for any reactions and document both positive and negative responses.
X. Observe the five "rights": give the right *dose* of the right *drug* to the right *client* at the right *time* by the right *route.*
Y. To ensure safety do not give a medication that someone else prepared. Institution policies may require having a colleague double check medications such as insulin and heparin. If you are unsure in any way, have a colleague verify.
Z. If using a computer-controlled dispensing system, follow agency policy for administration and documentation.

## Administration of Oral Medications

A. Special assessment: assess client's knowledge level, diet status, oral cavity, and ability to swallow medication.
B. Use agency equipment to crush tablets, if appropriate. In general, enteric-coated tablets should not be crushed. Only scored tablets can be broken.
C. With the exception of time-release capsules, capsule contents may be mixed with food to enhance swallowing.
D. Prepare solid medications (tablets, capsules, etc.).
   1. All solid medications can be placed in one medicine cup unless an assessment needs to be made before administering a particular medication (e.g., blood pressure, apical pulse).
   2. Unit dose containers can remain in original individual package.

   3. To reduce chance of contamination, place any removable lids open side up; place necessary medications into cap of container; transfer to med cup; replace lid and container.
E. Prepare liquid medications.
   1. Shake liquid medications, if necessary, to mix.
   2. Pour away from bottle label.
   3. Read liquid amount at meniscus of med cup at eye level to ensure accuracy.
   4. If needed, a syringe may be used to measure and administer liquid medications.
   5. Wipe lip of bottle with damp towel to prevent stickiness.
   6. Replace lid and container.
   7. Do not administer alcohol-based products, such as elixirs, to alcohol-dependent persons.
F. Sit client upright to enhance swallowing.
G. Have client swallow medication except with the following:
   1. Sublingual (SL) route: have client place medication under tongue (high rate of absorption). Do not allow fluids for 30 minutes following administration.
   2. Buccal route: have client place medication between gum and cheek. Do not allow fluids for 30 minutes following administration.
   3. Iron: have client use straw to prevent staining teeth.
H. Stay with client until medication is gone. Use gloves if you need to place your finger in client's mouth.
I. Special concerns
   1. Use a calibrated dropper, nipple, or syringe to give medications to an infant.
   2. Keep infant at 45° angle.
   3. See whether medication is available in liquid form if client is a child or unable to swallow solid medication.
   4. Be sure not to use a child's favorite food, as this may result in distrust.
   5. If using an NG or stomach tube for medication administration, check for correct placement before administration and follow medication with water. Be sure to check for food interaction.

## Administration of Rectal Drugs

A. Special assessment: assess client's bowel function and ability to retain suppository/enema.
B. Obtain suppository from storage area or refrigerator.
C. Provide privacy.
D. Position client left laterally.
E. Put on glove or finger cot.
F. Moisten suppository with water-soluble lubricant.

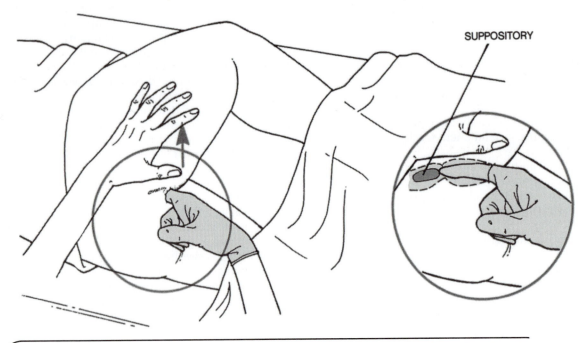

SUPPOSITORY

**Figure 2-1** A rectal suppository is inserted about 2 inches in adults so it will be placed in the internal anal sphincter

G. Insert suppository, tapered end first, approximately 2 inches (to pass internal sphincter) (Figure 2-1).
H. Hold buttocks together.
I. Encourage client to retain suppository for 10–20 minutes to allow suppository to melt.
J. If drug administered via enema, have client retain solution 20–30 minutes.

## Administration of Nasal Medications

A. Have client blow nose to clear mucus.
B. Position client so that head can be tilted back to aid in gravitational flow or in specific position to reach sinuses.
C. Push up on tip of nostril.
D. Place dropper or atomizer angled slightly upward just inside nostril; be careful not to touch nose with applicator.
E. Squeeze atomizer quickly and firmly or instill correct number of drops.
F. Remind client to keep head tilted for 5 minutes.
G. Inform client the drops may produce an unpleasant taste.
H. Leave tissues with client; instruct just to wipe nose, not blow, to allow for absorption.
I. Special concerns
   1. If client aspirates and begins to cough, sit client upright, stay until client's distress is relieved.
   2. If client is an infant, lay infant on its back.

## Administration of Inhalants

A. Special assessment: monitor vital signs before and after treatments.
B. Have client inhale and exhale deeply.
C. Have client place lips around mouthpiece without touching and inhale medication until lungs are fully inflated. Inhale slowly and deeply while depressing the top of the canister, close mouth, hold breath 10 seconds, then exhale. A specially designed spacer device is available to assist the client who may have difficulty with this.
D. Have client remove mouthpiece, hold breath as long as able, and then exhale completely.
E. If necessary, repeat procedure until medication is gone. Allow 2–5 minutes between inhalations.
F. Wash mouthpiece with warm water.
G. Special concerns
   1. Have tissues handy; encourage expectoration of sputum.
   2. Be sure client is aware that coughing is expected after treatment.
   3. If mouth is placed directly on inhaler, it is possible that the tongue will absorb medication, resulting in inadequate dosing and tongue irritation.

## Administration of Ophthalmic Medications

A. Check solution for color and clarity before administering.

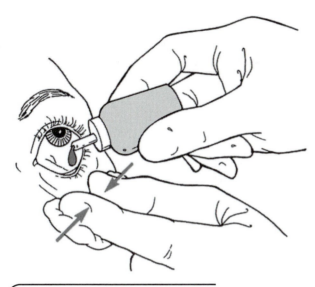

**Figure 2-2** Instilling eye drops

B. Warm solution in hands before administration.
C. Have client lie on back or sit with head turned to affected side to aid in gravitational flow.
D. Cleanse eyelid and eyelashes with sterile gauze pad soaked with physiologic saline. Assess eye condition.
E. Have client look up.
F. Assist client in keeping eye open by pulling down on cheekbone with thumb or forefinger and pulling up on eyelid. Be sure lower conjunctiva is exposed (Figure 2-2).
G. Place necessary number of drops into lower conjunctiva near outer canthus (less sensitive than cornea).
H. If using ointment, squeeze into lower conjunctiva moving from inner to outer canthus (Figure 2-3).
   1. Do not touch eye with applicator.
   2. Twist tube to break medication stream.
I. Have client blink 2–3 times.

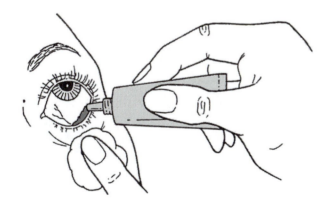

**Figure 2-3** Instilling eye ointment

J. Wipe away any excess medication starting from inner canthus.
K. Repeat if necessary using clean tissue.
L. Special concerns
   1. Ophthalmic medications are for individual clients; droppers and ointments should not be shared.
   2. Restrain infants and children if necessary.

## Administration of Otic Medications

A. Warm medication in hands prior to administration.
B. Put on gloves.
C. Have client turn to unaffected side to aid gravitational flow.
D. Clean outer ear using a wet gauze pad. Assess ear condition.
E. Straighten ear canal by pulling pinna up and back for adults or down and back for infants and children under 3 (Figure 2-4).

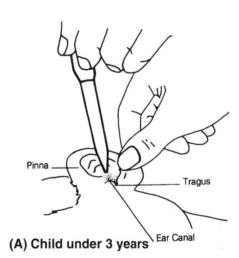

Pinna

Tragus

Ear Canal

**(A) Child under 3 years**

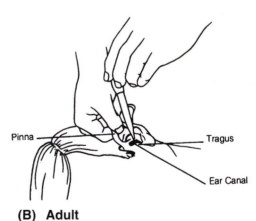

Pinna

Tragus

Ear Canal

**(B) Adult**

**Figure 2-4** Administering ear drops

F. Instill necessary number of drops along side of canal without touching ear with dropper.

G. Maintain position of ear until medication has totally entered canal.

H. Have client remain on side for 5–10 minutes to allow medication to reach inner ear.

I. Cotton may be used to keep medication in canal, but only if it is premoistened with medication.

J. Repeat procedure for other ear if necessary.

K. Special concern: restrain infants and children if necessary.

## Administration of Topical Agents

A. Provide privacy and expose only appropriate area to promote comfort.

B. Cleanse area of old medications using gauze pads with soap and warm water.

C. Use gloves and gauze, tongue depressor, or sterile applicator, if integument broken.

D. Assess area for any changes or contraindications of application.

E. Spread medication over site evenly and thinly.

F. If necessary, cover area loosely with a dressing.

G. Special concerns
   1. Clients often receive topical agents for image-altering problems. Applying the medication offers a good opportunity to talk about these problems and to share information about improvements.
   2. When applying nitroglycerin ointment, take client's blood pressure 5 minutes before and after application.
   3. Use gloves to administer medication to prevent self-absorption.
   4. When using transderm patches, use gloves to avoid inadvertent drug absorption. Remove backing and place patch in area with little hair. Press edges down to secure patch.

## Administration of Vaginal Medications

A. Provide privacy.

B. Put on gloves.

C. Have client void.

D. Place client on a bedpan in dorsal recumbent position with hips and knees flexed (Figure 2-5).

E. Cleanse perineum with warm, soapy water, working from outer to inner position.

F. Moisten applicator tip with water-soluble lubricant or just water.

G. Separate labia to insert applicator approximately 2 inches, angled downward and back.

H. Instill medication.

I. If giving douche, dry client's buttocks; otherwise have client remain in position approximately 15–20 minutes (there is no sphincter to hold suppository in place).

J. Wash applicator with warm, soapy water.

K. Provide client with pads if needed.

## Administration of Parenteral Medications

### General Principles

A. Special assessments for parenteral medications:
   1. Assess area for presence of lesions, rashes, or abscesses prior to administration.
   2. Assess for discomfort or impaired mobility, which may affect site selection.
   3. Assess client ability for self-injection, if appropriate.

B. Select appropriate needle size and syringe.
   1. Use tuberculin 1 mL syringe for volumes less than 1 mL.
   2. Needle lumen must be larger for solutions with increased viscosity.

C. When medication comes in a vial, cleanse rubber stopper with alcohol wipes/swab.

D. Without contaminating plunger, draw up air equal to the amount of medication needed.

E. Inject the air into the vial to prevent negative pressure and aid in aspirating medication.

F. Remove the appropriate amount of medication (the vial may be multidose).

G. Check to ensure no air bubbles are present; if bubbles are a problem, draw up slightly more medication than is needed, return all medication to vial, and withdraw medication again or tap syringe until air is all collected at top of barrel and can be expelled.

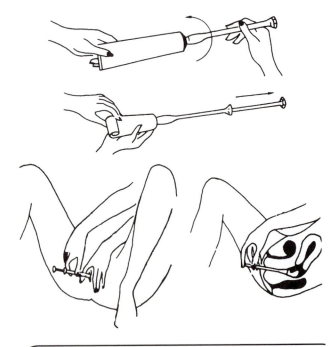

**Figure 2-5** The client should be in a dorsal recumbent position for the administration of vaginal creams

H. When using an ampule: tap neck to force medication into ampule, wrap neck with alcohol wipe/swab, snap off top away from self, place needle into ampule to withdraw medication. A filter needle should be used to avoid glass shards. Discard filter needle after use into sharps container.

I. When mixing a powder, use a filter needle when drawing up medication. Reconstitute according to manufacturer's recommendations.

J. Replace protective cover on needle before proceeding, using a one-hand scoop method.

K. Select appropriate site, avoiding bruised or tender areas; rotate sites as much as possible.

L. Cleanse site with alcohol wipe/swab to decrease contamination. Use gloves to avoid contact with blood.

M. Insert needle quickly with bevel up, leaving a small amount of needle showing, and release hold (to decrease pain).
　1. With the exception of heparin and insulin, aspirate to check for blood.
　2. If blood present, remove needle and start again.
　3. When giving medications IV, a blood return is desired.

N. Inject medication slowly.

O. Quickly withdraw needle and immediately place pressure over the site with a new swab. Massage area if giving Z-track injection.

P. Dispose of syringe in appropriate manner, but do not recap. Utilize safety cover for needle, if available, before placing in sharps container.

Q. Record site when documenting medication.

R. Variations on preparing medications
　1. Disposable injection systems have already-prepared cartridges with attached needle appropriate to route and viscosity. To add medication, add sterile air from cartridge to vial, then add medication from vial to cartridge.
　2. When combining two medications from an ampule and a vial, first determine appropriate volumes, as well as total volume. Withdraw appropriate volume of medication from vial, followed by medication in ampule.
　3. When combining medications from two vials, determine appropriate volume for each drug and total volume. Inject air into vial A, then into vial B. Withdraw medication from vial B, then return to vial A.

## Subcutaneous (SC) Administration

A. Use size 25 g to 27 g, ½–1-inch needle, maximum volume 1.5 mL.

B. Put on gloves.

C. Pinch skin to form SC fold.

D. Insert needle at 45° angle in thigh or arm or 90° angle in abdomen (to avoid entering muscle) (Figure 2-6).

E. Possible sites
　1. Lateral aspect of upper arm
　2. Anterior thigh
　3. Abdomen: 1 inch away from umbilicus
　4. Back, in scapular area

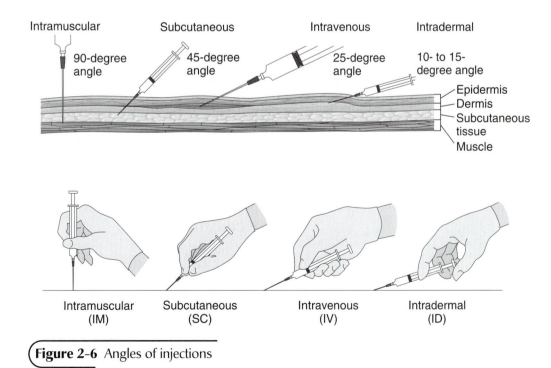

**Figure 2-6** Angles of injections

## Hypodermoclysis

**A.** A method of giving large volume solutions SC at a slow rate.

**B.** Reserved for clients unable to receive fluids IV.

**C.** Gloves must be worn.

## Intradermal Administration

**A.** Use size 26 g to 27 g, 1-inch needle on a 1 mL or tuberculin syringe (volume will be approximately 0.1 mL).

**B.** Put on gloves.

**C.** Stretch skin taut.

**D.** Insert needle at 10–15° angle approximately 1–2 mm depth with needle bevel upward.

**E.** Possible sites
   1. Ventral forearm
   2. Scapula
   3. Upper chest

**F.** When wheal appears, remove needle; do not massage site.

## Intramuscular (IM) Administration

**A.** Use size 18 g to 23 g, 1–2-inch needle, maximum volume 5 mL.

**B.** Put on gloves.

**C.** Stretch skin taut.

**D.** Insert needle at 90° angle.

**E.** Possible sites
   1. Gluteus minimus (ventrogluteal): landmarks are anterior-superior iliac spine, iliac crest, greater trochanter of femur.
   2. Vastus lateralis (anterior thigh) (Figure 2-7): a handbreadth above the knee and below greater trochanter; good site for children.

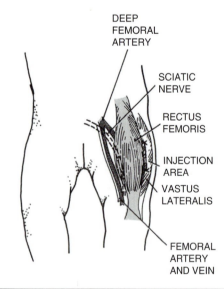

**Figure 2-7** Anterior view of the location of the vastus lateralis muscle in a young child

DEEP FEMORAL ARTERY
SCIATIC NERVE
RECTUS FEMORIS
INJECTION AREA
VASTUS LATERALIS
FEMORAL ARTERY AND VEIN

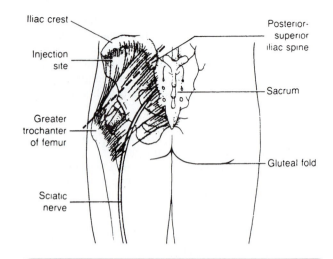

**Figure 2-8** When using the dorsogluteal site, injection is made into the gluteus medius muscle

Iliac crest
Injection site
Greater trochanter of femur
Sciatic nerve
Posterior-superior iliac spine
Sacrum
Gluteal fold

   3. Rectus femoris (medial thigh): a handbreadth above knee and below greater trochanter; good site for infants and self-injection.
   4. Gluteus medius (dorsogluteal) (Figure 2-8): landmarks are posterior superior iliac spine, iliac crest, greater trochanter of femur.
   5. Deltoid (Figure 2-9): landmarks are acromium process, axilla base; for small doses less than 2 mL only.

**F.** Z-track injection (IM variation) for irritating solutions.
   1. Needle size: replace needle used to draw up medication with one 2–3 inches long, 20–22 g.
   2. Pull skin away from site laterally with nondominant hand to ensure medication enters muscle.
   3. Wait 10 seconds after injecting medication before withdrawing needle.
   4. Release skin; do not massage (seals needle track).
   5. Encourage physical activity.
   6. Possible sites: gluteus medius best, but may use any IM site except deltoid.

**G.** A 45° angle may be sufficient for infants and children.

## Administration of Intravenous (IV) Medications

**A.** General principles
   1. Check site for complications (redness, swelling, tenderness).
   2. Check for blood return.
   3. Prepare medication according to manufacturer's specifications.
   4. Appropriate tubing selection varies according to institution policy. Generally, rates greater

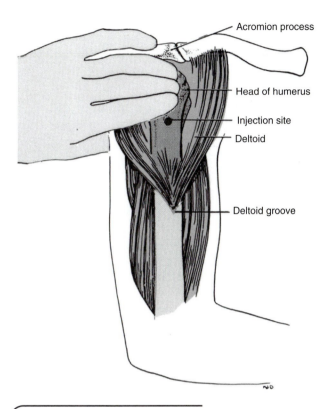

Acromion process

Head of humerus

Injection site

Deltoid

Deltoid groove

**Figure 2-9** Deltoid injection site

than or equal to 12 hours require macrotubing (60 gtts/mL), all others require macrotubing (10, 15, or 20 gtts/mL).

    5. Gloves should be worn when contact with blood or other body fluids is a possibility.

**B.** A scheduled routine flushing of the IV site is required to check for patency and if intravenous catheter is still in the vein. Flushing is also done before and after intermittent medications. Site may be called: male adapter, heplock, heparin lock, capped jelco, INT.

    1. Clean injection port with alcohol at each step.

    2. Use SASH method to give medication.

      **a.** S: flush with 2–3 mL saline.

      **b.** A: administer medication at prescribed rate using either the needleless system, a blunt needle, or a short needle with a gauge equal to or smaller than catheter (25 g ½ in).

      **c.** S: flush with 2–3 mL saline (maintain positive pressure to prevent blood back-up into catheter).

      **d.** If a central line (CVP) or PICC line is present, then an additional flush of Heplock flush is administered (to prevent blood clotting in line). Most facilities protocol require the use of 10-cc syringes for all flushes in CVPs or PICCs due to the less pressure force exerted on the lines.

**C.** Secondary piggyback/add-a-line (added to an existing IV line) (Figure 2-10).

    1. With regulator turned off, spike tubing into IV bag with medication.

    2. Squeeze drip chamber; fill halfway with solution.

    3. Run fluid through tubing.

    4. If using add-a-line tubing, lower main IV bag on hanger provided, otherwise hang bag at same level as primary bag.

    5. Swab most proximal port with alcohol for add-a-line systems, otherwise lower port is acceptable.

    6. Attach 20 g 1-inch needle to tubing, if a needleless system is not being used.

    7. Insert needle into injection port.

    8. Regulate rate with control and watch to count drops.

    9. When medication absorbed, main line will start to drip again.

    10. Turn off secondary tubing.

    11. Return main bag to original position.

    12. Special concerns

      **a.** Be sure to label tubing with date.

      **b.** Use new tubing every 24–72 hours (according to institution policy).

**D.** Intravenous push medications

    1. Using an appropriately sized needle, prepare medication as ordered.

    2. Cleanse injection port with alcohol or other appropriate cleanser.

    3. Unless otherwise recommended, turn off primary IV bag; flush with saline if indicated.

    4. Insert needle and administer medication at prescribed rate.

**E.** Electronic regulators

    1. Syringe infusers

      **a.** Check for drug compatibility, flush with saline if necessary.

      **b.** Place syringe into infuser and prime appropriate tubing with prepared medication.

      **c.** Secure unit and activate unit according to manufacturer's recommendations.

    2. Pumps and controllers

      **a.** Prime tubing according to manufacturer's recommendations; do not purge when attached to client.

      **b.** Prior to connecting IV to client, check to determine if tubing allows gravity free-flow. If it does, be sure to turn off regulator.

      **c.** Connect tubing to client and turn on electronic regulator.

      **d.** Confirm alarm function by keeping tubing clamped while machine is turned on. Do not turn off alarms.

      **e.** Follow manufacturer's directions for deactivating alarm and starting IV flow.

      **f.** Explain regulator and alarms to client.

      **g.** Confirm flow rate with hourly checks on client, fluid, and regulator.

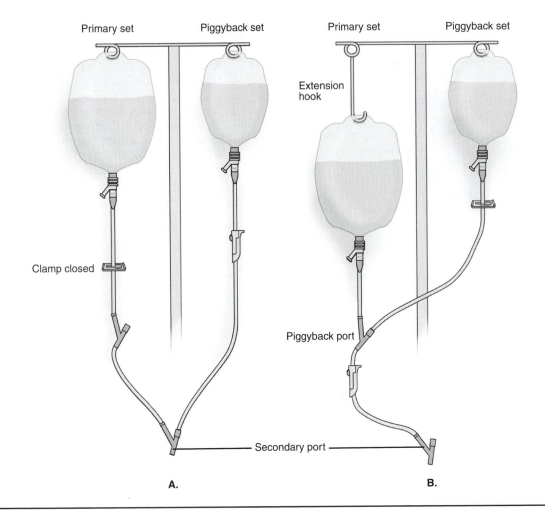

Primary set     Piggyback set         Primary set     Piggyback set

Extension hook

Clamp closed

Piggyback port

Secondary port

A.                  B.

**Figure 2-10** (A) In this setup, the tubing to the primary set is clamped to allow the piggyback unit to empty first. The tubing on the primary setup is unclamped once the piggyback unit empties. (B) In this setup, the primary bottle is hung on an extension hook to allow the piggyback unit to empty first. The primary unit then begins to empty

## MEDICATION CALCULATIONS

### Conversions

Conversions need to be made within systems (from one measurement to another) and also among systems (from apothecary to metric or household to metric).

### *Conversions within Systems*

A. Metric system
   1. Based on decimal system, basic unit is 10.

2. Units of measurement are
   a. Meter (m) for length
   b. Gram (g) for weight
   c. Liter (l or L) for volume
3. Multiples and fractions of 10 are identified by prefixes (Table 2–1).
   a. 0.001 liter would then be equal to 1 milliliter (mL).
   b. 1000 grams would be equal to a kilogram (kg).
4. Commonly used terms of weight include kilogram, gram, milligram, and microgram.

**Table 2-1** Metric Prefixes Denoting Multiples and Fractions of 10

| | **Multiples** | | | **Measure** | **Fractions** | | | **Micro** |
|---|---|---|---|---|---|---|---|---|
| Decimal Metric | 1000 Thousands Kilo– | 100 Hundreds Hecto– | 10 Tens Deka– | LGM | 0.1 Tenths Deci– | 0.01 Hundredths Centi– | 0.001 Thousandths Milli– | .000001 Millionths Micro– |

**Table 2-2** Household Units of Liquid Measure

60 drops (gtts) = 1 teaspoon (tsp)
3 tsp = 1 tablespoon (tbsp)
6 tsp = 1 ounce (oz)
2 tbsp = 1 oz
6 oz = 1 teacup
8 oz = 1 glass
8 oz = 1 measuring cup

**Table 2-3** Approximate Equivalents to Remember

| Household | Metric |
|---|---|
| 1 drop (gtt) | = .06 milliliter (mL) |
| 15 drops (gtt) | = 1 mL [1 cc] |
| 1 teaspoon (tsp) | = 5 (4) mL |
| 1 tablespoon (tbsp) | = 15 mL |
| 2 tbsp | = 30 mL |
| 1 ounce (oz) | = 30 mL |
| 1 teacup (6 oz) | = 180 mL |
| 1 glass (8 oz) | = 240 mL |
| 1 measuring cup (8 oz) | = 240 mL |
| 2 measuring cups (1 pint) | = 500 mL |

5. Commonly used terms of volume include liter and milliliter. *Note: A cube measuring 1 cm per side holds one milliliter, so a cubic centimeter (cc) equals a milliliter (mL): 1 cc = 1 mL.*
6. To convert within the metric system, set up a ratio with the conversion factor on the right and the desired information on the left, cross multiply, divide to find X, and complete needed math. Remember to keep ratios equal: whatever is done to one side must be done to the other.
7. Example: convert 5000 mg to g
   a. 1000 mg = 1 g
   b. $\frac{5000 \text{ mg}}{X} = \frac{1000 \text{ mg}}{1 \text{ g}}$
   c. (X) (1000 mg) = (5000 mg) (1 g)
   d. $\frac{(X) (1000 \text{ mg})}{(1000 \text{ mg})} = \frac{(5000 \text{ mg}) (1 \text{ g})}{(1000 \text{ mg})}$
   e. X = (5) (1 g)
   f. X = 5 g
   g. 5000 mg = 5 g
B. Household system
   1. Approximate measures that vary according to manufacturer, temperature.
   2. Common units include teaspoon (tsp), tablespoon (tbsp), ounce (oz), cup, and drop (gtt) (Table 2–2).
   3. Conversions within the system are the same.
   4. Example: convert 3 tsp to drops
      a. 60 drops = 1 tsp
      b. $\frac{3 \text{ tsp}}{X} = \frac{1 \text{ tsp}}{60 \text{ gtts}}$
      c. (1 tsp) (X) = (3 tsp) (60 gtts)
      d. $\frac{(1 \text{ tsp}) (X)}{1 \text{ tsp}} = \frac{(3 \text{ tsp}) (60 \text{ gts})}{1 \text{ tsp}}$
      e. X = 180 gtts

### Conversions from One System to Another

A. Conversions are done in the same manner. Some of the equivalents must be memorized (Table 2–3).
B. Example: convert 90 gtts to ml
   1. 15 gtts = 1 mL
   2. $\frac{90 \text{ gtts}}{X} = \frac{15 \text{ gtts}}{1 \text{ mL}}$
   3. (15 gtts) (X) = (90 gtts) (1 mL)

4. $\frac{(15 \text{ gtts}) (X)}{15 \text{ gtts}} = \frac{(90 \text{ gtts}) (1 \text{ mL})}{15 \text{ gtts}}$
5. X = 6 mL

## Dosage Calculations

A. Calibrated containers are available for oral liquids (Figure 2-11), and liquid injectables (Figure 2-12).
B. Formula for calculations
   $\frac{\text{ordered amount of drug}}{\text{amount of drug on hand}} = \frac{\text{unknown quantity needed (X)}}{\text{known quantity of drug}}$
C. Be sure all conversions are done first. The technique of using ratios is the same.

### Technique

A. Dosage calculation for scored tablet
   1. 2000 mg of a drug is ordered. It is available as a scored tablet containing 4 grams.
   2. Calculation
      a. Convert 4 grams into mg
         1. $\frac{4 \text{ g}}{X \text{ mg}} = \frac{1 \text{ g}}{1000 \text{ mg}}$
         2. 4000 = X   Therefore, 4 g = 4000 mg

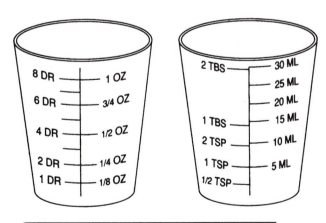

**Figure 2-11** Disposable medicine containers

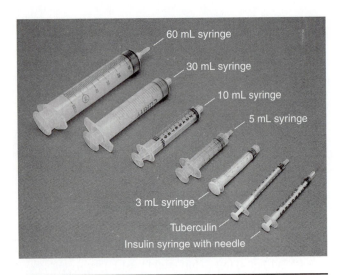

**Figure 2-12** Commonly used syringes (not to scale)

b. Now calculate dosage

1.
$$\frac{2000 \text{ mg (ordered amt)}}{4000 \text{ mg (amt on hand)}} = \frac{X \text{ (unknown quantity)}}{1 \text{ tablet (known quantity)}}$$

2. 2000 mg = 4000 mg X

Divide each by 4000

3. $\dfrac{2000 \text{ mg}}{4000 \text{ mg}} = \dfrac{4000 \text{ mg}}{4000 \text{ mg}}$

4. $\dfrac{2000 \text{ mg}}{4000 \text{ mg}} = X$

5. X = 0.5 tablet

3. Give ½ tablet.

B. Dosage calculation for liquid

1. The order is for potassium chloride (KCl) 20 mEq. The bottle is labeled KCl elixir 10 mEq/mL. How many mL will be given?

a. Ordered amount of drug is 20 mEq; amount of drug on hand is 10 mEq.

b. Unknown quantity is X; known quantity of drug on hand is 1 mL.

2. Calculations

a. $\dfrac{20 \text{ mEq}}{10 \text{ mEq}} = \dfrac{X}{1 \text{ mL}}$

b. (10 mEq) (X) = (20 mEq) (1 mL)

c. $\dfrac{(10 \text{ mEq}) (X)}{10 \text{ mEq}} = \dfrac{(20 \text{ mEq}) (1 \text{ mL})}{10 \text{ mEq}}$

d. X = 2 mL

3. Give 2 mL potassium chloride.

C. Dosage calculation for a capsule

1. The order reads: Phentoin Sodium capsules (Dilantin) gr V orally. Available is a bottle labeled Dilantin 100 mg per capsule. How many capsules will be given?

2. Calculations

a. First, convert gr 5 to mg

1) 1 gr = 60 mg

2) $\dfrac{5 \text{ gr}}{1 \text{ gr}} = \dfrac{X \text{ mg}}{60 \text{ mg}}$

3) X = 300 mg

b. Now calculate the dosage

1) $\dfrac{\text{ordered amt is 300 mg}}{\text{amt on hand 100 mg}} =$

$\dfrac{X \text{ (unknown) capsules}}{1 \text{ (known) capsules}}$

2) 300 mg = X

100 mg = 1

3) 100 X = 300

4) X = 3

3. Give 3 capsules.

D. Dosage calculation for parenteral medications

1. Order reads: Furosemide (Lasix) 35 mg IV. The vial is labeled 40 mg = 4 mL. How many mL should be given?

2. Calculations

a. $\dfrac{\text{(ordered amt) 35 mg}}{\text{(amt on hand) 40 mg}} = \dfrac{\text{(unknown quantity)}}{4 \text{ mL (known quantity)}}$

1) $\dfrac{35 \text{ mg}}{40 \text{ mg}} = \dfrac{X}{4 \text{ mL}}$

2) 40 X = 140

3) X = 3.5

b. Give 3.5 mL

c. Another method:

1) $\dfrac{\text{(ordered amt) (known quantity)}}{\text{(amt on hand)}}$

2) $\dfrac{(35 \text{ mg}) (4 \text{ mL})}{(40 \text{ mg})} = 3.5 \text{ mL}$

E. Dosage calculation for units (some medications such as heparin and penicillin are ordered in units)

1. The order is penicillin 750,000 units. The vial reads 300,000 units/2 mL. How many mL will be given?

2. Ordered amount of drug is 750,000 units; amount of drug on hand is 300,000 units.

3. Unknown quantity is X; known quantity is 2 mL.

4. Calculations

a. $\dfrac{750,000 \text{ units}}{300,000 \text{ units}} = \dfrac{X}{2 \text{ mL}}$

b. (300,000 units) (X) = (750,000 units) (2 mL)

c. $\dfrac{300,000 \text{ X}}{3,000,000 \text{ units}} = \dfrac{1,500,000}{300,000}$

d. $X = \dfrac{150}{30}$

e. X = 5 mL

5. Give 5 mL penicillin.

F. Dosage calculation for powders that need to be reconstituted by adding sterile water or normal saline solution (the total amount of solution is used for calculations)

1. Mefoxin 1 g is ordered; mefoxin 2 g is on hand. Add 4.3 mL to equal 5 mL solution.
2. Ordered amount of drug is 1 g; amount of drug on hand is 2 g.
3. Unknown quantity is X; known quantity is 5 mL.
4. Calculations
   a. $\dfrac{1\ g}{2\ g} = \dfrac{X}{5\ mL}$
   b. $(2\ g)\,(X) = (5\ mL)\,(1\ g)$
   c. $\dfrac{(2\ g)\,(X)}{2\ g} = \dfrac{(5\ mL)\,(1\ g)}{2\ g}$
   d. $X = 2.5\ mL$
5. Give 2.5 mL mefoxin.

G. Dosage calculation in children (pediatric dosages)
   1. Body surface area (BSA): most accurate method for calculating pediatric dosages
      a. West nomogram, Figure 2-13, if BSA is not known: draw a line from height on the nomogram; the point of intersection on surface area is the BSA.
      b. Formula using surface area ($m^2$)
         $$\dfrac{\text{surface area } (m^2)}{1.73\ m^2} \times \text{adult dose} = \text{child dose}$$
      c. Example of calculating a pediatric dosage using BSA:
         1) The adult dose is 100 mg Demerol; the child weighs 20 kg and is 40 inches tall.
         2) BSA is 0.77 $m^2$
         3) Calculations
            a) $\dfrac{0.77^2}{1.73\ m^2} \times 100\ mg = X$
            b) $0.45 \times 100\ mg = X$
            c) $45\ mg = X$
         4) Child's dose is 45 mg.
   2. Pediatric dosages may also be calculated by weight (mg/kg)
      a. Example: the order is for phenobarbital 2 mg/kg of body weight; the client weighs 25 kg.
      b. Calculations
         1) $\dfrac{2\ mg}{X} = \dfrac{1\ kg}{25\ kg}$
         2) $(1\ kg)\,(X) = (2\ mg)\,(25\ kg)$
         3) $\dfrac{(1\ kg)\,(X)}{1\ kg} = \dfrac{(2\ mg)\,(25\ kg)}{1\ kg}$
         4) $X = 50\ mg$
      c. Give 50 mg of phenobarbital.

H. Dosage calculation for IV medications
   1. Macrodrop
      a. More commonly used in adult IVF (intravenous fluid) administration
      b. In order to calculate the flow rate, need to know drop factor: 10, 15, or 20 gtt/mL

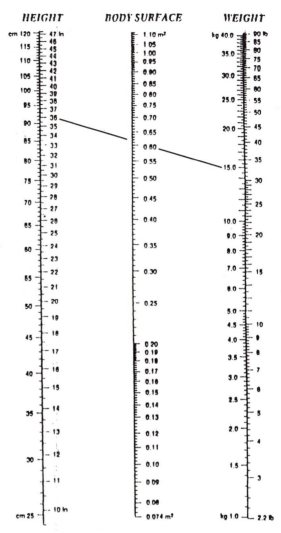

HEIGHT          BODY SURFACE          WEIGHT

Nomogram for determining body surface of children from height and weight. ($S = W^{0.425} \times H^{0.725} \times 71.84$, or log $S =$ log $W \times 0.425 +$ log $H \times 0.725 + 1.8564$ [$S =$ body surface in $cm^2$; $W =$ weight in kg; $H =$ height in cm]).

**Figure 2-13** Nomogram. In this example, a child who weighs 15 kilograms and is about 92 centimeters in height has a body surface area of .60 square meter. (Source: "A Formula to Estimate the Approximate Surface Area if Height and Weight Be Known" by D. Dubois and E. F. Dubois, 1916, *Archives of Internal Medicine*, 17, p. 863. Modified with permission.)

   2. Microdrop
      a. More commonly used for children, elderly or critically ill where exact control is required
      b. Drop factor is always 60 gtt/mL

3. Formula for calculation

$$\frac{\text{amount of solution}}{\text{time in minutes}} \times \text{Drop factor} = \text{gtt/min}$$

4. Example: the order is for 1000 mL NS over 8 hours; drop factor is 10 gtt/mL
   a. Calculation
      1) $\dfrac{1000 \text{ mL}}{480 \text{ min}} \times \dfrac{10 \text{ gtt/mL}}{\text{mL}} = X$
      2) $\dfrac{1000 \text{ mL/gtt}}{480 \text{ min}} = 20.8 \text{ gtt/min}$
      3) X = 20.8 gtt/min

5. The same formula can be used for IVs requiring microdrop rates, or the following formula can be used:
   mL/hour = microdrops/min
   This formula works because the drop factor for microdrop tubing is always 60 microgtts/mL and an hour is 60 minutes.
   a. Example: order is for 1000 mL D$_5$NS over 24 hours. Drop factor is 60 gtt/mL
   b. Calculation with the first formula
      1) $\dfrac{1000 \text{ mL}}{1440 \text{ min}} \times \dfrac{60 \text{ gtt}}{\text{mL}} = X$
      2) $\dfrac{(1000 \text{ mL}) \times (60 \text{ gtt})}{1440 \text{ min/mL}} = 41.66$
      3) X = 41.66 gtt/min
   c. Cannot give a partial drop, so rate is 42 gtt/min.
   d. Calculation with the second formula
      1) First determine the mL/hour:
         $\dfrac{\text{total volume}}{\text{total hours}}$
      2) $\dfrac{1000 \text{ mL}}{24 \text{ hours}} = 42 \text{ mL/hour} = 42 \text{ gtt/min}$

6. Readjusting IV rates may be necessary when the prescribed rate for an existing IV is changed
   a. Formula for calculation
      $\dfrac{\text{amount of solution remaining}}{\text{remaining hours in minutes}} \times \text{drop factor}$
   b. Example: the order is to infuse remaining 700 mL over 3 hours; drop factor is 15 gtt/mL.
   c. Calculation
      1) $\dfrac{700 \text{ mL}}{180 \text{ min}} \times \dfrac{15 \text{ gtt}}{\text{mL}} = X$
      2) $\dfrac{700 \text{ mL} \times 15 \text{ gtt}}{180} = 58.33$
      3) $\dfrac{700 \text{ gtt}}{12 \text{ min}} = 58.3 \text{ gtt/min}$
   d. Cannot give partial drop, so run IV at 58 gtt/min.

## Sample Questions

4. The order reads Digoxin 0.375 mg once daily. The bottle reads Digoxin 0.25 mg per tablet. How much should the nurse administer?

5. The order is chloral hydrate 200 mg. The bottle reads chloral hydrate 0.1 g/capsule. Give _____ capsules.

6. The order is penicillin 50,000 units. The vial reads penicillin 500,000 units. Add 4.3 mL to yield 5 mL. Give _____ mL.

7. The order is ampicillin 0.4 mg/kg. Client weighs 38.5 pounds. The bottle reads ampicillin 10 mg/mL. Give _____ mL.

8. Phenytoin (Dilantin) 5 mg/kg is ordered for a 40-pound child. It is to be administered in three equal doses. The drug is available in an oral suspension containing 125 mg/mL. How many ml should be administered per dose?

9. The order is for 1.2 million units of penicillin G (Bicillin) IM. Available is 600,000 units/mL. How much should the nurse administer?

10. Order is for 2500 mL D$_5$W over 24 hours. Drop factor is 15 gtt/mL. Run IV at _____ gtts/minute.

11. Order is for 2000 mL D$_5$W over 24 hours. Drop factor is 60 gtt/mL. Run IV at _____ gtt/minute.

12. Enoxaparin sodium (Lovenox) 25 mg SC q 12 hours is ordered. The label reads 30 mg /0.3 mL. How much should the nurse administer?

13. The order is for meperidine 50 mg IM q 4 hours prn. The label reads meperidine 75 mg/mL. How much should the nurse administer?

14. An adult is on continuous IV heparin therapy for thrombophlebitis. The IV contains 15,000 units of heparin in 500 mL of 5% dextrose (D$_5$W) at the rate of 20 mL per hr. How many units per hour is the client receiving?
    1. 60 units.
    2. 25 units.
    3. 600 units.
    4. 700 units.

15. The order is for Ancef 1 gram IV in 50 cc 5% dextrose ($D_5W$) to run in over 30 minutes every 6 hours. The administration set delivers 10 gtts/cc. What should the drip rate be?

   1.  8 gtt/min.

   2.  15 gtt/min.

   3.  17 gtt/min.

   4.  25 gtt/min.

 **Answers and Rationales**

4. 1.5 tablets. The formula to use is:

$$\frac{\text{ordered amt}}{\text{amt on hand}} \times \text{quantity}$$

$$\frac{0.375}{0.25} \times 1 \text{ tablet} = 1.5 \text{ tablets}$$

5. 2 capsules. First convert grams to mg.

1000 mg = 1 g

1000 mg × 0.1 = 100 mg

Then use ordered over amount on hand times quantity.

$$\frac{200 \text{ mg}}{100 \text{ mg}} \times 1 \text{ capsule} = 2 \text{ capsules}$$

6. 0.5 mL. The formula to use is ordered over amount on hand times volume.

$$\frac{50,000 \text{ units}}{500,000 \text{ units}} \times 5 \text{ mL} = 0.5 \text{ mL}$$

7. 0.7 mL. First convert pounds to kg. 38.5 pounds divided by 2.2 pounds/kg = 17.5 kg. Calculate total mg to be given.

$$\frac{0.4 \text{ mg}}{\text{kg}} \times 17.5 \text{ kg} = 7 \text{ mg}$$

Then use ordered over amount on hand times volume.

$$\frac{7 \text{ mg}}{10 \text{ mg}} \times 1 \text{ mL} = 0.7 \text{ mL}$$

8. 1.2 mL/dose. First convert pounds to kg. Divide 40 pounds by 2.2 pounds/kg for a weight of 18.18 kg. Multiply 5 mg/kg for a total daily dose of 91 mg. Calculate the dose using ordered over amount on hand times volume.

$$\frac{91 \text{ mg}}{125 \text{ mg}} \times 5 \text{ mL} = 3.6 \text{ mL total daily dose}$$

Divide 3.6 mL by 3 doses = 1.2 mL/dose.

9. 2 mL.

$$\frac{1,200,000 \text{ units}}{600,000 \text{ units}} \times 1 \text{ mg} = 2 \text{ mL}$$

10. 26 gtt/min. Divide 2500 mL by 24 hours. Then divide the result by 60 minutes per hour and multiply by 15 gtt/mL.

11. 83 gtt/min. Divide 2000 mL by 24 hours for 83 mL/hour. This is divided by 60 min/hour and multiplied by 60 gtt/mL for a total of 83 gtt/min.

12. 0.25 mL. Ordered amount is 25 mg. Available is 30 mg in 0.3 mL.

$$\frac{0.25 \text{ mg}}{0.30 \text{ mg}} \times 0.3 \text{ mL} = 0.25 \text{ mL}$$

13. 0.67 mL. Ordered amount is 50 mg. Available is 75 mg/mL.

$$\frac{50 \text{ mg}}{75 \text{ mg}} \times 1 \text{ mL} = 0.66667 \text{ mL}$$

14. 3. Divide 500 mL by 20 mL to determine the number of hours of the infusion: 25 hours. Next, divide 25 hours into 15,000 units to get units/hour: 600 units of heparin/hour.

15. 3.

$$\frac{\text{total volume infused}}{\text{time in minutes}} \times \text{drop factor} = \text{gtt per minute}$$

$$\frac{50 \text{ mL}}{30 \text{ minutes}} \times \frac{10 \text{ gtt}}{1 \text{ mL}} = 16.6 = 17 \text{ gtt/min}$$

 # Central Nervous System Drugs

## LOCAL ANESTHETICS

A.  Prototype: Lidocaine (Xylocaine)

    1.  Action. Amide-type anesthetic that blocks nerve conduction; metabolized by hepatic enzymes; produces temporary loss of sensation and motion in a limited area of the body.

    2.  Use. Topical anesthesia, regional anesthesia (Unit 4), antiarrhythmic (discussed in Cardiovascular Drugs).

3. Adverse effects. Drowsiness, dizziness, light-headedness, restlessness, numbness of lips and tongue; headache with spinal anesthesia; hypotension, bradycardia, cardiovascular collapse; convulsions; tinnitus; muscle weakness; anaphylaxis; respiratory depression.
4. Nursing implications
   a. Force fluids with spinal anesthesia.
   b. When used for spinal or epidural anesthesia, should be preservative free.
   c. Monitor VS, and keep siderails up.
   d. Epinephrine, a vasoconstrictor, may be added to lidocaine (Xylocaine).
   e. May interfere with swallowing reflex.
   f. Discard drug without preservatives after immediate use.
   g. Due to adverse effects, elderly clients should be closely monitored.
   h. Do not use discolored, cloudy solutions.
B. Related drugs. See Table 2-4.

 **Sample Questions**

16. Why is epinephrine added to local anesthetic preparations?
    1. Prolong anesthetic action.
    2. Lower blood pressure.
    3. Prevent arrhythmias.
    4. Increase blood flow to injection site.

17. A client complains of a severe sore throat after the extraction of 2 wisdom teeth. Viscous lidocaine (Xylocaine) is ordered. Which of the following should be included in client teaching concerning the use of viscous lidocaine (Xylocaine)?
    1. Take viscous lidocaine (Xylocaine) with fluids to soothe sore throat.
    2. Instruct client to use a humidifier while taking viscous lidocaine (Xylocaine).

**Table 2-4** Local Anesthetics

| Drug | Use | Adverse Effects | Nursing Implications |
|---|---|---|---|
| Procaine (Novocain) | Nerve block Spinal anesthesia Infiltration anesthesia | Anaphylaxis is seen more with ester-type anesthetics | • Procaine is an ester-type anesthetic metabolized by esterase found in plasma<br>• Emergency resuscitation equipment should be available<br>• Monitor VS (see lidocaine [Xylocaine]) |
| Benzocaine (Americaine) | Topical anesthesia | See procaine (Novocain) and lidocaine (Xylocaine) | • Benzocaine (Americaine) is similar to procaine (Novocain) and is an ester-type anesthetic<br>• Commonly found in OTC preparations to treat sunburn, rashes, sore throats, and hemorrhoids |
| Mepivacaine (Carbocaine) | Infiltration nerve block anesthesia | See lidocaine (Xylocaine) | • Amide-type local anesthetic that has two times the potency and toxicity of lidocaine |
| Bupivacaine (Marcaine) | Epidural blocks Infiltration anesthesia Peripheral nerve block | See lidocaine (Xylocaine) | • Long-acting amide-type anesthetic<br>• Toxicity seen more often in children and elderly |
| Etidocaine (Duranest) | Infiltration anesthesia Peripheral nerve block Central neural blocks | See lidocaine (Xylocaine) | • Analgesia effects last 1½–2 times longer than lidocaine |

3. Advise client to wait 60 minutes before eating after drug application.
4. Encourage client to take viscous lidocaine (Xylocaine) with food to reduce GI distress.

## Answers and Rationales

16. 1. Epinephrine prolongs anesthetic action, while shortening the onset of action and reducing blood flow to injection site.

17. 3. Viscous lidocaine (Xylocaine) can interfere with swallowing reflex and clients should wait at least 60 minutes after use before eating.

# NON-NARCOTIC ANALGESICS AND ANTIPYRETICS

A. Prototype: salicylates
Acetylsalicylic Acid (aspirin) (ASA)
  1. Action
     a. Analgesia: inhibits formation of prostaglandins involved with pain. Analgesia also occurs by action of hypothalamus and blocking generation of pain impulses.
     b. Antipyretic: inhibits formation of prostaglandins in production of fever. Aspirin acts on the hypothalamus to produce vasodilation.
     c. Anti-inflammatory: inhibits prostaglandin synthesis causing anti-inflammatory action.
     d. Antiplatelet action occurs when aspirin inhibits prostaglandin derivative, thromboxane $A_2$.
  2. Use. Mild to moderate pain; control of fever; inflammatory conditions; reduce TIA occurrence; reduce risk of MI in men with unstable angina.
  3. Adverse effects. Tinnitus, confusion, dizziness—all are symptoms of salicylism; drowsiness; epistaxis, bleeding, bruising; edema, hypertension; nausea, vomiting, diarrhea, gastritis; hypersensitivity; hypoglycemia, sweating; impaired renal function; respiratory alkalosis and metabolic acidosis are associated with aspirin toxicity.
  4. Nursing implications
     a. Clients with history of nasal polyps, asthma, rhinitis, chronic urticaria have high incidence of aspirin hypersensitivity.
     b. Clients with diabetes should have glucose monitored.
     c. Monitor CBC, prothrombin time, kidney and liver function studies for clients on long-term therapy.
     d. Additive effect for clients on anticoagulant.
     e. Stop therapy 1 week before surgery.
  5. Discharge teaching
     a. Drink plenty of fluids to prevent salicylate crystalluria.
     b. Take with glass of water, antacid, milk, or food to reduce gastric irritation.
     c. Parents should not give to children or adolescents with flu or chickenpox because Reye's syndrome may occur.
     d. Report signs of bleeding and bruising to physician.
     e. Discontinue use if tinnitus, dizziness, or GI distress occur.
     f. Pregnant women should not use.
     g. Do not crush enteric-coated tablets.
     h. Do not ingest large amounts of alcohol as this increases risk of GI bleeding.
B. Related drugs. See Table 2-5.
C. Prototype: acetaminophen (Tylenol)
  1. Action. Analgesic and antipyretic action (see aspirin); does not have anti-inflammatory or antiplatelet action.
  2. Use. Mild to moderate pain, fever control.
  3. Adverse effects. Rash, thrombocytopenia, liver toxicity. Toxicity can occur 2–24 hours after ingestion.
  4. Nursing implications
     a. Monitor liver and kidney function, and CBC periodically for clients on long-term therapy.
     b. Can cause psychologic dependence.
     c. Antidote: acetylcysteine (Mucomyst)
  5. Discharge teaching. Notify physician if no relief of symptoms within 5 days of therapy.

## Sample Questions

18. Which of the following should be included in teaching concerning the administration of indomethacin (Indocin)?
    1. Have periodic ophthalmic examinations.
    2. Take on an empty stomach.
    3. Take aspirin for headache relief.
    4. Eat high-fiber foods to prevent constipation.

19. In comparing aspirin to acetaminophen (Tylenol), what is true pertaining to Tylenol?
    1. It is contraindicated in clients with peptic ulcer disease.
    2. It is contraindicated in clients with asthma.
    3. It is as effective as aspirin for reducing fever.

**Table 2-5** Nonsteroidal Anti-Inflammatory Drugs (NSAIDs)*

| Drug | Use | Adverse Effects | Nursing Implications |
|---|---|---|---|
| Ibuprofen (Motrin, Advil) | Relief of mild to moderate pain<br>Primary dysmenorrhea<br>Rheumatoid and osteoarthritis | May cause sodium or water retention<br>Thrombocytopenia, hemolytic anemia<br>Acute renal failure, hematuria<br>Can elevate liver enzymes | • Do not take with aspirin<br>• Take with food or with milk to decrease GI distress<br>• Monitor liver enzymes |
| Naproxen (Naprosyn) | Rheumatoid and osteoarthritis<br>Ankylosing spondylitis<br>Primary dysmenorrhea<br>Acute gout attacks<br>Juvenile diabetes | See aspirin and ibuprofen (Motrin) | • See aspirin and ibuprofen (Motrin) |
| Indomethacin (Indocin) | Close patent ductus arteriosus in premature infant<br>Acute gouty arthritis<br>Moderate severe refractory rheumatoid and osteoarthritis<br>Ankylosing spondylitis | GI distress, anorexia<br>Severe headache<br>Corneal cloudiness, visual field changes | • Clients need to have periodic ophthalmic examinations<br>• Do not take aspirin; see aspirin |
| Piroxicam (Feldene) | Acute or long-term manage-ment of rheumatoid or osteoarthritis | Higher incidence of GI bleeding | • See aspirin, indomethacin (Indocin), and ibuprofen (Motrin) |
| Ketorolac (Toradol) | Short-term pain management | Risk of renal impairment and GI bleeding in prolonged use | • Do not give longer than 5 days<br>• Anaphylaxis can occur with first dose |
| Celecoxib (Celebrex) | Primary dysmenorrhea<br>Acute pain<br>Rheumatoid and osteoarthritis | Peripheral edema<br>Abdominal pain<br>Upper respiratory infection | • Separate administration with magnesium or aluminum containing antacids by 2 hours<br>• Monitor liver enzymes, renal function, H & H and electrolytes |
| Valdecoxib (Bextra) | Primary dysmenorrhea<br>Osteoarthritis<br>Adult rheumatoid arthritis | Anemia<br>Fluid retention<br>Increased blood pressure | • Can take without regard to food<br>• Do not take aspirin or other NSAIDs with this medication |

*NSAIDs are prostaglandin Inhibitors

4. It has a stronger anti-inflammatory effect than aspirin.

**20.** Which condition is an indication for aspirin use?
1. Asthma.
2. TIA.
3. Gout.
4. Nasal polyps.

**21.** Which drug is the drug of choice used to treat primary dysmenorrhea?
1. Acetaminophen (Tylenol).
2. Piroxicam (Feldene).
3. Indomethacin (Indocin).
4. Ibuprofen (Motrin).

18. **1.** Indomethacin (Indocin) may cause visual field changes or corneal cloudiness. Clients should have periodic ophthalmic examinations to monitor for visual change.

19. **3.** Acetaminophen (Tylenol) is as effective as aspirin in reducing fever. Both have similar antipyretic actions.

20. **2.** Due to aspirin's antiplatelet effect, aspirin can be used to decrease TIA.

21. **4.** Ibuprofen (Motrin) is the drug of choice to treat primary dysmenorrhea.

# NARCOTIC ANALGESICS

A. Prototype: morphine sulfate
   1. Action. Acts on opioid receptors in CNS and induces sedation, analgesia, and euphoria.
   2. Use. Relief of moderate to severe pain, preoperative and/or postoperative medication, pain relief in MI, relief of dyspnea occurring in pulmonary edema or acute left ventricular failure.
   3. Adverse effects. Sedation, confusion, euphoria, impaired coordination, dizziness; urinary retention, constipation, hyperglycemia; respiratory depression; hypotension, tachycardia, bradycardia; nausea, vomiting, decreased uterine contractility; allergic reactions; tolerance, physical and psychological dependence; pupil constriction.
   4. Nursing implications
      a. Assess client's pain before giving medication.
      b. Evaluate effectiveness of analgesic including onset and duration of response to medication.
      c. Observe for signs of tolerance with prolonged use.
         1) Tolerance means that a larger dose of narcotic analgesic is required to produce the original effect.
         2) The first sign of tolerance is usually a decreased duration of effect of the analgesic.
      d. Monitor respiratory rate and depth before giving drug, and periodically thereafter.
      e. Encourage sighing, coughing, and deep breathing.
      f. Warn ambulatory clients to avoid activities that require alertness.
      g. Advise client to change position slowly.
      h. Check for signs of urinary retention.
      i. Keep stool record and institute measures to prevent constipation; e.g., fluids, foods high in fiber, and activity as tolerated; administer stool softeners and laxatives as ordered.
      j. Have narcotic antagonist (naloxone [Narcan]) available for reversal of effects if necessary.
      k. Teach client not to drink alcoholic beverages while taking narcotics.
      l. Monitor for withdrawal symptoms and decrease dose slowly because these drugs may produce physical dependence.
      m. Use special caution with clients with increased intracranial pressure, chronic obstructive pulmonary disease (COPD), alcoholism, severe hepatic or renal disease, and in elderly or debilitated clients who may not metabolize the drug efficiently.
   5. Discharge teaching
      a. Take before pain intensifies to receive fullest analgesic effect.
      b. No alcohol or CNS depressants should be taken.
      c. No smoking or ambulating alone after drug has been taken.
      d. Avoid activities requiring alertness.
B. Related drugs. See Table 2-6.
C. Narcotic agonists/antagonists
   1. Examples: pentazocine (Talwin), nalbuphine (Nubain), butorphanol (Stadol), buprenorphine (Buprenex), fentanyl (Duragesic)
   2. Mechanism of action
      a. Term "agonist" refers to the fact that they bind to opioid receptors to produce analgesia.
      b. Term "antagonist" refers to the fact that they counteract the effects of the pure narcotic agonists (i.e., morphine, meperidine [Demerol]).
   3. Use. Relief of moderate to severe pain; may be used for clients who cannot tolerate pure narcotic agonists. Caution: May produce withdrawal in a client who has been taking pure narcotic agonists for a week or more.
   4. Adverse effects. Drowsiness, nausea, psychotomimetic effects, e.g., hallucinations; respiratory depression and constipation but less of a risk than with pure narcotic agonists such as butorphanol (Stadol), nalbuphine (Nubain), pentazocine (Talwin).
D. Combination drugs
   1. Some narcotics can be combined with other drugs.
   2. Examples of this would be codeine combined with Empirin, Fiorinal, or Tylenol.

**Table 2-6** Narcotic Analgesics

| Drug | Use | Comments |
|---|---|---|
| Codeine | Moderate to severe pain, cough relief | • Less potential for dependence than morphine sulfate<br>• Take oral form with food<br>• Monitor for cough suppression<br>• Smoking can reduce pain relief<br>• Cautious use with client on MAO inhibitor |
| Hydromorphone (Dilaudid) | Moderate to severe pain | • Take oral form with food<br>• Mix with 5 mL of sterile water or normal saline for IV use<br>• Smoking reduces pain relief |
| Meperidine (Demerol) | Moderate to severe pain, preoperative medication | • Take oral form with food<br>• PO dose <50% as effective as parenteral<br>• IM preferred route for duplicate doses |
| Methadone (Dolophine) | Severe pain, narcotic withdrawal | • IM preferred route |
| Oxycodone Hydrochloride (Percocet, Percodan) | Moderate to severe pain | • Monitor liver and blood studies<br>• Give oral form with food<br>• High abuse potential |
| Oxycontin | Moderate to severe pain | • Monitor respirations<br>• Take with food<br>• Not intended for use as an "as needed" analgesic (See also oxycodone) |

 **Sample Questions**

22. A client is 1 day post-op. She tells the nurse that she's worried she will become addicted to painkillers so she wants to wait for the pain to become very intense before she takes anything. What is the best response by the nurse?
    1. "Meperidine (Demerol) is very addicting. You shouldn't request pain medication unless you really need it."
    2. "Meperidine (Demerol) is not appropriate for you. I'll ask the physician to order a non-narcotic pain medication for you."
    3. "Meperidine (Demerol) will be most effective if you take it before your pain becomes severe. This will decrease your needing excess amounts of a narcotic."
    4. "Meperidine (Demerol) is ordered for you to help manage your pain. You really should take it."

23. Before administering meperidine (Demerol) to a client, which assessment is most important for the nurse to make?
    1. Apical pulse rate.
    2. Respiratory rate.
    3. Blood pressure.
    4. Level of consciousness.

24. Which adverse effect would the nurse expect to observe in a client receiving a narcotic analgesic?
    1. Urine retention.
    2. Diarrhea.
    3. Hypoglycemia.
    4. Hypertension.

 **Answers and Rationales**

22. **3.** Narcotic drugs should be taken before pain becomes intense so the client can receive the fullest analgesic effects. By adhering to this, the client will have good pain control and will not be requesting additional doses.

23. **2.** Respiratory rate needs to be assessed before giving the client a narcotic as narcotics can have a life-threatening effect.

24. **1.** An adverse side effect of narcotic analgesics is urinary retention. You would also monitor constipation, hyperglycemia, and hypotension.

## NARCOTIC ANTAGONISTS

A. Prototype: naloxone hydrochloride (Narcan)
   1. Action. Occupies opiate receptor sites and prevents or reverses effects of agonists such as morphine sulfate.
   2. Use. Postoperative respiratory depression caused by narcotics, therapy in suspected or confirmed narcotic overdose.
   3. Adverse effects. Excess dosage in narcotic depression: hypertension, tremors, reversal of

analgesia, hyperventilation, increases PTT. In too-quick reversal: nausea, vomiting; sweating, tachycardia.

    4. Nursing implications
      **a.** Emergency resuscitative equipment needs to be available.
      **b.** Monitor VS, especially respirations.
      **c.** Monitor client closely as activity of some narcotics last longer than that of naloxone hydrochloride (Narcan).
      **d.** Monitor surgical clients for bleeding.
      **e.** Withdrawal symptoms will be seen in client addicted to narcotics.
**B.** Related drug: naltrexone (Trexan)
    **1.** Used in narcotic detoxification and to prevent readdiction in drug users.
    **2.** Initial treatment of overdose is naloxone hydrochloride (Narcan) and then naltrexone (Trexan) is given as it has a longer duration of action.
**C.** Related drug: nalmefene (Revex)
    **1.** Used to treat opioid overdose.
    **2.** Can be given IM or SC if IV access is lost.

 ## Sample Questions

**25.** Which of the following observations by the nurse indicates an adverse effect of naloxone hydrochloride (Narcan) on the client?
    1. Hypotension.
    2. Bradycardia.
    3. Tremors.
    4. Increased urine output.

**26.** Which client should have cautious use of naloxone hydrochloride (Narcan)?
    1. Meperidine (Demerol) addict.
    2. Client with brittle diabetes.
    3. Client with asthma.
    4. Postoperative radical neck.

 ## Answers and Rationales

**25. 3.** Tremors are an adverse effect of naloxone hydrochloride (Narcan) and indicate an overdose of the drug.

**26. 1.** If naloxone hydrochloride (Narcan) is given to a client who is addicted to narcotics, the client will experience withdrawal syndrome. Thus, narcotic addicts should use this drug cautiously.

# SEDATIVES AND HYPNOTICS

**A.** Prototype for the Barbiturates: phenobarbital sodium (Luminal)
    **1.** Action. Hinders movement of impulses from the thalamus to the brain cortex, thus creating depression in the CNS, which can range from mild to severe. Considered a long-acting barbiturate.
    **2.** Use. Sedation, hypnosis, seizure disorders.
    **3.** Adverse effects. Dizziness, ataxia, drowsiness, "hangover," anxiety, irritability, hand tremors, vision difficulties, insomnia; bradycardia, low blood pressure; chest tightness, wheezing, apnea, respiratory depression; nausea, vomiting, constipation; hypersensitivity reactions.
    **4.** Nursing implications
      **a.** High doses for long periods of time can cause physical dependence.
      **b.** Drug has extended half-life so steady plasma level may take 3–4 weeks of medication before occurring.
      **c.** Give reconstituted solutions within 30 minutes of mixing.
      **d.** Give IM deeply in large muscle mass and observe IM sites.
      **e.** IV administration: client must be monitored constantly: take VS frequently; have emergency equipment available; monitor for extravasation at infusion site.
      **f.** Pill can be crushed and mixed with food or fluid.
      **g.** Will cause restlessness in client in pain.
      **h.** Geriatric, pediatric, and debilitated clients can have paradoxical reactions.
      **i.** Monitor liver and blood studies with long-term therapy.
      **j.** Schedule IV drug under Federal Controlled Substances Act.
      **k.** Many drug interactions.
    **5.** Discharge teaching
      **a.** Drowsiness occurs in first few weeks of therapy and will decrease.
      **b.** Avoid potentially dangerous activities until response to drug is known.
      **c.** Alcohol is prohibited.
      **d.** Do not alter dosing schedule or amount.
      **e.** Do not stop abruptly.
      **f.** Teratogenic. Prolonged use necessitates alternative contraception methods if taking birth control pills.
      **g.** Do not keep at bedside due to potential for overdosing.
**B.** Related drugs. See Table 2-7.
*Note: actions, adverse effects, and nursing implications are similar to phenobarbital sodium (Luminal).*

**Table 2-7** Barbiturates

| Drug | Use |
|---|---|
| Amobarbital sodium (Amytal) (intermediate acting) | Sedation, hypnosis, preoperative medication, labor, chronic and acute seizures |
| Butabarbital sodium (Butisol) (intermediate acting) | Sedation, hypnosis, preoperative medication |
| Pentobarbital sodium (Nembutal) (short acting) | Sedation, hypnosis, preoperative medication |
| Secobarbital sodium (Seconal) (short acting) | Hypnosis, preoperative medication |
| Thiopental sodium (Pentothal Sodium) (ultrashort acting) | Induction of general anesthesia, acute seizures, decrease of intracranial pressure in neurosurgery, narcoanalysis and narcosynthesis in psychiatry |

C. Prototype for Benzodiazepines (antianxiety agents): diazepam (Valium)
   1. Action. Not fully understood. Depresses the CNS at the limbic system and reticular formation.
   2. Use. Anxiety disorders, acute alcohol withdrawal, muscle relaxant, tetanus, convulsive disorders, preoperative medication.
   3. Adverse effects. Dry mouth, constipation, urinary retention, photophobia and blurred vision; for other effects see adverse effects listed under pentobarbital sodium (Luminal).
   4. Nursing implications
     a. Adverse effects typically dose related.
     b. Two weeks of therapy needed before steady plasma levels seen.
     c. Tablet can be crushed.
     d. Do not mix with other drugs in the same syringe.
     e. Cautious IV use as drug can precipitate in IV solutions.
     f. IM should be deep into large muscle mass; rotate IM sites.
     g. Parenteral administration can cause low blood pressure, increased heart rate, muscle weakness, and respiratory depression.
     h. For extended therapy, monitor liver and blood studies.
     i. Adverse effects more likely in geriatric clients.
     j. Monitor I&O.
     k. Schedule IV drug under Federal Controlled Substances Act.

   5. Discharge teaching
     a. Avoid alcohol.
     b. Avoid potentially dangerous activities until response to drug is known.
     c. Smoking decreases drug effect.
     d. Avoid abrupt discontinuance of drug.
     e. If pregnant or planning a pregnancy, discuss ending drug therapy with physician.
     f. Long-term high dose use can cause physical dependence.
D. Related drugs. See Table 2-8.
   *Note: actions, adverse effects, and nursing implications are similar to diazepam (Valium).*
E. Other sedative/hypnotic drugs
   1. Drugs which produce sedation and/or sleep that are not barbiturates or benzodiazepines.
   2. Examples
     a. Buspirone (BuSpar): used for anxiety disorders.
     b. Ethchlorvynol (Placidyl): used for short-term insomnia (lasting 1 week).
     c. Zolpidem (Ambien): used for short-term insomnia (lasting 1 week).

## Sample Questions

27. The nurse would monitor the client who has been given pentobarbital sodium (Nembutal) for which adverse effects?
   1. Tachycardia.
   2. Hypertension.
   3. Dry mouth.
   4. Anxiety.

**Table 2-8** Benzodiazepines

| Drug | Use |
|---|---|
| Alprazolam (Xanax) | Anxiety |
| Clorazepate (Tranxene) | Anxiety |
| Flurazepam (Dalmane) | Hypnosis |
| Midazolam (Versed) | Preoperative medication, conscious sedation |
| Triazolam (Halcion) | Hypnosis |
| Chlordiazepoxide (Librium) | Anxiety, alcohol withdrawal |
| Clonazepam (Klonopin) | Seizures, restless leg syndrome, panic attacks |
| Lorazepam (Ativan) | Anxiety, preoperative medication |

28. Which group should not receive barbiturates?
    1. Children <5 years of age.
    2. Pregnant women.
    3. Adults prone to seizures.
    4. Adults with bleeding ulcers.

## Answers and Rationales

27. **4.** Anxiety is an adverse side effect.

28. **2.** Barbiturates are teratogenic and are contraindicated for pregnant women.

# ANTICONVULSANTS

A. Several categories of drugs are used to treat seizure activity. Each group will be addressed and there will be no prototype.
   1. Barbiturates (phenobarbital)
      a. Used for generalized and absence seizures.
      b. Refer to discussion under sedatives and hypnotics on barbiturates.
   2. Benzodiazepines (Diazepam [Valium])
      a. Drug of choice for status epilepticus. Also used for absence seizures.
      b. Refer to discussion under Sedatives and Hypnotics on Benzodiazepines.
   3. Hydantoins (phenytoin [Dilantin])
      a. Action. Prevents dissemination of electrical discharges in motor cortex area of the brain.
      b. Use. Tonic-clonic and complex partial seizures, status epilepticus, prevention of seizures that accompany neurosurgery.
      c. Adverse effects. Confusion, slurred speech, slow physical movement; blood dyscrasias; nausea, vomiting, constipation; gingival hyperplasia; hirsutism; rash; acne; hypotension, circulatory collapse, cardiac arrest.
      d. Nursing implications
         1) May take 7–10 days to achieve therapeutic serum concentration.
         2) Tablet can be crushed and should be mixed with food or fluid.
         3) Suspension must be shaken well.
         4) Can turn urine pink, red, or red-brown.
         5) IM route not recommended.
         6) Do not mix with other drugs.
         7) Monitor CBC, liver, thyroid, and urine tests.
         8) Gingival hyperplasia seen most often in children and adolescents.
         9) Stop drug immediately if a measles-like rash occurs.
      e. Discharge teaching
         1) Relate signs of fatigue, dry skin, deepening voice with extended therapy as drug can mask decreased thyroid reserve.
         2) Report jaundice as drug is metabolized in the liver and liver dysfunction causes elevated blood levels of drug.
         3) Abrupt drug withdrawal can cause seizures or status epilepticus.
         4) Withdraw gradually.
         5) Avoid potentially dangerous activities until drug response is known.
         6) Alcohol use can cause drug toxicity.
         7) Cautious use in pregnancy and lactation.
         8) Flu shot during therapy can increase seizure occurrence.
         9) Family members need instruction in care of client during a seizure.
   4. Succinimides (ethosuximide [Zarontin]): used in treatment of absence seizures.
   5. Acetazolamide (Diamox): diuretic used as an adjunct or alone in treatment of absence, tonic-clonic, or myoclonic seizures.
   6. Carbamazepine (Tegretol)
      a. Chemically similar to tricyclic antidepressants.
      b. Used in treatment of tonic-clonic, complex partial, and mixed seizures.
   7. Adjunct anticonvulsants
      a. Valproic acid (Depakene)
         1) Used in treatment of absence seizures.
         2) Low incidence of side effects as compared to other anticonvulsants.
      b. Felbamate (Felbatol): used to treat Lennox-Gastaut Syndrome in children and partial seizures.
      c. Lamotrigine (Lamictal): used to treat partial seizures.
      d. Gabapentin (Neurontin): used to treat partial seizures.

## Sample Questions

29. The nurse should teach clients to watch for which common adverse effect of phenytoin (Dilantin)?
    1. Alopecia.
    2. Edema.
    3. Gingival hyperplasia.
    4. Hallucinations.

30. What is the drug of choice for status epilepticus?
    1. Phenytoin (Dilantin).
    2. Carbamazepine (Tegretol).
    3. Phenobarbital (Luminal).
    4. Diazepam (Valium).

## Answers and Rationales

29. **3.** Gingival hyperplasia is a common adverse effect of phenytoin (Dilantin) seen most often in children and adolescents.

30. **4.** Diazepam (Valium) is the drug of choice for status epilepticus.

# MUSCLE RELAXANTS

A. Various drugs used to treat musculoskeletal problems. Three common drugs will be discussed. There will be no prototype drug.
   1. Baclofen (Lioresal)
      a. Mechanism of action not known but drug inhibits nerve activity in the spinal cord, thus decreasing spasms of skeletal muscles.
      b. Used in multiple sclerosis and spinal cord injuries.
      c. Adverse effects. CNS depression ranging from sedation to coma and seizures; urinary frequency; hirsutism, photosensitivity, acne-like rash; nausea and vomiting.
      d. Nursing implications. May be taken with food, monitor ambulation, depressant effects will be increased if mixed with other CNS depressants, monitor VS, client should avoid potentially dangerous activities until response is known, do not abruptly withdraw.
   2. Carisoprodol (Soma)
      a. Mechanism of action not known but is believed due to drug's central depressant action.
      b. Used in cerebral palsy, muscle stiffness, and spasm found in various musculoskeletal disorders.
      c. Adverse effects. Sedation; headache; syncope, tachycardia, postural hypotension; nausea, vomiting; hiccups, allergic reactions.
      d. Nursing implications. May be taken with food, drowsiness is common effect and client may need dosage reduced, client should not take alcohol or other CNS depressants, do not abruptly stop, allergic reactions usually occur from the first to the fourth dose.
   3. Dantrolene (Dantrium)
      a. Interferes with calcium release from the muscle, which causes a decrease in muscle contraction.
      b. Used for muscle spasms associated with cerebral vascular accident, spinal cord injury, cerebral palsy, and multiple sclerosis. Also given intravenously for malignant hyperthermia.
      c. Adverse effects. Drowsiness; malaise, diarrhea; hepatotoxicity (in extended use at high doses).
      d. Nursing implications. Capsule can be opened and contents can be mixed with juice or other liquid, monitor ambulation, liver and kidney function tests should be monitored, monitor IV site for extravasation, should be withdrawn after 45 days if no improvement has been seen.
   4. Cyclobenzaprine (Flexeril)
      a. Acts on brainstem to reduce tonic somatic muscle activity.
      b. Used for managing acute and painful muscle spasm.
      c. Adverse effects. Dizziness, drowsiness, confusion, fatigue, headache, nervousness, blurred vision, arrhythmias, constipation, dyspepsia, nausea, unpleasant taste, urinary retention.
      d. Nursing implications. Take with food, CNS depressant, drowsiness is common.

## Sample Questions

31. Which statement indicates a need for more teaching about baclofen (Lioresal) by the nurse?
    1. "I'll take my pills with my meals."
    2. "I'll drive myself to work each day."
    3. "I won't have wine with dinner anymore."
    4. "I'll use sunscreen when I go outside."

## Answers and Rationales

31. **2.** Due to the depressant effects of baclofen (Lioresal), the client should not engage in any potentially dangerous activities until the client response to the drug is known.

# ANTIPSYCHOTIC AGENTS

A. Prototype: phenothiazines (Chlorpromazine [Thorazine])
   1. Action. Not fully understood, but is thought to block dopamine receptors in the brain.

Chlorpromazine causes a sedative effect known as a neuroleptic effect and antipsychotic effect. Also causes an anti-emetic effect by depressing the chemoreceptor trigger zone (CTZ). Potentiates the effects of other CNS depressant drugs. Blocks peripheral acetylcholine (Ach) receptors, histamine ($H_1$) receptors, and alpha-adrenergic receptors. These actions cause anticholinergic, alpha-anti-adrenergic, and antihistamine effects that can produce adverse effects.

2. Use. Management of acute and chronic schizophrenia, manic phase of bipolar disorder, management of nausea and vomiting, control of excessive anxiety before surgery, treatment of acute intermittent porphyria, treatment of intractable hiccups, tetanus.

3. Adverse effects. Extrapyramidal symptoms; dizziness, sedation, seizures; orthostatic hypotension, tachycardia, arrhythmias; cholestatic jaundice; agranulocytosis; photosensitivity; anticholinergic effects: "Red, Hot, Dry, Blind, Mad"; urticaria; changes in menses and libido; potentiates CNS effects of narcotic analgesics, sedatives, hypnotics, and alcohol; neuroleptic malignant syndrome.

4. Nursing implications
   a. Monitor blood pressure (standing, lying, and sitting), pulse, respirations, and I&O.
   b. Wear gloves when handling parenteral or liquid form to prevent contact dermatitis.
   c. Give deep IM injection into gluteal muscle and massage well.
   d. Monitor client for extrapyramidal symptoms, which can occur 1–60 days after therapy is begun. Tardive dyskinesia can occur several months or years after therapy.
   e. Monitor CBC, liver function studies, glucose levels, and urinalysis and encourage periodic ocular examinations.
   f. Supervise ambulation to prevent falls until client develops a tolerance.
   g. Protect drug from light.

5. Discharge teaching
   a. Take with food or milk to decrease GI distress.
   b. Take drug at bedtime.
   c. Wear protective clothing and/or sunscreen before exposure to sun.
   d. With initial therapy, change positions gradually to reduce orthostatic hypotension.
   e. Report fever, sore throat to physician.
   f. Stop or reduce cigarette smoking, as this shortens the half-life and higher doses may be needed.
   g. Mix liquid form in juice, water, milk, or baby food.

   h. With long-term therapy, drug is gradually reduced before discontinuing therapy.
   i. Incompatible with many drugs. *Note: also review the anticholinergic drug atropine sulfate for nursing implications and discharge teaching.*

B. Related drugs. See Table 2-9.

**Table 2-9** Phenothiazines

| Drug | Use | Comments |
|---|---|---|
| Promethazine (Phenergan) | Pre- and postoperative sedation Prophylaxis for nausea, vomiting, motion sickness Adjunct to analgesics Allergic conditions | • Rarely causes extrapyramidal symptoms |
| Thioridazine (Mellaril) | Psychotic disorders Short-term use in depression Attention deficit disorder | • Rarely causes extrapyramidal symptoms |
| Fluphenazine (Prolixin) (Prolixin Decanoate) | Psychotic disorders | • Clients at great risk for extrapyramidal symptoms • Most potent phenothiazine |
| Haloperidol (Haldol) | Psychotic disorders Tourette's syndrome Short-term treatment in hyperactive children | • Clients at great risk for extrapyramidal symptoms • Causes less sedation and hypotension |
| Mesoridazine (Serentil) | Schizophrenia Acute/chronic alcoholism | • Increased sedation but less risk of extrapyramidal symptoms |
| Thiothixene (Navane) | Psychotic disorders | • Clients at great risk for extrapyramidal symptoms |
| Pimozide (Orap) | Tourette's syndrome | • Decreased sedation but increased risk of extrapyramidal symptoms |
| Molindone (Moban) | Psychotic disorders | • Clients at low risk for sedation and extrapyramidal symptoms |

32. The psychiatrist orders chlorpromazine (Thorazine) IM. If the medication is not properly handled, what effect could this have on the nurse?
    1. Skin discoloration.
    2. Skin irritation.
    3. Headache.
    4. Dizziness.

33. Which of the following interventions should be included in a care plan concerning chlorpromazine (Thorazine) therapy?
    1. Supervise ambulation.
    2. Take a hot bath to reduce agitation.
    3. Restrict fluid intake to prevent edema.
    4. Discontinue drug if sedation occurs.

34. Which phenothiazine is used specifically as an antiemetic and rarely causes extrapyramidal symptoms?
    1. Thioridazine (Mellaril).
    2. Fluphenazine (Prolixin).
    3. Promethazine (Phenergan).
    4. Chlorpromazine (Thorazine).

35. Which antipsychotic agent is also used to treat Tourette's syndrome and causes less sedation than other phenothiazines?
    1. Haloperidol (Haldol).
    2. Thioridazine (Mellaril).
    3. Fluphenazine (Prolixin).
    4. Chlorpromazine (Thorazine).

## Answers and Rationales

32. **2.** Handling the parenteral or liquid forms of chlorpromazine (Thorazine) may cause contact dermatitis, so gloves should be worn.

33. **1.** Chlorpromazine (Thorazine) during initial use can cause orthostatic hypotension; ambulation should be supervised to prevent falls until tolerance develops.

34. **3.** Promethazine (Phenergan) is used as an antiemetic and rarely causes extrapyramidal symptoms.

35. **1.** Haloperidol (Haldol) is also used to treat Tourette's syndrome and causes fewer sedative effects than other phenothiazines.

## Antipsychotic Agents (Continued)

C. Prototype: lithium (lithium carbonate [Eskalith])
   1. Action. Exact mode of action unknown. Thought to alter neurotransmitters in CNS that produce antidepressant and antimanic effects.
   2. Use. Treatment and prophylaxis of manic phase of bipolar disorder.
   3. Adverse effects. Confusion, restlessness, fatigue, weakness, hand tremors; arrhythmias, circulatory collapse, palpitations, hypotension; blurred vision; dry mouth, thirst, weight gain; nausea, diarrhea; leukocytosis.
   4. Nursing implications
      a. Monitor serum lithium levels (blood tests usually done monthly).
      b. Monitor for lithium intoxication.
      c. Treatment for lithium intoxication includes IV therapy with normal saline, diuretics, and hemodialysis.
      d. Monitor thyroid function studies periodically.
      e. May take 1–2 weeks to achieve therapeutic effects.
   5. Discharge teaching
      a. Drink 2.5–3 liters of fluid per day to relieve thirst and dry mouth.
      b. Maintain sodium intake of 6–10 g daily to reduce lithium toxicity.
      c. Take with food to decrease GI distress.
      d. Do not drive or operate machinery until drug response established.
      e. Report to physician: nausea, vomiting, edema, weight gain, tremors, and drowsiness (may be signs of lithium toxicity or hypothyroidism).
      f. Record weight on a weekly basis.
D. Related drugs: lithium citrate (Cibalith-S): available in liquid form

## Sample Questions

36. Which of the following interventions should the nurse stress while a client is on lithium therapy?
    1. Weigh self once a month.
    2. Restrict fluid intake to prevent edema.
    3. Do not restrict sodium intake.
    4. Avoid eating cheese and bananas and drinking wine.

## Answers and Rationales

36. **3.** Clients need to maintain sodium intake (usually 6–10 g daily) to prevent lithium toxicity.

## Antipsychotic Agents (Continued)

E. Prototype: tricyclic antidepressants (imipramine [Tofranil])
   1. Action. Structurally related to phenathiazines. Blocks reuptake of the neurotransmitters norepinephrine and serotonin at the neuronal membrane, which increases and prolongs the response of the neurotransmitters.
   2. Use. Endogenous and reactive depression; childhood enuresis.
   3. Adverse effects. Sedation, confusion; anticholinergic effects; orthostatic hypotension, arrhythmias; clients recovering from an acute MI should not take drug; blood dyscrasias; extrapyramidal symptoms; gynecomastia; jaundice.
   4. Nursing implications
      a. May take 2–4 weeks to achieve therapeutic effects. Monitor for suicidal tendencies.
      b. Monitor CBC for clients on long-term therapy.
      c. Monitor I&O.
      d. Drug therapy is discontinued gradually.
   5. Discharge teaching
      Take with food to decrease GI distress
      *Note: review the anticholinergic atropine sulfate for further nursing implications and discharge teaching as imipramine (Tofranil) has anticholinergic adverse effects*
F. Related drugs
   1. Amitriptyline (Elavil)
   2. Nortriptyline (Aventyl): more useful in elderly clients due to fewer anticholinergic effects.
   3. Desipramine (Norpramin)
   4. Doxepin (Sinequan)
   5. Amoxapine (Asendin)

## Sample Questions

37. Which of the following is included in client teaching concerning imipramine (Tofranil)?
   1. Expect to see improvement of depression in 2–3 days.
   2. Stop taking drug if dizziness occurs.
   3. Do not drive or operate machinery.
   4. Take drug on an empty stomach.

38. When should the client expect to see improvement of depression while on imipramine (Tofranil)?
   1. 1–2 days.
   2. 1 week.
   3. Several weeks.
   4. Immediately after first dose.

## Answers and Rationales

37. **3.** Imipramine (Tofranil) can cause drowsiness; the client should avoid driving or operating machinery.

38. **3.** It takes several weeks (2–4 weeks) before clients may see improvement of depression.

## Antipsychotic Agents (Continued)

G. Prototype: monoamine oxidase inhibitors (MAO inhibitors) (phenelzine [Nardil])
   1. Action. Inhibits MAO, which increases neurotransmitter levels (dopamine, norepinephrine, serotonin).
   2. Use. Neurotic and atypical depression.
   3. Adverse effects. Orthostatic hypotension; dry mouth, blurred vision, constipation; hypertensive crisis; liver dysfunction; leukopenia.
   4. Nursing implications
      a. Monitor blood pressure while standing, sitting, and supine.
      b. Interacts with many drugs.
      c. Monitor I&O.
      d. Therapeutic effectiveness takes 2–4 weeks.
      e. Monitor liver function studies, glucose, and CBC.
   5. Discharge teaching
      a. Avoid foods or beverages containing tyramine or tryptophan including: caffeine beverages, soy sauce, red wine, beer, cheese, yogurt, sour cream, raisins, bananas, avocado, herring, beef and chicken liver, Italian green beans.
      b. Change position slowly.
H. Related drugs
   1. Tranylcypromine (Parnate): contraindicated in clients over age 60.
   2. Isocarboxazid (Marplan)

39. Which foods/beverages should be avoided while taking phenelzine (Nardil)?
    1. Cheese.
    2. Apples.
    3. Pasta.
    4. Cereal.

## Answers and Rationales

39. **1.** Foods such as cheese that contain tyramine or tryptophan should be avoided while taking MAO inhibitors to prevent hypertensive crisis.

## Antipsychotic Agents (Continued)

I. Prototype: selective serotonin reuptake inhibitors (fluoxetine [Prozac])
   1. Action. Blocks serotonin reuptake and increases transmission at serotonergic synapses.
   2. Use. Major depression; obsessive-compulsive disorder.
   3. Adverse effects. CNS stimulation, sexual dysfunction, nausea, headache, anorexia, weight loss, skin rash.
   4. Nursing implications
      a. Can take up to 4 weeks to achieve therapeutic effects.
      b. Interacts with warfarin (Coumadin).
      c. Cannot be combined with monoamine oxidase inhibitors.
   5. Discharge teaching
      a. Take in the morning.
      b. Report skin rash immediately.
J. Related drugs
   1. Paroxetine (Paxil)
   2. Sertraline (Zoloft)

3. Citalopram (Celexa)
4. Fluvoxamine (Luvox)
5. Escitalopram (Lexapro)
K. Miscellaneous antidepressants
   1. Bupropion (Wellbutrin)
   2. Venlafaxine (Effexor)
   3. Nefazodone (Serzone)
   4. Trazodone (Desyrel)
   5. Clozapine (Clozaril)
   6. Olanzapine (Zyprexa)
   7. Risperidone (Risperdal)

## Sample Questions

40. Which statement indicates a need for more teaching by the nurse concerning fluoxetine (Prozac) therapy?
    1. "I will take this medication in the morning."
    2. "I will use calamine lotion if I get a skin rash."
    3. "It will take a month before I feel better."
    4. "I will check with my physician before I take any other medications."

## Answers and Rationales

40. **2.** A skin rash resulting from use of fluoxetine (Prozac) indicates an allergic reaction and should be reported to the physician immediately.

# Autonomic Nervous System Drugs

## ADRENERGIC DRUGS

A. Prototype
Adrenergic drugs are divided into two groups, direct-acting and mixed-acting. The direct-acting contain most of the adrenergic drugs.

## Direct-Acting Adrenergics

### Nonselective (Alpha and Beta) Agonists

Prototype: Epinephrine (Adrenalin Chloride)
1. Action. Epinephrine (Adrenalin Chloride) has the same actions stimulated as the sympathetic nervous system. It increases the force of myocardial contraction; increases systolic blood pressure, cardiac rate and output; relaxes bronchial smooth muscle; inhibits histamine release; increases tidal volume and vital capacity; prevents insulin release and raises blood sugar; prevents uterine contractions and relaxes uterine smooth muscle; lowers intraocular pressure and decreases formation of aqueous humor; constricts arterioles in kidneys, mucous membranes, and skin; and dilates blood vessels in skeletal muscle.
2. Use. Treatment of anaphylaxis and bronchospasm, cardiac resuscitation, control or prevention of low blood pressure during spinal anesthesia, lengthening effects of local anesthesia, promotion of mydriasis, treatment of acute hypotension.
3. Adverse Effects. Systemic: anxiety, headache, fear, arrhythmias, hypertension, cerebral/subarachnoid hemorrhage, hemiplegia, pulmonary edema, insomnia, anginal pain in clients with angina pectoris, tremors, vertigo, sweating, nausea, vomiting, agitation, disorientation, paranoid delusions; prolonged use at high doses causes increased serum lactic acid levels, metabolic acidosis, and increased blood glucose. Local injection: necrosis at sites when injections are repeated. Nasal solution: stinging and burning locally, rebound congestion. Ophthalmic solutions: stinging on initial use, eye pain, headache, browache, blurred vision, photophobia, problems with night vision, pigment deposits in conjunctiva, cornea, and eyelids with prolonged use.

4. Nursing Implications
   a. Use great caution in preparing and calculating doses as this is a potent drug.
   b. Tolerance occurs with extended use.
   c. Solutions should be clear and colorless (except suspension for injection). Protect solutions from light, heat, and freezing.
   d. Suspension for injection must be shaken well.
   e. Rotate SC sites and monitor for necroses.
   f. Have a fast-acting alpha-adrenergic blocker such as phentolamine (Regitine) or vasodilator such as nitrite available for excessive hypertensive reaction.
   g. Have an alpha-adrenergic blocker available for pulmonary edema.
   h. Have a beta-adrenergic blocker available for cardiac arrhythmias.
   i. Monitor VS.
5. Discharge Teaching
   a. For inhalation products: do not exceed recommended dosage; take drug during second half of inspiration, take second inhalation 3–5 minutes after first dose.
   b. For nasal solutions: do not use for more than 3–5 days; burning and stinging may occur initially but are transient.
   c. For ophthalmic solution: slight stinging may occur initially but is usually transient; headache and browache are also transient.
   d. Do not take any OTC medications without physician approval.

Prototype: norepinephrine bitartrate (Levophed)
1. Action. Norepinephrine bitartrate (Levophed) is an alpha and beta-1 receptor agonist and has no effect on beta-2 receptors. Its biggest action is seen on the cardiovascular system, where the following happens: an increase in total peripheral resistance (vasopressor response); and increased force, rate, and impulse conduction of the heart, which is usually overridden by activation of baroreceptors, thus causing bradycardia. Other actions are mydriasis and elevated blood glucose and insulin.
2. Use. Revives blood pressure in acute hypotensive states (sympathectomy, spinal anesthesia, poliomyelitis, septicemia, blood transfusion, drug reactions); adjunct in treatment of cardiac arrest.
3. Adverse effects. Bradycardia; cardiac arrhythmias; headache.

4. Nursing implications
   a. Do not mix drug in 100% saline solutions (NS) as oxidation will occur. Mix in 5% dextrose solution or 5% dextrose in saline solution.
   b. Give into large vein to prevent extravasation.
   c. Do not infuse in femoral vein in elderly clients or those with occlusive vascular disease.
   d. Check blood pressure every 2 minutes after start of infusion until desired blood pressure is attained; then check blood pressure every 5 minutes if infusion continued.
   e. Monitor IV site for extravasation.
   f. Have phentolamine (Regitine) available in case of extravasation. 5–10 mg of phentolamine (Regitine) in 10–15 mL of saline should be infiltrated into area.
   g. Drug solution should be clear and colorless.

## Selective Alpha Agonists

Prototype: phenylephrine (Neo-Synephrine)
1. Action. Phenylephrine (Neo-Synephrine) produces vasoconstriction and increased blood pressure. Topical application produces vasoconstriction of mucous membranes. Application to eye causes mydriasis and vasoconstriction and promotes flow of aqueous humor.
2. Use. Stabilizes blood pressure during anesthesia; vascular failure in shock; subdues paroxysmal supraventricular tachycardia; rhinitis of allergy and common cold; sinusitis; wide-angle glaucoma; ophthalmoscopic examination or surgery; uveitis.
3. Adverse effects. Eye tearing and stinging, headache, browache, blurred vision, increased sensitivity to light; nasal rebound congestion; nasal burning, stinging, dryness, and sneezing; palpitations, tachycardia, bradycardia (overdose); hypertension; trembling, sweating, feeling of fullness in the head; sleeplessness, dizziness, light-headedness, tingling in extremities.
4. Nursing implications
   a. For IV infusion, check blood pressure, pulse, and central venous pressure every 2–5 minutes.
   b. IV overdose can cause ventricular arrhythmias.

   c. Phentolamine (Regitine) should be available for hypertensive crisis seen in IV administration.
   d. Levodopa (L-Dopa) is used to decrease excess mydriatic effect.
   e. If systemic adverse effects are seen from nasal and eye use, stop drug and notify physician.
   f. Apply pressure to lacrimal sac of eye during and for 1–2 minutes after administration of eye drops.
   g. Incompatible with butacaine, oxidizing agents, ferric salts, metals, and alkalies.
   h. Wash hands after handling drug as blurred vision and unequal pupil size can result if drug-contaminated finger rubs eye.
5. Discharge teaching
   a. Client should not change dose in any way.
   b. If drug has been taken for 5 days without relief, notify physician.
   c. Clear nasal passages before using nasal preparations.
   d. Wear sunglasses after eye administration if eyes sensitive to light.
   e. Call physician if eye sensitivity lasts more than 12 hours after drug has been given.
   f. Ophthalmic solutions can stain contact lenses.
   g. Tips and droppers of nasal solutions should be cleaned with hot water after each use.
   h. Do not touch droppers of eye solutions.
6. Related drugs
   a. Methoxamine (Vasoxyl): used for treating acute hypotension seen during surgery. It is given IV for immediate effect or IM for longer lasting effects.
   b. Agents found in OTC cough, cold, and allergy remedies and in eye decongestant products include naphazoline, oxymetazoline, tetrahydrozoline, xylometazoline.

## Nonselective Beta (Beta-1 and Beta-2) Agonists

Prototype: isoproterenol (Isuprel)
1. Action. Isoproterenol (Isuprel) has cardiovascular actions of vasodilation, which decreases diastolic blood pressure and peripheral resistance, and actions of increased cardiac output. Other actions are bronchodilation; raising levels of blood glucose, insulin, and free fatty acids; and causing release of renin from the kidney.

2. Use. Acute heart failure; management of intraoperative bronchospasm; additive treatment in cardiac arrest, AV heart block, Stokes-Adams syndrome; treatment of chronic bronchoconstriction; management of syncope; treatment of bronchospasm in COPD and asthma.
3. Adverse effects. Restlessness, anxiety, CNS stimulation, hyperkinesia, insomnia, tremors, irritability, vertigo, headache; arrhythmias, tachycardia, angina, blood pressure changes; pulmonary edema, respiratory difficulties; flushing, pallor, sweating; nausea, vomiting, heartburn.
4. Nursing implications
   a. Tolerance can develop with prolonged use.
   b. A beta-adrenergic blocker should be available if arrhythmias occur.
   c. Client needs continuous ECG monitoring during IV administration.
   d. IV infusion must be given via infusion pump with guidelines from the physician.
5. Discharge teaching
   a. Client should not alter dosage.
   b. Inhalation form should be taken during second half of inspiration; second inhalation should be taken 3–5 minutes later.
   c. Client should not chew or swallow sublingual tablets.
   d. Avoid OTC drugs unless approved by physician.
6. Related drugs
   a. Isoxsuprine hydrochloride (Vasodilan) is used in cerebrovascular insufficiency and peripheral vascular disease. It is given to adults IM or PO.
   b. Ritodrine (Yutopar) is used for management of preterm labor.

## Selective Beta-1 Agonists

Prototype: dopamine hydrochloride (Intropin)
1. Action. Dopamine hydrochloride (Intropin) increases cardiac output and systolic blood pressure. In low doses it reduces renal vascular resistance, which increases glomerular filtration rate and urinary output.
2. Use. Corrects hemodynamic imbalance in shock caused by myocardial infarction, trauma, septicemia, congestive heart failure, and open heart surgery.
3. Adverse effects. Tachycardia, palpitations, hypotension, vasoconstriction; nausea, vomiting; dyspnea, headache; piloerection.

4. Nursing implications
   a. Must be administered cautiously as even small errors can produce deleterious effects.
   b. Always dilute drug if not prediluted.
   c. Dose must be decreased by 1/10 in clients who have been receiving MAO inhibitors.
   d. Do not mix with other drugs.
   e. Protect drug from light.
   f. Infuse into large vein.
   g. Monitor for extravasation and have phentolamine (Regitine) available if this occurs.
   h. Closely check blood pressure, urine output, and cardiac output.
5. Related drugs: Dobutamine (Dobutrex) is used in treatment of acute heart failure. It is given to adults via IV infusion.

## Selective Beta-2 Agonists

All drugs in this group are similar so there will be no prototype. Two representative examples will be mentioned.
1. Metaproterenol sulfate (Alupent) is used to treat bronchial asthma and bronchospasm that accompanies emphysema and bronchitis. It is given orally and via metered-dose inhaler or inhalant solution to adults. Children 60 pounds or less receive syrup orally and children more than 12 years can receive inhalation therapy.
   a. Adverse effects. CNS stimulation; cardiac arrhythmias, tachycardia, palpitations, changes in blood pressure; respiratory difficulties; sweating, pallor, flushing; nausea, vomiting, heartburn.
   b. Nursing implications
      1. Tolerance can develop with prolonged use.
      2. Have a beta-adrenergic blocker available in case of arrhythmia.
      3. Give inhalant during second half of inspiration.
      4. Teach clients to not alter dose and not to take any OTC drugs without physician approval.
2. Terbutaline sulfate (Brethine): refer to data on metaproterenol sulfate (Alupent). It is given PO, SC, and via inhaler to adults and children more than 12 years.

## Mixed-Acting Adrenergics

Prototype: ephedrine (various products)
1. Action. Ephedrine's actions are similar to the peripheral autonomic effects of

norepinephrine. The main effects of the drug are reduced nasal congestion, increased blood pressure, bronchodilation, cardiac stimulation, and stimulation of the CNS.

2. Use. Relief of allergies and mild asthma; therapy in shock and hypotension.
3. Adverse effects. Systemic with increased doses: headache, insomnia, nervousness; palpitations, tachycardia, arrhythmias, urinary retention; nausea, vomiting, anorexia; sweating, thirst. Topical use: burning, stinging, sneezing, dry nasal mucosa, rebound congestion. Overdose: confusion, delirium, convulsions, pyrexia, coma; hypertension; respiratory depression; paranoid psychosis; auditory and visual hallucinations.
4. Nursing implications
   a. Parenteral solution must be clear and should be protected from light.
   b. Monitor urine output.
   c. Clients with cardiovascular problems need monitoring of cardiac response and blood pressure.
   d. Client receiving IV ephedrine needs close monitoring of vital signs.
5. Discharge teaching
   a. Client should not use nasal decongestant longer than 5 days.
   b. Anxiety reaction can occur with extended use of systemic ephedrine.
   c. Ephedrine is commonly abused. Client needs to be aware of adverse effects and proper use.
   d. Client should not take any OTC preparations without consulting physician.
   e. Insomnia is a common effect and doses should be spaced accordingly.
6. Related drugs: Metaraminol (Aramine): used for acute hypotension and can be given preoperatively to prevent hypotension; given SC, IM, or IV; given to adults and children.

## Sample Questions

41. What can the nurse expect if a low dose level of dopamine hydrochloride (Intropin) is given intravenously?
    1. A decrease in glomerular filtration rate.
    2. A decrease in the force of myocardial contractions.
    3. An increase in urine output.
    4. An increase in tactile sensation.

42. Which nursing action is contraindicated while receiving IV dopamine hydrochloride (Intropin)?
    1. The nurse will monitor vital signs frequently.
    2. The nurse will check the IV infusion site frequently for extravasation.
    3. The nurse will infuse the drug via macrodrip tubing and will adjust the rate manually.
    4. The nurse will check client extremities for temperature and color.

43. A client experiences extravasation at the insertion site of dopamine hydrochloride (Intropin) IV. The infusion is stopped. What should be done next?
    1. Warm compresses should be applied to the IV site.
    2. An ice pack should be applied to the IV site.
    3. The extremity with the IV site should be elevated on two pillows.
    4. The IV site should be infiltrated with phentolamine (Regitine).

44. When high doses of dopamine hydrochloride (Intropin) are given IV for treatment of shock, what effect would the nurse be looking for?
    1. Increased blood pressure.
    2. Decreased heart rate.
    3. Increased respirations.
    4. Elevated body temperature.

45. Which drug produces effects that closely mimic high doses of dopamine hydrochloride (Intropin)?
    1. Atropine sulfate.
    2. Ephedrine.
    3. Isoproterenol (Isuprel).
    4. Norepinephrine (Levophed).

## Answers and Rationales

41. **3.** Dopamine hydrochloride (Intropin) at low doses causes dilation of renal and mesenteric arteries, which in turn causes increased urine output.

42. **3.** Dopamine hydrochloride (Intropin) needs to be infused via a minidrip tubing and attached to an infusion pump for accurate administration.

43. **4.** If extravasation occurs when dopamine hydrochloride (Intropin) is administered, the IV site should be infiltrated with phentolamine (Regitine) immediately after discontinuing the infusion.

**44. 1.** High doses of dopamine hydrochloride (Intropin) stimulate alpha-adrenergic activity, which causes increased blood pressure.

**45. 4.** Dopamine hydrochloride (Intropin) given in high doses has effects that closely mimic norepinephrine (Levophed).

# ADRENERGIC BLOCKING AGENTS

A. Prototype for alpha-adrenergic blocking agents: phentolamine (Regitine)
   1. Action. Phentolamine (Regitine) blocks alpha-1 receptors, thus causing blood vessel dilation; decreased blood pressure; increased cardiac output; miosis; increased tearing, mucus secretion, gastric acid secretion, and gastrointestinal motility.
   2. Use. Diagnosis of pheochromocytoma; management of hypertensive episodes in pheochromocytoma; treatment of extravasation from norepinephrine (Levophed) or dopamine hydrochloride (Intropin); adjunctive therapy in cardiogenic shock or other situations of decreased cardiac output.
   3. Adverse effects. Hypotension, orthostatic hypotension; MI, cerebrovascular occlusion (these effects can occur with hypotensive states that can occur after parenteral administration); tachycardia, arrhythmias; dizziness, weakness, flushing; nausea, vomiting, diarrhea; nasal stuffiness.
   4. Nursing implications
      a. For parenteral administration client must be in supine position. Blood pressure and pulse should be checked every 2 minutes until stable.
      b. Use reconstituted solutions immediately.
      c. Have client lie down or put head down if feeling dizzy or light-headed.
      d. Treatment for overdose: keep client lying down with head lowered, supportive measures, IV infusion of levarterenol (norepinephrine).
B. Related drug: ergotamine tartrate (Ergomar)
   1. Along with adrenergic blocking activity, has a direct stimulatory effect on smooth muscle. It also decreases pulsation in cranial arteries and has emetic and oxytocic effects.
   2. Used for treatment of vascular headaches such as migraines or cluster headaches.
   3. Given to adults via sublingual or inhalation route.
   4. Adverse effects. Nausea, vomiting; numbness, tingling, and muscle pain in extremities; pulselessness in legs; precordial pain; transient tachycardia or bradycardia; ergotism (ergot poisoning); dependency and abuse.

5. Nursing implications
   a. Take drug at beginning of migraine attack.
   b. Avoid prolonged use.
   c. Give antiemetics for nausea and vomiting.
   d. Monitor extremities.
   e. Pregnant client should not receive this drug.
   f. Client should not increase dose of drug without consulting physician.
   g. Use lowest effective dose.

## Beta-Adrenergic Blocking Agents

*Note: Refer to Beta Blockers in the section on Cardiovascular Drugs.*

Timolol maleate (Timoptic) is an optic beta-adrenergic blocker. It decreases intraocular pressure whether glaucoma is present or not. It also decreases aqueous humor formation and increases aqueous humor outflow. It is used to treat glaucoma and hypertension. It is given orally and via eye drops to adult clients.

 **Sample Questions**

46. A client calls the physician's office and states that she has vomited each time she has taken ergotamine tartrate (Ergomar). What is the nurse's best response?
    1. "Vomiting is a common adverse effect. Tell the physician so he can prescribe an antiemetic for you."
    2. "Stop taking the drug immediately. Vomiting is a toxic drug effect."
    3. "You must be allergic to the drug. Notify the physician."
    4. "Vomiting is a transient effect and it will eventually go away."

47. Which group of individuals would be excluded from receiving ergotamine tartrate (Ergomar)?
    1. Clients with diabetes.
    2. Clients with asthma.
    3. Clients suffering from alcoholism.
    4. Pregnant women.

48. Which of the following information would be excluded from the client teaching about ergotamine tartrate (Ergomar)?
    1. Take the drug as soon as you feel a migraine headache coming on.
    2. Have your blood pressure checked routinely when taking this drug.
    3. Increase the dose as needed to help control your migraines.

4. Tell the physician if you have any numbness or tingling in your toes and fingers.

## Answers and Rationales

**46.** **1.** Ergotamine tartrate (Ergomar) has emetic effects; vomiting is a common side effect. The client needs an antiemetic to help control this problem.

**47.** **4.** Ergotamine tartrate (Ergomar) has oxytocic effects; it is contraindicated in pregnant women.

**48.** **3.** Ergotamine tartrate (Ergomar) is a drug that is abused by clients by altering dosage amount. Only the physician should change the dose of the drug.

## CHOLINERGICS

**A.** Prototype: acetylcholine chloride (Miochol)
  **1.** Action. A neurotransmitter that mediates synaptic activity in the nervous system; stimulates the vagus nerve and parasympathetic nervous system (PNS) causing vasodilation and cardiac depression; causes miosis of the eye as it contracts the iris sphincter muscle; contracts and relaxes the urinary bladder, causing micturition. Acetylcholine chloride (Miochol) is identical to synthesized acetylcholine (Ach).
  **2.** Use. To produce miosis in eye surgery.
  **3.** Adverse effects. Systemic absorption: hypotension, bradycardia; bronchospasm; flushing, sweating.
  **4.** Nursing implications
    **a.** Reconstitute vial just before use and discard unused portion.
    **b.** Shake vial gently to mix drug.
**B.** Related drugs: Bethanechol chloride (Urecholine)
  **1.** Used to treat postoperative urinary retention.
  **2.** See acetylcholine chloride (Miochol); also nausea, vomiting, diarrhea, abdominal cramping, dizziness, faintness; cholinergic crisis can occur with overdose.
  **3.** Nursing implications
    **a.** Monitor VS, breath sounds, and I&O.
    **b.** PO drug should be given one hour before meals or two hours after meals.
    **c.** Never give IM or IV as drug may cause life-threatening effects.
    **d.** Atropine sulfate is antidote.
  **4.** Discharge teaching
    **a.** Encourage client not to drive or operate heavy machinery while taking drug.
    **b.** Teach client to change positions slowly.
*Note: Carbachol (Isopto Carbachol) and pilocarpine (Almocarpine) are discussed under Miotics in section on Eye Drugs.*

**C.** Prototype: acetylcholinesterase inhibitors: Neostigmine (Prostigmin)
  **1.** Action. Neostigmine (Prostigmin) inhibits the neurotransmitter acetylcholine, which produces a cholinergic response, and produces reversible cholinesterase inactivation, which permits a prolonged effect of acetylcholine at cholinergic synapses.
  **2.** Use. Treatment and diagnosis of myasthenia gravis; prevention of postoperative abdominal distension; treatment and prevention of postoperative bladder distension; postoperative reversal of nondepolarizing muscle relaxants.
  **3.** Adverse effects. Nausea, vomiting, cramping, diarrhea, increased salivation; muscle tremor and weakness; dyspnea, bronchospasm, increased bronchial secretions, respiratory depression; hypo- or hypertension, arrhythmias, bradycardia; miosis; cholinergic crisis.
  **4.** Nursing implications
    **a.** Keep atropine and emergency resuscitation equipment readily available, especially for parenteral use.
    **b.** Monitor vital signs, breath sounds, I&O.
    **c.** Report to physician if client does not void within 1 hour after receiving dose.
  **5.** Discharge teaching
    **a.** Encourage client to take drug with food or milk if GI distress occurs.
    **b.** Instruct client to keep a record of response to drug.
    **c.** Instruct client to monitor and report adverse effects.
    **d.** Advise client to wear a medic alert bracelet (for myasthenia gravis).
    **e.** Instruct client to cough, breathe deeply, and perform range of motion exercises regularly.
**D.** Related drugs
  **1.** Pyridostigmine (Mestinon, Regonol): used to treat myasthenia gravis and postoperative reversal of nondepolarizing skeletal muscle relaxants. Additional adverse effects: rash; thrombophlebitis with IV use.
  **2.** Edrophonium chloride (Tensilon): used to diagnose myasthenia gravis.
  **3.** Tacrine (Cognex): used to treat mild to moderate Alzheimer's disease.
  **4.** Pilocarpine (Akarpine): used in open-angle glaucoma.
  **5.** Donepezil (Aricept): used in Alzheimer's disease.

## Sample Questions

**49.** The client is prescribed bethanechol chloride (Urecholine). What information about this drug is important for the nurse to know?

1. IM or IV is the preferred route.
2. Bethanechol chloride (Urecholine) should be given with food.
3. Breath sounds should be monitored.
4. Constipation is a frequent adverse effect.

50. Which drug would be given to treat neostigmine (Prostigmin) overdose?
    1. Acetylcholine acetate (Miochol).
    2. Atropine sulfate.
    3. Bethanechol (Urecholine).
    4. Lidocaine (Xylocaine).

 **Answers and Rationales**

**49. 3.** Breath sounds should be monitored to assess for wheezing and bronchospasm.

**50. 2.** Atropine sulfate, an anticholinergic, is the antidote for neostigmine (Prostigmin).

# ANTICHOLINERGICS

A. Prototype: atropine sulfate
   1. Action. Atropine sulfate is a plant alkaloid derived from the atropa belladonna plant that blocks the neurotransmitter acetylcholine and inhibits parasympathetic actions.
   2. Use. To produce mydriasis and cycloplegia for eye examinations; treat uveitis; preoperative medication to reduce secretions and bradycardia; treat sinus bradycardia or asystole; hypermotility of GU tract; adjunct in treating asthmatic bronchospasm; GI disorders, peptic ulcer, GI hypermotility and biliary colic; antidote for overdoses of parasympathomimetic drugs; prevention of adverse effects when reversing neuromuscular blockade postoperatively with acetylcholine inhibitor; antidote to organophosphate pesticides.
   3. Adverse effects. Disorientation, restlessness, hallucinations, headache, dizziness; palpitation, hypertension or hypotension, ventricular tachycardia; blurred vision, photophobia; suppression of sweating; urinary hesitancy and retention, constipation; dry mouth; flushed, dry skin.
   4. Nursing implications
      a. Do not give to clients with myasthenia gravis, acute glaucoma, prostatic hypertrophy.
      b. Monitor VS, especially pulse and blood pressure and I&O.
      c. Monitor for constipation and check bowel sounds.
      d. Monitor geriatric clients for CNS stimulation and heat stroke (infants and small children should also be monitored for heat stroke).
      e. Smaller doses usually are given to geriatric clients due to adverse effects.
   5. Discharge teaching
      a. Take drug 30 minutes before meals.
      b. Eat foods high in fiber and drink plenty of liquids to overcome constipation.
      c. Keep dental appointments as decreased salivation makes clients more prone to tooth decay.
      d. Use good oral hygiene, i.e., rinse mouth, brush teeth, hard candy, saliva substitute, fluids.
      e. Maintain periodic eye appointments to monitor for increased intraocular pressure.
      f. Avoid hot baths and showers, sun, and heat to prevent heat stroke.
      g. Change position gradually.
      h. Do not drive or operate machinery.
B. Related drugs. See Table 2-10.

**Table 2-10** Anticholinergics

| Drug | Use | Comments |
|---|---|---|
| Scopolamine | Preanesthetic medication (Transderm-scop) used for prophylaxis of motion sickness Mydriatic and cycloplegic for eye exam Irritable bowel syndrome, diverticulitis Management of postencephalitic parkinsonism | • Place transderm scop patch behind ear the night before trip. Replace patch after three days if more prolonged effects are needed. |
| Glycopyrrolate (Robinul) | Preanesthetic medication Adjunct in peptic ulcer disease therapy Reverse neuromuscular blockade | • Has fewer CNS effects than atropine. Do not mix with barbiturates or alkaline drugs. |

**Sample Questions**

51. Which of the following effects of atropine sulfate would the nurse expect a client to exhibit?
    1. Dry mouth.
    2. Increased bronchial secretions.
    3. Tachycardia.
    4. Miosis.

52. Which statement indicates that the client needs more teaching concerning the use of atropine sulfate?
    1. "I will brush my teeth and see my dentist regularly."
    2. "I will eat low-residue foods to prevent diarrhea."
    3. "I will take my medication at least a half hour before meals."
    4. "I will stay in my air conditioned house on hot and humid days."

 **Answers and Rationales**

51. **1.** Atropine sulfate causes dry mouth and decreases secretions, which is why it is given as a preanesthetic.

52. **2.** Atropine sulfate can cause constipation; high-fiber foods and fluids should be encouraged.

# ANTIPARKINSON AGENTS

## General Considerations

There are 2 major categories of antiparkinson's agents: (1) anticholinergics and (2) dopaminergic agents

A. Antiparkinson drugs control rather than cure symptoms of Parkinson's. Antiparkinson agents can cause or worsen other disorders, and clients, especially the elderly, need to be closely monitored for adverse effects. Antiparkinson drugs are initiated and discontinued gradually. Drugs should not be abruptly withdrawn. Antiparkinson agents are contraindicated in clients with glaucoma, prostatic hypertrophy, duodenal ulcers, tachycardia, and biliary obstruction.

B. Prototype: anticholinergics (trihexyphenidyl HCl [Artane]) This drug is similar to atropine sulfate.
    1. Action. Blocks the neurotransmitter acetylcholine at certain cerebral synapses and inhibits parasympathetic responses.
    2. Use. Treat Parkinson's disease, prevent or control antipsychotic drug-induced extrapyramidal tract symptoms.
    3. Adverse effects. Note phrase "Red, hot, dry, blind, mad"; dry mouth; constipation; tachycardia, hypotension; dizziness, drowsiness, confusion; decreased bronchial secretions; blurred vision, photophobia, acute glaucoma; urinary retention; suppression of sweating.
    4. Nursing implications
        a. Drug can be taken before or after meals.
        b. See atropine sulfate.
        c. Drug should be gradually withdrawn.
    5. Discharge teaching. See atropine.
C. Related drugs. See Table 2-11.
D. Prototype: dopaminergic agents (levodopa [Larodopa])
    1. Action. Levodopa (Larodopa) is a metabolic precursor of the catecholamine neurotransmitter dopamine that readily crosses the blood-brain barrier and restores dopamine levels in extrapyramidal centers.
    2. Use. Treat Parkinson's disease (except drug-induced Parkinson's).
    3. Adverse effects. Anorexia, nausea, vomiting; orthostatic hypotension, dizziness, headache; constipation, dry mouth; mydriasis; urinary retention, darkened urine; increase BUN, AST (SGOT), ALT (SGPT), LDH, bilirubin, alkaline phosphatase; decreased WBCs, hemoglobin, and hematocrit, decreased glucose tolerance; blurred vision; muscle twitching, blepharospasm, ataxia, increased hand tremors; disturbed breathing; confusion, anxiety, agitation.
    4. Nursing implications
        a. Monitor vital signs and client for adverse effects.
        b. Monitor client for behavior changes.
        c. Monitor CBC, glucose, and kidney and liver function studies.
        d. With long-term therapy levodopa (Larodopa) may lose its effectiveness and adjunctive drugs may be used.

**Table 2-11** Antiparkinson Agent (Anticholinergic)

| Drug | Use | Comments |
|---|---|---|
| Benztropine Mesylate (Cogentin) | Treat Parkinson's disease and as adjunct with trihexyphenidyl HCl (Artane) Prevent or control drug-induced extrapyramidal tract symptoms | • Longer lasting sedative effects and muscle relaxation than trihexyphenidyl HCl (Artane) |

5. Discharge teaching
   a. Restrict foods high in Vitamin $B_6$ (pyridoxine) (i.e., liver, green vegetables, fortified cereals, whole grain cereals). Vitamin $B_6$ reverses therapeutic effects of levodopa (Larodopa).
   b. Change positions gradually.
   c. Do not abruptly stop taking drug as sudden withdrawal can lead to parkinsonian crisis.

**Table 2-12** Antiparkinson Agents (Dopaminergic Agents)

| Drug | Use | Comments |
|---|---|---|
| Carbidopa/ Levodopa (Senemet) | Treatment of Parkinson's disease | • Carbidopa prevents metabolism of levodopa and allows more levodopa for transport to brain.<br>• Adverse CNS effects may occur sooner.<br>• Levodopa (Larodopa) should be discontinued 8 hours before starting Senemet. |
| Bromocriptine (Parlodel) | Parkinson's Treatment of amenorrhea, galactorrhea Female infertility Suppression of postpartum lactation Acromegaly | • Treat Parkinson's.<br>• Often given with levodopa (Larodopa) or carbidopa/ levodopa (Senemet).<br>• Give with food or milk.<br>• Contraindicated in clients with hypersensitivity to ergot alkaloids.<br>• Oral contraceptives antagonize effects of bromocriptine (Parlodel). Advise client to use another method of contraception.<br>• This drug causes increased fertility.<br>• Hypotension is a frequently seen adverse effect. |
| Ropinirole (Requip) | Idiopathic Parkinson's disease | • Directly stimulates dopamine receptors.<br>• Given alone in early stages of Parkinson's disease and with levodopa (Larodopa) in later stages.<br>• Give with food to decrease nausea.<br>• Must be discontinued gradually.<br>• Assess for hypotension as dose is increased.<br>• Assess liver and renal function during treatment. |

   d. Do not take OTC medications without consulting physician.
   e. Take drug between meals.
6. Related drugs. See Table 2-12.

 **Sample Questions**

53. Which adverse effect would be absent with trihexyphenidyl HCl (Artane) therapy?
    1. Dizziness.
    2. Dry mouth.
    3. Diarrhea.
    4. Suppression of sweating.

54. Which statement by the client indicates understanding of proper use of levodopa (Larodopa)?
    1. "If my symptoms get worse I will stop taking this drug."
    2. "I will not eat liver or boxed cereals."
    3. "If I have a cold I will take aspirin or a cold remedy."
    4. "I will eat foods low in residue to prevent diarrhea."

55. Which instruction should the nurse give to clients taking bromocriptine (Parlodel)?
    1. "Take 1 hour before meals."
    2. "Do not use birth control pills as contraceptives."
    3. "This drug causes infertility and use of contraceptives will not be necessary."
    4. "Adverse effects will be reduced if taken during the day."

 **Answers and Rationales**

53. **3.** Trihexylphenidyl HCl (Artane) is an anticholinergic that can cause constipation, not diarrhea.

54. **2.** Vitamin $B_6$ (pyridoxine) reverses the therapeutic effects of levodopa (Larodopa); clients should restrict their intake of foods high in vitamin $B_6$ such as whole-grain cereals, fortified cereals, liver, green vegetables.

55. **2.** Oral contraceptives antagonize the effects of bromocriptine (Parlodel). Another method of birth control should be used.

# Drugs Affecting the Endocrine System

Refer also to Table 4-24, Hormone Functions.

## ANTIDIABETIC AGENTS

A. Prototype: insulin
1. Action. Hormone that increases glucose transport across cell membranes; transforms glycogen into glucose, prevents breakdown of fats to fatty acids, and inhibits protein breakdown.
2. Use. Clients with Type 1 diabetes; Clients with Type 2 diabetes not controlled with oral hypoglycemic agents, diet, and exercise; Clients with Type 2 diabetes undergoing stressful situations: infection or surgery; pregnant women with diabetes emergency management of diabetic coma.
3. Adverse effects. Allergic reaction: local or systemic; hypoglycemia; ketoacidosis.
4. Nursing implications
   a. There is a difference between insulin injection and insulin injection concentrated, for which 500 units = 1 mL.
   b. Human insulins should only be mixed with each other.
   c. IV insulin can be absorbed by the container or tubing.
   d. Stable at room temperature for 1 month.
   e. Do not inject cold insulin, causes lipodystrophy.
   f. Drug solution should not be used if discolored or contains precipitate. Do not shake vial. Gently roll (all except regular insulin) vial between palms before drawing up medicine.
   g. Check expiration date.
   h. When mixing two insulins, rapid-acting insulin should be drawn up first.
   i. Syringe must coordinate with strength of insulin.
   j. Injection sites must be rotated.
   k. Treat severe hypoglycemic reaction with glucagon or 10–50% IV glucose.
   l. Treat ketoacidosis with IV insulin and IV fluids.
   m. Diet is prescribed by physician.
   n. Monitor blood glucose levels.
   o. Fixed-combination insulins such as "70/30 insulin" are available. Contains 70% NPH and 30% regular insulin. "50/50 insulin" is also available and contains 50% NPH and 50% regular insulin.
   p. Insulin analog: insulin lispro (Humalog) is a synthetic insulin with a faster onset and shorter duration of action than human insulin.
   q. Injections should be given immediately after mixing two insulins.
5. Discharge teaching
   a. Available without a prescription (except insulin injection, concentrated). Prescription is needed for needles and syringes (depending on state law).
   b. Change of insulin brand, type, etc., is done by physician.
   c. In initial period of dosage regulation client may have visual problems. Should not get lens changes until vision is balanced.
   d. Remove prefilled syringes from refrigerator 1 hour before administration.
   e. Inject at a 90° angle if you can pinch an inch, otherwise inject at a 45° angle.
   f. Report symptoms of reactions at injection site.
   g. Know symptoms of hypoglycemic reaction and have some type of fast-acting carbohydrate available at all times.
   h. If ill, continue taking insulin and drink freely noncaloric liquids. Notify physician if diet cannot be followed.
   i. Monitor blood glucose at home and instruct on use.
   j. Smoking decreases insulin absorption.
   k. When traveling, needs to have necessary supplies.
   l. Carry a medical identification card.

B. Refer to Table 4-25, Characteristics of Insulin Preparations, Unit 4.

## Sample Questions

56. The nurse is teaching the client about insulin injections. Which statement is correct?
   1. Insulin needs to be shaken well before being drawn up into the syringe.
   2. Long-acting insulins are clear in color.
   3. When putting regular and NPH insulin in the same syringe, draw regular insulin up first.
   4. NPH is compatible with regular and lente insulin.

57. What information will the nurse instruct the client about minimizing local skin reactions to insulin?

1. Injecting it slowly.
2. Always refrigerating it.
3. Giving it in divided doses.
4. Bringing it to room temperature before administering.

58. Which statement by the client indicates a need for further teaching by the nurse?
    1. "I will inject my insulin at a 90° angle."
    2. "I will take more insulin when I go to my exercise class."
    3. "I will always have some kind of sugar with me in case I have a hypoglycemic reaction."
    4. "I will carefully draw up my doses of insulin."

## Answers and Rationales

56. **3.** Regular insulin should be drawn up before NPH insulin when putting the two together in one syringe.

57. **4.** Insulin should be at room temperature before injecting to decrease occurrence of lipodystrophy.

58. **2.** Exercise increases glucose use in the body, so a decreased dose of insulin may be needed.

## Oral Hypoglycemic Agents

A. Prototype: tolbutamide (Orinase)
  1. Action. Lowers blood glucose concentrations by stimulating secretion of endogenous insulin from beta cells in the pancreas. Increases peripheral sensitivity to insulin. From the class of sulfonylureas.
  2. Use. Type 2 diabetes: not controlled by diet and exercise, used with insulin in client with Type 2 diabetes when neither insulin nor oral hypoglycemic agents work well alone.
  3. Adverse effects. Hypoglycemia; increased chance of cardiovascular disease; anorexia, nausea, vomiting, diarrhea; hemolytic anemia; allergic skin rashes; photosensitivity; inappropriate ADH secretion.
  4. Nursing implications
    a. Tablet can be crushed.
    b. Monitor closely during initial therapy.
    c. If client stabilized on tolbutamide (Orinase) is exposed to stress (infection, surgery), the oral agent may be discontinued and replaced by insulin.
    d. Can transfer from one sulfonylurea to another easily.

    e. Monitor and teach symptoms of hypoglycemic reactions and how to treat.
    f. Monitor blood and urine glucose levels.
  5. Discharge teaching
    a. Reinforce that drug is not "oral" insulin and will control diabetes.
    b. Use form of birth control other than oral contraceptives.
    c. Alcohol can trigger a hypoglycemic reaction.
    d. Cover body in sunshine. Use sunscreen.
    e. Weigh weekly and report progressive gain.
    f. Carry medical identification.
B. Refer to Table 4-26, Oral Hypoglycemic Agents, Unit 4.

## Sample Questions

59. The client tells the nurse that his brother has Type 1 diabetes and he takes insulin. The nurse is asked why his brother cannot take an oral antidiabetic agent. The nurse explains that oral antidiabetic agent. What explanation will the nurse give regarding oral antidiabetic agents in Type 1 diabetes?
    1. He has little or no endogenous insulin that can be released.
    2. He is allergic to oral antidiabetic agents.
    3. He would need so much of an oral antidiabetic agent that it would be financially prohibitive for him to take one.
    4. He would have more episodes of hypoglycemia with oral antidiabetic agents.

60. Tolbutamide (Orinase) should not be taken if a person is allergic to what substance?
    1. Penicillin.
    2. Insulin.
    3. Sulfa.
    4. Caffeine.

61. The client will need more teaching about tolbutamide (Orinase) if he makes which of the following statements?
    1. "I will get a medic alert bracelet that says I'm a diabetic taking tolbutamide (Orinase)."
    2. "I'm glad I can still have wine with my meals."
    3. "If I go outside, I'll stay out of the sun or use sunscreen."
    4. "I know that tolbutamide (Orinase) will help control my diabetic condition."

**59. 1.** Oral antidiabetic agents can only work when the client has endogenous insulin, which is not the case in Type 1 diabetes.

**60. 3.** Clients who are allergic to sulfa cannot take tolbutamide (Orinase), which is a sulfonylurea.

**61. 2.** Alcohol combined with an oral hypoglycemic agent can trigger a hypoglycemic reaction.

# PITUITARY HORMONES

A. Prototype: hormone corticotropin (ACTH) (cosyntropin [Cortrosyn])
  1. Action. Synthetic corticotropin that stimulates corticosteroid release from functional adrenal cortex.
  2. Use. As a diagnostic test to diagnose adrenal insufficiency.
  3. Adverse effects. (see Corticosteroids) Cushing's syndrome if given over a period of time, hypersensitivity reactions.
  4. Nursing implications. (see Corticosteroids) Administer deep IM.
B. Prototype: ADH (antidiuretic hormone) (vasopressin [Pitressin]).
  1. Action. Hormone released by posterior pituitary gland that regulates water metabolism and prevents dehydration. Has vasoconstrictor effect that elevates blood pressure. In diabetes insipidus a deficiency in ADH is characterized by polyuria and polydipsia. Vasopressin (Pitressin) acts as a replacement for ADH.
  2. Use. Replacement therapy for diabetes insipidus.
  3. Adverse effects. Hypersensitivity, anaphylaxis; water intoxication, hyponatremia; nausea, diarrhea, cramping; hypertension; nasal irritation, headache.
  4. Nursing implications
    a. Monitor BP, weight, and I&O.
    b. Vasopressin is available SC, IM, IV, and intra-arterially.
  5. Discharge teaching
    a. Keep record of I&O, weight.
    b. If URI and use drug intranasally, absorption may be affected.
    c. Report sudden changes in output.
    d. Drink water with dose to reduce GI distress.
C. Related Drugs

  1. Desmopressin (DDAVP)
    a. Can be given PO, SC, IV, or intranasally; monitor for extravasation.
    b. Keep refrigerated.
  2. Lypressin spray (Diapid): given intranasally.

**62.** Which of the following is the desired response of vasopressin (Pitressin)?
  1. Lower urine specific gravity.
  2. Lower urine output.
  3. Treat hypotension.
  4. Control polyphagia.

**63.** A client complains of GI distress following administration of vasopressin (Pitressin). What instructions should the nurse provide to the client?
  1. Eat crackers after taking the dose.
  2. Take a warm bath to reduce abdominal cramping.
  3. Lie down for 30 minutes following administration.
  4. Drink a glass of water with each dose.

**62. 2.** The goal of vasopressin (Pitressin) is to lower urine output; replacement for the ADH hormone.

**63. 4.** Drinking a glass of water with each dose will decrease GI distress.

# PITUITARY HORMONES (CONTINUED)

D. Prototype: somatotropin (growth hormone) (somatropin [Humatrope])
  1. Action. Somatotropin stimulates growth of skin, connective tissue, and long bones.
  2. Use. Replacement therapy in children with growth retardation caused by lack of somatotropin.
  3. Adverse effects. Hyperglycemia; pain at injection site; myalgia; headache; hypercalciuria; allergic reactions.
  4. Nursing implications
    a. Record height.
    b. Monitor blood glucose.
    c. Rotate IM sites. Do not give SC.
    d. Store in refrigerator.
    e. Discontinue if epiphyses have fused.
  5. Discharge teaching. Annual bone age assessment test.

# CORTICOSTEROIDS

## General Information

A. The adrenal cortex secretes three natural steroids: glucocorticoids, mineralcorticoids, and adrenal androgens and estrogens.
   1. Glucocorticoids (Cortisol)
      a. Have anti-inflammatory effects.
      b. Regulate carbohydrate, protein, and fat metabolism.
   2. Mineralcorticoids (Aldosterone, Desoxycorticosterone)
      Regulate water and electrolyte metabolism.
   3. Adrenal androgens and estrogens
      a. Supplement sex hormones from gonads.
      b. Corticosteroids suppress immune response and affect all body systems.
B. Prototype: hydrocortisone (Cortisol)
   1. Action. Glucocorticoid, mineralcorticoid, and immunosuppressive actions.
   2. Use. Replacement therapy for adrenocorticoid insufficiency; anti-inflammatory for many allergic, inflammatory, or immunoreactive disorders.
   3. Adverse effects. Increased susceptibility to infection; hypokalemia, hypocalcemia; sodium and fluid retention; increased appetite, nausea, peptic ulcer; headache, hypertension, congestive heart failure; osteoporosis; acne, impaired wound healing, hirsutism, skin thinning; ecchymosis, petechiae; hyperglycemia, impaired glucose metabolism, growth retardation, menstrual disorders; glaucoma, cataract formation; mental disturbances, insomnia; thrombophlebitis; masks symptions of infection.
   4. Nursing implications
      a. Observe for mental changes.
      b. Monitor BP, weight, I&O, blood glucose, and serum potassium.
      c. IM use: inject deep IM. Do not give SC.
      d. Corticosteroid doses are not interchangeable.
      e. Corticosteroids are not abruptly withdrawn. Doses are tapered to allow the adrenal gland to function independently.
   5. Discharge teaching
      a. Take drug before 9 A.M. (This causes less suppression on the adrenal cortex.)
      b. Take with food or milk to decrease GI effects.
      c. Never abruptly stop taking. This could precipitate acute adrenal crisis.
      d. Eat foods high in potassium.
      e. Avoid individuals with infections.
      f. Restrict sodium, alcohol, and caffeine intake.
      g. Carry Medic Alert card.
      h. Follow directions for topical use. Do not use an occlusive dressing, and apply ointment sparingly.
      i. Rinse mouth after using inhaled steroids.
C. Related drugs
   1. Dexamethasone (Decadron)
      a. Given IV to treat cerebral edema or allergic symptoms.
      b. Betamethasone (Celestone)
      c. Dexamethasone and betamethasone are 10–30 times more potent than hydrocortisone.
      d. Both drugs can be inhaled to treat asthma.
   2. Methylprednisolone (Solu-Medrol) (has little mineralcorticoid action)
      a. Prednisone (Deltasone)
      b. Prednisolone (Delta-Cortef)
      *Note: All of these drugs are 4–5 times as potent as hydrocortisone. Prednisone and prednisolone have half the mineral-corticoid action of hydrocortisone.*
   3. Fludrocortisone (Florinef)
      a. An oral synthetic mineralcorticosteroid.
      b. Used to treat Addison's disease.

 **Sample Questions**

64. Which statement should be included in teaching concerning hydrocortisone (Cortisol) therapy?
    1. Take aspirin to treat fever.
    2. Take hydrocortisone (Cortisol) before meals.
    3. Restrict caffeine and alcohol intake.
    4. Restrict potassium intake.

65. What occurrence is prevented by gradually discontinuing hydrocortisone (Cortisol)?
    1. Anaphylaxis.
    2. Diabetic coma.
    3. Adrenal insufficiency.
    4. Cardiovascular collapse.

 **Answers and Rationales**

64. **3.** Hydrocortisone (Cortisol) can cause GI distress and even lead to a peptic ulcer with long-term use. Caffeine and alcohol can further increase GI distress and should be restricted.

**65. 3.** Adrenal insufficiency can occur with abrupt removal of corticosteroids. Corticosteroids are gradually discontinued so that the adrenal glands can begin to secrete corticosteroids independently.

# THYROID HORMONES

A. Prototype: levothyroxine (Synthroid)
   1. Other various agents used to treat hypothyroid conditions include desiccated thyroid: thyroglobulin (Proloid); liotrix (Thyrolar); liothyronine sodium (Cytomel).
   2. Use. Replacement or substitution of diminished or absent thyroid function due to thyroid disease or thyroidectomy.
   3. Adverse effects. Headache, nervousness, insomnia, irritability; palpitations, increased blood pressure, tachycardia, dysrhythmias, angina; weight loss, nausea, vomiting; menstrual irregularities; allergic skin reaction; heat intolerance.
   4. Nursing implications
      a. Baseline weight and thyroid studies.
      b. Avoid aspirin use.
      c. Protect from light.
      d. Check pulse before taking.
   5. Discharge teaching
      a. Do not alter dosage.
      b. Carry Medic Alert card.

## Sample Questions

66. What action should the nurse perform before administering levothyroxine (Synthroid)?
    1. Check the client's pulse.
    2. Listen to the client's chest.
    3. Take the client's temperature.
    4. Assess the client's neuro status.

## Answers and Rationales

**66. 1.** An adverse effect of levothyroxine (Synthroid) is tachycardia; the nurse should check the client's pulse before administration.

# THYROID ANTAGONISTS

A. Prototype: propylthiouracil (PTU)
   1. Action. Prevents synthesis of thyroid hormones. Partially prevents peripheral conversion of $T_4$ to $T_3$.

   2. Use. Management of hyperthyroidism.
   3. Adverse effects. Hypothyroidism; agranulocytosis, thrombocytopenia, bleeding; nausea, vomiting, loss of taste; rash, urticaria, skin pigmentation; jaundice, hepatitis; nephritis.
   4. Nursing implications
      a. Take same time daily with respect to meals. Food can change absorption rate.
      b. Drug response occurs 2–3 weeks after starting drug.
      c. Therapy may last 6 months to several years with remission in 25% of clients.
      d. Can be given during pregnancy. Stopped 2–3 weeks before delivery.
      e. Do not nurse baby.
      f. Check pulse daily.
   5. Discharge teaching
      a. Report signs of agranulocytosis (fever, chills, sore throat).
      b. Report signs of bleeding promptly.
      c. Ask physician about use of iodized salt and seafood in diet.

B. Related drugs
   1. Methimazole (Tapazole): similar to propylthiouracil (PTU) except it is 10 times more potent. Given once daily due to long duration of action. Risk of hepatotoxicity is less.
   2. Iodines: cause dose-related effects on thyroid function. Low doses necessary for thyroid function. High amounts inhibit thyroid function. Used to decrease size and vascularity of the thyroid before thyroid surgery, management of thyroid storm, treatment of hyperthyroidism, and treatment of thyroid cancer. Adverse effect: GI distress.

## Sample Questions

67. The client calls the physician's office and complains of chills, fever, and sore throat. Which nursing action is appropriate?
    1. Tell the client it sounds like she has the flu and that she should drink lots of fluids, take aspirin, and get extra rest.
    2. Tell the client to come in immediately for a throat culture and blood work as this may be a serious drug reaction.
    3. Expect the physician to prescribe another thyroid antagonist drug as this is an allergic reaction.
    4. Tell the client that these are expected drug reactions and that they will subside in a few days.

**Answers and Rationales**

**67. 2.** Symptoms of chills, fever, and sore throat while receiving propylthiouracil (PTU) require throat culture and blood work right away.

# WOMEN'S AND MEN'S HEALTH AGENTS

A. Prototype: progesterone (Progestin)
   1. Action. Changes a proliferative endometrium into a secretory one; causes a change in consistency of cervical mucus; stops spontaneous uterine contractions.
   2. Use. Amenorrhea; abnormal uterine bleeding; endometrial cancer; prevention of conception.
   3. Adverse effects
      a. In parenteral administration: Breakthrough bleeding, spotting, dysmenorrhea, breast tenderness; headache, dizziness; edema, thromboembolism, hypertension; nausea, vomiting, bloating, weight gain; jaundice; rash, hirsutism, acne, oily skin; vision changes.
      b. Other effects: Hypertension; reduced glucose tolerance; thromboembolism in high doses in specific groups of women.
   4. Nursing implications
      a. Take oral forms with food.
      b. Monitor weight.
      c. Monitor BP.
      d. For intramuscular injection
         1) Inject deeply into gluteal muscle.
         2) Rotate injection sites.
         3) Shake vial to ensure uniform dispersion.
   5. Discharge teaching
      a. Client should not smoke.
      b. Client should have regular Pap tests and should do breast self-exam.
      c. Client should report calf pain, breast lumps, or severe headache.
B. Related drugs
   1. Hydroxyprogesterone (Delalutin), medroxyprogesterone (Provera), and megesterolacetate (Megace).
   2. Oral contraceptives
      a. Estrogen-progestin combinations
         1) Action. Suppress ovulation by preventing release of follicle-stimulating hormone (FSH) and luteinizing hormone (LH). Act directly on reproductive organs.
         2) Use. Prevention of pregnancy; amenorrhea; functional bleeding; endometriosis.
         3) Adverse effects. Same as for progesterone.

4) Nursing implications
   a) Stop taking 1 week before surgery to decrease risk of thromboembolism.
   b) If one menstrual period is missed and tablets were taken correctly, continue pills; if two periods are missed, stop pills and have pregnancy test; will need additional birth control method for first month of drug therapy.
   c) Smoking increases risk of thromboembolism.
   d) May take longer to conceive after stopping pills. See Nursing Implications for progesterone.
      b. Progestin-only preparations
         1) Referred to as "minipills."
         2) Less effective than estrogen-progestin combinations.
         3) Action not understood.
         4) Adverse effects and nursing implications are same as for estrogen-progestin combinations.
         5) If two consecutive doses are missed, client must stop drug, use alternative birth control, wait until menses occurs, and start therapy again.
C. Fertility agents
   1. Prototype: clomiphene citrate (Clomid) given PO.
   2. Menotropins (Pergonal) given IM.
   3. Chorionic gonadotropin (A.P.L.) given IM.
   4. Action. Increases the release of gonadotropins and stimulates the growth and maturation of ovum.
   5. Use. Infertility, induces ovulation.
   6. Adverse effects. Multiple births, headache, tachycardia, nausea, vomiting, constipation, anxiety, DVT, breast pain, diplopia.
   7. Nursing implications. Monitor for adverse effects, support client and partner throughout their attempt to achieve fertility.
D. Bisphosphonates
   1. Alendronate (Fosamax).
   2. Tiludronate (Skelid).
   3. Action. Bisphosphonates inhibit normal and abnormal bone resorption of bone by decreasing osteoclast activity.
   4. Use. Prevention and treatment of osteoporosis in men and postmenopausal women, and Paget's disease.
   5. Adverse effects. Flatus, gastritis, acid regurgitation, dysphagia, muscle pain, constipation or diarrhea, and headache.
   6. Nursing implications
      a. Alendronate: take in the morning with 8 ounces of water 30 minutes before meals or other medications. Sit upright after taking

for at least 30 minutes to prevent esophageal irritation.
      b. Tiludronate: take on an empty stomach at least 2 hours before or after eating.
  E. Selective estrogen receptor modulators (SERMs)
    1. Raloxifene (Evista): used to prevent postmenopausal osteoporosis.
    2. Tamoxifen (Novadex): used for prevention and treatment of breast cancer.
    3. Action. SERMs work by stimulating estrogen receptors on bone and blocking estrogen receptors on breast tissue.
    4. Adverse effects. Hot flashes and leg cramps; can increase the risk of thromboembolism.
    5. Nursing implications. Periodically monitor CBC and platelet counts.
  F. Men's health agents
    1. Androgens: testosterone, danazol (Danocrine), fluoxymesterone (Halotestin), methyltestosterone (Android).
    2. Action. Stimulate spermatogenesis and maintenance of secondary sex characteristics, and stimulate the formation and maintenance of muscular and skeletal protein.
    3. Use. Primarily for replacement therapy; treatment of breast cancer in women.
    4. Adverse effects. Fluid retention, headaches, nausea, vomiting, constipation or diarrhea, acne, gynecomastia, priapism, depression, jaundice, and bleeding.
    5. Nursing implications. Available PO. Testosterone also available IM and transdermally. Give with food to decrease GI upset. Transdermal testosterone: Matrix type placed on the scrotum; reservoir patch placed on the abdomen, back, thighs, or upper arms. Matrix type doesn't need to be removed for bathing, sexual activity, or swimming; reservoir patch needs to be removed for these activities. For IM use give deep IM in the gluteus. Therapeutic effects may take 3–4 months and should not be abruptly discontinued.
  G. Androgen inhibitors: 5-Alpha-Reductase Inhibitor: finasteride (Proscar)
    1. Given orally to treat BPH and may take up to 6 months before relief of BPH symptoms occurs. May cause impotency, decreased libido, or ejaculatory dysfunction.
  H. Phosphodiesterase inhibitor: Sildenafil (Viagra), tadalafil (Cialis), vardenafil (Levitra)
    1. Given orally to treat male erectile dysfunction.
    2. Contraindicated in clients taking nitrates. Sildenafil potentiates hypotensive effects of nitrates. Adverse effects: flushing, headache, GI upset.
    3. Nursing implications. Take 1 hour before sexual intercourse. Clients with a history of cardiac disease or angina should use cautiously.

## Sample Questions

68. The client calls the gynecology clinic and states she thinks she is pregnant even though she has consistently taken her birth control pills. What would be the nurse's best response?
    1. Continue taking the pills and see the physician.
    2. Stop taking the pills and see the physician.
    3. Continue taking the pills and see if menses occurs in the next cycle.
    4. Stop taking the pills for this cycle; wait 28 days and start them again.

69. Which conditions could be present in clients who are prescribed the medication danazol (Danocrine)?
    1. Infertility.
    2. Muscular dystrophy.
    3. Sexual dysfunction in men and women.
    4. Endometriosis and fibrocystic breast disease.

## Answers and Rationales

68. **2.** If the client is taking birth control pills and believes she is pregnant, she should stop taking the pills and see the physician.

69. **4.** Danazol is given in the treatment of endometriosis and helps relieve the symptoms of fibrocystic breast disease.

## OXYTOCICS

A. Prototype: oxytocin (Pitocin)
  1. Action. Posterior pituitary gland hormone that may initiate labor by stimulating uterine smooth muscle contractions. Releases milk from breast in breastfeeding women.
  2. Use. Labor induction; control postpartum bleeding; treatment of incomplete abortion; stimulate breast milk ejection.
  3. Dose. IV infusion: add 0.5–2 milliunits/min, increase by 1–2 milliunits/min every 15–60 minutes until contraction pattern (maximum 20 milliunits/min). IV for uterine bleeding: 10–40 units to 1 liter of dextrose or electrolyte solution.
     IM: 10 units after delivery of placenta.
  4. Adverse effects. Water intoxication, hypotension; postpartum hemorrhage; PVCs, cardiac arrhythmias; uterine rupture; nausea, vomiting; hypertension, cardiovascular

**Table 2-13** Oxytocin-Related Drugs

| Drug | Use | Adverse Effects | Nursing Implications |
|------|-----|-----------------|----------------------|
| Ergonovine (Ergotrate) Ergot Alkaloid (produce vasoconstriction and intense oxytocic effects) | Control late postpartum bleeding Treatment and prevention of postpartum and postabortion bleeding | Severe hypertension; bradycardia; nausea, vomiting; diarrhea | • Monitor BP, heart rate, and fundus<br>• Notify physician if BP increases<br>• Contraindicated to induce labor |
| Methylergonovine (Methergine) | Prophylaxis after delivery of placenta | Fewer adverse effects than ergonovine. See above. | • Never administer before delivery of placenta |
| Ergot Alkaloid (see above) | Management of postpartum bleeding | | • See above |

collapse; fetus: bradycardia, hypoxia, intracranial hemorrhage, death; anaphylactic reactions.
5. Nursing implications
    a. Infusion pump for IV infusion.
    b. Monitor BP, heart rate, I&O.
    c. Use fetal monitor to monitor fetal heart rate and uterine contractions.
    d. Notify physician and stop infusion if fetal or maternal distress. Place mother on left side.
    e. Drug IV line should be piggybacked into a primary infusion line.
    f. Physician should be readily available to manage maternal or fetal complications.
B. Related drugs. See Table 2-13.

 **Sample Questions**

70. The nurse sets up an oxytocin (Pitocin) infusion. Which of the following are nursing considerations in caring for clients receiving oxytocin infusions?
    1. The nurse should increase the infusion by 3 milliunits/min every 15 minutes until there is a pattern of contractions.
    2. Time-tape the solution and use a microdrop tubing to monitor the rate.

3. Use an infusion pump and piggyback infusion into primary infusion line.
4. Monitor client's temperature every 15 minutes.

71. Which statement is correct regarding the reason why Methylergonovine (Methergine) is given?
    1. To induce labor.
    2. In the first stage of labor.
    3. After placental delivery.
    4. IV prophylactically to prevent postpartum hemorrhage.

 **Answers and Rationales**

70. **3.** Oxytocin (Pitocin) infusion should be administered on an infusion pump and piggybacked into a primary infusion line to control rate of infusion and to minimize/prevent potentially dangerous adverse effects of oxytocin (Pitocin).

71. **3.** It is given after placental delivery because methylergonovine (Methergine) can cause uterine tetany.

 **Eye Drugs**

## MYDRIATICS AND CYCLOPLEGICS

A. Prototype: atropine (Isopto Atropine)
    1. Action. An anticholinergic that causes mydriasis (dilation) of the pupil and cycloplegia, which paralyzes the lens and eye muscles.
    2. Use. Facilitate eye exams and treat uveitis.
    3. Adverse effects. Photophobia, reduced lacrimation, impaired distant vision,

increased intraocular pressure, eye pain, blurred vision.
4. Nursing implications
   a. Sunglasses to reduce photophobia.
   b. Artificial tears for reduced lacrimation.
   c. Elderly clients should be screened prior to receiving atropine—can increase intraocular pressure.
   d. Should not drive until drug effects have worn off.
B. Related drugs
   1. Sympathomimetic agents:
      a. Apraclonidine (Iopidine)
      b. Dipivefrin (Propine)
   2. Cyclopentolate (Cyclogyl)

 **Sample Questions**

72. To reduce the chance of having systemic effects related to atropine, which intervention will be performed after administration?
    1. Place a warm compress over both eyes.
    2. Rinse the eye with water following instillation.
    3. Maintain pressure on inner canthus for 1–2 minutes.
    4. Have client wipe eyes with gauze after instillation.

73. Which of the following conditions should be assessed for prior to topical atropine application?
    1. Cataracts.
    2. Glaucoma.
    3. Uveitis.
    4. Conjunctivitis.

74. Which statement by the client indicates that he understands the instructions given following instillation of atropine?
    1. "My son will drive me home after the exam."
    2. "If my eyes itch it's OK to rub them."
    3. "I plan to go to the beach after this appointment."
    4. "I will mow the lawn as soon as I get home."

 **Answers and Rationales**

72. **3.** Applying pressure to the inner canthus (lacrimal sac) will reduce systemic effects.

73. **2.** Atropine can raise intraocular pressure. Clients with glaucoma have increased intraocular pressure and a further increase in intraocular pressure could lead to an acute crisis and blindness.

74. **1.** Vision is temporarily impaired following the examination. This client should not drive, as distant vision is impaired.

## MIOTICS

A. Prototype: acetylcholine (Miochol)
   1. Action. A cholinergic drug that causes miosis (contraction) of the pupil and contraction of the ciliary muscle in the eye.
   2. Use. Decreases intraocular pressure in glaucoma and achieves miosis in cataract surgery.
   3. Adverse effects. Low toxicity after systemic absorption; transient hypotension, decreased heart rate; bronchospasm; flushing, sweating.
   4. Nursing implications
      a. Reconstitute just before use due to instability of solution.
      b. Systemic reactions treated with intravenous atropine.
B. Related drugs
   1. Carbachol (Isopto Carbachol): Tell client of brief stinging in eye after use; symptoms of eye and brow pain, photophobia, and blurred vision will usually be lessened with prolonged use.
   2. Echothiophate (Phospholine Iodine): Solutions are unstable, client must wash hands before use.
   3. Pilocarpine (Pilocar, Isopto Carpine): Causes blurred vision and focusing difficulty. Client needs to understand that glaucoma treatment is long and needs adherence to prevent blindness; eyedropper tip should not be contaminated; clients with asthma and lung disorders should be observed for respiratory difficulties.
   4. Physostigmine (Isopto Eserine)
      a. Beta blockers
         1) Betaxolol (Beoptic)
         2) Timolol (Timoptic)
      b. Carbonic anhydrase inhibitors (CAIs): Indicated for treatment of glaucoma.
         1) Acetazolamide (Diamox)
         2) Dorzolamide (Trusopt)

## Sample Questions

75. Eye medication that treats glaucoma has what effect?
    1. Both mydriatic and miotic.
    2. Mydriatic.
    3. Miotic.
    4. Malaise.

76. Which statement made by the client indicates a need for more teaching about pilocarpine?
    1. "I know a side effect of pilocarpine is blurred vision."
    2. "I won't touch the eyedropper tip of the pilocarpine to my eye when instilling the drops."

    3. "I will stop the pilocarpine as soon as my vision improves."
    4. "I know that pilocarpine can cause side effects in my eye as well in other areas of my body."

## Answers and Rationales

75. **3.** Miotic eye medication causes a contraction of the eye pupil and contraction of the ciliary muscle, which helps to decrease intraocular pressure.

76. **3.** Treatment for glaucoma will continue throughout the client's life. Eye medication should not be discontinued.

# Cardiovascular Drugs

## CARDIAC GLYCOSIDES

A. Prototype: digoxin (Lanoxin)
   1. Action. Increases force of myocardial contraction (positive inotropic effect). Decreases rate of conduction (negative chronotropic effect) while increasing refractory period of the AV node. Positive inotropic effect improves blood supply to vital organs and kidneys, providing a diuretic effect. Has a slow onset and shorter duration of action than other cardiac glycosides. Is eliminated through the kidneys. Digoxin elixir is better absorbed by the GI tract than digoxin tablets.
   2. Use. Congestive heart failure (CHF); atrial fibrillation; atrial flutter; paroxysmal atrial tachycardia.
   3. Adverse effects. Cumulative with a narrow margin of safety. With toxicity there are many symptoms that make it difficult to distinguish from the condition being treated. Arrhythmias, bradycardia: arrhythmias more frequently seen in children; anorexia, nausea, vomiting, diarrhea; headaches, fatigue, confusion, insomnia, convulsions; visual disturbances: blurred vision, green or yellow tint or halos; hypersensitivity. Toxicity occurs more quickly in presence of a low serum potassium. Quinidine-digoxin reaction may occur. When digoxin is stabilized in clients receiving quinidine, serum digoxin levels could double, leading to possible toxicity.
   4. Nursing implications
      a. Half-life is longer in elderly.
      b. Monitor CBC, serum electrolytes, liver and renal function studies, and ECG.
      c. Hold if apical rate is below 60 or greater than 120 beats per minute in adults, below 90 beats per minute in infants, or below 70 beats per minute in children up to adolescence.
      d. Monitor I&O and daily weights; potassium levels. Encourage foods high in potassium.
      e. Monitor serum digoxin levels therapeutic range (0.5–2.0 ng/mL).
      f. Give after meals if GI distress.
      g. Do not confuse digoxin with digitoxin (Crystodigin) as they are not the same.
      h. IM injections are painful and absorption is erratic. Avoid IM injections if possible and give in large muscle mass.
      i. Digoxin antidote: Digoxin Immune Fab (Digi-bind).
   5. Discharge teaching
      a. Take radial pulse and notify physician if toxicity symptoms occur.
      b. Take dose the same time each day and do not skip or double up on dose.
      c. Daily weights.

**Table 2-14** Review of Antiarrhythmic Drugs

| Drug | Action | Adverse Effects | Nursing Implications |
|---|---|---|---|
| Quinidine | Depresses myocardial excitability; slows conduction time in atria and ventricles, prolongs P-R interval and QRS complex; prolongs refractory period; depresses myocardial contractility, reduces vagal tone. Used in atrial fibrillation and flutter ventricular tachycardia. | Hematologic/Dermatologic: Agranulocytosis; thrombocytopenia purpura; urticaria<br>CNS: vertigo; blurred vision; diplopia; confusion, syncope<br>GI: vomiting; cramping<br>CV: AV heart block; atrial or ventricular arrhythmias; hypotension; severe bradycardia; arterial embolism | • Administer drug with food to minimize GI symptoms (nausea and vomiting)<br>• Carefully monitor electrolyte levels, blood counts, and kidney and liver function<br>• Advise clients that diarrhea is common in early therapy and should disappear<br>• Encourage client to report dizziness or faintness immediately<br>• Instruct patient to avoid fatigue, excessive caffeine, alcohol, smoking, heavy meals, stressful situations, OTC medications |
| Procainamide (Pronestyl) | Depresses ectopic pacemakers; action on the heart similar to quinidine. Used to treat PVCs, ventricular tachycardia, and some atrial arrhythmias. | Same as quinidine, plus severe hypotension with parenteral use, possible development of a erythematosus-like syndrome in some clients | • Inform client that drug may cause light-headedness and dizziness<br>• Periodic ECG determinations and blood counts in clients on prolonged therapy |
| Lidocaine (Xylocaine) | Suppresses automaticity of ectopic pacemaker; shortens refractory period; decreases duration of action potential in Purkinje fibers; local anesthetic action. Used for acute ventricular arrhythmias. | CNS: dizziness; slurred speech; apprehension; muscle twitching; tremors; convulsions<br>CV: hypotension, bradycardia<br>Dermatologic: urticaria, peripheral edema | • Closely monitor IV flow rate to ensure maintenance of adequate plasma levels<br>• Observe carefully for signs of CNS toxicity (e.g., confusion, tremors), particularly during IV infusion<br>• Monitor cardiac function and blood pressure closely. IM use may increase CPK (creatine phosphokinase) levels |
| Disopyramide (Norpace) | Increases action potential duration and effective refractory period of the atria and ventricles which decreases automaticity and conduction velocity. Useful for PVCs and episodes of ventricular tachycardia. | CV: hypotension; precipitation or aggravation of CHF<br>GU: urinary hesitancy<br>CNS: dry mouth; blurred vision; fatigue, headache, malaise, dizziness<br>GI: nausea, constipation | • Caution client to avoid driving until effects of drug are known because dizziness may occur<br>• Monitor I&O because urinary retention may occur<br>• Encourage use of hard candy to relieve dry mouth |
| Verapamil (Calan, Isoptin)<br>Nifedipine (Procardia)<br>Diltiazem (Cardizem) | Calcium channel blockers inhibit the influx of extracellular calcium ions into cardiac and smooth muscle cells. Antianginal effects include dilation of coronary arteries and arterioles. Verapamil also decreases the influx of calcium into the cardiac contractile and conduction cells of the SA and AV node. Useful in management of chronic, stable angina and treatment of supraventricular tachyarrhythmias. | CV: hypotension, bradycardia; palpitations, peripheral edema<br>CNS: flushing; weakness; dizziness; light-headedness.<br>GI: nausea; cramping; heartburn; constipation with verapamil<br>Respiratory: dyspnea; cough; wheezing | • Carefully monitor blood pressure during initial therapy and whenever dosage changes are made because hypotension may occur<br>• Monitor liver enzymes periodically during therapy<br>• Be alert for signs of CHF, which can occur especially if client is also receiving a beta blocker |
| Digitalis | Stimulates the force of cardiac contraction with improvement of cardiac output. Decreases cardiac oxygen demands, diastolic heart size, and heart rate. Useful in treatment of CHF and certain arrhythmias, such as atrial fibrillation and atrial flutter. | Digitalis toxicity:<br>CNS: headache, fatigue, malaise, drowsiness, muscle weakness, insomnia, agitation, seizures, paresthesias of hands and feet, personality changes, impaired memory, hallucinations<br>CV: arrhythmias (all types are possible)<br>ENT: yellow-green halos<br>GI: anorexia, nausea and vomiting, abdominal distension and pain | • Closely observe client for signs of toxicity<br>• Check with physician regarding what pulse rates (both high and low) should be used as indicators for withholding medication<br>• Watch for changes in pulse rate (sudden increase above 120 or fall below 60)<br>• Recognize signs of hypokalemia, which increases the incidence of digitalis toxicity<br>• Encourage client to take digitalis at prescribed times only<br>• Advise client that protracted diarrhea or vomiting can create an electrolyte imbalance and lead to digitalis toxicity<br>• Recommend adherence to prescribed diet |

d. Avoid high-sodium foods. Increase dietary intake of potassium.

e. Separate digoxin from other pills in pillbox.

B. Related drugs: Phosphodiesterase inhibitors: milrinone (Primacor) and inamrinone (Inocor), used for short-term management of CHF. Also see Table 2-14.

 ## Sample Questions

77. What is the main action of cardiac glycosides?
    1. Release free calcium with cardiac muscle.
    2. Increase the rate of impulse formation at the SA node.
    3. Decrease the conduction of electrical impulses in the heart.
    4. Decrease the force of myocardial contractions.

78. What should the nurse teach the client about cardiac glycosides?
    1. Avoid fruits with potassium.
    2. How to monitor the radial pulse.
    3. Always take digoxin on an empty stomach.
    4. Return to the health care provider in 1 year.

79. Which lab value would be a concern to the nurse?
    1. 0.5 ng/mL
    2. 1.0 ng/mL
    3. 1.5 ng/mL
    4. 2.2 ng/mL

80. Which statement by the client will assure the nurse that the client understands teaching about the adverse effects of digoxin?
    1. "I'll call the physician if my pulse is below 70."
    2. "If a rash develops, I'll apply a topical cream."
    3. "I will call the physician daily to report my weight."
    4. "I will notify the health care provider if vomiting or diarrhea develops."

 ## Answers and Rationales

77. **1.** It is believed that free calcium is released within the cardiac muscle cell, potentiating the action of actin and myosin, which are the major proteins responsible for muscle contraction.

78. **2.** The client should be taught how to monitor the radial pulse, and to hold the medication if the pulse is less than 60 beats per minute for an adult, less than 70 for children, or less than 90 for an infant.

79. **4.** The normal range of digoxin is 0.5–2.0 ng/mL, with a toxic threshold of 2.5 ng/mL.

80. **4.** Vomiting and diarrhea are adverse effects of digoxin therapy and may also be symptoms of digoxin toxicity. The client should report this occurrence to the physician.

# ANTIANGINAL DRUGS

A. Prototype: nitrites and nitroglycerin (Nitro-bid, Nitrodur, Nitrostat IV)
   1. Action. Dilates the peripheral vascular smooth muscles of smaller vessels, which decreases cardiac preload and afterload leading to decreased myocardial oxygen needs. Selectively dilates large coronary arteries, which helps to decrease anginal pain and hypoxia of the myocardium. Given by many different routes of administration including PO, SL, buccal, topical, transdermal. Tolerance may develop with continued use.
   2. Use. Treatment and prophylaxis of angina pectoris. IV nitroglycerin manages congestive heart failure associated with acute MI and controls intraoperative hypotension or manages hypertension.
   3. Dose (adults)
      a. SL: 0.15–0.6 mg at onset of attack or anticipation of attack.
      b. PO: Sustained release 2.5–2.6 mg TID or QID. Topical ointment: 1–2 inches every 8 hours up to 4–5 inches every 4 hours.
      c. Transdermal: 0.1–0.6 mg/hr, can increase up to 0.8 mg/hr; patch worn 12–14 hours/day.
      d. Spray: 1–2 sprays, can repeat every 5 minutes for 15 minutes.
      e. Buccal: 1 mg every 5 hours; dose and frequency increased as needed.
      f. IV: 5 mcg/min in 5% dextrose in water or 0.9% sodium chloride and titrate every 3–5 minutes until response.
   4. Adverse effects. Headache, usually disappears with long-term therapy; flushing; hypotension, dizziness; reflex tachycardia; skin rash with ointment.
   5. Nursing implications
      a. No more than 3 tablets SL should be taken in a 15-minute period (1 tablet every 5 minutes). If pain not relieved by 3 tablets over 15 minutes, could indicate an acute MI and physician should be contacted.

b. Leave tablets at bedside and allocate a specific number of tablets in container. Instruct client to tell nurse when having an attack and number of tablets taken.

c. Sustained-release tablets or capsules should be taken 1 hour before meals or 2 hours after meals.

d. Nitroglycerin ointment should be applied to a hairless or shaved area to promote absorption. New site should be used with each new dose. Use ruled applicator paper that comes with ointment to measure dose. Wear gloves when applying ointment to applicator. Leave applicator paper on site. Cover the applicator paper with plastic wrap and secure with tape.

e. Transdermal nitroglycerin has aluminum backing and patch. Remove before defibrillation. Avoid standing near microwave ovens to prevent burns. Patches are usually applied in morning and removed in evening to prevent tolerance.

f. Dilute IV nitroglycerin in 5% dextrose or 0.9% sodium chloride. Avoid using polyvinyl chloride (PVC) plastic as it can absorb nitroglycerin. Non-PVC is provided by the manufacturer. IV use requires continuous hemodynamic monitoring.

6. Discharge teaching

a. Rise slowly to prevent dizziness.

b. Store in original dark glass container in a cool place. Date bottle when opening and discard after 3 months.

c. Headache will discontinue with long-term use.

d. Keep diary of the number of anginal attacks and tablets taken.

e. Do not drink alcohol.

B. Related drugs: Isosorbide dinitrate (Isordil): used to treat and prevent anginal attacks; given SL or PO.

 **Sample Questions**

81. The client states that he is getting headaches after taking nitroglycerin. How does the nurse interpret this occurrence?
   1. Toxic effect.
   2. Symptom of tolerance.
   3. Hypersensitivity reaction.
   4. Adverse effect.

82. The physician decides to order nitroglycerin transdermal patches. Which instruction is important?
   1. Remove patch when showering.

2. Replace the transdermal patch every 8 hours.
   3. Do not stand near microwave ovens while in use.
   4. Put on an extra transdermal patch if chest pain occurs.

83. Which of the following should the nurse include in teaching about taking sublingual nitroglycerin?
   1. To replace tablets on a yearly basis.
   2. Keep tablets in a moist warm environment.
   3. Take the tablet before exercise to prevent angina.
   4. Notify physician if after 5 consecutive doses the chest pain persists.

 **Answers and Rationales**

81. **4.** A headache is a frequently seen adverse effect that usually disappears with long-term therapy. The physician may order aspirin or acetaminophen for headache relief.

82. **3.** The back of a transdermal nitroglycerin patch contains aluminum, which could cause burns to clients standing near microwave ovens or if defibrillation is needed.

83. **3.** Nitroglycerin should be taken before exercise to prevent an anginal attack.

## ANTIANGINAL DRUGS (CONTINUED)

C. Prototype for Calcium Channel Blockers: verapamil (Calan, Isoptin)

1. Action. Inhibits myocardial oxygen demand by inhibiting the influx of calcium through muscle cell, which leads to reduced afterload and coronary vasodilation. Decreases myocardial contractility, causing peripheral vasodilation leading to decreased heart workload.

2. Use. Angina; essential hypertension (PO form); cardiac dysrhythmias (IV use).

3. Adverse effects. Constipation; nausea and vomiting; hypotension; bradycardia; AV block; dizziness.

4. Nursing implications
   a. Monitor VS, I&O, and ECG.
   b. Encourage high-fiber foods and increased fluid intake (condition permitting).

5. Discharge teaching
   a. Take radial pulse before taking verapamil.

**b.** Avoid caffeine.

**c.** Avoid driving or operating machinery/heavy equipment until response to drug is established.

**d.** Change positions slowly to decrease orthostatic hypotension.

**e.** Do not abruptly discontinue verapamil therapy as rebound angina could occur. Dose is generally tapered.

**f.** Continue with nitroglycerin therapy if prescribed.

**6.** Related drugs. See Table 2-14.

 **Sample Questions**

**84.** A client is taking nitroglycerin with verapamil (Isoptin). What occurrence should the nurse watch for?

1. Hyperkalemia.
2. Hypotension.
3. Seizures.
4. Insomnia.

**85.** Which statement by the client indicates understanding concerning the use of verapamil (Isoptin)?

1. "If I get dizzy I will stop taking the pills and call the physician."
2. "I'm glad that I can continue to drink coffee."
3. "I will only have to take the pills for a couple of weeks."
4. "I will take my pulse before taking my pill."

 **Answers and Rationales**

**84.** **2.** Verapamil (Isoptin) reduces afterload and with concurrent use of nitroglycerin can cause hypotension.

**85.** **4.** Clients should take pulse before taking verapamil (Isoptin) as this drug can cause bradycardia.

## PERIPHERAL VASODILATORS

**A.** Prototype: isoxsuprine HCl (Vasodilan)
Relaxation of the smooth muscle of blood vessels. Used to treat peripheral vascular disorders such as Raynaud's and Buerger's disease (thromboangitis obliterans), diabetic vascular disease, and varicose ulcers.

**B.** Antiplatelet agents

**1.** Dipyridamole (Persantine): Potent vasodilator that also decreases platelet aggregation and clotting time. Selectively dilates small resistance vessels of coronary vascular bed. Used in the prevention of thromboembolism in cardiac valve replacement surgery; also used in other thromboembolic disorders to decrease platelet aggregation. Adverse effects: headaches, dizziness, weakness, hypotension, GI distress, flushing, and skin rashes. Monitor BP. Other antiplatelets: Aspirin, cilostazol (Pletal), clopidogrel (Plavix), and teclopidine (Ticlid).

 **Sample Questions**

**86.** The client complains of nausea while taking isoxsuprine HCl (Vasodilan). What instruction will the nurse give the client?

1. Stop taking the medication and report this to the physician.
2. Take an antacid with the isoxsuprine HCl (Vasodilan).
3. Keep taking the drug as this effect is only transient.
4. Report this to the physician so he can reduce the dose of isoxsuprine HCl (Vasodilan).

 **Answers and Rationales**

**86.** **4.** Adverse effects of isoxsuprine HCl (Vasodilan) are dose related and can be dealt with by reduction of the dose.

## ANTIDYSRHYTHMICS

**A.** Prototype: quinidine (Quinaglute) class 1A

**1.** Action. Alkaloid from the bark of the cinchona tree. Related to quinine, an antimalarial drug. Decreases myocardial excitability and slows conduction velocity, while prolonging the refractory period. PR interval and QRS complex may be prolonged. Has anticholinergic effects that reduce vagus nerve activity, which slows AV conduction.

**2.** Use. Atrial dysrhythmias, atrial fibrillation, and atrial flutter; ventricular dysrhythmias.

**3.** Adverse effects. Cinchonism: GI distress, tinnitus, visual disturbances, dizziness, headache; AV block, hypotension; thrombocytopenia; hypersensitivity; nausea, vomiting, diarrhea.

**4.** Nursing implications
  **a.** Monitor ECG and VS, serum electrolytes, CBC, kidney and liver function.
  **b.** Monitor serum quinidine levels. Normal range 3–6 mcg/mL.
  **c.** Take an apical pulse.
  **d.** Take with food if GI upset.
  **e.** Clients taking digoxin and quinidine are more prone to digitalis toxicity.
**5.** Discharge teaching
  **a.** Take radial pulse before taking.
  **b.** Report symptoms of cinchonism, palpitations, faintness, or breathlessness.

**B.** Related drugs. See Table 2-14.
  **1.** Procainamide
  **2.** Disopyramide

 ## Sample Questions

**87.** Which of the following adverse effects is unique to quinidine (Quinaglute)?
  1. SLE (systemic lupus erythematosus).
  2. Agranulocytosis.
  3. Cinchonism.
  4. Hypoglycemia.

**88.** What client teaching should be included concerning quinidine administration?
  1. Drink plenty of orange juice.
  2. Maintain a high-fiber diet.
  3. Take Pepto Bismol if diarrhea occurs.
  4. Take medication with meals.

 ## Answers and Rationales

**87. 3.** Cinchonism is a syndrome seen specifically when using quinidine; manifested by tinnitus, GI distress, dizziness, visual disturbances, and headache.

**88. 4.** Taking quinidine with meals will decrease GI distress.

## ANTIDYSRHYTHMICS (CONTINUED)

**C.** Prototype: lidocaine (Xylocaine) class 1B
  **1.** Action. Prolongs refractory period in the myocardium and Purkinje fibers. Has little effect on atria. Depresses automaticity but therapeutic doses do not depress myocardial contractility. Also used as a local anesthetic.

**2.** Use. Ventricular arrhythmias, i.e., VT; VF; PVCs.
**3.** Dose (given parenterally only)
  **a.** Adult
    1) IV Bolus: 50–100 mg at a rate of 25–50 mcg/kg/minute; once arrhythmia controlled continue infusion of 1–4 mg/minute.
    2) IM: 200–300 mg and repeat in 60–90 minutes if needed.
  **b.** Pediatric:
    1) IV: 1 mg/kg followed by an infusion of 30 mcg/kg/minute.
**4.** Adverse effects. Drowsiness; CNS stimulation can develop leading to seizures; ventricular tachycardia, heart block, hypertension, bradycardia.
**5.** Nursing implications
  **a.** Monitor ECG, VS, neurologic status, and serum lidocaine levels.
  **b.** Therapeutic lidocaine levels range between 1.5–6 mcg/mL.
  **c.** Use an infusion pump.
  **d.** Cardiac IV lidocaine should not contain preservatives or epinephrine.
  **e.** Deltoid muscle is preferred for IM use.
  **f.** Do not mix with other drugs.

**D.** Related drugs
  **1.** Mexiletine (Mexitel): related to lidocaine
  **2.** Tocainide (Tonocard): related to lidocaine
  **3.** Phenytoin sodium (Dilantin)
  Also see Table 2-15.

**E.** Class IC drugs: Both drugs given orally to treat ventricular dysrhythmias.
  **1.** Flecainide (Tambocor)
  **2.** Propafenone (Rythmol)

**F.** Class I A, B, C drugs
  **1.** Moricizine (Ethmozine): a sodium channel blocker used to treat life-threatening ventricular dysrhythmias; given orally.

 ## Sample Questions

**89.** Which of the following statements is correct concerning the administration of phenytoin (Dilantin)?
  1. Phenytoin is administered by continuous infusion.
  2. Phenytoin can be mixed in dextrose solutions.
  3. 0.9% normal saline should be used to flush IV line and site before and after administration.
  4. Phenytoin is given by rapid IV push.

**Table 2-15** Drugs Related to Lidocaine

| Drug | Action | Use | Adverse Effects | Nursing Implications |
|------|--------|-----|-----------------|----------------------|
| Tocainide (Tonocard) | Oral analog of lidocaine (Xylocaine) | Ventricular arrhythmias | Drug-induced SLE; dyspnea; GI distress; see lidocaine | • Give with food to reduce GI distress<br>• Avoid driving or operating heavy machinery until drug response known<br>• Take radial pulse |
| Phenytoin sodium (Dilantin) | Also an antiepileptic drug; see lidocaine | Ventricular and supraventricular arrhythmias unresponsive to lidocaine or procainamide. Also used to treat digitalis-induced arrhythmias. | Drowsiness; slurred speech; ataxia; nystagmus; hypotension; agranulocytosis; rash; nausea, vomiting | • Should not be given with other antidysrhythmics<br>• IV: do not mix with dextrose as crystallization can occur. Flush IV line with saline before and after administration.<br>• Do not mix with other drugs<br>• Monitor CBC<br>• Therapeutic levels range between 10–20 mcg/mL |

 ## Answers and Rationales

89. **3.** Phenytoin (Dilantin) has a high alkalinity and can precipitate easily. Flushing the IV line and site with 0.9% normal saline will minimize venous irritation and prevent precipitation.

# ANTIDYSRHYTHMICS (CONTINUED)

F. Prototype: bretylium (Bretylol) class III
　　1. Action. An antifibrillatory drug. Initially releases norepinephrine to increase conduction velocity and strengthen the heartbeat.
　　2. Use. Life-threatening arrhythmias.
　　3. Adverse effects. Hypotension, dizziness; worsening arrhythmias, hypertension; nausea, vomiting, diarrhea.
　　4. Nursing implications
　　　　a. Monitor ECG, vital signs, I&O.
　　　　b. Gradually reduce dose.
　　　　c. Change position slowly.
G. Related drugs
　　1. Amiodarone (Cordarone)
　　　　a. Given orally to treat chronic recurrent ventricular tachycardia or ventricular fibrillation that is unresponsive to other drugs.
　　2. Ibutilide (Corvert): given parenterally to treat atrial dysrhythmias.
H. Unclassified antidysrhythmic: Adenosine (Adenocard) is given IV to treat PSVT.

 ## Sample Questions

90. Which adverse effect should the nurse monitor while a client is on maintenance bretylium therapy?
　　1. Hypotension.
　　2. Tachycardia.
　　3. Insomnia.
　　4. Hearing loss.

 ## Answers and Rationales

90. **1.** Hypotension occurs because after the initial release of norepinephrine, bretylium blocks further release of norepinephrine.

# BETA BLOCKERS (CLASS II)

A. Prototype: propranolol (Inderal)
　　1. Action. Beta-adrenergic blocker that decreases heart rate, force of contraction, myocardial irritability, and conduction velocity, and depresses automaticity.
　　2. Use. Cardiac arrhythmias caused by excessive cardiac stimulation of sympathetic nerve impulse; digitalis-induced arrhythmias; essential hypertension; angina pectoris; preoperative management of pheochromocytoma; prevention of migraine headaches.

2

3. Adverse effects. Dizziness, drowsiness, insomnia, depression; hypoglycemia; bronchospasm; bradycardia, heart block, hypotension; rash.
4. Nursing implications
   a. Take apical pulse.
   b. Monitor I&O, daily weights.
   c. Gradually reduce dose before discontinuing.
   d. Pulse rate may not rise following exercise or stress, due to beta-blocking effects.
5. Discharge teaching
   a. Take radial pulse before administering drug.
   b. Avoid alcoholic beverages.
   c. Avoid cold exposure to extremities.
   d. Change positions slowly.

B. Related drugs
   *Note: "olol" is present in generic names.*
   1. Esmolol (Brevibloc): class II antidysrhythmic, used to treat tachycardia, supraventricular tachycardia, atrial fibrillation, and atrial flutter.
   2. Nadolol (Corgard): used to treat essential hypertension and angina.
   3. Pindolol (Visken): used to treat essential hypertension.
   4. Timolol (Blocadren): used to treat essential hypertension.
   5. Atenolol (Tenormin): class II antidysrhythmic, also used to treat angina and hypertension.
   6. Metoprolol (Lopressor): class II antidysrhythmic, given after MI to decrease risk of sudden cardiac death, and also used to treat angina and hypertension.
   7. Sotalol (Betapase): class III antidysrhythmic, generally used to treat life-threatening ventricular dysrhythmias, i.e., ventricular tachycardia.

 **Sample Questions**

91. Which occurrence should clients be monitored for if taking beta-adrenergic blocking agents?
    1. Hyperglycemia.
    2. Heat intolerance.
    3. Respiratory difficulties, bradycardia.
    4. The development of arthritis.

 **Answers and Rationales**

91. **3.** Beta-adrenergic blocking agents reduce heart rate and force of contraction, as well as possibly causing bronchoconstriction.

# CARDIAC STIMULANTS

A. Cardiac stimulants are also autonomic nervous system drugs. The autonomic nervous system drugs are discussed in more detail in a previous section in this unit.
B. Representative drugs
   1. Atropine sulfate
      a. Blocks vagal stimulation of the SA node in the heart, thus increasing heart rate. Acts systemically to block cholinergic activity throughout the body.
      b. Cardiac uses: treatment of sinus bradycardia or asystole; management of symptomatic sinus bradycardia; diagnosis of sinus node dysfunction.
      c. Adverse effects are related to blocking of cholinergic activity in the body.
   2. Isoproteronol (Isuprel)
      a. Stimulates beta-1 adrenergic receptors in heart to increase cardiac output. Is also a bronchodilator.
      b. Cardiac uses: cardiac standstill; carotid sinus hypersensitivity; Stokes-Adams syndrome; ventricular arrhythmias.
      c. Adverse effects: headache, palpitations, dry mouth, flushing, sweating, and bronchial edema.

# ANTICOAGULANTS

A. Prototype: anticoagulants hinder one or more steps of the coagulation process. They do not dissolve existing blood clots but prevent further coagulation from occurring.
B. Related drugs: low-molecular-weight heparin (LMWH). See Table 2-16 comparing Heparin and Warfarin sodium (Coumadin).
   1. Enoxaparin (Lovenox)
   2. Dalteprin (Fragmin)
   3. Action. Enzymatically removes part of heparin molecule, making a smaller, more accurate heparin.
   4. Use. Prophylaxis in deep venous thrombosis (DVT) or pulmonary embolism (PE) especially after hip/knee or abdominal surgery.
   5. Adverse effects. Bleeding, anemia, and thrombocytopenia.
   6. Nursing implications. Assess and monitor for symptoms of bleeding. Special monitoring of bleeding times not necessary. Antidote: protamine sulfate.

**Table 2-16** Comparison of Heparin and Warfarin (Coumadin)

| | Heparin | Coumadin |
|---|---|---|
| **Action** | Blocks conversion of prothrombin to thrombin and fibrinogen to fibrin. Immediate action. | Blocks prothrombin synthesis. Action takes 12–24 hrs to occur. |
| **Use** | Prophylaxis and treatment of thrombosis and embolism. Anticoagulati on for vascular and cardiac surgery. Prevention of clotting in heparin lock sets, blood samples, and during dialysis. Treatment of disseminated intravascular clotting syndrome (DIC). Adjunctive treatment of coronary occlusion with acute MI. | Prophylaxis and treatment of thrombosis and embolism. Atrial fibrillation with embolization. Adjunct in treatment of coronary occlusion and small cell carcinoma of lung with chemotherapy and radiation. |
| **Dose** | **Adult:** SC (deep, intrafat): initially, 10,000–20,000 units, then 8000–10,000 units every 8 hours or 15,000–20,000 units every 12 hours or as determined by coagulation test results. Intermittent IV injection: 10,000 units initially followed by 5000–10,000 units every 4–6 hours. Continuous IV infusion: inject 5000 units initially followed by 20,000–40,000 units/day in 1000 mL of sodium chloride solution.<br><br>**Pediatric:** IV: Initially 50 units per kilogram. Maintenance: 50–100 units per kilogram IV drip every 4 hours. | **Adult:** Oral: 5–10 mg PO initially, then 2–10 mg PO per day based on PT or INR. |
| **Adverse Effects** | Hemorrhage, bruising, thrombocytopenia. Alopecia Osteoporosis Allergic reactions: fever, chills, urticaria, bronchospasm. Elevated AST (SGOT), ALT (SGPT). | Hemorrhage from any tissue or organ. Anorexia, nausea, vomiting, diarrhea. Hypersensitivity: dermatitis, urticaria, fever Jaundice, hepatitis Overdosage: petechicre, paralytic ileus; skin necrosis of toes (purple toes syndrome), and others tissues. |
| **Antidote** | Protamine sulfate<br>*Laboratory test used to monitor therapy:* partial thromboplastin time (PTT) | Vitamin K<br>*Laboratory tests used to monitor therapy:* prothrombin time (PT), INR |
| **Nursing Implications** | • Read label carefully as drug is supplied in differing strengths.<br>• Do not give IM.<br>• SC injection: given in fatty layer of abdomen or just above iliac crest; use 1/2″–5/8″ needle after drawing heparin into syringe; do not inject within 2 inches of umbilicus, scars, or bruises; do not aspirate; do not massage injection site; rotate injection sites and document.<br>• Continuous IV infusion should be given via IV volume control device.<br>• Observe needle sites daily for signs of hematoma.<br>• Monitor CBC, PTT and other coagulation tests.<br>• Test stool for occult blood daily.<br>• Have antidote protamine sulfate available.<br>• Monitor VS.<br>• Report: hematuria, bloody stools, hematemesis, bleeding gums, petechiae, nosebleed, bloody sputum.<br>• Alcohol and smoking alter drug response.<br>• Aspirin, antihistamines, ginseng, ginkgo biloba, and NSAIDS shouldn't be taken while on heparin therapy as these agents may cause platelet function interference.<br>• Do not abruptly withdraw.<br>• Generally followed with oral anticoagulant therapy. | • Known for highest adverse drug interactions of all groups.<br>• Tablet can be crushed and taken with any fluid.<br>• Monitor prothrombin time (PT) and INR.<br>• Have antidote vitamin K available.<br>• Many drug interactions.<br>• Smoking increases dose requirement. |
| **Discharge Teaching** | Heparin used only in hospital setting. | • Stress importance of not skipping doses.<br>• Client will need to report frequently for blood tests.<br>• Client shouldn't take any medication or herbals without checking first with physician.<br>• Client should report signs of bleeding.<br>• Use soft toothbrush; floss teeth with waxed floss.<br>• Shave with electric razor.<br>• Client should tell other health care personnel such as dentists, dental hygienists, etc., that he is taking Coumadin.<br>• Client should carry medical identification (Medic Alert) stating name of drug, name of physician, etc.<br>• Teach client measures to avoid venous stasis. |

## Sample Questions

92. Which action should the nurse perform while the client is on IV heparin?
    1. Protect the medication from light.
    2. Use IM route if there are frequent intravenous site changes.
    3. Attach the IV heparin to an infusion pump.
    4. Explain to the client that stools may turn gray.

93. What should the nurse have readily available for a heparin overdose?
    1. Platelets.
    2. Urokinase.
    3. Protamine sulfate.
    4. Vitamin K.

94. The client requests pain medication for a headache. The physician has ordered aspirin X grains PO every 4 hours for pain. What action should the nurse take?
    1. Substitute Tylenol for the aspirin.
    2. Give the aspirin as ordered.
    3. Call the physician for a different pain reliever.
    4. Give 5 grains of aspirin now and 5 grains in 2 hours.

95. The nurse is teaching about warfarin sodium (Coumadin) therapy. Which statement by the nurse needs correcting?
    1. "If you miss your daily dose of Coumadin, take 2 tablets the next day."
    2. "Use waxed dental floss while on Coumadin therapy."
    3. "Notify your physician before taking any other medication."
    4. "Avoid drinking alcohol in any form while on Coumadin therapy."

## Answers and Rationales

92. **3.** Continuous intravenous infusion of heparin needs constant monitoring to ensure accuracy in dose. An infusion pump or volume controller should be used for this purpose.

93. **3.** Protamine sulfate is the antidote for heparin overdose.

94. **3.** A client on heparin therapy should not take aspirin due to increased potential for bleeding. The nurse needs to contact the physician for a different pain medication.

95. **1.** Changing dose of warfarin sodium (Coumadin) by missing a dose on one day and doubling the dose on the following day is unacceptable as it will negatively affect blood coagulation.

# THROMBOLYTIC DRUGS

A. Prototype: streptokinase (Streptase)
   1. Action. Transforms plasminogen to plasmin which degrades fibrinogen, fibrin clots, and other plasma proteins.
   2. Use. Pulmonary emboli; coronary artery thrombosis; deep venous thrombosis; arteriovenous cannula occlusion.
   3. Adverse effects. Bleeding; allergic reaction; arrhythmias.
   4. Nursing implications
      a. Start therapy as soon as possible after thrombus appears as thrombi older than 7 days react poorly to streptokinase.
      b. When used in treatment of an acute MI, start therapy within 6 hours of attack. When used in treatment of a stroke, therapy should be started within a 3-hour window of the attack.
      c. Heparin is discontinued before streptokinase is started.
      d. Corticosteroids can be given to decrease allergic reaction.
      e. Reconstitute streptokinase with normal saline (preferred solution) or 5% dextrose solution.
      f. IM injections are contraindicated.
      g. Monitor blood coagulation studies and VS.
      h. Maintain bed rest while receiving drug.
      i. Monitor for excessive bleeding every 15 minutes for the first hour of treatment, every 30 minutes for second to eighth hours, then every 8 hours.
      j. Keep whole blood available.
      k. Aminocaproic acid is the antidote for streptokinase.
B. Related drugs
   1. Alteplase (Activase)
   2. Anistreplase (Eminase)
   3. Reteplase (Retavase)
   4. Tenecteplase (TNKase)
   5. Urokinase (Abbokinase)

96. What will the nurse assess during and after streptokinase treatment?
    1. Urticaria.
    2. Diarrhea.
    3. Sore throat.
    4. Peripheral edema.

 **Answers and Rationales**

96. 1. Streptokinase (Streptase) is a foreign protein and does cause allergic reactions. Urticaria would be a sign of this.

# ANTILIPEMIC AGENTS

A. Prototype: cholestyramine (Questran)
   1. Action. Prevents the metabolism of cholesterol in the body.
   2. Use. Type IIa hyperlipoproteinemia; pruritus caused by partial biliary obstruction.
   3. Adverse effects. Constipation, nausea, and vomiting; deficiencies in fat-soluble vitamins A, D, K; rash and skin irritation; osteoporosis; headache, dizziness, syncope; arthritis; fever.
   4. Nursing implications
      a. Monitor cholesterol and serum triglyceride levels.
      b. Assess preexisting constipation problems.
      c. Long-term use increases bleeding tendencies: oral vitamin K may be given prophylactically.
   5. Discharge teaching
      a. Take with water or preferred liquid and dissolve.
      b. Take before meals.
      c. Eat a high-bulk diet low in cholesterol and saturated fats with increased fluids.
      d. Do not omit doses or change dose intervals.
      e. Do not take cholestyramine (Questran) at the same time as other medications as there will be interference with absorption.
      f. Encourage exercise and weight loss.
      g. Give for several months or years if it is effective.
B. Related drugs
   1. Colestipol (Colestid) is similar in action, use, adverse effects, and nursing implications to cholestyramine (Questran).

2. Reductase inhibitors: Atorvastatin (Lipitor), fluvastatin (Lescol), lovastatin (Mevacor), pravastatin (Pravachol), and simvastatin (Zocor) decrease cholesterol levels by stopping the body from making its own cholesterol. Used to treat hypercholesterolemia types IIa and IIb. Adverse effects: headache; insomnia, fatigue, blurred vision, myalgias, nausea, hepatotoxicity, elevated CPK, alkaline phosphatase, and transaminase. Nursing implications: monitor renal and hepatic studies; take with meals to increase absorption.
3. Gemfibrozil (Lopid) decreases triglycerides and increases HDL cholesterol. May cause diarrhea or GI upset.
4. Niacin: vitamin $B_3$ (Nicobid): reduces liver synthesis and reduces cholesterol and total lipid levels. Used in treatment of hyperlipidemia. Adverse effects: tingling, flushing, jaundice, GI upset, pruritus. Nursing implications: dosage is individualized. Niacin is an OTC preparation that should be taken under a physician's care.

 **Sample Questions**

97. Which statement by the client indicates a need for more teaching about cholestyramine (Questran) by the nurse?
    1. "I will continue going to exercise class."
    2. "I will take the drug after meals."
    3. "I will dissolve the drug in liquid before taking it."
    4. "I will increase the fiber in my diet."

 **Answers and Rationales**

97. 2. Cholestyramine (Questran) should be taken before meals for better absorption.

# ANTIHYPERTENSIVES

## General Information for Administration of Antihypertensives

1. Primary objective of antihypertensive therapy is to control essential hypertension and maintain BP with minimal adverse effects.

2. Antihypertensives reduce peripheral resistance and decrease volume of circulating blood.
3. Orthostatic hypotension is a common adverse effect for all antihypertensives.
4. Should not be abruptly discontinued as rebound hypertension could occur.
5. Discharge instructions for all antihypertensives
   a. Have adverse effects that may affect client compliance in taking medication. It is important for client to receive thorough teaching and support to maintain compliance.
   b. Do not abruptly discontinue or skip doses of medications.
   c. Change positions gradually; avoid alcohol, hot showers and baths.
   d. Do not take OTC drugs without consulting physician.
   e. Monitor weight and eat low-sodium foods.
   f. Take BP and record in diary. Report changes to physician.
   g. Do not drive or operate heavy machinery until drug effects are established.
   *Note: thiazide diuretics are discussed under Renal Drugs; MAO (monamine oxidase inhibitors) are discussed under Central Nervous System Drugs; beta blockers are discussed under Antiarrhythmics; and calcium channel blockers are discussed under Antianginal Drugs.*
A. Prototype: central acting antihypertensives (clonidine [Catapres])
   1. Action. Blocks sympathetic nerve impulses in brain, which causes decreased sympathetic outflow leading to decreased BP, vasoconstriction, heart rate, and cardiac contractility.
   2. Use. Used either alone or in combination with other antihypertensives.
   3. Adverse effects. Orthostatic hypotension; drowsiness, behavior changes; peripheral edema, CHF; Raynaud's phenomenon; impotence, urinary retention; dry mouth, constipation.
   4. Nursing implications
      a. Monitor I&O, weight, and BP.
      b. Monitor clients with a history of mental depression.
   5. Discharge teaching. Take last dose of medication in the evening to minimize drowsiness during the day.
B. Related drugs. Methyldopa (Aldomet): may cause blood dyscrasias and hepatotoxicity; monitor blood work and liver function tests.
C. Prototype: alpha-adrenergic receptor blocker (prazosin [Minipress])

1. Action. Blocks alpha receptors in arterial smooth-muscle vasculature and mediates vasoconstriction.
2. Use. Essential hypertension and hypertension caused by pheochromocytoma.
3. Adverse effects. Postural hypotension and syncope with initial therapy; reflex tachycardia. See clonidine (Catapres).
4. Nursing implications. Monitor vital signs.
5. Discharge teaching
   a. Take with food to reduce dizziness, light-headedness.
   b. Take initial dose at bedtime to reduce effects of syncope.
   c. Report sexual difficulties.
6. Related drugs
   a. Doxazosin (Cardura)
   b. Terazosin (Hytrin)
D. Prototype: peripheral-acting antiadrenergic agents (reserpine [Serpalan])
   1. Action. Lowers BP by blocking norepinephrine in CNS and peripherally.
   2. Use. Rarely used due to its adverse effects and availability of other antihypertensives; agitated psychosis; essential hypertension with a diuretic; parenteral use to treat hypertensive emergencies.
   3. Adverse effects. Suicidal depression, drowsiness; nasal obstruction; increased incidence of breast cancer in women; impotence; decreased cardiac output, postural hypotension; diarrhea, increased gastric secretions.
   4. Nursing implications
      a. Monitor for depression; obtain a mental health history for depression.
      b. Assess for family history of breast cancer.
      c. Administer with meals to reduce GI distress.
      d. Monitor BP and I&O.
      e. Rinse mouth or use hard candy for dry mouth.
   5. Related drugs. Guanethidine (Ismelin): antihypertensive agent rarely used due to its adverse effect; affects sympathetic nerve endings by releasing norepinephrine; and then interferes with release of norepinephrine; with initial use may see transient hypertension and elevated heart rate.
E. Prototype: ACE inhibitor (angiotensin-converting enzyme inhibitor) (captopril [Capoten])
   1. Action. Lowers BP by inhibiting angiotensin-converting enzyme, which inhibits angiotensin II (vasoconstrictor) and indirectly reduces serum aldosterone levels.
   2. Use. Initial therapy of essential hypertension in clients with normal renal function; severe hypertension in clients with renal dysfunction; CHF.

3. Adverse effects. Blood dyscrasias; hypotension; proteinuria; hyperkalemia; rash; loss of taste perception.
4. Nursing implications
   a. Monitor CBC, electrolytes, and urinalysis.
   b. Administer 1 hour before meals.
5. Discharge teaching
   a. Report fever, sore throat, and rash.
   b. Use salt substitutes only if prescribed (many substitutes contain K+).
6. Related drugs
   a. Enalapril (Vasotec)
   b. Lisinopril (Zestril)
   c. Benezepril (Lotensin)
   d. Fosinopril (Monopril)
   e. Ramipril (Altace)
   f. Losarten (Cozaar) and valasartan (Diovan): angiotensin II receptor blockers
F. Prototype: direct-acting vasodilators (hydralazine [Apresoline])
   1. Action. Direct relaxation of arteriolar smooth muscle causing vasodilation.
   2. Use. Hypertension; parenteral hydralazine (Apresoline) is used in hypertensive emergencies.
   3. Adverse effects. Headache, dizziness, depression; tachycardia, angina, palpitations; lupus-like syndrome, rash, fever; weight gain, sodium retention; nausea, vomiting, anorexia.

4. Nursing implications
   a. Monitor CBC, ANA titer, and LE preparation.
   b. Clients receiving parenteral hydralazine (Apresoline) check BP and pulse every 5 minutes until stable while on parenteral agent.
5. Related drugs
   a. Minoxidil (Loniten)
      1) Has more adverse effects than hydralazine. May cause cardiac muscle lesions and hirsutism.
      2) Topical preparation (Rogaine) is available to treat baldness.
   b. Nitroprusside (Nipride)
      1) Given IV to treat hypertensive emergencies.
      2) Should be administered in an infusion pump. IV tubing and container should be wrapped in aluminum foil to protect from light. VS, neuro checks, and I&O should be closely monitored.
   c. Diazoxide (Hyperstat)
      1) Given IV to treat hypertensive emergencies.
      2) May cause hyperglycemia.
See Table 2-17.

**Table 2-17** Review of Antihypertensive Drugs

| Drug | Action | Adverse Effects | Nursing Implications |
|---|---|---|---|
| Diuretics<br>Thiazide diuretics<br>  Chlorothiazide<br>  (Diuril)<br>Hydrochlorothiazide<br>  (Esidrex, Hydro<br>  Diuril, Oretic)<br>Chlorthalidone<br>  (Hygroton)<br>Metolazone<br>  (Zaroxolyn) | Block sodium reabsorption in ascending tubule of kidney; water excreted with sodium, producing decreased blood volume | Hyperuricemia, hyperglycemia, hypercalcemia, elevated BUN; hypokalemia, orthostatic hypotension, anorexia, nausea, vomiting, light-headedness, headache, drowsiness, rash | • Monitor I&O and observe for excessive diuresis.<br>• Encourage client to make positional changes slowly to decrease occurrence of orthostatic hypotension.<br>• Perform baseline and periodic determinations of electrolytes, BUN, uric acid, blood sugar, weight, and blood pressure.<br>• If possible, administer in the morning to avoid nocturia.<br>• Administer with food to minimize gastric distress.<br>• Encourage inclusion of high-potassium foods in diet to decrease possibility of hypokalemia. Advise client to avoid high-sodium foods.<br>• Stress the importance of taking the drugs regularly as prescribed. |
| Loop (High-Ceiling) diuretics<br>Furosemide (Lasix)<br>Ethacrynic acid (Edecrin)<br>Bumetanide (Bumex) | Inhibit reabsorption of sodium and chloride at the proximal portion of ascending loop of Henle | Similar to thiazides but intensity differs. Hypocalcemia, hearing loss. | See above. |

*(continues)*

**Table 2-17** Review of Antihypertensive Drugs *(continued)*

| Drug | Action | Adverse Effects | Nursing Implications |
|---|---|---|---|
| Potassium-sparing diuretic Spironolactone (Aldactone) | Antagonizes the effect of aldosterone on the tubular cells of the kidney; sodium excreted in exchange for potassium | Hyperkalemia, gynecomastia, hirsutism, irregular menses, rash, drowsiness or confusion | • Monitor I&O, blood pressure, and weight regularly.<br>• Instruct client to be alert for signs of hyponatremia.<br>• Inform client that swelling and tenderness of the breasts occur most often with prolonged therapy.<br>• Monitor serum potassium levels daily during early stages of therapy.<br>• Advise client to avoid excessive intake of potassium-rich foods. |
| Drugs acting on the CNS Methyldopa (Aldomet) | Metabolized into a false neurotransmitter displacing norepinephrine from its receptor sites; sympathetic activity reduced | Orthostatic hypotension, sedation, weakness, drowsiness, dry mouth, liver damage | • Advise slow positional changes and avoid prolonged standing in one position.<br>• Inform client the drug may darken urine.<br>• Advise client to observe for signs of liver dysfunction. |
| Clonidine (Catapres) | Stimulates alpha-adrenergic receptor in brain, causing inhibition of sympathetic vasoconstriction | Orthostatic hypotension, sedation, drowsiness, dry mouth, anxiety, depression | • Closely observe clients with prior history of mental depression because the drug may cause depressive episodes.<br>• Advise slow positional changes.<br>• Encourage client to dangle feet for a few minutes before standing. |
| Beta-Adrenergic Blockers Propranolol (Inderal) Nadolol (Corgard) | Reversible competitive blocking action at beta-adrenergic receptor sites. Results in decreased heart rate and force of contraction, slowed AV conduction, decreased plasma renin, and lowered blood pressure | Drowsiness, light-headedness, lethargy, cramping, nausea, and bradycardia | • Record I&O and client's weight and notify physician of any significant changes.<br>• Advise client to rise slowly, avoid prolonged standing, and be careful when operating machinery.<br>• Inform client that smoking may reduce effectiveness of drug.<br>• Evaluate heart rate and rhythm before administration of the drug.<br>• Warn client that alcohol may enhance the hypotensive effect of the drug.<br>• Perform urinary protein estimates prior to therapy and at monthly intervals thereafter. |
| Drugs acting on renin-angiotensin system Captopril (Capoten) Enalapril (Vasotec) | Depresses the functioning of the renin-angiotensin-aldosterone mechanism by inhibiting angiotensin-converting enzyme (ACE) in the plasma | Rash, pruritus, proteinuria (mainly captopril), agranulocytosis (mainly captopril), excessive hypotension, blood dyscrasias | • Administer (captopril) one hour before meals.<br>• Instruct client to report blood dyscrasias (sore throat, fever) and excessive hypotension (dizziness) and rashes immediately. |
| Vasodilators Hydralazine (Apresoline) | Direct relaxation of arteriolar smooth muscle producing decreased peripheral resistance | Headache, nausea, vomiting, diarrhea, sweating, palpitations, and tachycardia. Systemic lupus-like symptoms (high doses). | • Advise client that headache and palpitations may occur during early stages of therapy.<br>• Perform periodic blood counts, LE cell preparations, and antinuclear antibody titer determinations.<br>• Advise client to make positional changes slowly.<br>• Observe clients receiving large amounts of hydralazine closely for signs of developing lupus-like reaction. |

## Sample Questions

**98.** A client is started on prazosin (Minipress) 1 mg PO daily. Which client teaching instruction should the nurse stress?
1. Rise slowly from a lying or sitting position.
2. Take the drug on an empty stomach.
3. Force fluids to 2 liters/day.
4. Take the medication in the morning.

**99.** Which of the following should the nurse specifically assess for prior to clients starting on captopril (Capoten) therapy?
1. Depression.
2. Renal dysfunction.
3. Liver disease.
4. Hyperglycemia.

**100.** Which antihypertensive drug may be linked to breast cancer and may cause suicidal depression?
1. Guanethidine (Ismelin).
2. Hydralazine (Apresoline).
3. Reserpine (Serpalan).
4. Clonidine (Catapres).

**101.** Which of the following actions should the nurse take when administering nitroprusside (Nipride)?
1. Mix the solution in normal saline.
2. Administer the drug by IV push.
3. Monitor neuro checks and VS every hour.
4. Wrap IV bottle and tubing with aluminum foil.

**102.** Which side effect should the client be aware of when taking clonidine (Catapres)?
1. Anxiety.
2. Diarrhea.
3. Dry mouth.
4. Irritability.

## Answers and Rationales

**98.** 1. As with most antihypertensives, initial therapy of prazosin (Minipress) may produce orthostatic hypotension; client should rise slowly.

**99.** 2. Renal damage is an adverse response to captopril (Capoten) that is more apt to occur in clients with renal dysfunction.

**100.** 3. Reserpine (Serpasil) has been known to cause suicidal depression; an increased incidence of breast cancer has also been noted with this drug.

**101.** 4. Nitroprusside (Nipride) is sensitive to light and becomes less active; therefore the IV tubing and container should be covered.

**102.** 3. Clonidine (Catapres) can cause dry mouth due to decreased salivary flow.

# Renal Drugs

## DIURETICS

**A.** Prototype: thiazide diuretics (hydrochlorothiazide (HCTZ) [Hydrodiurill])
1. Action. Blocks sodium reabsorption in the distal convoluted tubule, which prevents water reabsorption, increases urine output, and decreases blood volume. Potassium is also excreted.
2. Use. Essential hypertension; edema associated with CHF.
3. Adverse effects. Hypokalemia, hyponatremia; drowsiness; hyperglycemia; photosensitivity, hypersensitivity: thiazides are chemically related to sulfonamides; orthostatic hypotension, arrhythmias; anorexia, nausea, vomiting, diarrhea; agranulocytosis.
4. Nursing implications
Monitor I&O, weights, and serum electrolytes, glucose, and BUN.
5. Discharge teaching
   a. Take medication in the early morning and after meals to prevent GI distress.
   b. Report symptoms of agranulocytosis such as fever, sore throat.
   c. Change positions slowly.
   d. Eat foods high in potassium (i.e., oranges, bananas, strawberries).
   e. Take daily weights.

B. Related drugs
  1. Metolazone (Zaroxolyn)
  2. Chlorathiazide (Diuril)
  3. Chlorthalidone (Hygroton)
  4. Bendroflumethiazide (Naturetin)

## Sample Questions

103. Which statement by the client indicates that she needs more client teaching in regard to hydrochlorothiazide (Hydrodiuril) therapy?
  1. "I will take my medication with orange juice."
  2. "I will take my medication before going to bed."
  3. "I will take my medication after meals."
  4. "I will notify the physician if I have a sore throat."

## Answers and Rationales

103. **2.** Taking hydrochlorothiazide (Hydrodiuril) before going to bed may cause nocturia and interrupted sleep. The client needs to be taught to take the medication in the morning as the diuretic effect begins in 2 hours and peaks in 4 hours.

## DIURETICS (CONTINUED)

C. Prototype: loop diuretics (furosemide [Lasix])
  1. Action. Acts by inhibiting reabsorption of sodium and chloride at the proximal portion of the ascending loop of Henle, increasing water excretion. This drug is considered to be potent.
  2. Use. Hypertension, pulmonary edema, edema seen with congestive heart failure, cirrhosis, and renal disease.
  3. Adverse effects. Fluid and electrolyte imbalances: hypokalemia, hypochloremic alkalosis, hyperuricemia, hyponatremia, hypocalcemia, hypomagnesemia, hyperglycemia; nausea, vomiting, anorexia, constipation; diarrhea in children given high doses with sorbitol as the vehicle; jaundice, acute pancreatitis; polyuria, nocturia, urinary bladder spasm; dizziness, paresthesias, headache, blurred vision, irreversible hearing loss; leukopenia, anemia; orthostatic hypotension, cardiac arrhythmias; muscle spasms; photosensitivity, rash, pruritus.
  4. Nursing implications
    a. Can take with food.
    b. Monitor CBC, serum and urine electrolytes, BUN, blood glucose, uric acid.
    c. Monitor VS closely when client receiving IM or IV administration. Client should be switched to oral preparation when practical.
    d. IM injection is painful; use Z-track technique.
    e. Infusion rate must be closely monitored. Should not be more than 4 mg per minute.
    f. Elderly require close monitoring during active diuresis. Watch for fluid and electrolyte imbalances.
    g. Monitor I&O.
    h. Weigh client daily.
    i. Monitor for hearing loss.
    j. Monitor clients with diabetes closely.
    k. Tablets slightly discolored are still considered potent; discolored parenteral solutions should be discarded.
    l. Compatible with 5% dextrose in water, sodium chloride, and lactated Ringer's; use solution mixed with furosemide (Lasix) within 24 hours.
  5. Discharge teaching
    a. Take dose early in day to avoid nocturia.
    b. Usually allowed liberal salt intake; consult physician.
    c. Caution client about orthostatic hypotension if on high dose of furosemide (Lasix) or on other antihypertensive agents.
    d. Needs diet high in potassium and maybe a potassium supplement.
    e. Stay out of the sun and use sunscreen.
  6. Related drugs. Ethacrynic acid (Edecrin) and bumetanide (Bumex) are similar to furosemide (Lasix). Both drugs are used for treating edema and can be given orally and parenterally.

## Sample Questions

104. Which group of clients needs special monitoring by the nurse while receiving furosemide (Lasix) therapy?
  1. Premature infants.
  2. Client with diabetes.
  3. Client with asthma.
  4. Clients with peripheral vascular disease (PVD).

## Answers and Rationales

104. **2.** Furosemide (Lasix) can cause hyperglycemia. Clients with diabetes need close monitoring of urine and blood glucose while on furosemide therapy.

# DIURETICS (CONTINUED)

D. Prototype: carbonic anhydrase inhibitors (acetazolamide [Diamox])
   1. Action. Promotes renal excretion of sodium, potassium, bicarbonate, and water via reduction of hydrogen ion secretion in the renal tubule cells of the kidney.
   2. Use. Adjunct in treating congestive heart failure; adjunct in treating open-angle glaucoma to decrease intraocular pressure; acute mountain sickness; epilepsy.
   3. Adverse effects. Nausea, vomiting, anorexia, melena, constipation; hematuria, renal colic, renal calculi, crystalluria; liver damage; fatigue, nervousness, drowsiness, dizziness, depression, headache, tremor, convulsions; transient myopia; bone marrow depression; urticaria, pruritus, rash, photosensitivity; weight loss, fever, acidosis; increased excretion of calcium, potassium, magnesium, and sodium; hyperglycemia; hyperuricemia.
   4. Nursing implications
      a. Can be taken with food.
      b. Tablets (regular only, not sustained-release) can be crushed or dissolved in hot water. Will not dissolve in fruit juice.
      c. Give in morning to avoid interrupting sleep.
      d. Avoid IM route; alkalinity of solution causes pain.
      e. Monitor clients for metabolic acidosis.
      f. Monitor I&O and weight when using drug for edema.
      g. Maintain fluid intake to prevent kidney stones.
      h. Many adverse effects are dose related.
      i. Monitor diabetic clients.
      j. Potassium loss greatest in early treatment.
      k. Observe for signs of hypokalemia; those at high risk for this are clients receiving other diuretics or digitalis glycosides, and the elderly.
      l. Client may need a potassium supplement.
      m. Monitor serum electrolytes, blood gases, urinalysis.
      n. Parenteral solution should be used within 24 hours after reconstitution.
   5. Discharge teaching
      a. Do not interchange brands without asking physician.
      b. Avoid excess salt intake.
      c. Report any adverse effects.
      d. Do not drive or perform other activities if experiencing CNS effects.
      e. If taken in high doses or for long periods of time, client will need a diet high in potassium.
E. Prototype: potassium-sparing diuretics (spironolactone [Aldactone])
   1. Action. Acts by blocking aldosterone receptors in the kidney tubule, thus causing excretion of water and sodium and potassium retention.
   2. Use. Primary hyperaldosteronism; edema; treatment and prevention of hypokalemia; essential hypertension.
   3. Adverse effects. Hyperkalemia; hyponatremia; gynecomastia; thirst, dry mouth, diarrhea; impotence, irregular menses, hirsutism; headache, dizziness, drowsiness, confusion; rash, urticaria.
   4. Nursing implications
      a. Give with food.
      b. Tablet can be crushed.
      c. Monitor serum electrolytes.
      d. Diuretic effect may take until third day of therapy and may last 2–3 days after drug is stopped.
      e. Monitor I&O and check for edema.
      f. Weigh client daily.
      g. Monitor blood pressure.
      h. Adverse effects usually reversible if drug discontinued.
   5. Discharge teaching
      a. Teach signs of electrolyte imbalance and when to report.
      b. Consult physician concerning potassium and sodium intake. Usually client should avoid a high-potassium diet.
   6. Related drugs
      a. Triamterene (Dyrenium): prevents sodium reabsorption in the distal tubule of the kidney, which causes retention of potassium and sodium and water. It is used to treat edema, hypertension, and hypokalemia. Adverse effects: hyperkalemia, renal calculi, nausea, vomiting, anorexia, diarrhea, headache, fatigue, rash, photosensitivity, and blood dyscrasias. Nursing implications: give the drug with food to decrease GI upset; give the drug in the morning, monitor I&O, body weight, serum electrolytes, and BUN; client should avoid foods high in potassium.
      b. Amiloride (Midamor): resembles triamterene. The biggest difference is that it is much more potent than triamterene.
F. Prototype: osmotic diuretics (mannitol [Osmitrol])
   1. Action. Acts by increasing the osmotic pressure of the glomerular filtrate inside the renal tubules. This causes less reabsorption of fluid and electrolytes by the tubules and increased loss of fluid, chloride, and sodium.
   2. Use. Prevention and treatment of acute renal failure; reduction of intracranial pressure; reduction of intraocular pressure; urinary excretion of drug overdoses.
   3. Adverse effects. Nausea, anorexia, thirst; diuresis, urinary retention; dizziness, headache, convulsions; pulmonary

congestion; tachycardia, chest pain, high or low blood pressure; metabolic acidoses; hypokalemia, hyponatremia, hypochloremia, dehydration.

4. Nursing implications
   a. Test dose given to clients with advanced oliguria.
   b. Monitor serum and urine electrolytes, central venous pressure, and renal function.
   c. Accurate I&O every 30 minutes.
   d. Monitor VS.
   e. Monitor for signs of electrolyte imbalance.
   f. Weigh client daily.
   g. Avoid extravasation.
   h. Drug may crystallize if exposed to low temperatures. Warm solution to dissolve crystals.
   i. Solutions above 15% have tendency to crystallize. IV filter must be used for infusing solutions 15% and above.

 **Sample Questions**

105. A client is receiving mannitol. The nurse is aware that mannitol will help to decrease what condition?
   1. Hypertension.
   2. Hyperkalemia.
   3. Peripheral edema.
   4. Increased intracranial pressure.

 **Answers and Rationales**

105. 4. Mannitol is used primarily in the treatment of intracranial pressure, but also to treat acute renal failure, where rapid reduction of pressure and volume is required.

## POTASSIUM-REMOVING RESIN

A. There is one drug in this category, sodium polystyrene sulfonate (Kayexalate).
B. Characteristics of polystyrene sulfonate (Kayexalate)
   1. A resin that exchanges sodium ions for potassium ions in the large intestine.
   2. Used in the treatment of hyperkalemia.
   3. Given orally or rectally via high enema to both adults and children.
   4. Nursing implications
      a. Retain rectal suspension for at least 30–60 minutes.
      b. Monitor for electrolyte deficiency.
         1) Hypokalemia can occur.
         2) Magnesium and calcium can also be lost.
         3) Sodium may be retained.
      c. Constipation can occur with oral administration.
      d. Rectal administration helps prevent constipation.
      e. Mix resin with sorbitol and water (never with oil).
      f. Stop administration when serum potassium is 4–5 milliequivalents.

 # Respiratory Drugs

## ANTIASTHMATIC DRUGS

A. Prototype: theophylline
   1. Action. Classified as a methylxanthine; a bronchodilator that relaxes the bronchial smooth muscle cells. It also increases renal blood flow, thus producing a diuretic effect, and acts as a CNS stimulant.
   2. Use. Emphysema; chronic bronchitis; asthma; CHF.
   3. Adverse effects. CNS stimulation: irritability, nervousness, restlessness *(Note: children are more susceptible to developing CNS stimulation effects);* tachycardia, hypotension, palpitations *(Note: shouldn't be used in clients with cardiovascular disease);* tachypnea, flushing; nausea, vomiting, GI distress *(Note: should not be used in clients with peptic ulcer disease or hyperthyroidism);* rectal irritation with rectal suppository use.
   4. Nursing implications
      a. Monitor theophylline levels (10–20 mcg/mL).
      b. Monitor vital signs and symptoms of toxicity.

    c. Clients who smoke tobacco and marijuana require higher doses of theophylline.

    d. Administer with milk or meals if GI distress is present, otherwise give 1–2 hours before meals with water.

  5. Discharge teaching

    a. Consult with the physician before taking OTC drugs.

    b. Avoid excessive caffeine use.

    c. Do not crush or chew time-released or enteric-coated preparations.

**B.** Related drugs (See prototype: theophylline for adverse effects)

  1. Aminophylline (Somophyllin)

    a. Can be given PO, rectal, IV, or IM.

    b. IM injection is painful and generally avoided.

    c. IV infusion should not exceed 25 milligrams per minute.

    d. Vital signs should be monitored.

    e. Often used to treat severe bronchoconstriction.

    f. Avoid mixing with other medications as it is incompatible with many medications.

  2. Theo-dur

  3. Slow-Bid

  4. Quibron-T

  5. Elixophylline

*All of the above are derivatives of theophylline. Note: they are less potent than theophylline and dosage adjustments may be needed.*

**C.** Prototype: cromolyn sodium (Intal, Nasalcrom)

  1. Action. Acts on lung mucosa to prevent histamine release. Classified as a mast cell stabilizer.

  2. Use. Prophylactically to reduce the number of asthmatic attacks. It is not used in the treatment of acute asthmatic attacks; to treat allergic rhinitis; ophthalmically to treat allergic disorders.

  3. Adverse effects. Bronchoconstriction; cough; nasal congestion; rash.

  4. Discharge teaching

    a. Proper use of inhaler

      1) With spinhaler place capsule in container and exhale fully.

      2) Place mouthpiece between lips.

      3) Tilt head back.

      4) Inhale deeply and rapidly to cause the propeller to turn.

      5) Remove the inhaler.

      6) Hold breath a few seconds.

      7) Slowly exhale.

    b. Capsules should not be swallowed or opened.

    c. Rinsing or gargling may reduce irritation in the mouth.

    d. Discontinue use if an allergic reaction occurs.

**D.** Leukotriene inhibitors: Zileuton (Zyflo), zafirlukast (Accolate), and montelukast (Singulair), used to prevent asthma attacks.

## Sample Questions

**106.** Which statement by a client's mother best indicates her understanding of the use of cromolyn sodium?

  1. "I will have him take this medication during an asthma attack."

  2. "I will open the capsule and dilute it in juice."

  3. "I will tell him to take a puff of medication upon exhalation."

  4. "I will have him use this medication to prevent asthma attacks."

**107.** Which adverse effect should a client's mother be alert for when administering theophylline?

  1. Drowsiness.

  2. Irritability and restlessness.

  3. Constipation.

  4. Bradycardia.

**108.** Which of the following fluids should be avoided while taking theophylline?

  1. Ginger ale.

  2. Apple juice.

  3. Hot chocolate.

  4. Milk.

**109.** The client's mother asks the nurse the purpose of offering theophylline. What is the nurse's best response?

  1. "This drug decreases inflammation in the bronchi."

  2. "Theophylline's antihistamine effect will counteract bronchospasm."

  3. "This drug will help to facilitate removal of secretions."

  4. "Theophylline dilates the bronchial tree and will make breathing easier."

## Answers and Rationales

106. **4.** Cromolyn sodium is effective in preventing asthma attacks because it prevents histamine release.

107. **2.** Irritability and restlessness are symptoms of CNS stimulation, which could lead to seizures. Children are very prone to CNS stimulation with this drug.

108. **3.** Hot chocolate contains caffeine, which can further increase CNS effects of theophylline.

109. **4.** Theophylline dilates the smooth muscle cells in the bronchi, which enhances breathing and counteracts bronchial constriction.

# ANTIHISTAMINES

A. Antihistamines reduce histamine activity by blocking histamine receptor sites. They act within 15–30 minutes after administration but are eliminated slowly from the body. Antihistamines are used to suppress symptoms of histamine release in allergy. Other uses of antihistamines include rhinitis, colds, motion sickness, vertigo, Parkinson's disease, and as a sleep aid. It is important to remember to administer any antihistamine before an allergy attack to prevent histamine from occupying receptor sites and thus decreasing the severity of the attack. There are a few classes of drugs that contain antihistamine properties. Sedation is the most common adverse effect of antihistamines. Paradoxical excitation has been seen in children taking these drugs, and symptoms such as dizziness, confusion, sedation, and hypotension are seen in the elderly. There are also anticholinergic effects from antihistamines, which include dry nose, mouth, and throat; urinary retention; constipation; tachycardia; and blurred vision.

B. Chlorpheniramine maleate (Chlor-Trimeton): given PO, IM, SC, and IV. Available in a sustained-release form. There are increased depressant effects if taken with alcohol or other CNS depressants. Give oral forms with food if GI upset occurs.

C. Diphenhydramine HCl (Benadryl): given PO, IM, and IV. IM should be given deeply in a large muscle mass. Hypersensitivity reactions occur more with parenteral administration than with PO. Related drugs: Clemastine (Tavist) and dimenhydrinate (Dramamine).

D. Promethazine HCl (Phenergan): given PO, IM, rectally, and IV. Can be taken with food. Oral administration for allergy usually given before meals (ac) or at bedtime (hs) as a single dose. Monitor respiratory function especially in children as drug can suppress cough reflex and thicken bronchial secretions. Can cause photosensitivity.

E. Second generation non-sedating antihistamines
   1. Desloratadine (Clarinex)
   2. Fexofenadine (Allegra)
   3. Cetirizine (Zyrtec)

## Sample Questions

110. What would the nurse teach the client to do to lessen the sedation effects of antihistamines?
   1. Increase caffeine intake during the day.
   2. Take the antihistamine when going to bed.
   3. Take the antihistamine with a vitamin.
   4. Have a 2-hour nap in the morning and afternoon.

111. What is an adverse effect that is seen more often in children than adults who are taking antihistamines?
   1. Dizziness.
   2. Dry mucous membranes.
   3. Constipation.
   4. CNS excitement.

## Answers and Rationales

110. **2.** The sedation effects of antihistamines will be decreased if the client takes the drug at bedtime.

111. **4.** A side effect of antihistamines that is seen more commonly in children than adults is excitation of the central nervous system.

# MUCOLYTICS

A. Acetylcysteine (Mucomyst)
   1. Action. Reduces the viscosity of mucus in the bronchial tree.
   2. Use. Cystic fibrosis; acute and chronic bronchopulmonary diseases such as pneumonia, bronchitis, and emphysema; acetylcysteine is the antidote for acetaminophen (Tylenol) overdose.

3. Adverse effects. May cause bronchospasm in asthmatic clients and should be discontinued; stomatitis, nausea, vomiting.
4. Nursing implications
   a. Suction equipment should be readily available.
   b. Has a foul odor of "rotten eggs."
   c. Should rinse mouth after treatment.

## Sample Questions

112. Which of the following should be available for clients receiving acetylcysteine?
   1. A glass of water.
   2. Tracheostomy set-up.
   3. Suction set-up.
   4. Room deodorizer.

## Answers and Rationales

112. **3.** Acetylcysteine (Mucomyst) can cause an outpouring of copious secretions, which may cause gagging. Suction may be needed to facilitate the removal of secretions to prevent aspiration.

# EXPECTORANTS AND ANTITUSSIVES

A. Expectorants
   1. Expectorants reduce the viscosity of bronchial secretions, which allows for their removal from the lungs. They are used in the management of cough associated with the common cold and in the treatment of bronchitis.
   2. Guaifenesin (Robitussin): can be given to adults and children. It increases the respiratory tract fluid thus reducing viscosity of secretions. It is the most frequently used OTC expectorant medication. Client should be told to increase fluid intake and add humidification. A common adverse effect is gastric upset, which is caused by its stimulatory effect on gastric secretions.
   3. Terpin hydrate elixir: directly stimulates the bronchial secretory glands. Is often used as a vehicle for other cough medications. Terpin hydrate has a high alcohol content and shouldn't be given to alcoholics. Also shouldn't be given to children under 12 years.

B. Antitussives
   1. Antitussives are given to reduce the force and amount of coughing. They can act centrally by suppressing the cough center in the brain or peripherally to reduce the susceptibility of irritant receptors to activity. Some antitussives contain narcotics. The antitussives are given for the symptomatic relief of nonproductive cough.
   2. Dextromethorphan (Benylin DM, Pertussin): This is the most frequently used non-narcotic antitussive. Because of its safety record, it is used for children as well as adults. Common adverse effects are dizziness, drowsiness, and nausea. It shouldn't be given to clients receiving MAO inhibitors.
   3. Codeine: Due to its addicting capabilities, it should be given in the smallest dose possible to decrease adverse effects and tolerance. The client needs to be watched for signs of dependency. Common adverse effects are nausea, vomiting, and constipation. Encourage clients to increase fluid intake and take a laxative if constipation occurs. Provide for client safety due to codeine's sedative effects. If the client is taking other CNS depressants with codeine, there is an increased chance of CNS effects. Respiratory depression occurs at high doses. Observe respiratory rate and use cautiously in clients with asthma or emphysema.

## Sample Questions

113. Which of the following points should be made regarding guaifenesin by the nurse?
   1. Guaifenesin has a high incidence of adverse effects.
   2. Increase fluid intake to help liquefy and loosen secretions while taking guaifenesin.
   3. Guaifenesin has a high alcohol content.
   4. This drug can cause blood glucose level to rise.

114. In which situation would the use of an antitussive be inappropriate?
   1. The client's cough is interfering with eating meals.
   2. The client's cough is associated with a suppurative lung disorder.
   3. The client's cough is the source of a complication such as a rib fracture.
   4. The client's cough is irritating to the respiratory tract.

115. Which adverse effect is associated with the use of high doses of codeine as an antitussive?
1. Diarrhea.
2. Nasal congestion.
3. Respiratory depression.
4. Skin rash.

## Answers and Rationales

113. **2.** Clients taking guaifenesin (Robitussin) need to increase fluid intake daily to help thin and loosen secretions. This allows the drug to be more effective.

114. **2.** An antitussive is not appropriate for a client with lung disease accompanied by increased sputum as pneumonia or atelectasis could occur.

115. **3.** Respiratory depression is an adverse effect associated with use of codeine. It is a life-threatening effect.

# Gastrointestinal Tract Drugs

## HISTAMINE (H$_2$) ANTAGONISTS

A. Prototype: cimetidine (Tagamet)
1. Action. Decreases stomach acidity by impeding the action of histamine. Competes with histamine for occupancy of histamine (H$_2$) receptor sites on the parietal cells in the stomach and suppresses the release of gastric acid.
2. Use. Short-term treatment of active duodenal ulcer and benign gastric ulcer; decreased dose after ulcer has healed to inhibit reappearance; pathologic hypersecretory conditions, e.g., Zollinger-Ellison syndrome.
3. Adverse effects. Diarrhea, muscle pain, rash; CNS effects of dizziness, confusion, drowsiness, headache; changes in liver function studies; agranulocytosis and neutropenia; antiandrogenic effects (impotence and gynecomastia).
4. Nursing implications
   a. Oral form should be taken with meals.
   b. Antacids decrease absorption; give antacid 1 hour before or after administration.
   c. Usual course of treatment for ulcer disease is 4–6 weeks.
   d. Many drug interactions.
   e. Watch for CNS changes particularly in the elderly as confusion is a major toxic effect.
   f. Use cautiously with clients who have impaired renal or hepatic function.
   g. Monitor CBC and liver function studies.

5. Discharge teaching. Smoking decreases effectiveness of cimetidine.
6. Related drugs. See Table 2-18.
B. Proton pump inhibitors
1. Prototype: omeprazole (Prilosec)
2. Used to decrease gastric acid concentration in peptic ulcer and gastroesophageal reflux disease.
3. Nursing implications
   a. Do not chew, crush, or open capsule.
   b. Can be administered with antacids.
4. Related drugs. Esomeprazole (Nexium), lansoprazole (Prevacid), pantoprazole (Protonix), rabeprazole (Aciphex).
C. Peptic ulcers caused by *Helicobacter pylori* are commonly treated with a combination of two antibiotics, a bismuth compound and a histamine antagonist or proton pump inhibitor.

**Table 2-18** Other H$_2$ Antagonists

| Drug | Nursing Implications |
|---|---|
| Ranitidine (Zantac) | • Avoid administration of antacids at same time.<br>• Hemodialysis may reduce Zantac blood levels. |
| Famotidine (Pepcid) | • May be given with antacid dose.<br>• Dosage modifications not necessary in elderly except with renal impairment. |
| Nizatidine (Axid) | • Can elevate serum salicylate levels in clients taking high doses of aspirin. |

## Sample Questions

116. What is the primary action of cimetidine?
    1. Suppresses the action of acetylcholine at the receptor responsible for histamine release.
    2. Decreases the pH of gastric fluids.
    3. Antagonizes the action of histamine at its $H_2$ receptor site.
    4. Neutralizes gastric secretions.

117. An antacid is ordered in conjunction with the cimetidine. What instruction should the nurse give concerning concurrent use of an antacid with cimetidine?
    1. Take both drugs together.
    2. Take both drugs with milk.
    3. Take both drugs with meals.
    4. Take the drugs 1 hour apart.

118. Which statement made by the client best indicates his understanding of cimetidine therapy?
    1. "I will stop taking cimetidine when my stomach pain is gone."
    2. "I will stop smoking."
    3. "I will take cimetidine on an empty stomach."
    4. "I know that cimetidine will turn my stools black."

119. In elderly clients taking cimetidine, which adverse effect should the nurse be most concerned with?
    1. Confusion.
    2. Diarrhea.
    3. Muscle pain.
    4. Constipation.

## Answers and Rationales

116. **3.** Cimetidine (Tagamet) competes with histamine for occupancy of histamine ($H_2$) receptor sites on the parietal cells in the stomach.

117. **4.** Antacids decrease cimetidine absorption.

118. **2.** Smoking decreases the effectiveness of cimetidine (Tagamet) and is also contraindicated in ulcer disease.

119. **1.** Confusion is a major toxic effect in the elderly.

# GASTROINTESTINAL (GI) ANTICHOLINERGICS

With the advent of $H_2$ antagonists, gastrointestinal anticholinergics are rarely used. $H_2$ antagonists have a more prolonged action and fewer side effects, and are considered more effective in treating gastric ulcers. Gastrointestinal anticholinergics delay gastric emptying time, which prolongs the action of antacids.

# ANTACIDS

A. There are five antacid categories with the same action of neutralizing gastric acid. There are significant differences among each of the five categories; therefore, no individual antacid is considered a prototype. The categories are displayed in Table 2-19: magnesium, compounds of aluminum, sodium, calcium, alkaline, or a combination.
   1. Use. Control ulcer pain; peptic ulcer; esophageal reflux; prophylaxis for Curling's ulcer.
   2. Nursing implications for all antacids
      a. Shake liquid antacids prior to use.
      b. Liquids tend to be more effective than tablets.
      c. Tablets must be chewed completely before swallowing.
      d. Take a sip of water following antacid administration to ensure passage to the stomach.
      e. Large amounts of water will dilute the antacid.
      f. Aluminum and magnesium combinations to reduce the side effects of diarrhea and constipation.
      g. Do not take other oral drugs within 1–2 hours of an antacid.
      h. Can interfere with the intended response of enteric-coated medications.
B. See Table 2-19 for categories and adverse effects.

**Table 2-19** Antacids

| Drug Categories | Adverse Effects | Nursing Implications |
|---|---|---|
| Magnesium-containing antacids Magnesium Hydroxide (Milk of Magnesia) | Diarrhea | • Doses greater than 1.5 mL may have a laxative effect.<br>• Contraindicated in clients with renal failure.<br>• Monitor for symptoms of hypermagnesemia, CNS changes, hypotension, nausea, vomiting. |
| Aluminim-containing antacids Aluminum Hydroxide (Amphogel) | Constipation | • Check serum for hypophosphatemia.<br>• Monitor for fecal impaction and intestinal obstruction in elderly.<br>• Aluminum can accumulate in CNS causing toxic effects; not given over a long period of time. |
| Sodium Carbonate/Bicarbonate Dihydroxyaluminum Sodium Carbonate (Rolaids) | Constipation, sodium retention | • Must chew tablet.<br>• Not for long-term use. |
| Sodium Bicarbonate (Baking Soda) | Systemic alkalosis, bloating, sodium retention | • Contraindicated in congestive heart failure, hypertension, or sodium-restricted diets.<br>• Monitor for milk-alkali syndrome, nausea, vomiting, headache, hypercalcemia, hypercalciuria, hypophosphatemia. |
| Calcium Carbonate (Tums, Maalox) | Acid rebound, milk-alkali syndrome, hypercalcemia, constipation | • Monitor for milk-alkali syndrome.<br>• Not to be taken with milk or foods high in vitamin D. |
| Aluminum Magnesium combinations Magaldrate (Riopan) | Constipation or diarrhea, hypermagnesemia | • Other common antacids in this group are Maalox, DiGel, Gelusil.<br>• Use cautiously in clients with impaired renal function and monitor magnesium levels. |

 ## Sample Questions

120. Which antacid is LEAST LIKELY to cause adverse effects?
    1. Magnesium hydroxide (Milk of Magnesia).
    2. Aluminum hydroxide (Amphogel).
    3. Aluminum/magnesium combination (Maalox).
    4. Calcium carbonate (Tums).

121. What is one of the first effects that the nurse will tell the client to expect from taking Maalox?
    1. Constipation.
    2. Decrease of gastric acid secretions.
    3. Alleviation of burning pain.
    4. Diarrhea.

 ## Answers and Rationales

120. **3.** Antacid combinations containing aluminum and magnesium have reduced adverse effects as aluminum antacids cause constipation and magnesium antacids cause diarrhea.

121. **3.** Antacids such as Maalox neutralize gastric acidity, thus reducing pain. Constipation and diarrhea are adverse effects with antacids and may be decreased when taking a combination antacid acid such as Maalox.

## ANTIDIARRHEAL AGENTS

A. Antidiarrheal agents slow intestinal motility and propulsion. There are two categories of drugs to treat diarrhea.
    1. Absorbents: act by binding drugs, digestive enzymes, toxins, bacteria which may be causing diarrheal condition.

2. Opiates: act by reducing the propulsive movement of small intestine and colon, causing dehydration of intestinal contents.

B. Related drugs. See Table 2-20.

 **Sample Questions**

122. The physician orders Lomotil 5 mg PO QID for diarrhea. What adverse effect of Lomotil must the nurse be alert for?
   1. Urinary retention.
   2. Decreased peristalsis.
   3. Tinnitus.
   4. Diarrhea.

123. A client's daughter mentions to the nurse that her 6-year-old son often takes Pepto-Bismol for an upset stomach. What potential problem should the nurse reinforce that Pepto-Bismol could cause in children?
   1. Interacts with multivitamins.
   2. Will cause anorexia.
   3. Has an antibiotic effect.
   4. Contains salicylate.

 **Answers and Rationales**

122. **1.** Lomotil contains atropine, which is an anticholinergic that can cause urinary retention.

123. **4.** Pepto-Bismol contains small amounts of salicylate. Salicylates are connected with Reye's syndrome and are not recommended in children under the age of 18.

## LAXATIVES

A. Protype: Laxatives either stimulate or change the consistency of stools. Five of the most common categories of laxatives are used to induce 1 or more bowel movements per day.
   1. Use. Promote movement of feces through the bowel to prevent/treat constipation, prevent straining during defecation, or for preparation before diagnostic tests/surgery.
   2. Saline cathartics attract and hold large amounts of fluids thereby increasing the bulk of stools. The nurse needs to encourage fluid intake to prevent dehydration.

**Table 2-20** Antidiarrheals

| Category | Drug | Adverse Effects | Nursing Implications |
|---|---|---|---|
| Adsorbent | Bismuth subsalicylate (Pepto-Bismol) | Salicylate poisoning, impaction, darkening of stool and tongue | • Over-the-counter (OTC) preparation<br>• Use cautiously with aspirin or other aspirin-containing drugs |
| | Kaolin and Pectin (Kaopectate) | Constipation, fecal impaction | • OTC preparation<br>• Regular and concentrated suspensions<br>• Extended use can cause disruption of nutrient absorption in body. |
| Opiate | Loperamide Hydrochloride (Imodium) | Toxic megacolon in clients with ulcerative colitis; drowsiness, dizziness, abdominal discomfort, constipation | • Synthetically related to meperidine (Demerol)<br>• Shouldn't be taken together with other CNS depressants<br>• Treat overdose with slurry of activated charcoal and watch for CNS depression. |
| | Diphenoxylate Hydrochloride with Atropine (Lomotil) | Sedation, flushing, palpitations, blurred vision, dry mouth, urinary retention | • Withhold in severe dehydration or electrolyte imbalance<br>• Addiction possible in high doses and with prolonged use |
| | Opium Tincture (Paregoric) | Respiratory depression, physical and psychological dependence, mental impairment | • Reduced dose for elderly and clients with respiratory problems<br>• Safety precautions<br>• Give with 2–3 swallows of water to ensure passage to stomach |

**Table 2-21** Laxatives

| Category | Drug | Adverse Effects | Nursing Implications |
|---|---|---|---|
| Saline | Magnesium citrate (Citroma) | Hypermagnesia in renal failure, nausea | • Laxation in 2–6 hrs<br>• Available in effervescent form<br>• Most effective on empty stomach and followed with a glass of water |
| | Magnesium hydroxide (Milk of Magnesia) | See magnesium citrate | • Lower doses act as antacid<br>• Shake bottle before taking |
| | Glycerin (Glycerol) | Abdominal cramps, rectal discomfort | • Evacuation occurs in 15–30 minutes after enema/suppository |
| Bulk-forming | Methylcellulose (Citrucel, Cologel) | Fecal impaction, esophageal obstruction, nausea | • Laxation in 12–72 hrs<br>• Take with 1 glass of water to prevent fecal impaction<br>• Must not chew tablet form or take in dry powder form as it may cause esophageal obstruction |
| | Psyllium hydrophilic muciloid (Metamucil) | Same as above | Same as above |
| Lubricant | Mineral oil | Impairs absorption of fat-soluble vitamins and nutrients, lipid pneumonia | • Administer in an upright position<br>• Do not take with meals, first given in evening<br>• Retention enema is usually followed by a cleansing enema<br>• Keep in refrigerator |
| Stool softener | Ducosate sodium (Colace) | Rare: rash, abdominal cramps | • Effective in 12–72 hrs<br>• Take with plenty of fluids<br>• Use caution with clients on sodium-restricted diets |
| Stimulant | Bisacodyl (Dulcolax) | Rare | • Effect in 12 hr PO, and 15 min.–1 hour in rectal form<br>• PO drug given before breakfast or at bedtime<br>• Do not take tablets within 1 hour of antacid or milk administration |
| | Cascara Sagrada | Large doses can cause hypokalemia, glucose intolerance, calcium deficiency, anorexia | • Could discolor urine<br>• Effect in 6–12 hrs<br>• Prolonged use can cause rebound constipation |
| | Castor oil (Emulsoil, Neoloid) | Rebound constipation, abdominal cramps, nausea, vomiting | • Effect in 2–3 hrs<br>• Do not schedule within 2 hours of taking other oral drugs<br>• Shake emulsion well<br>• Give with juice or carbonated beverage to mask castor oil's unpleasant odor and taste |
| | Phenolphthalein (Ex-Lax, Feen-a-Mint, Correctol) | Rash, lupus-like syndrome | • Effect in 6–8 hrs<br>• Urine/feces may have reddish discoloration<br>• Usually given at bedtime<br>• Effect could last 3–4 days<br>• Discontinue if rash occurs |
| | Senna (Senokot) | Abdominal cramps, nausea | • Laxation in 6–10 hrs<br>• Administer at bedtime<br>• Urine/feces may have yellowish-brown or reddish-brown discoloration |

3. Bulk-forming laxatives increase the bulk of the feces by stimulating mechanical peristalsis and are considered the safest of all the laxative groups.
4. Lubricant laxatives coat the feces with an oil film and prevent the colon from reabsorbing water from the feces.
5. Stool softeners prevent straining during defecation and prevent constipation by decreasing surface tension of feces.
6. Stimulant laxatives stimulate peristalsis.
7. Should not be given to clients with symptoms of nausea, vomiting, abdominal pain, symptoms of appendicitis, or intestinal obstruction.
8. Used for a week or less to prevent rebound constipation and dependence.
9. Appropriate fluid intake and a diet high in fiber will help promote proper bowel function.

B. Related drugs. See Table 2-21.

## Sample Questions

124. What group of laxatives would the nurse tell the client is considered the safest and most natural?
    1. Saline-cathartics group.
    2. Lubricant-laxative group.
    3. Stool-softener group.
    4. Bulk-forming laxative group.

125. The nurse should withhold a laxative from the client that has what condition?
    1. Nausea.
    2. Excess body weight.
    3. Increase in appetite.
    4. Painful defecation.

## Answers and Rationales

124. **4.** Bulk-forming laxatives are considered the safest and most natural of all laxative groups because they are natural or semisynthetic substances, they produce stools that are formed normally, and are not absorbed systemically.

125. **1.** A client with nausea should never be given a laxative because this person is at risk for fluid and electrolyte imbalance.

## ANTIEMETICS

A. Protype: Antiemetics are given to prevent and treat nausea, vomiting, and nausea associated with motion sickness, CNS, disorders, administration of certain drugs, and radiation therapy. There are five categories of antiemetics:
    1. Antihistamines and anticholinergics: block acetylcholine and histamine $H_2$ receptors.
    2. Neuroleptics: bind with dopamine2
    3. Prokinetics: stimulate acetylcholine to increase gastric emptying.
    4. Serotonin-blocking agents: block transmission of afferent visceral and chemoreceptor triggers (mostly associated with chemotherapy).
    5. Substance P Neurokinin-1 receptor antagonist: used in conjunction with serotonin antagonists and a corticosteroid. See Table 2-22.

## Sample Questions

126. What nursing diagnosis would be appropriate for a client taking promethazine (Phenergan)?
    1. Disturbed body image.
    2. Diarrhea.
    3. Risk for injury.
    4. Chronic pain.

## Answers and Rationales

126. **3.** Due to the side effect of drowsiness, the client needs to refrain from driving or operating dangerous machinery while taking this medication.

## EMETICS

A. Prototype: ipecac syrup
Not fully known but probably stimulates the CTZ and irritates the GI tract to induce vomiting, thus delaying the absorption time of toxic substances. Emesis should occur within 20–30 minutes.
    1. Use. Stimulate vomiting for clients (in a hospital setting) who have taken toxic doses of oral medications, and poisons.
    2. Adverse effects. Fluid and electrolyte imbalance; stimulated and then suppressed nervous system; hypotension; persistent vomiting; aspiration.
    3. Nursing implications
        a. Should not be given after charcoal administration as it antagonizes the effects.
        b. Administer with water and monitor vital signs.
        c. Repeat dose once if vomiting does not occur.

**Table 2-22** Antiemetics

| Category | Drug | Adverse Effects | Nursing Implications |
|---|---|---|---|
| Antihistamines | Diphenhydramine (Benadry) Antivert | Dry mouth, drowsiness Promethazine HO Phenergan | • If preventing nausea, give 30 minutes prior to noxious stimuli<br>• Not compatible with lactated Ringer's IV solution |
| Anticholinergics | Scopolamine (Transderm-Scop) | Increased heart rate, disorientation | • Monitor VS |
| Neuroleptics | Chlorpromazine HCl (Thorazine) Prochlorperazine (Compazine) | Drowsiness, blurred vision, hypotension, Dizziness | • If IM, use large muscle<br>• Do not give SC |
| Prokinetic | Metoclopramide (Reglan) | Anxiety | • Monitor for dehydration |
| Serotonin blockers | Dolasetron mesylate (Anzement) Ondansetron HCL (Zofran) | Headache, hypotension, GI upset | • Monitor BP<br>• Give 30 min before chemo |
| Substance P neurokinin-1 receptor antagonist | Aprepitant | Asthenia, hiccups | • Give in morning<br>• Use additional contraception |

   **d.** If a client is younger than age 10 only one dose should be given.
   **e.** Should not be given to semiconscious or unconscious clients or clients having seizures.
   **f.** Should not be given if substance ingested is corrosive, petroleum-based, or cyanide.
   **g.** Not to be used in home setting.
**B.** Prototype: apomorphine HCl.
A CNS depressant and a controlled substance that is given subcutaneously. In adults is usually effective in 5–15 minutes. Clients who are allergic to morphine or other opiates should not take apomorphine.

 **Sample Questions**

**127.** What action should the client perform after an accidental poisoning?
   1. Drink milk.
   2. Drink water until vomiting occurs.
   3. Take laxatives.
   4. Call the Poison Control Center.

 **Answers and Rationales**

**127. 4.** The Poison Control Center should be called for instructions.

## SUCRALFATE (CARAFATE)

**A.** Prototype: sucralfate (Carafate)
   **1.** Action. Reacts with gastric acid to form a substance that adheres to the ulcer site to protect the ulcer from bile salts, pepsin, and acid. This permits healing.
   **2.** Use. Treatment of duodenal ulcer: short term (up to 8 weeks).
   **3.** Adverse effects. Diarrhea, constipation; gastric discomfort; dry mouth; pruritus, rash; back pain; dizziness, sleeplessness.
   **4.** Nursing implications
      **a.** Separate administration from other drugs by 2 hours to decrease chance of interaction.
      **b.** Take on an empty stomach.
      **c.** Antacids should not be given within 1/2 hour before or after sucralfate dose.
   **5.** Related drug. Misoprostol (Cytotec).

**a.** Protects stomach lining by increasing mucus and bicarbonate production and inhibiting secretion of gastric acid.

**b.** Used to prevent NSAID and aspirin-induced ulcers in clients at high risk of complications from gastric ulcers.

# Sample Questions

**128.** By what mechanism does sucralfate enable the client's ulcer to heal?

1. Coating the stomach mucosa, thus preventing gastric acid irritation.
2. Forming a paste-like substance at the ulcer site that serves as a protective barrier.
3. Binding with all gastric contents to inactivate their function in the stomach.
4. Attracting white and red blood cells to the stomach to increase circulation.

**129.** Which of the following teaching points about sucralfate should the nurse emphasize to ensure success with the therapy?

1. Discontinue the drug if indigestion occurs.
2. Use the drug on an as-needed basis if future ulcer problems occur.
3. Constipation may occur with long-term use.
4. Take the drug 1 hour before meals or 2 hours after meals and at bedtime.

# Answers and Rationales

**128. 2.** Sucralfate (Carafate) reacts with gastric acid and becomes a paste-like substance that forms a protective barrier at the ulcer site.

**129. 4.** Sucralfate is more active in the lower-pH environment of an empty stomach. By taking the drug 1 hour before meals or 2 hours after meals, the stomach is empty and optimal results will be obtained from the drug.

# Arthritis Drugs

## ARTHRITIS DRUGS

**A.** Prototype: auranofin (Ridaura)
  1. Action. Mechanism of action is unclear. This is the only group of drugs that may partially reverse or stop joint destruction.
  2. Use. These drugs are most effective early in rheumatoid arthritis.
  3. Adverse effects. Most common: skin rash, proteinura, blood dyscrasias, gastric irritation, diarrhea. Nitroid crisis is an anaphylactic reaction that resembles effects of a large dose of nitroglycerin: i.e., flushing, severe hypotension, tachycardia, light-headedness.
  4. Nursing implications
     **a.** Gold salts should not be given to clients with hepatic and renal disorders, hypertension, uncontrolled diabetes, or heart failure, or to clients receiving radiation therapy.
     **b.** Baseline CBC must be checked prior to administration and checked throughout therapy.
     **c.** Nitroid crisis is more apt to occur with IM injection of gold salts; therefore a test dose is given.
     **d.** VS should be monitored and resuscitation equipment should be readily available with test dose.
     **e.** Diarrhea is more severe with oral gold salts.
     **f.** Oral auranofin is less toxic and better tolerated than IM.
     **g.** Overdose of gold salts can be treated with dimercaprol (BAL).
     **h.** Gold salts given IM are best given in the gluteal muscle.
  5. Discharge teaching. Be aware that therapeutic effects may not be seen for several months.
**B.** Other gold salts
  1. Aurothioglucose (Solganol)
  2. Gold sodium thiomalate (Myochrysine)
  3. Both drugs are given IM only. Noncompliance can be a problem with both drugs as weekly injections may be needed for several months.
**C.** Antimalarials
  1. Chloroquine (Aralen)
  2. Hydroxychloroquine (Plaquenil)
  3. These drugs are used to treat malaria and rheumatoid arthritis that is unresponsive to NSAIDs.

4. Nursing implications
   a. The nurse needs to remind clients that frequent ophthalmic examinations are required as visual impairment can occur.
   b. The nurse must be alert for blood dyscrasia, GI distress, and dermatologic reactions.
D. Other drugs
   1. Adalimumab (Humira)
   2. Etanercept (Enbrel)
   3. Leflunomide (Avara)
   4. Infliximab (Remicade)
   5. Penicillamine (Cupriminel)
   6. These are newer antiarthritis agents used to treat rheumatoid arthritis that no longer responds to traditional therapy.

 **Sample Questions**

130. When a client comes to the office for monthly visits, which of the following would be excluded from the nurse's assessment?
   1. Assess client's skin.
   2. Examine client's oral cavity.
   3. Question client about any itching.
   4. Check client's blood sugar levels.

131. The client has been receiving auranofin for 2 months and is showing little clinical response to it; she is experiencing the following adverse effects of the drug: abdominal cramps, vomiting, diarrhea, and stomatitis. The physician decides to continue auranofin. What is the reason for this?
   1. Side effects of auranofin are rare and will pass quickly.
   2. It will take several months of therapy with auranofin to achieve therapeutic effects.
   3. The physician is not sure of the best effects from auranofin because it is such a new form of treatment.
   4. Side effects of auranofin always occur just before the beginning of a therapeutic response to the drug.

 **Answers and Rationales**

130. **4.** Skin rashes, pruritus, and mouth lesions are all adverse effects of gold salts and need to be monitored frequently. Hyperglycemia has not been associated with gold salt therapy.

131. **2.** It can take 6 months or longer for the gold salts to show a therapeutic response. Because of this, clients are left on gold salt therapy even though they are experiencing adverse effects before therapeutic response.

# ANTIGOUT DRUGS

A. Prototype: allopurinal (Zyloprim)
   1. Action. Prevents the production of uric acid by inhibiting the enzyme xanthine oxidose.
   2. Use. Used to manage primary or secondary gout and to prevent attacks; used to treat clients with recurrent calcium oxalate calculi.
   3. Adverse effects. GI symptoms: nausea, vomiting, diarrhea; skin rash, maculopapular; hepatomegaly; drowsiness.
   4. Nursing implications
      a. Discontinue use at first sign of skin rash.
      b. Force fluids (1–2 liters) to help prevent formation of uric acid kidney stones.
      c. Monitor liver function tests and CBC throughout therapy.
      d. Administer drug after meals.
   5. Discharge teaching. Advise client not to drive.
B. Prototype: colchicine (Novocolchine)
   1. Action. Drug of choice to treat acute gout attacks and prophylaxis of recurrent gout. It decreases the inflammatory response to deposition of monosodium urate crystals.
   2. Adverse effects. Nausea, vomiting, diarrhea, abdominal pain; bone marrow depression; hair loss; rash; thrombophlebitis if given IV.
   3. Nursing implications
      a. Do not give IM or SC as this causes severe irritation.
      b. Monitor IV site.
      c. Assess for rash.
      d. Monitor CBC.
      e. Take drug after meals.
      f. Hair loss is reversible when drug is stopped.
      g. During an acute attack is usually given every 1–2 hours until pain is relieved and should be stopped if nausea, vomiting, or diarrhea occurs.
      h. No more than 12 tablets should be given in a 24-hour period.

 **Sample Questions**

132. What instruction should the nurse give in regard to colchicine therapy?

1. The drug will be absorbed better if you take it on an empty stomach.
2. You should limit your fluid intake while you're on this drug.
3. No more than 12 colchicine tablets should be taken in a 24-hour period.
4. If you have another gout attack, you need to wait 12 hours before taking colchicine.

133. What client condition would alert the nurse to discontinue colchicine?
1. The client becomes dizzy.
2. Diarrhea or vomiting occurs.
3. Stools turn black.
4. Serum uric acid level is below normal.

134. In addition to treating gouty arthritis, which drug is also used to treat calcium oxalate stones?
1. Allopurinol (Zyloprim)
2. Colchicine (Novocholchine)
3. Naproxen (Naprosyn)
4. Sulindac (Clinoril)

 **Answers and Rationales**

132. **3.** In order for the client to be treated safely with colchicine (Novocolchine), not more than 12 tablets should be taken in a 24-hour period.

133. **2.** Diarrhea and vomiting are both early signs of colchicine toxicity. Other signs of early toxicity are anorexia, nausea, abdominal discomfort, and weakness. Colchicine should be stopped immediately before more serious toxicity occurs.

134. **1.** Allopurinol (Zyloprim) is used to manage and prevent gout attacks. A new use for this drug is treatment of calcium oxalate stones.

 # Antimicrobials

## GENERAL INFORMATION

A. Terminology
   1. Bacteriostatic: prevents multiplication and growth of bacterial organisms.
   2. Bactericidal: kills bacterial organisms.
B. Cultures need to be obtained before initiating therapy.
C. Sites of action
   1. Agents that suppress bacterial cell wall synthesis: action creates a defect in bacterial cell wall structure and death of organism.
   2. Agents that suppress protein synthesis within the bacterial cell: action interferes with normal growth and reproduction of bacterial cell, which eventually causes its eradication.
   3. Agents that interfere with bacterial cell membrane permeability: action causes intracellular parts to escape and leads to bacterial cell death.
   4. Agents with antimetabolite action: action causes interference with a necessary metabolic process that the bacterial cell needs for normal growth and function.
   5. Agents that inhibit nucleic acid synthesis: action involves the use of enzymes for reproduction that are not found in human cells.
D. Need to be administered at regular intervals so therapeutic blood levels can be maintained. This will prevent development of resistant strains of organisms. An order for QID administration means giving the drug at 6-hour intervals.
E. Peak and trough levels
   1. Blood levels need to be high enough to be therapeutic but not so high that severe toxicity is caused.
   2. Peak: client's blood is drawn 1 hour after IM or 30 minutes after IV administration.
   3. Trough: client's blood is drawn just before next dose of antibiotic is given.
F. Superinfection
   1. Infection occurring when client is receiving or has recently been given antibiotic treatment.
   2. Develops when normal bacterial flora are changed by the use of an antibiotic. Allows growth of bacteria that are resistant to the antibiotic being used.

3. Clients more susceptible when placed on broad-spectrum antibiotics.

G. Resistance
   1. Many bacteria have developed resistance to antibiotic therapy.
   2. Ways to prevent resistance
      a. Use antibiotics only when necessary.
      b. Do not use antibiotics to treat viral infections.
   3. Streptogramins: antibiotics to treat resistant strains of bacteria. Used to treat vancomycin resistant enterococcus (VRE) and methicillin resistant *S. aureus* (MRSA).
      a. Quinupristin/dalfopristin (Synercid)
      b. Linezolid (Zyvox)

## AMINOGLYCOSIDES

A. Prototype: gentamicin (Garamycin)
   1. Action. Acts by suppressing protein synthesis in bacterial cell. Bactericidal.
   2. Use. Serious gram-negative bacterial infections, eye infections.
   3. Adverse effects. Ototoxicity, nephrotoxicity, neuromuscular blockade, hypersensitivity, photosensitivity with topical preparations.
   4. Nursing implications
      a. Cautious use in clients with decreased renal function, reduced hearing, dehydration, neuromuscular disorders.
      b. Monitor hearing and balance.
      c. Monitor renal function tests and I&O.
      d. Client needs adequate hydration.
      e. Safety precautions if there are vestibular nerve effects.
      f. Monitor drug levels.
   5. Discharge teaching
      a. Full course of treatment is essential.
      b. Report problems with balance or hearing changes.
      c. Avoid sunlight.

B. Related drugs. Amikacin (Amikin), kanamycin (Kantrex), neomycin (Neobiotic), streptomycin, tobramycin (Nebcin), netilmicin (Netromycin), paromomycin (Humatin). Kanamycin (Kanrex) and neomycin (Neobiotic) are given orally to prepare the bowel for surgery. Neomycin (Neobiotic) is given to persons in hepatic failure to reduce ammonia levels.

 **Sample Questions**

135. What is the antibacterial action of gentamicin (Garamycin)?
   1. Anti-inflammatory.
   2. Bacteriostatic.
   3. Bactericidal.
   4. Anthelmintic.

136. The nurse will assess the client daily for which of the following adverse effects of gentamicin (Garamycin)?
   1. Constipation.
   2. Hearing loss.
   3. Tetany.
   4. Bradycardia.

137. The nurse needs to monitor the client daily for the presence of superinfection. How is a superinfection defined in relation to an infection?
   1. It has an increasing number of the organism's normal microbial competitors.
   2. It necessitates increased amount of antibiotics for treatment.
   3. It occurs if antibiotic therapy is abruptly stopped.
   4. It develops when an antibiotic alters the normal bacterial flora.

 **Answers and Rationales**

135. 3. Gentamicin (Garamycin) acts by suppressing protein synthesis in the bacterial cell. This effect is bactericidal.

136. 2. Gentamicin (Garamycin) can cause auditory and vestibular damage. The nurse must assess the client daily for hearing loss while on this drug.

137. 4. A superinfection occurs when normal bacterial flora are changed by the use of an antibiotic. This allows growth of bacteria that are resistant to the antibiotic currently being used.

## PENICILLINS

A. Prototype: penicillin G potassium (Pentids)
   1. Action. Inhibits cell wall synthesis of microorganisms. Bactericidal. Natural penicillin.
   2. Use. Systemic infections caused by gram-positive cocci; syphilis; prophylaxis for rheumatic fever and bacterial endocarditis.
   3. Adverse effects. Hypersensitivity reactions; GI upset; anemia, thrombocytopenia, leukopenia; nephritis; potassium poisoning; irritation at injection site.

**4.** Nursing implications

    **a.** Monitor client for allergic reactions. Have emergency equipment available.

    **b.** Clients with questionable serious penicillin allergy may be skin tested.

    **c.** Give oral form on empty stomach.

    **d.** Oral form should be taken with a full glass of water.

    **e.** Monitor CBC, BUN, and creatinine.

    **f.** Probenecid (Benemid) may be given to increase blood levels of penicillins.

    **g.** Monitor IV and IM injection sites.

    **h.** IV solutions are stable at room temperature for 24 hours only.

**5.** Discharge teaching

    **a.** Complete the therapy even if you feel well before the medicine is finished.

    **b.** Oral doses should be taken around the clock.

    **c.** Don't take for other infections.

**B.** Related drugs

  **1.** Penicillinase-resistant penicillins

    **a.** Used to treat infections caused by penicillinase-producing organisms.

    **b.** Examples: nafcillin sodium (Nafcil, Unipen), cloxacillin (Tegapen), dicloxacillin (Oxapen)

  **2.** Aminopenicillins

    **a.** Increased effectiveness against gram-negative organisms.

    **b.** Examples: ampicillin (Amcill, Polycillin), amoxicillin trihydrate (Amoxil), bacampicillin (Spectrobid)

  **3.** Extended-spectrum penicillins

    **a.** Structurally similar to ampicillin but have an increased spectrum of activity against gram-negative bacteria.

    **b.** Examples: carbenicillin sodium (Geocillin), piperacillin sodium (Pipracil), ticarcillin (Ticar), mezlocillin (Mezlin)

  **4.** Penicillin/beta-lactamase inhibitor combinations

    **a.** Combination of penicillin with beta-lactamase inhibitor which prevents destruction of penicillin by enzymes and extends the penicillin's spectrum of antimicrobial activity.

    **b.** Examples: Amoxicillin/potassium clavulanate (Augmentin), piperacillin/tazobactam (Zosyn), ampicillin/sublactam (Unasyn), ticarcillin/clavulanate (Timentin)

 **Sample Questions**

**138.** Before giving a prescription for penicillin V potassium, the nurse reviews basic information about penicillins. Which of the following statements is true?

  **1.** Penicillins are well absorbed from the gastrointestinal tract after oral ingestion.

  **2.** Penicillins have a long half-life due to their extended excretion time.

  **3.** Extended-spectrum penicillins have an increased ability to penetrate outer membranes of gram-negative bacteria.

  **4.** Penicillins easily enter bacterial cell membranes due to their lipid solubility.

**139.** Penicillin is ordered for a client. The physician also orders probenecid therapy. What will the nurse tell the client that the action of probenecid will do?

  **1.** Prevent a hypersensitivity reaction to the penicillin.

  **2.** Enhance metabolism of the penicillin.

  **3.** Stimulate the immune system.

  **4.** Increase blood levels of the penicillin.

 **Answers and Rationales**

**138. 3.** Extended-spectrum penicillins enter the membranes of gram-negative organisms more readily than other penicillin groups.

**139. 4.** Probenecid (Benemid) is given with penicillin to enhance therapeutic blood levels of the penicillin.

## CEPHALOSPORINS

**A.** Prototype for first-generation cephalosporins: cefazolin sodium (Ancef). *Note: The cephalosporins are divided into four groups or "generations" based on their spectrums of activity.*

  **1.** Action. Inhibits bacterial cell wall synthesis. Bactericidal.

  **2.** Use. Infections caused by gram-positive cocci; septicemia; bone, joint, and skin infections; prophylactic use in surgery; serious intra-abdominal infection.

  **3.** Adverse effects. Phlebitis at IV site; diarrhea, pseudomembranous colitis; hypersensitivity reactions; fungal overgrowth; discomfort at IM injection site; nephrotoxicity; hepatotoxicity; bone marrow depression.

  **4.** Nursing implications

    **a.** Give IM injections deeply into large muscle masses; rotate sites.

    **b.** Assess for history of penicillin allergy as there is a cross allergy between cephalosporins and penicillin.

c. Dose will be reduced with renal impairment and decreased liver function.
d. Increased risk of renal toxicity if given with other nephrotoxic drugs.
e. Monitor renal, liver function studies, and I&O.
f. Prolonged IV administration can cause thrombophlebitis. Assess and rotate IV sites.
g. Probenecid therapy will increase blood levels of cephalosporin.

5. Discharge teaching
   a. Finish full course of therapy even if you feel well.
   b. Promptly report diarrhea, rash, hives, difficulty breathing, unusual bleeding.
   c. Report signs of superinfection.
6. Related drugs. Cephalexin (Keflex), cephalothin sodium (Keflin), cephapirin sodium (Cefadyl), cepharadine (Velosef).

B. Prototype for second-generation cephalosporins: cefoxitin sodium (Mefoxin)
   1. Action. See action for cefazolin sodium (Ancef).
   2. Use. Infections caused by gram-negative and gram-positive bacteria; septicemia; pelvic, skin, and soft-tissue infections; prophylaxis in abdominal or pelvic surgery; gonorrhea.
   3. Adverse effects. See adverse effects for cefazolin sodium (Ancef).
   4. Nursing implications. Lidocaine used as diluent for IM injection and helps reduce pain of IM injection. See Nursing Implications and Discharge Teaching for cefazolin sodium (Ancef).
   5. Related drugs. Cefaclor (Ceclor), cefamandole naftate (Mandol), cefuroxime sodium (Ceftin), cefmetazole (Zefazone), cefonicid (Monocid), cefotetan (Cefotan), cefprozil (Cefzil), loracarbef (Lorabid).

C. Prototype for third-generation cephalosporins: cefotaxime (Claforan)
   1. Action. See action for cefazolin sodium (Ancef).
   2. Use. Serious infections caused by gram-negative and gram-positive bacteria; meningitis, especially in neonates; uncomplicated gonorrhea.
   3. Adverse effects. See adverse effects for cefazolin sodium (Ancef).
   4. Nursing implications
      a. Do not mix with aminoglycoside solutions. Give these drugs separately.
      b. Protect IV solutions from light. See Nursing Implications and Discharge Teaching for cefazolin sodium (Ancef).
   5. Related drugs. Ceftazidime (Fortaz), ceftizoxime sodium (Cefizox), ceftriaxone sodium (Rocephin), cefdinir (Omnicef), cefixime (Suprax), cefoperazone (Cefobid), cefotaxime (Claforan), cefpodoxime (Vantin), ceftibuten (Cedax).

D. Prototype for fourth-generation cephalosporins: cefepine (Maxipine).
   1. Action. See action for cefazolin sodium (Ancef).
   2. Use. Urinary tract infections caused by *E. coli* or *Klebsiella*; skin infections caused by *S. aureus*; pneumonia caused by *S. pneumoniae*, *Pseudomonas aeruginosa* or *Enterobacter*.
   3. Adverse effects. See adverse effects for cefazolin sodium (Ancef).
   4. Nursing implications. Have Vitamin K available if hypoprothrombinemia develops. See Nursing Implications and Discharge Teaching for cefazolin sodium (Ancef).
   5. Related drug. Cefditoren (Spectracef).

## Sample Questions

140. What action do penicillins and cephalosporins have on bacteria?
   1. Inhibiting bacterial cell wall synthesis.
   2. Preventing bacterial protein synthesis.
   3. Increasing permeability of bacterial membranes.
   4. Inhibiting metabolic processes in the bacterial cell.

141. Which medication will increase the chance of developing nephrotoxicity if the client is taking cefazolin sodium also?
   1. An antacid.
   2. Vitamin D.
   3. Dimenhydrinate (Dramamine).
   4. An aminoglycoside.

142. Which statement by the client indicates a need for more teaching about cephalosporins by the nurse?
   1. "I will take every bit of this medication even if I feel better."
   2. "I will tell the doctor if I have diarrhea, a rash, or any difficulty breathing."
   3. "I will continue to test my urine for glucose with Clinitest tablets."
   4. "I will tell the dentist that I'm taking a cephalosporin when I go for my appointment."

143. Which lab result is indicative of an adverse effect of cephalosporins?
  1. Increased potassium.
  2. Decreased AST (SGOT) and ALT (SGPT).
  3. Elevated hemoglobin.
  4. Increased BUN and creatinine.

 **Answers and Rationales**

140. **1.** Penicillins and cephalosporins have the same action on bacteria: inhibition of bacterial cell wall synthesis.

141. **4.** There is an increased risk of renal toxicity when cephalosporins are given with other nephrotoxic drugs such as diuretics and aminoglycosides.

142. **3.** A diabetic client who is taking a cephalosporin drug will get a false-positive glucose reaction if Clinitest tablets are used in urine testing. The client needs to use Clinistix or Tes Tape for urine testing.

143. **4.** Cephalosporins can cause renal toxicity for which an elevated BUN and creatinine would be indicative.

# MACROLIDES

A. Prototype: erythromycin base (E-Mycin)
  1. Action. Inhibits protein synthesis in bacterial cell. Bacteriostatic. Has broad spectrum of activity.
  2. Use. Persons allergic to penicillin; Legionnaire's disease; mycoplasma pneumonia; intestinal dysenteric amebiasis; acne; staphylococcal and streptococcal infections.
  3. Adverse effects. Gastrointestinal irritation, reversible hearing loss, hepatitis, allergic reactions, superinfections.
  4. Nursing implications
     a. Do not crush enteric-coated tablet.
     b. Take on empty stomach with a full glass of water.
     c. Do not give with acids.
     d. Monitor liver function tests.
     e. GI symptoms are dose related.
     f. Give IM deeply into a large muscle mass.
     g. IV must be diluted sufficiently and administered slowly to avoid venous irritation and thrombophlebitis.
B. Related drugs. Erythromycin estolate (Ilosone), erythromycin gluceptate (Ilotycin), erythromycin stearate, azithromycin (Zithromax), clarithromycin (Biaxin), dirithromycin (Dynabac).

 **Sample Questions**

144. The client is allergic to penicillin. What explanation will the nurse tell the client that he can be given erythromycin?
  1. Erythromycin is more easily absorbed from the GI tract than penicillin.
  2. Erythromycin has a spectrum of activity that is similar to penicillin.
  3. Erythromycin has fewer adverse effects than penicillin.
  4. Erythromycin is not as toxic to the body as penicillin.

145. Which statement by the client indicates a need for more teaching about erythromycin?
  1. "If I notice any change in my hearing I will call the doctor."
  2. "I will take the erythromycin with orange juice."
  3. "I won't take the erythromycin with meals."
  4. "I won't crush the erythromycin tablets, I'll swallow them whole."

 **Answers and Rationales**

144. **2.** Erythromycin and penicillin have a similar spectrum of activity; so individuals who are allergic to penicillin can take erythromycin.

145. **2.** Acidity decreases the activity of erythromycin; it should not be taken with acids such as fruit juices.

# TETRACYCLINES

A. Prototype: tetracycline hydrochloride (Achromycin V)
  1. Action. Broad-spectrum drug with bacteriostatic action and, at higher doses, bactericidal action. Inhibits bacterial wall synthesis. Reduces free fatty acids from triglycerides, thus reducing acne lesions.
  2. Use. Chlamydia, mycoplasma, rickettsia, acne vulgaris, gonorrhea, spirochetes.

**3.** Adverse effects. Headache, dizziness; neutropenia; nausea, vomiting, diarrhea, colitis, abdominal cramping; hepatotoxicity; photosensitivity, hypersensitivity; superinfections; chelating to teeth and new bone.
   **4.** Nursing implications
      **a.** Avoid use during pregnancy, in nursing women, and in children under age 8 as drug binds to calcium in teeth and new bone growth, which results in tooth discoloration of permanent teeth and retarded bone growth.
      **b.** Give deep IM.
      **c.** Monitor CBC and signs of liver toxicity.
   **5.** Discharge teaching
      **a.** Avoid use with calcium supplements, antacids, iron, or dairy products as these may reduce tetracycline absorption.
      **b.** Avoid the sun while taking drug and for a few days after therapy is terminated.
      **c.** Use meticulous hygiene to reduce superinfections.
      **d.** Complete prescribed course.
**B.** Related drugs
   **1.** Doxycycline (Vibramycin): can be administered with food. Safe to use in clients with renal impairment.
   **2.** Minocycline (Minocin): can be taken with food. Dizziness and fatigue may occur.
   **3.** Demeclocycline (Declomycin): administer on an empty stomach. Foods high in calcium and iron interfere with absorption.
   **4.** Oxytetracycline (Terramycin): administer on an empty stomach. Food disrupts extent and rate of absorption.

 **Sample Questions**

146. Which of the following should the nurse include in teaching about taking tetracyclines?
   1. Take tetracycline HCl with milk.
   2. Take tetracycline with food.
   3. Encourage sitting in sun to enhance tetracycline's effects.
   4. Take tetracycline before meals.

147. Which of the following adverse effects should the client report to the physician while taking tetracycline?
   1. Constipation.
   2. Hypertension.
   3. Tachycardia.
   4. Diarrhea.

 **Answers and Rationales**

146. **4.** Tetracycline is best absorbed on an empty stomach. Taking tetracycline with food or milk impairs absorption.

147. **4.** Diarrhea should be reported to the physician, who can rule out diarrhea as a symptom of superinfection or an adverse effect.

## CHLORAMPHENICOL

**A.** Prototype: chloramphenicol (Chloromycetin)
   **1.** Action. A synthetic broad-spectrum agent. Primarily bacteriostatic but is bactericidal in higher doses. Inhibits protein synthesis.
   **2.** Use. *Haemophilus influenzae* meningitis, rickettsia, salmonella typhi, mycoplasma, bacteroides, typhoid fever. *Note: chloramphenicol (Chloromycetin) used only in severe infections when other antibiotics cannot be used due to its severe adverse effect of aplastic anemia.*
   **3.** Adverse effects. Aplastic anemia; neurotoxicity; gray-baby syndrome (seen in premature infants, newborns, and children less than 2 years old. Abdominal distention, vomiting, pallor, irregular respirations, circulatory collapse, and death can occur due to the infant's immature liver function); hypersensitivity; nausea, vomiting, enterocolitis; superinfections; bitter taste especially after IV injection.
   **4.** Nursing implications
      **a.** Obtain and monitor baseline CBC, platelets, and serum iron.
      **b.** Monitor children less than 2 years old for gray-baby syndrome.
      **c.** Do not give by IM injection.
   **5.** Discharge teaching
      **a.** Inform physician immediately of fever, fatigue, sore throat, or bruising.
      **b.** Take drug on an empty stomach unless GI upset.
      **c.** Notify physician and discontinue drug if symptoms of hypersensitivity occur.

 **Sample Questions**

148. Which of the following changes in an infant should the nurse immediately report to the physician?
   1. Vomiting.
   2. Constipation.
   3. Flushing.
   4. Dry skin.

148. **1.** Abdominal distention and vomiting are early symptoms of gray-baby syndrome and should be reported immediately as this syndrome is life-threatening.

# SULFONAMIDES

A. Prototype: sulfisoxazole (Gantrisin)
   1. **Action.** Prevents conversion of para-aminobenzoic acid (PABA) to folic acid, which is required for bacterial growth. Effects are usually bacteriostatic but can be bactericidal in high urinary concentrations.
   2. **Use.** Urinary tract infections, otitis media, nocardiosis (occurs in the lungs and spreads to skin, brain, and other areas), systemic infections, vaginitis, superficial eye infections.
   3. **Adverse effects.** Hypersensitivity; Stevens-Johnson syndrome (acute onset of fever, bullae on skin and ulcers on mucous membranes of lips, eyes, mouth, nasal passages, and genitalia. Pneumonia, joint pain, and prostration are also seen); fever 7–10 days after starting therapy may indicate sensitization or hemolytic anemia; renal dysfunction; hematologic reaction; GI reaction; photosensitivity.
   4. **Nursing implications**
      a. Give oral form on empty stomach with full glass of water.
      b. Observe skin for presence of rash, ulcers.
      c. Monitor temperature.
      d. Monitor I&O; force fluids; check urine pH; cautious use in clients with renal dysfunction; monitor renal function tests.
      e. Monitor CBC.
   5. **Discharge teaching**
      a. Avoid direct sunlight.
      b. Complete full course of treatment.
      c. Diabetics who take oral hypoglycemic agents need to be aware of increased chance of hypoglycemic reactions with use of sulfonamides.
      d. Oral contraceptives may be unreliable while client is receiving sulfonamides. Alternate method of contraception should be used.
B. Related drugs
   1. Sulfasalazine (Azulfidine) used in treatment of ulcerative colitis. Contains aspirin, so is contraindicated in clients allergic to salicylates.
   2. Sulfamethorazole (Gantanol) can be given in combination with trimethoprin (Proloprim) as Septra or Bactrim. Used in treating urinary tract infections, bronchitis, and pneumocystis pneumonia.

### Sample Questions

149. Eight days after taking sulfisoxazole, a child develops a fever. When the child's mother calls the pediatrician's office about this, what instructions will the nurse provide?
   1. Reduce the dose of the sulfisoxazole.
   2. Have the child rest in bed.
   3. Call the pediatrician if more symptoms develop.
   4. Stop the sulfisoxazole and bring the child in to see the pediatrician today.

### Answers and Rationales

149. **4.** A fever 7–10 days after starting sulfisoxazole is an adverse effect of the drug that could indicate a sensitization to the drug or hemolytic anemia. The drug should be stopped and the client should see the physician as soon as possible.

# URINARY ANTI-INFECTIVES

A. The medications are dependent on the desired goal, whether the client has an acute, recurrent or chronic UTI.
   1. Urinary anti-infectives are structurally different so there will be no prototype drug
   2. See Table 2-23.

### Sample Questions

150. The client should be taught which of the following points about nitrofurantoin?
   1. Take it on an empty stomach.
   2. You may experience nausea and vomiting.
   3. You can crush the tablet if it's too hard to swallow whole.
   4. It doesn't interact with any other drugs.

**Table 2-23** Urinary Anti-Infectives

| Drug | Use | Adverse Effects | Nursing Implications |
|---|---|---|---|
| Methenamine (Hiprex; Mandelamine) | Converted to formaldehyde (which is bactericidal) in the presence of acidic urine. | Nausea, vomiting, diarrhea, abdominal discomfort. | • Give with food or milk to prevent GI upset.<br>• Avoid foods, fluids, and medications that alkalinize urine.<br>• Monitor I&O.<br>• Increase fluid intake.<br>• Monitor liver function tests. |
| Nalidixic Acid (Neg Gram) | Bactericidal effect on gram-negative bacteria by preventing transmission of genetic information. | Headache, dizziness, vertigo, visual disturbances, photosensitivity. | • Minor CNS reactions are common and should decrease in 48 hours.<br>• Client should wear sunglasses if bothered by bright lights.<br>• Client should avoid sun exposure, wear sunscreen and appropriate clothing.<br>• Give with food to decrease GI upset. |
| Nitrofurantoin (Macrodantin) | Interferes with carbohydrate metabolism of bacteria. Is bacteriostatic in low concentrations and bactericidal in high concentrations. | Pulmonary hypersensitivity, nausea, vomiting, lower extremity paresthesias. | • Monitor pulmonary status.<br>• Give drug with milk or meals.<br>• Monitor neurologic status.<br>• Avoid tooth staining by not crushing tablets, dilute suspension, and rinse mouth after taking drug. |
| Phenazopyridine (Pyridium) | An azo dye excreted in the urine which provides a topical analgesic effect to the urinary tract. | Rash, headache, GI disturbances, reddish–orange discoloration of urine. | • Give after meals to prevent GI upset.<br>• Tell client that urine may turn reddish–orange and can stain fabrics.<br>• Stop drug if skin or sclera turn yellow which is a sign of drug accumulation. |
| Cinoxacin (Cinobac) | Prevents protein synthesis and DNA replication in bacterial cell. | Dizziness, headache, nausea, tinnitus. | • No breastfeeding while taking this drug.<br>• Use carefully in clients with liver, kidney, and CNS disorders.<br>• Give at evenly spaced time periods during each 24 hours of drug administration. |

 **Answers and Rationales**

150. 2. GI irritation is the most frequent adverse effect of nitrofurantoin (Macrodantin).

# VANCOMYCIN HYDROCHLORIDE (VANCOCIN)

A. Prototype: vancomycin hydrochloride (Vancocin)
   1. Action. Interferes with cell membrane synthesis and exhibits a bactericidal and bacteriostatic effect.

2. Use. Staphylococcus infections, pseudomembranous colitis, gram-positive organisms. Penicillin-G and methicillin-resistant bacteria.
3. Adverse effects. Ototoxicity, nephrotoxicity, hypersensitivity, thrombophlebitis, red-neck syndrome (flushing and hypotension from rapid IV infusion), superinfections.
4. Nursing implications
   a. Monitor I&O.
   b. Obtain and monitor renal and auditory function tests.
   c. Administer IV slowly to prevent phlebitis, extravasation, red-neck syndrome.

151. Which of the following is an important nursing consideration when administering IV vancomycin hydrochloride (Vancocin)?
    1. Mix the dose in 50 mL of dextrose in water.
    2. Infuse over 30 minutes.
    3. Infuse over 60 minutes.
    4. Administer IV push.

## Answers and Rationales

151. 3. IV vancomycin hydrochloride (Vancocin) should be given over 1 hour to help prevent thrombophlebitis and red-neck syndrome.

# FLUOROQUINOLONES

A. Prototype: ciprofloxacin (Cipro)
   1. Action. Inhibits DNA-gyrase (an enzyme needed for replication of bacterial DNA). Bactericidal effect.
   2. Use. Pseudomonas infections, gram-negative urinary tract infections or gram-negative systemic infections.
   3. Adverse effects. Nausea, vomiting, diarrhea, flatulence; headache, tremors, confusion, dizziness, insomnia; fever; rash; elevated BUN, AST (SGOT), ALT (SGPT), creatinine; decreased WBC, hematocrit.
   4. Nursing implications
      a. Administer with a large glass of water to prevent crystalluria.
      b. Do not give with antacids.
      c. Give 2 hours after meals.
B. Related drugs. Norfloxacin (Noroxin), gatifloxacin (Tequin), levofloxacin (Levaquin), lomefloxacin (Maxaquin), moxifloxacin (Avelox), sparfloxacin (Zagam), trovafloxacin (Trevan).

## Sample Questions

152. Which statement by the client indicates that she understands correct use of ciprofloxacin (Cipro)?
    1. "I will take this drug with Maalox to prevent GI upset."
    2. "I will stop taking this drug when I no longer have pain upon urination."
    3. "I will drink an 8-oz glass of water with this drug."
    4. "I will take this drug with a cup of tea or coffee, as caffeinated beverages make this drug work more quickly."

## Answers and Rationales

152. 3. Taking an 8-oz glass of water will help to prevent crystalluria.

# ANTITUBERCULAR DRUGS

A. Prototype: isoniazid (INH)
   1. Action. Bacteriostatic and in high concentrations becomes bactericidal. Mechanism of action not known but is believed to interfere with lipid and nucleic acid biosynthesis in tubercle bacilli that are actively growing.
   2. Use. Initial treatment of tuberculosis; prophylactic treatment of tuberculosis in high-risk groups.
   3. Adverse effects. Peripheral neuritis; jaundice, elevation in liver function tests; nausea, vomiting; blood dyscrasias.
   4. Nursing implications
      a. Assess neuromuscular function and give pyridoxine (vitamin B$_6$) to treat and/or prevent problems.
      b. Regularly scheduled baseline liver function studies.
      c. Monitor for hepatic dysfunction.
      d. Take drug on empty stomach in a single daily dose.
      e. Give drug with meals and divide daily dose into 3 equal parts if GI upset occurs.
      f. Assess for bruising, bleeding, fever, sore throat.
      g. Monitor CBC.
   5. Discharge teaching
      a. Tyramine-containing foods may cause hypertensive crises, so should be avoided.
      b. Avoid histamine-containing foods as may cause an exaggerated drug response.
      c. Avoid use of alcohol.
      d. May cause a feeling of euphoria. Plan rest periods and don't overdo.
      e. Drug therapy must not be interrupted and must be continued for prescribed time.
B. Related drugs. See Table 2-24.

**Table 2-24** Drugs Commonly Used to Treat Tuberculosis

| Drug and Dosage | Adverse Effects | Nursing Implications |
|---|---|---|
| Isoniazid (INH) 10 to 20 mg/kg (up to 300 mg) PO or IM daily, or 15 mg/kg PO or IM twice a week | Peripheral neuritis, a numbness and tingling in hands and feet. Vitamin B6 (pyridoxine) may be given to prevent or treat this condition. Hepatitis, with the risk increasing with age. Liver enzymes may be routinely monitored in elderly or symptomatic clients. Hyperexcitability may occur with single 300 mg dose. | • Tell client to report signs of neuritis and hepatitis (anorexia, nausea, vomiting, jaundice, malaise, or dark urine). • Isoniazid may interfere with phenytoin (Dilantin) metabolism, requiring a lower dose of the TB medication; should be taken on an empty stomach, and the client should not drink alcohol while on therapy. |
| Ethambutol (Myambutol) 15 to 25 mg/kg PO daily, or 50 mg/kg PO twice weekly | Optic neuritis, a loss of red-green color discrimination, and decreased visual acuity can occur with dosages of 25 mg/kg. Reversible, if medication discontinued. Skin rash. | • Tell client to notify physician if vision blurs or if unable to see red or green. • Use the drug with caution if a visual exam cannot be done and in clients with renal impairment. |
| Rifampin (Rifadin, Rimactane) 10 to 20 mg/kg (up to 600 mg) PO daily, or 600 mg PO twice a week | Body fluids (urine, tears, saliva, etc.) may turn orange. Hepatitis Flu-like syndrome Purpura (rare) | • Tell clients to expect orange-tinged body fluids. • Tell clients to report anorexia, nausea, vomiting, jaundice, malaise, or dark urine. • Use the drug with caution in cases of liver disease. • Rifampin affects the actions of other drugs, including anticoagulants, oral hypoglycemics, corticosteroids, oral contraceptives, and methadone. |
| Streptomycin 15 to 20 mg/kg (up to 1 g) IM daily or 25 to 30 m/kg IM twice a week | Damage to cranial nerve VIII (vestibulocochlear). Damage to the vestibular portion causes dizziness, vertigo, tinnitus, and roaring in ears. Auditory damage causes loss of hearing at high frequency ranges. Renal toxicity. | • Baseline renal and audiology studies may be obtained before therapy begins. • Tell client to report any ringing, roaring, or fullness in ears. • Help coordinate outpatient arrangements for IM injections, if necessary. |
| Pyrazinamide 20 to 40 mg/kg (up to 2 g) PO daily | Excess uric acid levels, which can cause gout or hepatitis. | • Baseline uric acid and liver enzyme levels may be obtained; monitor uric acid and liver enzymes. • Instruct patient to report any signs of gout (painful swelling in joints, chills, fever) and hepatitis (anorexia, nausea, vomiting, jaundice, malaise, and dark urine). • Use with caution in clients who have liver disease, gout, or renal impairment. |

Other drugs used: capreomycin (Capastat), kanamycin (Kantrex), ethionamide (Trecator-SC), para-amino-salicylic acid, and cycloserine (Seromycin).

 **Sample Questions**

153. The nurse needs to tell the client which fact about rifampin?
    1. Rifampin increases the effectiveness of oral contraceptives.
    2. Rifampin may cause soft-contact lenses to be permanently discolored.
    3. Rifampin will increase the activity of coumarin-type oral anticoagulants.

4. Rifampin is taken in the usual adult dose of 60 mg daily.

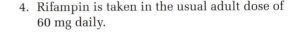 **Answers and Rationales**

153. **2.** Rifampin (Rimactane) discolors body secretions such as sweat, urine, feces, and tears a red-orange color.

# Antiviral Agents

## ACYCLOVIR (ZOVIRAX)

A. Prototype: acyclovir (Zovirax)
  1. Action. Inhibits viral DNA replication. Does not cure herpes infections but decreases the severity and duration of herpes.
  2. Use. Herpes simplex virus 1 and 2, initial treatment of genital herpes infection.
  3. Adverse effects. Nausea, vomiting, diarrhea; rash; headache, vertigo; crystalluria; phlebitis at injection site; transient burning with topical use.
  4. Nursing implications
      a. Do not give IV bolus. Give IV over 1 hour to prevent crystalluria and phlebitis.
      b. Clients should drink plenty of fluids.
  5. Discharge teaching
      a. Use topical preparation sparingly, and use rubber gloves when applying.
      b. Avoid sexual contact while lesions are visible.
      c. Drug does not cure herpes nor prevent transmission to others.
B. Related drugs
  1. Ribavirin (Virazole): Given by inhalation to treat respiratory syncytial virus (RSV) in hospitalized infants and small children. Inhalation of aerosol can be teratogenic.
  2. Zidovudine (AZT, Retrovir): Developed to control AIDS or ARC (AIDS-related complex) with *Pneumocystis carinii*. Causes leukocytopenia; monitor blood work.

  3. Rimantadine (Flumadine). Used in treatment and prevention of influenza A.
  4. Nevirapine (Viramune). Used with other antiviral agents to treat HIV in children and adults.
  5. Indinavir (Crixivan). Used to treat adults with HIV.
  6. Valacyclovir (Valtrex).

 ## Sample Questions

154. Which statement concerning the use of acyclovir is correct?
  1. Sexual relations can be resumed while using topical acyclovir.
  2. Acyclovir can be used for repeated genital herpes infections.
  3. Acyclovir should be given IV over 1 hour.
  4. Acyclovir prevents the recurrence of genital herpes.

## Answers and Rationales

154. **3.** IV acyclovir (Zovirax) should be given over 1 hour to prevent phlebitis and crystalluria.

 # Antifungal Agents

## ANTIFUNGALS

A. Prototype: amphotericin B (Fungizone)
  1. Action. Fungicidal or fungistatic. Alters the fungal cell membrane permeability by binding to sterols. Clients must be monitored due to many toxic effects.
  2. Use. Candida infections, histoplasmosis, coccidiomycoses, blastomycosis, cryptococcoses.
  3. Adverse effects. Febrile reactions, nausea, vomiting; nephrotoxicity, hypokalemia, azotemia; thrombophlebitis; hypotension, tachycardia, or cardiovascular collapse with rapid infusion; blood dyscrasia; hypersensitivity.
  4. Nursing implications
      a. Monitor CBC, BUN, creatinine, electrolytes.
      b. Administer analgesics, antihistamines, prior to infusion to minimize febrile reactions.
      c. Infuse drug slowly.
      d. Monitor VS frequently.

e. Monitor I&O.
f. Administer potassium supplements.
g. Do not mix with other drugs.
B. Related drugs
1. Nystatin (Mycostatin): Used to treat candida infections.
2. Griseofulvin (Grisactin): Used to treat ringworm infections. Adverse effects: headaches, blood dyscrasias, GI upset, rash from sunlight. Give on full stomach. Clients allergic to penicillin should use this drug with caution.
3. Fluconazole (Diflucan): Used to treat candida infections and cryptococcal meningitis.
4. Ketoconazole (Nizoral): Used to treat systemic fungal infections.
5. Terbinafine (Lamisil): Used to treat onychomycosis.

## Sample Questions

155. Which electrolyte imbalance should the nurse monitor for while a client is on amphotericin B therapy?
1. Hyponatremia.
2. Hypokalemia.
3. Hyperkalemia.
4. Hypercalcemia.

## Answers and Rationales

155. **2.** Hypokalemia can occur due to nephrotoxocity of this drug.

# Anthelmintic Agents

## ANTHELMINTICS

A. The anthelmintics are a group of drugs that affect various systems within the worms, causing them to die. Most of these drugs are poorly absorbed in the gastrointestinal tract. Approximately 98% of the drug remains effective as it passes through the GI tract and is excreted in the feces.

B. See Table 2-25.

**Table 2-25** Anthelmintics

| Drug | Action | Use | Adverse Effects | Nursing Implications |
|---|---|---|---|---|
| Pyrantel (Antiminth) | Paralyzes intestinal tract of worm. | Roundworm, pinworm, hookworm | Nausea, vomiting, anorexia, abdominal cramps, diarrhea. | • Give with milk or fruit juice.<br>• Entire dose must be taken at once.<br>• Offer frequent, small meals. |
| Mebendazole (Vermox) | Inhibits glucose and other nutrient uptake of helminth. | Pinworm, roundworm, threadworm, hookworm | Abdominal cramping, occasional fever. | • Can be taken with or without food.<br>• Tablet can be chewed or crushed.<br>• Examine stool for presence of worms. |
| Thiabendazole (Mintezol) | Interferes with parasitic metabolism. | Threadworm, pinworm | Dizziness, drowsiness, headache, anorexia, nausea, malodor of urine. | • Give with food.<br>• Chew tablets before swallowing.<br>• Avoid activities such as driving and working with machinery. |
| Praziquantel (Biltricide) | Enhances perme-ability of the cell membranes of the parasite to calcium. | Shistosomes and flukes | Headache, dizziness, abdominal pain, increased liver enzymes. | • Give with food or liquids.<br>• Do not chew.<br>• Do not breastfeed. |

**156.** How is mebendazole (Vermox) quite effective against pinworms?
1. It is active in the stomach where the pinworm eggs hatch.
2. It is poorly absorbed in the GI tract and kills the pinworms that infect the intestines.
3. Its systemic activity kills pinworms all over the body.
4. It stimulates peristalsis causing the pinworms to be expelled before they reproduce.

**156. 2.** Pinworms infect the intestines. Mebendazole (Vermox) is poorly absorbed in the GI tract and therefore is quite effective against these helminths.

 # Antineoplastic Agents

## ANTINEOPLASTIC AGENTS

A. General considerations
1. Combination of antineoplastic agents usually used to destroy cancer cells.
2. Clients must be closely monitored due to many toxic adverse effects.
3. Agents destroy cancer cells and may also kill normal cells.
B. General adverse effects. Nausea, vomiting, anorexia; diarrhea and constipation; stomatitis; alopecia; bone marrow depression (leukopenia, anemia, and thrombocytopenia); hepatic toxicity; hyperuricemia; fatigue.
C. Nursing implications
1. Handle antineoplastic agents carefully; mutagenic and possibly carcinogenic.
2. Nurses should wear gloves, long-sleeved cover gown, protective goggles, and mask as appropriate.
3. Monitor IV site closely to assess for extravasation and stop IV if it occurs.
4. Treat used equipment as hazardous waste.
5. Administer antiemetic if ordered prior to chemotherapy and up to 48 hours afterwards.
6. Monitor CBC.
7. Monitor I&O.
8. Monitor liver and renal function studies.
9. Inspect oral cavity daily.
D. Discharge teaching
1. Eat frequent, small portions of high-calorie, high-protein, bland, low-residue foods.
2. Avoid highly seasoned foods, drink clear liquids if nauseated.
3. Frequent rest periods.
4. Expect alopecia and purchase scarves or wigs.
5. Report fever, use good hand-washing technique, avoid individuals with upper respiratory infections.
6. Use soft toothbrush and baking soda rinse to minimize stomatitis.
7. Use progressive relaxation exercises or guided imagery to help cope with nausea.

## ALKYLATING AGENTS

A. Prototype: cyclophosphamide (Cytoxan)
1. Action. Produces cytoxic effects by damaging DNA and interfering with cell replication. Most effective against rapidly dividing cells.
2. Use. Leukemias; multiple myeloma; neuroblastoma; ovarian, breast, lung cancers; Hodgkin's disease; Ewing's sarcoma.
3. Adverse effects. Gonadal suppression, hemorrhagic and nonhemorrhagic cystitis.
4. Nursing implications
   a. Force fluids.
   b. Assess for signs and symptoms of unexplained bleeding.
   c. Assess leukocyte count frequently.
   d. Monitor CBC, uric acid, electrolytes, thrombocytes, and hepatic and renal function at least twice a week.
   e. Instruct client to report hematuria or dysuria immediately.
B. Related drugs. See Table 2-26.

**Table 2-26** Alkylating Agents

| Drug | Use | Comments |
|------|-----|----------|
| Cisplatin (Platinol) | Lymphoma; myeloma; melanoma; osteosarcoma; cervical, ovarian, testicular, lung, esophageal, prostatic cancers. | • Causes nephrotoxicity and ototoxicity, ensure adequate hydration and give diuretics prior to therapy.<br>• Have client void every hour or insert Foley catheter before initiating treatment.<br>• Assess for hearing deficits. |
| Busulfan (Myleran) | Polycythermia vera, chronic myelogenous leukemia. | • Discontinue drug when white blood cells (WBC) reach 15,000 mm$^3$.<br>• Monitor CBC as this drug can cause severe bone marrow depression. |
| Mechlorethamine HCl (Mustargen) | Hodgkin's disease, non-Hodgkin's lymphomas; lung cancer. | • Assess for edema, ascites, weight gain.<br>• Assess for signs and symptoms of dehydration.<br>• Wear gloves if applying solid preparation. |
| Thiotepa | Bladder, breast, and ovarian cancers. | • Decreased dose for renal or hepatic impairment and bone marrow depression.<br>• Only given parenterally. |
| Chlorambucil (Leukeran) | Breast and ovarian cancer; non-Hodgkin's lymphomas; chronic lymphocytic leukemia. | • Assess CBC, WBC, and serum uric acid levels routinely.<br>• Avoid IM injections when platelet count is low.<br>• Urge client to drink 10–12 glasses of fluid per day.<br>• Provide urine alkalinization if uric acid levels are increased. |

## Sample Questions

157. Which of the following should be included in client teaching about cyclophosphamide (Cytoxan) therapy?
    1. Omit dose if anorexic or nauseated.
    2. Drink plenty of water.
    3. Take cyclophosphamide with meals.
    4. Take cyclophosphamide before going to bed.

158. Which of the following medications might the physician order along with cyclophosphamide?
    1. Metoclopramide (Reglan).
    2. Diphenhydramine HCl (Benadryl).
    3. Minoxidil (Loniten).
    4. Dexamethasone (Decadron).

## Answers and Rationales

157. **2.** Hemorrhagic and nonhemorrhagic cystitis are related to cyclophosphamide (Cytoxan) therapy.

Drinking plenty of water and fluids reduces the risk of developing both types of cystitis.

158. **1.** Metaclopramide (Reglan) is an antiemetic used to treat the nausea and vomiting that are adverse effects seen with cyclophosphamide (Cytoxan) therapy.

## ANTIMETABOLITES

A. Prototype: methotrexate with leucovorin rescue
   1. Action. Leucovorin calcium is a folic acid analog that interferes with mitotic process by blocking folinic acid.
   2. Use. Acute lymphoblastic leukemia; cancer of breast, lung, testes, ovary, head, and neck; choriocarcinoma.
   3. Adverse effects. See General Considerations. Intrathecal use may cause fever, headache, and vomiting.
   4. Nursing implications. Leucovorin calcium is frequently given to prevent toxicity when high doses of methotrexate are given.
   5. Discharge teaching. See General Considerations. Instruct client to avoid self-medication with OTC vitamins (folic acid and derivatives may alter drug response).

**B.** Related drugs.
1. 5-Fluorouracil (5-FU)
2. Mercaptopurine (Purinethol)
3. Cytarabine (Cytosar-U)
4. Floxuridine (FUDR)
5. Fludarabine (Fludara)

## Sample Questions

159. Which of the following drugs is given to prevent methotrexate toxicity?
    1. Trimethobenzamide HCl (Tigan)
    2. Prednisone
    3. Allopurinol (Zyloprim)
    4. Leucovorin calcium

160. Which of the following agents should be avoided by clients on methotrexate therapy?
    1. Folic acid
    2. Vitamin C
    3. Iron
    4. Vitamin D

## Answers and Rationales

159. **4.** Leucovorin calcium is a reduced form of folic acid that takes up binding sites to prevent methotrexate toxicity.

160. **1.** Folic acid can alter methotrexate response.

# ANTIBIOTIC ANTINEOPLASTIC AGENTS

**A.** Prototype: doxorubicin HCl (Adriamycin)
1. Action. Attaches to DNA and prevents DNA synthesis in vulnerable cells.
2. Use. Cancer of thyroid, lung, bladder, breast, and ovary; acute leukemia; sarcoma; Ewing's sarcoma; neuroblastoma; lymphomas.
3. Adverse effects. Nausea, vomiting, stomatitis; ECG changes; agranulocytosis, leukopenia, thrombocytopenia; hyperpigmentation of skin and nails; alopecia.
4. Nursing implications
    a. Do not give SC or IM—local reaction and skin necrosis can occur.
    b. IV use: reconstitute with normal saline or sterile water; reconstituted solution stable for 24 hours at room temperature or 48 hours if refrigerated; protect from sunlight; do not infuse in less than 5 minutes; red streaking over vein and facial flushing are signs of too-rapid administration.
    c. Do not mix with other drugs.
    d. Monitor IV site; for local extravasation pour normal saline on area, apply a cold compress; infiltration with corticosteroid may be ordered.
    e. Monitor CBC, serum uric acid levels, cardiac output (listen for $S_3$), weight.
    f. Frequent mouth care.
    g. Client needs sufficient fluids to prevent hyperuricemia.
    h. Assist client with information on wigs and head coverings before hair loss starts.
    i. Offer support to client to deal with drug therapy and diagnosis.
    j. Wear gloves to prepare this drug. Wash skin with soap and water if powder or solution contacts skin.
    k. Urine is red colored for 1–2 days after administration. Clears within 48 hours.

**B.** Related drugs. See Table 2-27.

## Sample Questions

161. While the client is receiving intravenous doxorubicin the nurse should monitor which of the following?
    1. Chest X-rays.
    2. Sodium levels.
    3. Liver function studies.
    4. Electrocardiograms.

162. What complaints would alert the nurse to stop the infusion of doxorubicin?
    1. Headache and dizziness.
    2. Burning and pain at the infusion site.
    3. Upset stomach and heartburn.
    4. Light-headedness and confusion.

163. Which nursing action is NOT appropriate for the client receiving doxorubicin?
    1. Provide frequent mouth care for the client.
    2. Tell the client his urine will be red-tinged for the first couple of days after administration of the drug.
    3. Put the client on fluid restriction.
    4. Explain to the client he will lose his hair.

**Table 2-27** Antibiotic Antineoplastic Agents

| Drug | Action | Uses | Comments |
|------|--------|------|----------|
| Bleomycin Sulfate (Blenoxane) | Prevents DNA, RNA, and protein synthesis in cells. Cell cycle specific in G2 and M phases. | Lymphomas, melanoma, cancers of head, neck, esophagus, lung, skin, penis, testes, vulva, cervix, anus. | • Pulmonary side effects of dyspnea, fever, rales, cough. <br>• Febrile reaction usually occurs on first day of therapy. <br>• Monitor respiratory status. |
| Dactinomycin (Actinomycin D) | Prevents synthesis of messenger RNA; cell cycle nonspecific. | Testicular cancer, melanoma, choriocarinoma, Wilm's tumor, neuroblastoma, retinoblastoma, Ewing's sarcoma, Kaposi's sarcoma. | • Monitor IV site carefully. <br>• Do not expose drug solution to direct sunlight. |
| Daunorubicin (Daunomycin) | Inhibits DNA synthesis; cell cycle specific in S-phase of cell cycle. | Acute myelocytic and lymphocytic leukemia. | • ECG changes can occur. <br>• Urine turns red on day of administration. <br>• Monitor IV site carefully <br>• Never give IM or SC. <br>• Do not mix with heparin. |
| Mitomycin (Mutamycin) | Prevents DNA and protein synthesis in cells; cell cycle nonspecific | Cancer of gastrointestinal tract, breast, lung, bladder, cervix. | • See Prototype Drug |
| Plicamycin (Mithramycin) | Prevents DNA synthesis; decreases serum calcium by unknown action; blocks action of parathyroid hormone. | Testicular cancer, hypercalcemia. | • Side effect of bleeding. <br>• Monitor blood coagulation studies. <br>• Monitor client for signs of hypocalcemia. |

## Answers and Rationales

161. **4.** Doxorubicin (Adriamycin) can cause ECG changes; the nurse should monitor electrocardiograms while the client is receiving this drug.

162. **2.** Intravenous infusion of doxorubicin (Adriamycin) should be stopped if the client complains of burning and pain at the infusion site. These signs are indicative of extravasation, which could lead to skin necrosis.

163. **3.** Fluids should not be restricted for a client receiving doxorubicin; this drug can cause hyperuricemia if fluid intake is not sufficient.

## ANTINEOPLASTICS AFFECTING HORMONAL BALANCE

A. Mechanism of action of hormonal agents.
   1. Exact mechanism is not completely understood.

   2. Believed that hormonal agents hinder use of steroids necessary for cell growth.
   3. Hormonal therapy keeps cancer cells in resting phase, thus decreasing growth of tumor.
   4. No direct cytotoxic effect of hormonal agents so they are unable to cure cancer.
B. Estrogens (female hormones). See Table 2-28.
C. Androgens (male hormones) are also used as replacement therapy for growth and development of male sex organs and secondary sex characteristics in androgen-deficient males. See Table 2-29.
D. Antihormonal agents
   1. Antiestrogen: Tamoxifen (Nolvadex)
      a. Use. Advanced breast cancer in pre- and postmenopausal women.
      b. Adverse effects. Most common are similar to signs of menopause (hot flashes and flushing); nausea, vomiting; temporary bone and tumor pain; temporary drop in WBC count.
      c. Nursing implications. Monitor WBC count; tell premenopausal women to use contraception as short-term therapy causes ovulation.
   2. Antiadrenal: aminoglutethamide (Cytadren)
      a. Use. Adrenal and metastatic breast cancer.

**Table 2-28** Estrogens

| Drug | Use | Adverse Effects | Nursing Implications |
|---|---|---|---|
| Diethylstilbestrol (DES) | Breast and prostate cancer. | Headache; vertigo; insomnia; nausea; weight changes; phlebitis; edema; uterine bleeding; feminization in males; changes in calcium and folic acid metabolism | • Monitor calcium levels.<br>• Monitor males for signs of feminization.<br>• Monitor salt intake and keep it reduced.<br>• Weigh client daily. |
| Ethinyl Estradiol (Estinyl) | Breast and prostate cancer. | See Diethylstilbestrol (DES) | See Diethylstilbestrol (DES) |

**Table 2-29** Androgens

| Drug | Use | Adverse Effects | Nursing Implications |
|---|---|---|---|
| Fluoxymesterone (Halotestin) | Breast and renal cancer | Nausea; vomiting; weight gain; edema and fluid retention; vaginal dryness and itching; acne; hypercalcemia if bone cancer present; masculinization of females | • Monitor client for masculinizing effects.<br>• Monitor weight.<br>• Low salt intake.<br>• Restrict fluids if necessary.<br>• Monitor blood pressure. |
| Testosterone Cypionate (Depo-Testosterone) | Breast cancer | See Fluoxymesterone (Halotestin) | • IM must be given deeply into gluteal muscle.<br>• See Fluoxymesterone (Halotestin) |

    **b.** Adverse effects. Drowsiness; anorexia, nausea; vomiting, severe pancytopenia; rash; and adrenal insufficiency.

    **c.** Nursing implications. Possible replacement therapy with hydrocortisone and mineralocorticoids; monitor blood pressure, thyroid studies, and CBC; tell client that drug may cause drowsiness and orthostatic hypotension.

**3.** Gonadotropin releasing hormone: leuprolide (Lupron)

    **a.** Use. Prostate cancer.

    **b.** Adverse effects. Hot flashes, transient bone pain, rash, alopecia, cardiac arrhythmias, breathing difficulty, and hematuria.

    **c.** Nursing implications. Monitor and rotate injection sites; only use syringes provided with drug; provide comfort measures.

## Sample Questions

**164.** Which diagnostic test should the nurse monitor when the client is receiving diethylstilbestrol?

    1. Arterial blood gases.

    2. Liver enzymes.

    3. Serum potassium.

    4. Serum calcium.

**165.** Which statement about diethylstilbestrol made to a male client by the nurse is incorrect?

    1. "You may develop signs of increased masculinity while taking diethylstilbestrol."

    2. "You need to decrease your salt intake while taking diethylstilbestrol."

    3. "You will need to weigh yourself each day while taking diethylstilbestrol."

    4. "You can experience vascular problems while taking diethylstilbestrol."

## Answers and Rationales

**164. 4.** Diethylstilbestrol (DES) can cause hypercalcemia; serum calcium levels need to be monitored.

**165. 1.** Diethylstilbestrol (DES) can cause signs of feminization in males, not increased masculinity in males.

**Table 2-30** Mitotic Inhibitors

| Drug | Use | Adverse Effects | Nursing Implications |
|------|-----|-----------------|----------------------|
| Etoposide (VP-16; VePesid) | Lymphomas; acute nonlymphocytic leukemia; cancer of lung, testes, bladder, prostate, liver, uterus | Myelotoxic; nausea; vomiting; diarrhea; somnolence; peripheral neuropathy; hepatotoxicity | • Do not give IM or SC as will cause tissue necrosis.<br>• Do not give IV push.<br>• Avoid skin contact with this drug.<br>• Hypotension can occur during administration; monitor blood pressure. |
| Vinblastine (Velban) | Lymphomas; cancer of testes, breast, kidney, head and neck, Kaposi's sarcoma | Peripheral neuropathies, parethesias, neuritis, muscle pain and weakness, pain in tumor site, urinary retention | • Monitor CBC and platelets.<br>• Frequent neuro checks.<br>• Monitor for extravasation.<br>• Monitor I&O. |
| Pacitaxel (Taxol) | Advanced ovarian cancer | Severe allergic reactions, bone marrow suppression, peripheral neuropathy, muscle pain | • Wear gloves when handling.<br>• Premedicate client with a steroid and an H-1 and H-2 antagonist before administration.<br>• Check blood pressure and pulse during administration. |

## MITOTIC INHIBITORS

A. Prototype: vincristine (Oncovin)
　1. Action. Acts on cells undergoing mitosis, thus stopping cell division.
　2. Use. Acute leukemia; lymphomas; cancer of brain, breast, cervix, testes; Wilm's tumor.
　3. Adverse effects. Peripheral neuropathy; paresthesias; loss of deep tendon reflexes; jaw pain; cramps; muscle weakness; constipation; nausea, vomiting, stomatitis; phlebitis; alopecia; hyponatremia; leukopenia; photosensitivity.
　4. Nursing implications
　　a. Do not give IM or SC as tissue necrosis can occur.
　　b. For IV use, inject solution directly into vein or into tubing of running IV infusion. Infusion can be given over 1 minute.
　　c. Monitor bowel function.
　　d. Frequent neuro checks.
　　e. Monitor CBC and platelets.
　　f. Advise client to avoid overexposure to sun.
B. Related drugs. See Table 2-30.

 **Sample Questions**

166. The client requests information about the adverse effects of vincristine. Which statement by the nurse would need correcting?
　1. "You may experience muscle cramps and muscle weakness."

2. "You won't lose any hair."
3. "You may have constipation."
4. "You won't have any breathing problems."

 **Answers and Rationales**

166. 2. Alopecia is an adverse effect of vincristine (Oncovin).

## MISCELLANEOUS ANTINEOPLASTIC AGENTS

A. L-Asparaginase (Elspar)
　1. Action. Enzyme that destroys asparagine, an amino acid necessary for protein synthesis of leukemia cells. Causes death to leukemia cells.
　2. Use. Acute lymphocytic leukemia.
　3. Adverse effects. Anorexia, nausea, vomiting, azotemia, hemorrhagic pancreatitis, rash, hyperglycemia, increased serum ammonia, anaphylaxis, and hepatotoxicity.
　4. Nursing implications
　　a. Monitor CBC, platelets, renal and pancreatic enzymes, coagulation studies, uric acid, blood glucose, and serum albumin.
　　b. Don't shake vial.
　　c. Only give drug in a clear solution; chance of hypersensitivity is increased with each dose.
B. Hydroxyurea (Hydrea)
　1. Action. Urea derivative that kills granulocytes. Prevents DNA synthesis in cell cycle.

2. Use. Chronic myelogenous leukemia; malignant melanoma and cancers of the head, neck, ovary, and colon; sickle cell crisis.
3. Adverse effects. Anemia, leukopenia, megaloblastosis, thrombocytopenia, anorexia, nausea, vomiting, and diarrhea.
4. Nursing implications. Monitor CBC, platelets, liver and renal enzymes; encourage fluids.
C. Procarbazine (Matulane)
   1. Action. Similar to alkylating agents; inhibits RNA, DNA, and protein synthesis in the cell.
   2. Use. Hodgkin's disease, multiple myeloma, malignant melanoma, lung cancer, and brain tumors.
   3. Adverse effects. Anorexia, nausea, vomiting, leukopenia, thrombocytopenia, and altered reproductive potential.
   4. Nursing implications
      a. Advise client to avoid alcohol, sedatives, narcotics, and tricyclic antidepressants (drug is an MAO inhibitor).
      b. Restrict foods high in tyramines.
      c. Monitor CBC, platelets, and liver enzymes.

## Sample Questions

167. Your client is receiving L-asparaginase (Elspar) and complains of stomach pain. You will need to evaluate which laboratory test?
    1. Platelet count.
    2. BUN.
    3. Serum amylase.
    4. Serum potassium.

## Answers and Rationales

167. **3.** Stomach pain may be a sign of pancreatitis, which is an adverse effect of L-asparaginase (Elspar). The nurse should monitor serum amylase as an elevation of this enzyme indicates a need to discontinue the drug.

# Immunosuppressants

## AZATHIOPRINE (IMURAN)

A. Prototype: azathioprine (Imuran)
   1. Action. Purine analog and derivative of mercaptopurine that antagonizes purine metabolism, interferes with nucleic acid synthesis, and alters antibody production. Immunosuppressant action not fully understood.
   2. Use. Adjunct to prevent rejection of renal transplants; severe rheumatoid arthritis.
   3. Adverse effects. Hypotension, pulmonary edema; hepatotoxicity; nausea, vomiting, diarrhea, stomatitis, anorexia; alopecia; bone marrow suppression, leukopenia, thrombocytopenia; hypersensitivity pancreatitis, skin rash; secondary infection.
   4. Nursing implications
      a. Monitor CBC, liver and kidney function studies.
      b. Monitor for symptoms of infection.
      c. Monitor for symptoms of rejection.
   5. Discharge teaching
      a. Take with food.
      b. Report signs of infection and bruising.

      c. Use good handwashing and hygiene and avoid individuals with URIs.
B. Related drugs
   1. Mycophenolate (CellCept)
      a. Used to prevent and treat rejection of renal transplants.
      b. Given orally.

## Sample Questions

168. Which statement by the client indicates a need for further teaching in regard to azathioprine therapy?
    1. "I will take one daily dose 1 hour before breakfast."
    2. "I should avoid individuals who have the flu or a cold."
    3. "I will notify the physician if I notice any bruising."
    4. "I will try to maintain good personal hygiene."

2

168. 1. Azathioprine (Imuran) should be taken with food and in divided doses to reduce GI upset.

## CYCLOSPORINE (SANDIMMUNE)

A. Prototype: cyclosporine (Sandimmune)
  1. Action. Exact immunosuppressant action unknown. Interferes with T-lymphocyte activity.
  2. Use. Prophylaxis for recipients of kidney, heart, and liver transplants to prevent organ rejection.
  3. Adverse effects. Nephrotoxicity; hepatotoxicity; hypertension; infections; tremors; leukopenia; diarrhea, nausea, vomiting; anaphylaxis in IV use; gum hyperplasia.
  4. Nursing implications
     a. Monitor CBC, liver and kidney function studies.
     b. With IV use epinephrine; resuscitation equipment should be available.
     c. Protect IV infusion from light.
     d. Mix PO medication in milk or orange juice at room temperature. Stir and drink immediately and rinse glass with more milk or juice to ensure that entire dose has been taken.

e. Notify physician if bruising present or oliguria.
  5. Discharge teaching. See Azathioprine (Imuran).
B. Related drugs
  1. Tacrolimus (Prograf)
     a. Used to prevent rejection with kidney, heart, and liver transplants.
     b. Given orally or IV.

## Sample Questions

169. Which lab values should be monitored in clients receiving cyclosporine?
  1. Electrolytes.
  2. Glucose.
  3. BUN and creatinine.
  4. Serum amylase.

## Answers and Rationales

169. 3. Cyclosporine (Sandimmune) has nephrotoxic effects; therefore, BUN and creatinine levels should be monitored.

# Vitamins and Minerals

Vitamins and some minerals are vital substances needed by the human body. Because nutrition plays an important role, they are primarily discussed in the nutrition section, Unit 4. Excessive quantities of vitamins can cause adverse effects. Treatment of poisonous minerals is included here as is fluoride, a treatment for prevention of dental caries.

## VITAMINS

A. General considerations related to vitamins.
  1. Vitamins are necessary for body metabolism of carbohydrates, protein, and fat.
  2. Dosage of vitamins is stated in RDAs—recommended daily allowances.
  3. Fat-soluble vitamins accumulate in the body; therefore excessive amounts should not be taken.

B. See Table 4-3, Vitamins, Unit 4.

## Sample Questions

170. A client admits to taking Vitamin A in excess of 50,000 units daily. The nurse explains that this is considered an overdose and that he can get adequate amounts of vitamin A in his diet. What is an example of a good dietary source of vitamin A?
  1. Spinach.
  2. Pork.
  3. Nuts.
  4. Tomatoes.

## Answers and Rationales

**170. 1.** Dark green vegetables such as spinach are good food sources of vitamin A.

## MINERALS

**A.** General considerations related to minerals.
  1. Minerals are essential components of living tissues.
  2. Dosage of minerals is stated in RDAs.
  3. Minerals are divided into 2 groups, major elements and micronutrients.
      a. Major elements: calcium, phosphorus, magnesium, sodium, potassium, chloride, and sulfur.
      b. Micronutrients: iron, copper, iodine, manganese, zinc, fluorine, cobalt, chromium, molybdenum, and selenium.
**B.** See Table 4-2, Minerals, Unit 4.

## Sample Questions

**171.** What information should the nurse provide the client regarding iron administration?
  1. Take it with milk.
  2. Take it with meals.
  3. Take after meals with an antacid.
  4. Take with orange juice between meals.

## Answers and Rationales

**171. 4.** Orange juice contains vitamin C which helps to absorb iron. Iron should be taken between meals for maximum absorption. *Note: sometimes iron is given with meals to decrease GI side effects, but absorption is reduced.*

## HEAVY METAL ANTAGONISTS

**A.** Heavy metals such as lead, iron, arsenic, gold, and mercury can have toxic effects. Heavy metal antagonists prevent or reverse poisoning by neutralizing the heavy metals. Toxic effects or poisoning can occur from drug overdose (e.g., gold salts or iron), or accidental ingestion of lead chips from lead-containing paint, or pesticide ingestion.
**B.** Examples of heavy metal antagonists
  1. Deferoxamine mesylate for iron intoxication
      a. May turn urine red.
      b. When given IV, use an infusion pump and monitor blood pressure frequently.
      c. May cause hypotension, tachycardia, allergic reactions, and pain on injection.
  2. Edetate calcium disodium (Calcium EDTA). For lead poisoning; can cause renal toxicity. May increase intracranial pressure: do not give IV if lead encephalopathy.
  3. Dimercaprol (BAL in oil). Given IM in combination with calcium EDTA to treat lead poisoning. Also used to treat arsenic, mercury, and gold toxicity. Painful on injection and can cause hypertension and tachycardia in large doses.
  4. Edetate disodium (Disodium EDTA) for hypercalcemic crisis.

## Sample Questions

**172.** What should be monitored when administering calcium EDTA for lead poisoning?
  1. Liver function studies.
  2. Kidney function.
  3. Hemoglobin and hematocrit.
  4. Glucose levels.

## Answers and Rationales

**172. 2.** Calcium EDTA can cause renal toxicity.

# Herbs and Herbal Health Products

## HISTORY

A. Eighty percent of the world's population currently use herbs for some aspect of primary health care.
B. Plants and plant products are still a common element today in the healing disciplines of ayurvedic (homeopathic) medicine, naturopathic (traditional oriental) medicine, and Native American groups.
C. Americans embrace the use of herbs/herbal health products and spend approximately $5 billion dollars a year on "natural" herbal products.
D. Americans who use herbs/herbal health products are generally better educated and are holistically health oriented. These individuals are more likely to discuss and report their overall health status to their health care provider. Americans are also reluctant to tell health care providers of their herb use, are risking adverse interactions between herbs and their prescriptions, and are putting themselves at risk for surgery or any invasive procedure without disclosure of their herbs/herbal health products use.

## SOURCE AND USE

A. Herbs are flowering plants, shrubs, trees, moss ferns, fungus, seaweed or algae plants, or plant parts that are valued for medicinal qualities. Herbs and herbal health products are used in all shapes and forms.
B. Common uses include infusions, teas, tablets (pills), lozenges, extracts, salves, balms, ointments, and oils.

## NATURAL PHARMACY

A. Herbs are considered to be pharmacologic remedies that are readily available over-the-counter for general use. Herbs/herbal health products may be natural but not necessarily safe.
B. Herbs are chemical compounds that are biologically active and as such require review and safety education before their use.
C. Currently there is a lack of standardized and scientific data to support the general use of the herbs/herbal health products that are sold as nutritional supplements.
D. These do not require FDA approval. The FDA requirements for the strength and purity of the supplement on the label are in the early stages.

## COMPLICATIONS

A. Toxic impurities and incorrectly mixed herbs have resulted in kidney failure and death.
B. Allergic reactions and interaction with prescription drugs have also been reported.
C. The FDA has become involved with herbs/herbal health products when there have been serious health issues and deaths as in the case of ephedra and cascara sagrada. See Table 2-31 for commonly used herbs and the possible side effects.

## PROFESSIONAL RESPONSIBILITIES

The nurse, as a professional, should provide for clients the resources and client education materials that include common names and uses and side effects of herbs and herbal health products. The nurse must include in the health assessment interview open-ended questions regarding use of herbal supplements and OTC medications. The nurse must be aware of common herbs/herbal health products and their interaction with commonly prescribed medications.

## Table 2-31 Commonly Used Herbs

| Common Herbs | Common Use | Possible Clinical Side Effects |
|---|---|---|
| Ginko | Improve memory; increase blood circulation (peripheral and to the brain); treat bronchial, asthmatic, and pulmonary conditions | • Increased risk of bleeding<br>• Changes in hemodynamic monitoring<br>• Interference with antiseizure medications<br>• GI distress |
| St. John's Wort | Antianxiety, anti-inflammatory, antidepressive, and sedative agent | • Decreased effectiveness of digoxin<br>• Intensify or prolong effects of narcotics and anesthetic agents<br>• Large doses may result in photosensitivity<br>• Potential for constipation, abdominal cramps, dry mouth, fatigue, dizziness, insomnia, or restlessness |
| Ginseng | Increase physical stamina and mental concentration, enhance general health, stimulate CNS, decrease the advances of Alzheimer's disease, reduce tinnitus for those with chronic ringing in the ear | • Potential to falsely increase digoxin levels<br>• Potential for bleeding in postmenopausal females<br>• Potential for hypertension when combined with caffeine<br>• May result in increased heart rates<br>• Contraindicated in pregnancy and lactation |
| Garlic | Lower cholesterol and triglyceride levels and blood pressure; currently looked at for antioxidant, fibrinolytic, and antimicrobial properties destroying bacteria, fungi, and parasites | • Potential for dangerously low blood sugars when combined with diabetes medication<br>• Potential for headaches and potentiate myalgia and fatigue<br>• Potential for increased bleeding and bruising, especially for individuals taking anticlotting medications |
| Feverfew | Prevent migraine headaches; decrease the number and severity of headaches; arthritis and rheumatic disease | • Potential for allergic reactions with allergies to ragweed, asters, chrysanthemums, or daisies<br>• Potential for abdominal pain, glossitis, stomatitis, and allergic dermatitis; GI upsets and nervousness<br>• Potential for interaction with thrombolytics, anticoagulants, and aspirin, increasing bleeding<br>• Potential for dangerously high levels of heart rate and blood pressure if combined with Imitrex or other migraine medication<br>• Potential for withdrawal syndrome in abrupt withdrawal, including rebound headaches, insomnia, fatigue, and nervousness<br>• Contraindicated in pregnancy and lactation |
| Kava Kava | Nervousness, anxiety, or restlessness; used as a muscle relaxant, antispasmodic, anticonvulsant—psychotropic treatment for cystitis | • Potential for increased effects of certain antiseizure medications, intensifying psychoactive agents<br>• Potentiate barbiturates and prolong effects of certain anesthetics<br>• Potential for increased alcohol effects with risk of toxicity<br>• Potential for allergic reactions—rash, GI discomfort, changes in ocular movement, and hepatotoxicity<br>• Potential for increased risk of suicide for people with endogenous depression<br>• Contraindicated in pregnancy and lactation |
| Licorice | Treat coughs and chills; expectorant; anti-inflammatory; antiallergic; treatment of, preventing, and healing stomach ulcers | • Potential for hypertension, swelling, or electrolyte imbalance<br>• Potential for headaches, lethargy, and sodium and water retention in long-term use<br>• Potential for potassium loss and possible heart failure |

*(continues)*

**Table 2-31** Commonly Used Herbs *(continued)*

| Common Herbs | Common Use | Possible Clinical Side Effects |
|---|---|---|
| Ginger | Motion sickness, nausea, vomiting, and vertigo, stomachaches, to aid digestion, a mild stimulant to help promote circulation | • Potential for increased bleeding in clients already taking certain anticlotting medications, anyone at risk for hemorrhage<br>• Contraindicated for treating morning sickness associated with pregnancy<br>• Potential for CNS depression or dysrhythmia in overdose |
| Saw Palmetto | Enlarged prostate and urinary inflammations; mild diuretic | • Potential for GI upset, nausea, abdominal pain, hypertension, headache, urinary retention, and back pain<br>• Potential for effects with other hormone therapies such as adrenergic drugs and oral contraceptives; may result in oral contraceptive failure<br>• Reduces absorption of iron<br>• Potential for false-positive prostate specific antigen test results<br>• Contraindicated in pregnancy and lactation due to its hormonal effects |
| Valerian | Mild sleep aid, muscle relaxant, for relief of nervous stomachs, for stress relief, or as a sedative; decrease time to sleep, does not result in sleep hangover | • Potential for GI complaints, headache<br>• Potential for excitatory effects, cardiac function disorders, and restless-sleepless states<br>• Potential for increased effects of certain antiseizure medications<br>• Potential for prolonging the effects of certain anesthesia agents<br>• Potential for increased sedative effects of barbiturates<br>• Potential to demonstrate an additive effect when used with benzodiazepines<br>• Potential for hepatomegaly when combined with other herbs such as skullcap and mistletoe<br>• Contraindicated in infants and pregnant women |

# Vaccines and Toxoids

## VACCINES AND TOXOIDS

A. Vaccines and toxoids: general information
1. Given to prevent some infectious diseases and diseases transferred by animal bites and injuries.
2. Vaccine is composed of weakened or dead microorganisms that cause antibody formation.
3. Toxoid is a bacterial toxin that has reduced toxicity but can cause antibody formation.
4. Immunity is the ability to fight or conquer infection.
   a. Natural immunity exists from birth and is a basic form of resistance to disease.
   b. Acquired immunity occurs after birth. Can be active or passive. Involves the manufacture of antibodies against antigens in the body. Takes time to develop and considered to be permanent. Acquired by the person having a specific disease or by inoculation with toxoid or vaccines. Passive immunity involves the individual receiving antibodies against antigens that have been formed someplace other than within the person. Is immediate but effects are short-lived. Is acquired through injection of serum containing antibodies.
5. If immunosuppressed, receiving corticosteroid therapy, or has an active infection, should not be inoculated.
B. Specific vaccines and toxoids
1. DPT (Diphtheria, Tetanus Toxoid, and Pertussis Vaccine). Produces active immunity by forming antibodies.

a. DTwP Vaccine (Tri-Immunol). Contains diphtheria and tetanus toxoids and whole-cell pertussis vaccine.

b. DTaP Vaccine (Tripedia, Acel-Imune, Certiva, Infanix). Contains diphtheria and tetanus toxoids and acellular pertussis vaccine. Has fewer side effects and is more effective than DTwP. Recommended for all children, including those who began the series with DTwP.

c. Doses are given at 2 months, 4 months, 6 months, between 15 and 18 months, and 4 and 6 years.

2. MMR (Measles, Mumps, Rubella). Contains live attenuated virus. Should not be given during pregnancy. Give with caution to children who have a history of thrombocytopenia and anaphylactic-like reactions to eggs, neomycin, and gelatin.

a. Give between 12 and 15 months and 4 and 6 years. Second dose must be given before age 12.

b. DPT can be given with MMR.

3. Inactivated Polio Vaccine (IPV). Contains inactivated viruses of all three polio serotypes. Four doses are given: at 2 months, at 4 months, between 6 and 18 months, and between 4 and 6 years. Has no serious adverse effects.

4. Bacillus Calmette-Guerin Vaccine (BCG). Produces active immunity to tuberculosis (TB). Give to infants in countries where TB is endemic. Persons who have had BCG will have a positive purified protein derivative (PPD) test.

a. Also used to stimulate the immune system in treating cancer.

b. Should not be given to persons taking antituberculosis drugs.

5. Hepatitis B Vaccine (Engerix-B). Effective against all types of hepatitis B and recommended for individuals at risk to contract hepatitis B. Now recommended for all children.

a. Does not prevent an unrecognized infection already present.

b. Two IM doses are given 1 month apart and a third dose is given 6 months after the first dose.

6. Hemophilus Influenza B (Hibtiter). Given at 2, 4, and 6 months and booster at 15 months.

7. Td (Adult Tetanus Toxoid and Diphtheria Toxoid). Give at age 14–16 years and repeated every 10 years.

8. Varicella Virus Vaccine (Varivax). Contains live, attenuated varicella viruses. Has no serious adverse effects. A single dose should be given to children 12 to 18 months of age.

9. Hepatitis A Vaccine (Havrix). Contains inactivated hepatitis A virus. Recommended where there is high risk for disease. Has no

serious adverse effects. First dose given at 12 months of age and second dose 6–12 months after.

10. Refer to Table 5-5, Recommended Schedule for Immunization, Unit 5.

 ## Sample Questions

173. A 4-month-old child is brought to the clinic for the next set of immunizations. Which of the following would contraindicate receiving immunizations at this time?
   1. Delayed development.
   2. Weight loss.
   3. Anorexia.
   4. Active infection.

 ## Answers and Rationales

173. **4.** Any evidence of an active infection contraindicates immunization. Other contraindications for immunization are immunosuppression and corticosteroid therapy.

## IMMUNE SERUMS

A. Immune serums

1. Provide passive immunity. They are antibodies that are formed in another person or animal and then given to the client. Offer immediate immunity but duration is short. Treatment considered to be only moderately effective.

2. Hepatitis B immune globulin, human. Given as a prophylactic treatment after exposure to hepatitis B. Needs to be given to adults within 7 days of exposure and repeated in 28–30 days. Newborns are immunized at birth and then again at 3 and 6 months. Cautious use in persons with hypersensitivity to immune globulins. Adverse effects: tenderness at injection site and urticaria.

3. Immune serum globulin (immunoglobulin). Given to nonimmunized persons to prevent or reduce severity of various infectious diseases and prophylactically in primary immune deficiencies. Adverse effects: pain and redness at the injection site.

4. Tetanus immune globulin, human (Hypertet). Used if wound more than 24 hours old or if client has fewer than two previous tetanus toxoid injections. Is considered to be better

than antitoxin. Adverse effect: discomfort at the injection site.

5. Rho (D) immune globulin, human (RhoGAM). Given to Rh-negative mothers with Rh-positive fetus, and also given to Rh-negative women who have miscarriages or abortions. Must be given within 72 hours of delivery. Contraindicated in hypersensitivity to immune globulin. Adverse effect: local tenderness.

 **Sample Questions**

174. The client is given the hepatitis B immune globulin serum, which will provide passive immunity. What is an advantage of passive immunity?
    1. It has effects that last a long time.
    2. It is highly effective in treatment of disease.
    3. It offers immediate protection.
    4. It encourages the body to produce antibodies.

175. What common adverse effects will the nurse tell the client may be experienced after being given hepatitis B immune globulin?
    1. Tachycardia and chest tightness.
    2. Heartburn and diarrhea.
    3. Dyspnea and upper respiratory infection.
    4. Pain and tenderness at the injection site.

 **Answers and Rationales**

174. **3.** Passive immunity provides immediate protection. Passive immunity is also short-lived, is limited in effectiveness, and does not stimulate the body to produce antibodies.

175. **4.** The most common adverse effects of hepatitis B immune globulin are pain and tenderness at the injection site.

## REFERENCES AND SUGGESTED READINGS

Abrams, A. (2006). *Clinical drug therapy; Rationales for nursing practice* (8th ed.). Philadelphia: Lippincott Williams & Wilkins.

Aschenbrenner, D., Cleveland, L., & Venable, S. (2005). *Drug therapy in nursing* (2nd ed.). Philadelphia: Lippincott Williams & Wilkins.

Barnes, P. M., & Powell-Griner, E. (2004). Complementary and alternative medicine use among adults: United States, 2002. U.S. Department of Health and Human Services.

Curren, A. M. (2008). *Math for meds: Dosage and solutions* (10th ed.). Clifton Park, NY: Delmar Cengage Learning.

Deglin, J. H., & Vallerand, A. H. (2008). *Davis's drug guide for nurses* (11th ed.). Philadelphia: F. A. Davis.

Dubois, D., & Dubois, E. F. (1916). A formula to estimate the approximate surface area if height and weight be known. *Archives of Internal Medicine, 17,* 863.

Gutierrez, K., & Queener, S. (2003). *Pharmacology for nursing practice.* St. Louis, MO: Mosby.

Hodgson, B., & Kizor, R. J. (2008). *Saunders nursing drug handbook* (12th ed.). St. Louis, MO: Saunders.

Karch, A. (2006). *Focus on nursing pharmacology* (4th ed.). Philadelphia: Lippincott Williams & Wilkins.

Lehne, R. (2007). *Pharmacology for nursing care* (6th ed.). Philadelphia: Elsevier Science.

Micozzi, M. S. (2005). *Fundamentals of complementary and alternative medicine* (3rd ed.). New York: Elsevier Health Science.

National Council of State Boards of Nursing, Inc. (2008). NCLEX-RN® Examination. Chicago: Author.

Pickar, G. D. (2007). *Dosage calculations, a ratio-proportion approach* (2nd ed.). Clifton Park, NY: Delmar Cengage Learning.

Saxton, D., O'Neill, N. E., & Glavinspiehs, C. (2005). *Math and meds for nurses* (2nd ed.). Clifton Park, NY: Delmar Cengage Learning.

Spratto, G. R., & Woods, A. L. (2009). *Delmar nurse's drug handbook 2009.* Clifton Park, NY: Delmar Cengage Learning.

Wilson, B., Shannon, M., & Stang, C. (2008). *Nurse's drug guide 2008.* Upper Saddle River, NJ: Prentice Hall.

# UNIT 3

# UNIVERSAL PRINCIPLES OF NURSING CARE MANAGEMENT

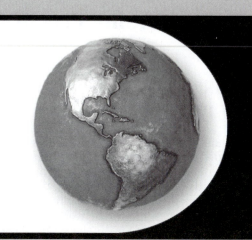

Nurses must frequently apply various management principles while caring for their clients in various health care settings. This unit has been crafted to clarify these issues. It begins with a comprehensive view of nursing practice standards as well as legal and ethical aspects of nursing.

Client care management issues such as determining priorities, working with the health care team, making assignments, delegating to unlicensed assistive personnel, and coordinating client care as the client progresses from admission through discharge have been described along with valuable principles to facilitate the nurse's application of this information.

Safety considerations regarding fire, disaster management, electricity, equipment, and the use of physical restraints have been incorporated.

This unit also includes selected principles and interventions related to specific aspects of care such as body mechanics, transfer techniques, positioning, the hazards and prevention of immobility, application of cold and heat, asepsis, and the care of clients who develop or are at risk for pressure ulcers. Additionally, a section on cultural diversity in health practices explores key issues related to cultural, religious, food, and death practices in the process of nursing care delivery.

## UNIT OUTLINE

# Nursing Practice Standards

## NURSING: SCOPE & STANDARDS OF PRACTICE (2004)

Standards are authoritative statements by which the nursing profession describes the responsibilities for which its practitioners are accountable. Consequently, standards reflect the values and priorities of the profession. Standards provide direction for professional nursing practice and a framework for the evaluation of practice. Written in measurable terms, standards also define the nursing profession's accountability to the public and the client outcomes for which nurses are responsible.

*Nursing: Scope & Standards of Practice* describes a competent level of nursing practice and professional performance that is common to all registered nurses. The scope of the practice statement articulates the who, what, when, where, and how of practice, for nursing organizations, policy makers and the nurse's accountability to the public. The practice part of the statement consists of 2 components: Standards of Practice, which contains 6 standards and Standards of Professional Performance, which contains 9 standards. These are presented in the following section (ANA, 2004).

*Nursing: Scope & Standards of Practice* is used in conjunction with *Nursing's Social Policy Statement* (ANA, 2003) and the *Guide to the Code of Ethics for Nurses: Interpretation and Application* (ANA, 2008). Together these resources provide a complete and definitive description that best serves the public's health and the nursing profession. There are additional scope of practice statements specific to those registered nurses in the specialty practices, but have been omitted from this text because the emphasis of this text is preparation of the nurse generalist (one who has graduated from a diploma, associates or baccalaureate level program).

## STANDARDS OF PRACTICE

(Reprinted with permission from American Nurses Association, *Nursing: Scope and Standards of Practice*, ©2004 nursebooks.org, American Nurses Association, Silver Spring, MD)

### Standard 1. Assessment

**Registered nurse collects comprehensive data pertinent to the client's health or the situation.**

### Measurement Criteria

A. Data collection process:
   1. Systematic
   2. Ongoing
B. Holistic data collection involves:
   1. Client
   2. Family
   3. Other health care providers as appropriate
   4. Environment
C. Priority of data collection activities determined by:
   1. Client's immediate condition
   2. Anticipated needs of the client or situation
D. Uses appropriate evidence-based:
   1. Assessment techniques
   2. Instruments
E. Uses analytical models and problem-solving tools
F. Synthesizes available relevant data, information, and knowledge to identify patterns and variances
G. Relevant data documented in a retrievable format

### Standard 2. Diagnosis

**Registered nurse analyzes the assessment data to determine the diagnoses or issues.**

### Measurement Criteria

A. Diagnoses or issues from assessment data
B. Diagnoses are validated with:
   1. Client
   2. Family
   3. Other health care providers, when possible and appropriate
C. Diagnoses or issues documented to facilitate determination of:
   1. Expected outcomes
   2. Plan of care

### Standard 3. Outcomes Identification

**Registered nurse identifies expected outcomes for a plan individualized to the client or the situation.**

### Measurement Criteria

A. Outcomes are formulated with:
   1. Client
   2. Family
   3. Other health care providers, when possible and appropriate
B. Culturally appropriate expected outcomes derived from diagnoses
C. Considers associated risks, benefits, costs, current scientific evidence, and clinical expertise

**D.** Defines expected outcomes considering associated risks, benefits and costs, and current scientific evidence, in terms of:
   1. Client
   2. Client values
   3. Ethical considerations
   4. Environment
   5. Situation
**E.** Outcomes include a time estimate for attainment
**F.** Outcomes provide direction for continuity of care
**G.** Modifies outcomes based on:
   1. Changes in the status of the client
   2. Evaluation of the situation
**H.** Documents expected outcomes as measurable goals

## Standard 4. Planning

**Registered nurse develops a plan that prescribes strategies and alternatives to attain expected outcomes.**

### Measurement Criteria

**A.** Develops individualized plan considering client characteristics or the situation, including:
   1. Age
   2. Culturally appropriate
   3. Environmentally sensitive
**B.** Plan is developed with:
   1. Client
   2. Family
   3. Others, as appropriate
**C.** Plan includes strategies that address:
   1. Each of identified diagnoses or issues
   2. Promotion and restoration of health
   3. Prevention of illness, injury, and disease
**D.** Provides for continuity within the plan
**E.** Incorporates a time line within the plan
**F.** Establishes the plan priorities with:
   1. Client
   2. Family
   3. Others, as appropriate
**G.** Utilizes the plan to provide direction to health care team
**H.** Plan reflects current statutes, rules and regulations, and standards
**I.** Integrates current trends and research affecting care
**J.** Considers the economic impact of the plan
**K.** Plan uses standardized language/recognized terminology

## Standard 5. Implementation

**Registered nurse implements the identified plan.**

### Measurement Criteria

**A.** Implements plan in safe and timely manner
**B.** Documents implementation of the identified plan, including:
   1. Any modifications
   2. Changes
   3. Omissions

**C.** Uses evidence-based interventions and treatments specific to the diagnosis or problem
**D.** Uses community resources and systems to implement plan
**E.** Collaborates with nursing colleagues and others

## Standard 5a. Coordination of Care

**Registered nurse coordinates care delivery.**

### Measurement Criteria

**A.** Coordinates implementation of the plan
**B.** Employs strategies to promote health and a safe environment
**C.** Documents the coordination of the care

## Standard 5b. Health Teaching and Health Promotion

**Registered nurse employs strategies to promote health and a safe environment.**

### Measurement Criteria

**A.** Provides health teaching that addresses:
   1. Healthy lifestyles
   2. Risk-reducing behaviors
   3. Developmental needs
   4. Activities of daily living
   5. Preventive self-care
**B.** Uses health promotion and health-teaching methods appropriate to:
   1. Situation
   2. Client's developmental level
   3. Learning needs
   4. Readiness
   5. Ability to learn
   6. Language preference
   7. Culture
**C.** Seeks opportunities for feedback/evaluation of effectiveness of strategies

## Standard 6. Evaluation

**Registered nurse evaluates progress toward attainment of outcomes.**

### Measurement Criteria

**A.** Evaluation of outcomes is:
   1. Systematic
   2. Ongoing
   3. Criterion-based
   4. Related to structures and processes in the plan and time line
**B.** Client and other care providers are involved in process, as appropriate
**C.** Effectiveness of planned strategies evaluated by:
   1. Client responses
   2. Attainment of expected outcomes

D. Documents the results of the evaluation
E. Uses ongoing assessment data to revise (as needed):
  1. Diagnoses
  2. Outcomes
  3. Plan
  4. Implementation
F. Disseminates results (as appropriate, in accordance with state and federal laws and regulations) to:
  1. Client
  2. Others involved in the care or situation

# STANDARDS OF PROFESSIONAL PERFORMANCE

## Standard 7. Quality of Practice

**Registered nurse systematically enhances the quality and effectiveness of nursing practice.**

### Measurement Criteria

A. Documents application of the nursing process in a responsible, accountable, and ethical manner
B. Uses the results of quality improvement activities to initiate changes in:
  1. Nursing practice
  2. Health care delivery system
C. Uses creativity and innovation in nursing practice to improve care delivery
D. Participates in activities to improve quality and effectiveness of nursing practice. May include:
  1. Identifying aspects of practice important for monitoring
  2. Using indicators for monitoring
  3. Collecting data to monitor quality and effectiveness
  4. Analyzing quality data to identify opportunities for improvement
  5. Making recommendations to improve nursing practice or outcomes
  6. Implementing activities to enhance the quality of nursing practice
  7. Developing, implementing, and evaluating policies, procedures, and/or guidelines to improve the quality of practice
  8. Participating on interdisciplinary teams to evaluate clinical care or health services
  9. Participating in efforts to minimize costs and unnecessary duplication
  10. Analyzing factors related to safety, satisfaction, effectiveness, and cost/benefit options
  11. Analyzing organizational systems for barriers
  12. Implements processes to remove or decrease barriers within organizational systems
  13. Incorporates new knowledge to initiate changes in nursing practice if desired outcomes not achieved

## Standard 8. Education

**Registered nurse attains knowledge and competency that reflects current nursing practice.**

### Measurement Criteria

A. Participates in ongoing educational activities related to knowledge bases and professional issues
B. Demonstrates a commitment to lifelong learning:
  1. Self-reflection
  2. Inquiry to identify learning needs
C. Seeks experiences that reflect current practice to maintain skills and competence in clinical practice or role performance
D. Acquires knowledge and skills appropriate to the specialty area, practice setting, role, or situation
E. Maintains records that provide evidence of competency and lifelong learning
F. Seeks experiences and formal and independent learning activities to maintain and develop clinical and professional skills and knowledge

## Standard 9. Professional Practice Evaluation

**Registered nurse evaluates one's own nursing practice in relation to professional practice standards and guidelines, relevant statutes, rules, and regulations.**

### Measurement Criteria

A. Provides age-appropriate care in a culturally and ethnically sensitive manner
B. Engages in self-evaluation on a regular basis by identifying:
  1. Areas of strength
  2. Areas for further professional development
C. Obtains informal feedback regarding own practice from clients, peers, colleagues, and others
D. Participates in systematic peer review, as appropriate
E. Takes action to achieve goals identified during the evaluation process
F. Provides rationales for practice beliefs, decisions, and actions as part of the informal and formal evaluation processes

## Standard 10. Collegiality

**Registered nurse interacts with and contributes to the professional development of peers and colleagues.**

### Measurement Criteria

A. Shares knowledge and skills with peers and colleagues (i.e., client care conferences, presentations, or formal or informal meetings)
B. Provides peers with feedback regarding their practice/role performance
C. Interacts with peers and colleagues to enhance own professional nursing practice/role performance
D. Maintains compassionate and caring relationships with peers and colleagues

E. Contributes to an environment conducive to education of health care professionals

F. Contributes to a supportive and healthy work environment

## Standard 11. Collaboration

**Registered nurse collaborates with client, family, and others in the conduct of nursing practice.**

### Measurement Criteria

A. Communicates with client, family, and health care providers regarding client care and the nurse's role in the provision of that care

B. Collaborates with appropriate individuals in creating a documented plan focused on outcomes with decisions related to care and delivery of services that indicate communication

C. Partners with others to effect change and generate positive outcomes through knowledge of the client or situation

D. Documents referrals, including provisions for continuity of care

## Standard 12. Ethics

**Registered nurse integrates ethical provisions in all areas of practice.**

### Measurement Criteria

A. Uses current *Code of Ethics for Nurses with Interpretive Statements* (ANA) to guide practice

B. Delivers care in a way that preserves and protects client autonomy, dignity, and rights

C. Maintains client confidentiality within regulatory parameters

D. Serves as a client advocate and fosters skills for self-advocacy

E. Maintains a therapeutic/professional client-nurse relationship with appropriate role boundaries

F. Demonstrates commitment to practicing self-care, managing stress, and connecting with self and others

G. Contributes to resolving ethical issues of clients, colleagues, or systems (i.e., ethics committees)

H. Reports illegal, incompetent, or impaired practices

## Standard 13. Research

**Registered nurse integrates research findings into practice.**

### Measurement Criteria

A. Utilizes the best available evidence, including research findings, to guide practice decisions

B. Actively participates in research activities at various levels appropriate to the nurse's level of education and position. Such activities may include:

1. Identifying clinical problems specific to nursing research (client care and nursing practice)
2. Participating in data collection (surveys, pilot projects, formal studies)
3. Participating in a formal committee or program
4. Sharing research activities and/or findings with peers and others
5. Conducting research
6. Critically analyzing and interpreting research for application to practice
7. Using research findings in development of policies, procedures, and standards of practice in client care
8. Incorporating research as a basis for learning

## Standard 14. Resource Utilization

**Registered nurse considers factors related to safety, effectiveness, cost, and impact on practice in the planning and delivery of nursing services.**

### Measurement Criteria

A. Evaluates factors such as safety, effectiveness, availability, cost and benefits, efficiencies, and impact on practice when choosing practice options that would result in the same expected outcome

B. Assists client and family to identify and secure appropriate/available services to address health-related needs

C. Assigns or delegates tasks, based on needs and condition of the client, potential for harm, stability of the client's condition, complexity of the task, and predictability of the outcome

D. Assists client and family to become informed consumers about options, costs, risks, and benefits of treatment and care

## Standard 15. Leadership

**Registered nurse provides leadership in the professional practice setting and the profession.**

### Measurement Criteria

A. Engages in teamwork as a team player and a team builder

B. Works to create and maintain healthy work environments in local, regional, national, or international communities

C. Displays ability to define a clear vision, associated goals, and a plan to implement and measure progress

D. Demonstrates a commitment to continuous, lifelong learning for self and others

E. Teaches others to succeed by mentoring and other strategies

F. Exhibits creativity and flexibility through times of change

G. Demonstrates energy, excitement, and a passion for quality work

3

**H.** Accepts mistakes by self and others to create a culture where risk-taking is not only safe but expected

**I.** Inspires loyalty through valuing people as the most precious asset in organization

**J.** Directs coordination of care across settings and among caregivers, including oversight of licensed and unlicensed personnel in any assigned or delegated tasks

**K.** Serves in key roles in work setting (committees, councils, and administrative teams)

**L.** Promotes advancement of profession via participation in professional organizations

# Legal and Ethical Aspects of Nursing

## OVERVIEW

It is important for nurses to recognize that nursing practice is guided by legal restrictions and professional obligations. Legal responsibilities are regulated by state nurse-practice acts and may vary from state to state. In addition, general standards for the practice of nursing have been developed and published by the American Nurses' Association, which has also developed a code of ethics.

Nurses need to be aware of these standards, as well as legal and ethical concepts and principles, because nurses are accountable for their actions in all these areas in their professional role.

### Ethical Concepts That Apply to Nursing Practice

**A.** *Ethics*: rules and principles that guide nursing decisions or conduct in terms of the rightness/wrongness of that decision or action.

**B.** *Morals*: personally held beliefs, opinions, and attitudes that guide our actions.

**C.** *Values*: appraisal of what is "good."
   1. Dilemmas may occur when different values conflict.
   2. Example: client's right to refuse treatment may be in conflict with nurse's obligation to benefit client and to carry out treatment.

**D.** *Ethical dilemma*: a problem in making a decision because there is no clearly correct or right choice. This may result in having to choose an action that violates one principle or value in order to promote another.

**E.** *Autonomy*: an individual has the right to make his or her own decision regarding treatment and care.

**F.** *Paternalism*: another person makes decisions about what is right or best for the individual.

**G.** *Beneficence*: promoting good or doing no harm to another.

**H.** *Right to know*: right to knowledge necessary or helpful in making an informed decision.

**I.** *Principle of double effect*: promoting good may involve some expected harm, such as adverse side effects of medication.

**J.** *Distributive justice*: allocation of goods and services and how or to whom they are distributed.
   1. Equality: everyone receives the same.
   2. Need: greater services go to those with greater needs (e.g., critically ill client receives more intensive nursing care).
   3. Merit: services go to more deserving (used as a criterion for transplant recipients).

## GUIDE TO THE CODE OF ETHICS FOR NURSES: INTERPRETATION AND APPLICATION (ANA, 2001)*

*The Guide to the Code of Ethics for Nurses: Interpretation and Application* contains the full text of the *Code of Ethics for Nurses with Interpretative Statements (ANA, 2001)*, in addition to a history, purpose, application, case studies and examples. This guide is used as a tool for teaching employees and students how to apply the values in the *Code of Ethics*.

The *Code of Ethics for Nurses* serves the following purposes:

- It is a succinct statement of the ethical obligations and duties of every individual who enters the nursing profession.
- It is the profession's non-negotiable ethical standard.
- It is an expression of nursing's own understanding of its commitment to society.

### Code of Ethics for Nurses

**A.** The nurse, in all professional relationships, practices with compassion and respect for the inherent dignity, worth, and uniqueness of every individual, unrestricted by considerations of social or economic status, personal attributes, or the nature of health problems.

*Reprinted with permission from American Nurses' Association, *Guide to the Code of Ethics for Nurses: Interpretation and Application*, © 2001. nursebooks.org, American Nurses' Association, Silver Spring, MD.

B. The nurse's primary commitment is to the client, whether an individual, family, group, or community.

C. The nurse promotes, advocates for, and strives to protect the health, safety, and rights of the client.

D. The nurse is responsible and accountable for individual nursing practice and determines the appropriate delegation of tasks consistent with the nurse's obligation to provide optimum client care.

E. The nurse owes the same duties to self as to others, including the responsibility to preserve integrity and safety, to maintain competence, and to continue personal and professional growth.

F. The nurse participates in establishing, maintaining, and improving health care environments and conditions of employment conducive to the provision of quality health care and consistent with the values of the profession through individual and collective action.

G. The nurse participates in the advancement of the profession through contributions to practice, education, administration, and knowledge development.

H. The nurse collaborates with other health professionals and the public in promoting community, national, and international efforts to meet health needs.

I. The profession of nursing, as represented by associations and their members, is responsible for articulating nursing values, for maintaining the integrity of the profession and its practice, and for shaping social policy.

## Legal Concepts That Apply to Nursing Practice

A. *Standards*: identify the minimal knowledge and conduct expected from a professional practitioner. Standards are applied as they relate to a practitioner's experience and educational preparation. For example, any nurse would be expected to be certain that an ordered medication was being given to the correct client. However, more complex nursing actions, such as respirator monitoring, would require supervised experience and/or continuing education.

B. *Negligence*: lack of reasonable conduct or care. Omitting an action expected of a prudent person in a particular circumstance is considered negligence, as is committing an action that a prudent person would not.

C. *Malpractice*: professional negligence, misconduct, or unreasonable lack of skill resulting in injury or loss to the recipient of the professional services.

D. *Competence*: ability or qualification to make informed decisions.

E. *Informed consent*: agreement to the performance of a procedure/treatment based on knowledge of facts, risks, and alternatives.
  1. Simple: having capacity to give consent for the treatment or procedure.

  2. Valid: having capacity to give consent and also demonstrating an understanding of the nature of the treatment, expected effects, possible side effects, and alternatives to treatment.

F. *Assault*: unjustifiable threat or attempt to touch or injure another.

G. *Battery*: unlawful touching or injury to another.

H. *Crime*: act that is a violation of duty or breach of law, punishable by the state by fine or imprisonment (see Table 3-1).

I. *Tort*: a legal wrong committed against a person, his or her rights, or property; intentional, willfully committed without just cause (see Table 3-1). The person who commits a tort is liable for damages in a civil action.
  1. Negligence and malpractice are torts.
  2. Victims of malpractice are entitled to receive monetary awards (damages) to compensate for their injury or loss.

J. *Good Samaritan doctrine*: rescuer is protected from liability when assisting in an emergency situation or rescuing a person from imminent and serious peril, if attempt is not reckless and person's condition is not made worse.

K. *Licensure*: Granted by states to protect public
  1. Purposes
    a. Standards for entry into practice
    b. Defines what licensed person can do (e.g., Nurse Practice Acts)
  2. License revocation/suspension
    a. Criteria vary in each state.
    b. Licensed nurses should be aware of their state's Nurse Practice Act.
    c. Nurses who are disciplined in one state may also be disciplined in another state in which they hold a license.

**Table 3-1** Examples of Crimes and Torts

| Crimes | Torts |
| --- | --- |
| Assault and battery | Assault and battery |
| Involuntary manslaughter: committing a lawful act that results in the death of a client | False imprisonment: intentional confinement of a client without consent |
| Illegal possession or sale of a controlled substance | Fraud |
| | Negligence/malpractice: |
| | • Medication errors |
| | • Carelessness resulting in loss of client's property |
| | • Burns from hot water bottles, heating pads, hot soaks |
| | • Failure to prevent falls by not using bed rails |
| | • Incompetence in assessing symptoms (shock, chest pain, respiratory distress) |
| | • Administering treatment to wrong client |

### Legal Concepts Related to Psychiatric-Mental Health Nursing

**A.** *Voluntary commitment*: client consents to hospital admission.
  1. Client must be released when he no longer chooses to remain in the hospital.
  2. State laws govern how long a client must remain hospitalized prior to release.
  3. Client has the right to refuse treatment.

**B.** *Involuntary commitment*: client is hospitalized without consent.
  1. Most states require that the client be mentally ill and be a danger to others/self (includes being unable to meet own basic needs such as eating or protection from injury).
  2. In most states the client who has been involuntarily committed may *not* refuse treatment.

**C.** *Insanity*: a legal term for mental illness in which an individual cannot be held responsible for or does not understand the nature of his or her acts.

**D.** *Insanity defenses*: not guilty by reason of insanity.
  1. M'Naghten rule ("right and wrong test"): the accused is not legally responsible for an act if, at the time the act was committed, the person did not, because of mental defect or illness, know the nature of the act or that the act was wrong.
  2. Irresistible impulse: the accused, because of mental illness, did not have the will to resist an impulse to commit the act, even though able to differentiate between right and wrong.
  3. Individuals who commit crimes and successfully plead insanity defenses may be involuntarily committed to psychiatric hospitals under civil commitment laws. There is presently a trend toward finding individuals insane and guilty.

**E.** *Rights of clients*: rights that each state may grant to its residents committed to a psychiatric hospital.
  1. Right to receive treatment and not just be confined
  2. Right to the least restrictive alternative (locked vs unlocked units, inpatient vs outpatient care)
  3. Right to individualized treatment plan and to participation in the development of that plan and to an explanation of the treatment
  4. Right to confidentiality of records
  5. Right to visitors, mail, and use of telephone
  6. Right to refuse to participate in experimental treatments
  7. Right to freedom from seclusion or restraints
  8. Right to an explanation of rights and assertion of grievances
  9. Right to due process

## Legal Responsibilities of the Nurse

A nurse is expected to:
**A.** Be responsible for his or her own acts
**B.** Protect the rights and safety of patients
**C.** Witness, but not obtain, informed consent for medical procedures
**D.** Document and communicate information regarding client care and responses
**E.** Refuse to carry out orders that the nurse knows/believes are harmful to the client
**F.** Perform acts allowed by that nurse's state nurse practice act
**G.** Reveal client's confidential information only to appropriate persons
**H.** Perform acts for which the nurse is qualified by either education or experience
**I.** Witness a will (this is not a legal obligation, but the nurse may choose to do so)
**J.** Restrain clients only in emergencies to prevent injury to self/others. Clients have the right to be free from unlawful restraint.

# Managing Client Care

## PRIORITIES OF CLIENT CARE

### For One Client

**A.** Maslow's Hierarchy of Needs (1954) (see Table 3-2)
  1. Principles
    **a.** An individual's needs are depicted in ascending levels on the hierarchy.
    **b.** Needs on one level must be (at least partially) met before one can focus on a higher-level need

**Table 3-2** Maslow's Hierarchy of Needs

**Maturity**

Growing Toward

Self-Actualization
Self-Esteem/Respect Needs
Affection or Belonging Needs
Safety and Security Needs
Physiologic/Survival Needs

Adaptation based on Maslow's Hierarchy of Needs.

2. Levels of Maslow's Hierarchy
  a. Physiologic/survival needs: basic human needs (e.g., oxygen, water, food, elimination, physical and mental rest, activity, and avoidance of pain)
  b. Safety and security needs
    1) Protection from physical harm (e.g., mechanical, thermal, chemical, or infectious)
    2) Interpersonal, economic, and emotional security
  c. Affection or belonging needs
    1) Giving and receiving of affection
    2) Sense of belonging (e.g., including client/family in planning of care)
  d. Self-esteem/respect needs
    1) Feeling of self-worth
    2) Need for recognition
  e. Self-actualization
    1) Highest level: not reached by all
    2) Independence
    3) Feeling of achievement or competency
B. Application of Maslow's Hierarchy in health care
  1. Client care
    a. Basic physiologic needs should take precedence over higher-level needs and on up the continuum accordingly.
    b. Professional nurse often delivers care at multiple levels simultaneously (e.g., while feeding a client, you position them to prevent aspiration and converse with them).
    c. Tool to guide decision making of priorities in emergencies and time management of care.
  2. Also applies to families, staff, and yourself

## For Multiple Clients

A. Maslow's Hierarchy applies (e.g., more critically ill clients will require more care to meet their physiologic/survival needs)
B. Organizing multiple client assignments
  1. Analyze and plan for entire shift.
  2. Develop a working plan so that priorities get accomplished and all clients receive optimal care.
  3. First consider schedules for nursing activities (e.g., meds, treatments, VS, mealtimes, client appointments, I&Os, etc.).
  4. Then work in the nonscheduled activities that need to be accomplished to meet care plan goals (e.g., supporting family, teaching client, meeting with other departments about scheduling, writing care plan, discharge planning).

# ASSIGNMENT METHODS FOR DELIVERY OF CARE

## Principles

A. Registered nurse (RN) is the decision maker/delegator
  1. Assesses each client. Determines appropriate plan of care.

2. Assesses available staff and their job descriptions. Decides how to use human resources to accomplish care.
B. Typical levels of staff
  1. Nursing Assistants
    a. Unlicensed assistive personnel (UAP)
    b. Assign to majority of the "routine" procedures (e.g., baths, bed making, routine VS, etc.)
  2. Licensed Practical Nurse (LPN)/Licensed Vocational Nurse (LVN)
    a. LPN/LVNs work under the direction of a registered nurse or a physician.
    b. Performs most patient care except in some specialty areas.
    c. Some states prohibit IV push medications or to hang the first unit of blood.
  3. Registered Nurse (RN)
    a. Performs the most complex procedures (e.g., starting IVs, developing the plan of care, interpreting ECGs, correlating laboratory results with client status)
    b. Applies the nursing process for each client
    c. Coordinates the medical plan with the nursing care plan
    d. Coordinates client activities
      1) Other departments
      2) Health care workers
      3) Community
    e. Performs client/family teaching
    f. Ensures documentation of care and outcomes
    g. Directs and supervises care given by LPNs and ancillary personnel
    h. Acts as a client advocate; supporting, pleading, or arguing in favor of the client regarding:
      1) Client rights
      2) Facility policy
      3) Treatment/care issues
      4) Personnel issues

## Delegation to Unlicensed Assistive Personnel (UAP)

A. *Delegation* is the transfer of authority to a competent individual to perform a selected nursing task in a selected situation.
  1. Based on principle of public safety.
  2. RN has ultimate accountability for the provision and management of nursing care (includes delegation decisions).
  3. When done correctly, it allows more care to be provided in a given time period by distributing the workload and allowing better use of the RN's time.
B. Five Rights of Delegation
  1. Right Task
    a. Often defined by state's Nurse Practice Act
    b. Facility policy

c. Job description of UAP, or specific role delineation for a specific UAP
d. Tasks appropriate for consideration:
1) Repetitive custodial nature
2) Not require UAP to make clinical judgment
3) Not require complex steps or decisions
4) Results predictable
5) Potential risk is minimal
6) Uses standard unchanging procedure

2. Right Circumstances
a. Assess the client's condition and stability.
b. Identify the environment/setting (e.g., ICU vs. long-term care).
c. Identify the collective nursing care needs of the whole assignment.
d. Assess the client's plan of care and goals.
e. Provide the appropriate skill-mix and lines of reporting.
f. Provide the needed supplies and equipment.
g. Match complexity of the task with the UAP's competence and level of supervision available.
h. Identify any infection control or safety issues.

3. Right Person
a. Organization's standards for competency of UAPs.
b. Instruct or assess the UAP's competence on a client-specific basis.
c. Perform UAP evaluations based on the standards.

4. Right Direction/Communication
a. Communicate the task(s) clearly and on client-specific and UAP-specific bases.
b. Use oral and/or written vehicles to communicate, depending on the circumstances.
c. Communicate specific information to be reported, specific data to collect, and time lines for reporting.
d. Communicate specific tasks to be performed and any client-specific instruction or limitations.
e. Expected outcomes or potential complications and when to communicate this information.
f. What signs and symptoms to be alert for and how to report it.
g. Communicate availability of support.
h. Verify understanding.

5. Right Supervision/Evaluation
a. Supervision may be provided by the delegating nurse or other designated staff.
b. Supervising nurse must know the expected method for supervision (direct or indirect), the competency of the UAP, nature of the delegated tasks, and the stability of the client condition.
c. Ensure adequate time is allotted to providing needed supervision.

d. Supervise or assign supervision to other appropriate licensed nurses.
e. Monitor performance, and get and provide feedback as indicated (check intermittently).
f. Intervene as needed.
g. Provide education as needed.
h. Ensure clear documentation.
i. Evaluate the client outcome.
j. Evaluate your delegation practice.

C. Other considerations
1. Plan and start delegating before you get too busy.
2. The delegation relationship takes time to build.
3. Select the UAP for the task, if possible (e.g., one UAP might do best with a large, faster-paced assignment, while another may do better with clients who can benefit by a slower conversational approach).
4. Allow flexibility where possible.
5. Use positive feedback.
6. Give credit.

## Admission of Client to Hospital

A. Room assignment
1. Check available data (e.g., diagnosis, age, pertinent history)
2. Does client need to be close to nurses' station for optimal monitoring?
3. Does client need isolation or special precautions?
4. Who will be the client's roommate?
5. Consider the physical layout of available rooms and bathrooms. What would be best for the client based on his or her functional status?

B. Perform a baseline admission assessment per facility procedure.
C. Obtain needed equipment (e.g., urinal, denture cup, etc.).
D. Explain and document the disposition of valuables per facility policy.
E. Orient to facility/policies (e.g., visiting hours, parking, telephone, chaplaincy services, TV, mealtimes, electrical equipment, etc.).
F. Orient to unit (e.g., layout, lounges, smoking policy, activities, menu selection, medication times, straight vs. prn orders, mealtimes, unit personnel, etc.).
G. Orient to room (e.g., roommate; bedside stand, table, and closet; call light, bathroom call system, bed operation, TV, telephone, etc.).

## Caring for the Client Who Leaves the Unit

A. Coordinate scheduling to consider client's diagnosis, activity/test to be performed, and client's other therapeutic goals.
B. Prepare client physically and psychologically as indicated.

C. Consider the client's condition; medication, diet, and treatment regimes; as well as specific precautions and adjust the client's schedule as needed.
D. Communicate pertinent information to other departments/personnel.

## Discharge of Client from the Hospital

A. Discharge to home
   1. Begin discharge plan on admission.
   2. Teach client/significant other about disease process, needed precautions, restrictions, treatments, and medications.
   3. Assess and document knowledge of disease and home-care regimen and ability to perform safely.
   4. Make referrals as needed for added support and care (e.g., community/home health nurses, home health aide, community support groups, social worker, physical therapist, etc.).
   5. Arrange for client to obtain needed equipment/supplies (e.g., bedside commode, ostomy supplies, dressings, etc.).
   6. Ensure that client has needed prescriptions.
   7. Provide written/audio/visual educational materials at the level of the client's ability and appropriate community resource contact information.
   8. Schedule or direct client to arrange for appropriate follow-up.
   9. Communicate with individuals/agency(ies) responsible for follow-up care.
B. Discharge of client to long-term care facility: communicate with facility nursing staff
   1. Client's functional abilities and limitations
   2. Present medical regime and schedule
   3. Mental and behavioral status
   4. Family support/involvement
   5. Nursing care plan and response
   6. Existing advance directives
   7. Recent medication administration records
   8. History and physical
   9. Pertinent diagnostic reports
   10. Other: requirements per insurance

 **Safety**

## FIRE SAFETY/PREPAREDNESS PRACTICES

A. Be aware of hazards and report immediately.
B. Locate and remember:
   1. Escape routes
   2. Fire drill procedures
   3. Use of available equipment
      a. Fire escapes
      b. Fire doors
      c. Fire alarms
      d. Fire sprinkler controls
      e. Fire extinguishers
      f. Shut-off valves for $O_2$ and/or medical air
   4. Keep fire exits clear.
C. Fire safety
   1. Prevention is everyone's responsibility.
   2. Three elements needed for a fire to start
      a. Fuel: substance that will burn
      b. Heat: flame or spark
      c. Oxygen: room air contains 21% $O_2$
   3. See Table 3-3.
D. In the event of a fire:
   1. Follow the RACE acronym:
      **R** = Remove all persons in immediate danger to safety
      **A** = Active alarm and have someone call 911

**Table 3–3** Fire Hazards and Prevention

| Fire Hazards | Fire Prevention |
| --- | --- |
| Faulty electrical equipment and wiring | Report frayed or exposed electrical wires<br>Report sparks or excessive heat coming from electrical equipment |
| Overloaded circuits | Avoid overloaded circuits<br>Don't use adaptors or extension cords |
| Plugs that are not properly grounded | Use only 3-pronged grounded plugs<br>Do not allow electrical equipment from outside the institution to be used until it is checked by the maintenance department |
| Clutter | Avoid clutter |
| Unsafe practices when $O_2$ in use | No open flames or smoking in the area<br>Remove flammable liquids from the area<br>Post "Oxygen in Use" signs as per institutional policy<br>Secure $O_2$ storage per institutional policy |
| Smoking | Remove cigarettes and matches from room<br>Report suspicious odors of smoke or burning immediately<br>Control smoking practices per institutional policy<br>Limit smoking to designated areas<br>No smoking in bed<br>Directly supervise smoking of selected clients<br>Ensure use of safe ashtrays/metal receptacles |
| Spontaneous combustion | Dispose of chemicals, rags, and combustible substances in proper containers |

**C** = Close doors to prevent spread of smoke and fire

**E** = Extinguish the fire using the PASS acronym:

   **P** = Pull the pin

   **A** = Aim on the base of fire

   **S** = Squeeze the handle

   **S** = Sweep from side to side

2. Shut off piped-in $O_2$ and/or medical air.
3. Follow institutional policy concerning announcing the fire and location and notifying fire company.
4. Avoid use of elevators.
5. Follow institutional evacuation plan as needed.

## EQUIPMENT

A. Follow facility procedure when using various equipment.
B. Unfamiliar equipment
   1. Contact your staff development department or supervisor for information.
   2. Read available manufacturer's literature.
C. Suspected malfunction (i.e., equipment that does not do its task consistently or correctly, makes unusual noises, or gives off an unusual odor or extreme temperature)
   1. Don't try to repair.
   2. Replace it immediately.
   3. Contact maintenance department so that it can be checked out safely and repaired.

## RESTRAINTS

A. Physical restraints should be used only if necessary to prevent injury to the client or others.
   1. Signed, dated, physician's order needs to be written specifying the form of restraint and a time limit for restraint use. (At that time the client will be reevaluated for restraint need to determine if a less restrictive method is appropriate.)
   2. Least restrictive form of restraint should be used
      a. Maintain functional abilities
      b. Decrease risk of complications
      c. Minimize behavioral reaction
   3. Remove restraints for 10 min q2h for ROM, repositioning/ambulation, toileting, and preventative skin care.
   4. Document rationale for restraint, other measures tried in lieu of restraint (e.g., distraction, family notification, environmental modifications), client response, and preventative care.

# PRINCIPLES AND INTERVENTIONS FOR SPECIFIC ASPECTS OF CARE

## Body Mechanics

A. Safe and efficient use of appropriate muscle groups to do the job
B. Principles for the safe movement of clients
   1. Keep your back straight.
   2. Ensure a wide base of support (keep your feet separated).
   3. Bend from the hips and knees (not the waist).
   4. Use the major muscle groups (strongest).
   5. Use your body weight to help push or pull.
   6. Avoid twisting (pivot the whole body).
   7. Hold heavy objects close to your body.
   8. Push or pull objects instead of lifting.
   9. Ask for help as needed.
   10. Synchronize efforts with client and other staff.
   11. Use turning or lifting sheets as needed.
   12. Use mechanical devices as needed.

## Transfer and Movement Principles and Techniques

A. From bed to chair or wheelchair
   1. Identify client's strongest side.
   2. Place chair beside bed, on same side as client's strongest side, so it faces the foot of bed. Stabilize chair and lock wheels.
   3. Lower bed, lock wheels, and elevate head of bed.
   4. If assistance is needed:
      a. Place one arm under client's shoulders. The other arm should be placed over and around the knees.
      b. Bring legs over the side of bed while raising the client's shoulders off the bed.
      c. Dangle client and watch for signs of fainting or dizziness. (Stand in front of client for protection in case of balance problems.)
      d. Protect paralyzed arm during transfer. (Use sling or clothing for support.)
      e. Place client's feet flat on the floor. (If client has a weak leg, use your leg and foot to brace the weak foot and knee.)
      f. Face the client and grasp firmly by placing your arms under the armpits. Have client lean forward so that your control of the client's upper body is stabilized.
      g. Using a wide base of support and bending at your knees, coach the client to assist as much as possible by using verbal instruction and counting.
      h. Stand client (if weight bearing is permitted) by pivoting the feet, legs, and hips to a standing position.
      i. Continue the slow pivotal movement until client is positioned over chair. Lower client into chair.

**B.** Log rolling

   1. Performed when spinal column must be kept straight (post-injury or surgery).
   2. Two or more persons needed
      a. Both staff should be on side opposite where client is to be turned.
         1) One staff places hands under client's head and shoulders.
         2) One staff places hands under client's hips and legs.
         3) Move client as a unit toward you.
         4) Cross arms over chest and place pillow between legs.
         5) Raise side rail.
      b. Both staff move to side of bed to which client is being turned.
         1) One staff should be positioned to keep client's shoulders and hips straight.
         2) One staff should be positioned to keep thighs and lower legs straight.
         3) At the same time the client is drawn toward both staff in a single unified motion. The client's head, spine, and legs are kept in a straight position.
      c. Position with pillows for support and raise side rails.

## Positioning of the Client

**A.** General principles
   1. Privacy/draping
   2. Universal precautions as needed
   3. Knowledge of client's condition when moving client (e.g., paresis or paralysis of a limb; need to support joints or limbs in a specific manner; awareness of pressure points)
   4. Good posture and body alignment
   5. Use of added supports as needed (e.g., pillows, wedge cushions, handrolls, foot boards)
   6. Comfort: reduce pressure and strain on body parts
   7. Safety
   8. Bed in a low position once repositioned
   9. Access to personal items and care (e.g., call bell, drinking water, tissues, telephone, etc.)
   10. Clients should change position fairly frequently (at least every 2 hours).

**B.** Positions
   1. Semi-Fowler's (see Figure 3-1A)
      a. Backrest elevated at 45° angle
      b. Knees supported in slight flexion
      c. Arms rest at sides
   2. High Fowler's (see Figure 3-1B)
      a. Backrest elevated at 90° angle (right angle)
      b. Knees slightly flexed
      c. Arms supported on pillows or bedside table
      d. Allows for good chest expansion in clients with cardiac or respiratory problems

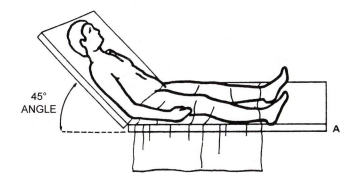

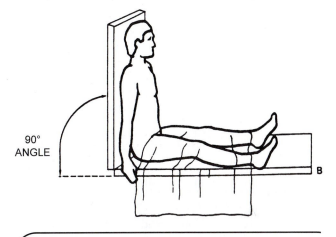

**Figure 3-1** (A) Semi-Fowler's position, (B) high Fowler's position

   3. Supine (dorsal/horizontal recumbent)
      a. Client lies on back.
      b. Client's head and shoulders slightly elevated with pillow (modified per client condition, physician order, or agency policy regarding spinal injury, surgery or post spinal anesthesia)
      c. Small pillow under lumbar curvature
      d. Prevent external rotation of legs with supports placed laterally to trocanters
      e. Knees slightly flexed
      f. Prevent footdrop with foot board, rolled pillow or high top sneakers (depends on persistence of client condition)
   4. Prone (see Figure 3-2)
      a. Client lies on abdomen.
      b. Head turned to one side on small pillow or on flat surface.
      c. Small pillow just below diaphragm to support lumbar curve, facilitate breathing, and decrease pressure on female breasts.
      d. Pillow under lower legs to reduce plantar flexion and flex knees.
      e. May be modified in amputees where flexion of hips and knees may be contraindicated.

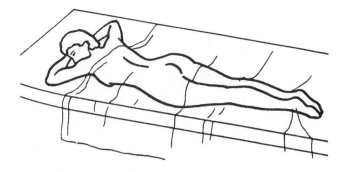

**Figure 3-2** Prone position

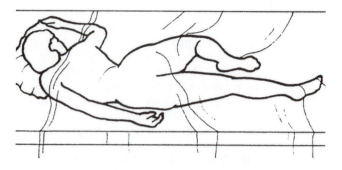

**Figure 3-3** Sims' position

5. Trendelenburg
   a. Client lies on back with head lower than rest of body.
   b. Enhances circulation to the heart and brain. Sometimes used when shock is present.
   c. In emergencies, the entire lower bed may be elevated on "shock blocks."
   d. May be used for prolapsed cord outside of the hospital.
6. Modified Trendelenburg
   a. Client is positioned with legs elevated to an angle of approximately 20°, knees straight, trunk horizontal, and head slightly elevated.
   b. Used for persons in shock to improve cerebral circulation and venous return to the heart without compromising respiration. (Contraindicated when head injury is present.)
7. Lateral (side-lying)
   a. Client lies on side.
   b. Pillow under head to prevent lateral neck flexion and fatigue.
   c. Both arms are slightly flexed in front of the body. Pillow under the upper arm and shoulder provides support and permits easier chest expansion.
   d. Pillow under upper leg and thigh prevents internal rotation and hip adduction.
   e. Rolled pillow behind client's back.
8. Sims' (semiprone; see Figure 3-3)
   a. Similar to lateral, but with weight supported on *anterior* aspects of the ilium, humerus, and clavicle.
   b. Used for vaginal and rectal exams, enema administration, and drainage of oral secretions from the unconscious client. Comfortable for the client in the last trimester of pregnancy.
   c. Client placed on side (left side for enema or rectal exam) with head turned to side on a pillow.
   d. Lower arm is extended behind the body.
   e. Upper arm flexed in front of body and supported by a pillow.
   f. Upper leg is sharply flexed over pillow with the lower leg slightly bent.

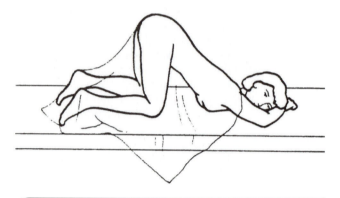

**Figure 3-4** The knee-chest position

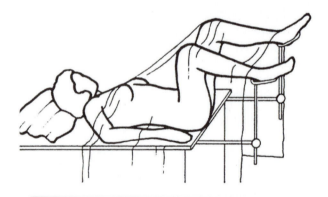

**Figure 3-5** Dorsal lithotomy position

9. Knee-chest (see Figure 3-4)
   a. Client first lies on abdomen with head turned to one side on a pillow.
   b. Arms flexed on either side of head.
   c. Finally the client is assisted to flex and draw knees up to meet the chest.
   d. Difficult position to be maintained—do not leave client alone. Used for rectal and vaginal exams.
10. Dorsal lithotomy (see Figure 3-5)
    a. Used for female pelvic exam.
    b. Have client void before assuming this position.

**c.** Client lies on back with the knees well flexed and separated.

**d.** Frequently stirrups are used. (Adjust for proper feet and lower leg support.)

**e.** If prolonged use of stirrups, be alert to signs of clot formation in the pelvis and lower extremities.

## Immobility

**A.** Definition: inability to move in environment freely

    **1.** May be prescribed to limit movement of body/body part(s) as part of treatment/care plan

        **a.** Bed rest objectives may be:

           **1)** Reduce physical activity

           **2)** Allow rest

           **3)** Reduce oxygen needs

           **4)** Allow to regain strength

           **5)** Prevent further injury

           **6)** Promote healing

           **7)** Restrict movement of specific body part(s)

    **2.** May be related to physical inactivity, cognitive, and/or emotional changes

**B.** Conditions that may require bed rest include cardiovascular, neurological, musculoskeletal, cancer, AIDS, etc.

**C.** Factors affecting immobility

    **1.** Length of immobility

    **2.** Severity of illness or injury

    **3.** Premorbid physical condition

    **4.** Emotional state

**D.** Hazards of immobility (see Table 3-4)

## Cold Application

**A.** Systemic

    **1.** Lowers metabolic rate

        **a.** Client lies on top of one, or between two, cooling blankets. Blanket(s) are attached to a machine that circulate(s) coolant solution.

           **1)** Follow agency policy/procedure for care of client treated with hypothermia blanket(s).

           **2)** Monitor VS (T, P, R, and BP) regularly and frequently.

           **3)** Attention to skin hygiene and protection with oil as required.

           **4)** Frequent repositioning and assessment of body surface areas.

           **5)** Observe for signs of tissue damage and frostbite (pale areas).

           **6)** Assist client in basic needs (e.g., hygiene, elimination, nutrition, etc.).

           **7)** Identify client temperature at which to cease the treatment (temperature may continue to drift downward). Monitor VS frequently until stable for 72 hours.

    **2.** Alcohol or sponge bath (tepid solutions, 85°–100° F)

        **a.** Alcohol bath—combination of alcohol and water (alcohol has a drying effect on skin—used less frequently). Alcohol increases heat loss by evaporation.

        **b.** Sponge bath—cool or tepid (not cold) water.

        **c.** Frequent and regular VS monitoring (T, P, R, and BP).

        **d.** Large areas sponged at one time allowing for transfer of body heat to the cooling solution.

        **e.** Wet cloths applied to forehead, ankles, wrists, armpits, and groin where blood circulates close to skin surface.

        **f.** Identify temperature to cease treatment due to potential for continued downward temperature drift.

    **3.** Discontinue systemic cold applications and report and document findings if:

        **a.** Shivering occurs (this mechanism will raise body temperature);

        **b.** Cyanosis of the lips or nails occurs; or

        **c.** Accelerated weak pulse occurs.

**B.** Local

    **1.** Purposes

        **a.** Control bleeding by constriction of blood vessels.

        **b.** Reduce inflammation:

           **1)** Inhibit swelling.

           **2)** Decrease pain.

           **3)** Reduce loss of motion at site of inflammation.

        **c.** Control accumulation of fluid.

        **d.** Reduce cellular activity (e.g., check bacterial growth in local infections).

        **e.** Effective *initial* treatment after trauma (24-48 hours). This application of cold is then frequently followed by a phase of application of heat.

    **2.** Ice caps or ice collars

        **a.** Covered with cotton cloth, flannel, or towel to absorb moisture from condensation. Change as needed.

        **b.** Not left on for longer than 1 hour.

        **c.** Cease treatment and report if client complains of cold or numbness, or if area appears mottled.

    **3.** Cold compresses

        **a.** Use sterile technique for open wounds. Check site of application after 5–10 minutes for signs of intolerance (cyanosis, blanching, mottling, maceration, or blisters).

        **b.** Remove after prescribed treatment period (usually 20 minutes).

**C.** Special considerations

    **1.** Elderly clients and clients with impaired circulation have decreased tolerance to cold.

    **2.** Moist application of cold penetrates better than dry application.

**Table 3-4** Hazards of Immobility

| Potential Negative Effects of Immobility | Nursing Interventions |
|---|---|
| **Cardiovascular:** | |
| *Orthostatic hypotension:* Impaired ability to equalize blood supply upon assuming an upright position (BP drop, weakness, dizziness, or fainting) | • Monitor VS<br>• Dangle client's legs 2-3 times/day, if appropriate<br>• Tilt tables<br>• Encourage progressive weight-bearing, as indicated<br>• Monitor for change in lying and sitting/standing BP |
| *Increased cardiac workload:* Blood volume redistributes and increases circulating volume (increased heart rate) | • Monitor tolerance for various ADLs<br>• Monitor characteristics of pulses |
| *Valsalva maneuver:* Holding breath and fixing thorax, breath forced against closed glottis during movement | • Teach to exhale rather than hold breath when moving in bed<br>• Overhead trapeze for repositioning |
| *Thrombus formation:* Venous stasis, external pressure against veins | • Proper positioning<br>• Assess for Homan's sign<br>• Elastic stockings, sequential compression devices, etc.<br>• Ensure adequate hydration<br>• Anticoagulants |
| **Respiratory:** | |
| *Limited chest expansion* | • Monitor respiratory rate and depth<br>• Monitor for use of accessory muscles |
| *Decreased movement and pooling of secretions* | • Check breath sounds in all lobes and for degree of aeration<br>• Teach to perform deep breathing and coughing exercises |
| *Impaired oxygen exchange* | • Assess for effective cough<br>• Note any evidence of adventitious lung sounds |
| **Metabolic:** | |
| *Reduced metabolic rate (except with fever)* | • Encourage to be up and about during day, if possible |
| *Tissue atrophy and protein catabolism* | • Provide diet with increased protein and calories<br>• Nutritional supplements<br>• Check weights |
| *Bone demineralization* | • Watch for peripheral edema |
| *Fluid and electrolyte imbalances* | • Monitor laboratory studies |
| **Gastrointestinal:** | |
| *Slower peristalsis (risk for constipation/nausea and vomiting, fecal impaction)* | • Monitor frequency and consistency of BMs<br>• Check for bowel sounds in all four quadrants of abdomen<br>• Prevent or treat constipation<br>• Assess for signs of fecal impaction |
| **Urinary Elimination:** | |
| *Stasis of urine (risk of infection)* | • Monitor I&O<br>• Assist client to empty bladder |
| *Renal calculi* | • Assess for signs of urinary tract infection and renal calculi |
| **Musculoskeletal:** | |
| *Decreased strength* | • Consult PT and OT, as indicated and endurance<br>• Rehab techniques as indicated |
| *Muscle atrophy* | - Active and passive ROM |
| *Contractures* | - Isokinetic/resistive |
| *Osteoporosis* | - Stretch and flexibility<br>• Change position at least q of 2 h<br>• Monitor height over time<br>• Restorative nursing care<br>• Check ROM |

*(continues)*

**Table 3-4** Hazards of Immobility *(continued)*

| | |
|---|---|
| Pressure Ulcers:<br>*Prolonged pressure on area disturbs blood supply and nutrition to a body part* | • Monitor skin condition<br>• Use pressure reduction/relieving devices<br>• Position to avoid injury to tissues and promote lung expansion<br>• Check intertriginous areas for accumulation of sweat and loss of fluid |
| Psychological:<br>*Depression, disorientation, social isolation, altered body concept, anxiety, etc.*<br>*Sleep disturbances- disrupted sleep and wake cycles* | • Provide education<br>  Consult other interdisciplinary team members, as needed<br>• Encourage participation as capable in ADLs<br>• Provide emotional support<br>• Create pleasant environment<br>• Coordinate care to allow client to get through sleep cycles<br>• Provide orienting materials  (e.g., clocks, newspapers, eyeglasses, hearing aids, etc.) |

## Application of External Heat

A. Rationale
1. Relaxes muscles in spasm.
2. Softens exudates for easy removal.
3. Hastens healing due to vasodilation.
4. Localization of infection. *Note: Do not apply heat to the abdomen with suspected appendicitis as it may precipitate rupture.*
5. Hastens suppuration.
6. Warms a body part.
7. Reduces congestion of an underlying organ.
8. Increases peristalsis.
9. Reduces pressure from accumulated fluids.
10. Comforts and relaxes.
B. Dry heat
1. Hot water bottle/bag, electric heating pad, lamp, cradle, or aquamatic pad.
2. Deeper tissue penetration modes: ultrasound, and shortwave and microwave diathermy (administered by Licensed Physical Therapist).
3. Follow agency policy for heat application mode ordered:
   a. Check temperature of water and machine setting carefully;
   b. Assess site of application frequently for signs of tissue damage or burns; and
   c. Be alert to potential bleeding resulting from vasodilation.
C. Moist heat
1. Soaks, compresses, hot packs
   a. Follow agency policy.
   b. Check temperature of application.
   c. Use sterile technique for open wounds.
   d. Assess skin condition after 5 minutes for increased swelling, excessive redness, blistering, maceration, pronounced pallor, or if the client reports pain or discomfort.
   e. Remove the device after 15–25 minutes or as ordered/necessary.
D. Special considerations
1. Moist heat penetrates deeper than dry and is usually better tolerated.
2. The skin area involved may vary in any individual depending on the number of heat receptors present.
3. Heat is less tolerated in the very young, elderly, and clients with circulatory problems.

## Asepsis

A. Defined as the absence of disease-producing organisms.
B. Medical asepsis
1. Practices to reduce the number of microorganisms after they leave the body or to reduce transmission.
2. Often referred to as *clean technique*.
3. Includes:
   a. Hand washing/decontamination
   b. Standard precautions
   c. Isolation technique (i.e., contact, droplet, airborne)
   d. Cleaning/disinfecting of equipment
C. Surgical asepsis
1. Practices aimed at destroying pathological organisms before they enter the body through an open wound.
2. Referred to as *sterile technique*.
3. Includes:
   a. Physical barriers: gloves, masks, gowns, drapes, protective eyewear
   b. High-risk procedures:
      1) Catheter insertion
      2) Surgical wound dressing changes
      3) Administration of injections

c. Associated with populations with high risk for infection. The clients in this category are:
   1) Transplant recipients
   2) Burn victims
   3) Neonates
   4) Immunosuppressed/AIDS, clients with cancer receiving chemotherapy
4. Principles of surgical asepsis
   a. Sterile field: area where sterile materials for a sterile procedure are placed (e.g., a table covered with sterile drape).
   b. Sterile field remains sterile throughout procedure.
   c. Movement in and around field must not contaminate it.
   d. Keep hands in front of you and above your waist (never reach across the field with unsterile items).
   e. Barrier techniques (gown, gloves, masks, and drapes are used as indicated to decrease transmission).
   f. Edges of sterile containers are not sterile once opened.
   g. Dry field is necessary to maintain sterility of field.

# UNIVERSAL/CLINICAL ISSUES

## Pressure Ulcer (Dermal Ulcer, Decubitis Ulcer)

A. Any lesion caused by unrelieved pressure that causes local interference with circulation and subsequent tissue damage.
B. Risk factors
   1. Immobility (e.g., bed- and chair-bound clients as well as those with impaired ability to reposition themselves)
   2. Incontinence
   3. Impaired nutritional status/intake
   4. Impaired level of consciousness
   5. Impaired physical condition (e.g., stability of condition, chronicity, and severity)
   6. Skin condition impaired (e.g., nourishment, turgor, integrity)
   7. Predisposing conditions (e.g., diabetes mellitus, neuropathy, vascular disease, anemia, cortisone therapy)
C. General prevention, care, and treatment
   1. Inspect skin and document status and interventions daily.
   2. Cleanse when soiling occurs (e.g., avoid hot water, harsh or drying cleansing agents).
   3. Minimize dry skin (e.g., avoid cold or dry air and use moisturizers as needed).
   4. Minimize moisture from irritating substances (e.g., urine, feces, perspiration, wound drainage).

   a. Cleanse immediately and apply protective barrier as indicated.
   5. Avoid massage over bony prominences. (Massage around but not directly over pressure sites.)
   6. Change position frequently, every 15 minutes to 2 hours, to decrease prolonged pressure.
   7. Reduce friction and shearing (e.g., promote lifting rather than dragging).
   8. Support surfaces:
      a. Pressure relieving: static surfaces (e.g., air, gel, foam, or a combination)
      b. Pressure reducing: dynamic surfaces (e.g., low air-loss systems or air fluidized beds)
   9. Positioning devices.
   10. Nutritional intake (especially calories, protein, and fluids if not contraindicated). Also vitamin A and C, iron, zinc, and arginine supplemental products.
   11. ROM, ambulation, or activities as appropriate to promote increased circulation.
   12. Avoid pressure from appliances and care equipment.
D. Staging of pressure ulcers
   1. Stage I
      a. Observable pressure-related alteration of intact skin as compared to adjacent or opposite area on body
      b. May include changes in color (red, blue, purple tones), temperature (warmth or coolness), skin stiffness (hardness, edema) and/or sensation (pain) (Temporary blanching from pressure can last up to 30 minutes.)
   2. Stage II
      a. Partial thickness loss of skin involving epidermis and/or dermis.
      b. Superficial breakdown characterized by blister, abrasion, or shallow crater. Wound base is pink and moist, painful, and free from necrosis.
   3. Stage III
      a. Full thickness skin loss involving subcutaneous damage or necrosis. May extend to but not through underlying fascia.
      b. Infection is generally present.
      c. Characterized by deep crater or eschar. May include undermining and exudate. Wound base is not usually painful.
   4. Stage IV
      a. Full thickness loss of skin with severe destruction, tissue necrosis, or damage to muscle, bone, or supporting structures (e.g., tendon or joint capsule).
      b. Infection, undermining, and sinus tracts are frequently present.
   5. If wound contains necrotic tissue or eschar, accurate staging cannot be confirmed until wound base is visible.

E. Specific wound care treatments
  1. Goals
     a. Support moist wound healing
     b. Prevent or treat infection
     c. Avoid trauma of tissue and surrounding skin
     d. Comfort
  2. Solutions
     a. Cleansing products
     b. Control of bacteria
  3. Dressings or coverings
     a. Damp to dry dressing (e.g., gauze dressing put on damp and removed at tacky dry status) debrides slough and eschar.
        1) If dries completely and adheres to *viable* tissue, moisten dressing before removal.
     b. Nonadherent dressing impregnated with sodium chloride to draw in wound exudate and decrease bacteria.
        1) Change at least daily.
     c. Transparent films, semipermeable membrane to promote moist healing by gas exchange and prevention of bacterial and fluid penetration.
        1) Change when seal is lost or excessive amount of fluid collected underneath.
     d. Hydrocolloid wafers contain water-loving colloids. Wound exudate mixes with wafer to form a gel, moist environment, and nonsurgical debridement.
        1) Wafers are occlusive and should not be used on infected wounds.
     e. Gels/hydrogels available in sheets or gels and are nonadherent. They provide a moist environment and some absorption of bacteria and exudate from the wound.
        1) Not highly absorptive
           a) Do not use on wounds with copious exudate.
           b) Be alert to maceration of periwound areas. (Use moisture barriers.)
     f. Exudate absorptive dressings, beads, pastes, or powders, which, when mixed, conform to the wound shape. Attracts debris, exudate, and bacteria via osmosis.
        1) Removed only by irrigation. Do not use with deeply undermined wounds or tracts.
     g. Foams create a moist environment and absorption.
        1) Nonadherent to wound. Many require a secondary dressing to secure.
     h. Calcium alginate pads or ropes made from seaweed that convert to a firm substance when mixed with exudate.
        1) Highly absorptive: will dry out wounds that have little exudate.
     i. Moisture barrier (e.g., A & D ointment) protects high-risk skin from moisture and breakdown.
     j. Skin sealant protects high-risk skin from moisture and/or chemical breakdown.
  4. Debridement: Removal of necrotic devitalized tissue (eschar or slough). Necrotic tissue provides nutrients for bacterial growth and needs to be removed for healing to occur.
     a. Methods of debridement
        1) Enzymatic/chemical
        2) Mechanical
        3) Surgical
        4) Physiologic/autolytic
     b. Be alert to bleeding and damage to adjacent viable tissue.
  5. Miscellaneous
     a. Whirlpool: for cleansing.
     b. Hyperbaric $O_2$: application of high $O_2$ concentration for healing.
     c. Electrical stimulation: stimulates healing.
     d. Growth factor: cell growth stimulation.
     e. Vacuum-assisted closure (VAC): uses negative pressure.
F. Documentation
  1. Interventions and response to interventions
  2. Address:
     a. Location of lesions
     b. Dimensions: measure and record size (length, width, and depth in cm)
        1) Measuring guides with concentric circles available.
        2) Use sterile applicator to determine accurate depth.
        3) Photographs: need client's written permission.
     c. Stage
     d. Undermining, pockets, or tracts (e.g., measuring underdetermined areas of a wound by length, width, depth)
     e. Condition of tissue
        1) Granulation: red, moist, beefy.
        2) Epithelialized: new pink, shiny epidermis.
        3) Necrotic tissue: avascular.
           a) Slough: yellow, green, gray, brown.
           b) Eschar: hard, black, leathery.
     f. Drainage
        1) Volume (scant, small, moderate, copious, number of soaked dressings)
        2) Color
        3) Consistency
        4) Odor
     g. Periwound condition and wound margins (e.g., erythema, crepitus, induration, maceration, hematoma, desiccation, blistering, denudation, pustule, tenderness, temperature)
     h. Pain: related to procedures or constant, location, severity

# Cultural Diversity in Health Practices

A. Culture: socially transmitted behavioral patterns, rules of conduct, arts, values, beliefs, customs, rituals, lifeways, and products of existence that guide the worldview and decision making

B. Key component of the nursing assessment process in order to plan care in a manner that is sensitive and respectful of the individual needs of the client/significant others

C. Cultural considerations
   1. An individual may not necessarily identify strongly with a specific group just because he/she was born into it.
   2. An individual may identify with more than one group.
   3. Clients may choose to practice selected customs of a group while not honoring others.
   4. How a client identifies with a culture, ethnic group, or religion may affect his/her health practices and care up to the end of life.
   5. Rituals tend to become most important to individuals at times of significant life transitions.
   6. When ethical dilemmas arise, the leader of the spiritual or cultural group might be consulted.

D. Assessment
   1. Does the client identify strongly with a specific group or groups?
   2. What are the beliefs, customs, practices, and rules that are most important to the client?
   3. How can the health care team support the client and plan care that will address these needs? Are there special wishes/needs?
   4. Is the client part of a community, congregation, or extended family structure? Does this play an important part in his/her life?
   5. How do the identified culture(s) influence feelings about health and care? It is important to assess areas related to the situation (e.g., for a client newly diagnosed with AIDS: What gives the client's life meaning? What does pain mean to this client?).

E. Selected examples of diverse cultures that might influence health care practices
   1. Jehovah's Witness
      a. Urge members to refuse blood transfusions.
   2. Christian Scientists, Orthodox Jews, Greeks, and some Spanish-speaking societies may not allow organ donation because of their belief that the body needs to remain intact and whole.
   3. Native Americans believe that health is universal. It is a balancing of mind, body, spirit, and nature.
      a. May choose medicine people or local healers for one problem and modern medicine for others.
   4. Seventh-Day Adventists
      a. Prohibit consumption of pork, shellfish, alcohol, coffee, and tea (all meat and fish avoided by the most devout).
   5. Hindus
      a. Prohibit consumption of beef (all meat and alcohol are avoided by the most devout).
      b. Food is eaten with right hand (regarded as clean).
   6. Muslims
      a. Prohibit consumption of pork and pork products (e.g., lard) and alcohol. Consumption of blood is forbidden; therefore, all meat and poultry are cooked to well done.
      b. Bread is required with each meal (a gift from God).
      c. Food is eaten with the right hand (regarded as clean).
      d. Beverages are not consumed until after the meal (some believe it unhealthy to eat and drink at the same time). Some Muslims do not mix hot and cold foods at the same meal.
      e. Fasting as the start of a remedy: Prophet Mohammed said the "stomach is the house of every disease."
      f. High concern for ingredients in mouthwash, non–home-prepared food, medication (gelatin capsules derived from pig, insulin, etc.).
      g. Special daily prayer times
         1) Need basin of water to wash before praying
         2) Bed or chair facing Mecca
         3) Read or listen to the Qur'an
      h. Death is God's will and foreordained. The worldly life is preparation for eternal life.
      i. Death rituals
         1) Body washed three times by a Muslim of the same gender and wrapped in white
         2) Buried as soon as possible in a brick- or cement-lined grave with the body facing Mecca (no cremation and typically no autopsy)
   7. Roman Catholic
      a. Anointing of the Sick (Last Rites) for the seriously ill. This Sacrament of Healing discusses God's grace and brings physical and spiritual strength.

8. Jewish
   a. Prohibit the consumption of pork and shellfish.
   b. Kosher means properly preserved.
      1) Properly slaughtered, prepared, and served
      2) Do not mix dairy products and meat in the same meal
      3) Plates and utensils for preparation and serving of meat and dairy products kept separate
   c. Death rituals
      1) Death is expected part of the life cycle; after death the soul continues to flourish
      2) Respectful to stay with a dying person
      3) No autopsy, cremation, or embalming (keep the body whole, no desecration)
      4) Burial as soon as possible
      5) Shiva: Immediate family "sits Shiva" for 7 days beginning with the burial; the mourners do not work; they think about the deceased; they cover the mirrors of the home, receive visitors, and conduct an evening service
9. Male circumcision is religiously practiced by the followers of Judaism and Islam.
   a. Ceremony, with great festivities, usually conducted 8 days after birth for Jews and within the early few years of age among Muslims

## Sample Questions

1. A female client tells the nurse that she has tested positive for HIV, but she does not want the nurse to tell anyone. What is the best action for the nurse to take?
   1. Document this information on the client's chart.
   2. Tell the client's physician.
   3. Inform the health care team who will come in contact with the client.
   4. Encourage the client to disclose this information to her physician.

2. A young woman who has tested positive for HIV tells her nurse that she has had many sexual partners. She tells her nurse that she believes that she will die soon. What would be the best response for the nurse to make?
   1. "Where there's life there's hope."
   2. "Would you like to talk to the nurse who works with HIV-positive clients?"
   3. "You are a long way from dying."
   4. "Not everyone who is HIV positive will develop AIDS and die."

3. An adult is offered the opportunity to participate in research on a new therapy. The researcher asks the nurse to obtain the client's consent. What is the most appropriate action for the nurse to take?
   1. Be sure the client understands the project before signing the consent form.
   2. Read the consent form to the client and give him/her an opportunity to ask questions.
   3. Refuse to be the one to obtain the client's consent.
   4. Give the form to the client and tell him/her to read it carefully before signing it.

4. An adult has signed the consent form for a research study but has changed her mind. The nurse tells the client that she has the right to change her mind based upon which of the following principles?
   1. Paternalism and justice.
   2. Autonomy and informed consent.
   3. Beneficence and double effect.
   4. Competence and right to know.

5. The nurse is preparing to move an adult who has right-sided paralysis from the bed into a wheelchair. Which statement describes the best action for the nurse to take?
   1. Position the wheelchair on the left side of the bed.
   2. Keep the head of the bed elevated 10°.
   3. Protect the client's left arm with a sling during the transfer.
   4. Bend at the waist while helping the client into a standing position.

6. An adult has experienced a cerebrovascular accident that has resulted in right-sided weakness. The nurse is preparing to move the client to the right side of the bed so that he may then be turned to his left side. What is an important principle when moving the client in bed?
   1. To keep the feet close together.
   2. To bend from the waist.
   3. To use body weight when moving objects.
   4. A twisting motion will save steps.

7. Which statement by the nurse best indicates a correct understanding of "log rolling" when moving a client?
   1. One nurse may perform this task alone.
   2. Pillows are needed for positioning in order to provide support.
   3. The legs should be moved before the head is moved.
   4. Keeping the neck in a straight position is the primary concern.

8. The nurse is caring for a client who has a temperature of 105°F (40.5°C). The physician orders the application of a cooling blanket. The nurse should know that which of the following statements is true about the use of a cooling blanket?
   1. Cold application will increase the metabolic rate.
   2. Vital signs should be monitored every 8 hours.
   3. The client should remain in one position to conserve energy.
   4. Skin hygiene and protection of body surface areas is essential.

9. Topical heat is ordered for all of the following clients. The order should be questioned for which client?
   1. A teenager who is active and rapidly growing.
   2. A new mother who is breastfeeding.
   3. A middle-aged adult with a cardiac dysrhythmia.
   4. An adult with arteriosclerosis obliterans.

10. The nurse is preparing to administer a sponge bath to an infant with a high fever. What should be included in the administration of the bath?
    1. Large amounts of alcohol to increase evaporation of heat.
    2. Adjustment of the water temperature to 60°–70°F.
    3. Wet cloths applied to all areas where blood circulates close to skin surfaces.
    4. Small areas of the body sponged at a time to avoid rapid heat loss.

11. The nurse is instructing the family of a homebound, bedridden client in the general prevention of pressure sores. What should be included in the teaching?
    1. Promoting lifting rather than dragging when turning the client.
    2. Massaging directly over pressure sites.
    3. Changing the client's position every 4 hours.
    4. Cleaning soiled areas with hot water.

12. A nurse is assessing a client with a Stage I pressure ulcer. Which finding would be noted?
    1. Superficial skin breakdown.
    2. Deep pink, red, or mottled skin.
    3. Subcutaneous damage or necrosis.
    4. Damage to muscle or bone.

13. An adult has developed a stage II pressure ulcer. He is scheduled to receive wet to dry dressings every shift. What will the nurse state is the purpose of receiving this type of dressing?
    1. Draw in wound exudate and decrease bacteria.
    2. Debride slough and eschar.
    3. Promote healing by gas exchange.
    4. Promote a moist environment and soften exudate.

14. The nurse is performing a wound irrigation and dressing change. Which action, if taken by the nurse, would be a break in technique?
    1. Consistently facing the sterile field.
    2. Washing hands before opening the sterile set.
    3. Opening the bottle of irrigating solution and pouring directly into a container on the sterile field.
    4. Opening the sterile set so that the initial flap is opened away from the nurse.

15. An adult is homeless and has gangrene on his foot. The physician has recommended hospitalization and surgery. The client has refused. The nurse knows which of the following is true?
    1. The client can be restrained if one physician declares him incompetent.
    2. The client can be hospitalized against his will.
    3. The client cannot choose which treatment to refuse.
    4. The client may sign against medical advice (AMA).

16. An adult has been medicated for her surgery. The operating room (OR) nurse, when going through the client's chart, realizes that the consent form has not been signed. Which of the following is the best action for the nurse to take?
    1. Assume it is emergency surgery and the consent is implied.
    2. Get the consent form and have the client sign it.
    3. Tell the physician that the consent form is not signed.
    4. Have a family member sign the consent form.

17. A licensed nurse in one state receives a job offer as a nurse in an adjoining state. Which of the following should the nurse do first?
    1. Contact the first state's board of nursing to cancel the 1st received license.
    2. Contact the hospital the nurse wants to work in and ask them to contact its state board of nursing.

3. Contact the new state's board of nursing and ask for reciprocity.

4. Take the examining test in the new state.

18. An adult has just returned to the unit from surgery. The nurse transferred him to his bed but did not put up the siderails. The client fell and was injured. What kind of liability does the nurse have?

1. None.

2. Negligence.

3. Intentional tort.

4. Assault and battery.

19. The nurse is in the hospital's public cafeteria and hears two nursing assistants talking about the client in 406. They are using the client's name and discussing intimate details about the client's illness. Which of the following actions is best for the nurse to take?

1. Go over and tell the nursing assistants that their actions are inappropriate, especially in a public place.

2. Wait and tell the assistants later that they were overheard discussing the client. Otherwise, they might be embarrassed.

3. Tell the nursing assistants' supervisor about the incident. It is the supervisor's responsibility to address the issue.

4. Say nothing. It is not the nurse's job or responsibility for the assistants' actions.

20. The nurse is about to medicate a woman for breast cancer lumpectomy. The client says, "I'll be glad when the surgery is over. It will eliminate all the cancer from my body." Which of the following is the best action for the nurse to take?

1. Medicate the client and tell the physician.

2. Correct the client's misconceptions.

3. Call the doctor without medicating the client.

4. Give the medication to the client and note her comment in the chart.

21. A client on your medical-surgical unit has a cousin who is a physician and wants to see the chart. Which of the following is the best response for the nurse to take?

1. Hand the cousin the client's chart to review.

2. Ask the client to sign an authorization, and have someone review the chart with the cousin.

3. Call the attending physician and have the doctor speak with the cousin.

4. Tell the cousin that the request cannot be granted.

22. A nurse comes upon a motor vehicle accident when driving to work. The nurse administers care to the people involved. Under the Good Samaritan Act, for what could the nurse be liable?

1. For nothing, any action is covered.

2. For gross negligence.

3. For not providing the standard of care found in a hospital.

4. For not stopping and offering care.

23. The nurse is supervising a newly trained certified nurse aide (CNA). An adult has just arrived on the unit after surgery. Which of the following is the most appropriate task for the nurse to delegate to the CNA?

1. Taking the client's vital signs while the nurse watches.

2. Suctioning the client's tracheostomy and reporting back to the nurse.

3. Changing the client's postoperative (post-op) surgical dressing then describing it to the nurse.

4. Testing urine with a reactant strip, and recording and reporting the results.

24. The nurse is making the assignment for the floor. There is one LPN and three RNs. Which of the following clients should the LPN be assigned to?

1. A client who is intubated and a newly diagnosed diabetic.

2. A recent ICU transfer and a person with AIDS.

3. A client awaiting a nursing home bed and a client 1 day post-hernia repair.

4. A new admission for cholecystectomy and a client 1 day post-op mastectomy.

25. Which of the following clients should the nurse provide care to first?

1. A client who needs her dressing changed.

2. A client who needs to be suctioned.

3. A client who needs to be medicated for incisional pain.

4. A client who is incontinent and needs to be cleaned.

26. Which of the following clients should the nurse see first?

1. A client who has just returned from the OR.

2. A client whose call light is not working.

3. A client with Alzheimer's disease.

4. A client who is receiving a heating pad treatment.

27. Four clients have signaled with their call bells for the nurse. Who should be seen first?
    1. A client who needs to use the toilet.
    2. A client who does not have his glasses or hearing aid.
    3. A client who has just been given morphine.
    4. A client in a geri chair with a restraint vest on.

28. An adult who is in the terminal stages of AIDS is admitted to the floor. During the admission assessment, the nurse would ask her if she brought with her which of the following?
    1. A will.
    2. Funeral instructions.
    3. An organ donation card.
    4. Health care proxy.

29. The nurse enters a room and finds a fire. Which is the best initial action?
    1. Evacuate any people in the room, beginning with the most ambulatory and ending with the least mobile.
    2. Activate the fire alarm or call the operator, depending on the institution's system.
    3. Get a fire extinguisher and put out the fire.
    4. Close all the windows and doors, and turn off any oxygen or electrical appliances.

30. The nurse is unfamiliar with a new piece of OR equipment that is scheduled to be used today. What is the best course of action?
    1. Ask another nurse for instructions on how to use it.
    2. Wait until she has attended a class on using the equipment before using it.
    3. Get another nurse who is familiar with the equipment to operate it.
    4. Read the instructions provided with the equipment.

31. It is the first home care visit to an adult who is in an electric hospital bed with an oxygen tank behind it. The bed's three-prong, grounded electric cord is connected to a frayed, two-prong extension cord. What is the most appropriate action for the nurse to take?
    1. Turn off the oxygen supply, so as not to accelerate any spark into a fire.
    2. Turn off the electricity, so as to maintain the oxygen supply to the client.
    3. Tell the family to replace the extension cord as soon as possible.
    4. Unplug the bed after turning off the power.

32. Which action by the CNA demonstrates the best understanding of the use of restraints?
    1. Placing all clients in bed with the siderails up.
    2. Applying a jacket restraint for the client who pulls out IV lines.
    3. Fastens the ends of the restraint(s) to the siderails.
    4. Fastens the restraints with a half bow knot to an area the client cannot reach.

33. An adult has had both wrists restrained because she is agitated and pulls out her IV lines. Which of the following would the nurse observe if the client is not suffering any ill effects from the restraints?
    1. She cannot reach her water pitcher.
    2. She is sleeping with her hands by her side.
    3. Her capillary refill is less than 2 seconds.
    4. Her feet restraints are tied to the bed.

34. An adult is to be placed in a knee-chest position for an exam by a new staff member. Which of the following should the nurse observe?
    1. The arms are at the client's side.
    2. The head and upper chest are supported with a pillow.
    3. The lower legs are supported with a pillow.
    4. The back supports the client's weight.

35. An adult has been placed in Sims' position by the CNA. Which of the following should the nurse observe?
    1. The right arm is flat under the hip.
    2. The left leg is flexed at the hip and knee.
    3. The right leg is flexed at the hip and knee.
    4. A pillow under lower legs to reduce plantar flexion.

36. The nurse is evaluating whether the CNAs are correctly log rolling an adult in bed. Which action by the CNA should be observed by the nurse?
    1. Use a draw sheet to aid the turning.
    2. Do not place a pillow behind the head.
    3. Do not put a pillow between the client's legs.
    4. Place the bed in the lowest position.

37. An adult is supine. Which of the following can the nurse do to prevent external rotation of the legs?
    1. Put a pillow under the client's lower legs.
    2. Place a pillow directly under the client's knees.
    3. Use a trochanter roll alongside the client's upper thighs.
    4. Lower the client's legs so that they are below the hips.

38. A C4 quadriplegic has slid down in the bed. Which of the following is the best method for the nurse to use to reposition him?
    1. One nurse lifting under his buttocks while he uses the trapeze.
    2. Two people lifting him up in bed with a draw sheet.
    3. Two people log rolling the client from one side to the other.
    4. One nurse lifting him under his shoulders from behind.

39. A woman is to have a pelvic exam. Which of the following should the nurse have the client do first?
    1. Remove all her clothes and her socks and shoes.
    2. Go to the bathroom and void, saving a sample.
    3. Assume a lithotomy position on the exam table.
    4. Have the client sign the consent form.

40. An adult had a left, above-the-knee amputation 2 weeks ago. For what reason should a nurse place the client in a prone position three times a day?
    1. Prevents pressure ulcers on the sacrum.
    2. Helps the prosthesis to fit correctly.
    3. Prevents flexion contractures.
    4. Allows better blood flow to the heart.

41. An adult has a chest tube placed and is in a semi-Fowler's position. Why would the nurse place the client in this position?
    1. It is necessary to prevent pulmonary emboli.
    2. It allows the nurse to have access to the chest tube.
    3. It promotes comfort and drainage.
    4. It is the only position a chest tube will work in.

42. An adult is to have a rectal examination. In which of the following positions should the nurse position the client?
    1. Supine.
    2. Prone.
    3. Sims'.
    4. Right lateral.

43. An adult has just returned to the unit from the OR where he spent more than 2 hours in the lithotomy position. Which of the following assessments should the nurse make because of the positioning during the surgery?
    1. Lower extremity pulses, paresthesias, and pain.
    2. The presence of bowel sounds.
    3. Upper extremity pulses, paresthesias, and pain.
    4. Ability to walk.

44. A man who has been in a motor vehicle accident is going into shock. Before placing the client in a modified Trendelenburg position, what problem would the nurse assess for first?
    1. Long bone fractures.
    2. Air embolus.
    3. Head injury.
    4. Thrombophlebitis.

45. The client has been placed in the Trendelenburg position. The nurse knows the effects of this position on the client include which of the following?
    1. Increased blood flow to the feet.
    2. Decreased blood pressure.
    3. Increased pressure on the diaphragm.
    4. Decreased intracranial pressure.

46. What is the difference between the left lateral and the Sims' position?
    1. Sims' position is semiprone, halfway between lateral and prone.
    2. Lateral position places the client's weight on the anterior upper chest and the left shoulder.
    3. Sims' position places the weight on the right shoulder and hip.
    4. Lateral position places the weight on the right hip and shoulder.

47. A woman needs to be placed in position for a pelvic exam. Which of the following describes how the nurse should position the client?
    1. Supine with knees and hips bent and thighs abducted.
    2. Lying on her back, extremities moderately flexed.
    3. Kneeling with arms, upper chest, and head resting on a pillow.
    4. Lying on her left side with right knee and thigh flexed toward her chest.

48. An adult is bedridden. The nurse knows which of the following should be included in the plan of care?
    1. Asking the client about comfort prior to positioning.
    2. Instituting a 4-hour turning schedule.
    3. Planning range of motion exercises every 2 hours.
    4. Using support devices to maintain alignment.

49. The nurse of a bedridden woman is evaluating whether the family members understand how to position the client correctly. Which of the following should the nurse observe?

1. Lower arm and leg are always supported in the lateral positions.
2. The extremities should always be extended to prevent contractures.
3. The spine should have maximal lordosis in almost all positions.
4. The family should change the position at least every 2 hours.

50. A victim of a motor vehicle accident is brought to the emergency room via ambulance in hypovolemic shock. When placing the client in a modified Trendelenburg position, how will the nurse place the client?

1. Legs out straight and elevated approximately 20°.
2. Supine, with the head of the bed lowered.
3. Prone, with the head of the bed elevated.
4. Supine, tilting the bed so the head is above the heart.

51. A bedridden woman is positioned on her right side. There is a pillow beneath her head. Her right arm is extended near her hip. Her left leg is extended and parallel with the right leg. Which of the following is correct?

1. The client's right leg should be flexed at the hip and knee.
2. The client's right arm should be flexed at the shoulder and elbow.
3. There should not be a pillow under her head.
4. She should be semiprone with the weight on her upper chest.

52. The nurse uses a wide stance when moving a heavy box of supplies. Which of the following is the best reason the nurse would do this?

1. Avoids back strain.
2. Contracts the muscles.
3. Lowers the center of gravity.
4. Increases stability.

53. A woman who is brought in after a motor vehicle accident has suffered a head injury and possible spinal injury. What action should the nurse perform when moving her from the stretcher to the bed?

1. Have the client move segmentally.
2. Sit the woman up and transfer her to the bed.
3. Move the woman with a draw sheet.
4. Log roll the client.

54. Which of the following techniques would the nurse in a nursing home use to transfer a C4 quadriplegic from bed to wheelchair?

1. One nurse dangling the client, then using a transfer belt.
2. Two people, one at the client's knees, the other under his arms.
3. Two nurses using a mechanical lifting device (Hoya).
4. Two nurses, one on either side, lifting the client with a sheet.

55. The nurse will be dangling an adult prior to transferring her from the bed to a wheelchair. Which of the following actions is essential for the nurse to make before moving the client?

1. Assess blood pressure and heart rate.
2. Ensuring that the bed is in the highest position.
3. Assessing the client's height and range of motion.
4. Enlisting the help of another nurse or a CNA.

56. An adult has just been admitted for acute asthma exacerbation and placed in a high Fowler's position. For what reason does the nurse know that this is the best position?

1. Facilitates maximal ventilation.
2. Is required for the aerosol treatments to work.
3. Allows for chest physiotherapy.
4. Is the position for the chest X-ray.

57. An older adult is to go home with her family. The nurse is evaluating that the family members can correctly move the client from the bed to a chair. Which of the following should be seen?

1. The transfer belt is placed loosely around the waist.
2. There is no pause while the client is standing.
3. The family member leans forward from the waist.
4. The client and family member have one foot slightly in front of the other.

58. An adult suffered a stroke and has right-sided hemiparesis. The nurse is going to transfer her from bed to wheelchair. Which of the following is the best method?

1. Have the client put her arms around the nurse's neck.
2. Position the wheelchair closer to the weaker foot.
3. Place the wheelchair about a foot away from the bed on the right side.
4. Put the wheelchair at a 45° angle to the bed on the left side.

59. The nurse knows which of the following is the proper technique for medical asepsis?
    1. Gloving for all client contact.
    2. Changing hospital linen weekly.
    3. Using your hands to turn off the faucet after handwashing.
    4. Gowning to care for a 1-year-old child with infectious diarrhea.

60. The nurse is conducting a class on aseptic technique and standard precautions. Which of the following statements is correct and should be included in the discussion?
    1. Standard precautions destroy the number of potentially infectious agents.
    2. Medical asepsis is designed to decrease exposure to bloodborne pathogens.
    3. Medical asepsis is designed to confine microorganisms to a specific area, limiting the number, growth, and transmission of microorganisms.
    4. The term standard precautions is synonymous with disease or category-specific isolation precautions.

61. The nurse is to open a sterile package from central supply. Which is the correct direction to open the first flap?
    1. Toward the nurse.
    2. Away from the nurse.
    3. To the nurse's left or right.
    4. It does not matter as long as the nurse only touches the outside edge.

62. For which procedure would the nurse use aseptic technique and which would require the nurse to use sterile technique?
    1. Aseptic technique for changing the client's linen and sterile technique for placing a central line.
    2. Aseptic technique for urinary catheterization in the hospital and sterile technique for cleaning surgical wounds.
    3. Aseptic technique for a spinal tap and sterile technique for surgery.
    4. Aseptic technique for food preparation and sterile technique for starting an IV line.

63. An adult has a draining pressure ulcer on her sacrum and is to be discharged to her daughter's care. The nurse has taught the client's daughter to perform dressing changes. Which observation by the nurse indicates that the daughter's technique is done correctly?
    1. She uses only sterile gloves to remove the old dressing.
    2. She irrigates the wound from the bottom up.
    3. She places the forceps used to remove the old dressing on the sterile field.
    4. She washes her hands before each gloving and after the procedure is done.

64. A woman is transferred to a skilled nursing facility from the hospital because she is unable to ambulate due to a left femoral fracture. Which client description gives a greater risk factor for developing a pressure ulcer?
    1. 5 ft 4 in tall, 130 lb, and eats more than half of most meals.
    2. Apathetic but oriented to person, place, and time.
    3. Slightly limited mobility and needs assistance to move from bed to chair.
    4. Good skin turgor, no edema, and her capillary refill is less than 3 seconds.

65. An elderly male client is transferred to a skilled nursing facility from the hospital because he is unable to ambulate due to a left femoral fracture. When doing a skin assessment, the nurse notices a 3-cm, round area partial thickness skin loss that looks like a blister on the client's sacrum. Which stage is apparent?
    1. Stage I pressure ulcer.
    2. Stage II pressure ulcer.
    3. Stage III pressure ulcer.
    4. Stage IV pressure ulcer.

66. When planning for the care of a client with a pressure ulcer on the sacrum, the nurse would include which of the following?
    1. Positioning the client with a donut around the area to relieve pressure on the ulcer.
    2. Massaging the sacrum, concentrating on the bony prominences and reddened areas.
    3. Using a heat lamp twice a day to dry the wound.
    4. Having a pressure-relieving device such as an air mattress or gel flotation pad.

67. The nurse is to apply a dressing to a stage II pressure ulcer. Which of the following dressings is best?
    1. Dry gauze dressing.
    2. Wet gauze dressing.
    3. Wet to dry dressing.
    4. Moisture-vapor permeable dressing.

**68.** A client with a hip fracture has a sacral pressure ulcer. Which of the following would indicate the best response to treatment?
1. The client's nutritional status including: adequate protein; carbohydrates; fats; vitamins A, B, C, and K; and minerals, including copper, iron, and zinc.
2. The client's skin status, including length, width, depth, condition of the wound margins, and stage of the ulcer as well as the integrity of the surrounding skin.
3. Increased mobility including the ability to reposition self in bed or wheelchair and walking with assistance.
4. Absence of clinical signs of infection including redness, warmth, swelling, pain, odor, and exudate.

**69.** An adult who has a disorder of the hypothalamus is on a hypothermia blanket. The nurse should make which of the following assessments?
1. Document the client's ability to sweat.
2. Ensure the client's skin is warm and dry.
3. Record baseline vital signs, neurologic status, and skin integrity.
4. Confirm that the client is alert and oriented.

**70.** The nurse notices that a Jewish client did not eat any of their food on the meal tray. What would be the nurse's first best action?
1. Request the client's family to bring food in for the client.
2. Request a kosher meal from the dietary department.
3. Instruct the client that food will facilitate the healing process.
4. Ask the client why the food has not been eaten.

**71.** The physician's orders for an adult include warm compresses to the left leg three times a day for treatment of an open wound. What action will the nurse perform?
1. Use medical aseptic techniques throughout the procedure.
2. Wet the compress and apply it directly to the area.
3. Place both a dry covering and waterproof material over the compress.
4. Remove the compress after about 5 minutes.

**72.** An adult is receiving a hot soak to her right arm. What assessment will the nurse make?
1. The water temperature at the start of the treatment is 120°F (48°C).
2. That the water basin is placed at shoulder height.

3. Throughout the treatment, the water remains at approximately the same temperature.
4. The client's baseline and after-treatment temperature.

**73.** An adult has chronic lower back pain and receives hot packs three times a week. The nurse knows the treatment is given for which of the following reasons?
1. To help remove debris from the wound.
2. To keep the client warm and raise his temperature.
3. To improve the client's general circulation.
4. To relieve muscle spasm and promote muscle relaxation.

**74.** While giving an adult a tepid sponge bath to reduce his temperature, the nurse notes that the client is shivering. How does the nurse interpret this action?
1. Sponge bath is being given too slowly.
2. Client has a decreased metabolic demand.
3. Body is trying to warm itself.
4. Temperature of the water is below 90°F (32°C).

**75.** A caregiver is giving a tepid sponge bath to her invalid mother who has a fever. When evaluating the caregiver to ensure the procedure is being given correctly, the nurse would note the caregiver performing which of the following?
1. Tests the water temperature on the inside of her wrist.
2. Rubs each area with the wet sponge.
3. Sponges one part of the body, and then another.
4. Rubs her mother's skin dry after each area is sponged.

**76.** An adult is to have a tepid sponge bath to lower his fever. What temperature should the nurse make the water?
1. 65°F (188°C).
2. 90°F (32°C).
3. 110°F (43°C).
4. 105°F (40.5°C).

**77.** A man has sprained his ankle. Why would the nurse apply cold therapy to the injured area?
1. Reduce the body's temperature.
2. Increase circulation to the area.
3. Aid in reabsorbing the edema.
4. Relieve pain and control bleeding.

**78.** An adult is going home from the emergency room with directions to apply a cold pack to his ankle sprain. He asks how he will know if the cold pack has worked. What information would the nurse provide to the client?

1. After the first application, the swelling will be decreased.
2. He will notice the red-blue bruises will turn purple.
3. There should be less pain after applying the cold pack.
4. That the skin will be blanched and numb afterward.

79. The nurse is caring for a client who has recently immigrated from India. Which action is most appropriate when developing the nursing care plan?

1. Ask the client if any special needs are present.
2. Order a diet with no pork products.
3. Assign the client to an east-facing room.
4. Perform a cultural needs assessment.

80. An unconscious adult is admitted to the emergency department in hypovolemic shock. The client's spouse says that the client is a Jehovah's Witness and should not receive a blood transfusion. The physician orders a transfusion. What should the nurse do?

1. Inform the physician of the family's request and encourage exploration of other volume expander options.
2. Call the hospital attorney to get an authorization to administer the transfusion.
3. Discuss the urgent need for a transfusion with the client's spouse.
4. Give the emergency transfusion as ordered.

81. A client of the Muslim faith is admitted with insulin-dependent diabetes mellitus and pneumonia. Which aspects of the client's care would be of greatest concern to the nurse? Select all that apply.

1. _____ Well-done roast beef on the lunch tray.
2. _____ Order for porcine insulin.
3. _____ Chicken for Friday's meal.
4. _____ Medication in a capsule.
5. _____ Elixir of terpin hydrate.

 **Answers and Rationales**

1. 4. A nurse is legally obliged to protect a client's right to privacy. The second point in the ANA Code is the ethical obligation.

2. 2. This provides the client with expert care. Standard 5b provides for client participation in gaining knowledge and for promotion of health.

3. 3. Nurses cannot obtain consent. They may legally witness consent to medical procedures. When the consent is for a research study, the research team is responsible for obtaining consent.

4. 2. Autonomy is the ethical right to decide what treatment you will or will not receive. Informed consent can be withdrawn; it includes the right to know and competence.

5. 1. Place the wheelchair beside the bed, on the client's strongest side, so that it faces the foot of the bed.

6. 3. Objects should be pushed or pulled instead of lifted. Using the body weight to push or pull prevents strain to muscles and joints.

7. 2. A pillow should be placed between the knees/legs for support while the client is being turned.

8. 4. Assessment of the skin, protection of the skin surfaces with oil, and repositioning are all vital to prevent skin breakdown.

9. 4. Heat is not well tolerated in clients with circulatory impairment. If topical heat application is to be carried out in a client with circulatory impairment, the nurse should assess the site frequently for signs of tissue damage.

10. 3. Wet cloths should be applied to forehead, ankles, wrists, axilla, and groin. These are the areas where blood circulates closest to the skin surface.

11. 1. Promoting lifting rather than dragging when turning or moving the client will reduce friction and shearing. This will assist in preventing pressure sores.

12. 2. Stage I pressure ulcers show discoloration of skin to a deep pink, red, or mottled appearance.

13. 2. In a wet to dry dressing, the wet gauze dressing either covers the wound or is packed into the wound and covered with a dry dressing. The dry layer creates a wick and pulls moisture (drainage) from the wound, debriding slough and bacteria.

14. 3. After opening a sterile bottle, the edge of the bottle is considered to be contaminated. The nurse should pour a little solution out first to wash away organisms on the lip of the opening and then pour from the same side of the bottle into the sterile container on the sterile field.

15. **4.** A competent client may decide which treatments and procedures to accept or refuse.

16. **3.** It is the physician's responsibility to obtain the consent and to ensure that the signer is competent. A medicated client generally is not deemed competent and the surgery may have to be postponed.

17. **3.** Endorsement (reciprocity) from one state to another is usually done when the nurse is licensed.

18. **2.** The nurse has been negligent and can be liable for malpractice.

19. **1.** The client has a right to confidentiality and her case should not be discussed in a public place.

20. **3.** The client does not clearly understand the procedure. Medicating the client can cloud her judgment and should be withheld. The doctor is the person to clarify the misconceptions.

21. **2.** The client must agree to and sign an authorization before others can review the chart, including insurance companies. Most institutions require someone on staff to review the chart with the client or client representative.

22. **2.** Actions that a reasonable, prudent person with the same level of skill and training would have provided are covered, but gross negligence is not.

23. **4.** Testing urine via reactant strips (Dip stix) and recording the results is usually within the scope of a CNA's training. The CNA should also report the results to the nurse, especially if they are abnormal.

24. **3.** These clients are the least sick and require the least amount of highly skilled nursing care.

25. **2.** Any client with a potential compromise of the airway should be dealt with first.

26. **1.** A client who has just returned from the OR is at highest risk for potential problems.

27. **3.** An adverse reaction to any drug can be life-threatening and should be dealt with first.

28. **4.** A living will, durable power of attorney for health care, or a health care proxy is an important part of an admission assessment, especially for a terminally ill client.

29. **1.** Rescue and evacuate any people in the room first. Begin with those who are able to walk, then those in wheelchairs, finally those who are nonambulatory in stretchers or beds.

30. **3.** Only those with knowledge of the equipment should operate it.

31. **4.** Because any electrical (or gas) appliance is a hazard around oxygen, it is better to unplug the dangerous cord after turning off the power.

32. **4.** The half bow knot is a secure knot that will not loosen but can be easily released by the nurse in an emergency.

33. **3.** A normal capillary refill is less than 3 seconds, which would indicate good circulation. Answers 1 and 2 are expected, not ill effects.

34. **2.** A pillow can be placed under the head or chest.

35. **3.** The correct position is with the right leg flexed, left arm extended at side, right arm and head on pillow.

36. **1.** A draw sheet helps to maintain tension along the back and allows the body to be turned as one.

37. **3.** A blanket roll along the side of the hips down to the midthighs helps to prevent external rotation.

38. **2.** A draw sheet is the easiest and most effective method to lift a quadriplegic client up in bed.

39. **2.** The client should have an empty bladder, reserving a sample for analysis if needed.

40. **3.** Flexion contractures can be prevented by placing the client in a prone position and by exercising.

41. **3.** This position facilitates drainage and is generally most comfortable.

42. **3.** The rectum is easily accessed when the hip is bent at a right angle.

43. **1.** The lithotomy position places pressure on the nerves and blood vessels of the legs.

44. **3.** Head injuries and chest injuries are contraindications for the Trendelenburg position.

45. **3.** The chest cavity is pushed by the pressure from the abdominal contents.

46. **1.** The Sims' position is halfway between the left lateral position and the prone position.

47. **1.** The dorsal lithotomy position is used for most pelvic exams.

48. **4.** Support devices such as pillows, special mattresses, trochanter rolls, and foot boards help to maintain alignment and prevent contractures.

49. **4.** Position changes should occur at least every 2 hours, more often if needed.

50. **1.** The modified Trendelenburg position raises the legs only.

51. **2.** The lower arm should be flexed, so the body does not rest on it.

52. **4.** The greater the stability, the less chance of injury. When increasing the base of support, the nurse helps to maintain balance.

53. **4.** Log rolling a client would protect the spinal column and keep the body in alignment.

54. **3.** A mechanical lifting device (Hoya, Hoyer) helps to transfer clients and prevents back injury to the nurses.

55. **1.** The client may experience a drop in blood pressure and should be assessed before and after dangling, especially if standing will be included.

56. **1.** A high Fowler's position allows maximal chest expansion and decreases hypoxia.

57. **4.** Both the family member and the client should have one foot slightly in front of the other. This allows for a greater base of support and helps when rocking to achieve a standing position.

58. **4.** This position is best for clients who have difficulty walking. The client can pivot into the chair and lessen the amount of body rotation. The chairs should be on the strong side.

59. **4.** Gowns should be worn when the nurse's clothing is likely to be soiled by infected material.

60. **3.** Medical asepsis should be practiced everywhere. It includes such things as handwashing.

61. **2.** This allows for the least possible potential for contamination while opening the package.

62. **1.** Changing linen should be done with aseptic technique, whereas putting in central lines requires sterile technique.

63. **4.** Handwashing should occur before donning the nonsterile gloves, when changing from nonsterile

to sterile gloves, and after the procedure. This prevents the spread of microorganisms.

64. **3.** The fact that the client is chair-bound has the greatest impact on her developing pressure ulcers.

65. **2.** A stage II pressure ulcer may look like a blister, abrasion, or shallow crater and only involve a partial thickness skin loss of the epidermis and/or dermis.

66. **4.** Any supportive device that protects bony prominences aids in relieving pressure. This can include gel flotation devices, sheepskins, alternating pressure mattresses, and various air loss beds.

67. **4.** Moisture-vapor permeable dressings help stage II ulcers heal faster than saline dressings.

68. **2.** The best clinical indicator of healing is observation of the skin and evaluation of the pressure ulcer.

69. **3.** Baseline vital sign assessment is necessary to document against those taken during and after the treatment.

70. **4.** Assessment should be performed first to determine why the client is not eating, which may be due to illness, medication, or cultural beliefs.

71. **3.** The layers act as insulators and prevent moisture loss. Some nurses prefer placing the waterproof layer next to the compress and then covering with a dry cover, whereas others reverse the order, putting the waterproof layer on the outside.

72. **3.** The nurse should check the temperature every 5 minutes or so, and replace some of the water with a hotter solution. Care should be taken to stir the basin while adding the additional water so as not to burn the client.

73. **4.** Most people with chronic lower back pain find relief with applications of heat.

74. **3.** Shivering indicates that the body is trying to warm itself and conserve heat.

75. **3.** Each area is sponged slowly and gently. The face and forehead, the neck, arms, and legs for 3–5 minutes, and the back for 10 minutes.

76. **2.** Unlike a cooling sponge bath where the temperature begins at this point and gradually is lowered to 65°F (18°C) at the end, this is the

temperature that the water begins and ends for a tepid sponge bath.

77. **4.** Cold will produce an anesthetic effect and help to reduce pain as well as control bleeding by constricting blood vessels.

78. **3.** Cold produces an anesthetic effect and can relieve pain.

79. **4.** The nurse should perform a cultural needs assessment. Just because the client is a recent immigrant from India does not mean that the client belongs to a particular religion.

80. **1.** The client's next of kin has stated that the client should not get a transfusion. Jehovah's Witnesses prohibit blood transfusions. The client's family has a right to refuse the treatment. There are other volume expanders that could be tried.

81. **2, 4, 5.** Muslims do not put pork products in their bodies. Porcine insulin is a pork product. Gelatin capsules may come from pork. An elixir is made of alcohol. A devout Muslim does not drink alcohol.

## REFERENCES AND SUGGESTED READINGS

Daniels, R., Nosek, L., & Nicoll, L. (2007). *Contemporary medical-surgical nursing.* Clifton Park, NY: Delmar Cengage Learning.

Delane, S., & Ladner, P. (2006). *Fundamentals of nursing* 3E. Clifton Park, NY: Delmar Cengage Learning.

*Federal requirements for Medicare/Medicaid interpretive guidelines.* (2003). Washington, DC: Department of Health and Human Services, Health Care Financing Administration.

Maslow, A. H. (1970). *Motivation and personality* (2nd ed.). New York: Harper & Row.

Mazanec, P., & Tyler, M. (2003). Cultural considerations in end-of-life care. *American Journal of Nursing*, 103(3), 50–59.

McNeill, L., & Schanne, L. (2003, May). Combating the effects of immobility. *Nursing Spectrum*, 22.

National Pressure Ulcer Advisory Panel Fifth National Conference. (2007). Washington, D.C: Author.

Nursesbooks.org. American Nurses Association (2004). *Nursing: Scope and Standards of Practice.* Silver Spring MD: American Nurses Association.

Purnell, L., & Paulanka, B. (2003). *Transcultural health care.* (2nd, ed) Philadelphia: F. A. Davis.

# UNIT 4
# ADULT NURSING

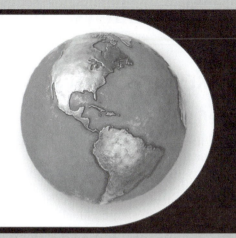

Nursing care of the adult client in today's changing health care environment is a challenge to the skill and knowledge of the professional nurse. Holistic care requires that nurses not only meet a client's physical needs through technical skills and sound clinical judgment, they also must be aware of a client's psychosocial needs. The role of client advocate puts the nurse in a unique position to help clients achieve the highest level of wellness.

This unit presents a comprehensive review of nursing care of adult clients with specific health problems. It begins with a section on multisystem stressors (such as infection, pain, and surgery). These stressors are common to many areas of nursing practice and may be applied to clients with various levels of health care needs. Issues related to aging are also presented.

The unit is further divided according to specific body systems. For each system there is a review of anatomy and physiology. Each step of the nursing process (assessment, analysis, planning, intervention, and evaluation) is then reviewed for the system, followed by consideration of the major health problems of that system. A discussion of complementary and alternative therapies is also included at the end of this unit. Congenital disorders will be discussed in Unit 5.

## UNIT OUTLINE

# Multisystem Stressors

## STRESS AND ADAPTATION

### Definitions

A. Stress: tension resulting from changes in the internal or external environment; either physiologic, psychologic, developmental, or social
B. Stressors: agents or forces threatening an individual's ability to meet his or her needs
C. Adaptation: an individual's (or the body's) reaction to and attempt to deal with stress

### General Characteristics

A. A certain amount of stress is necessary for life and growth, but excessive and continuous stress can be detrimental.
B. Success of adaptation depends on perception of stressor(s), the individual's coping mechanisms, and biologic adaptive resources.
C. Types of stressors: physical, chemical, microbiologic, psychologic, social, and age-related growth and development.

### General Adaptation Syndrome

#### Response to Stress

A. Caused by release of certain adaptive hormones
B. Three stages
  1. Alarm reaction
    a. Sympathetic nervous system is activated (fight-or-flight response)
    b. Results in increased heart rate, blood pressure, and respirations; dilated pupils; increased state of alertness; increased blood sugar and coagulability; increased tension of skeletal muscles
  2. Resistance: body adapts to stressor; uses physical, physiologic, and psychologic coping mechanisms.
  3. Exhaustion: adaptive resources are depleted, overwhelmed, or insufficient; if stress is excessive and continues, death will occur without support.

#### Stress Management/Nursing Responsibilities

A. Instruct the client concerning ways to manage stress
  1. Eat a well-balanced diet.
  2. Get sufficient amount of rest.
  3. Exercise regularly.
  4. Use relaxation methods and techniques: such as deep breathing, guided imagery, progressive muscle relaxation, relaxation response, meditation, yoga, biofeedback.
  5. Engage in a social support system.

## INFLAMMATORY RESPONSE

A reaction of the body at the cellular level in response to injury or noxious stimuli.

### Causes

A. Physical irritants (e.g., trauma or a foreign body)
B. Chemical irritants (e.g., strong acids or alkalis)
C. Microorganisms (e.g., bacteria and viruses)

### Components

A. Vascular response: transitory period of localized vasoconstriction, followed by vasodilation, increased capillary permeability, and blood stasis
B. Formation of inflammatory exudate
  1. Composition: water, colloids, ions, and defensive cells
  2. Functions: dilution of toxins, transportation of nutrients to area of injury for tissue repair, transportation of protective cells that phagocytize and destroy bacteria
C. Defense cell response: migration of leukocytes to affected area for phagocytosis of foreign bodies and dead cells
D. Healing: resolution of inflammation and regeneration of tissue or replacement with scar tissue

### Assessment Findings

A. Local: pain, swelling, heat, redness, and impaired function of part (five cardinal signs of inflammation)
B. Systemic (appear with moderate to severe response): fever, leukocytosis, chills, sweating, anorexia, weight loss, general malaise

## IMMUNE RESPONSE

The essence of the immune system response is recognition, neutralization, elimination, and metabolism of foreign substance with or without injury to the body's own tissue.

## Functions of the Immune System

A. Defense: protection against antigens. An *antigen* is a protein or protein complex recognized as nonself.
B. Homeostasis: removal of worn out or damaged components (e.g., dead cells).
C. Surveillance: ability to perceive or destroy mutated cells or nonself cells.

## Alterations in Immune Functioning

See Table 4-1.

## Types of Immunity

There are two major types of immunity: natural (or innate) and acquired.
A. Natural (innate) immunity: immune responses that exist without prior exposure to an immunologically active substance. Genetically acquired immunity is natural immunity.
B. Acquired immunity
   1. Immune responses that develop during the course of a person's lifetime.
   2. Acquired immunity may be further classified as naturally or artificially acquired, active or passive. Active immunity results when the body produces its own antibodies in response to an antigen. Passive immunity results when an antibody is transferred artificially.
      a. Naturally acquired active immunity: results from having the disease and recovering successfully
      b. Naturally acquired passive immunity: antibodies obtained through placenta or breast milk
      c. Artificially acquired active immunity: conferred by immunization with an antigen
      d. Artificially acquired passive immunity: antibodies transferred from sensitized person (e.g., immune serum globulin [gamma globulin])

## Components of Immune Response

A. Located throughout the body
B. Organs include thymus, bone marrow, lymph nodes, spleen, tonsils, appendix, Peyer's patches of small intestine.
C. Main cell types are WBCs (especially lymphocytes, plasma cells, and macrophages); all originate from the same stem cell in bone marrow, then differentiate into separate types.
   1. Granulocytes
      a. Eosinophils: increase with allergies and parasites
      b. Basophils: contain histamine and increase with allergy and anaphylaxis
      c. Neutrophils: involved in phagocytosis
   2. Monocytes (macrophages) (e.g., histiocytes, Kupffer cells): involved in phagocytosis
   3. Lymphocytes (T cells and B cells): involved in cellular and humoral immunity

## Classification of Immune Responses

### Cellular Immunity

A. Mediated by T cells: persist in tissues for months or years
B. Functions: transplant rejection, delayed hypersensitivity, tuberculin reactions, tumor surveillance/destruction, intracellular infections

### Humoral Immunity

A. Mediated by B cells
   1. Production of circulating antibodies (gamma globulin)
   2. Only survive for days
B. Functions: bacterial phagocytosis, bacterial lysis, virus and toxin neutralization, anaphylaxis, allergic hay fever and asthma

**Table 4-1** Alterations in Immune Functioning

| Immune Function | Hypofunction | Hyperfunction |
|---|---|---|
| Defense | Immunosuppression with increased susceptibility to infection; includes disorders such as neutropenia, AIDS, immunosuppression secondary to drugs and hypo- or agammaglobulinemia. | Inappropriate and abnormal response to external antigens; an allergy. |
| Homeostasis | No known effect | Abnormal response where antibodies react against normal tissues and cells; an *autoimmune disease*. |
| Surveillance | Inability of the immune system to perceive and respond to mutated cells, suspected mechanism in cancer. | No known effect. |

# NUTRITION

## Basic Concepts

### Principles

A. Essential nutrients: carbohydrates, fats, proteins, minerals, vitamins, and water that must be supplied to the body in specified amounts.

B. Foods: the sources of nutrients, provide energy to help build, repair, and maintain tissue and regulate body processes.

C. Malnutrition: results from deficiency, excess, or imbalance of required nutrients.

### Carbohydrates (Sugars and Starches)

A. Major source of food energy; 4 kcal/g; composed of carbon, hydrogen, and oxygen

B. Classification
1. Monosaccharides: simplest form of carbohydrate
   a. Glucose (dextrose): found chiefly in fruits and vegetables; oxidized for immediate energy
   b. Fructose: found in honey and fruits
   c. Galactose: not free in nature; part of milk sugar
2. Disaccharides: double sugars
   a. Sucrose: found in table sugar, syrups, and some fruits and vegetables
   b. Lactose: found in milk
   c. Maltose: intermediate product in the hydrolysis of starch
3. Polysaccharides: composed of many glucose molecules
   a. Starch: found in cereal grains, potatoes, root vegetables, and legumes
   b. Glycogen: synthesized and stored in the liver and skeletal muscles
   c. Cellulose, hemicellulose, pectins, gums, and mucilages: indigestible polysaccharides
4. Dietary fiber: includes several polysaccharides plus other substances that are not digestible by GI enzymes.
   a. Dietary fiber (roughage) holds water so that stools are soft and bulky; increases motility of the small and large intestine and decreases transit time; reduces intraluminal pressure in the colon.
   b. Sources: wheat bran, unrefined cereals, whole wheat, raw fruits and vegetables, dried fruits.

C. Functions of carbohydrates
1. Cheapest and most abundant source of energy; only source of energy for central nervous system
2. To spare protein for tissue building when sufficient carbohydrate is present
3. Necessary for the complete oxidation of fats (to prevent ketosis)

D. Dietary sources: grains, fruits, vegetables, nuts, milk, sugars ("empty calories," contain few nutrients)

### Lipids (Fats)

A. Most concentrated source of energy in foods; 9 kcal/g; contain carbon, hydrogen, oxygen

B. Include fats, oils, resins, waxes, and fatlike substances such as glycerides, phospholipids, sterols, and lipoproteins

C. Fatty acids
1. Saturated fatty acids: usually solid at room temperature; predominantly present in animal fats
2. Monounsaturated fatty acids: present in oleic acid found in olive oil, peanut oil
3. Polyunsaturated fatty acids: usually liquid at room temperature; predominantly present in plant fats and fish
4. Essential fatty acids: cannot be manufactured by the body (e.g., linoleic fatty acid)
5. Nonessential fatty acids: can be synthesized by the body

D. Functions of lipids
1. Most concentrated source of energy
2. Insulation and padding of body organs
3. Component of the cell membrane
4. Carrier of the fat-soluble vitamins A, D, E, K
5. Help maintain body temperature

E. Dietary sources: oil from seeds of grains, nuts, vegetables; milk fat, butter, cream cheese; fat in meat; lard, bacon fat; fish oil; egg yolk

F. Cholesterol: essential constituent of body tissues
1. A component of cell membranes
2. A precursor of steroid hormones
3. Can be manufactured in the body
4. Present in animal fats
5. Dietary sources: egg yolk, brains, liver, butter, cream, cheese, shellfish

G. Indications for low-fat diet
1. Cardiovascular disease
2. Gallbladder disease
3. Malabsorption syndromes, cystic fibrosis, pancreatitis

### Proteins

A. Organic compounds that may be composed of hundreds of amino acids; 4 kcal/g; contain nitrogen in addition to carbon, hydrogen, and oxygen

B. Classification
1. Complete protein: contains all the essential amino acids; usually from animal food sources.
2. Incomplete protein: lacks one or more essential amino acids; usually from plant food sources.

C. Amino acids
1. Essential amino acids: eight amino acids that cannot be synthesized in the body and must be taken in food.
2. Nonessential amino acids: 12 amino acids that can be synthesized in the body.
D. Functions of proteins
1. Necessary for growth and continuous replacement of cells throughout life
2. Play a role in the immune processes
3. Participate in regulating body processes such as fluid balance, muscle contraction, mineral balance, iron transport, buffer actions
4. Provide energy if necessary
E. Dietary sources: meat, fish, eggs, milk, cheese, poultry, grains, nuts, legumes (soybeans, lentils, peanuts, peanut butter)
F. Deficiencies
1. Conditions
a. Kwashiorkor (protein depletion that develops over short period of time)
b. Marasmus (severe tissue wasting from inadequate intake of calories and proteins)
2. Manifestations
a. Generalized weakness
b. Weight loss
c. Lowered resistance to infection
d. Slow wound healing and prolonged recovery from illness
e. Growth failure
f. Brain damage to fetus or infant
g. Edema due to decreased albumin in blood
h. Anemia in severe deficiency
i. Fatty infiltration of liver and liver damage
3. Risk factors
a. Chronically ill
b. Elderly on fixed incomes
c. Low-income families
d. Strict vegetarians
G. Indications for high-protein diet
1. Burns, massive wounds when tissue building desired
2. Mild to moderate liver disease for organ repair when liver is still functioning
3. Malabsorption syndromes such as cystic fibrosis
4. Undernutrition
5. Pregnancy to meet needs of mother and developing fetus
6. Pregnancy-induced hypertension to replace protein lost in urine
7. Nephrosis to replace protein lost in urine
8. Deficiencies
H. Indications for low-protein diet
1. Liver failure (liver does not metabolize protein causing nitrogen toxicity to brain)
2. Kidney failure (kidneys can no longer excrete nitrogenous waste products causing toxic nitrogen levels in the brain)

I. Nursing interventions for clients needing low-protein diet
1. Increase carbohydrates so energy needs will be met by carbohydrates, not by breakdown of proteins
2. Protein intake that is allowed will be complete proteins (animal sources)

## Energy Metabolism

A. Measurement of energy expressed in terms of heat units called kilocalories (kcal): amount of heat required to raise 1 kg water by 1°C
B. Energy expenditure
1. Basal metabolism
a. Amount of energy expended to carry on the involuntary work of the body while at rest
b. Factors influencing basal metabolic rate (BMR): body surface area, sex, age, body temperature, hormones, pregnancy, fasting, malnutrition
2. Physical activity: amount of energy expended depends upon the type of activity, the length of time involved, and the weight of the person
C. Factors determining total energy needs
1. Amount necessary for BMR
2. Amount required for physical activity
3. Specific dynamic action of food ingested
4. Growth
5. Climate

## Minerals

Inorganic compounds that yield no energy; essential structural components involved in many body processes (see Table 4-2).

## Vitamins

Organic compounds necessary in small quantities for cellular functions of the body; do not give energy; necessary in many enzyme systems (see Table 4-3).
A. Fat-soluble vitamins (A, D, E, K): can be stored in body; toxic in large amounts.
B. Water-soluble vitamins ($B_1$ [thiamin]; $B_2$ [riboflavin]; $B_6$ [pyridoxine]; $B_{12}$ [hydroxycobalamin]; C [ascorbic acid]; folacin; niacin): cannot be stored in body so must be ingested daily; dissolves in cooking water, toxicity unlikely.

## Water

A. Distribution: present in all body tissues; accounts for 50–60% total body weight in adults and 70–75% in infants.
1. Intracellular fluid: exists within the cells.
2. Extracellular fluid: includes plasma fluid, interstitial fluid, lymph, and secretions.

Table 4-2 Minerals

| Mineral | Functions | Deficiency Syndrome | Food Sources | Comments |
|---------|-----------|---------------------|--------------|----------|
| Calcium | Development of bones and teeth<br>Transmission of nerve impulses<br>Muscle contraction<br>Permeability of cell membrane<br>Catalyze thrombin formation<br>Maintenance of normal heart rhythm | Rickets, osteoporosis, osteomalacia, stunted growth, fragile bones, tetany, occurs when parathyroids removed | Dairy products; dark green leafy vegetables; broccoli; canned-fish with bones (sardines, salmon) clams, oysters; cooked dried beans; peas | Needs vitamin D, magnesium, and parathormone for utilization. Acid, lactose, and vitamin D favor absorption. Inverse relationship to phosphorus. |
| Phosphorus | Development of bones and teeth<br>Transfer of energy in cells (ATP)<br>Cell permeability<br>Buffer salts<br>Component in phospholipids | Rickets, stunted growth, poor bone mineralization, muscle weakness | Milk, cheese, meat, fish, poultry, eggs, legumes, nuts, whole-grain cereals | Factors that affect calcium absorption also affect phosphorus. Inverse relationship to calcium. |
| Magnesium | Constituent of bones and teeth<br>Cation in intracellular fluid<br>Muscle and nerve irritability<br>Activate enzymes in carbohydrate metabolism | Tremor observed in severe alcoholism, diabetic acidosis, severe renal disease | Milk, cheese, meat, nuts, legumes, green leafy vegetables, whole-grain cereals, seafood | Absorption similar to calcium. |
| Sulfur | Constituent of keratin in hair, skin, and nails<br>Detoxification reactions<br>Constituent of thiamin, biotin, insulin, coenzyme A, melanin, glutathione | None | Protein foods, eggs, meat, fish, poultry, milk, cheese, nuts | Diet adequate in protein provides sufficient sulfur. |
| Iron | Constituent of hemoglobin, myoglobin, oxidative enzymes | Anemia | Liver, organ meats, meat, poultry, egg yolk, whole-grain cereals, legumes, dark green vegetables, dried fruit | Ascorbic acid enhances absorption. |
| Iodine | Constituent of thyroxine<br>Regulate rate of energy metabolism | Simple goiter, creatinism, myxedema | Iodized salt, seafood | Allergies to iodine-rich foods may indicate allergy to iodine dyes used in diagnostic tests. |
| Sodium | Principle cation of extracellular fluid<br>Osmotic pressure<br>Fluid balance<br>Regulate nerve irritability and muscle contraction<br>Pump for active transport of glucose | Rare, seen in persons with SIADH | Table salt, processed meats, canned soups and vegetables | Diet usually provides excess.<br>Increase in clients with cystic fibrosis and persons taking lithium.<br>Decrease intake in clients with hypertension, congestive heart failure, renal failure, and edema. |

*(continues)*

**Table 4-2** Minerals (continued)

| Mineral | Functions | Deficiency Syndrome | Food Sources | Comments |
|---|---|---|---|---|
| Potassium | Principal cation of intracellular fluid<br>Osmotic pressure<br>Fluid balance<br>Acid-base balance<br>Regular heart rhythm<br>Nerve irritability and muscle contraction | Muscle weakness, arrhythmias<br>Deficiency may occur with diabetic acidosis<br>Deficiency may occur with thiazide and loop diuretics | Oranges, bananas, dried fruits, melons, apricots, most fruits and vegetables, whole-grain cereals | Readily absorbed.<br>Increase intake in clients taking thiazide and loop diuretics.<br>Decrease intake for clients in renal failure. |
| Chlorine | Chief anion of extracellular fluid<br>Constituent of gastric juice<br>Acid-base balance<br>Activate salivary amylase | Seen only after prolonged vomiting | Table salt, processed meats, fish, fruits (dates, bananas) | Rapidly absorbed. |

**Table 4-3** Vitamins

| Vitamin | Functions | Deficiency Syndrome | Food Sources | Comments |
|---|---|---|---|---|
| *Fat Soluble*<br>Vitamin A (retinol) | Maintenance of mucous membranes<br>Visual acuity in dim light, growth and bone development | Night blindness, xerophthalmia, keratinization of epithelium, poor bone and tooth development | Fish liver oils, liver, butter, cream, whole milk, egg yolk, dark green vegetables, yellow vegetables, yellow fruits, fortified margarine | Bile necessary for absorption.<br>Large amounts are toxic. |
| Vitamin D (cholecalciferol) | Increase absorption of calcium and phosphorus<br>Bone mineralization | Rickets, osteomalacia, enlarged joints, muscle spasms, delayed dentition | Fish liver oils, fortified milk | Synthesized in skin by activity of ultraviolet light.<br>Large amounts are toxic. |
| Vitamin E (tocopherol) | Reduces oxidation of vitamin A, phospholipids, and polyunsaturated fatty acids | Hemolysis of red blood cells, deficiency not likely | Vegetable oils, wheat germ, nuts, legumes, green leafy vegetables | Not toxic. |
| Vitamin K (phylloquinone) | Formation of prothrombin and other clotting proteins | Prolonged clotting time, hemorrhagic disease in newborn and liver disease | Green leafy vegetables, cabbage, liver, alfalfa | Bile necessary for absorption; injectable form may be given in gallbladder and liver disease. Large amounts are toxic. |
| *Water Soluble*<br>Vitamin $B_1$ (thiamine) | Involved in carbohydrate metabolism<br>Thiamine pyrophosphate (TPP) | Beriberi, mental depression, polyneuritis, cardiac failure | Enriched cereals, whole grains, meat, organ meats, pork, fish, poultry, legumes, nuts | Very little storage. |
| Vitamin $B_2$ (riboflavin) | Coenzyme for transfer and removal of hydrogen<br>Flavin adenine dinucleotide (FAD) | Cheilosis, photophobia, burning and itching of eyes, sore tongue and mouth | Milk, eggs, organ meats, green leafy vegetables | Limited storage. |

(continues)

**Table 4-3** Vitamins (continued)

| Vitamin | Functions | Deficiency Syndrome | Food Sources | Comments |
|---------|-----------|---------------------|--------------|----------|
| Vitamin $B_6$ (pyridoxine, pyridoxal, pyridoxamine) | Coenzyme for transamination, transsulfuration, and decarboxylation | Convulsions, dermatitis, nervous irritability | Meat, poultry, fish, vegetables, potatoes | Converts glycogen to glucose. Given with isoniazid (INH) to prevent INH side effect of peripheral neuropathy. |
| Vitamin $B_{12}$ (hydroxy-cobalamin) | Formation of mature red blood cells Synthesis of DNA and RNA | Pernicious anemia, neurologic degeneration, macrocytic anemia | Animal foods only | Intrinsic factor is necessary for absorption. |
| Vitamin C (ascorbic acid) | Synthesis of collagen Formation of intercellular cement Facilitation of iron absorption | Scurvy, bleeding gums, poor wound healing, cutaneous hemorrhage, capillary fragility | Citrus fruits, tomatoes, melon, raw cabbage, broccoli, strawberries | Most easily destroyed vitamin. Very little storage in body. |
| Folacin (folic acid) | Maturation of red blood cells, interrelated with vitamin $B_{12}$ | Megaloblastic anemia, tropical sprue | Organ meats, muscle meats, poultry, fish, eggs, green leafy vegetables | Ascorbic acid necessary for utilization. |
| Niacin (nicotinamide) | Coenzyme to accept and transfer hydrogen, coenzyme for glycolysis | Pellagra, dermatitis, neurologic degeneration, glossitis, diarrhea | Meat, poultry, fish, whole grains, enriched breads, nuts, legumes | Amino acid tryptophan is a precursor. |

B. Functions: the medium of all body fluids
   1. Necessary for many biologic reactions.
   2. Acts as a solvent.
   3. Transports nutrients to cells and eliminates waste.
   4. Body lubricant.
   5. Regulates body temperature.
C. Sources
   1. Ingestion of water and other beverages
   2. Water content of food eaten
   3. Water resulting from food oxidation
D. Recommended daily intake
   1. Replacement of losses through the kidneys, lungs, skin, and bowel
   2. Thirst usually a good guide
   3. Approximately 48 oz/day of water from all sources is adequate; requirement is higher if physical activity is strenuous or if sweating is profuse.

## Dietary Guides

A. Food pyramid
   1. Foods are grouped by composition and nutrient value: grains; vegetable group; fruit group; meat, poultry, fish, dry beans, eggs and nut group; and milk, yogurt and cheese group.
   2. Greater emphasis on fruits and vegetables with less emphasis on meats and fats than with basic four.
   3. Recommends using fats and sweets sparingly.

B. Recommended daily allowances: established by the Food and Nutrition Board of the National Academy of Science; recommended nutrient intake is provided for infants, children, men, women, pregnant and lactating women; recommendations are stated for protein, kcal, and most vitamins and minerals.
C. Food composition tables: helpful in calculating the nutritive value of the daily diet; list nutrient content of foods.
D. Height and weight charts: ideal or desirable body weight for both men and women at specified heights with a small, medium, or large frame.
E. Exchange lists for meal planning
   1. Foods are separated into six exchange lists.
   2. Specific foods on each list are approximately equal in carbohydrate, protein, fat, and kcal content.
   3. Individual foods on the same list may be exchanged for each other at the same meals.
   4. Food lists are helpful in planning diets for weight control or diabetes.

# Nutritional Assessment

## Health History

A. Presenting problem
   1. Weight changes
      a. Usual body weight 20% above or below normal standards.

**b.** Recent loss or gain of 10% of usual body weight.
   2. Appetite changes: may increase or decrease from usual.
   3. Food intolerances: allergies, fluids, fat, salt, seafood
   4. Difficulty swallowing
   5. Dyspepsia or indigestion
   6. Bowel dysfunction: record frequency, consistency, color of stools.
      **a.** Constipation
      **b.** Diarrhea
**B.** Lifestyle: eating behaviors such as fast foods, "junk foods," and skipping meals; cultural/religious concerns (vegetarian, kosher foods, exclusion of certain food groups); alcohol, socioeconomic status, living conditions (alone or with family).
**C.** Use of medications: vitamin supplements, antacids, antidiarrheals, laxatives, diuretics, antihypertensives, immunosuppressants, oral contraceptives, antibiotics, antidepressants, digitalis, anti-inflammatory agents, catabolic steroids.
**D.** Medical history: gastrointestinal diseases; endocrine diseases; hyperlipidemia; coronary artery disease; malabsorption syndrome; circulatory problems or heart failure; cancer; radiation therapy; chronic lung, renal, or liver disease; food allergies; recent major surgery; eating disorders; obesity.
**E.** Family history: obesity, allergies, cardiovascular diseases, diabetes, thyroid disease.
**F.** Dietary history: evaluation of the nutritional adequacy of diet
   1. 24-hour recall
   2. Food diary for a given number of days

### Physical Examination

**A.** Assess for alertness and responsiveness
**B.** Record weight in relation to height, body build, and age
**C.** Inspect posture, muscle tone, skeleton for deformities
**D.** Elicit reflexes
**E.** Auscultate heart rate, rhythm; blood pressure
**F.** Inspect hair, skin, nails, oral mucosa, tongue, teeth
**G.** Inspect for swelling of legs or feet
**H.** Anthropometric measurements: indicators of available stores in muscle and fat compartments of body
   1. Height/weight ratio (Body Mass Index [BMI])
   2. Midarm muscle circumference
   3. Skinfold thickness (triceps, biceps, subscapular, abdominal, hip, pectoral, or calf)

### Laboratory/Diagnostic Tests

**A.** Blood studies: serum albumin, iron-binding capacity, hemoglobin, hematocrit, lymphocyte count, blood sugar, total cholesterol, high-density lipids, low-density lipids, triglycerides, serum electrolytes
**B.** Urine studies, urinalysis, glucose, ketones, albumin, 24-hour creatinine
**C.** Nitrogen balance studies
**D.** Feces, hair
**E.** Intradermal delayed hypersensitivity testing

## Analysis

Nursing diagnoses for the client with a nutritional dysfunction may include:
**A.** Imbalanced nutrition: less than body requirements
**B.** Imbalanced nutrition: more than body requirements
**C.** Risk for imbalanced nutrition: more than body requirements
**D.** Impaired oral mucous membrane
**E.** Self-care deficit, feeding
**F.** Disturbed sensory perceptions
**G.** Risk for impaired skin integrity
**H.** Impaired swallowing
**I.** Impaired tissue integrity
**J.** Activity intolerance
**K.** Disturbed body image
**L.** Constipation
**M.** Diarrhea
**N.** Deficient fluid volume
**O.** Excess fluid volume
**P.** Delayed growth and development
**Q.** Risk for infection
**R.** Deficient knowledge
**S.** Noncompliance

## Planning and Implementation

### Goals

**A.** Normal weight will be achieved and maintained.
**B.** Integrity of oral cavity will be maintained.
**C.** Client will feed self or receive help with feeding.
**D.** Normal skin integrity will be achieved/maintained.
**E.** Client will not aspirate.
**F.** Normal tissue integrity will be achieved/maintained.
**G.** Client will be able to exercise normally.
**H.** Client will maintain/develop satisfactory self-image.
**I.** Normal bowel functioning will be maintained.
**J.** Fluid and electrolyte balance will be achieved/maintained.
**K.** Client will have normal growth and development patterns.
**L.** Client will not develop infection.
**M.** Client will demonstrate knowledge of special dietary needs/prescriptions.
**N.** Client will comply with special diet.

# Interventions

## Care of the Client on a Special Diet

A. General information: therapeutic diets involve modifications of nutritional components necessitated by a client's disease state or nutritional status or to prepare a client for a procedure.

B. Nursing care in relation to special diets
   1. Assess client's mental, emotional, physical, and economic status; appropriateness of diet to client's condition; and ability to understand diet and comply with it.
   2. Maintain appropriate diet and teach client.
   3. Changing diet means changing lifelong patterns.
   4. Teach client importance of adhering to special diets that are long term.

## Weight Control Diets

A. Underweight: 10% or more below individual's ideal weight
   1. Causes: failure to ingest enough kcal, excess energy expenditure, irregular eating habits, GI disturbances, mouth sores, cancer, endocrine disorders, emotional disturbances, lack of education, economic problems.
   2. Treatment: diet counseling, correction of underlying disease, nutritional supplements, behavioral therapy, social service referral.

B. Overweight: 10% or more above individual's ideal weight

C. Obesity: 20% or more above individual's ideal weight
   1. Causes: overeating, underactivity, genetic factors, fat cell theory, alteration in hypothalamic function, endocrine disorders, emotional disturbances.
   2. Treatment: diet counseling, nutritionally balanced diet, behavior modification, increased physical activity, medical treatment of any underlying disease, appropriate referrals.

D. Nursing care
   1. Explain dietary instructions.
      a. Reducing fats and "empty calories" reduces caloric intake without sacrificing nutritional intake
      b. Increasing exercise increases metabolism
   2. Caution against fad diets that may be nutritionally inadequate.
   3. Encourage support groups if indicated.

## Diabetic Diet (Consistent carbohydrates)

A. Prescribed for clients with diabetes mellitus.

B. Purposes include: attain or maintain ideal body weight, ensure normal growth, maintain plasma glucose levels as close to normal as possible.

C. Principles
   1. Distribution of kcal: protein 12–20%; carbohydrates 55–60%; fats (unsaturated) 20–25%.
   2. Daily distribution of kcal: equally divided among breakfast, lunch, supper, snacks.
   3. Use foods high in fiber and complex carbohydrates.
   4. Avoid simple sugars, jams, honey, syrup, frosting.

D. Teach client to utilize exchange lists.

E. New recommendations include low-fat, high fiber diet.

## Low-Sodium Diet (No-added-salt diet)

A. Purpose is to restrict sodium intake to less than 2300 mg of sodium per day for clients with hypertension or cardiac disease.

B. One method is the DASH (Dietary Approaches to Stop Hypertension) Eating Plan.

C. Food choices
   1. Choose and prepare food with little salt.
   2. Continue to meet potassium requirement of 4700 mg/day.
   3. Avoid table salt, processed meats, canned soups, snack food containing salt.
   4. Teach client to read labels of prepared food.

## Protein-Modified Diets

A. Gluten-free diet
   1. Purpose is to eliminate gluten (a protein) from the diet.
   2. Indicated in malabsorption syndromes such as sprue and celiac disease.
   3. Eliminate all barley, rye, oats, and wheat (BROW).
   4. Avoid: cream sauces, breaded foods, cakes, breads, muffins.
   5. Allow corn, rice, and soy flour.
   6. Teach client to read labels of prepared foods.

B. PKU (Phenylketonuria) diet
   1. Purpose is to control intake of phenylalanine, an amino acid that cannot be metabolized.
   2. Diet will be prescribed until at least age 6 to prevent brain damage and mental retardation.
   3. Avoid: breads, meat, fish, poultry, cheeses, legumes, nuts, eggs.
   4. Give Lofenalac formula.
   5. Teach family to use low-protein flour for baking.
   6. Sugar substitutes such as Nutrasweet contain phenylalanine and must not be used.

C. Low-purine diet
   1. Indicated for gout, uric acid kidney stones, and uric acid retention.
   2. Purpose is to decrease the amount of purine, a precursor to uric acid.

3. Teach client to avoid: organ meats, other meats, fowl, fish and lobster, lentils, dried peas and beans, nuts, oatmeal, whole wheat.
4. Eggs are not high in purine.

## Fat-Restricted Diets

Purpose is to restrict amount of fats ingested for clients with chronic pancreatitis, malabsorption syndromes, gallbladder disease, cystic fibrosis, and hyperlipidemia, and to control weight.

## Bariatric Diet

A. Prescribed for clients after bariatric weight loss surgeries for obesity.
B. After surgery, small stomach will hold about 1 oz.
   1. First week: nutritious liquids; Second week: Pureed, high-protein foods
   2. Avoid high carbohydrates
   3. Possible complication: Dumping Syndrome (nausea, hypotension, hypoglycemia)
   4. Client is educated before surgery about post-operative diet.

## Renal Diet

A. Prescribed for clients with end-stage renal disease (ESRD).
B. Principles
   1. Prevent accumulation of protein waste between dialysis treatments.
   2. Potassium is restricted to 3000–4000 mg/day. (Restrict milk intake to ½ cup/day due to high potassium content.)
   3. Limit sodium to 3 grams/day (No-added-salt diet).
   4. Teach client to measure proper food choices and to measure fluid intake and output.

## Consistency Modifications

A. Clear liquid diet
   1. Purpose is to rest GI tract and maintain fluid balance.
   2. Indications include difficulty chewing or swallowing; before certain diagnostic tests to reduce fecal material; immediate postoperative period (until bowel sounds have returned) to maintain electrolyte balance; and nausea, vomiting, and diarrhea.
   3. Foods allowed: "see-through foods" include water, tea, broth, jello, apple juice, clear carbonated beverages, and frozen ice pops.
   4. Not nutritionally adequate.
B. Full liquid diet
   1. Used as a transition diet between clear liquid and soft diet; usually short term.
   2. Foods allowed: clear liquids, milk and milk products, all fruit juices, cooked and strained cereals.
   3. Can be nutritionally adequate.
C. Soft diet
   1. Used as a transition diet between full liquid and regular diet.
   2. Indications include postoperatively, mild GI disturbances, chewing difficulties from lack of teeth or oral surgery.
   3. Foods allowed: foods low in fiber, connective tissue and fat (full liquid diet, pureed vegetables, eggs cooked any way except fried, tender meat, potatoes, cooked fruit).
   4. Nutritionally adequate.
D. Bland diet
   1. Promotes healing of the gastric mucosa and is chemically and mechanically nonstimulating.
   2. Foods allowed: soft diet without spices.
E. Low-residue diet
   1. Residue is the indigestible substances left in digestive tract after food has been digested.
   2. Indications include colon, rectal, or perineal surgery to reduce pressure on the operative site; prior to examination of the lower bowel to enhance visualization; internal radiation for cancer of the cervix; Crohn's disease or regional enteritis; ulcerative colitis to reduce irritation of the large bowel; and diarrhea.
   3. Teach client to avoid foods high in fiber, foods having skins and seeds, and milk and milk products.

## Evaluation

A. Client's weight is within normal limits.
B. No lesions in oral cavity.
C. Client feeds self or receives needed assistance with feeding.
D. Skin and tissue integrity is maintained.
E. Client demonstrates ability to exercise.
F. Client makes positive statements about self-image.
G. Client's bowel functioning is normal.
H. Serum electrolytes are within normal limits.
I. Client will exhibit growth and development patterns appropriate for age.
J. Client shows no evidence of infection.
K. Client states reason for special diet.
L. Client describes foods allowed and not allowed on prescribed diet.
M. Client adheres to prescribed diet.

## Enteral Nutrition

Preferred method for nutritional support for the malnourished client whose GI system is intact.

## Oral Feeding

A. Always the first choice.
B. Oral formula supplements may be used between meals to provide added kcal and nutrients.
   1. Offer small quantities several times a day.
   2. Vary flavors, avoid taste fatigue.
   3. Chill and serve over ice.

## Tube Feeding

A. Used for clients who have a functioning GI tract but cannot ingest food orally
   1. Feeding tubes
      a. Short term: nasogastric tube
      b. Long term: esophagostomy, gastrostomy, or enterostomy tube
   2. Formulas: nutritionally adequate, tolerated by client, easily prepared, easily digested, usual concentration 1 kcal/mL
   3. Feeding schedules
      a. Intermittent: usually 4–6 times per day, volumes up to 400 mL, by slow gravity drip over 30–60 minutes
      b. Continuous: usually administered by pump through a duodenal or proximal jejunostomy feeding tube
   4. Nursing responsibilities
      a. Administer formulas at room temperature (refrigerate unused portion).
      b. Gradually increase rate and concentration until desired amount is attained if there are no signs of intolerance (e.g., gastric residual greater than 120 mL, nausea, vomiting, diarrhea, distention, diaphoresis, increased pulse, glycosuria, aspiration).
      c. Check tube placement and elevate head of bed (see also Nasogastric Tubes).
      d. Monitor I&O, serum electrolytes, fractional urines, serum glucose, daily weights; keep a stool record as well as an ongoing assessment of tolerance.

## Parenteral Nutrition

Nutrients are infused directly into a vein for clients who are unable to eat or digest food through the GI tract, who refuse to eat, or who have inadequate oral intake.

### Total Parenteral Nutrition (TPN)

A. Involves the infusion of nutrients through a central vein catheter. A central vein is needed because its larger caliber and higher blood flow will quickly dilute the hypertonic hyperalimentation solution to isotonic concentrations.
B. Hyperalimentation solutions
   1. Hypertonic glucose of 20–70%, amino acids, water, vitamins, and minerals with lipid emulsions given in a separate solution.
   2. Three-in-one solutions
      a. Lipids mixed with dextrose and amino acids in pharmacy.
      b. Prepared by pharmacy in a 3-liter container and administered over 24 hours.
C. Nursing responsibilities
   1. For details of nursing care of the client with a central venous line, see IV Therapy.
   2. Inspect solution before hanging.

a. Check for correct solution and additives against physician's order.
      b. Check expiration date.
      c. Observe fluid for cloudiness or floating particulate matter.
   3. Control flow rate of solution.
      a. Verify order and monitor flow rate.
      b. Administration via pump is required.
      c. Tubing with in-line filter is required.
      d. Never attempt to speed up or slow down infusion rate.
         1) Speeding up infusion causes large amounts of glucose to enter body, causing hyperosmolar state.
         2) Slowing down infusion can cause hypoglycemic state, as it takes time for the pancreas to adjust to reduced glucose level.
   4. Monitor fluid balance.
   5. Assess client for signs and symptoms of infection (fever, chills, elevated WBC count).
   6. Obtain fractional urines or Accu-Chek every 6 hours.
   7. Administer sliding scale insulin for hyperglycemia, as ordered.
   8. Provide psychological support.
   9. Encourage exercise regimen.

### IV Lipid Emulsions

A. May be given through a central vein or peripherally in order to prevent essential fatty acid deficiency in long-term TPN clients, or to provide supplemental kcal IV.
B. Nursing care
   1. Protect the stability of the emulsion.
      a. Administer in its own separate IV bottle and IV tubing, and piggyback the emulsion into the Y connector closest to the catheter insertion. Follow hospital policy and manufacturer's recommendations for specific products. Some hospital facilities combine TPN and lipid into one bag.
      b. Inspect solution for evidence of separation of oil, frothiness, inconsistency, particulate matter; discard solution if any of these signs of instability occur.
      c. Do *not* shake the bottle; this might cause aggregation of fat globules.
      d. Discard partially used bottles.
   2. Control the infusion rate accurately and safely.
      a. If using gravity method, lipid emulsion must hang higher than hyperalimentation to prevent backflow.
      b. Pump is preferred but may not be possible due to viscous nature of emulsion.
   3. Prevent and assess for adverse reactions.
      a. Administer slowly according to package insert over first 30 minutes; if no adverse reactions, increase rate to complete

infusion over the specified number of hours.

    **b.** Obtain baseline vital signs; repeat after first 30 minutes, and then every 4 hours until completion.

    **c.** Acute reactions may include: fever, chills, dyspnea, nausea, vomiting, headache, lethargy, syncope, chest or back pain, hypercoagulability, thrombocytopenia.

  **4.** Evaluate tolerance and client response.

### Peripheral Vein Parenteral Nutrition (PPN)

**A.** Can be used for short-term support, when the central vein is not available, and as a supplemental means of obtaining nutrients. Client must be able to tolerate a relatively high fluid volume.

**B.** Solution contains the same components as central vein therapy, but lower concentrations (less than 20% glucose).

**C.** Care is the same as for the client receiving hyperalimentation centrally.

**D.** Phlebitis and thrombosis are common and IV sites will need frequent changing.

# INFECTION

Infection is an invasion of the body by pathogenic organisms that multiply and produce injurious effects. Communicable disease is an infectious disease that may be transmitted from one person to another.

## Chain of Events

**A.** Causative agent: invading organism (e.g., bacteria, virus)

**B.** Reservoir: environment in which the invading organism lives and multiplies

**C.** Portal of exit: mode of escape from reservoir (e.g., respiratory tract, GI tract)

**D.** Mode of transmission: method by which invading organism is transported to new host (e.g., direct contact, air, food)

**E.** Portal of entry: means by which organism enters new host (e.g., respiratory tract, broken skin)

**F.** Susceptible host: susceptibility determined by factors such as number of invading organisms, duration of exposure, age, state of health, nutritional status

## Nursing Responsibilities in Prevention of Spread of Infection

**A.** Maintain an environment that is clean, dry, and well ventilated.

**B.** Use proper handwashing before and after client contact and after contact with contaminated material.

**C.** Disinfect and handle wastes and contaminated materials properly.

**D.** Prevent transmission of infectious droplets.

  **1.** Teach clients to cover mouth and nose when sneezing or coughing.

  **2.** Place contaminated tissues and articles in paper bag before disposing.

**E.** Institute proper isolation techniques as required by specific disease

**F.** Use surgical aseptic technique when appropriate: caring for open wounds, irrigating, or entering sterile cavities.

**G.** Practice standard precautions when caring for all clients regardless of their diagnosis in order to minimize contact with blood and body fluids and prevent the transmission of specific infections such as hepatitis B and human immunodeficiency virus (HIV).

  **1.** Hands must always be washed before and after contact with clients even when gloves have been used.

  **2.** If hands come in contact with blood, body fluids, or human tissue they should be immediately washed with soap and water.

  **3.** Gloves should be worn before touching blood or body fluids, mucous membranes, or nonintact skin.

  **4.** Gloves should be changed between each client contact and as soon as possible if torn.

  **5.** Wear masks and protective eyewear during procedures that are likely to generate splashes of blood or other body fluids.

  **6.** Wear gowns during procedures that are likely to generate splashes of blood or other body fluids and when cleaning spills from incontinent clients or changing soiled linen.

  **7.** Disposable masks should be used when performing CPR.

  **8.** Dispose of used needles properly. They should be promptly placed in a puncture-resistant container (i.e., sharps container). They *should not* be recapped, bent, broken, or removed from syringes.

# PAIN

Pain is an unpleasant sensation, entirely subjective, that produces discomfort, distress, or suffering. "Pain is what the person says it is and exists when the person says it does." It is considered the "fifth vital sign" and is included in the routine patient assessment (Daniels, et al.)

## Gate Control Theory

**A.** Substantia gelatinosa in the dorsal horn of the spinal cord acts as a gate mechanism that can close to keep pain impulses from reaching the brain, or can open to allow pain impulses to ascend to the brain.

**B.** Most pain impulses are conducted over small-diameter nerve fibers; if predominant nerve message is pain, the gate opens and allows pain impulses to reach the brain.

**C.** The gate can be closed by conflicting impulses from the skin conducted over large-diameter nerve fibers, by impulses from the reticular formation in the brainstem, or by impulses from the entire cerebral cortex or thalamus.

## Acute Pain and Chronic Pain

**A.** Acute pain
1. Short duration; may last from split second to about 6 months.
2. Serves the purpose of warning the client that damage or injury has occurred in the body that requires treatment.
3. Subsides as healing occurs.
4. Usually associated with autonomic nervous system symptoms, e.g., increased pulse and blood pressure, sweating, pallor.

**B.** Chronic pain
1. Prolonged duration; lasts for 6 months or longer.
2. Serves no useful purpose.
3. Persists long after injury has healed.
4. Rarely accompanied by autonomic nervous system activity.

## Assessment of Pain

See Table 4-4.

## General Nursing Interventions

**A.** Establish nurse-client relationship.
1. Let the client know that you believe that his pain is real.

---

**Table 4–4** Pain Assessment

*Influencing factors*
- Past experience with pain
- Age (tolerance generally increases with age)
- Culture and religious beliefs
- Level of anxiety
- Physical state (fatigue or chronic illness may decrease tolerance)

*Characteristics of pain*
- Location
- Quality
- Intensity
- Timing and duration
- Precipitating factors
- Aggravating factors
- Alleviating factors
- Interference with activities of daily living
- Patterns of response

---

2. Respect the client's attitudes and behavioral responses to pain using a standardized pain scale appropriate to age and condition.
3. Document effectiveness of interventions in a timely manner.

**B.** Assess characteristics of pain and evaluate client's response to interventions.

**C.** Promote rest and relaxation.
1. Prevent fatigue.
2. Teach relaxation techniques, e.g., slow, rhythmic breathing, guided imagery.

**D.** Institute comfort measures.
1. Positioning: support body parts.
2. Decrease noxious stimuli such as noise or bright lights.

**E.** Provide cutaneous stimulation: massage, pressure, baths, vibration, heat, cold packs; increased input of large-diameter fibers closes gate.

**F.** Relieve anxiety and fears.
1. Spend time with client.
2. Offer reassurance, explanations.

**G.** Provide distraction and diversion, e.g., music, puzzles.

**H.** Administer pain medication as needed.
1. Administer pain medication in early stages before pain becomes severe.
2. Administer pain medication prior to procedure that produces discomfort.
3. If pain is present most of the day, a preventative approach may be used, e.g., an around-the-clock schedule may be ordered in place of a prn schedule.
4. Document effectiveness of intervention.

**I.** Teach client about pain and pain control measures, e.g., relaxation techniques, cutaneous stimulation.

## Specific Medical and Surgical Therapies for Pain

See also Narcotic and Nonnarcotic Analgesics in Unit 2.

### Nonnarcotic Analgesics

**A.** Salicylates (ASA, aspirin [Ecotrin] choline magnesium trisalicylate [Trillisate], diflunisal [Dolobid], salsalate [Disalcid])
**B.** Acetaminophen (Datril, Tylenol)
**C.** Nonsteroidal anti-inflammatory drugs (NSAIDs: ibuprofen [Motrin], indomethacin [Indocin], piroxicam [Feldene]) (See Table 2-5).

### Adjuvants

**A.** Includes several classes of drugs that may either:
1. Potentiate the effects of narcotic or nonnarcotic analgesics, e.g., hydroxyzine (Vistaril, Atarax)

2. Have independent analgesic properties in certain situations, e.g., tricyclic antidepressants such as amitriptyline (Elavil) for neuropathic pain
3. Help control signs and symptoms associated with pain, e.g., anxiety, depression, nausea, and insomnia

## Patient-Controlled Analgesia (PCA)

A. Type of intravenous pump that allows the client to administer narcotic analgesic (e.g., morphine) on demand within preset dose and frequency limits.
B. Goal is to achieve more constant level of analgesia as compared to prn IM injections; also, in general, causes less sedation and lower risk of respiratory depression.
C. Used most often for postoperative pain management; also used for intractable pain in terminal illness.
D. PCA pump may be used solely on PCA mode or may be combined with a continuous basal mode where client is receiving continuous infusion of narcotic in addition to self-administered bolus injections.
E. The dose of the analgesic bolus and the time interval between boluses (lockout period) is preset on the pump by the RN according to physician's orders.
F. Nursing Interventions
   1. Instruct client in use of PCA pump
      a. Demonstrate how to push control button.
      b. Explain concept of client-controlled analgesia.
   2. Assess client's level of consciousness, respiratory rate, and degree of pain relief frequently.
   3. Keep control button within client reach.
   4. Educate the family to contact the nurse if client's pain is not controlled, instead of family members pushing the button.

## Intraspinal Narcotic Infusion

A. Involves intraspinal infusion of narcotics or local anesthetic agents for relief of acute or chronic pain.
B. Medication is infused through catheter placed in the subarachnoid (intrathecal) or epidural space in the thoracic or lumbar area.
C. Repeated injections of narcotics produce analgesia without many of the side effects associated with systemic narcotics (e.g., sedation).
D. Indications
   1. Temporary intraspinal narcotic therapy is used most frequently for postoperative pain.
   2. For chronic pain, e.g., management of chronic cancer pain, the catheter may be tunneled under the skin and implanted subcutaneously in the abdomen; an implantable infusion device may be used to provide continuous narcotic infusion.

E. Nursing interventions
   1. Monitor client closely for respiratory depression especially during initiation of treatment. (May be reversed with naloxone [Narcan]).
   2. Assess for other side effects:
      a. Urinary retention: Foley catheter may be used in post-op client until infusion is discontinued
      b. Pruritus: may be treated with antihistamine or medication rate reduction
      c. Nausea and vomiting
   3. Check insertion site frequently for signs of infection.

## Electrical Stimulation Techniques for Pain Control

A. Transcutaneous electrical nerve stimulator (TENS)
   1. Noninvasive alternative to traditional methods of pain relief
   2. Used in treating acute pain (e.g., post-op pain) and chronic pain (e.g., chronic low back pain)
   3. Consists of impulse generator connected by wires to electrodes on skin; produces tingling, buzzing sensation in the area.
   4. Mechanism based on gate-control theory: electrical impulse stimulates large diameter nerve fibers to "close the gate."
   5. Nursing responsibilities
      a. Do not place electrodes over incision site, broken skin, carotid sinus, eyes, laryngeal or pharyngeal muscles.
      b. Do not use in client with cardiac pacemaker.
      c. Provide skin care.
         1) Remove electrodes once a day; wash area with soap and water and air dry.
         2) Wipe area with skin prep pad before reapplying electrode.
         3) Assess area for signs of redness; reposition electrodes if redness persists for more than 30 minutes.
B. Dorsal column stimulator
   1. Used in selected clients for whom conventional methods of pain relief have not been effective.
   2. Electrode is surgically placed over the dorsal column of the spinal cord via laminectomy; connected by wires to a transmitter that may be worn externally or be implanted subcutaneously.

## Neurosurgical Procedures for Pain Control

A. Performed for persistent intractable pain of high intensity
B. Involves surgical destruction of nerve pathways to block transmission of pain

C. Types
1. Neurectomy: interruption of cranial or peripheral nerves by incision or injection
2. Rhizotomy: interruption of posterior nerve root close to the spinal cord
   a. Laminectomy is necessary.
   b. Results in permanent loss of sensation and position sense in affected parts.
3. Chordotomy: interruption of pain-conducting pathways within the spinal cord
   a. Laminectomy usually required.
   b. May be done by percutaneous needle insertion.
   c. Interrupts conduction of pain and temperature sense in affected parts.
4. Sympathectomy: interruption of afferent pathways in the sympathetic division of the autonomic nervous system; used to control pain from causalgia and peripheral vascular disease.
D. Nursing responsibilities
1. Provide pre- and post-op care for a laminectomy.
2. Assess extremities for sensation (e.g., touch, pain, temperature, pressure, position sense) and movement.
3. Provide safety measures to protect client from injury and carefully monitor skin for signs of damage or pressure.
4. Teach client ways to compensate for loss of sensation in affected parts.
   a. Visually inspect skin for signs of injury or pressure.
   b. Check temperature of bath water.
   c. Avoid use of hot water bottles, heating pads.
   d. Avoid extremes of temperature.

## Acupuncture

A. A Chinese technique of pain control by insertion of fine needles at various points on the body to promote the flow of chi (life energy).
B. Based on Eastern philosophy where insertion of needles is thought to block energy flow and restore the body's harmony
C. Mechanism of action: two theories
1. Trigger points: the needles stimulate hypersensitive areas in muscle that produce local and referred pain. Extinction of the trigger point alleviates the referred pain.
2. Endorphin system: needle insertion activates production of endorphins (body's natural opiates).
D. Acupressure: a less invasive variation; uses finger pressure and massage

## Hypnosis

A. Has been used in dental procedures, labor and delivery, pain control in cancer.

B. Mechanism is thought to be related to positive suggestions that alter client's perception of pain.

## Behavioral Techniques

A. Types
1. Operant conditioning: based on decreasing positive reinforcement for pain behaviors
2. Biofeedback: teaches clients to control physiologic responses to pain (e.g., muscle tension, heart rate, blood pressure) and to replace them with a state of relaxation.
B. Work best in conjunction with other types of pain management and stress reduction techniques.

# FLUIDS AND ELECTROLYTES

## Basic Principles

### Fluids

A. Water constitutes over 50% of individual's weight; largest single component.
B. Body water divided into two compartments
1. Intracellular: within cells
2. Extracellular: outside cells, further divided into interstitial and intravascular fluid
C. Fluids in two compartments move among cells, tissue spaces, and plasma.

### Electrolytes

A. Salts or minerals in extracellular or intracellular body fluids
B. If positively charged, called cations; if negatively charged, called anions
C. Common electrolytes and normal blood values
1. Sodium (Na)—135–148 mEq/liter
2. Potassium (K)—3.5–5 mEq/liter
3. Calcium (Ca)—8.5–10.5 mg/dL
4. Magnesium (Mg)—1.8–2.7 mEq/liter
5. Chloride (Cl)—98–106 mEq/liter

## Movement of Fluids and Electrolytes

A. Diffusion: movement of particles from an area of greater concentration to an area of lesser concentration as part of random activity
B. Active transport: movement across cell membranes requiring energy from an outside source
C. Osmosis: movement of water through a semipermeable membrane
D. Osmolality: concentration of body fluids

## Fluid and Electrolyte Imbalances

See Table 4-5.
A. Hypovolemia: extracellular fluid volume deficit
B. Hypervolemia: extracellular fluid volume excess

**Table 4-5** Fluid and Electrolyte Imbalances

| Imbalance | Causes | Assessment Findings | Nursing Interventions |
|---|---|---|---|
| Hypovolemia (extracellular fluid volume deficit) | Hemorrhage, diarrhea, vomiting, kidney disease, diaphoresis, burns, fever, draining fistulas, sequestration of fluids (peritonitis, edema associated with burns) | Nausea and vomiting, weakness, weight loss, anorexia, longitudinal wrinkles of the tongue, dry skin and mucous membranes, decreased fullness of neck veins, postural hypotension, oliguria to anuria, shock | Measure I&O. Weigh daily. Monitor closely and regulate isotonic IV infusion. Monitor blood pressure (determine lying down, sitting, and standing). Report urine output less than 30 mL/hr. Carefully assess skin and mucous membranes. Monitor for signs of shock. |
| Hypervolemia (extracellular fluid volume excess) | Excess or too rapid administration of any isotonic solution; side effect of corticosteroid administration; cardiac, liver, or renal disease; cerebral damage; stress | Weight gain, pitting edema, dyspnea, cough, diaphoresis, frothy or pink-tinged sputum, edema of the eyelids, distended neck veins, elevated blood pressure, moist rales (crackles) | Weigh daily. Measure I&O. Regulate IV fluids/administration of diuretics strictly and monitor carefully. Monitor abdominal girth. Assess for pitting edema. Restrict sodium and water intake. |
| Water excess syndromes | Excessive intake of water, inability to excrete water due to kidney or brain damage, excessive administration of electrolyte-free solutions, poor salt intake, use of diuretics, irrigation of nasogastric tube with plain water, administration of excessive amount of ice chips to a vomiting client or one with a nasogastric tube | Polyuria (in absence of renal disease), oliguria (with renal disease), twitching, hyper irritability, disorientation, coma, convulsions, abdominal cramps | Measure I&O. Weigh daily. Restrict oral and IV intake. Replace fluid losses with isotonic solutions. Use normal saline solution for nasogastric tube irrigation. |
| Water deficit syndromes | Increased water output due to watery diarrhea, diabetic acidosis, excess TPN; dysphagia; impaired thirst mechanism; coma; general debility; diaphoresis; excess protein intake without sufficient water intake | Thirst, poor skin turgor, dry skin and mucous membranes, dry furrowed tongue, sunken eyeballs, weight loss, elevated temperature, apprehension, oliguria to anuria | Measure I&O. Weigh daily. Assess skin frequently. Ensure that clients with a high solute intake receive adequate water. Assess vital signs frequently, particularly temperature. Monitor TPN infusions accurately. |
| Hyperkalemia | Renal insufficiency, adrenocortical insufficiency, cellulose damage (burns), infection, acidotic states, rapid infusion of IV solutions with potassium, overzealous administration of potassium-conserving diuretics | Thready, slow pulse; shallow breathing; nausea and vomiting; diarrhea; intestinal colic, irritability; muscle weakness, numbness, flaccid paralysis; tingling; difficulty with phonation, respiration | Administer Kayexalate as ordered. Administer/monitor IV infusion of glucose and insulin. Control infection. Provide adequate calories and carbohydrates. Discontinue IV or oral sources of potassium. |

*(continues)*

**Table 4-5** Fluid and Electrolyte Imbalances *(continued)*

| Imbalance | Causes | Assessment Findings | Nursing Interventions |
|---|---|---|---|
| Hypokalemia | Anorexia, alcoholism, gastric and intestinal suction, GI surgery, vomiting, diarrhea, laxative abuse, thiazide diuretics, steroid therapy, stress, alkalotic states | Thready, rapid, weak pulse; faint heart sounds; decreased blood pressure; skeletal muscle weakness; decreased or absent reflexes; shallow respirations; malaise; apathy; lethargy; loss of orientation; anorexia, vomiting, weight loss, gaseous intestinal distention | Be especially cautious if administering drugs that are not potassium sparing. Administer potassium supplements to replace losses. Monitor acid-base balance. Monitor pulse, blood pressure, and ECG. |
| Hypernatremia | Excessive/rapid IV administration of normal saline solution, inadequate water intake, kidney disease | Dry, sticky mucous membranes; flushed skin; rough, dry tongue; firm skin turgor; intense thirst; edema; oliguria to anuria | Weigh daily. Assess degree of edema frequently. Measure I&O. Assess skin frequently and institute nursing measures to prevent breakdown. Encourage sodium-restricted diet. |
| Hyponatremia | Decreased sodium intake, increased sodium excretion through diaphoresis or GI suctioning, adrenal insufficiency | Nausea and vomiting; abdominal cramps; weight loss; cold, clammy skin; decreased skin turgor; fingerprinting over the sternum; shrunken tongue; apprehension; headache; convulsions; confusion; weakness; fatigue; postural hypotension; rapid, thready pulse | Provide foods high in sodium. Administer normal saline solution IV. Assess blood pressure frequently (measure lying down, sitting, and standing). |
| Hypercalcemia | Hyperparathyroidism, immobility, increased vitamin D intake, osteoporosis and osteomalacia (early stages) | Nausea and vomiting, anorexia, constipation, headache, confusion, lethargy, stupor, decreased muscle tone, deep bone and/or flank pain | Encourage mobilization. Limit vitamin D and calcium intake. Administer diuretics. Protect from injury. |
| Hypocalcemia | Acute pancreatitis, diarrhea, hypoparathyroidism, lack of vitamin D in diet, long-term steroid therapy | Painful tonic muscle spasms, facial spasms, fatigue, laryngospasm, positive Trousseau's and Chvostek's signs, convulsions, dyspnea | Administer oral calcium lactate or IV calcium chloride or gluconate. Provide safety by padding side rails. Administer dietary sources of calcium. Provide quiet environment. |
| Hypermagnesemia | Renal insufficiency, dehydration, excessive use of magnesium-containing antacids or laxatives | Lethargy, somnolence, confusion, nausea and vomiting, muscle weakness, depressed reflexes, decreased pulse and respirations | Withhold magnesium-containing drugs/foods. Increase fluid intake (unless contraindicated). |
| Hypomagnesemia | Low intake of magnesium in diet, prolonged diarrhea, massive diuresis, hypoparathyroidism | Paresthesias, confusion, hallucinations, convulsions, ataxia, tremors, hyperactive deep reflexes, muscle spasm, flushing of the face, diaphoresis | Provide good dietary sources of magnesium. |

C. Water excess: hypo-osmolar imbalances; water intoxication or solute deficit
D. Water deficit: hyperosmolar imbalances; water depletion or solute excess
E. Hyperkalemia: potassium excess, serum potassium above 5.5 mEq/liter
F. Hypokalemia: potassium deficit, serum potassium below 3.5 mEq/liter
G. Hypernatremia: sodium excess, serum sodium level above 148 mEq/liter
H. Hyponatremia: sodium deficit, serum sodium level below 135 mEq/liter
I. Hypercalcemia: calcium excess, serum calcium level above 10.5 mg/dL
J. Hypocalcemia: calcium deficit, serum calcium level below 8.5 mg/dL
K. Hypermagnesemia: magnesium excess, serum magnesium level above 2.7 mEq/liter
L. Hypomagnesemia: magnesium deficit, serum magnesium level below 1.8 mEq/liter

# ACID-BASE BALANCE

## Basic Principles

A. Normal pH of the body is 7.35–7.45.
B. Buffer or control systems maintain normal pH. In acidic state, kidneys excrete acids and reabsorb bicarbonate while the respiratory system gives off carbon dioxide. In alkalotic states, the kidneys excrete bicarbonate and the respiratory system retains carbonic acid.
See Table 4-6.

**Table 4-6** Normal Blood Gas Values

| pH | PaCO$_2$ | PaO$_2$ | HCO$_3$ |
|---|---|---|---|
| 7.35–7.45 | 35–45 mm Hg | 80–100 mm Hg | 22–26 mEq/L |

## Acid-Base Imbalances

See Table 4-7.
A. Metabolic acidosis: a primary deficit in the concentration of base bicarbonate in the extracellular fluid; decreased pH and bicarbonate, decreased pCO$_2$ (if respiratory compensation)
B. Metabolic alkalosis: a primary excess of base bicarbonate in the extracellular fluid; elevated pH and bicarbonate, elevated pCO$_2$ (if respiratory compensation)
C. Respiratory acidosis: a primary excess of carbonic acid in the extracellular fluid; decreased pH, elevated pCO$_2$ and bicarbonate (if renal compensation)
D. Respiratory alkalosis: a primary deficit of carbonic acid in the extracellular fluid; elevated pH, decreased pCO$_2$ and bicarbonate (if renal compensation)

**Table 4-7** Acid-Base Imbalances

| Imbalance | Causes | Assessment Findings | Nursing Interventions |
|---|---|---|---|
| Metabolic acidosis | Diabetic ketoacidosis, uremia, starvation, diarrhea, severe infections, renal tubular acidosis | Headache, nausea and vomiting, weakness, lethargy, disorientation, tremors, convulsions, coma | Administer sodium bicarbonate as ordered and monitor for signs of excess. Monitor for signs of hyperkalemia. Provide alkaline mouthwash (baking soda and water) to neutralize acids. Lubricate lips to prevent dryness from hyperventilation. Measure I&O. Institute seizure precautions. Monitor arterial blood gases and electrolytes. |
| Metabolic alkalosis | Severe vomiting, nasogastric suctioning, diuretic therapy, excessive ingestion of sodium bicarbonate, biliary drainage | Nausea and vomiting, diarrhea, numbness and tingling of extremities, tetany, bradycardia, decreased respirations | Replace fluid and electrolyte losses (potassium and chloride). Institute seizure precautions. Measure I&O. Assess for signs of hypokalemia. Monitor arterial blood gases and electrolytes. |

*(continues)*

**Table 4–7** Acid-Base Imbalances *(continued)*

| Imbalance | Causes | Assessment Findings | Nursing Interventions |
|---|---|---|---|
| Respiratory acidosis | COPD, barbiturate or sedative overdose, acute airway obstruction, weakness of respiratory muscles | Headache, weakness, visual disturbances, rapid respirations, confusion, drowsiness, tachycardia, coma | Place in semi-Fowler's position. Maintain patent airway. Turn, cough, and deep breathe. Perform postural drainage. Administer fluids to help liquefy secretions (unless contraindicated). Administer low-concentration oxygen therapy. Monitor arterial blood gases and electrolytes. Administer prophylactic antibiotics as ordered. |
| Respiratory alkalosis | Hyperventilation, mechanical overventilation, encephalitis | Numbness and tingling of mouth and extremities, inability to concentrate, rapid respirations, dry mouth, coma | Offer reassurance. Encourage breathing into a paper bag or voluntary breath holding. Ensure adequate rest. Provide sedation as ordered. Monitor mechanical ventilation, arterial blood gases, and electrolytes. |

E.  Compensation
   1.  If the metabolic system is causing the problem, the respiratory system attempts to correct the problem or compensate.
       a.  Compensation for metabolic acidosis is known as Kussmaul or "air hunger" respirations in which client breathes deeply to blow off acid ($CO_2$).
       b.  Compensation for metabolic alkalosis is slow breathing to conserve $CO_2$.
   2.  If the respiratory system is causing the problem, the metabolic system attempts to correct the problem or compensate.
       a.  Compensation for respiratory acidosis is a rise in $HCO_3$.
       b.  Respiratory alkalosis is such a rapid process there might not be significant compensation.

# INTRAVENOUS THERAPY

## Purposes

A.  Maintenance of fluid and electrolyte balance
B.  Replacement of fluid and electrolyte loss
C.  Provision of nutrients
D.  Provision of a route for medications

## Nursing Interventions

A.  Select correct solution after checking physician's order.
B.  Note clarity of solution.
C.  Calculate flow rate (Intravenous Calculations, Unit 2). Time-tape bag to assist in monitoring flow rate.
D.  Assess infusion rate and site at least hourly.
E.  Use infusion pump if administering medications (e.g., aminophylline, heparin, insulin).
F.  Maintain I&O record.
G.  Provide tubing change and IV site change according to hospital policy. Intravenous Nurses Society standards recommend IV site and tubing change every 48 hours.
H.  Discontinue IV if complications occur.

## Complications of Intravenous Therapy

See Table 4-8.

## Central Lines

### Uses

A.  Administration of TPN
B.  Measurement of central venous pressure (CVP)
C.  IV therapy when suitable peripheral veins are not available
D.  Long-term antibiotic therapy
E.  Chemotherapy

**Table 4–8** Complications of IV Therapy

| Complication | Nursing Manifestation | Interventions |
|---|---|---|
| Infiltration | Blanching of skin, swelling, pain at site; cool to touch; decreased infusion rate | Discontinue IV. Restart in a new site. May apply warm compresses to increase fluid absorption. |
| Extravasation | Infusion of a vesicant into the surrounding tissue; redness, heat, pain at site | Discontinue IV. Restart in a new site. May apply warm compress. |
| Phlebitis | Redness, heat, and swelling at site; possible pain and red line along course of vein | Discontinue IV. Restart in new site. Apply warm compresses to site. |
| Pyrogenic reaction | Fever, chills, general malaise, nausea, vomiting, headache, backache | Discontinue infusion immediately. Monitor vital signs and notify physician. Retain IV equipment for culture/lab study. |
| Air embolism | Dyspnea, cyanosis, hypotension, tachycardia, loss of consciousness | Stop infusion immediately. Turn client on left side with his head down. Administer oxygen. Notify physician. |
| Circulatory overload | Apprehension, shortness of breath, coughing, frothy sputum, crackles, engorged neck veins, increased blood pressure and pulse | Slow down IV rate. Monitor vital signs. Notify physician. |

## Types

A. Nontunneled catheters: inserted into subclavian vein for short-term access
   1. Subclavian catheters: single lumen
   2. Multilumen catheters: double, triple, or quadruple lumens for simultaneous infusion of fluids or for blood drawing with fluid infusion.
B. Tunneled catheters: long, silicone catheter threaded through subcutaneous layer to prevent infection with long-term use; catheter tip is located in the superior vena cava.
   1. Hickman/Broviac catheters: single- or double-lumen catheters with external presentation; need to be flushed daily with a heparinized saline solution and must be clamped when not in use; repair kit available.
   2. Groshong catheters: similar to Hickman/Broviac; difference is in valve at closed distal end of catheter that opens when used and remains closed at other times, preventing blood backup into catheter; no clamping is necessary; flushing is done daily with saline in a vigorous manner.
   3. Implantable ports (portacath): totally internal device consists of subcutaneous self-sealing injection port and a tunneled catheter; flushing is done with a heparinized saline solution every 28 days; access must be with a special noncoring needle.
   4. Peripherally inserted central catheter (PICC): short-term long lines that can be inserted by qualified nurses; inserted via a vessel in the antecubital fossa (median or cephalic); flushing is with a heparinized saline solution.

## Care of the Client with a Central Venous Line (CVL)

A. Assist physician with placement; catheters should initially be flushed with saline. Have fluids or cap and flush available (heparin or saline).
B. Confirm placement in superior vena cava by X-ray prior to catheter use.
C. Institute nursing measures to prevent infection (particularly important with TPN because high concentration of glucose encourages growth of bacteria).
   1. Change dressings
      a. Usually 3 times per week and as needed (e.g., when loose or wet) but agency policies may vary.
      b. Use sterile technique and apply sterile occlusive dressing.
   2. Monitor for signs of infection: redness, drainage, odor at site, or elevated temperature.
   3. Do not piggyback anything into a TPN infusion line except intralipids.
D. Monitor for infiltration: check for swelling of neck, face, and shoulder, and pain in upper arm.
E. Prevent catheter occlusion.
   1. Keep infusion continuous.
   2. Use infusion pump.
   3. Check for kinks in tubing.
   4. Evaluate for catheter migration or dislodgment.
F. Prevent air embolism.
   1. Tighten and tape all tubing connections to prevent accidental disconnection.

2. Clamp catheter (except Groshong) and instruct client to perform Valsalva maneuver when changing or detaching tubing.
3. Check tubing for cracks or perforations.
G. Maintain proper infusion rate.
    1. Monitor rate closely to prevent clotting, fluid depletion, or fluid overload.
    2. Never attempt to speed up or slow down infusion.
H. With a multilumen catheter, flush ports not being used to prevent clotting (per agency's protocol).
I. With Hickman/Broviac catheters, Groshongs, PICCs, and implanted port provide other specific care according to agency protocol.
J. If clotting occurs, try to aspirate or add a declotting agent according to agency protocol. Do not irrigate. Do not use force to flush.
    1. Streptokinase requires 1 hour waiting time to achieve results.
    2. Urokinase requires 10 minutes waiting time to achieve results.
K. When drawing blood specimens, discard initial sample of 10 mL prior to drawing required volume for specimens. Flush with saline prior to flushing with heparinized saline solution or continuing fluids.

## Blood Transfusions

See Blood Transfusions.

## SHOCK

An abnormal physiologic state in which an imbalance between the amount of circulating blood volume and the size of the vascular bed results in circulatory failure and oxygen and nutrient deprivation of tissues. See Table 4-9 for classification of shock.

### Body's Response to Shock

A. Hyperventilation leading to respiratory alkalosis
B. Vasoconstriction: shunts blood to heart and brain
C. Tachycardia
D. Fluid shifts: intracellular to extracellular shift to maintain circulating blood volume
E. Impaired metabolism: tissue anoxia leads to anaerobic metabolism causing increased capillary permeability and lactic acid buildup, resulting in metabolic acidosis
F. Impaired organ function

**Table 4-9** Classification of Shock

| Type | Characteristics | Causes |
|---|---|---|
| Hypovolemic | Decreased circulating blood volume | Blood loss<br>Plasma loss (e.g., burns)<br>Fluid loss (e.g., excessive vomiting or diarrhea) |
| Cardiogenic | Failure of the heart to pump properly | Myocardial infarction<br>Congestive heart failure<br>Cardiac arrhythmias<br>Pericardial tamponade<br>Tension pneumothorax |
| Septic | Factors favoring septic shock:<br>• Development of antibiotic-resistant organisms<br>• Invasive procedures such as urinary tract instrumentation<br>• Immunosuppression and old age<br>• Trauma: presence of blood in peritoneal cavity greatly increases likelihood of peritonitis | Release of bacterial toxins that act directly on the blood vessels producing massive vasodilation and pooling of blood; results most frequently from gram-negative septicemia. |
| Neurogenic | Failure of arteriolar resistance, leading to massive vasodilation and pooling of blood | Interruption of sympathetic impulses from:<br>• Exposure to unpleasant circumstances<br>• Extreme pain<br>• Spinal cord injury<br>• High spinal anesthesia<br>• Vasomotor depression<br>• Head injury |
| Anaphylactic | Massive vasodilation resulting from allergic reaction causing release of histamine and related substances | Allergic reaction to:<br>• Insect venom or snake venom<br>• Medications or food<br>• Dyes used in radiologic studies |

1. Kidney: decreased perfusion can result in renal failure.
2. Lung: shock lung (adult respiratory distress syndrome [ARDS])

## Assessment Findings

A. Skin
   1. Cool, pale, moist in hypovolemic and cardiogenic shock
   2. Warm, dry, pink in septic and neurogenic shock
B. Pulse
   1. Tachycardia, due to increased sympathetic stimulation
   2. Weak and thready
C. Blood pressure
   1. Early stages: may be normal due to compensatory mechanisms
   2. Later stages: systolic and diastolic blood pressure drops
D. Respirations: rapid and shallow, due to tissue anoxia and excessive amounts of $CO_2$ (from metabolic acidosis)
E. Level of consciousness: restlessness and apprehension, progressing to coma
F. Urinary output: decreases due to impaired renal perfusion
G. Temperature: decreases in severe shock (except septic shock).

## Nursing Interventions

A. Maintain patent airway and adequate ventilation.
   1. Establish and maintain airway.
   2. Administer oxygen as ordered.
   3. Monitor respiratory status, blood gases.
   4. Start resuscitative procedures as necessary.
B. Promote restoration of blood volume; administer fluid and blood replacement as ordered.
   1. Crystalloid solutions: Ringer's lactate, normal saline
   2. Colloid solutions: albumin, plasmanate, dextran
   3. Blood products: whole blood, packed red blood cells, fresh frozen plasma
C. Administer drugs as ordered (see Table 4-10).
D. Minimize factors contributing to shock.
   1. Elevate lower extremities to 45° to promote venous return to heart, thereby improving cardiac output.
   2. Avoid Trendelenburg's position: increases respiratory impairment.
   3. Promote rest by using energy-conservation measures and maintaining as quiet an environment as possible.
   4. Relieve pain by cautious use of narcotics.
      a. Because narcotics interfere with vasoconstriction, give only if absolutely necessary, IV and in small doses.
      b. If given IM or subcutaneously, vasoconstriction may cause incomplete

absorption; when circulation improves, client may get overdose.
   5. Keep client warm.
E. Maintain continuous assessment of the client.
   1. Check vital signs frequently.
   2. Monitor urine output: report urine output of less than 30 mL/hour.
   3. Observe color and temperature of skin.
   4. Monitor CVP.
   5. Monitor ECG.
   6. Check lab studies: CBC, electrolytes, BUN, creatinine, blood gases.
   7. Monitor other parameters such as arterial blood pressures, cardiac output, pulmonary artery pressures, pulmonary artery wedge pressures.
F. Provide psychologic support: reassure client to relieve apprehension, and keep family advised.

**Table 4-10** Drugs Used to Treat Shock

| Generic (Trade) Name | Action |
| --- | --- |
| Dopamine (Intropin) | *Low dosage:* Dilates renal, mesenteric, and splanchnic vessels, which in turn increases perfusion of kidneys and urine output. *High dosage:* Increases cardiac contractility; causes vasoconstriction (often given with nitroprusside [Nipride]). |
| Dobutamine (Dobutrex) | Increases myocardial contractility; vasodilator. |
| Isoproterenol (Isuprel) | Increases myocardial contractility; decreases peripheral resistance by dilating peripheral vascular bed; usefulness is limited by the tachycardia it produces. |
| Norepinephrine (Levophed) | Improves cardiac contractility and cardiac output; potent vasoconstrictor. |
| Sodium nitroprusside (Nipride) | Vasodilator; decreases peripheral resistance and workload of heart, thereby increasing cardiac output; used in cardiogenic shock and hypertensive emergencies. |
| Digitalis preparations | Improves cardiac performance. |
| Corticosteroids | Used especially in septic shock; helps to protect cell membranes and decreases the inflammatory response to stress. |
| Antibiotics | Used in treating infectious processes related to septic shock. |

***Note:*** Vasopressors such as Levophed can cause almost complete occlusion of arterioles, causing a decrease of blood flow to larger tissue areas. Therefore, if blood pressure is adequate, a vasodilator such as Nipride could probably be given as well, to modify the vasoconstrictor effects.

# MULTIPLE TRAUMA

## Assessment and Emergency Care

### Airway

A. Assess, establish, and maintain an adequate airway.
 1. Do not hyperextend the neck in a client with suspected cervical spine injury.
 2. Use jaw thrust instead.
B. Administer artificial resuscitation if necessary.
C. Observe for chest trauma such as open sucking wounds or flail chest (see Chest Trauma).
D. Administer high-flow oxygen 85–100% to achieve maximum cellular oxygenation. Monitor for $CO_2$ retention in clients with COPD.
E. Draw blood samples for ABGs.

### Hemorrhage and Shock

A. Deep wounds with pulsating blood flow
 1. Apply firm pressure over the wound with a sterile dressing.
 2. If wound is on a limb, elevate the extremity.
 3. Apply pressure with three fingers over appropriate pressure point.
 4. Once bleeding is controlled, apply a pressure dressing.
 5. Tourniquets should be used only when all other methods have failed.
B. Venous bleeding: apply direct pressure to bleeding site.
C. Never remove any foreign object, such as a knife, from the client; immobilize the object with packing.
D. Assess for and treat shock (see Shock).
E. Administer tetanus booster as ordered.

### Neurologic Injuries

A. Establish a baseline level of consciousness and reassess frequently.
B. Inspect the scalp, head, face, and neck for abrasions, hematomas, and lacerations.
C. Gently palpate the head for any injuries.
D. Inspect the nose and ears for leakage of cerebrospinal fluid.
E. Evaluate pupillary size, shape, equality, and reaction to light.
F. Assess for sensation and motor abilities.
G. Observe for signs of increased intracranial pressure.
H. For additional details of care (see Head Injury and Spinal Cord Injury).

### Abdominal Injuries

A. Keep client NPO.
B. Assist with insertion of nasogastric tube (for assessment of stomach bleeding and aspiration of stomach contents, which prevents vomiting).
C. Inspect abdomen for injuries.
D. Auscultate bowel sounds.
E. Do not palpate the abdomen (could aggravate possible internal injuries).
F. Prepare client for peritoneal lavage if indicated.
G. Insert Foley catheter.
 1. Measure urine output every 15 minutes.
 2. Assess for hematuria.

### Musculoskeletal Injuries

A. Observe for sign of fracture: pain, swelling, tenderness, ecchymosis, crepitation (grating sound), loss of function, exposed bone fragments.
B. Cover open fracture with sterile dressing to prevent infection.
C. Immobilize any suspected fractures by splinting the joint above and below the injury.
D. Perform neurovascular check of area distal to fracture: assess for color, temperature, capillary refill, sensation, movement, pulses.

 **Sample Questions**

1. A client is admitted for treatment of Crohn's disease. Which information is most significant when the nurse assesses nutritional health?
 1. Anthropometric measurements.
 2. Bleeding gums.
 3. Dry skin.
 4. Facial rubor.

2. Total parenteral nutrition (TPN) is ordered for an adult client. Which statement is true regarding TPN?
 1. It contains 20–70% glucose.
 2. The RN will mix the lipids into the TPN bag before administration.
 3. When the client's blood glucose runs high, decrease the TPN rate.
 4. Check the client's potassium level every 6 hours.

3. The nurse has administered analgesia, but the client continues to complain of severe pain. Which of the following actions should be most appropriate for the nurse to take first?
 1. Contact the physician to request additional medication.
 2. Assist the client to a comfortable position and help her relax.
 3. Administer a narcotic analgesic.
 4. Inform the client that she may request additional pain medication in 3 hours.

4. Acetylsalicylic acid is being administered to an adult client. What is the most common mechanism of action for nonnarcotic analgesics?
   1. To inhibit prostaglandin synthesis.
   2. To alter pain perception in the cerebellum.
   3. To directly affect the central nervous system.
   4. To target the pain-producing effect of kinins.

5. An adult has been taking acetylsalicylic acid (ASA) 650 mg four times a day for chronic back pain. What complication is possible due to this level of ASA ingestion?
   1. Liver failure.
   2. Paralytic ileus.
   3. Gastrointestinal bleeding.
   4. Retinal detachment.

6. Ibuprofen (Motrin) is prescribed for an adult with chronic pain. The nurse must teach the client to observe which dietary precaution while taking ibuprofen?
   1. Eat a high-fiber diet.
   2. Drink citrus juices daily.
   3. Take the medication with milk.
   4. Omit spinach and other green leafy vegetables from the client's diet.

7. A post-op surgical client is ordered patient-controlled analgesia (PCA). Which statement by the RN will help reduce anxiety about receiving adequate pain relief?
   1. "A PCA is almost always effective."
   2. "Your comfort will be assessed frequently."
   3. "Have your family push the button for you."
   4. "We will have Narcan available if you get too much."

8. Preoperative teaching for an adult who is to have patient controlled analgesia (PCA) following surgery includes telling the client:
   1. "You will not be drowsy."
   2. "You will experience no pain."
   3. "Pain control will be adequate."
   4. "You will not have incisional pain but you may have muscle pain."

9. The client's family expresses concern that the client could overdose with a PCA. What protective mechanism prevents drug overdose with a PCA?
   1. The nurse controls the amount administered with each dose.
   2. Extensive client teaching precedes its use.
   3. The client can stop drug administration but not initiate it.

4. After a bolus is administered, there is a mandatory waiting period before another dose is given.

10. A nurse is the first professional to arrive at the scene of a multivehicle accident. An adult was riding a motorcycle. Upon impact, he fell off the bike and it fell back on his legs. What should be the RN's priority action?
    1. Assessing blood loss.
    2. Monitoring respiratory status.
    3. Obtaining vital signs.
    4. Removing the bike off him.

11. A nurse stops to help at a motorcycle accident in which an adult is bleeding profusely from a 4-inch gash on the left knee. Which of the following is the best approach for the nurse to take to stop the bleeding?
    1. Apply direct pressure to the wound.
    2. Move the motorcycle off his legs.
    3. Raise the extremity.
    4. Wrap a tourniquet above the wound.

12. The nurse is caring for a client who is receiving IV fluids. Which observation by the nurse indicates the IV has infiltrated?
    1. Pain at the site.
    2. A change in flow rate.
    3. Coldness around the insertion site.
    4. Redness around the insertion site.

13. The nurse is caring for a client whose arterial blood gases indicate metabolic alkalosis. Which of the following is most likely to cause metabolic alkalosis?
    1. Nasogastric suctioning.
    2. Diabetic ketoacidosis.
    3. COPD.
    4. Renal failure.

14. An adult client is admitted with metabolic acidosis. Which set of arterial blood gases should the nurse expect to find in a client with metabolic acidosis?
    1. pH 7.28; $PCO_2$–55; $HCO_3$–26.
    2. pH 7.50; $PCO_2$–40; $HCO_3$–31.
    3. pH 7.48; $PCO_2$–30; $HCO_3$–22.
    4. pH 7.30; $PCO_2$–36; $HCO_3$–18.

15. A elderly client is hospitalized for the treatment of gastroenteritis complicated by dehydration and hyponatremia. What is an early symptom of hyponatremia that the nurse would expect from this client?
    1. Ataxia.
    2. Hunger.

3. Thirst.

4. Weakness.

16. An adult has just been brought in by ambulance after a motor vehicle accident and has moderate anxiety. When assessing the client, the nurse would expect which of the following from sympathetic nervous system stimulation?

1. A rapid pulse and increased respiratory rate.

2. Decreased physiologic functioning.

3. Rigid posture and altered perceptual focus.

4. Increased awareness and attending.

17. An adult has received an injection of immunoglobulin. The nurse knows that the client will develop which of the following types of immunity?

1. Active natural immunity.

2. Active artificial immunity.

3. Passive natural immunity.

4. Passive artificial immunity.

18. The nurse knows which of the following is true about immunity?

1. Antibody-mediated defense occurs through the T-cell system.

2. Cellular immunity is mediated by antibodies produced by the B-cells.

3. Antibodies are produced by the B-cells.

4. Lymphocytes increase with an allergic response.

19. An adult is on a clear liquid diet. Which food item can be offered?

1. Milk.

2. Jello.

3. Orange juice.

4. Ice cream.

20. An adult is being taught about a healthy diet. How can the food pyramid help guide the client on his diet?

1. By indicating exactly how many servings of each group to eat.

2. By calculating how many calories the client should have.

3. By suggesting daily food choices.

4. By dividing the food into four basic groups.

21. Before administering a tube feeding the nurse knows to perform which of the following assessments?

1. The gastrointestinal (GI) tract, including bowel sounds, last BM, and distention.

2. The client's neurologic status, especially gag reflex.

3. The amount of air in the stomach.

4. That the formula is used directly from the refrigerator.

22. Which food choice contains the highest kilocalorie?

1. Apple.

2. Bacon.

3. Chicken.

4. Bread.

23. The nurse knows that a client understands a low residue diet when he selects which of the following from a menu?

1. Rice and lean chicken.

2. Strawberry pie.

3. Pasta with vegetables.

4. Tuna casserole.

24. An adult is receiving total parenteral nutrition (TPN). The nurse knows which of the following assessments is essential?

1. Evaluation of the peripheral intravenous (IV) site.

2. Confirmation that the tube is in the stomach.

3. Assessment of the GI tract, including bowel sounds.

4. Fluid and electrolyte monitoring.

25. The nurse knows which of the following statements about TPN and peripheral parenteral nutrition (PPN) is true?

1. TPN is usually indicated for clients needing short-term (less than 3 weeks) nutritional support, whereas PPN is for long-term maintenance.

2. A client needing more than 3000 calories would receive PPN, whereas TPN is given to those requiring less than 3000 calories.

3. TPN is often given to those with fluid restrictions, whereas PPN is used for those without constraints on their fluid intake.

4. TPN is given to those who need to augment oral feedings, whereas PPN is used for those who are nothing by mouth (NPO).

26. What is an important consideration regarding TPN administration?

1. IV site is kept aseptic while infusing the solution.

2. Feeding is poured into a pouch and then infused.

3. Solution is only hung for a maximum of 8 hours at a time.

4. New formula is added as needed so the line does not run dry.

27. An adult has been treated for pulmonary tuberculosis (TB) and is being discharged home with his wife and two young children. His wife asks how TB is passed from one person to another so she can prevent anyone else from catching it. How should the nurse respond?
    1. "You should wear gloves when handling his linen and bedding."
    2. "You should keep the windows and doors closed so as not to spread the droplets."
    3. "He must be careful to cough into a handkerchief that is washed in hot water or discarded."
    4. "Make sure to boil all water before drinking or using it."

28. The nurse evaluates a certified nursing assistant (CNA). Which of the following actions by the CNA demonstrates understanding of standard precautions?
    1. Wears gloves during all client contact.
    2. Cleans blood spills with soap and water.
    3. Pours bulk blood and other secretions down a drain connected to a sanitary sewer.
    4. Carries blood sample to the lab in an open basket.

29. An adult is on long-term aspirin therapy and is experiencing tinnitus. What is the best interpretation of this occurrence?
    1. The aspirin is working correctly.
    2. The client has a metal taste in their mouth.
    3. The client has an upper GI bleed.
    4. The client is experiencing a mild overdosage.

30. An adult is receiving a nonsteroidal anti-inflammatory drug (NSAID). Which of the following would the nurse include in the teaching about this medication?
    1. Take the NSAID with ASA for full effect.
    2. Take the NSAID with meals.
    3. Orange juice will help potential the action of the medication.
    4. The NSAID will coat the stomach lining.

31. An adult is to receive an intramuscular (IM) injection of morphine for post-op pain. Which of the following is necessary for the nurse to assess prior to giving a narcotic analgesic?
    1. The client's level of alertness and respiratory rate.
    2. The last time the client ate or drank something.
    3. The client's bowel habits and last bowel movement.
    4. The client's history of addictions.

32. An adult is to receive narcotic analgesic via a patient-controlled analgesia (PCA). The nurse is evaluating the client's understanding of the procedure. Which of the following statements by the client indicates that she understands PCA?
    1. "When I press this button the machine will always give me more medicine."
    2. "I will press the button whenever I begin to experience pain."
    3. "I should press this button every hour so the pain doesn't come back."
    4. "With this machine I will experience no more pain."

33. An adult suffered second- and third-degree burns over 20% of his body 2 days ago. What is the best way to assess the client's fluid balance?
    1. Maintain strict records of intake and output.
    2. Weigh the client daily.
    3. Monitor skin turgor.
    4. Check for edema.

34. A 78-year-old male has been working on his lawn for 2 days, although the temperature has been above 90°F. He has been on thiazide diuretics for hypertension. His lab values are: K 3.7 mEq/L, Na 129 mEq/L, Ca 9.9 mg/dL, and Cl 95 mEq/L. What would be a priority action for this man?
    1. Make sure he drinks eight glasses of water a day.
    2. Monitor for fatigue, muscle weakness, restlessness, and flushed skin.
    3. Look for signs of hyperchloremia.
    4. Observe for neurologic changes.

35. An adult who has gastroenteritis and is on digitalis has lab values of: K 3.2 mEq/L, Na 136 mEq/L, Ca 8.8 mg/dL, and Cl 98 mEq/L. The nurse puts which of the following on the client's plan of care?
    1. Stop digitalis therapy.
    2. Avoid foods rich in potassium.
    3. Observe for digitalis toxicity.
    4. Observe for Trousseau's and Chvostek's signs.

36. A client on hemodialysis is complaining of muscle weakness and numbness in his legs. His lab results are: Na 136 mEq/L, K 5.9 mEq/L, Cl 100 mEq/L, Ca 8.5 mg/dL. Which electrolyte imbalance is the client suffering from?
    1. Hyperkalemia.
    2. Hypernatremia.
    3. Hypocalcemia.
    4. Hypochloremia.

37. A client has cancer that has metastasized to her bones. She is complaining of increased thirst, polyuria, and decreased muscle tone in the legs. Her lab values are: Na 139 mEq/L, K 4.0 mEq/L, Cl 103 mEq/L, and Ca 8.0 mg/dL. What electrolyte imbalance is present?

    1. Hypocalcemia.
    2. Hypercalcemia.
    3. Hyperkalemia.
    4. Hypochloremia.

38. An adult who is anxious and hyperventilating has blood gases of: pH 7.47, $PaCO_2$ 33. What is the best initial action for the nurse to take?

    1. Try to have the client breathe slower or into a paper bag.
    2. Monitor the client's fluid balance.
    3. Give $O_2$ via nasal cannula.
    4. Administer sodium bicarbonate.

39. An adult has had gastroenteritis with vomiting for 3 days. He has taken baking soda without relief. His blood gases are as follows: pH 7.49, $PaCO_2$ 45, and $HCO_3$ 30. The nurse would expect which of the following to be included in the plan of care?

    1. Have the client drink at least eight glasses of water in the first day.
    2. Administer $NaHCO_3$ IV as per physician's orders.
    3. Continue sodium bicarbonate for nausea.
    4. Monitor electrolytes for hypokalemia and hypocalcemia.

40. An adult's blood gas results are: pH 7.31, $PaCO_2$ 49, and $HCO_3$ 24. What does the nurse interpret this as?

    1. Respiratory acidosis.
    2. Respiratory alkalosis.
    3. Metabolic acidosis.
    4. Metabolic alkalosis.

41. An adult who has diabetes has infectious diarrhea. His arterial blood gases are: pH 7.30, $PaCO_2$ 35, and $HCO_3$ of 19. The nurse would monitor the client for which of the following?

    1. Trousseau's sign.
    2. Hypokalemia.
    3. Hypoglycemia.
    4. Respiratory changes.

42. An adult has an IV line in the right forearm infusing D5 ½ NS with 20 mEq of potassium at 75 mL/h. Which statement would be a correct report from the RN?

    1. The potassium bag is piggybacked into the dextrose at 75 mL/h.
    2. The clamp should be closed below the D5 ½ NS bag.
    3. Potassium is on the secondary line.
    4. 75 mL will infuse in 1 hour.

43. An adult has a central venous line. Which of the following should the nurse include in the care plan?

    1. Complete blood count (CBC) and electrolytes.
    2. Regular serial chest X-rays to ensure proper placement of the central line.
    3. Continuous infusion of a solution at a keep vein open rate.
    4. Any signs of infection, air embolus, and leakage or puncture.

44. An adult has a Hickman-type central venous catheter and needs to have blood drawn from it. Which of the following is the nurse going to do first?

    1. Use sterile technique to assemble the supplies needed.
    2. Aspirate and discard the first 10 mL of the blood.
    3. First flush the catheter with heparinized solution, then withdraw the blood.
    4. Remove the cap on the catheter and replace it with a new one.

45. An adult has a central line in his right subclavian vein. The nurse is to change the tubing. Which of the following should be done?

    1. Use the present solution with the new tubing.
    2. Connect the new tubing to the hub prior to running any fluid through the tubing.
    3. Close the roller clamp on the new tubing after priming it.
    4. Have the client roll to the right side to prevent an air embolus.

46. An adult suffered a diving accident and is being brought in by an ambulance intubated and on a backboard with a cervical collar. What is the first action the nurse would take on arrival in the hospital?

    1. Take the client's vital signs.
    2. Insert a large bore IV line.
    3. Check the lungs for equal breath sounds bilaterally.
    4. Perform a neurologic check using the Glasgow scale.

47. An adult has been shot. His vital signs are blood pressure (BP) 90/60, pulse (P) 120 weak and thready, respirations (R) 20. During the initial assessment, he is placed in a modified Trendelenburg position. What desired effect should the position have on the client?
   1. An increase in the client's blood pressure.
   2. An increase in the client's heart rate.
   3. An increase in the client's respiratory rate.
   4. A decrease in blood loss.

48. An adult has been stung by a bee and is in anaphylactic shock. An epinephrine (adrenaline) injection has been given. The nurse would expect which of the following if the injection has been effective?
   1. The client's breathing will become easier.
   2. The client's blood pressure will decrease.
   3. There will be an increase in angioedema.
   4. There will be a decrease in the client's level of consciousness.

49. An adult who was in a motor vehicle accident, has been brought to the emergency department. She has a 4-in laceration on her forehead that is bleeding profusely. Her left ankle has an obvious deformity and is splinted. Her vital signs are BP 100/60, P 110, and R 16. What is the first action the nurse should take?
   1. Start an IV line for fluids.
   2. Place a Foley catheter.
   3. Get an ECG.
   4. Check her neurologic status.

50. An adult is brought in by ambulance after a motor vehicle accident. He is unconscious, on a backboard with his neck immobilized. He is bleeding profusely from a large gash on his right thigh. What is the first action the nurse should take?
   1. Stop the bleeding.
   2. Check his airway.
   3. Take his vital signs.
   4. Find out what happened from eyewitnesses.

 **Answers and Rationales**

1. **1.** Anthropometric measurements are the prime parameters used to evaluate fat and muscle stores in the body.

2. **1.** The concentration for dextrose in TPN can range from 20–70%.

3. **2.** Medication is usually more effective with relieving techniques. Many basic nursing measures reduce or eliminate discomfort. Administering analgesia alone does not replace thoughtful, comprehensive pain management.

4. **1.** Nonnarcotic analgesics inhibit prostaglandin synthesis. Prostaglandins increase the sensitivity of peripheral pain receptors to endogenous pain-producing substances.

5. **3.** High doses of aspirin are associated with GI bleeding.

6. **3.** NSAIDs such as ibuprofen are very irritating to the GI tract and should always be taken with milk or food to minimize the possibility of bleeding.

7. **2.** Pain is an individual experience. It is important to reassure the client that assessments will be made frequently and that drug dosages will be adjusted according to the amount of pain the client perceives.

8. **3.** Clients should be told that they will be able to control their pain.

9. **4.** Immediately after a bolus dose of medication is administered the device enters a mandatory lockout mode where no other boluses of medication can be delivered.

10. **2.** In the presence of multiple traumas, maintenance of a patent airway must always be the priority in the sequence of care delivery.

11. **1.** Direct pressure to the wound will aid in the development of a blood clot, which is the first step in wound healing and will prevent hemorrhage.

12. **3.** Coldness, pallor, and swelling around the insertion site are the best indicators that the fluid has infiltrated into subcutaneous tissue.

13. **1.** One cause of metabolic alkalosis is removal of $H^+$ and $Cl^-$ from the stomach through emesis or gastric suction, resulting in an excess of base.

14. **4.** The pH is below the normal range of 7.35–7.45. The $PCO_2$ is within the normal range of 35–45, and the $HCO_3$ is below the normal limits of 21–28. These values indicate a metabolic problem because the $PCO_2$ is within normal limits. It is the low $HCO_3$ that is causing acidosis.

15. **3.** Thirst is the body's attempt to restore blood volume depletion that occurs in hyponatremia.

16. **1.** The sympathetic nervous system during moderate anxiety will increase the pulse and respirations.

17. **4.** Passive artificial immunity occurs when antibodies are produced by another person or animal and injected into the recipient.

18. **3.** Antibodies or immunoglobulins are produced by the B cells and are part of the body's plasma proteins.

19. **2.** Plain gelatins can be given on a clear liquid diet, as well as tea, coffee, ginger ale, or lemon-lime soda.

20. **3.** The pyramid helps to guide the client in choosing a variety of foods to obtain the nutrients needed. It also aids in eating more of some groups (bread, cereal, rice, and pasta) and less of others (fats, oils, and sweets).

21. **1.** The GI tract should be assessed before each feeding to ensure functioning and minimal problems.

22. **2.** Bacon contains the highest kilocalorie, as it is from the fat group. Fats yield 9 kcal/g, whereas the other choices, from the carbohydrate and protein groups only yield 4 kcal/g.

23. **1.** A low-residue diet includes rice, lean meats, and eggs.

24. **4.** Clients receiving TPN can experience electrolyte imbalances, hypo- or hyperglycemia, as well as difficulties with fluid balance.

25. **3.** TPN can provide a greater concentration of calories than PPN. Therefore, TPN is given to those with fluid restrictions.

26. **1.** The IV site is kept aseptic by an occlusive dressing. It is a central line and the TPN with its high concentration of glucose provides an ideal medium for pathogens.

27. **3.** TB is spread through residue of evaporated droplets and may remain in the air for long periods of time. Thus care should be given when coughing or sneezing.

28. **3.** Bulk blood and other secretions like suctioned fluids are carefully poured down a drain connected to a sanitary sewer.

29. **4.** Tinnitus is a classic sign of aspirin overdosages, either from too much ingestion or limited excretion.

30. **2.** NSAIDs should be taken with food, milk, or antacid to prevent nausea or vomiting.

31. **1.** A decreasing level of alertness can signal early respiratory depression and a significant drop in the respiratory rate is a warning sign. Both should be taken prior to giving the medication for baseline purposes.

32. **2.** PCA allows the client to administer more analgesic before the pain becomes severe, thus allowing better pain control.

33. **2.** This is the best way to assess fluid balance, especially acute changes in those with large losses or acutely ill.

34. **4.** Neurologic changes can occur from hyponatremia. They include confusion, disorientation, lethargy, seizures, and coma.

35. **3.** Hypokalemia enhances digitalis toxicity and must be observed for carefully.

36. **1.** Potassium is normally 3.5–5.5 mEq/L. Clients with renal failure are prone to hyperkalemia.

37. **1.** The client's calcium is low. The normal values are 8.5–10.5 mg/dL. Hypocalcemia is common among those with bone cancer.

38. **1.** The client is in respiratory alkalosis and needs to increase the carbon dioxide. The easiest way to do this is to try and calm the client and/or have him breathe in and out of a paper bag, thus inhaling the exhaled carbon dioxide.

39. **4.** Hypokalemia and hypocalcemia are both common with metabolic alkalosis as a result of cellular buffering.

40. **1.** A low pH indicates acidosis, whereas the high $PaCO_2$ indicates the problem is respiratory rather than metabolic.

41. **4.** The client is in metabolic acidosis and the body will try to compensate through the respiratory system (with deep breaths), although it cannot completely correct the problem.

42. **4.** The IV fluids will infuse 75 mL/h, as the rate states. The potassium has already been mixed in the bag from pharmacy and infuses from one bag.

43. **4.** All of these are potential problems for those with a central line, which the nurse needs to be observant for.

44. **2.** The first 10 mL are drawn off and discarded. Lab values can be altered by the solution remaining in the catheter from the infusion or flush.

45. **3.** The roller clamp should be closed after priming, otherwise the fluid will continue to flow. Open the roller clamp after inserting the tubing into the hub.

**46. 3.** The airway is provided by the endotracheal tube. The nurse should assess breathing, the next step in the ABCs.

**47. 1.** The Trendelenburg position increases the blood return from the legs, thereby raising the blood pressure.

**48. 1.** The epinephrine would help to ease the client's respiratory distress.

**49. 1.** Her vital signs indicate that she is probably going into shock. Fluids are the first action to do after assessing ABCs.

**50. 2.** Airway is the first step of ABCs.

# Aging

## GENERAL INFORMATION

Aging is a normal developmental process occurring throughout the human life span that causes a mild progressive decline in body system functioning. The older client is generally regarded as one who is 65 years of age or older.

## Biologic Theories of Aging

**A.** Immune system theory
  **1.** The two primary immune organs, the thymus and bone marrow, are affected by the aging process, which contributes to a decline in T-cell production and stem cell efficiency.
  **2.** Increase of infections, autoimmune disease, and cancer with aging.
**B.** Cross-linking theory
  **1.** Cross-linking is a chemical reaction that binds glucose to protein, which causes abnormal division of DNA, interfering with normal cell functioning and intracellular transport over a lifetime.
  **2.** Eventually causes tissue and organ failure.
**C.** Free radical theory
  **1.** Molecules that are highly reactive as a result of oxygen metabolism in the body.
  **2.** Over time, cause physical decline by damaging proteins, enzymes, and DNA.
  **3.** Beta-carotene and vitamins C and E are naturally occurring antioxidants that counteract the free radicals.
**D.** Stress theory (wear and tear)
  **1.** The body, like any machine, will eventually "wear out" secondary to repetitive usage, damage, and stress.
  **2.** While this theory is seen as having some merit, individuals react differently to stress (positive and negative), causing controversy over the concept.
**E.** Genetics theory
  **1.** Preprogrammed life expectancy. Cells can only divide a specific number of times.
  **2.** Life expectancies among family members is similar, i.e., if the parents died over the age of 80, the children are more likely to live to that age.
**F.** Neuroendocrine theories
  **1.** Anterior pituitary hormones are thought to contribute to the aging process.
  **2.** An imbalance of certain chemicals in the brain may contribute to altered cell division within the body.

## Age-Related Changes

See Table 4-11.

## Psychosocial Changes in the Older Adult

**A.** A successful aging process includes physical, psychological, social, and cultural factors.
  **1.** Some cultures have a great respect for older persons.
  **2.** In the United States, much value is placed on youth.
  **3.** Be aware of ageism (discrimination against the older adult simply because of age).
**B.** Developmental tasks for the older adult
  **1.** Ego integrity vs. despair (Erikson)
    **a.** With ego integrity, the person's life is felt to have meaning and accomplishment.
    **b.** With despair, there are feelings of worthlessness for a life not well lived.
  **2.** Other possible developmental tasks
    **a.** Successfully adjusting to retirement.
    **b.** Making safe and satisfactory living arrangements.
    **c.** Adjusting to reduced income.
    **d.** Keeping socially active.
    **e.** Maintaining contact with friends and family.
    **f.** Making safe decisions about driving a car.
    **g.** Adjusting to death of spouse/significant other.
    **h.** Adjusting to idea of one's own death.

4

**Table 4-11** Age-Related Changes

| System | Change | Nursing Interventions |
|---|---|---|
| **Special Senses** | | |
| *Vision* | Presbyopia: decreased ability to focus on near objects (often requiring reading glasses)<br>Decreased lacrimal secretions—chronic dry eye, scratchiness<br>Pupils: smaller—decreased peripheral vision and ability to adapt to the dark; increased sensitivity to glare<br>Lens: larger, more rigid, and discolored (yellow opacity)—decreased depth perception and ability to focus<br>Colors distorted, especially blue/green<br>Red/orange more pleasing | Provide increased illumination without glare.<br>Provide safe environment by orienting client to surroundings and removing potential hazards.<br><br>Use sunglasses outdoors.<br>Use large-print books.<br>Avoid night driving. |
| *Hearing* | Presbycusis: decreased ability to hear pitch or level of sound (first high, then low and background)<br>Tinnitus—"ringing in the ear"; results from decreased blood supply to neurosensory receptors in ear; problems distinguishing horns/sirens | Look directly at the client when speaking and speak clearly and slowly; low-pitched voice heard best.<br>Decrease background noise. |
| *Taste/Smell* | Olfactory fibers atrophy—decreased sense of smell, decreased appetite/ability to enjoy foods | Provide attractive meals in comfortable social setting.<br>Vary taste, textures, and colors of foods.<br>Be alert for difficulty chewing or swallowing when selecting foods. |
| *Touch* | Sensory nerve receptors less acute—requires stronger stimuli, increased pain tolerance, skin tears, more difficult to distinguish hot, cold, or pressure<br>Fine discrimination abilities impaired, especially hands and feet | Protect skin from injury.<br>Lower bath water temperature to 100–105°F.<br>Provide for safety around hot liquids at mealtimes. |
| Nervous | Overall intellect remains the same<br>Fewer neurons and reduced blood flow to brain—some short-term memory loss and learning ability slowed<br>Myelin sheath degenerates—decreased reaction time, reduced deep tendon reflexes, and increased time to respond to stimuli<br>Change in sleep patterns | Promote independence in daily activities.<br>Allow ample time for completion of tasks.<br>Offer back rub or warm milk at bedtime.<br>Provide recreational and diversional activities.<br>Maintain environmental stability, minimize frequency of transfers. |
| Integumentary | Sweat glands diminish—decreased thermoregulation<br>Collagen and subcutaneous fat decreases (subcutaneous medications absorb more slowly)—wrinkles, poor turgor (poor estimate of hydration)<br>Hair follicles decrease/produce less melanin—baldness/gray hair<br>Vascular supply to nailbeds reduced—dull, brittle nails—hard to cut!<br>Delayed wound healing | Provide adequate warmth.<br>Maintain adequate hydration.<br>Avoid overexposure to the sun.<br>Provide adequate heat and humidity in environment.<br>Keep skin clean, dry, lubricated, and pressure free.<br>Decrease frequency of baths.<br>Refer to podiatrist. |
| Musculoskeletal | Muscle fibers decrease and muscles atrophy—decreased strength and endurance<br>Bone density decreases—osteoporosis, increased fractures<br>Ligaments and tendons lose elasticity—decreased ROM in joints<br>Intervertebral disks narrow—increased spine curves, balance diminishes (center of gravity) | Encourage exercise program.<br>Promote optimum physical activity within level of ability.<br>Maintain optimum nutrition, especially intake of protein, calcium, and vitamins.<br>Encourage use of appropriate adaptive or assistive devices to enhance mobility. |

*(continues)*

**Table 4-11** Age-Related Changes *(continued)*

| System | Change | Nursing Interventions |
|---|---|---|
| Cardiovascular | Increased peripheral resistance/increased blood pressure, especially systolic<br>Baroreceptors less sensitive—decreased sensitivity to change in positions (orthostatic hypotension)<br>Decreased venous valve competency—increased dependent edema<br>Mitral/aortic valves thicker and more rigid—more murmurs without disease<br>Decreased stroke volume and cardiac output<br>Decreased pacemaker cells—possible dysrhythmias | Assess symptoms and make appropriate modifications in care.<br>Teach client to change positions slowly to avoid falls.<br>Minimize edema and fatigue with rest periods and elevation of legs.<br>Teach energy conservation methods in daily activities. |
| Respiratory | Muscles weaken and atrophy, rib cage calcifies, barrel-shaped chest—increased energy to expand lungs, harder to cough and deep breathe<br>Less tidal volume and increased residual volume secondary to cell fibrosis<br>Alveoli decrease and thicken—less sensitive to hypoxia and hypercapnia<br>Atrophy of cilia—slowed cough reflex, increased risk of infection | Manipulate environment to enhance ventilation.<br>Position client to promote optimum ventilation.<br>Encourage exercises and prescribed pulmonary exercises.<br>Encourage annual influenza vaccines and one-time pneumococcal vaccine. |
| Gastrointestinal | Decreased smooth muscle tone, difficulty in swallowing (minor) and decreased peristalsis—decreased esophageal motility, increased heartburn and constipation<br>Decrease in digestive enzymes—altered absorption of fats, protein, $B_{12}$, folic acid, calcium, iron, medications<br>Decreased saliva, loss of teeth<br>Decreased sphincter tone—impactions, incontinence | Assess condition of teeth and mouth, fit and comfort of dentures, and ability to chew.<br>Encourage fluids and foods high in fiber.<br>Encourage optimal activity.<br>Promote independence and privacy in use of bathroom.<br>Keep stool record and observe for constipation. |
| Renal | Decreased GFR secondary to decreased kidney size and number of nephrons and decreased renal blood flow—ability to concentrate/dilute urine decreased, decreased excretion of medications<br>Decreased bladder capacity and weakened bladder and pelvic muscles—frequency, urgency, nocturia, incontinence, retention, infections<br>Prostate enlargement/obstruction (retention), dribbling, overflow incontinence | Assess voiding patterns.<br>Provide adequate fluids.<br>Establish a bladder program to promote continence (assist to bathroom or offer bedpan every 2–3 hours).<br>Avoid catheterization unless comatose, skin breakdown, or bladder outlet obstruction. |
| Reproductive<br>*Female* | Diminished vaginal secretions secondary to decreased estrogen—painful intercourse, infections | Promote good perineal care, treat with prescribed creams (e.g., estrogen).<br>Use vaginal lubricant as needed. |
| *Male* | Slower erections and ejaculations secondary to sclerosis of penile veins and arteries—decrease in sexual activity | Provide encouragement and discuss modifications of sexual expression as necessary; rest before and after sexual activity. |

# Psychologic/Social Theories of Aging

A. Activity theory
   1. Maintaining a level of active involvement in life helps the older adult stay psychologically and socially healthy.
   2. As life roles or physical capacity are lost, the older adult will substitute new roles or intellectual activities.
B. Continuity or developmental theory
   1. Adjustment to old age is impacted by individual personality, and the older adult

will exhibit similar choices and decisions to younger years.
2. This theory allows for great variation in successful aging, as individual habits and preferences are unique.

C. Disengagement theory
1. Gradual mutual withdrawal between the individual and society as the aging process continues.
2. While this theory was a major milestone in aging research, it is now felt to be flawed, as many older adults remain engaged in psychosocial aspects of life.

# PATTERNS OF HEALTH AND DISEASE IN THE OLDER ADULT

A. Diseases that occur to varying degrees in most older adults
1. Cataracts
2. Arteriosclerosis
3. Benign prostatic hypertrophy (males)

B. Diseases with increased incidence with advancing age
1. Neoplastic disease
2. Diabetes mellitus
3. Dementia disorders

C. Diseases that have more serious consequences in the elderly and make homeostasis more difficult to maintain
1. Pneumonia
2. Influenza
3. Trauma

D. Chronic disease very common
1. Seventy-nine percent of noninstitutionalized persons over age 70 have at least one chronic disease.
2. Most common chronic diseases: arthritis, hypertension, heart disease, cancer.
3. Most hospital visits for persons over 65 are for chronic diseases.

E. Functional disability (inability to perform activities of daily living [ADL])
1. Thirty-two percent of persons over 65 have some limitation of functions.
2. Twenty-five percent of persons over 65 require help with at least one ADL or IADL (instrumental activities of daily living; e.g., shopping, paying bills).

F. Chronic vs. acute diseases (see Table 4-12).

# ASSESSMENT

## Health History and Gerontologic Focus

A. Assessment of the older adult client is complex
1. Allow sufficient time to conduct a thorough health history interview.

**Table 4-12** Chronic Disease vs. Acute Disease

| Characteristic | Chronic Diseases | Acute Diseases |
|---|---|---|
| Cause | Multiple causes; often related to lifestyle | Specific etiologies |
| Onset | Slow, insidious | Rapid |
| Duration | Indeterminate; remissions and exacerbations | Short |
| Understanding of disease | Often difficult because of indeterminate course, remissions, and exacerbations | Simpler because symptoms more overt |
| Outcomes | Somewhat predictable but often debilitating and associated with long periods of illness<br>Management of condition<br>Lifestyle changes required<br>Individual with disease must assume control of disease | Symptoms resolve with cure of disease<br>Outcomes usually favorable; cures<br>Health care provider directs care and cure |

2. Depending on the client's stability, the interview may take more than one session.

B. Presenting problem
1. Assess client systematically depending upon the presenting problem.
2. Typical presentations of disease may change with age (i.e., client may not exhibit chest pain with a myocardial infarction).
3. The problem is likely to have multiple contributing factors and affect the client's functional abilities.

C. Mental status and mental health
1. It is important to obtain a baseline for orientation, memory, level of alertness, and decision-making capabilities.
2. Assess the client for quality of life issues, mood, affect, and anxiety.

D. Lifestyle and function
1. Often, there is little correlation between diseases and functional abilities.
2. The functional assessment provides a clearer picture of physical, psychologic, and social health.
3. Use the client's own baseline from previous assessments to determine any changes in function.
4. Have the client demonstrate function wherever possible (i.e., observe gait and balance, drinking a glass of water, dressing self).

E. Medication usage
   1. Ask for information about all types of medications that the client is taking, including prescription medications, nonprescription medications (especially analgesics and laxatives), vitamin supplements, and herbal medications.
   2. Be sure the client understands the purpose, dosage, side effects, and any special considerations or interactions for all medications.
   3. Discuss the client's abilities to obtain medications (i.e., renewing prescriptions, paying for medications).
   4. Polypharmacy is often present. Average older adult takes 11 prescription medications per day.
F. Nutrition and hydration
   1. Obtain food/fluid intake profile (either 24 hours or 3 days).
   2. Determine any difficulties ingesting food/fluids (chewing, salivation, swallowing, manual dexterity, tremors).
   3. Any foods the client is unable to eat (dairy products, sodium, sugar) or foods the client should eat (potassium- or calcium-rich foods/fluids).
   4. Inquire if an adequate amount of water is taken daily to stay hydrated.
   5. Inquire if able to afford/purchase/prepare food.
G. Past medical history
   1. Inquire about all chronic diseases and conditions. Be aware that the client may not even consider certain conditions treatable and therefore does not mention them, e.g., urinary incontinence or pain from arthritis.
   2. Obtain information about previous illnesses, hospitalizations, and surgeries.

## Physical Examination

A. Assess body systems as indicated.
B. Note physical changes in the older adult (see Table 4-11).

## Laboratory/Diagnostic Tests

A. Laboratory tests as indicated according to symptoms of individual client.
B. Interpret lab test results with aging changes in mind.

## ANALYSIS

Nursing diagnoses for older adult clients may include:
A. Activity intolerance
B. Bowel incontinence, constipation, diarrhea
C. Acute or chronic pain
D. Anxiety or death anxiety
E. Deficient fluid volume
F. Risk for infection
G. Impaired memory
H. Impaired physical mobility
I. Impaired oral mucous membrane
J. Imbalanced nutrition: less or more than body requirements
K. Ineffective airway clearance or breathing pattern, or impaired gas exchange
L. Self-care deficits: feeding, bathing/hygiene, dressing/grooming, toileting
M. Disturbed body image or ineffective role performance
N. Disturbed sensory perception
O. Sexual dysfunction
P. Impaired skin integrity
Q. Disturbed sleep pattern
R. Disturbed thought processes
S. Ineffective tissue perfusion
T. Impaired urinary elimination
U. Deficient diversional activity
V. Wandering
W. Impaired social interaction
X. Risk for other-directed violence
Y. Risk for falls or injury
Z. Relocation stress syndrome
AA. Impaired home maintenance

## PLANNING AND IMPLEMENTATION

### Goals

Client will maintain:
A. Maximum functional independence
B. Normal bowel and bladder elimination patterns
C. Sufficient communication skills
D. Positive self-concept
E. Freedom from injury and infection
F. Optimal cognitive functioning
G. Adequate nutritional status and fluid balance
H. A restful sleep pattern
I. Social contacts and interpersonal needs
J. Treatment regimens as prescribed

## INTERVENTIONS

### Pharmacotherapy in the Older Adult

A. General information
   1. Decreased body weight, dehydration, alterations in fat to muscle ratio, and slowed organ functioning may cause accumulation of a drug in the body due to higher concentrations in the tissues and slowed metabolism and excretion of the drug.
   2. Multiple chronic diseases affecting older adults may also cause changes in the metabolism and excretion of medications.

3. Medication errors among older community-dwelling adults are estimated to be 25–50%.
4. Drug-drug interactions are increased secondary to older adults often having more than one prescribing health care provider.

B. Nursing care
1. Conduct a "brown bag" evaluation to assess all prescription, over-the-counter, and herbal medications the client may be taking.
2. Assess the client's understanding of the reasons for the drug therapy.
3. Assess the client's vision, memory, judgment, reading level, hand dexterity, and motivation to determine ability to self-medicate.
4. Provide instructions in large-print, premeasured syringes, memory aids, and daily drug dose containers to enhance self-medicating abilities.
5. Check with the pharmacist for any drug-drug interactions if unsure.
6. Before beginning a medication, obtain baseline vital signs, mental status, vision, and bowel/bladder function.
7. Drug-induced side effects may present as confusion, incontinence, falls, or immobility.
8. Assess the client's ability to pay for the prescriptions.
9. If the client requires assistance in taking medications, teach family members. Proper techniques for administering oral medications include: position head forward with neck slightly flexed to facilitate swallowing and avoid risk of aspiration.
10. If client has swallowing difficulties, obtain liquid forms of oral medications wherever possible.
11. Assess client for effectiveness of medications and any adverse reactions.

# EVALUATION

A. Client performs self-care activities or caregiver provides assistance as needed.
B. Client is continent of bowel and bladder; voids in adequate amounts and has regular bowel movements.
C. Client is able to successfully communicate needs and concerns.
D. Client makes positive statements about self.
E. Client/caregiver modifies environment to support safety.
F. Client is alert, calm, and oriented, if possible.
G. Skin is intact without pressure ulcers.
H. Client eats a nutritionally balanced diet and maintains a stable weight.
I. Client maintains friends, social interactions, and sexual function.
J. Client describes and adheres to treatment plan.

# CONDITIONS

## Senile Dementia, Alzheimer's Disease

See also Unit 7.
A. General information
1. In dementia, the elderly client is alert with a progressive decline in memory and cognition accompanied by personality and behavioral changes.
2. Alzheimer's disease accounts for 60–75% of all dementias and is the number one reason for institutionalization of the elderly.
3. Other types of dementias include:
   a. Vascular: small infarctions in the brain result in dementia. Risk factors include hyperlipidemia, hypertension, and smoking.
   b. Frontoparietal: atrophy of neurons in the frontal lobes of the brain. Early symptoms are behavioral rather than cognitive abnormalities. (Pick's disease is most common.)
B. Medical management
1. Rule out other conditions that might be causing symptoms. A definitive diagnosis of Alzheimer's disease can only be made upon autopsy.
2. Medications for treatment include tacrine (Cognex), donepezil (Aricept), rivastigmine (Exelon), or galantamine (Reminyl).
   a. Used in mild to moderate stages of the disease: 25% of clients show symptom improvement, and 80% of clients show a delay in decline of cognition.
   b. Nursing considerations: Monitor for bradycardia and GI side effects, including anorexia and weight loss.
3. Treatment goals are to minimize behavioral symptoms, i.e., agitation, and maximize quality of life.
C. Assessment findings
1. Early in the disease process, may become depressed or anxious. Increased risk of suicide at this time.
2. See Table 4-13, for stages of Alzheimer's disease.
D. Nursing interventions
1. Provide a safe environment, e.g., bed in lowest position; check on client frequently; avoid restraints (increases agitation); use night-lights.
2. Provide structured environment and simple routines, e.g., lowered noise levels; appropriate lighting; confined area for wandering.
3. Enlist caregiver's assistance in assessing routine and establishing plan of care.

**Table 4-13** Stages of Alzheimer's Disease

| Stage | Timeframe | Clinical Manifestations |
|---|---|---|
| Early | 2–4 years | Forgetfulness; poor memory (may compensate by using notes)<br>Declining interest in people, environment, and current events<br>Impaired acquisition of new information<br>Impaired judgment; mild cognitive changes<br>   job performance declines; may lose job<br>May be apathetic, irritable, or show signs of depression<br>Normal EEG and CT |
| Middle | 2–12 years | Progressive memory loss<br>Disorientation to time, place, and events<br>Impaired ability to follow simple directions or simple math<br>Significant impairment of cognitive function and judgment<br>Wanders at night due to sleep-wake cycle disturbance<br>Neglects personal hygiene and activities of daily living<br>Becomes increasingly irritable, evasive, and anxious<br>May experience episodes of violent behavior<br>EEG–slowing; CT–normal or dilated ventricles |
| Late | 8–12 years | Extreme weight loss secondary to lack of eating<br>Severe impairment of all cognitive functions<br>Unable to communicate (verbal or written)<br>Dependent on others for activities of daily living<br>Incontinent of urine and feces<br>Pathological reflexes can be elicited<br>Motor skills are lost; becomes bedridden<br>EEG–diffuse slowing<br>CT–dilated ventricles and sulcal enlargement |

4. Use touch and a calm, relaxed manner in approaching the client.
5. Facilitate effective communication.
   a. Face the client and speak clearly using simple words and short sentences.
   b. Keep directions simple and choices to a minimum (e.g., "Do you want to eat chicken or fish?").
   c. Allow ample time for responses.
6. Encourage orientation with use of calendars and clocks; constantly reorienting the client is frustrating to all; consider validation therapy.
7. Have family bring items that stimulate memory, e.g., photographs and personal belongings, to the room.
8. Encourage mobility and provide opportunities for exercise, including walking and range of motion.
9. Avoid isolating the client; provide some stimulation such as soft music or television.
10. Provide nutritious, high-fiber foods and adequate fluids to maintain weight and hydration. Finger foods are a good choice.
11. Promote bowel and bladder continence by toileting at regular intervals.
12. Provide a simple bedtime routine that facilitates sleep, and encourage daytime activities to avoid excess napping.

# ELDER MISTREATMENT

A. General information
1. Elder mistreatment can take the form of abuse or neglect.
2. Abuse may be actual injury inflicted or verbal insults, the use of physical or chemical restraints, financial abuse of money or assets, withholding food/fluids/medications, sexual abuse, or abandonment.
3. The most common type of neglect is self-neglect in which the older adult is unable or unwilling to provide for him/herself. The responsible caregiver may also neglect by not providing necessary services or care.
4. A range of 4–10% of the older population experience elder mistreatment.
B. Assessment findings
1. Identify individuals at risk.
   a. Women over 75 years old who live with relatives and are physically, socially, and/or financially dependent.
   b. Persons whose primary caregivers express resentment, anger, or frustration with the older adult.
2. Clues to mistreatment
   a. Signs and symptoms may include poor hygiene and grooming, failure to thrive

4

(malnutrition), oversedation, depression, and/or fearfulness.

    **b.** Skin provides objective evidence. Look for bruises, burns, lacerations, or pressure ulcers.

  **3.** When assessing for mistreatment, the nurse should consider:

    **a.** Is the person in immediate danger of bodily harm?

    **b.** Is the person competent to make decisions regarding self care?

    **c.** What is the degree and significance of the person's functional impairments?

    **d.** What specific services might help to meet the unmet needs?

    **e.** Who in the family is involved and to what extent?

    **f.** Are the client and family willing to accept interventions?

**C.** Nursing interventions

  **1.** Report suspected mistreatment to adult protective services.

  **2.** Obtain client's consent for treatment.

  **3.** Document nursing assessments of client's physical and emotional status.

# OSTEOPOROSIS (See Unit 6)

# CEREBRAL VASCULAR ACCIDENT
(See Cerebrovascular Accident [CVA])

# BENIGN PROSTATIC HYPERTROPHY
(See Disorder of the Male Reproductive System)

# CATARACTS (See Disorders of the Eye)

# GLAUCOMA (See Disorders of the Eye)

 **Sample Questions**

**51.** What pulmonary function is common in elderly clients?

  1. Reduction in vital capacity.

  2. A decrease in residual volume.

  3. An increase in functional alveoli.

  4. Blood gases that reflect mild acidosis.

**52.** Which is a normal sign of aging in the renal system?

  1. Intermittent incontinence.

  2. Concentrated urine.

  3. Microscopic hematuria.

  4. A decreased glomerular filtration rate.

**53.** An elderly client reports using more salt in food to enhance flavor. What explains the reason for this action?

  1. A decreased number of taste buds.

  2. Confusion because of advanced age.

  3. A need for more sodium to ensure renal function.

  4. An attempt to compensate for lost fluids.

**54.** Which assessment finding in the elderly is caused by decreased vessel elasticity and increased peripheral resistance?

  1. Confusion and disorientation.

  2. An irregular peripheral pulse rate.

  3. An increase in blood pressure.

  4. Wide QRS complexes on the ECG.

**55.** Which action by the CNA would the nurse correct in the care of the older client with a hearing problem?

  1. Facing the client, speaking slowly and clearly.

  2. Examining the ear for cerumen accumulation.

  3. Assisting the client with hearing aid placement.

  4. Speaking loudly when talking to the client.

**56.** An elderly client repeatedly talks about how he wishes he was as strong and energetic as he was when he was younger. In planning care for this client, the nurse should include which of the following?

  1. Use of the intervention reminiscence.

  2. Confrontation of the client about being so grim.

  3. Changing the topic whenever he brings it up.

  4. Incorporation of a humorous view of the normal loss of strength.

**57.** An elderly woman is hospitalized for dehydration. During the admission interview, she admits to the nurse that she is depressed. The nurse would expect this client to exhibit which of the following symptoms?

  1. Increased energy level.

  2. Increased anxiety.

  3. Increased autonomy.

  4. Increased socialization.

**58.** Knowing the difference between normal age-related changes and pathologic findings, which finding should the nurse identify as pathologic in a 74-year-old client?

  1. Increase in residual lung volume.

  2. Decrease in sphincter control of the bladder.

  3. Increase in diastolic blood pressure.

  4. Decreased response to touch, heat, and pain.

59. A sexually active 63-year-old client complains of painful intercourse secondary to vaginal dryness. Which information is most important for the nurse to include in a teaching plan for this client?
   1. Discuss with the client all the medications being taken, including over-the-counter drugs, in order to determine a possible etiology for the dryness.
   2. Teach the client alternative methods of intimacy in the form of touch.
   3. Instruct the client to use an artificial water-based lubricant in the vagina to decrease the discomfort of intercourse.
   4. Prepare the client for a vascular work-up because the dryness is often related to vascular deficiencies.

60. An older client, who has medically controlled manic-depression and asthma has been prescribed cardiac medications for congestive heart failure. He complains to the home care nurse that he is nauseated. It would be justifiable for the nurse to reach which of the following conclusions as to the cause of the client's nausea?
   1. The reaction between the new medication regime and the foods caused the nausea.
   2. The problem of polypharmacy may exist as the client symptomatology may be a result of multiple drug interactions.
   3. The nausea could be psychosomatic and related to the client's depression over having to take new medications.
   4. The client may be taking too much of his new medications, which may contribute to his symptoms.

61. An older client has several medications ordered and has difficulty swallowing them. What strategy should the nurse use to administer these medications?
   1. Hide the medication by placing them in meat.
   2. Crush the medication and mix them with soft foods.
   3. Substitute injectable medications.
   4. Dissolve medications in liquid.

62. Which of the following measures is necessary to incorporate into a plan of care for a client who is diagnosed with senile dementia?
   1. Because these clients are easily bored, they need to be challenged with new activities.
   2. Environmental stimuli need to be eliminated.
   3. Communicate in simple words, short sentences, and a calm tone of voice.
   4. Schedule more demanding activities later in the day.

63. A 76-year-old man who is a resident in an extended care facility is in the late stages of Alzheimer's disease. He tells his nurse that he has sore back muscles from all the construction work he has been doing all day. Which response by the nurse is most appropriate?
   1. "You know you don't work in construction anymore."
   2. "What type of motion did you do to precipitate this soreness?"
   3. "You're 76 years old and you've been here all day. You don't work in construction anymore."
   4. "Would you like me to rub your back for you?"

64. An 86-year-old male with senile dementia has been physically abused and neglected for the past two years by his live-in caregiver. He has since moved and is living with his son and daughter-in-law. Which response by the client's son would cause the nurse great concern?
   1. "How can we obtain reliable help to assist us in taking care of Dad? We can't do it alone."
   2. "Dad used to beat us kids all the time. I wonder if he remembered that when it happened to him?"
   3. "I'm not sure how to deal with Dad's constant repetition of words."
   4. "I plan to ask my sister and brother to help my wife and me with Dad on the weekends."

65. An alert and oriented 84-year-old client is receiving home care services following a cerebrovascular accident (CVA) that has left her with right-sided hemiparesis. She lives with her middle-aged daughter and son-in-law. The nurse suspects she is being physically abused by her daughter. To elicit information effectively, the nurse should do which of the following?
   1. Directly ask the client if she has been physically struck or hurt by anyone.
   2. Wait until enough trust has been developed to enable the client to approach the nurse first.
   3. Confront the daughter with the suspicions.
   4. Interview the son-in-law to gain his perspective of the situation.

## Answers and Rationales

51. **1.** Muscles weaken reducing capability to cough or deep breathe, which reduces total lung capacity.

52. **4.** The glomerular filtration rate is decreased dramatically in the elderly due to changes in the renal tubules.

**53. 1.** The taste buds begin to atrophy at age 40, and insensitivity to taste qualities occurs after age 60. Studies related to diminished taste indicate that there are changes in the salt threshold for some elderly individuals.

**54. 3.** The blood pressure increases in response to the thickening of vessels and less distensible arteries and veins. There is also impedance to blood flow and increased systemic vascular resistance, contributing to hypertension.

**55. 4.** Raising the voice to speak loudly only increases the emission of higher frequency sounds, which the elderly client with presbycusis (a progressive bilateral perceptive loss of hearing in the older individual that occurs with the aging process) will have difficulty hearing.

**56. 1.** Assisting the older adult in reminiscing, or engaging in a "life review" process, is one way to assist the individual to accomplish developmental tasks. One such task, adjusting to decreasing physical strength, needs to be met to establish and preserve ego integrity.

**57. 2.** Many psychosocial symptoms occur with depression, including feelings of hopelessness, helplessness, and increased anxiety, which contributes to despair rather than ego integrity.

**58. 3.** A modest increase in systolic blood pressure, not diastolic blood pressure, is an expected age-related change due to an increase in vascular resistance and vessel rigidity. An increase in diastolic blood pressure, however, is not an expected age-related change. It is pathologic and needs to be monitored.

**59. 3.** The decrease in vaginal secretions, which contributes to vaginal dryness and subsequent painful intercourse, is a normal age-related change. Using a lubricant will decrease or eliminate this discomfort.

**60. 2.** Polypharmacy is the prescription, use, or administration of five or more medications. If not coordinated, different physicians, each focusing on a specific disease process, contribute to polypharmacy.

**61. 2.** Medications, crushed and mixed with soft foods, are easier to digest for persons who have difficulty swallowing.

**62. 3.** Keep communications simple and concrete. Close-ended questions are more beneficial than open-ended questions, which may require complex answers that serve only to confuse the client. Even if the client isn't able to fully comprehend communications, a calm tone of voice may alleviate any stress.

**63. 4.** In the late stages of Alzheimer's disease, it is better to go along with the client's reality rather than confront him with logic and reasoning. Asking close-ended, simple questions that relate to his reality is nonthreatening and calming. Note that the nurse responds in a way that is congruent with his main concern, which is his sore back.

**64. 2.** This statement is a cause for concern. Abusive patterns are highly likely to be passed from parents to children. When children grow up and move into positions where they are caring for their aged parents (role reversal), the abusive behavior can surface.

**65. 1.** Direct questioning, in an open and accepting manner, is important. Abused elders are often reluctant to report abuse and will not volunteer the information on their own. Clients need to feel free to indicate the existence of an activity about which they may feel embarrassment and shame.

# Perioperative Nursing

## OVERVIEW

### Effects of Surgery on the Client
*Physical Effects*

A. Stress response (neuroendocrine response) is activated.

B. Resistance to infection is lowered due to surgical incision.
C. Vascular system is disturbed due to severing of blood vessels and blood loss.
D. Organ function may be altered due to manipulation.

## *Psychologic Effects*

Common fears: pain, anesthesia, loss of control, disfigurement, separation from loved ones, alterations in roles or lifestyle.

## Factors Influencing Surgical Risk

A. Age: very young and elderly are at increased risk.
B. Nutrition: malnutrition and obesity increase risk of complications.
C. Fluid and electrolyte balance: dehydration, hypovolemia, and electrolyte imbalances can pose problems during surgery.
D. General health status: infection, cardiovascular disease, pulmonary problems, liver dysfunction, renal insufficiency, or metabolic disorders create increased risk.
E. Medications
    1. Anticoagulants (including aspirin and NSAIDs) predispose to hemorrhage; discontinue use according to physician's orders.
    2. Tranquilizers (e.g., phenothiazines) may cause hypotension and potentiate shock.
    3. Antibiotics: aminoglycosides may intensify neuromuscular blockade of anesthesia with resultant respiratory paralysis.
    4. Diuretics: may cause electrolyte imbalances.
    5. Antihypertensives: can cause hypotension and contribute to shock.
    6. Long-term steroid therapy: causes adrenocortical suppression; may need increased dosage during perioperative period.
F. Type of surgery planned: major surgery (e.g., thoracotomy) poses greater risk than minor surgery (e.g., dental extraction).
G. Psychologic status of client: excessive fear or anxiety may have adverse effect on surgery.

# PREOPERATIVE PERIOD

## Psychologic Support

A. Assess client's fears, anxieties, support systems, and patterns of coping.
B. Establish trusting relationship with client and significant others.
C. Explain routine procedures, encourage verbalization of fears, and allow client to ask questions.
D. Demonstrate confidence in surgeon and staff.
E. Provide for spiritual care if appropriate.

## Preoperative Teaching

A. Frequently done on an outclient basis.
B. Assess client's level of understanding of surgical procedure and its implications.
C. Answer questions, clarify and reinforce explanations given by surgeon.
D. Explain routine pre- and post-op procedures and any special equipment to be used.
E. Teach coughing and deep-breathing exercises, splinting of incision, turning side to side in bed, and leg exercises; explain their importance in preventing complications; provide opportunity for return demonstration.
F. Assure client that pain medication will be available post-op.

## Physical Preparation

A. Obtain history of past medical conditions, surgical procedures, allergies, dietary restrictions, and medications.
B. Perform baseline head-to-toe assessment, including vital signs, height, and weight.
C. Ensure that diagnostic procedures are performed as ordered. Common tests are:
    1. CBC (complete blood count)
    2. Electrolytes
    3. PT/PTT (prothrombin time; partial thromboplastin time)
    4. Urinalysis
    5. ECG (electrocardiogram)
    6. Type and crossmatch
    7. Chest X-ray
D. Prepare client's skin.
    1. Shower with antibacterial soap to cleanse skin if ordered; client may do this at home the night before surgery if outpatient admission.
    2. Skin prep if ordered: shave or clip hairs and cleanse appropriate areas to reduce bacteria on skin and minimize chance of infection.
E. Administer enema if ordered (usually for surgery on GI tract, gynecologic surgery).
F. Promote adequate rest and sleep.
    1. Provide back rub, clean linens.
    2. Administer bedtime sedation.
G. Instruct client to remain NPO after midnight to prevent vomiting and aspiration during surgery.

## Legal Responsibilities

A. Surgeon obtains operative permit (informed consent).
    1. Surgical procedure, alternatives, possible complications, disfigurements, or removal of body parts are explained.
    2. It is part of the nurse's role as client advocate to confirm that the client understands information given.
B. Informed consent is necessary for each operation performed, however minor. It is also necessary for major diagnostic procedures, e.g., bronchoscopy, thoracentesis, etc., where a major body cavity is entered.

C. Adult client (over 18 years of age) signs own permit unless unconscious or mentally incompetent.
   1. If unable to sign, relative (spouse or next of kin) or guardian will sign.
   2. In an emergency, permission via telephone or telegram is acceptable; have a second nurse verify by phone the telephone permission; both nurses will sign the consent form.
   3. Consents are not needed for emergency care if all four of the following criteria are met.
      a. There is an immediate threat to life.
      b. Experts agree that it is an emergency.
      c. Client is unable to consent.
      d. A legally authorized person cannot be reached.
D. Minors (under 18) must have consent signed by an adult (i.e., parent or legal guardian). An emancipated minor (married, college student living away from home, in military service, any pregnant female or any who has given birth) may sign own consent.
E. Witness to informed consent may be nurse, another physician, or other authorized person.
F. If nurse witnesses informed consent, specify whether witnessing explanation of surgery or just signature of client.

## Preparation Immediately before Surgery

A. Obtain baseline vital signs; report elevated temperature or blood pressure.
B. Provide oral hygiene and remove dentures.
C. Remove client's clothing and dress in clean gown.
D. Remove nail polish, cosmetics, hair pins, contact lenses, prostheses, and any body jewelry.
E. Instruct client to empty bladder.
F. Check identification band.
G. Administer pre-op medications as ordered.
   1. Narcotic analgesics (meperidine [Demerol], morphine sulfate) relax client, reduce anxiety, and enhance effectiveness of general anesthesia.

2. Sedatives (secobarbital sodium [Seconal]), sodium pentobarbital [Nembutal] decrease anxiety and promote relaxation and sleep.
3. Anticholinergics (atropine sulfate, scopolamine [Hyoscine]) and glycopyrrolate (Robinul) decrease tracheobronchial secretions to minimize danger of aspirating secretions in lungs, decrease vagal response to inhibit undesirable effects of general anesthesia (bradycardia).
4. Droperidol, fentanyl, or a combination may be ordered; should not be given with sedatives because of danger of respiratory depression; also helpful in control of postoperative nausea and vomiting.
H. Elevate side rails and provide quiet environment.
I. Prepare client's chart for OR, including operative permit and complete pre-op check list.
J. Stay with client after pre-op medications have been given and assist with bedpan for toileting needs.

# INTRAOPERATIVE PERIOD

## Anesthesia

### General Anesthesia

A. General information
   1. Drug-induced depression of CNS; produces decreased muscle reflex activity and loss of consciousness.
   2. Balanced anesthesia: combination of several anesthetic drugs to provide smooth induction, appropriate depth and duration of anesthesia, sufficient muscle relaxation, and minimal complications.
B. Stages of general anesthesia: induction, excitement, surgical anesthesia, and danger stage (see Table 4-14).
C. Agents for general anesthesia
   1. Inhalation agents may be gas or liquid.
   2. IV anesthetics: used as induction agents because they produce rapid, smooth

**Table 4-14** Stages of Anesthesia

| Stage | From | To | Client Status |
|---|---|---|---|
| Stage I (induction) | Beginning administration of anesthetic agent | Loss of consciousness | May appear euphoric, drowsy, dizzy. |
| Stage II (delirium or excitement) | Loss of consciousness | Relaxation | Breathing irregular; may appear excited; very susceptible to external stimuli. |
| Stage III (surgical anesthesia) | Relaxation | Loss of reflexes and depression of vital functions | Regular breathing pattern; corneal reflexes absent; papillary constriction. |
| Stage IV (danger stage) | Vital functions depressed | Respiratory arrest; possible cardiac arrest | No respirations; absent or minimal heartbeat; dilated pupils. |

induction; may be used alone in short procedures such as endoscopies.
  a. Common IV anesthetics: methohexital (Brevital), sodium thiopental (Pentathol), midazolam hydrochloride (Versed)
  b. Disadvantages: poor relaxation; respiratory and myocardial depression in high doses; bronchospasm, laryngospasm; hypotension, respiratory depression
3. Dissociative agents: produce state of profound analgesia, amnesia, and lack of awareness without loss of consciousness; used alone in short surgical and diagnostic procedures or for induction prior to administration of more potent general anesthetics.
  a. Agent: ketamine (Ketalar)
  b. Side effects: tachycardia, hypertension, respiratory depression, hallucinations, delirium
  c. Precautions: decrease verbal, tactile, and visual stimulation during recovery period
4. Neuroleptics: produce state of neuroleptic analgesia characterized by reduced motor activity, decreased anxiety, and analgesia without loss of consciousness; used alone for short surgical and diagnostic procedures, as premedication or in combination with other anesthetics for longer anesthesia.
  a. Agent: fentanyl citrate with droperidol (Innovar)
  b. Side effects: hypotension, bradycardia, respiratory depression, skeletal muscle rigidity, twitching
  c. Precautions: reduce narcotic doses by ½ to ⅓ for at least 8 hours postanesthesia as ordered to prevent respiratory depression.
D. Adjuncts to general anesthesia: neuromuscular blocking agents: used with general anesthetics to enhance skeletal muscle relaxation.
  1. Agents: pancuronium (Pavulon), succinylcholine (Anectine), tubocurarine, atracurium besylate (Tracrium), vecuronium bromide (Norcuron)
  2. Precaution: monitor client's respirations for at least 1 hour after drug's effect has worn off.

## Regional Anesthesia

A. General information (see also Table 4-15).
  1. Produces loss of painful sensation in one area of the body; does not produce loss of consciousness
  2. Uses: biopsies, excision of moles and cysts, endoscopies, surgery on extremities; childbirth
  3. Agents: lidocaine (Xylocaine), procaine (Novocain), tetracaine (Pontocaine)

## Conscious Sedation

A. General information
  1. Intravenous conscious sedation is induced by pharmacologic agents.

**Table 4-15** Regional Anesthesia

| Types | Method |
| --- | --- |
| Topical | Cream, spray, drops, or ointment applied externally, directly to area to be anesthetized. |
| Local infiltration block | Injected into subcutaneous tissue of surgical area. |
| Field block | Area surrounding the surgical site injected with anesthetic. |
| Nerve block | Injection into a nerve plexus to anesthetize part of body. |
| Spinal | Anesthetic introduced into subarachnoid space of spinal cord producing anesthesia below level of diaphragm. |
| Epidural | Anesthetic injected extradurally to produce anesthesia below level of diaphragm; used in obstetrics. |
| Caudal | Variation of epidural block; produces anesthesia of perineum and occasionally lower abdomen; commonly used in obstetrics. |
| Saddle block | Similar to spinal, but anesthetized area is more limited; commonly used in obstetrics. |

2. Sedative and analgesic medications are used to achieve an altered state of consciousness with minimal risk, relief of anxiety, an amnestic state, and pain relief from noxious stimuli.
3. These agents may include a combination of a benzodiazepine (midazolam, diazepam) and a narcotic (fentanyl, morphine).
4. This provides a safe and effective option for clients undergoing minor surgical and diagnostic procedures such as, but not limited to, endoscopic procedures, breast biopsy, dental surgery, and plastic surgery.
5. Conscious sedation is extremely safe when administered by qualified providers.
  a. Certified registered nurse anesthetists (CRNAs), anesthesiologists, dentists, oral surgeons, and other physicians are qualified providers of conscious sedation.
  b. Specifically trained registered nurses may assist in the administration of conscious sedation.
6. Verbal communication with the client can be maintained throughout the procedure, client may have a brief period of amnesia which may erase any memory of the procedure.
7. This will provide reassurance to a cooperative client and help monitor intact neurological status.
8. Supplemental oxygen should always be given to a client receiving conscious sedation.

9. Constant vigilance in monitoring of cardiorespiratory status (heart rate and rhythm, blood pressure, respiratory rate, and pulse oximetry) is crucial.
10. The provider who monitors the client receiving conscious sedation should have no other responsibilities during the procedure and should never abandon that client for any reason.

# POSTOPERATIVE PERIOD

## Postoperative Care

### Recovery Room (Immediate Postoperative Care)

A. Assess for and maintain patent airway.
   1. Position unconscious or semiconscious client on side (unless contraindicated) or on back with head to side and chin extended forward.
   2. Check for presence/absence of gag reflex.
   3. Maintain artificial airway in place until gag and swallow reflex have returned.
B. Administer oxygen as ordered.
C. Assess rate, depth, and quality of respirations.
D. Check vital signs every 15 minutes until stable, then every 30 minutes.
E. Note level of consciousness; reorient client to time, place, and situation.
F. Assess color and temperature of skin, color of nailbeds, and lips.
G. Monitor IV infusions: condition of site, type, and amount of fluid being infused and flow rate.
H. Check all drainage tubes and connect to suction or gravity drainage as ordered; note color, amount, and odor of drainage.
I. Assess dressings for intactness, drainage, hemorrhage.
J. Monitor and maintain client's temperature; may need extra blankets.
K. Encourage client to cough and deep breathe after artificial airway is removed.
L. If spinal anesthesia used, maintain flat position and check for sensation and movement in lower extremities.

### Care on Surgical Floor

A. Monitor respiratory status and promote optimal functioning.
   1. Encourage client to cough (if not contraindicated) and deep breathe every 1–2 hours.
   2. Instruct client to splint incision while coughing.
   3. Assist client to turn in bed every 2 hours.
   4. Encourage early ambulation.
   5. Encourage use of incentive spirometer every 2 hours: causes sustained, maximal inspiration that inflates the alveoli.
   6. Assess respiratory status and auscultate lungs every 4 hours; be alert for any signs of respiratory complications.
B. Monitor cardiovascular status and avoid post-op complications.
   1. Encourage leg exercises every 2 hours while in bed.
   2. Encourage early ambulation.
   3. Apply antiembolism stockings as ordered.
   4. Assess vital signs, color and temperature of skin every 4 hours.
C. Promote adequate fluid and electrolyte balance.
   1. Monitor IV and ensure adequate intake.
   2. Measure I&O.
   3. Irrigate NG tube properly, using normal saline solution.
   4. Observe for signs of fluid and electrolyte imbalances.
D. Promote optimum nutrition.
   1. Maintain IV infusion as ordered.
   2. Assess for return of peristalsis (presence of bowel sounds and flatus); peristalsis may take hours to return.
   3. Add progressively to diet as ordered and note tolerance.
E. Monitor and promote return of urinary function.
   1. Measure I&O.
   2. Assess client's ability to void.
   3. Report to surgeon if client has not voided within 8 hours after surgery.
   4. Check for bladder distention.
   5. Use measures to promote urination (e.g., assist male to sit on side of bed, pour warm water over female's perineum).
F. Promote bowel elimination.
   1. Encourage ambulation.
   2. Provide adequate food and fluid intake when tolerated.
   3. Keep stool record and note any difficulties with bowel elimination.
G. Administer post-op analgesics as ordered; provide additional comfort measures.
H. Encourage optimal activity, turning in bed every 2 hours, early ambulation if allowed (generally client will be out of bed within 24 hours; have client dangle legs before getting out of bed).
I. Provide wound care.
   1. Check dressings frequently to ensure they are clean, dry, and intact.
   2. Observe aseptic technique when changing dressings.
   3. Encourage diet high in protein and vitamin C.
   4. Report any signs of infection: redness, drainage, odor, fever.
J. Provide adequate psychologic support to client/significant others.
K. Provide appropriate discharge teaching: dietary restrictions, medication regimen, activity limitations, wound care, and possible complications.

# Postoperative Complications

## Respiratory System

Common post-op complications of respiratory tract are atelectasis and pneumonia.

A. Predisposing factors
   1. Type of surgery (e.g., thoracic or high abdomen surgery)
   2. Previous history of respiratory problems
   3. Age: greater risk over age 40
   4. Obesity
   5. Smoking
   6. Respiratory depression caused by narcotics
   7. Severe post-op pain
   8. Prolonged post-op immobility
B. Prevention: see Care on Surgical Floor.

## Cardiovascular System

Common post-op complications of the cardiovascular system are deep vein thrombosis, pulmonary embolism, and shock.

A. Predisposing factors to deep venous thrombosis (DVT)
   1. Lower abdominal surgery or septic diseases (e.g., peritonitis)
   2. Injury to vein by tight leg straps during surgery
   3. Previous history of venous problems
   4. Increased blood coagulability due to dehydration, fluid loss
   5. Venous stasis in the extremity due to decreased movement during surgery
   6. Prolonged post-op immobilization
B. Predisposing factors to pulmonary embolism: may occur as a complication of DVT.
C. Most common causes of shock during post-op period
   1. Hemorrhage
   2. Sepsis
   3. Myocardial infarction and cardiac arrest
   4. Drug reactions
   5. Transfusion reactions
   6. Pulmonary embolism
   7. Adrenal failure
D. Prevention of DVT, pulmonary embolism, and shock: see Care on Surgical Floor.

## Genitourinary System

Post-op complications of the genitourinary system often include urinary retention and urinary tract infection.

A. Predisposing factors to urinary retention include:
   1. Anxiety
   2. Pain
   3. Lack of privacy
   4. Narcotics and certain anesthetics that diminish client's sense of a full bladder
B. Prevention and nursing interventions for urinary retention: see Care on Surgical Floor.

C. Post-op urinary tract infections are most commonly caused by catheterization; prevention consists of using strict sterile technique when inserting a catheter, and appropriate catheter care (every 8 hours or according to agency protocol).

## Gastrointestinal System

An important GI post-op complication is paralytic ileus (paralysis of intestinal peristalsis).

A. Predisposing factors
   1. Temporary: anesthesia, manipulation of bowel during abdominal surgery
   2. Prolonged: electrolyte imbalance, wound infection, pneumonia
B. Assessment findings
   1. Absent bowel sounds
   2. No passage of flatus
   3. Abdominal distention
C. Nursing interventions
   1. Assist with insertion of nasogastric or intestinal tube with application of suction as ordered.
   2. Keep client NPO.
   3. Maintain IV therapy as ordered.
   4. Assess for bowel sounds every 4 hours; check for abdominal distention, passage of flatus.
   5. Encourage ambulation if appropriate.

## Wound Complications

A. Wound infection
   1. Predisposing factors
      a. Obesity
      b. Diabetes mellitus
      c. Malnutrition
      d. Elderly clients
      e. Steroids and immunosuppressive agents
      f. Lowered resistance to infection, as found in clients with cancer
   2. Assessment findings: redness, tenderness, drainage, heat in incisional area; fever; usually occurs 3–5 days after surgery.
   3. Prevention: see Care on Surgical Floor.
   4. Nursing interventions
      a. Obtain culture and sensitivity of wound drainage (*S. aureus* most frequently cultured).
      b. Perform cleansing and irrigation of wound as ordered.
      c. Administer antibiotic therapy as ordered.
B. Wound dehiscence and evisceration
   1. Dehiscence: opening of wound edges
   2. Evisceration: protrusion of loops of bowel through incision; usually accompanied by sudden escape of profuse, pink serous drainage
   3. Predisposing factors to wound dehiscence and evisceration
      a. Wound infection
      b. Faulty wound closure
      c. Severe abdominal stretching (e.g., coughing, retching)

4. Nursing interventions for wound dehiscence
   a. Apply Steri-Strips to incision.
   b. Notify physician.
   c. Promote wound healing.
5. Nursing interventions for wound evisceration
   a. Place client in supine position.
   b. Cover protruding intestinal loops with sterile moist normal saline soaks.
   c. Notify physician.
   d. Check vital signs.
   e. Observe for signs of shock.
   f. Start IV line.
   g. Prepare client for OR for surgical closure of wound.

## Sample Questions

66. An adult man is in the postanesthesia care unit (PACU) following a hemicolectomy. How often will the nurse monitor the vital signs?
    1. Continuously.
    2. Every 5 minutes.
    3. Every 15 minutes.
    4. On a prn basis.

67. An adult who has had general anesthesia for major surgery is in the PACU. Which of the following indicates the artificial airway should be removed?
    1. Gagging.
    2. Restlessness.
    3. An increase in pain.
    4. Clear lungs on auscultation.

68. An adult is 6 days post abdominal surgery. Which sign alerts the nurse to wound evisceration?
    1. Acute bleeding.
    2. Protruding intestines.
    3. Purple drainage.
    4. Severe pain.

69. An adult client's wound has eviscerated. Why would the respiratory status need to be assessed?
    1. Dehiscence elevates the diaphragm.
    2. Coughing increases intestine protrusion.
    3. Respiratory arrest commonly accompanies wound dehiscence.
    4. Splinting the wound will compromise respiratory status.

70. An adult client has acute leukemia and is scheduled for a Hickman catheter insertion under local anesthesia. What is a major advantage to the client for having regional anesthesia?
    1. Retains all reflexes.
    2. Remains conscious.
    3. Has retroactive amnesia.
    4. Is in the OR for a short period of time.

71. An adult male is scheduled for surgery and the nurse is assessing for risk factors. Which of the following are the greatest risk factors?
    1. He is 5 ft 4 in tall and weighs 125 lb.
    2. He expresses a fear of pain in the post-op period.
    3. He is 5 ft 4 in tall, weighs 360 lb, and has diabetes.
    4. He expresses a fear of the unknown.

72. The nurse in an outclient department is interviewing an adult 1 week prior to her scheduled elective surgery. In planning for the surgery, which of the following should the nurse include in her teaching?
    1. Detailed information about the procedure.
    2. Limitations of oral intake the day of the procedure.
    3. Writing a list for postoperative complications.
    4. The client should not take any of her routine medications the morning of the surgery.

73. The nurse enters a woman's room to administer the ordered pre-op medication for her hysterectomy. During the conversation, the client tells the nurse that she and her husband are planning to have another child in the coming year. The best action for the nurse to take is which of the following?
    1. Do not administer the pre-op medication, notify the nursing supervisor and the physician.
    2. Go ahead and administer the medication as ordered.
    3. Check to see if the client has signed a surgical consent.
    4. Send the client to the operating room (OR) without the medication.

74. The nurse administers 10 mg intramuscular (IM) morphine as a pre-op medication, and then discovers that there is no signed operative permit. What is the best action for the nurse to take?
    1. Send the client to surgery as scheduled.
    2. Notify the nursing supervisor, the OR, and the physician.
    3. Cancel the surgery immediately.
    4. Obtain the needed consent.

75. An adult received atropine sulfate (Atropine) as a pre-op medication 30 minutes ago and is now complaining of dry mouth and her pulse rate is higher than before the medication was administered. What is the nurse's best interpretation of these finding?
    1. The client is having an allergic reaction to the drug.
    2. The client needs a higher dose of this drug.
    3. This is a normal side effect of Atropine.
    4. The client is anxious about the upcoming surgery.

76. An adult who has chronic obstructive pulmonary disease (COPD) is scheduled for surgery and the physician has recommended an epidural anesthetic. Why would an epidural anesthetic be used instead of general anesthesia?
    1. There is too high a risk for pressure sores developing.
    2. There is less effect on the respiratory system with epidural anesthesia.
    3. Central nervous system control of vascular constriction would be affected with general anesthesia.
    4. There is too high a risk of lacerations to the mouth, bruising of lips, and damage to teeth.

77. An adult had a bunion removed under an epidural block. In the immediate post-op period, the nurse plans to assess the client for side effects of the epidural block that include which of the following?
    1. Headache.
    2. Hypotension, bradycardia, nausea, and vomiting.
    3. Hypertension, muscular rigidity, fever, and tachypnea.
    4. Urinary retention.

78. An adult received droperidol and fentanyl (Innovar) during surgery. In planning postoperative care, the nurse will need to monitor for which of the following during the immediate post-op period?
    1. Restlessness and anxiety.
    2. Delirium.
    3. Dysrhythmias.
    4. Respiratory depression.

79. An adult has just arrived on the general surgery unit from the postanesthesia care unit (PACU). Which of the following needs to be the initial intervention the nurse takes?
    1. Assess the surgical site, noting the amount and character of drainage.
    2. Assess for amount of urinary output and the presence of any distention.
    3. Allow the family to visit with the client to decrease the anxiety of the client.
    4. Take vital signs, assessing first for a patent airway and the quality of respirations.

80. An adult is receiving morphine via a PCA pump after her surgery. What statement by the nurse would best evaluate the level of pain being experienced?
    1. "Please rate your pain on a scale of 1–10."
    2. "Is the morphine working for you?"
    3. "Are you feeling any pain?"
    4. "Do you need the morphine level increased?"

81. A 58-year-old smoker underwent major abdominal surgery 2 days ago. During the respiratory assessment, the nurse notes he is taking shallow breaths and breath sounds are decreased in the bases. What is the best interpretation for these findings?
    1. Pneumonia.
    2. Atelectasis.
    3. Hemorrhage.
    4. Thromboembolism.

82. To prevent thromboembolism in the post-op client the nurse should include which of the following in the plan of care?
    1. Place a pillow under the knees and restrict fluids.
    2. Use strict aseptic technique including handwashing and sterile dressing technique.
    3. Assess bowel sounds in all four quadrants on every shift and avoid early ambulation.
    4. Assess for Homan's signs on every shift, encourage early ambulation, and maintain adequate hydration.

83. It is 2200 and the nurse notes that an adult male who returned from the PACU at 1400 has not voided. The client has an out of bed order, but has not been up yet. What is the best action for the nurse to take?
    1. Insert a Foley catheter into the client.
    2. Straight-catheterize the client.
    3. Assist the client to stand at the side of his bed and attempt to void into a urinal.
    4. Encourage the client to lie on his left side in bed and attempt to void into a urinal.

84. When assessing a post-op client, the nurse notes a nasogastric tube to low constant suction, the absence of a bowel movement since surgery, and

no bowel sounds. Based on these findings, what would be the most appropriate plan of action?

1. Increase the client's mobility and ensure he is receiving adequate pain relief.
2. Increase coughing, turning, and deep breathing exercises.
3. Discontinue the nasogastric tube as the client does not need it any more.
4. Assess for bladder pain and distention.

85. Preoperatively, the client's blood pressure was 110/70. In PACU, the vitals signs are assessed and the blood pressure is now 150/90. The client is complaining of severe pain. What is the nurse aware of due to this finding?

1. Pain does not affect the blood pressure.
2. The blood pressure elevation is an indication of hypovolemic shock.
3. Pain may cause elevated blood pressure.
4. The client needs a medication to lower the blood pressure.

##  Answers and Rationales

66. **3.** While in the postanesthesia care unit (PACU) the client's vital signs are assessed every 15 minutes.

67. **1.** The return of the gag reflex usually indicates that the client is able to manage his own secretions and maintain a patent airway.

68. **2.** Evisceration is the actual intestinal contents protruding through the abdominal wall.

69. **2.** Coughing increases intra-abdominal pressure, which could force loops of bowel out through the open wound.

70. **2.** The client receiving regional anesthesia has nerve impulses blocked but does not lose consciousness.

71. **3.** Obesity and diabetes are major risk factors with the potential for complications related to anesthesia.

72. **2.** Instructions should be given to the client regarding limitations of oral intake to avoid nausea and vomiting from the anesthesia.

73. **1.** No client should be administered the pre-op medication until the informed consent has been obtained. Informed consent means that the client understands the information about the surgery.

Even if the consent form is signed, the nurse should withhold sedating medication. This client clearly does not understand the planned procedure.

74. **2.** If a narcotic, sedative, or tranquilizing drug has been administered before signing of the consent, the drug's effects must be allowed to wear off before consent can be given.

75. **3.** These are normal side effects of an anticholinergic drug; adverse side effects would include ECG changes, constipation, and urinary retention.

76. **2.** Epidural anesthesia does not cause respiratory depression, but general anesthesia can, especially in a client with COPD.

77. **2.** These are all symptoms of sympathetic nervous system blockade, so the client should be closely monitored for these.

78. **4.** Depression of respiratory rate has been reported and tends to last longer than the analgesic effect when Innovar is used during surgery.

79. **4.** A specific assessment priority is the evaluation of a patent airway and respiratory and circulatory adequacy.

80. **1.** The client should obtain relief from pain, and using a scale to assess this is a more objective measure.

81. **2.** Atelectasis occurs commonly after abdominal surgery, especially in smokers. This occurs when mucus blocks the bronchioles and causes decreased breath sounds and shallow breathing.

82. **4.** Thromboembolism can be related to dehydration and immobility. These measures help prevent hypovolemia and subsequent sludging of cells. A positive Homan's sign is often associated with thromboembolism.

83. **3.** Nursing interventions to facilitate voiding include ambulation and normal positioning for voiding. The normal voiding position for the male is standing.

84. **1.** Paralytic ileus can be related to immobility and inadequate pain medication as well as bowel manipulation and the anesthetic used during surgery.

85. **3.** Physical pain may increase circulating catecholamines, resulting in hypertension. The nurse should assess the pain, provide comfort measures and analgesia, and then reassess the blood pressure.

# Oncologic Nursing

## PATHOPHYSIOLOGY AND ETIOLOGY OF CANCER

### Evolution of Cancer Cells

A. All cells constantly change through growth, degeneration, repair, and adaptation. Normal cells must divide and multiply to meet the needs of the organism as a whole, and this cycle of cell growth and destruction is an integral part of life processes. The activities of the normal cells in the human body are all coordinated to meet the needs of the organism as a whole, but when the regulatory control mechanisms of normal cells fail, and growth continues in excess of the body's needs, neoplasia results.

B. The term neoplasia refers to both benign and malignant growths, but malignant cells behave very differently from normal cells and have special features characteristic of the cancer process.

C. Because the growth control mechanism of normal cells is not entirely understood, it is not clear what allows the uncontrolled growth, therefore no definitive cure has been found.

### Characteristics of Malignant Cells

#### Differentiation

A. Cancer cells are mutated stem cells that have undergone structural changes so that they are unable to perform the normal functions of specialized tissue (un- or dedifferentiation).

B. They may function in a disorderly way or cease normal function completely, only functioning for their own survival and growth.

C. The most undifferentiated cells are also called anaplastic.

#### Rate of Growth

A. Cancer cells have uncontrolled growth or cell division.

B. Rate at which a tumor grows involves both increased cell division and increased survival time of cells.

C. Malignant cells do not form orderly layers, but pile on top of each other to eventually form tumors.

### Spread (Invasion and Metastasis)

A. Cancer cells are less adhesive than normal cells, more easily dissociated from their location.

B. Lack of adhesion and loss of contact inhibition make it possible for a cancer to spread to distant parts of the body (metastasis).

C. Malignant tumors are not encapsulated and expand into surrounding tissue (invasion).

### Etiology (Carcinogenesis)

Actual cause of cancer is unknown but there are a number of theories; it is currently thought that there are probably multiple etiologies.

#### Environmental Factors

A. Majority (over 80%) of human cancers related to environmental carcinogens

B. Types
  1. Physical
     a. Radiation: X-rays, radium, nuclear explosion or waste, ultraviolet
     b. Trauma or chronic irritation
  2. Chemical
     a. Nitrites and food additives, polycyclic hydrocarbons, dyes, alkylating agents
     b. Drugs: arsenicals, stilbestrol, urethane
     c. Cigarette smoke
     d. Hormones

#### Genetics

A. Some cancers show familial pattern.

B. May be caused by inherited genetic defects.

#### Viral Theory

A. Viruses have been shown to be the cause of certain tumors in animals.

B. Oncoviruses (RNA-type viruses) thought to be culprit.

C. Viruses (HTLV-I, Epstein-Barr, Human Papilloma Virus) linked to human tumors.

#### Immunologic Factors

A. Failure of the immune system to respond to and eradicate cancer cells

B. Immunosuppressed individuals more susceptible to cancer

# DIAGNOSIS OF CANCER

## Classification and Staging

### Tissue of Origin

A. Carcinoma: arises from surface, glandular, or parenchymal epithelium.
   1. Squamous cell carcinoma: surface epithelium
   2. Adenocarcinoma: glandular or parenchymal tissue
B. Sarcoma: arises from connective tissue.
C. Leukemia: starts in blood-forming tissues (i.e., bone marrow)
D. Lymphoma and multiple myeloma: starts in cells of immune system

### Stages of Tumor Growth

A. Several staging systems, important in selection of therapy
   1. TNM system: uses letters and numbers to designate the extent of the tumor.
      a. T: stands for primary growth; 1–4 with increasing size. T1S indicates carcinoma in situ.
      b. N: stands for lymph node involvement; 0–4 indicates progressively advancing nodal disease.
      c. M: stands for metastasis; 0 indicates no distant metastases, 1 indicates presence of metastases.
   2. Stages 0-IV: all cancers divided into five stages incorporating size, nodal involvement, and spread.
B. Cytologic diagnosis of cancer (e.g., Pap smear)
   1. Involves study of shed cells
   2. Classified by degree of cellular abnormality
      a. Normal
      b. Probably normal (slight changes)
      c. Doubtful (more severe changes)
      d. Probably cancer or precancerous
      e. Definitely cancer

## Client Factors

Early detection of cancer is crucial in reducing morbidity and mortality. Clients need to be taught about:
A. Seven warning signs of cancer (see Table 4-16).
B. Breast self-examination (BSE).
C. Importance of rectal exam for those over age 40
D. Hazards of smoking
E. Oral self-examination as well as annual exam of mouth and teeth
F. Hazards of excess sun exposure
G. Importance of Pap smear
H. Physical exam with lab work-up: every 3 years ages 20–40; yearly age 40 and over
I. Testicular self-examination (TSE)
   1. Testicular cancer: Most common cancer in young men between the ages of 15 and 34.

**Table 4-16** Seven Warning Signs of Cancer (Caution)

C – Change in bowel or bladder habits
A – A sore that doesn't heal
U – Unusual bleeding or discharge
T – Thickening or lump in breast (or elsewhere)
I – Indigestion or dysphagia
O – Obvious change in wart or mole
N – Nagging cough or hoarseness

Most testicular cancers are found by men themselves, by accident or when doing TSE.
   2. Testicular self-examination: Ideally, should be performed monthly, after a warm shower or bath, when the skin of the scrotum is relaxed. Standing in front of a mirror, the man should gently roll each testicle between the thumb and fingers of both hands. The testes are smooth, oval-shaped, and rather firm.
   3. Warning signs that men should look for:
      a. Painless swelling
      b. Feeling of heaviness
      c. Hard lump (size of a pea)
      d. Sudden collection of fluid in the scrotum
      e. Dull ache in the lower abdomen or in the groin
      f. Pain in a testicle or in the scrotum
      g. Enlargement or tenderness of the breasts

# TREATMENT OF CANCER

## Chemotherapy

### Principles

A. Based on ability of drug to kill cancer cells; normal cells may also be damaged, producing side effects. Effect is greatest on rapidly dividing cells, such as bone marrow cells, the GI tract, and hair.
B. Different drugs act on tumor cells in different stages of the cell growth cycle.

### Types of Chemotherapeutic Drugs

See Unit 2.
A. Antimetabolites: foster cancer cell death by interfering with cellular metabolic process.
B. Alkylating agents: act with DNA to hinder cell growth and division.
C. Plant alkaloids: obtained from the periwinkle plant; makes the host's body a less favorable environment for the growth of cancer cells.
D. Antitumor antibiotics: affect RNA to make environment less favorable for cancer growth.
E. Steroids and sex hormones: alter the endocrine environment to make it less conducive to growth of cancer cells.

## Major Side Effects and Nursing Interventions

A. GI System
   1. Nausea and vomiting
      a. Administer antiemetics routinely every 4–6 hours as well as prophylactically before chemotherapy is initiated.
      b. Withhold foods/fluids 4–6 hours before chemotherapy.
      c. Provide bland foods in small amounts after treatments.
   2. Diarrhea
      a. Administer antidiarrheals.
      b. Maintain good perineal care.
      c. Give clear liquids as tolerated.
      d. Monitor potassium, sodium, and chloride levels.
   3. Stomatitis
      a. Provide and teach the client good oral hygiene, including avoidance of commercial mouthwashes.
      b. Rinse with viscous lidocaine before meals to provide an analgesic effect.
      c. Perform a cleansing rinse with plain water or dilute a water-soluble lubricant such as hydrogen peroxide after meals.
      d. Apply water-soluble lubricant such as K-Y jelly to lubricate cracked lips.
      e. Advise client to suck on Popsicles to provide moisture.
B. Hematologic System
   1. Thrombocytopenia
      a. Teach client the importance of avoiding bumping or bruising the skin.
      b. Protect client from physical injury.
      c. Avoid aspirin or aspirin products.
      d. Avoid giving IM injections.
      e. Monitor blood counts carefully.
      f. Assess for and teach signs of increased bleeding tendencies (epistaxis, petechiae, ecchymoses).
   2. Leukopenia
      a. Use careful handwashing technique.
      b. Maintain reverse isolation if white blood cell count drops below 1000/mm$^3$.
      c. Assess for signs of respiratory infection.
      d. Instruct client to avoid crowds/persons with known infection.
   3. Anemia
      a. Provide for adequate rest periods.
      b. Monitor hemoglobin and hematocrit.
      c. Protect client from injury.
      d. Administer oxygen as necessary.
C. Integumentary System—Alopecia
   1. Explain that hair loss is not permanent.
   2. Offer support and encouragement.
   3. Scalp tourniquets or scalp hypothermia via ice pack may be ordered to minimize hair loss with some agents.
   4. Advise client to obtain a wig before initiating treatments.

D. Renal System
   1. May cause direct damage to kidney by excretion of metabolites; encourage fluids and frequent voiding to prevent accumulation of metabolites in bladder.
   2. Increased excretion of uric acid may damage kidneys.
   3. Administer allopurinol (Zyloprim) as ordered to prevent uric acid formation; encourage fluids when administering allopurinol.
E. Reproductive System
   1. Damage may occur to both men and women resulting in infertility and/or mutagenic damage to chromosomes.
   2. Banking sperm often recommended for men before chemotherapy.
   3. Clients and partners advised to use reliable methods of contraception during chemotherapy.
F. Neurologic System
   1. Plant alkaloids (vincristine) cause neurologic damage with repeated doses.
   2. Peripheral neuropathies, hearing loss, loss of deep tendon reflexes, and paralytic ileus may occur.

# Radiation Therapy
## Principles

A. Radiation therapy uses ionizing radiation to kill or limit the growth of cancer cells, may be internal or external.
B. It not only injures the cell membrane, but destroys or alters DNA so that the cells cannot reproduce.
C. Like chemotherapy, effect cannot be limited to cancer cells only; all exposed cells, including normal ones, will be injured, causing side effects. Localized effects are related to area of body being treated; generalized effects may be related to cellular breakdown products.
D. Types of energy emitted:
   1. Alpha: particles cannot pass through skin, rarely used
   2. Beta: particles cannot pass through skin, somewhat more penetrating than alpha, generally emitted from radioactive isotopes, used for internal source
   3. Gamma rays (electromagnetic or X-rays): penetrate deeper areas of body, most common form of external radiotherapy

## Methods of Delivery

A. External radiation therapy: beams high-energy rays directly to the affected area.
B. Internal radiation therapy: radioactive material is injected or implanted in the client's body for a designated period of time.
   1. Sealed implants: a radioisotope enclosed in a container so it does not circulate in

the body; client's body fluids should not become contaminated with radiation.

2. Unsealed sources: a radioisotope that is not encased in a container and does circulate in the body and contaminates body fluids.

## Factors Controlling Exposure

A. Half-life: time required for half of radioactive atoms to decay
   1. Each radioisotope has a different half-life.
   2. At the end of the half-life, the danger from exposure decreases.
B. Time: the shorter the duration, the less the exposure
C. Distance: the greater the distance from the radiation source the less the exposure
D. Shielding: all radiation can be blocked; rubber gloves stop alpha and usually beta rays; thick lead or concrete stops gamma rays
E. These factors affect health care worker's exposure as well as client's.
   1. Health care worker at greater risk from internal than external sources
   2. Film badge can measure the amount of exposure received
   3. No pregnant nurses or visitors permitted near radiation source

## Side Effects of Radiation Therapy and Nursing Interventions

A. Skin: itching, redness, burning, oozing, sloughing
   1. Keep skin free from foreign substances.
   2. Avoid use of medicated solutions, ointments, or powders that contain heavy metals such as zinc oxide.
   3. Avoid pressure, trauma, infection to skin; use bed cradle.
   4. Wash affected areas with plain water and pat dry; avoid soap.
   5. Use cornstarch, olive oil for itching; avoid talcum powder.
   6. If sloughing occurs, use a sterile dressing with micropore tape.
   7. Teach client to avoid exposing skin to heat, cold, or sunlight and to avoid constricting or irritating clothing.
B. Anorexia, nausea, and vomiting
   1. Arrange mealtimes so they do not directly precede or follow therapy.
   2. Encourage bland foods.
   3. Provide small, attractive meals.
   4. Avoid extremes of temperature.
   5. Administer antiemetics as ordered before meals.
C. Diarrhea
   1. Encourage low-residue, bland, high-protein foods.
   2. Administer antidiarrheal drugs as ordered.
   3. Provide good perineal care.
   4. Monitor electrolytes, particularly sodium, potassium, and chloride.

D. Anemia, leukopenia, and thrombocytopenia
   1. Isolate from those with known infections.
   2. Provide frequent rest periods.
   3. Encourage high-protein diet.
   4. Instruct client to avoid injury.
   5. Assess for bleeding.
   6. Monitor CBC, leukocytes, and platelets.

# Bone Marrow Transplant

A. General information
   1. Treatment alternative for a variety of diseases
      a. Malignancies including several types of leukemias
      b. Blood disorders including severe aplastic anemia, thalassemia
      c. Solid tumors such as breast cancer and brain tumors; treatment for these diseases frequently causes bone marrow destruction; autologous bone marrow transplant may be indicated (Bone marrow harvested before chemotherapy or radiation destroys it and infused after therapy completed)
      d. Other conditions including malignant infantile osteopetrosis, some inherited metabolic disorders
   2. Types
      a. Autologous: client transplant with own harvested marrow
      b. Syngeneic: transplant between identical twins
      c. Allogeneic: transplant from a genetically nonidentical donor
         1) Most common transplant type
         2) Sibling most common donor
   3. Procedure
      a. Donor suitability determined through tissue antigen typing; includes human leukocyte antigen (HLA) and mixed leukocyte culture (MLC) typing.
      b. Donor bone marrow is aspirated from multiple sites along the iliac crests under general anesthesia.
      c. Donor marrow is infused IV into the recipient.
   4. Early evidence of engraftment seen during the second week post-transplant; hematologic reconstitution takes 4–6 weeks; immunologic reconstitution takes months.
   5. Hospitalization of 2 or 3 months required.
   6. Prognosis is highly variable depending on indication for use.
B. Complications
   1. Failure of engraftment
   2. Infection: highest risk in first 3–4 weeks
   3. Pneumonia: nonbacterial or interstitial pneumonias are principal cause of death during first 3 months post-transplant

4. Graft vs. host disease (GVHD): principal complication; caused by an immunologic reaction of engrafted lymphoid cells against the tissues of the recipient
    a. Acute GVHD: develops within first 100 days post-transplant and affects skin, gut, liver, marrow, and lymphoid tissue
    b. Chronic GVHD: develops 100–400 days post-transplant; manifested by multiorgan involvement
5. Recurrent malignancy
6. Late complications such as cataracts, endocrine abnormalities

C. Nursing care: pretransplant
1. Recipient immunosuppression attained with total body irradiation (TBI) and chemotherapy to eradicate existing disease and create space in host marrow to allow transplanted cells to grow.
2. Provide protected environment.
    a. Client should be in a laminar airflow room or on strict reverse isolation; surveillance cultures done twice a week.
    b. Objects must be sterilized before being brought into the room.
    c. When working with children introduce new people where they can be seen, but outside child's room so child can see what they look like without isolation garb.
3. Monitor central lines frequently; check patency and observe for signs of infection (fever, redness around site).
4. Provide care for the client receiving chemotherapy and radiation therapy to induce immunosuppression.
    a. Administer chemotherapy as ordered, assist with radiation therapy if required.
    b. Monitor side effects and keep client as comfortable as possible.
    c. Monitor carefully for potential infection.
    d. Client will become very ill; prepare client and family.

D. Nursing care: post-transplant
1. Prevent infection.
    a. Maintain protective environment.
    b. Administer antibiotics as ordered.
    c. Assess all mucous membranes, wounds, catheter sites for swelling, redness, tenderness, pain.
    d. Monitor vital signs frequently (every 1–4 hours as needed).
    e. Collect specimens for cultures as needed and twice a week.
    f. Change IV setups every 24 hours.
2. Provide mouth care for stomatitis and mucositis (severe mucositis develops about 5 days after irradiation).
    a. Note tissue sloughing, bleeding, changes in color.
    b. Provide mouth rinses, viscous lidocaine, and antibiotic rinses.
    c. Do not use lemon and glycerin swabs.
    d. Administer parenteral narcotics as ordered if necessary to control pain.
    e. Provide care every 2 hours or as needed.
3. Provide skin care: skin breakdown may result from profuse diarrhea from the TBI.
4. Monitor carefully for bleeding.
    a. Check for occult blood in emesis and stools.
    b. Observe for easy bruising, petechiae on skin, mucous membranes.
    c. Monitor changes in vital signs.
    d. Check platelet count daily.
    e. Replace blood products as ordered (all blood products should be irradiated).
5. Maintain fluid and electrolyte balance and promote nutrition.
    a. Measure I&O carefully.
    b. Provide adequate fluid, protein, and caloric intake.
    c. Weigh daily.
    d. Administer fluid replacement as ordered.
    e. Monitor hydration status: check skin turgor, moisture of mucous membranes, urine output.
    f. Check electrolytes daily.
    g. Check urine for glucose, ketones, protein.
    h. Administer antidiarrheal agents as needed.
6. Provide client teaching and discharge planning concerning:
    a. Home environment (e.g., cleaning, pets, visitors)
    b. Diet modifications
    c. Medication regimen: schedule, dosages, effects, and side effects
    d. Communicable diseases and immunizations
    e. Daily hygiene and skin care
    f. Fever
    g. Activity

## Sample Questions

86. A woman is undergoing chemotherapy treatment for uterine cancer. She asks the nurse how chemotherapeutic drugs work. The most accurate explanation would include which statement?
1. They affect all rapidly dividing cells.
2. Molecular structure of the DNA segment is altered.
3. Chemotherapy only kills cancer cells.
4. The cancer cells are sensitive to drug toxins.

**4**

87. An adult experiences severe vomiting from cancer chemotherapy drugs. Which acid-base imbalance should the nurse anticipate?
    1. Ketoacidosis.
    2. Metabolic acidosis.
    3. Metabolic alkalosis.
    4. Respiratory alkalosis.

88. A woman loses most of her hair as a result of cancer chemotherapy. The nurse understands that which of the following is true about chemotherapy-induced alopecia?
    1. New hair will be gray.
    2. Avoid the use of wigs.
    3. The hair loss is temporary.
    4. Pre-chemo hair texture will return.

89. An adult is diagnosed with Hodgkin's disease Stage 1A. He is being treated with radiation therapy. To minimize skin damage from radiation therapy, the nursing care plan should include which of the following?
    1. Avoid washing with water.
    2. Apply a heating pad to the site.
    3. Cover the area with an airtight dressing.
    4. Avoid applying creams and powders to the area.

90. An adult develops a second-degree or second-level skin reaction from radiation therapy. When evaluating his symptoms, which of the following would not be present?
    1. Scaly skin.
    2. An itchy feeling.
    3. Dry desquamation.
    4. Reddening of the skin.

91. The nurse is teaching the client about signs of radiation-induced thrombocytopenia. Which symptom would be included in the teaching?
    1. Fatigue.
    2. Shortness of breath.
    3. Elevated temperature.
    4. A tendency to bruise easily.

92. The nurse is caring for a client who is receiving radiation therapy. Which activity by the client indicates further instruction on the side effects of radiation therapy?
    1. Using an electric razor.
    2. Eating a high-protein diet.
    3. Taking his children to see Santa at the mall.
    4. Calling the doctor for a temperature of 101°F (38.3°C).

93. A man says to the nurse, "I don't understand how my wife could have come down with cancer. She doesn't smoke or drink. How do people get cancer?" Which of the following should be included in the nurse's response? Select the one or all that apply.
    ___ Bacteria.
    ___ Viruses.
    ___ Dietary factors.
    ___ Genetic factors.

94. A woman has breast cancer. Her physician has just told her that her cancer has been staged as "T2, N1, M0," and the client asks the nurse what this means. What is the nurse's best response?
    1. "The primary tumor is 2 cm in diameter, she has one positive lymph node, and no metastasis."
    2. "There are two primary tumors, one involved lymph node chain, and no metastasis."
    3. "The primary tumor is between 2 cm and 5 cm in size, she has metastasis to one movable lymph node, and no distant metastasis."
    4. "There is carcinoma in situ, no regional lymph node metastasis, and the presence of distant metastasis cannot be assessed."

95. The nurse at a senior citizen center is teaching a class on the early warning signals of cancer. Which of the following will be a part of the teaching plan for this class?
    1. Reduction in the amount of dietary fat.
    2. Stop cigarette smoking.
    3. Avoid overexposure to the sun.
    4. Practice monthly breast self-exam (BSE).

96. Which statement tells the nurse that a man needs further information about testicular self-examination (TSE)?
    1. "The best time to perform TSE is immediately before sexual intercourse."
    2. "It's normal to find one testis lower than the other."
    3. "I should have my doctor examine any lumps I find, even though they might be benign."
    4. "That cord-like thing that I feel on the top and back of the testicle is not something to be worried about."

97. Which of the following actions is vital for the nurse to perform when assessing a client receiving chemotherapy?
    1. Checking complete vital signs every 8 hours.
    2. Taking rectal temperatures every 4 hours to check for infection.

3. Testing emesis for blood.
4. Avoiding fresh fruits and vegetables if absolute white blood count (WBC) is less than 1000/mm$^3$.

98. An adult asks the nurse how the chemotherapy that she is receiving for her lung cancer works. What is the nurse's best response?
    1. Block the sodium-potassium pump in the cell wall and cause cellular death due to an excess of intracellular potassium.
    2. Prevent the entry of oxygen into the cell and cause cellular death due to cellular anoxia.
    3. Shrink the size of the existing tumor, which causes the release of antitumor metabolites that are toxic to further tumor cell growth.
    4. Destroy enough of the tumor so that the body's immune system can eradicate the remaining cells.

99. An adult, diagnosed with multiple myeloma, is receiving cyclophosphamide (Cytoxan). The nurse must include which of the following interventions in the nursing care plan of this client?
    1. High-flow oxygen delivery to combat interstitial pneumonitis, which routinely develops with cyclophosphamide therapy.
    2. Encouraging the client to empty his bladder every 2 to 3 hours to prevent development of hemorrhagic cystitis.
    3. Application of an ice cap to reduce or prevent alopecia.
    4. Antiemetic therapy for 7–10 days after cyclophosphamide administration, or until blood studies show nadir is reached.

100. An adult is receiving cancer chemotherapy and demonstrates alteration in her oral mucous membranes. Which of the following should be included in her plan of care?
    1. Brushing teeth and flossing after every meal and at bedtime.
    2. Using normal saline mouth rinses every 2 hours while awake.
    3. No use of dentures until mucous membranes have healed.
    4. Bland, mechanical, soft diet until mucous membranes have healed.

101. Ten days ago, a client received chemotherapy for his non-Hodgkin's lymphoma, stage IV. Drugs administered through his vascular access device ("Port-a-cath") included doxorubicin, cyclophosphamide, vincristine, and prednisone (CHOP protocol). This morning, his blood work is as follows: WBC: 1500/mm$^3$; hemoglobin (Hgb): 7.6 gm/dl; RBC 3,000,000/mm$^3$; hematocrit (Hct) 22.3%; platelets 20,000/mm$^3$. The nurse knows that the client's plan of care will include which of the following interventions?
    1. Insertion of two extra IV lines for blood administration.
    2. Cutting fingernails and toenails to prevent scratching that could lead to bleeding or infection.
    3. Providing the client with a low-residue diet.
    4. Using a soft toothbrush and avoiding dental floss.

102. An adult who is receiving external radiation therapy for Hodgkin's disease makes all of the following statements to her nurse. Which statement tells the nurse that the client needs further teaching about the care she requires because of her radiation therapy?
    1. "I will check my mouth frequently for signs of irritation."
    2. "I know that if I get tired easily, it may be from the radiation and doesn't necessarily mean my Hodgkin's disease is getting worse."
    3. "I will use a good quality lotion on my skin to keep the radiation from burning it."
    4. "I may lose some of my hair during radiation and foods may not taste right."

103. A client asks the nurse to explain how the radiation therapy she will be receiving for her neck cancer is effective. What is the nurse's best response?
    1. Radiation causes breakage in the strands of the DNA helix, which leads to cell death.
    2. Radiation is antagonistic to glucose, which cells need for energy and replication; radiation prevents glucose from entering cells, leading to cell death.
    3. Cell walls are broken down by gamma rays during radiation therapy, leading to cell death.
    4. Oxygen cannot enter cells that have been irradiated, so the cell converts to anaerobic metabolism that causes its death.

104. The nurse manager on the oncology unit is assessing the knowledge level of the staff in regard to safety requirements for the client receiving internal radiation therapy. Which observation by the nurse manager indicates that further instruction is necessary?
    1. The physical therapist is ambulating the client in the hall.
    2. The nurse uses rubber gloves when emptying the bedpan.

3. The dietitian provides a low-residue diet for the client.

4. The housekeeping staff calls for Radiation Safety personnel to inspect the room before the client is discharged.

105. A woman is receiving internal radiation therapy for cancer of the cervix. Which statement indicates to the nurse that the client understands precautions necessary during her treatment?

   1. "I should get out of bed and walk around in my room at least every other hour."

   2. "My seven-year-old twins should not come to visit me while I'm receiving treatment."

   3. "I will try not to cough, because the force might make me expel the applicator."

   4. "I know that my primary nurse has to wear one of those badges like the people in the X-ray department wear, but they aren't necessary for anyone else who comes in here."

106. An adult is receiving internal radiation therapy for cancer of the cervix. Her radiation source, a rod, becomes dislodged. What will be the nurse's first action?

   1. Notify the Radiation Safety personnel at once and await further information.

   2. Use long-handled forceps to remove the rod and place in a lead-lined container.

   3. Apply two sets of rubber gloves and pick up the rod; place it in a white plastic "biohazard" bucket and call Radiation Safety personnel for a special pick-up.

   4. Use long-handled forceps to pick up rod; clean with normal saline, and reinsert into client's vagina, stopping when the rod meets resistance. This indicates that it is against the cervix.

107. In caring for the client receiving external radiation therapy, the nurse assesses for which of the following side effects?

   1. Extravasation injury at the IV site used for contrast media injection.

   2. Generalized or local edema.

   3. Infection and bleeding.

   4. Allergic reactions, particularly anaphylaxis.

## Answers and Rationales

86. **1.** There are numerous mechanisms of action for cancer chemotherapeutic drugs, but most affect rapidly dividing cells. The drugs interfere with cell division and prevent rapid division of cells.

87. **3.** Severe vomiting results in a loss of hydrochloric acid and acids from extracellular fluids, leading to metabolic alkalosis.

88. **3.** Alopecia from chemotherapy is only temporary.

89. **4.** Creams and powders, many of which contain heavy metals, will further irritate skin sensitized by radiation therapy and reduce the effectiveness of therapy by blocking radiation.

90. **4.** Reddening of the skin will not be seen in a second-level or second-degree reaction. A second-degree skin reaction would be evidenced by scaly skin, an itchy feeling, and dry desquamation.

91. **4.** Clients with decreased platelet count (thrombocytopenia) bleed easily. Thrombocytes are clotting cells.

92. **3.** People being treated with radiation therapy should avoid crowds because of the increased risk of infection. Crowds at Christmastime can be very large and children are frequent carriers of infection.

93. Bacteria should be marked. *Helicobacter pylori*, which causes stomach ulcers, has been linked to stomach cancer.

   Viruses should be marked. Viruses are thought to insinuate themselves into the genetic structure of cells, thereby altering future generations of that cell. Epstein-Barr is strongly implicated in the development of Burkitt's lymphoma. Some types of human papilloma virus, which causes genital warts, cause cancer of the cervix.

   Dietary factors should be marked. Approximately 40–60% of all environmental cancers are thought to have links to dietary factors such as fats, alcohol, foods containing nitrates/nitrites, and salt-cured and smoked meats.

   Genetic factors should be marked. Genetics are involved in cancer cell development. Damage to the DNA in certain populations of cells may lead to mutant cells being transmitted to future generations. Examples of cancers associated with familial inheritance include breast, colon, and rectal cancers.

94. **3.** In the TNM staging classification system, T refers to the primary tumor, and T2 is between 2 cm and 5 cm without extension to chest wall or skin. The N refers to regional lymph node involvement, with N1 indicating spread to an ipsilateral movable node. N0 indicates no regional lymph node spread; N2 indicates metastasis to an ipsilateral axillary node fixed to another node or other structure. M refers to distant metastasis,

with MX indicating that metastasis cannot be assessed, M0 that there is no distant spread, and M1 that there is spread present.

95. **4.** Only this answer, practicing breast self-exam, will yield a "warning signal of cancer" (i.e., a breast lump). Be certain that your response answers the question, not just that it contains factual information.

96. **1.** The man is mistaken (and needs more teaching) if he says that testicular self-exam should be performed immediately prior to sexual intercourse. The best time to do TSE is when the scrotum is relaxed, such as after a warm bath or shower.

97. **3.** Because of the bleeding disorders common in clients receiving chemotherapy, all body secretions, including emesis, should be assessed for obvious and occult blood.

98. **4.** Each time the tumor is exposed to the chemotherapeutic drug, a certain percentage of cells are killed. (The exact percentage is determined by the drug dosage used.) Because a *percentage* of tumor is killed, a part of tumor will remain after therapy. It is up to the body's immune system to destroy the remaining tumor, which an intact immune system may be able to do if the tumor is made small enough.

99. **2.** If the metabolites of cyclophosphamide are allowed to accumulate in the bladder, the subsequent irritation of the bladder wall capillaries will cause hemorrhagic cystitis. This condition is preventable; if it develops, one of its serious sequelae is bladder fibrosis. In addition to monitoring BUN and creatinine prior to administration, the nurse must promote hydration of at least 3 liters a day and frequent voiding.

100. **2.** The client will use normal saline mouth rinses every 2 hours while awake and every 6 hours at night to aid in the removal of thick secretions, debris, and bacteria.

101. **4.** By using a soft toothbrush and avoiding dental floss, the client promotes a healthy oral cavity without risking bleeding or disruption of skin integrity, which could lead to infection.

102. **3.** It is important to protect skin from irritation, and lotions, creams, powders, and ointments can all contribute to skin problems. Clients are advised to consult their radiation oncologists for troublesome skin problems and should be advised that after treatment, reepithelialization will occur.

103. **1.** There are two types of ionizing radiation: electromagnetic rays and particulate radiation. Either of these can cause tissue disruption, the most harmful of which is the alteration in the structure of the cell's DNA molecules; this will lead to cell death.

104. **1.** The client will be restricted to her room to minimize exposure of staff, visitors, and other clients to the radiation source.

105. **2.** Visitors younger than 18 years of age, and pregnant visitors, are not allowed during internal radiation therapy.

106. **2.** Long-handled forceps and a lead-lined container (sometimes called a "lead pig") must be kept in the room of any client receiving internal radiation therapy for this very occurrence.

107. **3.** If bone marrow-producing sites are included in the field being irradiated, anemia, leukopenia (low white blood cells), and thrombocytopenia (low platelets) may occur; these may lead to infection and/or bleeding.

# The Neurosensory System

## OVERVIEW OF ANATOMY AND PHYSIOLOGY

### The Nervous System

The functional unit of the nervous system is the nerve cell, or neuron. The nervous system consists of the central nervous system (CNS), which includes the brain and spinal cord, and the peripheral nervous system (PNS), which includes the cranial nerves and the spinal nerves. The autonomic nervous system (ANS) is a subdivision of the PNS that automatically controls body functions such as breathing and heartbeat. It is further divided into the sympathetic and parasympathetic nervous systems. The special senses of vision and hearing are also covered in this section.

## Neuron

A. Primary component of the nervous system; composed of cell body (gray matter), axon, and dendrites

B. *Axon:* elongated process or fiber extending from the cell body; transmits impulses (messages) away from the cell body to dendrites or directly to the cell bodies of other neurons; neuron usually has only one axon.

C. *Dendrites:* short, branching fibers that receive impulses and conduct them toward the nerve cell body. Neurons may have many dendrites.

D. *Synapse:* junction between neurons where an impulse is transmitted

E. *Neurotransmitters:* chemical agents (e.g., acetylcholine, norepinephrine) involved in the transmission of impulse across synapse

F. *Myelin sheath:* a wrapping of myelin (a whitish, fatty material) that protects and insulates nerve fibers and enhances the speed of impulse conduction
   1. Both axons and dendrites may or may not have a myelin sheath (myelinated/unmyelinated)
   2. Most axons leaving the CNS are heavily myelinated by Schwann cells

### Functional Classification

A. Afferent (sensory) neurons: transmit impulses from peripheral receptors to the CNS

B. Efferent (motor) neurons: conduct impulses from CNS to muscles and glands

C. Internuncial neurons (interneurons): connecting links between afferent and efferent neurons

## Central Nervous System: Brain and Spinal Cord

### Brain

A. *Cerebrum:* outermost area (cerebral cortex) is gray matter; deeper area is composed of white matter
   1. Two hemispheres: right and left
   2. Each hemisphere divided into four lobes; many of the functional areas of the cerebrum have been located in these lobes (see Figure 4-1).
      a. Frontal lobe
         1) Personality, behavior
         2) Higher intellectual functioning
         3) Precentral gyrus: motor function
         4) Broca's area: specialized motor speech area
      b. Parietal lobe
         1) Postcentral gyrus: registers general sensation (e.g., touch, pressure)
         2) Integrates sensory information
      c. Temporal lobe
         1) Hearing, taste, smell
         2) Wernicke's area: sensory speech area (understanding/formulation of language)
      d. Occipital lobe: vision

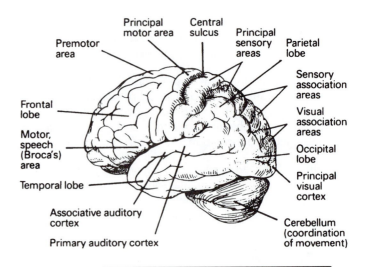

**Figure 4-1** Side view of the brain, showing principal functional areas

   3. Corpus callosum: large fiber tract that connects the two cerebral hemispheres
   4. Basal ganglia: islands of gray matter within white matter of cerebrum
      a. Regulate and integrate motor activity originating in the cerebral cortex
      b. Part of extrapyramidal system

B. Diencephalon: connecting part of the brain, between the cerebrum and the brain stem. Contains several small structures; the thalamus and hypothalamus are most important.
   1. Thalamus
      a. Relay station for discrimination of sensory signals (e.g., pain, temperature, touch).
      b. Controls primitive emotional responses (e.g., rage, fear).
   2. Hypothalamus
      a. Found immediately beneath the thalamus.
      b. Plays major role in regulation of vital functions such as blood pressure, sleep, food and water intake, and body temperature.
      c. Acts as control center for pituitary gland and affects both divisions of the autonomic nervous system.

C. Brain stem
   1. Contains midbrain, pons, and medulla oblongata.
   2. Extends from the cerebral hemispheres to the foramen magnum at the base of the skull.
   3. Contains nuclei of the cranial nerves and the long ascending and descending tracts connecting the cerebrum and the spinal cord.
   4. Contains vital centers of respiratory, vasomotor, and cardiac functions.

D. Cerebellum: coordinates muscle tone and movements and maintains position in space (equilibrium).

## Spinal Cord

A. Serves as a connecting link between the brain and the periphery.

B. Extends from foramen magnum to second lumbar vertebra.

C. H-shaped gray matter in the center (cell bodies) surrounded by white matter (nerve tracts and fibers).

D. Gray matter
   1. Anterior horns: contain cell bodies giving rise to efferent (motor) fibers
   2. Posterior horns: contain cell bodies connecting with afferent (sensory) fibers from dorsal root ganglion
   3. Lateral horns: in thoracic region, contain cells giving rise to autonomic fibers of sympathetic nervous system

E. White matter
   1. Ascending tracts (sensory pathways)
      a. Posterior columns: carry impulses concerned with touch, pressure, vibration, and position sense.
      b. Spinocerebellar: carry impulses concerned with muscle tension and position sense to cerebellum.
      c. Lateral spinothalamic: carry impulses resulting in pain and temperature sensations.
      d. Anterior spinothalamic: carry impulses concerned with crude touch and pressure.
   2. Descending tracts (motor pathways)
      a. Corticospinal (pyramidal, upper motor neuron): conduct motor impulses from motor cortex to anterior horn cells (cross in the medulla).
      b. Extrapyramidal: help to maintain muscle tone and to control body movement, especially gross automatic movements such as walking.

F. Reflex arc
   1. Reflex consists of an involuntary response to a stimulus occurring over a neural pathway called a reflex arc.
   2. Not relayed to and from brain; takes place at cord levels.
   3. Components
      a. Sensory receptor: receives/reacts to a stimulus.
      b. Afferent pathway: transmits impulses to spinal cord.
      c. Interneuron: synapses with a motor neuron (anterior horn cell).
      d. Efferent pathway: transmits impulses from motor neuron to effector.
      e. Effector: muscle or organ that responds to stimulus.

## Supporting Structures

A. Skull
   1. Rigid; numerous bones fused together.
   2. Protects and supports the brain.

B. Spinal column
   1. Consists of 7 cervical, 12 thoracic, and 5 lumbar vertebrae, as well as sacrum and coccyx.
   2. Supports the head and protects the spinal cord.

C. Meninges
   1. Membranes between the skull and brain and the vertebral column and spinal cord.
   2. Layers
      a. Dura mater: outermost layer, tough, leathery
      b. Arachnoid mater: middle layer, weblike
      c. Pia mater: innermost layer, delicate, clings to surface of brain
   3. Area between arachnoid and pia mater is called subarachnoid space.

D. Ventricles
   1. Four fluid-filled cavities connecting with one another and the spinal canal.
   2. Produce and circulate cerebrospinal fluid.

E. Cerebrospinal fluid (CSF)
   1. Surrounds brain and spinal cord.
   2. Offers protection by functioning as a shock absorber.
   3. Allows fluid shifts from the cranial cavity to the spinal cavity.
   4. Carries nutrients to and waste products away from nerve cells.

F. Vascular supply
   1. Two internal carotid arteries anteriorly.
   2. Two vertebral arteries leading to basilar artery posteriorly.
   3. These arteries communicate at the base of the brain through the circle of Willis.
   4. Anterior, middle, and posterior cerebral arteries are the main arteries for distributing blood to each hemisphere of the brain.
   5. Brain stem and cerebellum are supplied by branches of the vertebral and basilar arteries.
   6. Venous blood drains into dural sinuses and then into internal jugular veins.

G. Blood-brain barrier: protective barrier preventing harmful agents from entering the capillaries of the CNS; protects brain and spinal cord.

## Peripheral Nervous System

### Spinal Nerves

A. 31 pairs: carry impulses to and from spinal cord.

B. Each segment of the spinal cord contains a pair of spinal nerves (one for each side of the body).

C. Each nerve is attached to the spinal cord by two roots.
   1. Dorsal (posterior) root: contains afferent (sensory) nerve whose cell body is in the dorsal root ganglion.
   2. Ventral (anterior) root: contains efferent (motor) nerve whose nerve fibers originate in the anterior horn cell of the spinal cord (lower motor neuron).

## Table 4-17 Cranial Nerves

| Name and Number | Function |
|---|---|
| Olfactory: cranial nerve I | Sensory: carries impulses for sense of smell |
| Optic: cranial nerve II | Sensory: carries impulses for vision |
| Oculomotor: cranial nerve III | Motor: muscles for pupillary constriction, elevation of upper eyelid; 4 out of 6 extraocular movements |
| Trochlear: cranial nerve IV | Motor: muscles for downward, inward movement of eye |
| Trigeminal: cranial nerve V | Mixed: impulses from face, surface of eyes (corneal reflex); muscles controlling mastication |
| Abducens: cranial nerve VI | Motor: muscles for lateral deviation of eye |
| Facial: cranial nerve VII | Mixed: impulses for taste from anterior tongue; muscles for facial movement |
| Acoustic: cranial nerve VIII | Sensory: impulses for hearing (cochlear division) and balance (vestibular division) |
| Glossopharyngeal: cranial nerve IX | Mixed: impulses for sensation to posterior tongue and pharynx; muscles for movement of pharynx (elevation) and swallowing |
| Vagus: cranial nerve X | Mixed: impulses for sensation to lower pharynx and larynx; muscles for movement of soft palate, pharynx, and larynx; parasympathetic |
| Spinal accessory: cranial nerve XI: | Motor: movement of sternomastoid muscles and upper part of trapezius muscles |
| Hypoglossal: cranial nerve XII | Motor: movement of tongue |

### Cranial Nerves

A. 12 pairs: carry impulses to and from brain (see Table 4-17).
B. May have sensory, motor, or mixed functions.

### Autonomic Nervous System

A. Part of the peripheral nervous system
B. Includes those peripheral nerves (both cranial and spinal) that regulate functions occurring automatically in the body; ANS regulates smooth muscle, cardiac muscle, and glands.
C. Components
   1. Sympathetic nervous system: generally accelerates some body functions in response to stress; "fight or flight"
   2. Parasympathetic nervous system: controls normal body functioning
D. Effects of ANS activity: see Table 4-18.

## Vision

### External Structures of Eye

A. Eyelids (palpebrae) and eyelashes: protect the eye from foreign particles
B. Conjunctiva
   1. Palpebral conjunctiva: pink; lines inner surface of eyelids.
   2. Bulbar conjunctiva: white with small blood vessels, covers anterior sclera.
C. Lacrimal apparatus (lacrimal gland and its ducts and passages): produces tears to lubricate the eye and moisten the cornea; tears drain into the nasolacrimal duct, which empties into nasal cavity.
D. Movement of the eye is controlled by six extraocular muscles.

### Internal Structures of Eye

A. Three layers of the eyeball
   1. Outer layer
      a. Sclera: tough, white connective tissue ("white of the eye"); located anteriorly and posteriorly
      b. Cornea: transparent tissue through which light enters the eye; located anteriorly
   2. Middle layer
      a. Choroid: highly vascular layer, nourishes retina; located posteriorly
      b. Ciliary body: anterior to choroid, secretes aqueous humor; muscles change shape of lens
      c. Iris: pigmented membrane behind cornea, gives color to eye; located anteriorly. Pupil is a circular opening in the middle of the iris that constricts or dilates to regulate amount of light entering eye.
   3. Inner layer: retina
      a. Light-sensitive layer composed of rods and cones (visual cells)
         1) Cones: specialized for fine discrimination and color vision
         2) Rods: more sensitive to light than cones, aid in peripheral vision
      b. Optic disk: area in retina for entrance of optic nerve, has no photoreceptors
B. Lens: transparent body that focuses image on retina
C. Fluids of the eye
   1. Aqueous humor: clear, watery fluid in anterior and posterior chambers in anterior part of eye; serves as refracting medium and provides nutrients to lens and cornea; contributes to maintenance of intraocular pressure.
   2. Vitreous humor: clear, gelatinous material that fills posterior cavity of eye; maintains transparency and form of eye.

**Table 4-18** Effects of Autonomic Nervous System Activity

| Effector | Sympathetic (Adrenergic) Effects | Parasympathetic (Cholinergic) Effects |
|---|---|---|
| Eye | Dilates pupil (mydriasis) | Constricts pupil (miosis) |
| Glands of head Lacrimal | No effect | Stimulates secretion |
| Salivary | Scanty thick, viscous secretions, dry mouth | Copious thin, watery secretions |
| Heart | Increases rate and force of contraction | Decreases rate |
| Blood vessels | Constricts smooth muscles of skin, abdominal blood vessels, and cutaneous blood vessels. Dilates smooth muscle of bronchioles, blood vessels of heart, and skeletal muscles | No effect |
| Lungs | Bronchodilation | Bronchoconstriction |
| GI tract | Decreases motility. Constricts sphincters. Possibly inhibits secretions. Inhibits activity of gallbladder and ducts. Inhibits glycogenolysis in liver | Increases motility. Relaxes sphincters. Stimulates secretion. Stimulates activity of gallbladder and ducts |
| Adrenal gland | Stimulates secretion of epinephrine and norepinephrine | No effects |
| Urinary tract | Relaxes detrusor muscle. Contracts trigone sphincter (prevents voiding) | Contracts detrusor muscle. Relaxes trigone sphincter (allows voiding) |

## Visual Pathways

A. Retina (rods and cones) translates light waves into neural impulses that travel over the optic nerves.
B. Optic nerves for each eye meet at the optic chiasm.
   1. Fibers from median halves of the retinas cross here and travel to the opposite side of the brain.
   2. Fibers from lateral halves of retinas remain uncrossed.
C. Optic nerves continue from optic chiasm as optic tracts and travel to the cerebrum (occipital lobe), where visual impulses are perceived and interpreted.

## Hearing

### External Ear

A. Auricle (pinna): outer projection of ear composed of cartilage and covered by skin; collects sound waves.
B. External auditory canal: lined with skin; glands secrete cerumen (wax), providing protection; transmits sound waves to tympanic membrane.
C. Tympanic membrane (eardrum): at end of external canal; vibrates in response to sound and transmits vibrations to middle ear.

### Middle Ear

A. Ossicles
   1. 3 small bones: malleus (hammer) attached to tympanic membrane, incus (anvil), stapes (stirrup)
   2. Ossicles are set in motion by sound waves from tympanic membrane.
   3. Sound waves are conducted by vibration to the footplate of the stapes in the oval window (an opening between the middle ear and the inner ear).
B. Eustachian tube: connects nasopharynx and middle ear; brings air into middle ear, thus equalizing pressure on both sides of eardrum.

### Inner Ear

A. Cochlea
   1. Contains organ of Corti, the receptor end-organ for hearing.
   2. Transmits sound waves from the oval window and initiates nerve impulses carried by cranial nerve VIII (acoustic branch) to the brain (temporal lobe of cerebrum).
B. Vestibular apparatus
   1. Organ of balance.
   2. Composed of three semicircular canals and the utricle.

## ASSESSMENT

## Health History

### Nervous System

A. Presenting problem: symptoms may include behavior changes, memory loss, mood changes, nervousness or anxiety, headache, seizures, syncope, vertigo, loss of consciousness; problems with speech, vision, or smell; motor problems (paralysis, tremor); sensory problems (pain, paresthesias)
B. Lifestyle: drug and alcohol intake, exposure to toxins, recent travel, employment, stressors
C. Use of medications: prescribed and over-the-counter (OTC)

**D.** Past medical history
  1. Perinatal exposure to toxic agents, X-rays; difficult labor and delivery
  2. Childhood and adult: history of systemic diseases; seizures; loss of consciousness; head trauma
**E.** Family history: may uncover diseases with hereditary or congenital background

## Eye

**A.** Presenting problem: symptoms may include blurred vision, decreased vision, or blind spots; pain, redness, excessive tearing; double vision (diplopia); drainage
**B.** Use of eyeglasses, contact lenses; date of last eye exam
**C.** Lifestyle: occupation (exposure to fumes, smoke, or eye irritant); use of safety glasses
**D.** Use of medications: cortisone preparations may contribute to formation of glaucoma and cataracts
**E.** Past medical history: systemic diseases; previous childhood or adult eye disorders, eye trauma
**F.** Family history: many eye disorders may be inherited

## Ear

**A.** Presenting problem: symptoms may include hearing loss, tinnitus (ringing in ear), dizziness or vertigo, pain, drainage
**B.** Lifestyle: occupation (exposure to excessive noise levels), swimming habits
**C.** Use of medications: ototoxic drugs; aspirin (tinnitus)
**D.** Past medical history
  1. Perinatal: rubella in first trimester of pregnancy
  2. Childhood and adult: otitis media, perforated eardrum, measles, mumps, allergies, tonsillectomy, and adenoidectomy
**E.** Family history: hearing loss in family members

## Physical Examination

### Nervous System

**A.** Neurologic examination
  1. Mental status exam (cerebral function); see also Unit 7.
    **a.** General appearance and behavior
    **b.** Level of consciousness; see Neuro Check.
    **c.** Intellectual function: memory (recent and remote), attention span, cognitive skills
    **d.** Emotional status
    **e.** Thought content
    **f.** Language/speech
      1) Expressive aphasia: inability to speak
      2) Receptive aphasia: inability to understand spoken words

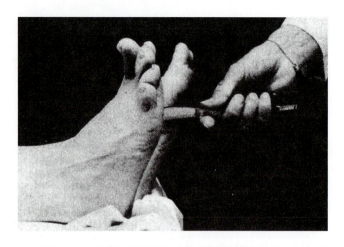

**Figure 4-2** Pathologic reflex (Babinski)

      3) Dysarthria: difficult speech due to impairment of muscles involved with production of speech
  2. Cranial nerves (see Table 4-17)
  3. Cerebellar function: posture, gait, balance, coordination
  4. Motor function: muscle size, tone, strength; abnormal or involuntary movements
  5. Sensory function: light touch, superficial pain, temperature, vibration, and position sense
  6. Reflexes
    **a.** Deep tendon: grade from 0 (no response) to 4 (hyperactive); 2 is normal
    **b.** Superficial
    **c.** Pathologic: Babinski's reflex (dorsiflexion of great toe with fanning of other toes) indicates damage to corticospinal tracts (see Figure 4-2)
**B.** Neuro check
  1. Level of consciousness (LOC)
    **a.** Orientation to time, place, and person
    **b.** Speech: clear, garbled, rambling
    **c.** Ability to follow commands
    **d.** If client does not respond to verbal stimuli, apply a painful stimulus (e.g., pressure on nailbeds, squeeze trapezius muscle); note response to pain:
      1) Appropriate: withdrawal, moaning
      2) Inappropriate: nonpurposeful
    **e.** Abnormal posturing (may occur spontaneously or in response to stimulus)
      1) Decorticate posturing: extension of legs, internal rotation and adduction of arms with flexion of elbows, wrists, and fingers (damage to corticospinal tracts; cerebral hemispheres)
      2) Decerebrate posturing: back arched, rigid extension of all four extremities with hyperpronation of arms and plantar flexion of feet (damage to upper brain stem, midbrain, or pons)

| Subscale | Response | Score |
|---|---|---|
| Best eye opening (E) | Spontaneous | 4 |
| | To voice | 3 |
| | To pain | 2 |
| | None | 1 |
| Best verbal response (V) | Oriented | 5 |
| | Confused conversation | 4 |
| | Inappropriate words | 3 |
| | Incomprehensible sounds | 2 |
| | None | 1 |
| Best motor response, upper limb (M) | Obeys commands | 6 |
| | Localizes to pain | 5 |
| | Flexor withdrawal (decorticate posturing) | 4 |
| | Abnormal flexion (decerebrate posturing) | 3 |
| | Extension | 2 |
| | Flaccid | 1 |

**Figure 4-3** Glasgow Coma Scale

2. Glasgow coma scale (see Figure 4-3)
   a. Objective evaluation of LOC, motor/verbal response; a standardized system for assessing the degree of neurologic impairment in critically ill clients.
   b. Cannot replace a complete neurologic check, but can be used as an aid in evaluation and to eliminate ambiguous terms such as stupor and lethargy.
   c. A score of 15 indicates client is awake and oriented; the lowest score, 3, is deep coma; a score of 7 or below is considered coma.
3. Pupillary reaction and eye movements
   a. Observe size, shape, and equality of pupils (note size in millimeters)
   b. Reaction to light: pupillary constriction
   c. Corneal reflex: blink reflex in response to light stroking of cornea
   d. Oculocephalic reflex (doll's eyes): present in unconscious client with intact brain stem
4. Motor function
   a. Movement of extremities (paralysis)
   b. Muscle strength
5. Vital signs: respiratory patterns (may help localize possible lesion)
   a. Cheyne-Stokes respiration: regular, rhythmic alternating between hyperventilation and apnea; may be caused by structural cerebral dysfunction or by metabolic problems, such as diabetic coma.
   b. Central neurogenic hyperventilation: sustained, rapid, regular respirations (rate of 25/minute) with normal blood oxygen levels; usually due to brain stem dysfunction.
   c. Apneustic breathing: prolonged inspiratory phase, followed by a 2- to 3-second pause; usually indicates dysfunction of respiratory center in pons.
   d. Cluster breathing: clusters of irregular breathing, irregularly followed by periods of apnea; usually caused by a lesion in upper medulla and lower pons.
   e. Ataxic breathing: breathing pattern completely irregular; indicates damage to respiratory centers of the medulla.

## Eye

A. Visual acuity: Snellen chart
B. Visual fields (peripheral vision)
   1. Confrontation method
   2. Perimetry: more precise method
C. External structures
   1. Position and alignment of eyes
   2. Eyebrows, eyelids, lacrimal apparatus, conjunctiva, sclera, cornea, iris, pupils (size, shape, equality, and reaction to light)
D. Extraocular movements; note paralysis, nystagmus (rapid, abnormal movement of the eyeball)
E. Corneal reflex

## Ear

A. Inspection and palpation of auricle, preauricular area, and mastoid area
B. Hearing acuity
   1. Whispered voice or ticking watch tests: gross estimation
   2. Audiometry: more precise method
C. Tuning fork tests distinguish between sensorineural and conductive hearing loss.
   1. Conductive hearing loss: secondary to problem in external or middle ear; transmission of sound waves to inner ear impaired
   2. Sensorineural (perceptive) hearing loss: disease of inner ear or cranial nerve VIII (acoustic branch)
   3. Weber's test: handle of vibrating tuning fork placed on midline of client's skull, sound should be heard equally in midline or in both ears; in conductive hearing loss, sound is louder in poorer ear; in sensorineural hearing loss, sound is louder in better ear.
   4. Rinne's test: tuning fork placed on mastoid process (bone conduction) until sound no longer heard, then placed in front of the ear (air conduction); sound should be heard longer (almost twice as long) with air conduction than with bone conduction; bone conduction greater than air conduction indicates conductive hearing deficit.

# Laboratory/Diagnostic Tests

## Nervous System

A. Lumbar puncture (LP)
1. A hollow spinal needle introduced into subarachnoid space of spinal canal between $L_4/L_5$ for diagnostic or therapeutic reasons
2. Purposes
   a. Measures CSF pressure (normal opening pressure 60–150 mm $H_2O$)
   b. Obtain specimens for lab analysis (protein [normally not present], sugar [normally present], cytology, C&S)
   c. Check color of CSF (normally clear) and check for blood
   d. Inject air, dye, or drugs into the spinal canal
3. Nursing care: pretest
   a. Have client empty bladder.
   b. Position client in lateral recumbent position with head and neck flexed onto the chest and knees pulled up.
   c. Explain the need to remain still during the procedure.
4. Nursing care: posttest
   a. Ensure labeling of CSF specimens in proper sequence.
   b. Keep client flat for 12–24 hours as ordered.
   c. Force fluids.
   d. Check puncture site for bleeding, leakage of CSF.
   e. Assess sensation and movement in lower extremities.
   f. Monitor vital signs.
   g. Administer analgesics for headache as ordered.
B. X-rays of skull and spine
1. Used to detect atrophy, erosion, or fractures of bones; calcifications
2. Pretest nursing care: remove hairpins, glasses, hearing aids.
C. Computerized tomography (CT scan)
1. Skull/spinal cord are scanned in successive layers by a narrow beam of X-rays; computer uses information obtained to construct a picture of the internal structure of the brain; contrast medium may or may not be used.
2. Used to detect intracranial and spinal cord lesions and monitor effects of surgery or other therapy.
3. Nursing care
   a. Explain appearance of scanner.
   b. Instruct client to lie still during procedure.
   c. Check for allergy to iodine if contrast material is used.
   d. Remove hairpins, etc.
D. Magnetic resonance imaging (MRI)
1. Also known as nuclear magnetic resonance (NMR)
2. Computer-drawn, detailed pictures of structures of the body through use of large magnet, radio waves
3. Used to detect intracranial and spinal abnormalities associated with disorders such as cerebrovascular disease, tumors, abscesses, cerebral edema, hydrocephalus, multiple sclerosis
4. Nursing care
   a. Instruct client to remove jewelry, hairpins, glasses, wigs (with metal clips), and other metallic objects.
   b. Be aware that this test cannot be performed on anyone with orthopedic hardware, intrauterine devices, pacemaker, internal surgical clips, or other fixed metallic objects in the body.
   c. Inform client of need to remain still while completely enclosed in scanner throughout the procedure, which lasts 45–60 minutes.
   d. Teach relaxation techniques to assist client to remain still and to help prevent claustrophobia.
   e. Warn client of normal audible humming and thumping noises from the scanner during test.
   f. Have client void before test.
   g. Sedate client if ordered.
E. Brain scan
1. Injection of radioactive isotope, followed by scanning of head; isotopes will accumulate in abnormal lesions and be recorded by the scanner.
2. Used to detect intracranial masses, vascular lesions, infarcts, hemorrhage
3. Nursing care: check for allergy to iodine.
F. Myelography
G. Cerebral angiography
1. Injection of radiopaque substance into the cerebral circulation via carotid, vertebral, femoral, or brachial artery followed by X-rays
2. Used to visualize cerebral vessels and detect tumors, aneurysms, occlusions, hematomas, or abscesses
3. Nursing care: pretest
   a. Explain that client may have warm, flushed feeling and salty or metallic taste in mouth during procedure.
   b. Check for allergy to iodine.
   c. Keep NPO after midnight or offer clear liquid breakfast only.
   d. Take baseline vital signs and neuro check.
   e. Administer sedation if ordered.
4. Nursing care: posttest
   a. Maintain pressure dressing over site if femoral or brachial artery used; apply ice as ordered.

  **b.** Maintain bed rest until next morning or as ordered.
  **c.** Monitor vital signs and neuro checks frequently; report any changes immediately.
  **d.** Check site frequently for bleeding or hematoma; if carotid artery used, assess for swelling of neck, difficulty swallowing or breathing.
  **e.** Check pulse, color, and temperature of extremity distal to site used.
  **f.** Keep extremity extended and avoid flexion.
**H.** Echoencephalography: use of ultrasound to detect midline shift of intracranial contents due to brain tumors, hematomas.
**I.** Electroencephalography (EEG)
 **1.** Graphic recording of electrical activity of the brain by several small electrodes placed on the scalp
 **2.** Used to detect focus or foci of seizure activity and to quantitatively evaluate level of brain function (determine brain death)
 **3.** Pretest nursing care: withhold sedatives, tranquilizers, stimulants for 2–3 days.
 **4.** Posttest nursing care: remove electrode paste with acetone and shampoo hair.

## Eye

**A.** Ophthalmoscopic exam
**B.** Refraction: detects refractive errors and provides information for prescription of eyeglasses and contact lenses
**C.** Perimetry: assesses peripheral vision, visual fields
**D.** Tonometry: measures intraocular pressure (normal: 12–20 mm Hg)

## Ear

**A.** Otoscopic exam
**B.** Audiometry: screening test for hearing loss and diagnostic test to determine degree and type of hearing loss
**C.** Vestibular function
 **1.** Caloric test
 **2.** Electronystagmography (ENG)

## ANALYSIS

Nursing diagnoses for clients with disorders of the neurosensory system may include:
**A.** Imbalanced nutrition: less than body requirements
**B.** Ineffective thermoregulation
**C.** Autonomic dysreflexia
**D.** Constipation
**E.** Bowel incontinence
**F.** Impaired urinary elimination
**G.** Urinary retention
**H.** Ineffective tissue perfusion: cerebral
**I.** Ineffective airway clearance
**J.** Ineffective breathing pattern
**K.** Risk for injury
**L.** Risk for aspiration
**M.** Risk for disuse syndrome
**N.** Risk for impaired skin integrity
**O.** Impaired verbal communication
**P.** Sexual dysfunction
**Q.** Impaired physical mobility
**R.** Feeding self-care deficit
**S.** Impaired swallowing
**T.** Bathing/hygiene self-care deficit
**U.** Dressing/grooming self-care deficit
**V.** Toileting self-care deficit
**W.** Disturbed sensory perception: visual, auditory, kinesthetic, gustatory, tactile, olfactory
**X.** Unilateral neglect
**Y.** Disturbed thought processes

## PLANNING AND IMPLEMENTATION

### Goals

**A.** Nutritional state will be optimal.
**B.** Normal body temperature will be maintained.
**C.** Complications will be recognized early and treated promptly.
**D.** Adequate bowel and bladder elimination will be maintained.
**E.** Cerebral perfusion will be improved.
**F.** Adequate respiratory function will be maintained.
**G.** Client will remain free from any injury resulting from neurosensory deficits.
**H.** Client's skin integrity will be maintained.
**I.** Client's ability to communicate will be improved.
**J.** Sexual health will return to optimal level.
**K.** Mobility will be restored to optimal level.
**L.** Maximum independence in self-care activities will be attained.
**M.** Sensory perception will be improved.
**N.** Optimal cognitive functioning will be attained.

### Interventions

#### Care of the Unconscious Client

**A.** Maintain a clear, patent airway.
 **1.** Place client in a side-lying or three-quarters prone position to prevent tongue from obstructing airway.
 **2.** If tongue is obstructing, insert oral airway.
 **3.** Prepare for insertion of a cuffed endotracheal or tracheostomy tube as the client's condition requires.
 **4.** Suction as needed.
 **5.** Check respiratory rate, depth, and quality every 1–2 hours and as needed.

6. Auscultate breath sounds for crackles (rales), rhonchi, or absent breath sounds every 4 hours and before and after suctioning.
B. Take vital signs and perform neuro checks at specified intervals as ordered; report any significant changes immediately.
C. Maintain fluid and electrolyte balance and ensure adequate nutrition.
  1. Administer IV fluids, nasogastric tube feedings as ordered.
  2. Maintain accurate I&O.
  3. Assess client's hydration status: skin turgor, check for dry mucous membranes.
  4. Provide mouth care to keep mucous membranes clean, moist, and intact.
D. Provide for client's safety.
  1. Keep side rails up at all times.
  2. Avoid restraints if at all possible.
  3. Observe client carefully for seizures and intervene to avoid precipitating factors: fever, hypoxia, electrolyte imbalance.
  4. Protect client if seizure occurs.
  5. Speak softly and use client's name during nursing care.
  6. Touch client as gently as possible.
  7. Protect client's eyes from corneal irritation.
    a. Check for corneal reflex.
    b. Instill artificial tears as ordered; patch eye.
E. Prevent complications of immobility.
  1. Keep skin clean, dry, and pressure free.
  2. Turn and reposition client every 2 hours.
  3. Perform passive range-of-motion (ROM) exercises every 4 hours.
  4. Use nursing measures to prevent deformities: footboard/high-topped sneakers to prevent footdrop, splint to prevent wrist drop.
F. Maintain adequate bladder and bowel elimination.
  1. Urinary: indwelling catheter (may use external device in male)
  2. Bowel: stool softeners and suppositories as ordered

## Care of the Client with Increased Intracranial Pressure (ICP)

A. General information
  1. An increase in intracranial bulk due to an increase in any of the major intracranial components: brain tissue, CSF, or blood.
  2. Increased ICP may be caused by tumors, abscesses, hemorrhage, edema, hydrocephalus, inflammation.
  3. Untreated increased ICP can lead to displacement of brain tissue (herniation).
  4. Presents life-threatening situation because of pressure on vital structures in the brain stem, nerve tracts, and cranial nerves.

B. Assessment findings
  1. Earliest sign: decrease in LOC; progresses from restlessness to confusion and disorientation to lethargy and coma
  2. Changes in vital signs (may be a late sign)
    a. Systolic blood pressure rises while diastolic pressure remains the same (widening pulse presence)
    b. Pulse slows
    c. Abnormal respiratory patterns (e.g., Cheyne-Stokes respirations)
    d. Elevated temperature
  3. Pupillary changes
    a. Ipsilateral (same side) dilation of pupil with sluggish reaction to light from compression of cranial nerve III
    b. Pupil eventually becomes fixed and dilated.
  4. Motor abnormalities
    a. Contralateral (opposite side) hemiparesis from compression of corticospinal tracts
    b. Decorticate or decerebrate rigidity
  5. Headache, projectile vomiting, papilledema (edema of the optic disc)
C. Nursing care
  1. Maintain patent airway and adequate ventilation.
    a. Prevention of hypoxia and hypercarbia (increased $CO_2$) important: hypoxia may cause brain swelling and hypercarbia causes cerebral vasodilation, which increases ICP.
    b. Before and after suctioning, hyperventilate the client with a resuscitator bag connected to 100% oxygen. Limit suctioning to 10–15 seconds.
    c. Assist with mechanical hyperventilation as indicated: produces hypocarbia (decreased $CO_2$) causing cerebral vasoconstriction and decreased ICP.
  2. Monitor vital signs and neuro checks frequently to detect rises in ICP.
  3. Maintain fluid balance: fluid restriction to 1200–1500 mL/day may be ordered.
  4. Position client with head of bed elevated to 30–45° and neck in neutral position unless contraindicated (improves venous drainage from brain).
  5. Prevent further increases in ICP.
    a. Maintain quiet, comfortable environment.
    b. Avoid use of restraints.
    c. Prevent straining at stool; administer stool softeners and mild laxatives as ordered.
    d. Prevent vomiting; administer antiemetics as ordered.
    e. Prevent excessive coughing.
    f. Avoid clustering nursing care activities together.
  6. Prevent complications of immobility.
  7. Administer medications as ordered.

a. Hyperosmotic agents (mannitol [Osmitrol]) to reduce cerebral edema; monitor urine output every hour (should increase).

b. Corticosteroids (dexamethasone [Decadron]); anti-inflammatory effect reduces cerebral edema

c. Diuretics (furosemide [Lasix]) to reduce cerebral edema.

d. Anticonvulsants (phenytoin [Dilantin]) to prevent seizures.

e. Analgesics for headache as needed
   1) Small doses of codeine
   2) Stronger opiates may be contraindicated since they potentiate respiratory depression, alter LOC, and cause pupillary changes.

8. Assist with ICP monitoring when indicated.

a. ICP monitoring records the pressure exerted within the cranial cavity by the brain, cerebral blood, and CSF.

b. Types of monitoring devices
   1) Intraventricular catheter: inserted in lateral ventricle to give direct measurement of ICP; also allows for drainage of CSF if needed
   2) Subarachnoid screw (bolt): inserted through skull and dura mater into subarachnoid space
   3) Epidural sensor: least invasive method; placed in space between skull and dura mater for indirect measurement of ICP

c. Monitor ICP pressure readings frequently and prevent complications.
   1) Normal ICP reading is 0–15 mm Hg; a sustained increase above 15 mm Hg is considered abnormal.
   2) Use strict aseptic technique when handling any part of the monitoring system.
   3) Check insertion site for signs of infection; monitor temperature.
   4) Assess system for CSF leakage, loose connections, air bubbles in lines, and occluded tubing.

9. Provide intensive nursing care for client treated with barbiturate therapy or administration of paralyzing agents.

a. Intravenous administration of barbiturates may be ordered to induce coma artificially in the client who has not responded to conventional treatment.

b. Paralytic agents such as vecuronium bromide (Norcuron) may be administered to paralyze the client.

c. Reduces cellular metabolic demands that may protect the brain from further injury.

d. Constant monitoring of the client's ICP, arterial blood pressures, pulmonary pressures, arterial blood gases, serum barbiturate levels, and ECG is necessary.

e. EEG monitoring as necessary.

f. Provide appropriate nursing care for the client on a ventilator.

10. Observe for hyperthermia secondary to hypothalamus damage.

## Care of the Client with Hyperthermia

A. General information
   1. Abnormal elevation of body temperature to 41°C (106°F) or above
   2. Caused by dysfunction of hypothalamus (temperature regulating center) from edema, head injury, hemorrhage, CVA, brain tumor, or intracranial surgery
   3. Hyperthermia increases cerebral metabolism; predisposes to seizures; may cause neurologic damage if prolonged

B. Nursing care
   1. Remove blankets and excess clothing if temperature rises above 38.4°C (101°F).
   2. Maintain room temperature at 21.1°C (70°F).
   3. Administer antipyretic drugs (acetaminophen [Tylenol]) orally or rectally every 4 hours as ordered.
   4. Increase fluid intake to 3000 mL/day unless contraindicated (in increased ICP).
   5. Monitor vital signs, especially temperature, every 2–4 hours (more often if hypothermia is used).
   6. Monitor urine output and urine specific gravity and assess for signs of dehydration.
   7. Observe for seizure activity and protect client if seizures occur.
   8. Change linen frequently if client is diaphoretic (sweating profusely).
   9. Apply methods for inducing hypothermia as ordered: cool or tepid sponge baths, fans, hypothermia blanket. (See also Unit 3.)
   10. Provide special care for the client with a hypothermia blanket. (See also Unit 3.)
      a. Reduce temperature gradually to prevent shivering and serious dysrhythmias; chlorpromazine (Thorazine) may be given for shivering.
      b. Provide frequent skin care to prevent breakdown.
         1) Check every hour for signs of tissue damage or frostbite.
         2) Apply lotion to skin to prevent drying.
         3) Turn every 2 hours if not contraindicated because of increased intracranial pressure.
      c. Monitor core body temperature.

## Care of the Client with Diminished Eyesight

A. Always speak and identify yourself upon entering the room to prevent startling the client.

B. Orient the client to his surroundings.
  1. Walk the client around the room and have him touch the objects in the room, e.g., table, chair.
  2. Keep personal belongings and objects in the room in the same place in order to increase client's independence and sense of security.
  3. Explain noises or other activities going on in the room.
C. Provide safety measures.
  1. Keep call bell nearby.
  2. Keep at least one side rail up.
  3. Keep the room orderly and free of clutter.
D. Assist the client in walking by having him take your arm; walk a half step in front of the client.
E. Offer explanations to the client and tell him what to expect next.
F. Provide mental stimulation and prevent sensory deprivation by providing frequent contacts with the staff, visitors, use of radio, TV, etc.

### Communicating with the Client with Impaired Hearing

A. Attract the client's attention by raising an arm or hand.
B. Face the client directly when speaking.
C. Do not obscure the client's view of your mouth in any way.
D. Initially state the topic or subject of your conversation to give the client clues as to what you are going to say.
E. Speak slowly and distinctly, but do not overaccentuate words.
F. Speak in a normal tone of voice; do not shout.
G. Verify that the client has understood you, if necessary.

### Irrigation of the Ear

A. Introduction of fluid into external auditory canal for cleansing purposes; may be used to apply antiseptic solutions.
B. Nursing care
  1. Explain procedure to the client.
  2. Prepare supplies needed: irrigating solution (about 500 mL normal saline at body temperature), irrigating syringe, basin, towel, cotton-tipped applicators, cotton balls.
  3. Assist client to a sitting or lying position with head tilted toward the affected ear.
  4. Straighten ear canal by pulling auricle upward and backward (down and backward on a child under 3 years).
  5. Insert tip of syringe into auditory meatus and direct the solution gently upward toward the top of the canal.
  6. Collect returning fluid in basin.
  7. Dry the outer ear with cotton balls.
  8. Instruct client to lie on affected side to encourage drainage of solution.
  9. Record the procedure and results.

## EVALUATION

A. Client maintains normal weight; no evidence of malnutrition.
B. Client's temperature is maintained within normal limits.
C. Dysreflexia will be prevented or recognized early and treated promptly.
D. Client has regular bowel movements.
E. Client has adequate patterns of urinary elimination.
F. Neuro checks are within normal limits.
G. Client maintains patent airway and has effective respiratory patterns.
H. Client remains free from injuries.
I. Client remains free from aspiration and complications of immobility.
J. Client's skin remains clear and intact.
K. Client communicates effectively, responds appropriately to others.
L. Client experiences satisfying sexual activity/expression.
M. No contractures or limitations in motor function have occurred or loss of mobility has been kept to a minimum.
N. Client attains independence in self-care activities; uses assistive devices as necessary.
O. Sensory dysfunction is corrected or compensated for.
P. Client is oriented to time, place, and person; memory is intact; able to evaluate reality.

## DISORDERS OF THE NERVOUS SYSTEM

### Headache

A. General information
  1. Diffuse pain in different parts of the head
  2. Types
    a. Functional
      1) Tension (muscle contraction): associated with tension or anxiety
      2) Migraine: recurrent throbbing headache
        a) Often starts in adolescence
        b) Affects women more than men
        c) Vascular origin: vasoconstriction or spasm of cerebral blood vessels (producing an aura) then vasodilation
      3) Cluster: similar to migraine (vascular origin); recur several times a day over a period of weeks followed by remission lasting for weeks or months
    b. Organic: secondary to intracranial or systemic disease (e.g., brain tumor, sinus disease)
B. Assessment findings
  1. Tension headache: pain usually bilateral, often occurring in the back of the neck and extending diffusely over top of head

2. Migraine headache: severe, throbbing pain, often in temporal or supraorbital area, lasting several hours to days; may be an aura (e.g., visual disturbance) preceding the pain; nausea and vomiting; pallor; sweating; irritability

3. Cluster headache: intense, throbbing pain, usually affecting only one side of face and head; abrupt onset, lasts 30–90 minutes; eye and nose water on side of pain; skin reddens

4. Diagnostic tests may be used to rule out organic causes.

C. Nursing interventions
1. Carefully assess details regarding the headache.
2. Provide quiet, dark environment.
3. Administer medications as ordered.
   a. Symptomatic during acute attack
      1) Nonnarcotic analgesics (aspirin, acetaminophen [Tylenol])
      2) Fiorinal (analgesic-sedative/tranquilizer combination)
      3) For migraines, ergotamine tartrate (Gynergen) or ergotamine with caffeine (Cafergot); vasoconstrictors given during aura may prevent the headache
      4) Midrin (vasoconstrictor and sedative)
      5) Sumatriptan (Imitrex) causes vasoconstriction in cerebral arteries; given via cutaneous injection.
   b. Prophylactic to prevent migraine attacks
      1) Methysergide maleate (Sansert): after 6 months' use, drug should be discontinued for a 2-month period before resuming
      2) Propranolol (Inderal) and amytriptyline (Elavil): have also been used in migraine prevention
4. Provide additional nursing interventions for pain.
5. Provide client teaching and discharge planning concerning:
   a. Identification of factors including diet that appear to precipitate attacks
   b. Examination of lifestyle, identification of stressors, and development of more positive coping behaviors
   c. Importance of daily exercise and relaxation periods
   d. Relaxation techniques
   e. Use and side effects of prescribed medications
   f. Alternative ways of handling the pain of headache: meditation, relaxation, self-hypnosis, yoga

## Meningitis

A. General information
1. Inflammation of the meninges of the brain and spinal cord

2. Caused by bacteria, viruses, or other microorganisms
3. May reach CNS
   a. Via the blood, CSF, lymph
   b. By direct extension from adjacent cranial structures (nasal sinuses, mastoid bone, ear, skull fracture)
   c. By oral or nasopharyngeal route
4. Most common organisms: meningococcus, pneumococcus, *H. influenzae*, streptococcus

B. Assessment findings
1. Headache, photophobia, malaise, irritability
2. Chills and fever
3. Signs of meningeal irritation
   a. Nuchal rigidity: stiff neck
   b. Kernig's sign: contraction or pain in the hamstring muscle when attempting to extend the leg when the hip is flexed
   c. Opisthotonos: head and heels bent backward and body arched forward
   d. Brudzinski's sign: flexion at the hip and knee in response to forward flexion of the neck
4. Vomiting
5. Possible seizures and decreasing LOC
6. Diagnostic test: lumbar puncture (measurement and analysis of CSF shows increased pressure, elevated WBC and protein, decreased glucose and culture positive for specific microorganism)

C. Nursing interventions
1. Administer large doses of antibiotics IV as ordered.
2. Enforce respiratory isolation for 24 hours after initiation of antibiotic therapy for some types of meningitis (consult hospital's infection control manual for specific directions).
3. Provide nursing care for increased ICP, seizures, and hyperthermia if they occur.
4. Provide nursing care for delirious or unconscious client as needed.
5. Provide bed rest; keep room quiet and dark if client has headache or photophobia.
6. Administer analgesics for headache as ordered.
7. Maintain fluid and electrolyte balance.
8. Prevent complications of immobility.
9. Monitor vital signs and neuro checks frequently.
10. Provide client teaching and discharge planning concerning:
    a. Importance of good diet: high protein, high calorie with small, frequent feedings.
    b. Rehabilitation program for residual deficits.

## Encephalitis

A. General information
1. Inflammation of the brain caused by a virus, e.g., herpes simplex (type I) or arbovirus (transmitted by mosquito or tick)

2. May occur as a sequela of other diseases such as measles, mumps, chickenpox.
B. Assessment findings
   1. Headache
   2. Fever, chills, vomiting
   3. Signs of meningeal irritation
   4. Possibly seizures
   5. Alterations in LOC
C. Nursing interventions
   1. Monitor vital signs and neuro checks frequently.
   2. Provide nursing measures for increased ICP, seizures, hyperthermia if they occur.
   3. Provide nursing care for confused or unconscious client as needed.
   4. Provide client teaching and discharge planning: same as for meningitis.

## Brain Abscess

A. General information
   1. Collection of free or encapsulated pus within the brain tissue
   2. Usually follows an infectious process elsewhere in the body (ear, sinuses, mastoid bone)
B. Assessment findings
   1. Headache, malaise, anorexia
   2. Vomiting
   3. Signs of increased ICP
   4. Focal neurologic deficits (hemiparesis, seizures)
C. Nursing interventions
   1. Administer large doses of antibiotics as ordered.
   2. Monitor vital signs and neuro checks.
   3. Provide symptomatic and supportive care.
   4. Prepare client for surgery if indicated (see Craniotomy).

## Brain Tumors

A. General information
   1. Tumor within the cranial cavity; may be benign or malignant
   2. Types
      a. Primary: originates in brain tissue (e.g., glioma, meningioma)
      b. Secondary: metastasizes from tumor elsewhere in the body (e.g., lung, breast)
B. Medical management
   1. Craniotomy: to remove the tumor when possible
   2. Radiation therapy and chemotherapy: may follow surgery; also for inaccessible tumors and metastatic tumors
   3. Drug therapy: hyperosmotic agents, corticosteroids, diuretics to manage increased ICP
C. Assessment findings

1. Headache: worse in the morning and with straining and stooping
2. Vomiting
3. Papilledema
4. Seizures (focal or generalized)
5. Changes in mental status
6. Focal neurologic deficits (e.g., aphasia, hemiparesis, sensory problems)
7. Diagnostic tests
   a. Skull X-ray, CT scan, MRI, brain scan: reveal presence of tumor
   b. Abnormal EEG
   c. Brain biopsy
D. Nursing interventions
   1. Monitor vital signs and neuro checks; observe for signs and symptoms of increased ICP.
   2. Administer medications as ordered.
      a. Drugs to decrease ICP, e.g., dextromethasone (Decadron)
      b. Anticonvulsants, e.g., phenytoin (Dilantin)
      c. Analgesics for headache, e.g., acetaminophen (Tylenol)
   3. Provide supportive care for any neurologic deficit (see Cerebrovascular Accident).
   4. Prepare client for surgery (see Craniotomy).
   5. Provide care for effects of radiation therapy or chemotherapy (see Oncologic Nursing).
   6. Provide psychologic support to client/significant others.
   7. Provide client teaching and discharge planning concerning
      a. Use and side effects of prescribed medications.
      b. Rehabilitation program for residual deficits.

## Cerebrovascular Accident (CVA)

A. General information
   1. Destruction (infarction) of brain cells caused by a reduction in cerebral blood flow and oxygen
   2. Affects men more than women; incidence increases with age
   3. Caused by thrombosis, embolism, hemorrhage
   4. Risk factors
      a. Hypertension, diabetes mellitus, arteriosclerosis/atherosclerosis, cardiac disease (valvular disease/replacement, chronic atrial fibrillation, myocardial infarction)
      b. Lifestyle: obesity, smoking, inactivity, stress, use of oral contraceptives
   5. Pathophysiology
      a. Interruption of cerebral blood flow for 5 minutes or more causes death of neurons in affected area with irreversible loss of function
      b. Modifying factors
         1) Cerebral edema: develops around affected area causing further impairment

2) Vasospasm: constriction of cerebral blood vessel may occur, causing further decrease in blood flow
3) Collateral circulation: may help to maintain cerebral blood flow when there is compromise of main blood supply

6. Stages of development
    a. Transient ischemic attack (TIA)
        1) Warning sign of impending CVA
        2) Brief period of neurologic deficit: visual loss, hemiparesis, slurred speech, aphasia, vertigo
        3) May last less than 30 seconds, but no more than 24 hours with complete resolution of symptoms
    b. Stroke in evolution: progressive development of stroke symptoms over a period of hours to days
    c. Completed stroke: neurologic deficit remains unchanged for a 2- to 3-day period.

B. Assessment findings
    1. Headache
    2. Generalized signs: vomiting, seizures, confusion, disorientation, decreased LOC, nuchal rigidity, fever, hypertension, slow bounding pulse, Cheyne-Stokes respirations
    3. Focal signs (related to site of infarction): hemiplegia, sensory loss, aphasia, homonymous hemianopsia
    4. Diagnostic tests
        a. CT and brain scan: reveal lesion
        b. EEG: abnormal changes
        c. Cerebral arteriography: may show occlusion or malformation of blood vessels

C. Nursing interventions: acute stage
    1. Maintain patent airway and adequate ventilation.
    2. Monitor vital signs and neuro checks and observe for signs of increased ICP, shock, hyperthermia, and seizures.
    3. Provide complete bed rest as ordered.
    4. Maintain fluid and electrolyte balance and ensure adequate nutrition.
        a. IV therapy for the first few days
        b. Nasogastric tube feedings if client unable to swallow
        c. Fluid restriction as ordered to decrease cerebral edema
    5. Maintain proper positioning and body alignment.
        a. Head of bed may be elevated 30–45° to decrease ICP
        b. Turn and reposition every 2 hours (only 20 minutes on the affected side)
        c. Passive ROM exercises every 4 hours.
    6. Promote optimum skin integrity: turn client and apply lotion every 2 hours.
    7. Maintain adequate elimination.
        a. Offer bedpan or urinal every 2 hours, catheterize only if absolutely necessary.

b. Administer stool softeners and suppositories as ordered to prevent constipation and fecal impaction.
8. Provide a quiet, restful environment.
9. Establish a means of communicating with the client.
10. Administer medications as ordered.
    a. Hyperosmotic agents, corticosteroids to decrease cerebral edema
    b. Anticonvulsants to prevent or treat seizures
    c. Thrombolytics given to dissolve clot (hemorrhage must be ruled out)
        1) Tissue plasminogen activator (tPA, Alteplase)
        2) Streptokinase, urokinase
        3) Must be given within 3 hours of episode
    d. Anticoagulants for stroke in evolution or embolic stroke (hemorrhage must be ruled out)
        1) Heparin
        2) Warfarin (Coumadin) for long-term therapy
        3) Aspirin and dipyridamole (Persantine) to inhibit platelet aggregation in treating TIAs
    e. Antihypertensives if indicated for elevated blood pressure

D. Nursing interventions: rehabilitation
    1. Hemiplegia: results from injury to cells in the cerebral motor cortex or to corticospinal tracts (causes contralateral hemiplegia because tracts cross in medulla)
        a. Turn every 2 hours (20 minutes only on affected side).
        b. Use proper positioning and repositioning to prevent deformities (foot drop, external rotation of hip, flexion of fingers, wrist drop, abduction of shoulder and arm).
        c. Support paralyzed arm on pillow or use sling while out of bed to prevent subluxation of shoulder.
        d. Elevate extremities to prevent dependent edema.
        e. Provide active and passive ROM exercises every 4 hours.
    2. Susceptibility to hazards
        a. Keep side rails up at all times.
        b. Institute safety measures.
        c. Inspect body parts frequently for signs of injury.
    3. Dysphagia (difficulty swallowing)
        a. Check gag reflex before feeding client.
        b. Maintain a calm, unhurried approach.
        c. Place client in upright position.
        d. Place food in unaffected side of mouth.
        e. Offer soft foods.
        f. Give mouth care before and after meals.
    4. Homonymous hemianopsia: loss of right or left half of each visual field

a. Approach client on unaffected side.
   b. Place personal belongings, food, etc., on unaffected side.
   c. Gradually teach client to compensate by scanning, i.e., turning the head to see things on affected side.
5. Emotional lability: mood swings, frustration
   a. Create a quiet, restful environment with a reduction in excessive sensory stimuli.
   b. Maintain a calm, nonthreatening manner.
   c. Explain to family that the client's behavior is not purposeful.
6. Aphasia: most common in right hemiplegics; may be receptive/expressive
   a. Receptive aphasia
      1) Give simple, slow directions.
      2) Give one command at a time; gradually shift topics.
      3) Use nonverbal techniques of communication (e.g., pantomime, demonstration).
   b. Expressive aphasia
      1) Listen and watch very carefully when the client attempts to speak.
      2) Anticipate client's needs to decrease frustration and feelings of helplessness.
      3) Allow sufficient time for client to answer.
7. Sensory/perceptual deficits: more common in left hemiplegics; characterized by impulsiveness, unawareness of disabilities, visual neglect (neglect of affected side and visual space on affected side)
   a. Assist with self-care.
   b. Provide safety measures.
   c. Initially arrange objects in environment on unaffected side.
   d. Gradually teach client to take care of the affected side and to turn frequently and look at affected side.
8. Apraxia: loss of ability to perform purposeful, skilled acts
   a. Guide client through intended movement (e.g., take object such as washcloth and guide client through movement of washing).
   b. Keep repeating the movement.
9. Generalizations about clients with left hemiplegia versus right hemiplegia and nursing care
   a. Left hemiplegia
      1) Perceptual, sensory deficits; quick and impulsive behavior
      2) Use safety measures, verbal cues, simplicity in all areas of care
   b. Right hemiplegia
      1) Speech-language deficits; slow and cautious behavior
      2) Use pantomime and demonstration

# Cerebral Aneurysm

A. General information
   1. Dilation of the walls of a cerebral artery, resulting in a sac-like outpouching of vessel
   2. Caused by congenital weakness in the vessel, trauma, arteriosclerosis, hypertension
   3. Pathophysiology
      a. Aneurysm compresses nearby cranial nerves or brain substance, producing dysfunction.
      b. Aneurysm may rupture, causing subarachnoid hemorrhage or intracerebral hemorrhage.
      c. Initially a clot forms at the site of rupture, but fibrinolysis (dissolution of the clot) tends to occur within 7–10 days and may cause rebleeding.
B. Assessment findings
   1. Severe headache and pain in the eyes
   2. Diplopia, tinnitus, dizziness
   3. Nuchal rigidity, ptosis, decreasing LOC, hemiparesis, seizures
C. Nursing interventions
   1. Maintain a patent airway and adequate ventilation.
      a. Instruct client to take deep breaths but to avoid coughing.
      b. Suction only with a specific order.
   2. Monitor vital signs and neuro checks and observe for signs of vasospasm, increased ICP, hypertension, seizures, and hyperthermia.
   3. Enforce strict bed rest and provide complete care.
   4. Keep head of bed flat or elevated to 20–30° as ordered.
   5. Maintain a quiet, darkened environment.
   6. Avoid taking temperature rectally and instruct client to avoid sneezing, coughing, and straining at stool.
   7. Enforce fluid restriction as ordered; maintain accurate I&O.
   8. Administer medications as ordered.
      a. Antihypertensive agents to maintain normotensive levels
      b. Corticosteroids to prevent increased ICP
      c. Anticonvulsants to prevent seizures
      d. Stool softeners to prevent straining
      e. Aminocaproic acid (Amicar) to decrease fibrinolysis of the clot (administered IV)
   9. Prevent complications of immobility.
   10. Institute seizure precautions.
   11. Provide nursing care for the unconscious client if needed.
   12. Prepare the client for surgery if indicated (see Craniotomy).

# Parkinson's Disease

A. General information
   1. A progressive disorder with degeneration of the nerve cells in the basal ganglia resulting in

generalized decline in muscular function; disorder of the extrapyramidal system

2. Usually occurs in the older population
3. Cause unknown; predominantly idiopathic, but sometimes disorder is postencephalitic, toxic, arteriosclerotic, traumatic, or drug induced (reserpine, methyldopa [Aldomet], haloperidol [Haldol], phenothiazines)
4. Pathophysiology
   a. Disorder causes degeneration of the dopamine-producing neurons in the substantia nigra in the midbrain.
   b. Dopamine influences purposeful movement.
   c. Depletion of dopamine results in degeneration of the basal ganglia.

B. Assessment findings
1. Tremor: mainly of the upper limbs, "pill-rolling," resting tremor; most common initial symptom
2. Rigidity: cogwheel type
3. Bradykinesia: slowness of movement
4. Fatigue
5. Stooped posture; shuffling, propulsive gait (see Figure 4-4)
6. Difficulty rising from sitting position
7. Masklike face with decreased blinking of eyes
8. Quiet, monotone speech
9. Emotional lability, depression
10. Increased salivation, drooling
11. Cramped, small handwriting
12. Autonomic symptoms: excessive sweating, seborrhea, lacrimation, constipation; decreased sexual capacity

C. Nursing interventions
1. Administer medications as ordered
   a. Levodopa (L-dopa)
      1) Increases level of dopamine in the brain; relieves tremor, rigidity, and bradykinesia.
      2) Side effects: anorexia; nausea and vomiting; postural hypotension; mental changes such as confusion, agitation, and hallucinations; cardiac arrhythmias; dyskinesias.
      3) Contraindications: narrow-angle glaucoma; clients taking MAO inhibitors, reserpine, guanethidine, methyldopa, antipsychotics; acute psychoses.
      4) Avoid multiple vitamin preparations containing vitamin $B_6$ (pyridoxine) and foods high in vitamin $B_6$.
      5) Be aware of any worsening of symptoms with prolonged high-dose therapy: "on-off" syndrome.
      6) Administer with food or snack to decrease GI irritation.
      7) Inform client that urine and sweat may be darkened.
   b. Carbidopa-levodopa (Sinemet): prevents breakdown of dopamine in the periphery and causes fewer side effects.
   c. Amantadine (Symmetrel): used in mild cases or in combination with L-dopa to reduce rigidity, tremor, and bradykinesia.

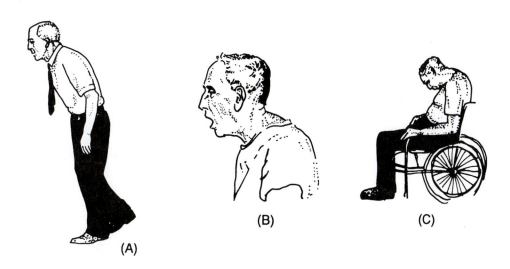

**Figure 4-4** The shuffling gait and early postural changes of Parkinson's disease shown in (A). (B) and (C) show an advanced stage of the disease with head held forward, mouth open, and inability to stand.

d. Anticholinergic drugs: benztropine mesylate (Cogentin), procyclidine (Kemadrin), trihexyphenidyl (Artane)
   1) Inhibit action of acetylcholine
   2) Used in mild cases or in combination with L-dopa
   3) Relieve tremor and rigidity
   4) Side effects: dry mouth, blurred vision, constipation, urinary retention, confusion, hallucinations, tachycardia
e. Antihistamines: diphenhydramine (Benadryl)
   1) Decrease tremor and anxiety
   2) Side effect: drowsiness
f. Bromocriptine (Parlodel)
   1) Stimulates release of dopamine in the substantia nigra.
   2) Often employed when L-dopa loses effectiveness.
g. Eldepryl (Selegilene) a MAO inhibitor inhibits dopamine breakdown and slows progression of disease
h. Tricyclic antidepressants given to treat depression commonly seen in Parkinson's disease
2. Provide a safe environment.
   a. Side rails on bed; rails and handlebars in toilet, bathtub, and hallways; no scatter rugs
   b. Hard-back or spring-loaded chair to make getting up easier
3. Provide measures to increase mobility.
   a. Physical therapy: active and passive ROM exercises; stretching exercises; warm baths
   b. Assistive devices
   c. If client "freezes," suggest thinking of something to walk over.
4. Encourage independence in self-care activities: alter clothing for ease in dressing; use assistive devices; do not rush client.
5. Improve communication abilities: instruct client to practice reading aloud, to listen to own voice, and enunciate each syllable clearly.
6. Refer for speech therapy when indicated.
7. Maintain adequate nutrition.
   a. Cut food into bite-sized pieces.
   b. Provide small, frequent feedings.
   c. Allow sufficient time for meals, use warming tray.
8. Avoid constipation and maintain adequate bowel elimination.
9. Provide psychologic support to client/significant others; depression is common due to changes in body image and self-concept.
10. Provide client teaching and discharge planning concerning
    a. Nature of the disease
    b. Use of prescribed medications and side effects

c. Importance of daily exercise: walking, swimming, gardening as tolerated; balanced activity and rest
d. Activities/methods to limit postural deformities: firm mattress with a small pillow; keep head and neck as erect as possible; use broad-based gait; raise feet while walking
e. Promotion of active participation in self-care activities

## Multiple Sclerosis (MS)

A. General information
   1. Chronic, intermittently progressive disease of the CNS, characterized by scattered patches of demyelination within the brain and spinal cord
   2. Incidence
      a. Affects women more than men
      b. Usually occurs from 20–40 years of age
      c. More frequent in cool or temperate climates
   3. Cause unknown; may be a slow-growing virus or possibly of autoimmune origin
   4. Signs and symptoms are varied and multiple, reflecting the location of demyelination within the CNS
   5. Characterized by remissions and exacerbations
B. Assessment findings
   1. Visual disturbances: blurred vision, scotomas (blind spots), diplopia
   2. Impaired sensation: touch, pain, temperature, or position sense; paresthesias such as numbness, tingling
   3. Euphoria or mood swings
   4. Impaired motor function: weakness, paralysis, spasticity
   5. Impaired cerebellar function: scanning speech, ataxic gait, nystagmus, dysarthria, intention tremor
   6. Bladder: retention or incontinence
   7. Constipation
   8. Sexual impotence in the male
   9. Diagnostic tests:
      a. CSF studies: increased protein and IgG (immunoglobulin)
      b. Visual evoked response (VER) determined by EEG: may be delayed
      c. CT scan: increased density of white matter
      d. MRI: shows areas of demyelination
C. Nursing interventions
   1. Assess the client for specific deficits related to location of demyelinization.
   2. Promote optimum mobility.
      a. Muscle-stretching and strengthening exercises
      b. Walking exercises to improve gait: use wide-based gait
      c. Assistive devices: canes, walker, rails, wheelchair as necessary

3. Administer medications as ordered.
    a. For acute exacerbations: corticosteroids (ACTH [IV], prednisone) to reduce edema at sites of demyelinization
    b. For spasticity: baclofen (Lioresal), dantrolene (Dantrium), diazepam (Valium)
    c. Beta interferon (Betaseron) to alter immune response
4. Encourage independence in self-care activities.
5. Prevent complications of immobility.
6. Institute bowel program.
7. Maintain urinary elimination.
    a. Urinary retention
        1) Administer bethanecol chloride (Urecholine) as ordered.
        2) Perform intermittent catheterization as ordered.
    b. Urinary incontinence
        1) Establish voiding schedule.
        2) Administer propantheline bromide (Pro-Banthine) if ordered.
    c. Force fluids to 3000 mL/day.
    d. Promote use of acid-ash foods like cranberry or grape juice.
8. Prevent injury related to sensory problems.
    a. Test bath water with thermometer.
    b. Avoid heating pads, hot-water bottles.
    c. Inspect body parts frequently for injury.
    d. Make frequent position changes.
9. Prepare client for plasma exchange (to remove antibodies) if indicated.
10. Provide psychologic support to client/significant others.
    a. Encourage positive attitude and assist client in setting realistic goals.
    b. Provide compassion in helping client adapt to changes in body image and self-concept.
    c. Do not encourage false hopes during remission.
    d. Refer to multiple sclerosis societies and community agencies.
11. Provide client teaching and discharge planning concerning
    a. General measures to ensure optimum health
        1) Balance between activity and rest
        2) Regular exercise such as walking, swimming, biking in mild cases
        3) Use of energy conservation techniques
        4) Well-balanced diet
        5) Fresh air and sunshine
        6) Avoiding fatigue, overheating or chilling, stress, infection
    b. Use of medications and side effects
    c. Alternative methods for sexual gratification; refer for sexual counseling if indicated.

# Myasthenia Gravis

A. General information
    1. A neuromuscular disorder in which there is a disturbance in the transmission of impulses from nerve to muscle cells at the neuromuscular junction, causing extreme muscle weakness
    2. Incidence
        a. Highest between ages 15 and 35 for women, over 40 for men.
        b. Affects women more than men
    3. Cause: thought to be autoimmune disorder whereby antibodies destroy acetylcholine receptor sites on the postsynaptic membrane of the neuromuscular junction.
    4. Voluntary muscles are affected, especially those muscles innervated by the cranial nerves.
B. Medical management
    1. Drug therapy
        a. Anticholinesterase drugs: ambenonium (Mytelase), neostigmine (Prostigmin), pyridostigmine (Mestinon)
            1) Block action of cholinesterase and increase levels of acetylcholine at the neuromuscular junction
            2) Side effects: excessive salivation and sweating, abdominal cramps, nausea and vomiting, diarrhea, fasciculations (muscle twitching)
        b. Corticosteroids: prednisone
            1) Used if other drugs are not effective
            2) Suppress autoimmune response
    2. Surgery (thymectomy)
        a. Surgical removal of the thymus gland (thought to be involved in the production of acetylcholine receptor antibodies)
        b. May cause remission in some clients especially if performed early in the disease
    3. Plasma exchange
        a. Removes circulating acetylcholine receptor antibodies
        b. Use in clients who do not respond to other types of therapy
C. Assessment findings
    1. Diplopia, dysphagia
    2. Extreme muscle weakness, increased with activity and reduced with rest
    3. Ptosis, masklike facial expression
    4. Weak voice, hoarseness
    5. Diagnostic tests
        a. Tensilon test: IV injection of Tensilon provides spontaneous relief of symptoms (lasts 5–10 minutes)
        b. Electromyography (EMG): amplitude of evoked potentials decreases rapidly
        c. Presence of antiacetylcholine receptor antibodies in the serum

**D.** Nursing interventions
1. Administer anticholinesterase drugs as ordered.
   a. Give medication exactly on time.
   b. Give with milk and crackers to decrease GI upset.
   c. Monitor effectiveness of drugs: assess muscle strength and vital capacity before and after medication.
   d. Avoid use of the following drugs: morphine and strong sedatives (respiratory depressant effect), quinine, curare, procainamide, neomycin, streptomycin, kanamycin and other aminoglycosides (skeletal muscle blocking effects).
   e. Observe for side effects.
2. Promote optimal nutrition.
   a. Mealtimes should coincide with the peak effects of the drugs: give medications 30 minutes before meals.
   b. Check gag reflex and swallowing ability before feeding.
   c. Provide a mechanical soft diet.
   d. If the client has difficulty chewing and swallowing, do not leave alone at mealtimes; keep emergency airway and suction equipment nearby.
3. Monitor respiratory status frequently: rate, depth; vital capacity; ability to deep breathe and cough.
4. Assess muscle strength frequently; plan activity to take advantage of energy peaks and provide frequent rest periods.
5. Observe for signs of myasthenic or cholinergic crisis.
   a. Myasthenic crisis
      1) Abrupt onset of severe, generalized muscle weakness with inability to swallow, speak, or maintain respirations
      2) Caused by undermedication, physical or emotional stress, infection
      3) Symptoms will improve temporarily with Tensilon test
   b. Cholinergic crisis
      1) Symptoms similar to myasthenic crisis and, in addition, the side effects of anticholinesterase drugs (e.g., excessive salivation and sweating, abdominal cramps, nausea and vomiting, diarrhea, fasciculations)
      2) Caused by overmedication with the cholinergic (anticholinesterase) drugs
      3) Symptoms worsen with Tensilon test; keep atropine sulfate and emergency equipment on hand
   c. Nursing care in crisis
      1) Maintain tracheostomy or endotracheal tube with mechanical ventilation as indicated (see Mechanical Ventilation).
      2) Monitor arterial blood gases and vital capacities.
      3) Administer medications as ordered.
         a) Myasthenic crisis: increase doses of anticholinesterase drugs as ordered.
         b) Cholinergic crisis: discontinue anticholinesterase drugs as ordered until the client recovers.
      4) Establish a method of communication.
      5) Provide support and reassurance.
6. Provide nursing care for the client with a thymectomy.
7. Provide client teaching and discharge planning concerning
   a. Nature of the disease
   b. Use of prescribed medications, their side effects and signs of toxicity
   c. Importance of checking with physician before taking any new medications including OTC drugs
   d. Importance of planning activities to take advantage of energy peaks and of scheduling frequent rest periods
   e. Need to avoid fatigue, stress, people with upper-respiratory infections
   f. Use of eye patch for diplopia (alternate eyes)
   g. Need to wear Medic-Alert bracelet
   h. Myasthenia Gravis Foundation and other community agencies

## Epilepsy

See Unit 5.

## Head Injury

**A.** General information
1. Usually caused by car accidents, falls, assaults
2. Types
   a. Concussion: severe blow to the head jostles brain, causing it to strike the skull; results in temporary neural dysfunction
   b. Contusion: results from more severe blow that bruises the brain and disrupts neural function
   c. Hemorrhage
      1) Epidural hematoma: accumulation of blood between the dura mater and skull; commonly results from laceration of middle meningeal artery during skull fracture; blood accumulates rapidly
      2) Subdural hematoma: accumulation of blood between the dura and arachnoid; venous bleeding that forms slowly; may be acute, subacute, or chronic
      3) Subarachnoid hematoma: bleeding in subarachnoid space

4) Intracerebral hematoma: accumulation of blood within the cerebrum

d. Fractures: linear, depressed, comminuted, compound

B. Assessment findings (depend on type of injury)
1. Concussion: headache, transient loss of consciousness, retrograde or posttraumatic amnesia, nausea, dizziness, irritability
2. Contusion: neurologic deficits depend on the site and extent of damage; include decreased LOC, aphasia, hemiplegia, sensory deficits
3. Hemorrhages
   a. Epidural hematoma: brief loss of consciousness followed by lucid interval; progresses to severe headache, vomiting, rapidly deteriorating LOC, possible seizures, ipsilateral pupillary dilation
   b. Subdural hematoma: alterations in LOC, headache, focal neurologic deficits, personality changes, ipsilateral pupillary dilation
   c. Intracerebral hematoma: headache, decreased LOC, hemiplegia, ipsilateral pupillary dilation
4. Fractures
   a. Headache, pain over fracture site
   b. Compound fractures: rhinorrhea (leakage of CSF from nose); otorrhea (leakage of CSF from ear)
5. Diagnostic tests
   a. Skull X-ray: reveals skull fracture or intracranial shift
   b. CT scan: reveals hemorrhage

C. Nursing interventions (see also Care of the Unconscious Client and Care of the Client with Increased ICP)
1. Maintain a patent airway and adequate ventilation.
2. Monitor vital signs and neuro checks; observe for changes in neurologic status, signs of increased ICP, shock, seizures, and hyperthermia.
3. Observe for CSF leakage.
   a. Check discharge for positive Testape or Dextrostix reaction for glucose; bloody spot encircled by watery, pale ring "halo" on pillowcase or sheet.
   b. Never attempt to clean the ears or nose of a head-injured client or use nasal suction unless cleared by physician.
4. If a CSF leak is present:
   a. Instruct client not to blow nose.
   b. Elevate head of bed 30° as ordered.
   c. Observe for signs of meningitis and administer antibiotics to prevent meningitis as ordered.
   d. Place a cotton ball in the ear to absorb otorrhea; replace frequently.
   e. Gently place a sterile gauze pad at the bottom of the nose for rhinorrhea; replace frequently.

5. Prevent complications of immobility.
6. Prepare the client for surgery if indicated.
   a. Depressed skull fracture: surgical removal or elevation of splintered bone; debridement and cleansing of area; repair of dural tear if present; cranioplasty (if necessitated for large cranial defect)
   b. Epidural or subdural hematoma: evacuation of the hematoma
7. Provide psychologic support to client/significant others.
8. Observe for hemiplegia, aphasia, and sensory problems, and plan care accordingly (see Cerebrovascular Accident).
9. Provide client teaching and discharge planning concerning rehabilitation for neurologic deficits; note availability of community agencies.

## Intracranial Surgery

A. Types
1. Craniotomy: surgical opening of skull to gain access to intracranial structures; used to remove a tumor, evacuate blood clot, control hemorrhage, relieve increased ICP
2. Craniectomy: excision of a portion of the skull; sometimes used for decompression
3. Cranioplasty: repair of a cranial defect with a metal or plastic plate
B. Nursing interventions: preoperative
1. Routine pre-op care (see Perioperative Nursing).
2. Provide emotional support; explain post-op procedures and that client's head will be shaved, there will be a large bandage on head, possibly temporary swelling and discoloration around the eye on the affected side, and possible headache.
3. Shampoo the scalp and check for signs of infection.
4. Shave hair.
5. Evaluate and record baseline vital signs and neuro checks.
6. Avoid enemas unless directed (straining increases ICP).
7. Give pre-op steroids as ordered to decrease brain swelling.
8. Insert Foley catheter as ordered.
C. Nursing interventions: postoperative
1. Provide nursing care for the unconscious client.
2. Maintain a patent airway and adequate ventilation.
   a. Supratentorial incision: elevate head of bed 15–45° as ordered; position on back (if intubated or conscious) or on unaffected side; turn every 2 hours to facilitate breathing and venous return.
   b. Infratentorial incision: keep head of bed flat or elevate 20–30° as ordered; do not flex head on chest; turn side to side every

2 hours using a turning sheet; check respirations closely and report any signs of respiratory distress.

   c. Instruct the conscious client to breathe deeply but not to cough; avoid vigorous suctioning.

3. Check vital signs and neuro checks frequently; observe for decreasing LOC, increased ICP, seizures, hyperthermia.

4. Monitor fluid and electrolyte status.

   a. Maintain accurate I&O.

   b. Restrict fluids to 1500 mL/day or as ordered to decrease cerebral edema.

   c. Avoid overly rapid infusions.

   d. Watch for signs of diabetes insipidus (severe thirst, polyuria, dehydration) and inappropriate ADH secretion (decreased urine output, hunger, thirst, irritability, decreased LOC, muscle weakness).

   e. For infratentorial surgery: may be NPO for 24 hours due to possible impaired swallowing and gag reflexes.

5. Assess dressings frequently and report any abnormalities.

   a. Reinforce as needed with sterile dressings.

   b. Check dressings for excessive drainage, CSF, infection, displacement and report to physician.

   c. If surgical drain is in place, note color, amount, and odor of drainage.

6. Administer medications as ordered.

   a. Corticosteroids: to decrease cerebral edema

   b. Anticonvulsants: to prevent seizures

   c. Stool softeners: to prevent straining

   d. Mild analgesics

7. Apply ice to swollen eyelids; lubricate lids and areas around eyes with petrolatum jelly.

8. Refer client for rehabilitation for residual deficits.

# Spinal Cord Injuries

A. General information

1. Occurs most commonly in young adult males between ages 15 and 25

2. Common traumatic causes: motor vehicle accidents, diving in shallow water, falls, industrial accidents, sports injuries, gunshot or stab wounds

3. Nontraumatic causes: tumors, hematomas, aneurysms, congenital defects (spina bifida)

4. Classified by extent, level, and mechanism of injury

   a. Extent of injury

      1) May affect the vertebral column: fracture, fracture/dislocation

      2) May affect anterior or posterior ligaments, causing compression of spinal cord

      3) May be to the spinal cord and its roots: concussion, contusion, compression or laceration by fracture/dislocation or penetrating missiles

   b. Level of injury: cervical, thoracic, lumbar

   c. Mechanisms of injury

      1) Hyperflexion

      2) Hyperextension

      3) Axial loading (force exerted straight up or down spinal column as in a diving accident)

      4) Penetrating wounds

5. Pathophysiology: hemorrhage and edema cause ischemia, leading to necrosis and destruction of the cord

B. Medical management: immobilization and maintenance of normal spinal alignment to promote fracture healing

1. Horizontal turning frames (Stryker frame)

2. Skeletal traction: to immobilize the fracture and maintain alignment of the cervical spine

   a. Cervical tongs (Crutchfield, Gardner-Wells, Vinke): inserted through burr holes; traction is provided by a rope extended from the center of tongs over a pulley with weights attached at the end.

   b. Halo traction

      1) Stainless steel halo ring fits around the head and is attached to the skull with four pins; halo is attached to plastic body cast or plastic vest

      2) Permits early mobilization, decreased period of hospitalization and reduces complications of immobility

3. Surgery: decompression laminectomy, spinal fusion

   a. Depends on type of injury and the preference of the surgeon

   b. Indications: unstable fracture, cord compression, progression of neurologic deficits

C. Assessment findings

1. Spinal shock

   a. Occurs immediately after the injury as a result of the insult to the CNS

   b. Temporary condition lasting from several days to 3 months

   c. Characterized by absence of reflexes below the level of the lesion, flaccid paralysis, lack of temperature control in affected parts, hypotension with bradycardia, retention of urine and feces

2. Symptoms depend on the level and the extent of the injury.

   a. Level of injury

      1) Quadriplegia: cervical injuries ($C_1$–$C_8$) cause paralysis of all four extremities; respiratory paralysis occurs in lesions above $C_6$ due to lack of innervation to

the diaphragm; (phrenic nerves at the $C_4$–$C_5$ level).

   2) Paraplegia: thoraco/lumbar injuries ($T_1$–$L_4$) cause paralysis of the lower half of the body involving both legs

  **b.** Extent of injury

    1) Complete cord transection

      **a)** Loss of all voluntary movement and sensation below the level of the injury; reflex activity below the level of the lesion may return after spinal shock resolves.

      **b)** Lesions in the conus medullaris or cauda equina result in permanent flaccid paralysis and areflexia.

    2) Incomplete lesions: varying degrees of motor or sensory loss below the level of the lesion depending on which neurologic tracts are damaged and which are spared.

**3.** Diagnostic test: spinal X-rays may reveal fracture.

**D.** Nursing interventions: emergency care

  **1.** Assess airway, breathing, circulation

    **a.** Do not move the client during assessment.

    **b.** If airway obstruction or inadequate ventilation exists: do not hyperextend neck to open airway, use jaw thrust instead.

  **2.** Perform a quick head-to-toe assessment: check for LOC, signs of trauma to the head or neck, leakage of clear fluid from ears or nose, signs of motor or sensory impairment.

  **3.** Immobilize the client in the position found until help arrives.

  **4.** Once emergency help arrives, assist in immobilizing the head and neck with a cervical collar and place the client on a spinal board; avoid any movement during transfer, especially flexion of the spinal column.

  **5.** Have suction available to clear the airway and prevent aspiration if the client vomits; client may be turned slightly to the side if secured to a board.

  **6.** Evaluate respiration and observe for weak or labored respirations.

**E.** Nursing interventions: acute care

  **1.** Maintain optimum respiratory function.

    **a.** Observe for weak or labored respirations; monitor arterial blood gases.

    **b.** Prevent pneumonia and atelectasis: turn every 2 hours; cough and deep breathe every hour; use incentive spirometry every 2 hours.

    **c.** Tracheostomy and mechanical ventilation may be necessary if respiratory insufficiency occurs.

  **2.** Maintain optimal cardiovascular function.

    **a.** Monitor vital signs; observe for bradycardia, arrhythmias, hypotension.

    **b.** Apply thigh-high elastic stockings or Ace bandages.

    **c.** Change position slowly and gradually elevate the head of the bed to prevent postural hypotension.

    **d.** Observe for signs of deep-vein thrombosis.

**3.** Maintain fluid and electrolyte balance and nutrition.

  **a.** Nasogastric tube may be inserted until bowel sounds return.

  **b.** Maintain IV therapy as ordered; avoid overhydration (can aggravate cord edema).

  **c.** Check bowel sounds before feeding client (paralytic ileus is common).

  **d.** Progress slowly from clear liquid to regular diet.

  **e.** Provide diet high in protein, carbohydrates, calories.

**4.** Maintain immobilization and spinal alignment always.

  **a.** Turn every hour on turning frame.

  **b.** Maintain cervical traction at all times if indicated.

**5.** Prevent complications of immobility; use footboard/high-topped sneakers to prevent footdrop; provide splint for quadriplegic client to prevent wrist drop.

**6.** Maintain urinary elimination.

  **a.** Provide intermittent catheterization or maintain indwelling catheter as ordered.

  **b.** Increase fluids to 3000 mL/day.

  **c.** Provide acid-ash foods/fluids to acidify urine and prevent infection.

**7.** Maintain bowel elimination: administer stool softeners and suppositories to prevent impaction as ordered.

**8.** Monitor temperature control.

  **a.** Check temperature every 4 hours.

  **b.** Regulate environment closely.

  **c.** Avoid excessive covering or exposure.

**9.** Observe for and prevent infection.

  **a.** Observe tongs or pin site for redness, drainage.

  **b.** Provide tong- or pin-site care. Cleanse with antiseptic solution according to agency policy.

  **c.** Observe for signs of respiratory or urinary infection.

**10.** Observe for and prevent stress ulcers.

  **a.** Assess for epigastic or shoulder pain.

  **b.** If corticosteroids are ordered, give with food or antacids; administer $H_2$ blocker as ordered.

  **c.** Check nasogastric tube contents and stools for blood.

**F.** Nursing interventions: chronic care

  **1.** Neurogenic bladder

    **a.** Reflex or upper motor neuron bladder; reflex activity of the bladder may occur after spinal shock resolves; the bladder is unable to store urine very long and empties involuntarily

b. Nonreflexive or lower motor neuron bladder: reflex arc is disrupted and no reflex activity of the bladder occurs, resulting in urine retention with overflow

c. Management of reflex bladder
   1) Intermittent catheterization every 4 hours and gradually progress to every 6 hours.
   2) Regulate fluid intake to 1800–2000 mL/day.
   3) Bladder taps or stimulating trigger points to cause reflex emptying of the bladder.

d. Management of nonreflexive bladder
   1) Intermittent catheterization every 6 hours.
   2) Credé maneuver or rectal stretch.
   3) Regulate intake to 1800–2000 mL/day to prevent overdistention of bladder.

e. Management depends on lifestyle, age, sex, home care, and availability of caregiver.

2. Spasticity
   a. Return of reflex activity may occur after spinal shock resolves; severe spasticity may be detrimental
   b. Drug therapy: baclofen (Lioresal), dantrolene (Dantrium), diazepam (Valium)
   c. Physical therapy: stretching exercises, warm tub baths, whirlpool
   d. Surgery: chordotomy

3. Autonomic dysreflexia
   a. Rise in blood pressure, sometimes to fatal levels
   b. Occurs in clients with cord lesions above $T_6$ and most commonly in clients with cervical injuries
   c. Reflex response to stimulation of the sympathetic nervous system
   d. Stimulus may be overdistended bladder or bowel, decubitus ulcer, chilling, pressure from bedclothes
   e. Symptoms: severe headache, hypertension, bradycardia, sweating, goose bumps, nasal congestion, blurred vision, convulsions
   f. Interventions
      1) Raise client to sitting position to decrease BP.
      2) Check for source of stimulus (bladder, bowel, skin).
      3) Remove offending stimulus (e.g., catheterize client, digitally remove impacted feces, reposition client).
      4) Monitor blood pressure.
      5) Administer antihypertensives (e.g., hydralazine HCl [Apresoline]) as ordered.

G. Nursing interventions: general rehabilitative care
   1. Provide psychologic support to client/significant others.
      a. Support during grieving process.
      b. Assist client to adjust to effects of injury.
      c. Encourage independence.
      d. Involve the client in decision making.
   2. Provide sexual counseling.
      a. Work with the client and partner.
      b. Explore alternative methods of sexual gratification.
   3. Initiate rehabilitation program.
      a. Physical therapy
      b. Vocational rehabilitation
      c. Psychologic counseling
      d. Use of braces, electronic wheelchair, and other assistance devices to maximize independence

## Specific Disorders of the Peripheral Nervous System

### Trigeminal Neuralgia (Tic Douloureux)

A. General information
   1. Disorder of cranial nerve V causing disabling and recurring attacks of severe pain along the sensory distribution of one or more branches of the trigeminal nerve
   2. Incidence increased in elderly women
   3. Cause unknown

B. Medical management
   1. Anticonvulsant drugs: carbamazepine (Tegretol), phenytoin (Dilantin)
   2. Nerve block: injection of alcohol or phenol into one or more branches of the trigeminal nerve; temporary effect, lasts 6–18 months
   3. Surgery
      a. Peripheral: avulsion of peripheral branches of trigeminal nerve
      b. Intracranial
         1) Retrogasserian rhizotomy: total severance of the sensory root of the trigeminal nerve intracranially; results in permanent anesthesia, numbness, heaviness, and stiffness in affected part; loss of corneal reflex
         2) Microsurgery: uses more precise cutting and may preserve facial sensation and corneal reflex
         3) Percutaneous radio-frequency trigeminal gangliolysis: current surgical procedure of choice; thermally destroys the trigeminal nerve in the area of the ganglion; provides permanent pain relief with preservation of sense of touch, proprioception, and corneal reflex; done under local anesthesia
         4) Microvascular decompression of trigeminal nerve: decompresses the trigeminal nerve; craniotomy

necessary; provides permanent pain relief while preserving facial sensation

C. Assessment findings
   1. Sudden paroxysms of extremely severe shooting pain in one side of the face
   2. Attacks may be triggered by a cold breeze, foods/fluids of extreme temperature, toothbrushing, chewing, talking, or touching the face
   3. During attack: twitching, grimacing, and frequent blinking/tearing of the eye
   4. Poor eating and hygiene habits
   5. Withdrawal from interactions with others
   6. Diagnostic tests: X-rays of the skull, teeth, and sinuses may identify dental or sinus infection as an aggravating factor.

D. Nursing interventions
   1. Assess characteristics of the pain including triggering factors, trigger points, and pain management techniques.
   2. Administer medications as ordered; monitor response.
   3. Maintain room at an even, moderate temperature, free from drafts.
   4. Provide small, frequent feedings of lukewarm, semiliquid, or soft foods that are easily chewed.
   5. Provide the client with a soft washcloth and lukewarm water and perform hygiene during periods when pain is decreased.
   6. Prepare the client for surgery if indicated.
   7. Provide client teaching and discharge planning concerning
      a. Need to avoid outdoor activities during cold, windy, or rainy weather
      b. Importance of good nutrition and hygiene
      c. Use of medications, side effects, and signs of toxicity
      d. Specific instructions following surgery for residual effects of anesthesia and loss of corneal reflex
         1) Protective eye care
         2) Chew on unaffected side only
         3) Avoid hot fluids/foods
         4) Mouth care after meals to remove particles
         5) Good oral hygiene; visit dentist every 6 months
         6) Protect the face during extremes of temperature

## Bell's Palsy

A. General information
   1. Disorder of cranial nerve VII resulting in the loss of ability to move the muscles on one side of the face
   2. Cause unknown; may be viral or autoimmune
   3. Complete recovery in 3–5 weeks in majority of clients

B. Assessment findings
   1. Loss of taste over anterior two-thirds of tongue on affected side
   2. Complete paralysis of one side of face
   3. Loss of expression, displacement of mouth toward unaffected side, and inability to close eyelid (all on affected side)
   4. Pain behind the ear

C. Nursing interventions
   1. Assess facial nerve function regularly (see Table 4-16).
   2. Administer medications as ordered.
      a. Corticosteroids: to decrease edema and pain
      b. Mild analgesics as necessary
   3. Provide soft diet with supplementary feedings as indicated.
   4. Instruct to chew on unaffected side, avoid hot fluids/foods, and perform mouth care after each meal.
   5. Provide special eye care to protect the cornea.
      a. Dark glasses (cosmetic and protective reasons) or eyeshield
      b. Artificial tears to prevent drying of the cornea
      c. Ointment and eye patch at night to keep eyelid closed
   6. Provide support and reassurance.

## Guillain-Barré Syndrome

A. General information
   1. Symmetrical, bilateral, peripheral polyneuritis characterized by ascending paralysis
   2. Can occur at any age; affects women and men equally
   3. Cause unknown; may be an autoimmune process
   4. Precipitating factors: antecedent viral infection, immunization
   5. Progression of disease is highly individual; 90% of clients stop progression in 4 weeks; recovery is usually from 3–6 months; may have residual deficits

B. Medical management
   1. Mechanical ventilation if respiratory problems present
   2. Plasmapheresis to reduce circulating antibodies
   3. Continuous ECG monitoring to detect alteration in heart rate and rhythm
   4. Propranolol to prevent tachycardia
   5. Atropine may be given to prevent episodes of bradycardia during endotracheal suctioning and physical therapy

C. Assessment findings
   1. Mild sensory changes; in some clients severe misinterpretation of sensory stimuli resulting in extreme discomfort
   2. Clumsiness: usually first symptom

3. Progressive motor weakness in more than one limb (classically is ascending and symmetrical)
4. Cranial nerve involvement (dysphagia)
5. Ventilatory insufficiency if paralysis ascends to respiratory muscles
6. Absence of deep tendon reflexes
7. Autonomic dysfunction
8. Diagnostic tests
    a. CSF studies: increased protein
    b. EMG: slowed nerve conduction
D. Nursing interventions
1. Maintain adequate ventilation.
    a. Monitor rate and depth of respirations; serial vital capacities.
    b. Observe for ventilatory insufficiency.
    c. Maintain mechanical ventilation as needed; keep airway free of secretions and prevent pneumonia.
2. Check individual muscle groups every 2 hours in acute phase to check for progression of muscle weakness.
3. Assess cranial nerve function: check gag reflex and swallowing ability; ability to handle secretions; voice.
4. Monitor vital signs and observe for signs of autonomic dysfunction such as acute periods of hypertension fluctuating with hypotension, tachycardia, arrhythmias.
5. Administer corticosteroids to suppress immune reaction as ordered.
6. Administer antiarrhythmic agents as ordered.
7. Prevent complications of immobility.
8. Promote comfort (especially in clients with sensory changes): foot cradle, sheepskin, guided imagery, relaxation techniques.
9. Promote optimum nutrition.
    a. Check gag reflex before feeding.
    b. Start with pureed foods.
    c. Assess need for nasogastric tube feedings if unable to swallow.
10. Provide psychologic support and encouragement to client/significant others.
11. Refer for rehabilitation to regain strength and to treat any residual deficits.

### Amyotrophic Lateral Sclerosis (Lou Gehrig's Disease)

A. General information
1. Progressive motor neuron disease, which usually leads to death in 2–6 years
2. Onset usually between ages 40 and 70; affects men more than women
3. Cause unknown
4. There is no cure or specific treatment; death usually occurs as a result of respiratory infection secondary to respiratory insufficiency
B. Assessment findings
1. Progressive weakness and atrophy of the muscles of the arms, trunk, or legs

2. Dysarthria, dysphagia
3. Fasciculations
4. Respiratory insufficiency
5. Diagnostic tests: EMG and muscle biopsy can rule out other diseases
C. Nursing interventions
1. Provide nursing measures for muscle weakness and dysphagia.
2. Promote adequate ventilatory function.
3. Prevent complications of immobility.
4. Encourage diversional activities; spend time with the client.
5. Provide compassion and intensive support to client/significant others.
6. Provide or refer for physical therapy as indicated.
7. Promote independence for as long as possible.

## DISORDERS OF THE EYE

### Cataracts

A. General information
1. Opacity of the ocular lens
2. Incidence increases with age
3. May be caused by changes associated with aging ("senile" cataract); may be congenital; or may develop secondary to trauma, radiation, infection, certain drugs (corticosteroids)
B. Assessment findings
1. Blurred vision
2. Progressive decrease in vision
3. Glare in bright lights
4. Pupil may develop milky-white appearance
5. Diagnostic test: ophthalmoscopic exam confirms presence of cataract
C. Nursing interventions: prepare client for cataract surgery.

### Cataract Surgery

A. General information
1. Performed when client can no longer remain independent because of reduced vision
2. Surgery performed on one eye at a time; usually in a same-day surgery unit
3. Local anesthesia and intravenous sedation usually used
4. Types
    a. Extracapsular extraction: lens capsule is excised and the lens is expressed; posterior capsule is left in place (may be used to support new artificial lens implant).
    b. Phacoemulsification: a type of extracapsular extraction; a hollow needle capable of ultrasonic vibration is inserted into lens, vibrations emulsify the lens, which is then aspirated.
    c. Intracapsular extraction: lens is totally removed within its capsule, may be

delivered from eye by cryoextraction (lens is frozen with a metal probe and removed).

    **5.** Peripheral iridectomy may be performed at the time of surgery; small hole cut in iris to prevent development of secondary glaucoma

    **6.** Intraocular lens implant often performed at the time of surgery.

**B.** Nursing interventions: preoperative (see also Perioperative Nursing)

    **1.** Assess vision in the unaffected eye since the affected eye will be patched post-op.

    **2.** Provide pre-op teaching regarding measures to prevent increased intraocular pressure post-op.

    **3.** Administer medications as ordered.

        **a.** Topical mydriatics and cycloplegics to dilate the pupil

        **b.** Topical antibiotics to prevent infection

        **c.** Acetazolamide (Diamox) and osmotic agents (oral glycerin or IV mannitol) to decrease intraocular pressure to provide a soft eyeball for surgery

**C.** Nursing interventions: postoperative

    **1.** Reorient the client to surroundings.

    **2.** Provide safety measures: elevate side rails, provide call bell, assist with ambulation when fully recovered from anesthesia.

    **3.** Prevent increased intraocular pressure and stress on the suture line.

        **a.** Elevate head of bed 30–40°.

        **b.** Have client lie on back or unaffected side.

        **c.** Avoid having client cough, sneeze, bend over, or move head too rapidly.

        **d.** Treat nausea with antiemetics as ordered to prevent vomiting.

        **e.** Give stool softeners as ordered to prevent straining.

        **f.** Observe for and report signs of increased intraocular pressure: severe eye pain, restlessness, increased pulse.

    **4.** Protect eye from injury.

        **a.** Dressings are usually removed the day after surgery.

        **b.** Eyeglasses or eye shield used during the day.

        **c.** Always use eye shield during the night.

    **5.** Administer medications as ordered.

        **a.** Topical mydriatics and cycloplegics to decrease spasm of ciliary body and relieve pain

        **b.** Topical antibiotics and corticosteroids

        **c.** Mild analgesics as needed

    **6.** Provide client teaching and discharge planning concerning

        **a.** Technique of eyedrop administration

        **b.** Use of eye shield at night

        **c.** No bending, stooping, or lifting

        **d.** Report signs or symptoms of complications immediately to physician: severe eye pain, decreased vision, excessive drainage, swelling of eyelid.

        **e.** Cataract glasses/contact lenses

            **1)** If a lens implant has not been performed, the client will need glasses or contact lenses.

            **2)** Temporary glasses are worn for 1–4 weeks, then permanent glasses fitted.

            **3)** Cataract glasses magnify objects by ⅓ and distort peripheral vision; have client practice manual coordination with assistance until new spatial relationships become familiar; have client practice walking, using stairs, reaching for articles.

            **4)** Contact lenses cause less distortion of vision; prescribed at 1 month.

## Glaucoma

**A.** General information

    **1.** Characterized by increased intraocular pressure resulting in progressive loss of vision; may cause blindness if not recognized and treated

    **2.** Risk factors: age over 40, diabetes, hypertension, heredity; history of previous eye surgery, trauma, or inflammation

    **3.** Types

        **a.** Chronic (open-angle) glaucoma: most common form, due to obstruction of the outflow of aqueous humor, in trabecular meshwork or canal of Schlemm

        **b.** Acute (closed-angle) glaucoma: due to forward displacement of the iris against the cornea, obstructing the outflow of the aqueous humor; occurs suddenly and is an emergency situation; if untreated, blindness will result

        **c.** Chronic (closed-angle) glaucoma: similar to acute (closed-angle) glaucoma, with the potential for an acute attack

    **4.** Early detection is very important; regular eye exams including tonometry for persons over age 40 is recommended.

**B.** Medical management

    **1.** Chronic (open-angle) glaucoma

        **a.** Drug therapy: one or a combination of the following

            **1)** Miotic eyedrops (pilocarpine) to increase outflow of aqueous humor

            **2)** Epinephrine eyedrops to decrease aqueous humor production and increase outflow

            **3)** Acetazolamide (Diamox): carbonic anhydrase inhibitor to decrease aqueous humor production

            **4)** Timolol maleate (Timoptic): topical beta-adrenergic blocker to decrease intraocular pressure

        **b.** Surgery (if no improvement with drugs)

1) Filtering procedure (trabeculectomy, trephining) to create artificial openings for the outflow of aqueous humor
2) Laser trabeculoplasty: noninvasive procedure performed with argon laser that can be done on an outclient basis; produces similar results as trabeculectomy

2. Acute (closed-angle) glaucoma
   a. Drug therapy (before surgery)
      1) Miotic eyedrops (e.g., pilocarpine) to cause pupil to contract and draw iris away from cornea
      2) Osmotic agents (e.g., glycerin [oral], mannitol [IV]) to decrease intraocular pressure
      3) Narcotic analgesics for pain
   b. Surgery
      1) Peripheral iridectomy: portion of the iris is excised to facilitate outflow of aqueous humor
      2) Argon laser beam surgery: noninvasive procedure using laser that produces same effect as iridectomy; done on an outclient basis
      3) Iridectomy usually performed on second eye later because a large number of clients have an acute attack in the other eye

3. Chronic (closed-angle) glaucoma
   a. Drug therapy: miotics (pilocarpine)
   b. Surgery: bilateral peripheral iridectomy to prevent acute attacks

C. Assessment findings
   1. Chronic (open-angle) glaucoma: symptoms develop slowly; impaired peripheral vision (tunnel vision); loss of central vision if unarrested; mild discomfort in the eyes; halos around lights
   2. Acute (closed-angle) glaucoma: severe eye pain; blurred, cloudy vision; halos around lights; nausea and vomiting; steamy cornea; moderate pupillary dilation
   3. Chronic (closed-angle) glaucoma: transient blurred vision; slight eye pain; halos around lights
   4. Diagnostic tests
      a. Visual acuity: reduced
      b. Tonometry: reading of 24–32 mm Hg suggests glaucoma; may be 50 mm Hg or more in acute (closed-angle) glaucoma
      c. Ophthalmoscopic exam: reveals narrowing of small vessels of optic disk, cupping of optic disk
      d. Perimetry: reveals defects in visual fields
      e. Gonioscopy: examine angle of anterior chamber

D. Nursing interventions
   1. Administer medications as ordered.
   2. Provide quiet, dark environment.

3. Maintain accurate I&O with the use of osmotic agents.
4. Prepare the client for surgery if indicated.
5. Provide post-op care (see Cataract Surgery).
6. Provide client teaching and discharge planning concerning
   a. Self-administration of eyedrops
   b. Need to avoid stooping, heavy lifting, or pushing, emotional upsets, excessive fluid intake, constrictive clothing around the neck
   c. Need to avoid the use of antihistamines or sympathomimetic drugs (found in cold preparations) in closed-angle glaucoma because they may cause mydriasis
   d. Importance of follow-up care
   e. Need to wear Medic-Alert tag

## Detached Retina

A. General information
   1. Detachment of the sensory retina from the pigment epithelium of the retina
   2. Caused by trauma, aging process, severe myopia, postcataract extraction, severe diabetic retinopathy
   3. Pathophysiology: tear in the retina allows vitreous humor to seep behind the sensory retina and separate it from the pigment epithelium

B. Medical management
   1. Bed rest with eyes patched and detached areas dependent to prevent further detachment
   2. Surgery: necessary to repair detachment
      a. Photocoagulation: light beam (argon laser) through dilated pupil creates an inflammatory reaction and scarring to heal the area
      b. Cryosurgery or diathermy: application of extreme cold or heat to the external globe; inflammatory reaction causes scarring and healing of area
      c. Scleral buckling: shortening of sclera to force pigment epithelium close to retina

C. Assessment findings
   1. Flashes of light, floaters
   2. Visual field loss, veil-like curtain coming across field of vision
   3. Diagnostic test: ophthalmoscopic examination confirms diagnosis

D. Nursing interventions: preoperative
   1. Maintain bed rest as ordered with head of bed flat and detached area in a dependent position.
   2. Use bilateral eye patches as ordered; elevate side rails to prevent injury.
   3. Identify yourself when entering the room.
   4. Orient the client frequently to time, date, and surroundings; explain procedures.
   5. Provide diversional activities to provide sensory stimulation.

E. Nursing interventions: postoperative (see also Cataract Surgery)
  1. Check orders for positioning and activity level.
     a. May be on bed rest for 1–2 days.
     b. May need to position client so that detached area is in dependent position.
  2. Administer medications as ordered: topical mydriatics, analgesics as needed.
  3. Provide client teaching and discharge planning concerning
     a. Technique of eyedrop administration
     b. Use of eye shield at night
     c. No bending from waist; no heavy work or lifting for 6 weeks
     d. Restriction of reading for 3 weeks or more
     e. May watch television
     f. Need to check with physician regarding combing and shampooing hair and shaving
     g. Need to report complications such as recurrence of detachment

## Eye Injuries/Emergency Care

A. Removal of loose foreign body from conjunctiva
  1. Foreign bodies, e.g., sand, dust, may cause pain and lacrimation.
  2. Instruct client to look upward.
  3. Evert lower lid to expose the conjunctival sac.
  4. Gently remove the particle with a cotton applicator dipped in sterile normal saline using a twisting motion.
  5. If particle is not found, examine the upper lid.
  6. Place cotton applicator stick or tongue blade horizontally on outer surface of upper lid; grasp under eyelashes with fingers of other hand and pull the upper lid outward and upward over the applicator stick.
  7. Gently remove the particle as previously described.
B. Penetrating injuries to the eye
  1. Examples: darts, scissors, flying metal.
  2. Do not attempt to remove object.
  3. Do not allow client to apply pressure to the eye.
  4. Cover eye lightly with sterile eye patch for embedded objects, e.g., metal; apply protective shield, e.g., paper cup, for impaled objects such as darts.
  5. Cover uninjured eye to prevent excessive movement of injured eye.
  6. Refer the client to an emergency room immediately.
C. Chemical burns
  1. Flush eye immediately with copious amounts of water for 15–20 minutes.
     a. Have client hold head under faucet to let water run over eye to thoroughly wash it out; may need to forcibly separate eyelids during flush
     b. If available, flush eye with syringe
  2. After flushing, refer client to an emergency room immediately.

# DISORDERS OF THE EAR

## Otosclerosis

A. General information
  1. Formation of new spongy bone in the labyrinth of the ear causing fixation of the stapes in the oval window; this prevents transmission of auditory vibration to the inner ear
  2. Found more often in females
  3. Cause unknown, but there is a familial tendency
B. Medical management: stapedectomy is the procedure of choice.
C. Assessment findings
  1. Progressive loss of hearing
  2. Tinnitus
  3. Diagnostic tests
     a. Audiometry: reveals conductive hearing loss
     b. Weber's and Rinne's tests: show bone conduction is greater than air conduction
D. Nursing interventions: see Stapedectomy.

## Stapedectomy

A. General information
  1. Removal of diseased portion of stapes and replacement with a prosthesis to conduct vibrations from the middle ear to inner ear; usually performed under local anesthesia
  2. Used to treat otosclerosis
B. Nursing interventions: preoperative
  1. Provide general pre-op nursing care, including an explanation of post-op expectations.
  2. Explain to the client that hearing may improve during surgery and then decrease due to edema and packing.
C. Nursing interventions: postoperative
  1. Position the client according to the surgeon's orders (possibly with operative ear uppermost to prevent displacement of the graft).
  2. Have client deep breathe every 2 hours while in bed, but no coughing.
  3. Elevate side rails; assist the client with ambulation and move slowly (may have some vertigo).
  4. Administer medications as ordered: analgesics, antibiotics, antiemetics, anti-motion-sickness drugs.
  5. Check dressings frequently for excessive drainage or bleeding.
  6. Assess facial nerve function, i.e., ask client to wrinkle forehead, close eyelids, puff out cheeks, smile and show teeth; check for any asymmetry.
  7. Question client about pain, headache, vertigo, and unusual sensations in the ear; report existence to physician.

8. Provide client teaching and discharge planning concerning
   a. Warnings against blowing nose or coughing; sneeze with the mouth open
   b. Need to keep ear dry in the shower; no shampooing until allowed
   c. No flying for 6 months, especially if an upper respiratory tract infection is present
   d. Placement of cotton ball in auditory meatus after packing is removed; change twice a day

## Ménière's Disease

A. General information
   1. Disease of the inner ear resulting from dilation of the endolymphatic system and increased volume of endolymph; characterized by recurrent and usually progressive triad of symptoms: vertigo, tinnitus, and hearing loss
   2. Incidence highest between ages 30 and 60
   3. Cause unknown; theories include allergy, toxicity, localized ischemia, hemorrhage, viral infection, or edema
B. Medical management
   1. Acute: atropine (decreases autonomic nervous system activity), diazepam (Valium), fentanyl, and droperidol (Innovar)
   2. Chronic
      a. Drug therapy: vasodilators (nicotinic acid), diuretics, mild sedatives or tranquilizers (diazepam [Valium]), antihistamines (diphenhydramine [Benadryl], meclizine [Antivert])
      b. Low-sodium diet, restricted fluid intake, restrict caffeine and nicotine.
   3. Surgery
      a. Surgical destruction of labyrinth causing loss of vestibular and cochlear function (if disease is unilateral)
      b. Intracranial division of vestibular portion of cranial nerve VIII
      c. Endolymphatic sac decompression or shunt to equalize pressure in endolymphatic space
C. Assessment findings
   1. Sudden attacks of vertigo lasting hours or days; attacks occur several times a year
   2. Nausea, tinnitus, progressive hearing loss
   3. Vomiting, nystagmus
   4. Diagnostic tests
      a. Audiometry: reveals sensorineural hearing loss
      b. Vestibular tests: reveal decreased function
D. Nursing interventions
   1. Maintain bed rest in a quiet, darkened room in position of choice; elevate side rails as needed.
   2. Only move the client for essential care (bath may not be essential).
   3. Provide an emesis basin for vomiting.

4. Monitor IV therapy; maintain accurate I&O.
5. Assist with ambulation when the attack is over.
6. Administer medications as ordered.
7. Prepare the client for surgery as indicated (post-op care includes using above measures).
8. Provide client teaching and discharge planning concerning
   a. Use of medication and side effects
   b. Low-sodium diet and decreased fluid intake
   c. Importance of eliminating smoking

## Sample Questions

108. An adult has a medical diagnosis of increased intracranial pressure and is being cared for on the neurology unit. The nursing care plan includes elevating the head of the bed and positioning the client's head in proper alignment. What is the reason for these actions?
    1. Makes it easier for the client to breathe.
    2. Prevents a Valsalva maneuver.
    3. Promotes venous drainage.
    4. Reduces pain.

109. A client begins to have Cheyne-Stokes respirations. What is the correct explanation for this occurrence?
    1. Completely irregular breathing pattern with random deep and shallow respirations.
    2. Prolonged inspirations with inspiratory and/or expiratory pauses.
    3. Rhythmic waxing and waning of both rate and depth of respiration with brief periods of interspersed apnea.
    4. Sustained, regular, rapid respirations of increased depth.

110. Which of the following reduces cerebral edema by constricting cerebral veins?
    1. Dexamethasone (Decadron).
    2. Mechanical hyperventilation.
    3. Mannitol (Osmitrol).
    4. Ventriculostomy.

111. The nurse is caring for an adult client who was admitted unconscious. The initial assessment utilized the Glasgow Coma Scale. The nurse knows that of the following, which are included when assessing a client using the Glasgow Coma Scale? Select all that apply.
    ____ Eye opening.
    ____ Motor response.
    ____ Pupillary reaction
    ____ Verbal performance.

112. Utilizing the Glasgow Coma Scale, which score would be indicative of coma?
    1. 0
    2. 2
    3. 6
    4. 10

113. When the nurse tested an unconscious client for noxious stimuli, the client responded with decorticate rigidity or posturing. What is the best description for this action?
    1. Flexion of the upper and lower extremities into a fetal-like position.
    2. Rigid extension of the upper and lower extremities and plantar flexion.
    3. Complete flaccidity of both upper and lower extremities and hyperextension of the neck.
    4. Flexion of the upper extremities, extension of the lower extremities, and plantar flexion.

114. An adult male is receiving cryotherapy for repair of a detached retina. When taking a history from him, which symptom should the nurse expect him to have?
    1. Diplopia.
    2. Severe eye pain.
    3. Sudden blindness.
    4. Bright flashes of light.

115. An adult who has a detached retina asks the nurse what may have contributed to the development of his detached retina. What is a risk factor associated with this condition?
    1. Hypertension.
    2. Nearsightedness.
    3. Cranial tumors.
    4. Sinusitis.

116. The nurse is explaining cryotherapy to a client who has a detached retina. What would be a major purpose for the procedure?
    1. Create a scar that promotes healing.
    2. Disintegrate debris in the eye.
    3. Freeze small blood vessels.
    4. Halt secretions of the lacrimal duct.

117. An adult client has a stapedectomy. Which of the following is most important for the nurse to include in the post-op care plan?
    1. Checking the gag reflex.
    2. Encouraging independence.
    3. Instructing the client not to blow the nose.
    4. Positioning the client on the operative side.

118. The nurse is assessing reflexes on a client. Which of the following correctly describes this reflex?
    1. Extension of the elbow and contraction of the triceps tendon.
    2. Supination and flexion of the forearm.
    3. Dorsiflexion of the great toe with fanning of the other toes.
    4. Flexion of the arm at the antecubital fossa and contraction of the biceps.

119. The nurse is assessing the optic nerve of a client. Which of the following is a correct method to evaluate cranial nerve (CN) II, the optic nerve?
    1. Inspect the pupils for reaction.
    2. Test extraocular movements.
    3. Use of a Snellen chart.
    4. Test for a corneal reflex.

120. Which of the following tests or tools could the nurse use to assess CN VIII, the acoustic nerve?
    1. Romberg.
    2. Rosenbaum chart.
    3. Inspection of pupils.
    4. Audiometry.

121. A nurse is obtaining a Glasgow Coma Score on a client. The score is as follows:
    Best eye opening 3
    Best motor response 6
    Best verbal response 4
    How would the nurse interpret this score?
    1. Opens eyes to speech, obeys verbal commands, and is confused.
    2. Opens eyes to pain, decorticates to pain, and does not speak.
    3. Opens eyes to pain, no motor response, and has inappropriate speech.
    4. Opens eyes spontaneously, obeys verbal commands, and is oriented × 3.

122. A nurse is preparing a client for an MRI. Which factor would exclude the client from the test?
    1. Wearing jewelry.
    2. Cardiac pacemaker.
    3. Claustrophobia.
    4. Allergy to iodine.

123. A nurse is assessing a client who has returned from a cerebral arteriogram. The left carotid was the site punctured. Which of the following indicates complications?
    1. Difficulty in swallowing.
    2. Puncture site is dry and red.

3. BP 120/82, HR 86, RR 22.

4. No swelling or hematoma at the site.

124. A client with a closed head injury is confused, drowsy, and has unequal pupils. Which of the following nursing diagnosis is *most important* at this time?

1. Altered level of cognitive function.
2. High risk for injury.
3. Altered cerebral tissue perfusion.
4. Sensory perceptual alteration.

125. A client is admitted with a head injury. To monitor hypothalamic function, the nurse should monitor what parameters?

1. Temperature and urinary output.
2. Gastric aspirate and BP.
3. Heart rate and pupillary responses.
4. Respiratory rate and skin integrity.

126. Which of the following is the best way for the nurse to assist a blind client in ambulation?

1. Allow client to take nurse's arm with the nurse walking slightly ahead of the client.
2. Allow client to walk beside the nurse with the nurse's hand on the client's back.
3. Allow client to walk down the hall with his or her hand along the wall.
4. Push the client in a wheelchair.

127. Which of the following is the best way for the nurse to communicate with the hearing impaired client?

1. Talk directly into the impaired ear.
2. Speak directly and clearly facing the person.
3. Shout into the good ear.
4. Write out all communication.

128. A nurse is assessing a client who is unable to extend the legs without pain, has a temperature of 103°F, and on flexion of the neck also flexes the hip and knee. Based on this assessment, What condition does the nurse suspect?

1. Meningitis.
2. Brain abscess.
3. Brain tumor.
4. Epilepsy.

129. A client has a fever of 103°F, nuchal rigidity, pain on extension of the legs, and opisthotonos. What would be the priority nursing diagnosis?

1. Acute pain.
2. Ineffective tissue perfusion
3. Anxiety.
4. Risk for injury.

130. A client presents with symptoms of increased intracranial pressure, papilledema, and headache. No history of trauma is found. Vital signs are: BP 110/60, HR 80, T 98.9°F, RR 24. What condition does the nurse suspect?

1. Brain tumor.
2. Meningitis.
3. Skull fracture.
4. Encephalitis.

131. What should the nurse include in the plan of care for a newly admitted client with an infratentorial craniotomy for a brain tumor?

1. Keep the head of the bed elevated 30–45°; and a large pillow under the client's head and shoulder.
2. Keep the head of the bed flat with a small pillow under the nape of the neck.
3. Assess vital signs and pupils every four hours.
4. Flex neck every 2 hours to prevent stiffness.

132. The home health nurse observes an aide who is transferring a client with hemiplegia from a sitting position in the bed to the wheelchair. Which action by the aide requires correction?

1. Grasping the client's arms to pull the client to a standing position.
2. Reminding the client to lean forward before rising.
3. Moving the client toward the unaffected side.
4. Bracing the affected knee and foot to assist the client to stand.

133. When comparing a cerebrovascular accident (CVA) to a transient ischemic attack (TIA), what is unique about the TIA?

1. It has permanent long-term focal deficits.
2. It is intermittent with spontaneous resolution of the neurologic deficit.
3. It is intermittent with permanent motor and sensory deficits.
4. It has permanent long-term neurologic deficits.

134. The nurse is teaching a client with transient ischemic attacks about aspirin therapy. Which statement by the client indicates understanding of the reason for his aspirin therapy?

1. "I must take the aspirin regularly to prevent the headache that many people have with this disorder."
2. "If I take aspirin, I am less likely to develop bleeding in my brain."
3. "The aspirin will help to prevent me from having a stroke."
4. "Taking aspirin regularly will reduce my chances of having a heart attack."

135. A client with Parkinson's disease is receiving combination therapy with levodopa (L-dopa) and carbidopa (Sinemet). Which of the following manifestations indicates to the nurse that an adverse drug reaction is occurring?
   1. Involuntary head movement.
   2. Bradykinesia.
   3. Shuffling gait.
   4. Depression.

136. A nurse is teaching the family of a client with Parkinson's disease. Which of the following statements by the family reflects a need for more education?
   1. "We can buy lots of soups for Dad."
   2. "We are teaching Dad posture exercises."
   3. "Dad is going to do his range of motion (ROM) exercises three times a day."
   4. "The bath bars will be installed before Dad comes home."

137. A 36-year-old female reports double vision, visual loss, muscular weakness, numbness of the hands, fatigue, tremors, and incontinence. Based on this report, what does the nurse suspect?
   1. Parkinson's disease.
   2. Myasthenia gravis (MG).
   3. Amyotrophic lateral sclerosis (ALS).
   4. Multiple sclerosis (MS).

138. Which nursing diagnosis is of the *highest priority* when caring for a client with myasthenia gravis (MG)?
   1. Pain.
   2. Risk for injury.
   3. Ineffective coping.
   4. Ineffective airway clearance.

139. The nurse has explained the use of neostigmine methylsulfate (Prostigmin) to a client with myasthenia gravis. Which comment by the client indicates the need for further instruction?
   1. "I need to take the medication regularly, even when I feel strong."
   2. "I should take the medication once daily at bedtime."
   3. "If I take too much medication, I can become weak and have breathing problems."
   4. "I may have difficulty swallowing my saliva if I take too much medication."

140. A nurse is assessing a client with a head injury. The client has clear drainage from the nose and ears. How can the nurse determine if the drainage is cerebrospinal fluid (CSF)?
   1. Measure the pH of the fluid.
   2. Measure the specific gravity of the fluid.
   3. Test for glucose.
   4. Test for chloride.

141. The nurse is caring for a confused client who sustained a head injury resulting in a subdural hematoma. The client's blood pressure is 100/60 mm Hg and he is unresponsive. Select the most effective position for the client as the nurse transports him to the operating room.
   1. Semi-Fowler's.
   2. Trendelenburg.
   3. High-Fowler's.
   4. Supine.

142. A client who has been treated in the emergency room for a head injury is preparing for discharge. The nurse is teaching the family about the signs of complications that may occur within the first 24 hours and the appropriate action to take if a complication is suspected. Which statement by the client's spouse would require further teaching by the nurse?
   1. "I'm not looking forward to checking on my husband all night long."
   2. "If he can just get a long nap, I'm sure that my husband will be fine."
   3. "I'll call the doctor immediately if my husband starts to vomit."
   4. "If my husband has trouble talking, I'll bring him to the hospital."

143. A client is admitted postcraniotomy. Decadron 4 mg IV is ordered every 6 hours. What is the purpose for this medication?
   1. Stabilize the blood sugar.
   2. Decrease cerebral edema.
   3. Prevent seizures.
   4. Maintain the integrity of the gastric mucosa.

144. A client is admitted with a $C_7$ complete transection. What must the nurse plan for in the immediate post-injury period?
   1. Bladder and bowel training.
   2. Possible ventilatory support.
   3. Complications of autonomic dysreflexia.
   4. Diaphragmatic pacing.

145. A client fell backward over a stair rail to the floor below and is not breathing. After calling for assistance, how should the nurse proceed?
   1. Initiate rescue breathing by performing a chin tilt maneuver and administering two breaths.

2. After determining absence of breathing, administer 15 chest compressions at the rate of 60 per minute.

3. Initiate rescue breathing by performing a jaw thrust maneuver and administering two breaths.

4. After determining pulselessness, administer five chest compressions at the rate of 60 per minute.

146. A client with a cervical spine injury was placed in Halo traction yesterday. When the client complains of discomfort around the pins, what action should the nurse take?

1. Carefully loosen the pins and notify the physician immediately.

2. Cleanse the skin around the pin sites and dry the area thoroughly.

3. Give the ordered analgesic and reassure the client that the pain is temporary.

4. Loosen the pins immediately and maintain the head in a neutral position.

147. A client with a C6 spinal cord injury 2 months ago now complains of a pounding headache. The pulse is 64 and the blood pressure is 220/110 mm Hg. Which of the following actions should the nurse take first?

1. Give the analgesic as ordered.

2. Check the client's output.

3. Elevate the client's head and lower the legs.

4. Notify the physician.

148. The nurse is evaluating the ability of a client with trigeminal neuralgia to implement the treatment that has been suggested. Which of the following behaviors by the client will be most effective in controlling manifestations?

1. Exercise the facial muscles at least twice daily.

2. Put the affected arm through full range of motion daily.

3. Avoid extremes in temperature of food and drink.

4. Use proper body mechanics in sitting and bending.

149. A client with Bell's palsy asks the nurse why artificial tears were ordered by the physician. Select the best reply by the nurse.

1. "When your affected eye fails to make tears, the eye can become irritated and ulcerated."

2. "Because your eye remains closed, foreign matter can be trapped beneath the lid."

3. "Artificial tears will remove the purulent drainage from your eye, which speeds healing."

4. "Because you cannot blink the affected eye, it can become dry and irritated."

150. A nurse is caring for a client with Guillain-Barré syndrome. Which of the following strategies is of the *most importance* in the plan of care?

1. Range of motion exercises three to four times per day.

2. Frequent measurement of vital capacity.

3. Use of artificial tears.

4. Starting an enteral feeding.

151. The nurse has presented information about amyotrophic lateral sclerosis (ALS) to a newly diagnosed client. Which question by the client indicates that he understands the nature of the disease?

1. "How can I avoid infecting my family with the virus?"

2. "How can I execute a living will?"

3. "How can I prevent an exacerbation of the disease?"

4. "How many people achieve remission with chemotherapy?"

152. A client reports gradual painless blurring of vision. On assessment, the nurse notes a cloudy opaque lens. What condition does the nurse suspect?

1. Glaucoma.

2. Cataracts.

3. Retinal detachment.

4. Diabetic retinopathy.

153. Which of the following risk factors would the nurse assess for in a client with glaucoma?

1. Family history, increased intraocular pressure, and age of 45–65.

2. History of diabetes and age greater than 50.

3. Female gender, cigarette smoking, age greater than 65.

4. Myopia, history of diabetes, and sudden severe physical exertion.

154. The nurse has been planning for home care with the family of a client who will undergo extracapsular lens extraction with an intraocular lens implant. Because the client and family speak very little English, the nurse takes extra care to evaluate their understanding. Which behavior by the client and/or family shows progress in understanding post-op home care instructions?

1. Using a chart showing various sleeping positions, the client points to a person lying on the affected side.

2. The family demonstrates that the eye should be cleaned with a washcloth, soap, and water.

3. The client demonstrates medication instillation by carefully dropping the solution on the cornea.

4. The family shows the nurse the sunglasses they have purchased for the client to wear post-op.

155. A nurse is admitting a client who reports vision loss. What additional information will be reported for the nurse to suspect glaucoma?
   1. Seeing floating spots.
   2. Eye pain.
   3. Seeing flashing lights.
   4. Sudden loss of vision.

156. Which of the following techniques should the nurse use to evaluate a client's understanding of self-care for chronic (primary) open-angle glaucoma?
   1. The nurse asks for the client's weekly blood pressure readings.
   2. The nurse asks if the client avoids watching television.
   3. The nurse observes the client's technique for monitoring blood glucose.
   4. The nurse observes the client's administration of eye drops.

157. A client is admitted with a detached retina of the left eye. The nurse patches both eyes. What is the rationale for patching both eyes?
   1. To prevent eye infections.
   2. To decrease eye movement.
   3. To prevent photophobia.
   4. To prevent nystagmus.

158. A neighbor splashes chlorine bleach in her eyes and calls the nurse for immediate help. What should be the nurse's first action?
   1. Lift the upper lid over the lower lid of each eye.
   2. Close and patch both eyes with a loose bandage.
   3. Continuously flush the eyes with tap water for 20 minutes.
   4. Instill an over-the-counter anti-irritant solution, such as Visine.

159. A client reports bilateral hearing loss. On assessment of the ear, the nurse observes chalky white plaques on the eardrum and the eardrum appears pinkish orange in color. The Rinne test

favors bone conduction. What condition does the nurse suspect?
   1. Cholesteatoma.
   2. Actinic keratosis.
   3. External otitis.
   4. Otosclerosis.

160. The nurse is teaching a post-op stapedectomy client. What should be included in the teaching?
   1. Work can be resumed the next day.
   2. Gently sneeze or cough with the mouth closed.
   3. Avoid airline flight for 6 months.
   4. Resume exercise in 1 week.

161. A client reports very loud, overpowering ringing in the ears, fluctuating hearing loss on the right side with severe vertigo accompanied by nausea and vomiting, What condition does the nurse suspect?
   1. Ménière's disease.
   2. Acoustic neuroma.
   3. Otosclerosis.
   4. Cholesteatoma.

162. What is the *priority* nursing diagnosis for a client with very loud overpowering ringing in his ears, fluctuating hearing loss on the right side with severe vertigo accompanied by nausea and vomiting and a feeling of fullness in the right ear?
   1. Knowledge deficit related to the disease process.
   2. Anxiety.
   3. Impaired physical mobility.
   4. Pain.

 **Answers and Rationales**

108. **3.** It has been demonstrated that positioning the client with the head elevated to 30° decreases ICP by promoting venous drainage from the head by gravity. Pronounced angulation of the head can obstruct venous return and increase ICP.

109. **3.** Cheynes-Stokes respirations are a pattern of breathing in which phases of hyperapnea regularly alternate with apnea. The pattern waxes (crescendo) and wanes (decrescendo).

110. 2. Mechanical hyperventilation to reduce $CO_2$ levels to 25 mm Hg produces cerebral vasoconstriction and thereby decreases ICP.

111. *Eye opening* should be selected. The Glasgow Coma Scale is a practical scale that independently evaluates three features: eye opening, motor response in the upper limb, and verbal performance.
*Motor response* should be selected. The Glasgow Coma Scale is a practical scale that independently evaluates three features: eye opening, motor response in the upper limb, and verbal performance.
*Verbal performance* should be selected. The Glasgow Coma Scale is a practical scale that independently evaluates three features: eye opening, motor response in the upper limb, and verbal performance.

112. 3. A score of 7 or less defines coma. The lowest achievable score is 3, which indicates deep coma. Fifteen is a perfect score.

113. 4. Decorticate rigidity or posturing is best described as an abnormal flexor response in the arm with extension and plantar flexion in the lower extremities.

114. 4. Momentary bright flashes of light are a common symptom of retinal detachment.

115. 2. Myopia or nearsightedness is a predisposing factor in the development of a retinal tear.

116. 1. Cryotherapy is used to produce a chorioretinal adhesion or scar that allows the retina to return to its normal position.

117. 3. The client should be taught to avoid blowing the nose because this action could increase the pressure in the eustachian tube and dislodge the surgical graft.

118. 3. The response describes the Babinski reflex. It is abnormal in an adult, signifying an upper motor neuron lesion.

119. 3. To correctly test cranial nerve II, the optic nerve, use a Snellen chart to assess visual acuity.

120. 4. An audiometry test tests different pitches and sounds.

121. 1. Three points are given for opening eyes to speech, 6 points are given for obeying verbal commands related to motor response, and 4 points are given for best verbal response when client is confused.

122. 2. Pacemakers and cerebral aneurysm clips are the exclusions for an MRI.

123. 1. Difficulty swallowing occurs from a hematoma developing and pushing on the trachea.

124. 3. The client is manifesting symptoms of increased intracranial pressure.

125. 1. Increased intracranial pressure causes hypothalamic dysfunction creating hypo/hyperthermia, SIADH, and diabetes insipidus. The hypothalamus regulates body temperature, osmolality of body fluids, hunger, and satiety.

126. 1. This method allows the client to have a feeling of control.

127. 2. Facing the person and speaking clearly is the best way to communicate with the hearing impaired.

128. 1. These are some of the symptoms of meningitis.

129. 2. The ineffective tissue perfusion is related to the increased intracranial pressure and inflammatory process.

130. 1. These findings are consistent with a brain tumor.

131. 2. This is the correct position for an infratentorial approach.

132. 1. Pulling the client's paralyzed arm can result in shoulder subluxation and pain. The client's unaffected hand must be free to reach for the arm of the wheelchair.

133. 2. A TIA is a temporary loss of function due to cerebral ischemia.

134. 3. Platelet-inhibiting drugs such as aspirin are taken prophylactically to prevent cerebral infarction secondary to embolism and thrombosis.

135. 4. Depression, confusion, and hallucinations are adverse effects that can occur after prolonged use of L-dopa. A "drug holiday" under medical supervision may restore drug effectiveness.

136. 1. The client should have semisolid, thickened food. Soup is thin in texture and could be aspirated by the client.

137. **4.** These are the symptoms of MS, which is more common in women ages 20–40.

138. **4.** Clients with MG have respiratory muscle failure.

139. **2.** The client is confused about the timing of medication administration. The anticholinesterase medication should be taken 30 minutes prior to meals to enhance the muscle strength needed for chewing and swallowing.

140. **3.** Cerebrospinal fluid is positive for glucose.

141. **1.** The client's head should be elevated about 30° to lower the intracranial pressure, which may be dangerously elevated in a subdural hematoma. The venous blood pressure begins to decline as intracranial pressure rises.

142. **2.** The wife may not understand that she must interrupt the client's sleep to detect early signs of increased intracranial pressure caused by contusion or hematoma development.

143. **2.** Cerebral edema is common after surgery. Decadron (a corticosteroid) is given to decrease the edema.

144. **2.** Edema above the area of the lesion can cause respiratory depression and arrest.

145. **3.** When initiating rescue breathing for a client with a suspected spinal injury, the jaw thrust maneuver is used with rescue breathing at the rate of 12 breaths per minute.

146. **3.** Discomfort at the pin sites is expected for several days after application of the Halo device. The pain can be controlled with mild analgesic medication. The client can benefit from the reassurance that the pain will not continue for the weeks that the traction will be in place.

147. **3.** The client is showing signs of autonomic dysreflexia. Placing the client in a sitting position will allow blood to pool in the legs, which should lower the blood pressure and prevent possible hypertensive hemorrhage.

148. **3.** Extremes of temperature of food or drink can trigger paroxysms of severe facial pain along the pathways of the trigeminal nerve. Meals are better tolerated if served at room temperature.

149. **4.** Bell's palsy may cause paralysis of the eyelid and loss of the blink reflex on the affected side.

The eye may not close completely. These problems render the eye susceptible to drying and irritation from dust or other debris.

150. **2.** Clients with Guillain-Barré have respiratory muscle weakness and respiratory failure.

151. **2.** Clients with ALS often experience respiratory failure as the disease progresses and need to communicate their wishes regarding ventilator support. The nurse should explore the client's wishes and facilitate discussion within the family. Arranging for the client to sign a living will, if the client wishes to do so, is also a nursing responsibility.

152. **2.** These are the assessment findings of cataracts.

153. **1.** These are common risk factors for glaucoma.

154. **4.** Sunglasses should be worn post-op for comfort and protection when outdoors.

155. **2.** Eye pain is present with open- and narrow-angle glaucoma, but not with a detached retina.

156. **4.** Glaucoma is usually treated with eye drops, such as betaxolol (Timoptic), a beta-adrenergic antagonist. The eye can be damaged when eye drops are used incorrectly.

157. **2.** Eye movements can increase the amount of detachment.

158. **3.** Immediate irrigation with copious amounts of water or normal saline solution may reduce alkaline burns of the cornea and conjunctiva. Any delay in initiating the irrigation can result in serious damage to eye structures.

159. **4.** These are classic signs of otosclerosis.

160. **3.** The client should avoid flying to prevent pressure changes in the ear at higher altitudes.

161. **1.** These are classic signs of Ménière's disease.

162. **1.** This client most likely has Ménière's disease. In Ménière's disease, client education is paramount. The client needs to be taught that with the increased volume of hydrolymph, excessive fluid intake increases the volume even more and exacerbates the disease. They should also be taught not to ambulate or make extreme movements during the acute attacks.

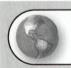

## OVERVIEW OF ANATOMY AND PHYSIOLOGY

The cardiovascular system consists of the heart, arteries, veins, and capillaries. The major functions are circulation of blood, delivery of oxygen and other nutrients to the tissues of the body, and removal of carbon dioxide and other products of cellular metabolism.

## Heart

The heart is a muscular pump that propels blood into the arterial system and receives blood from the venous system.

### Heart Wall

A. Pericardium: composed of fibrous (outermost layer) and serous pericardium (parietal and visceral); a sac that functions to protect the heart from friction.
B. Epicardium: covers surface of heart, becomes continuous with visceral layer of serous pericardium.
C. Myocardium: middle, muscular layer.
D. Endocardium: thin, inner membranous layer lining the chambers of the heart.
E. Papillary muscles: arise from the endocardial and myocardial surface of the ventricles and attach to the chordae tendinae.
F. Chordae tendinae: attach to the tricuspid and mitral valves and prevent eversion during systole.

### Chambers

A. Atria: two chambers, function as receiving chambers, lie above the ventricles
   1. Right atrium: receives systemic venous blood through the superior vena cava, inferior vena cava, and coronary sinus.
   2. Left atrium: receives oxygenated blood returning to the heart from the lungs through the pulmonary veins.
B. Ventricles: two thick-walled chambers; major responsibility for forcing blood out of the heart; lie below the atria.
   1. Right ventricle: contracts and propels deoxygenated blood into the pulmonary circulation via the pulmonary artery.
   2. Left ventricle: propels blood into the systemic circulation via the aorta during ventricular systole.

### Valves

See Figure 4-5.
A. Atrioventricular (AV) valves
   1. Mitral valve: located between the left atrium and left ventricle; contains two leaflets attached to the chordae tendinae.
   2. Tricuspid valve: located between the right atrium and right ventricle; contains three leaflets attached to the chordae tendinae.
   3. Functions
      a. Permit unidirectional flow of blood from specific atrium to specific ventricle during ventricular diastole.
      b. Prevent reflux flow during ventricular systole.
      c. Valve leaflets open during ventricular diastole and close during ventricular systole; valve closure produces first heart sound ($S_1$).
B. Semilunar valves
   1. Pulmonary valve: located between right ventricle and pulmonary artery
   2. Aortic valve: located between left ventricle and aorta
   3. Functions
      a. Permit unidirectional flow of blood from specific ventricle to arterial vessel during ventricular systole.

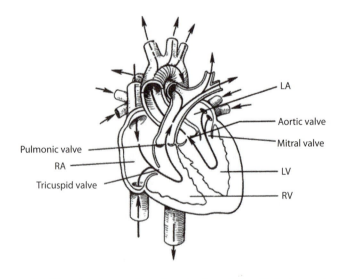

**Figure 4-5** The valves of the heart; arrows indicate the direction of blood flow.

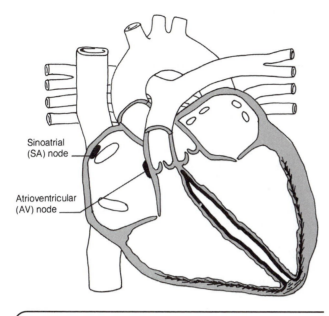

**Figure 4-6** Conduction system of the heart

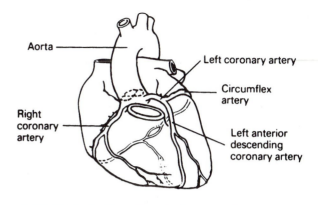

**Figure 4-7** Coronary circulation

    **b.** Prevent reflux blood flow during ventricular diastole.
    **c.** Valves open when ventricles contract and close during ventricular diastole; valve closure produces second heart sound ($S_2$).

## Conduction System

See Figure 4-6.
**A.** Sinoatrial (SA) node: the pacemaker of the heart; initiates the cardiac impulse, which spreads across the atria and into AV node.
**B.** Atrioventricular (AV) node: delays the impulse from the atria while the ventricles fill.
**C.** Bundle of His: arises from the AV node and conducts impulse to the bundle branch system.
    **1.** Right bundle branch: divided into anterior, lateral, and posterior; transmits impulses down the right side of the interventricular septum toward the right ventricular myocardium
    **2.** Left bundle branch: divided into anterior and posterior
        **a.** Anterior portion transmits impulses to the anterior endocardial surface of the left ventricle.
        **b.** Posterior portion transmits impulses over the posterior and inferior endocardial surfaces of the left ventricle.
**D.** Purkinje fibers: transmit impulses to the ventricles and provide for depolarization after ventricular contraction.
**E.** Electrical activity of heart can be visualized by attaching electrodes to the skin and recording activity by electrocardiograph.

## Coronary Circulation

See Figure 4-7.
**A.** Coronary arteries: branch off at the base of the aorta and supply blood to the myocardium and the conduction system; two main coronary arteries are right and left.
**B.** Coronary veins: return blood from the myocardium back to the right atrium via the coronary sinus.

# Vascular System

The major function of the blood vessels is to supply the tissues with blood, remove wastes, and carry unoxygenated blood back to the heart.

## Types of Blood Vessels

**A.** Arteries: elastic-walled vessels that can stretch during systole and recoil during diastole; they carry blood away from the heart and distribute oxygenated blood throughout the body.
**B.** Arterioles: small arteries that distribute blood to the capillaries and function in controlling systemic vascular resistance and, therefore, arterial pressure.
**C.** Capillaries: the following exchanges occur in the capillaries
    **1.** Oxygen and carbon dioxide
    **2.** Solutes between the blood and tissues
    **3.** Fluid volume transfer between the plasma and interstitial spaces
**D.** Venules: small veins that receive blood from the capillaries and function as collecting channels between the capillaries and veins.
**E.** Veins: low-pressure vessels with thin walls and less muscle than arteries; most contain valves that prevent retrograde blood flow; they carry deoxygenated blood back to the heart. When skeletal muscles surrounding veins contract, the veins are compressed, promoting movement of blood back to the heart.

## ASSESSMENT

### Health History

A. Presenting problem
   1. Nonspecific symptoms may include fatigue, shortness of breath, cough, dizziness, syncope, headache, palpitations, weight loss/gain, anorexia, difficulty sleeping.
   2. Specific signs and symptoms
      a. Chest pain: note character, quality, location, radiation, frequency, and whether it is associated with precipitating factors (exertion, eating, excitement).
      b. Dyspnea (shortness of breath): note kind and extent of precipitating activities.
      c. Orthopnea (form of dyspnea that develops when client lies down): determine how many pillows are used when sleeping; note any paroxysmal nocturnal dyspnea (PND) (client awakens suddenly in the night, breathing with difficulty).
      d. Palpitations (awareness of heartbeat, fluttering feeling): assess precipitating factors (anxiety, caffeine, nicotine, stress); ask client to tap out the rhythm.
      e. Edema (abnormal accumulation of fluid in tissues): note whether unilateral/bilateral, location, time of day when most apparent.
      f. Cyanosis (dusky, bluish coloration to the skin): note whether peripheral or central.
B. Lifestyle: occupation, hobbies, financial status, stressors, unusual life patterns, relaxation time, exercise, living conditions, smoking, sleep habits
C. Use of medications: OTC drugs, cardiac drugs, oral contraceptives, or estrogen replacement therapy
D. Personality profile: Type A, manic-depressive, anxieties
E. Nutrition: dietary habits; calorie, cholesterol, salt intake; alcohol consumption
F. Past medical history
   1. Heart murmurs, rheumatic fever, sexually transmitted diseases, angina, myocardial infarction (MI), hypertension, CVA, alcoholism, obesity, hyperlipidemia, varicose veins, claudication
   2. Pregnancies, contraceptive use
G. Family history: heart disease (congenital, acute, chronic); risk factors (diabetes, hypertension, obesity)

### Physical Examination

A. Skin and mucous membranes: note color/texture, temperature, hair distribution on extremities, atrophy or edema, venous pattern, petechiae, lesions, ulcerations or gangrene; examine nails.
B. Peripheral pulses: palpate and rate all arterial pulses (temporal, carotid, brachial, radial, femoral, popliteal, dorsalis pedis, and posterior tibial) on scale of: 0 = absent, 1 = palpable, 2 = normal, 3 = full, 4 = full and bounding.
C. Assess for arterial insufficiency and venous impairment.
D. Measure and record blood pressure.
E. Inspect and palpate the neck vessels.
   1. Jugular veins: note location, characteristics; measure jugular venous pressure.
   2. Carotid arteries: note location, characteristics
F. Precordium
   1. Inspect and palpate sternoclavicular, aortic, pulmonic, Erb's point, tricuspid, apical, epigastric sites.
   2. Note point of maximum impulse (PMI), pulsations, thrills.
G. Auscultate aortic, pulmonic, Erb's point, tricuspid, mitral or apical, xiphoid areas; note heart rate and rhythm (see Figure 4-8).
   1. Normal heart sounds ($S_1$ and $S_2$): note location, intensity, splitting
   2. Abnormal heart sounds ($S_3$, $S_4$): note location, occurrence in cardiac cycle
   3. Murmurs: note location, occurrence in cardiac cycle
   4. Friction rubs

### Laboratory/Diagnostic Tests

A. Blood chemistry and electrolyte analysis
   1. Serial cardiac enzymes (protein assays) will be evaluated with symptoms of acute coronary

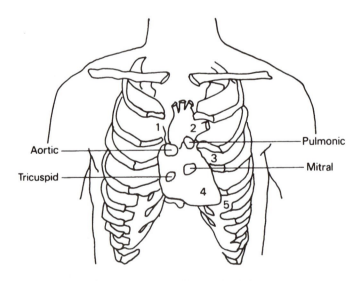

**Figure 4-8** Heart valves and areas of auscultation: (1) aortic area; (2) pulmonic area; (3) Erb's point; (4) tricuspid area; (5) mitral area

syndrome, chest pain/ischemia with and without infection, congestive heart failure, post cardiac surgical intervention, and post chest trauma.

    a. Nonspecific enzymes, elevated in myocardial injury and with other systems:

      1) Creatine kinase (CK); normally 50–325 million units/mL

      2) Myoglobin

      3) LDH

      4) AST (SGOT); normally 7–40 units/mL

    b. Specific cardiac isoenzymes, elevated in myocardial injury:

      1) Creatine kinase-MB (CKMB); normally 0%

      2) LDH1 and LDH2

      3) Troponin I or cardiac troponin T (currently used in place of LDH isoenzymes)

    c. Specific enzymes, elevations correlated with vascular inflammation, irritability of atherosclerotic plaque, and future coronary risk:

      1) Ischemic modified albumin (IMA)

      2) Serum lipids (HDLs, LDLs, VDRLs)

      3) C-reactive protein (CRP)

      4) Lipoprotein phospholipase A2 (PLAQ test)

    d. Specific cardiac proteins, elevated in congestive heart failure:

      1) B-type natriuretic peptide and N-terminal proB-type natriuretic peptide (BNP)

**B.** Hematologic studies

  1. CBC (see Hematologic system for values)

  2. Coagulation time: 5–15 min.; increased levels indicate bleeding tendency, used to monitor heparin therapy

  3. Prothrombin time (PT) 9.5–12 sec.; INR 1.0, increased levels indicate bleeding tendency, used to monitor warfarin therapy

  4. Activated partial thromboplastin time (APTT) 20–45 sec., increased levels indicate bleeding tendency, used to monitor heparin therapy

  5. Erythrocyte sedimentation rate (ESR) < 20 mm/hr; increased level indicate inflammatory process

**C.** Urine studies: routine urinalysis

**D.** Electrocardiogram (ECG or EKG)

  1. Noninvasive test that produces a graphic record of the electrical activity of the heart. In addition to determining cardiac rhythm, pattern variations may reveal pathologic processes (MI and ischemia, electrolyte and acid-base imbalance, chamber enlargement, block of the right or left bundle branch); see also Cardiac Monitoring.

  2. Portable recorder (Holter monitor) provides continuous recording of ECG for up to 24 hours; client keeps a diary noting presence of symptoms or any unusual activities.

**E.** Stress tests may show heart disease when resting ECG does not. Stress test types:

  1. Exercise: treadmill or bicycle

  2. Chemical: Persantine, Dobutamine, Adenosine

**F.** Cardiac nuclear scan: Radionucleotide imaging to identify ischemic/infracted tissue.

**G.** Phonocardiogram: noninvasive device to amplify and record heart sounds and murmurs.

**H.** Echocardiogram: noninvasive recording of the cardiac structures using ultrasound.

**I.** Cardiac catheterization: invasive, but often definitive test for diagnosis of cardiac disease.

  1. A catheter is inserted into the right or left side of the heart to obtain information.

    a. Right-sided catheterization: the catheter is inserted into an antecubital vein and advanced into the vena cava, right atrium, and right ventricle with further insertion into the pulmonary artery.

    b. Left-sided catheterization: performed by inserting the catheter into a brachial or femoral artery; the catheter is passed retrograde up the aorta and into the left ventricle.

  2. Purpose: to measure intracardiac pressures and oxygen levels in various parts of the heart; with injection of a dye, it allows visualization of the heart chambers, blood vessels, and course of blood flow (angiography).

  3. Nursing care: pretest

    a. Confirm that informed consent has been signed.

    b. Ask about allergies, particularly to iodine, if dye being used.

    c. Keep client NPO for 8–12 hours prior to test.

    d. Temporarily suspend metformin for dye and surgical procedures; do not restart until oral intake has resumed and renal function is normal.

    e. Record height and weight, take baseline vital signs, and monitor peripheral pulses.

    f. Inform client that a feeling of warmth and fluttering sensation as catheter is passed is common.

  4. Nursing care: posttest

    a. Assess circulation to the extremity used for catheter insertion.

    b. Check peripheral pulses, color, sensation of affected extremity every 15 minutes for 4 hours.

    c. If protocol requires, keep affected extremity straight for approximately 8 hours.

    d. Observe catheter insertion site for swelling and bleeding; a sandbag or pressure dressing may be placed over insertion site.

    e. Assess vital signs and report significant changes from baseline.

J. Aortography
1. Injection of radiopaque contrast medium into the aorta to visualize the aorta, valve leaflets, and major vessels on a movie film.
2. Purpose: to determine and diagnose aortic valve incompetence, aneurysms of the ascending aorta, abnormalities of major branches of the aorta.
3. Nursing care: pretest
   a. Confirm that informed consent has been signed.
   b. Inform client that a dye will be injected and to report any dyspnea, numbness, or tingling.
4. Nursing care: posttest
   a. Assess the puncture site frequently for bleeding or inflammation.
   b. Assess peripheral pulses distal to the injection site every hour for 4–8 hours posttest.
K. Coronary arteriography
1. Visualization of coronary arteries by injection of radiopaque contrast dye and recording on a movie film.
2. Purpose: evaluation of heart disease and angina, location of areas of infarction and extent of lesions, ruling out coronary artery disease in clients with myocardial disease.
3. Nursing care: same as for Aortography.

## ANALYSIS

Nursing diagnoses for the client with a cardiovascular dysfunction may include:

A. Excess fluid volume
B. Decreased cardiac output
C. Ineffective tissue perfusion
D. Impairment of skin integrity
E. Activity intolerance
F. Pain
G. Ineffective individual coping
H. Fear
I. Anxiety

## PLANNING AND IMPLEMENTATION

### Goals

A. Fluid imbalance will be resolved, edema minimized.
B. Cardiac output will be improved.
C. Cardiopulmonary and peripheral tissue perfusion will be improved.
D. Adequate skin integrity will be maintained.
E. Activity tolerance will progressively increase.

F. Pain in the chest or in the affected extremity will be diminished.
G. Client will use effective coping techniques.
H. Client's level of fear and anxiety will be decreased.

## Interventions

### Cardiac Monitoring

A. The cardiac monitor provides continuous information regarding the cardiac rhythm and rate (ECG). Constant surveillance and understanding of the basic electrocardiographic system is imperative to avoid/treat arrhythmias (see Figure 4-9).
1. ECG strip: each small square represents 0.04 second, each large square 0.2 second.
2. P wave: produced by atrial depolarization; indicates SA node function.
3. P-R interval
   a. Indicates atrioventricular conduction time or the time it takes an impulse to travel from the atria down and through the AV node
   b. Measured from beginning of P wave to beginning of QRS complex
   c. Normal: 0.12–0.20 second.
4. QRS complex
   a. Indicates ventricular depolarization
   b. Measured from onset of Q wave to end of S wave
   c. Normal: 0.06–0.10 seconds
5. ST segment
   a. Indicates time interval between complete depolarization of ventricles and repolarization of ventricles
   b. Measured after QRS complex to beginning of T wave
6. T wave
   a. Represents ventricular repolarization
   b. Follows ST segment

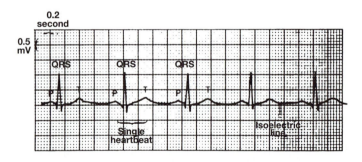

**Figure 4-9** A typical ECG; all beats appear as a similar pattern, equally spaced, and have three major units: P wave, QRS complex, and T wave

## Hemodynamic Monitoring (Swan-Ganz Catheter)

A. A pulmonary artery (PA) catheter with a balloon tip that is advanced through the superior vena cava into the right atrium, right ventricle, and pulmonary artery. When it is wedged it is in the distal arterial branch of the pulmonary artery.

B. Purposes
   1. Proximal port: measures right atrial pressure
   2. Distal port
      a. Measures pulmonary artery (PA) pressure (reflects left and right heart pressures) and pulmonary capillary wedge pressure (PCWP) (reflects left atrial and left ventricular end diastolic pressure)
      b. Normal values: PA systolic 15–30 mm Hg and diastolic 4–12 mm Hg; PCWP 6–12 mm Hg
   3. Balloon port: inflated with 1–1.5 cc air to obtain PCWP
   4. Thermistor lumen: used to measure cardiac output if ordered.

C. Nursing care
   1. A sterile dry dressing should be applied to site and changed every 24 hours; inspect site daily and report signs of infection.
   2. If catheter is inserted via an extremity, immobilize extremity to prevent catheter dislodgment or trauma.
   3. Observe catheter site for leakage.
   4. Ensure that balloon is deflated with a syringe attached, except when PCWP is read.
   5. Continuously monitor PA systolic and diastolic pressures and report significant variations.
   6. Maintain client in same position for each reading.
   7. Maintain pressure bag at 300 mm Hg.
   8. Record PA systolic and diastolic readings at least every hour and PCWP as ordered, noting position of client.

## Central Venous Pressure (CVP)

A. Obtained by inserting a catheter into the external jugular, antecubital, or femoral vein and threading it into the vena cava. The catheter is attached to an IV infusion and $H_2O$ manometer by a three-way stopcock or electronic transducer.

B. Purposes
   1. Reveals right atrial pressure, reflecting alterations in the right ventricular pressure
   2. Provides information concerning blood volume and adequacy of central venous return

   3. Provides an IV route for drawing blood samples, administering fluids or medication, and possibly inserting a pacing catheter

C. Normal range is 4–10 cm $H_2O$ or 2–6 mm Hg; elevation indicates hypervolemia, decreased level indicates hypovolemia.

D. Nursing care
   1. Ensure client is relaxed.
   2. Maintain zero point of manometer always at level of right atrium (midaxillary line).
   3. Determine patency of catheter by opening IV infusion line.
   4. Turn stopcock to allow IV solution to run into manometer to a level of 10–20 cm above expected pressure reading.
   5. Turn stopcock to allow IV solution to flow from manometer into catheter; fluid level in manometer fluctuates with respiration.
   6. Stop ventilatory assistance during measurement of CVP.
   7. After CVP reading, return stopcock to IV infusion position.
   8. Record CVP reading and position of client.
   9. Electronic transducer
      a. Ensure client is relaxed.
      b. Make sure transducer is zeroed and calibrated.
      c. If CVP line is in use, turn stopcock to allow pressure measurement from transducer, which will temporarily stop infusion.
      d. Ensure that infusion is reinitiated upon completion of reading.
      e. Record CVP.

# EVALUATION

A. Resolution of peripheral edema and neck vein distention; weight stable; lungs clear.
B. Capillary refill is less than 3 seconds; balanced I&O with urine output at least 30 mL/hour; hemodynamic measurements within normal range; usual mental status.
C. Stable vital signs; skin warm and dry; peripheral pulses present, equal, and strong; absence of edema; increased tolerance to activity; usual mentation; absence of pain.
D. Client's skin warm and dry, shows absence of redness and irritation; healing of lesions.
E. Progressive increase in tolerance for activity with heart rate and blood pressure stable; absence of pain.
F. Client expresses relief from pain; relaxed facial expression; stable vital signs; progressive increase in activity tolerance.
G. Demonstrates the use of effective coping skills and problem-solving techniques.
H. Verbalizes awareness of feelings of fear and anxiety. Client reports fear/anxiety as reduced/controlled.

# DISORDERS OF THE CARDIOVASCULAR SYSTEM

## The Heart

### Coronary Artery Disease (CAD)

A. General information
1. CAD refers to a variety of pathologic conditions that cause narrowing or obstruction of the coronary arteries, resulting in decreased blood supply to the myocardium.
2. Atherosclerosis (deposits of cholesterol and lipids within the walls of the artery) is the major causative factor.
3. Occurs most often between ages 30 and 50; men affected more often than women; nonwhites have higher mortality rates.
4. May manifest as angina pectoris or MI.
5. Risk factors: family history of CAD, elevated serum lipoproteins, cigarette smoking, diabetes mellitus, hypertension, obesity, sedentary and/or stressful/competitive lifestyle, elevated serum uric acid levels.

B. Medical management, assessment findings, and nursing interventions: see Angina Pectoris and Myocardial Infarction.

### Angina Pectoris

A. General information
1. Transient, paroxysmal chest pain produced by insufficient blood flow to the myocardium resulting in myocardial ischemia
2. Risk factors: CAD, atherosclerosis, hypertension, diabetes mellitus, thromboangiitis obliterans, severe anemia, aortic insufficiency
3. Precipitating factors: physical exertion, consumption of a heavy meal, extremely cold weather, strong emotions, cigarette smoking, sexual activity
4. Two main types:
   a. Stable angina: chest pain occurs with increased oxygen demand; relieved when precipitating factor is removed or with nitroglycerin.
   b. Unstable angina chest pain increases in frequency, duration, and intensity at low levels of activity or at rest; often a precursor to MI.

B. Medical management
1. Drug therapy: nitrates, beta-adrenergic blocking agents, and/or calcium-blocking agents, lipid reducing drugs if cholesterol elevated
2. Modification of diet and other risk factors
3. Surgery: coronary artery bypass surgery
4. Percutaneous transluminal coronary angioplasty (PTCA)

C. Assessment findings
1. Pain: substernal with possible radiation to the neck, jaw, back, and arms; may be relieved by rest
2. Palpitations, tachycardia
3. Dyspnea
4. Diaphoresis
5. Increased serum lipid levels
6. Diagnostic tests
   a. ECG may reveal ST segment depression and T-wave inversion during chest pain.
   b. Stress test may reveal an abnormal ECG during exercise.

D. Nursing interventions
1. Administer oxygen.
2. Give prompt pain relief with nitrates or narcotic analgesics as ordered.
3. Monitor vital signs, status of cardiopulmonary function.
4. Monitor ECG.
5. Place client in semi- to high-Fowler's position.
6. Provide emotional support.
7. Provide client teaching and discharge planning concerning
   a. Proper use of nitrates
      1) Nitroglycerin tablets (sublingual)
         a) Allow tablet to dissolve.
         b) Relax for 15 minutes after taking tablet to prevent dizziness.
         c) If no relief with 1 tablet, take additional tablets at 5-minute intervals, but no more than 3 tablets within a 15-minute period, reassess blood pressure after each tablet dissolved.
         d) Know that transient headache is a frequent side effect.
         e) Keep pills in original bottle, tightly capped and prevent exposure to air, light, and heat.
         f) Ensure tablets are within reach at all times.
         g) Check shelf life, expiration date of tablets.
      2) Nitroglycerin ointment (topical)
         a) Rotate sites to prevent dermal inflammation.
         b) Remove previously applied ointment.
         c) Avoid massaging/rubbing as this increases absorption and interferes with the drug's sustained action.
   b. Ways to minimize precipitating events
      1) Reduce stress and anxiety (relaxation techniques, guided imagery)
      2) Avoid overexertion and smoking
      3) Maintain low-cholesterol, low-saturated fat diet and eat small, frequent meals
      4) Avoid extremes of temperature
      5) Dress warmly in cold weather

    **c.** Gradual increase in activities and exercise
      **1)** Participate in regular exercise program
      **2)** Space exercise periods and allow for rest periods
  **8.** Instruct client to notify physician immediately if pain occurs and persists, despite rest and medication administration.

## Dysrhythmias

A dysrhythmia, often called an arrhythmia, is a disruption in the normal events of the cardiac cycle. It may take a variety of forms. Treatment varies depending on the type of dysrhythmia; commonly used drugs are summarized in Table 2-14.

### Sinus Tachycardia

**A.** General information
  **1.** A heart rate of over 100 beats/minute, originating in the SA node
  **2.** May be caused by fever, apprehension, physical activity, anemia, hyperthyroidism, drugs (epinephrine, theophylline), myocardial ischemia, caffeine

**B.** Assessment findings
  **1.** Rate: 100–160 beats/minute
  **2.** Rhythm: regular
  **3.** P wave: precedes each QRS complex with normal contour
  **4.** P-R interval: normal (0.08 second)
  **5.** QRS complex: normal (0.06 second)

**C.** Treatment: correction of underlying cause, elimination of stimulants; sedatives, propranolol (Inderal).

### Premature Atrial Complex (PAC)

**A.** General information
  **1.** Physical appearance: single ECG complex that occurs early
  **2.** Causes: nicotine, alcohol, anxiety, low potassium level, hypovolemia, myocardial ischemia

**B.** Assessment findings
  **1.** Ventricular and atrial rate dependent on underlying rhythm
  **2.** Rhythm; irregular due to premature complexes
  **3.** QRS shape; usually normal
  **4.** P wave: morphology may be the same, different, or absent
  **5.** P-R interval: may be shorter but within limits (0.12–0.20 second)
  **6.** P-QRS: 1:1

### Sinus Bradycardia

**A.** General information
  **1.** A slowed heart rate initiated by SA node
  **2.** Caused by excessive vagal or decreased sympathetic tone, MI, intracranial tumors, meningitis, myxedema, cardiac fibrosis; a normal variation of the heart rate in well-trained athletes

**B.** Assessment findings
  **1.** Rate: less than 60 beats/minute
  **2.** Rhythm: regular
  **3.** P wave: precedes each QRS with a normal contour
  **4.** P-R interval: normal
  **5.** QRS complex: normal

**C.** Treatment: usually not needed; if cardiac output is inadequate, atropine and isoproterenol (Isuprel) are usually prescribed; if drugs are not effective, a pacemaker may need to be inserted.

### Atrial Tachycardia

**A.** General information
  **1.** A heart rate above 160–250, originates in the SA node
  **2.** May be drug induced (including substance abuse), caused by fever, severe blood loss, thyroid storm, electrolyte imbalances, severe hypoxia

**B.** Assessment findings
  **1.** Rate: 160–250 beats/minute
  **2.** Rhythm: regular
  **3.** P Wave: precedes each QRS complex with normal contour
  **4.** P-R interval: normal (0.08 second)
  **5.** QRS complex: normal (0.06 second)

**C.** Treatment: correction of underlying problem, beta-blockers, calcium channel blocker, amniodarone

### Atrial Flutter

**A.** General information
  **1.** Atrial rate between 250 and 400, ventricular rate between 75 and 150
  **2.** May be idiopathic, associated with advanced age, valvular disease, HTN, cardiomyopathy, pulmonary disease, hyperthyroidism, moderate-to-heavy alcohol consumption

**B.** Assessment findings
  **1.** Rate: 250–400 beats/minute
  **2.** Rhythm: irregular
  **3.** P Wave: varies to QRS
  **4.** P-R interval: difficult to distinguish due to rate
  **5.** QRS complex: normal or abnormal

**C.** Treatment: correction of underlying problem, beta-blockers, calcium channel blocker, amniodarone, digitalis

### Atrial Fibrillation

**A.** General information
  **1.** An arrhythmia in which ectopic foci in the atria cause rapid, irregular contractions of the heart
  **2.** Commonly seen in clients with rheumatic mitral stenosis, thyrotoxicosis,

cardiomyopathy, hypertensive heart disease, pericarditis, and coronary heart disease

B. Assessment findings
  1. Rate
     a. Atrial: 350–600 beats/minute
     b. Ventricular: varies between 100–160 beats/minute
  2. Rhythm: atrial and ventricular regularly irregular
  3. P wave: no definite P wave; rapid undulations called fibrillatory (f) waves
  4. P-R interval: not measurable
  5. QRS complex: generally normal
C. Treatment: digitalis preparations, propranolol, verapamil in conjunction with digitalis; direct-current cardioversion

### Premature Ventricular Contractions (PVCs)

A. General information
  1. Irritable impulses originate in the ventricles
  2. Caused by electrolyte imbalance (hypokalemia); digitalis drug therapy; myocardial disease; stimulants (caffeine, epinephrine, isoproterenol); hypoxia; congestive heart failure
B. Assessment findings
  1. Rate: varies according to number of PVCs
  2. Rhythm: irregular because of PVCs
  3. P wave: normal; however, often lost in QRS complex
  4. P-R interval: often not measurable
  5. QRS complex: wide and distorted in shape, greater than 0.12 second
C. Treatment
  1. IV push of lidocaine (50–100 mg) followed by IV drip of lidocaine at rate of 1–4 mg/minute
  2. Procainamide (Pronestyl), quinidine
  3. Treatment of underlying cause

### Ventricular Tachycardia

A. General information
  1. A run of three or more consecutive PVCs; occurs from repetitive firing of an ectopic focus in the ventricles
  2. Caused by acute MI, CAD, digitalis intoxication, hypokalemia
B. Assessment findings
  1. Rate
     a. Atrial: 60–100 beats/minute
     b. Ventricular: 110–250 beats/minute
  2. Rhythm: atrial (regular), ventricular (occasionally irregular)
  3. P wave: often lost in QRS complex
  4. P-R interval: usually not measurable
  5. QRS complex: greater than 0.12 second, wide
C. Treatment
  1. IV push of lidocaine (1 mg/kg for a dose of 50–100 mg), then IV drip of lidocaine 1–4 mg/minute

  2. Procainamide via IV infusion of 2–6 mg/minute
  3. Direct-current cardioversion
  4. Bretylium, propranolol (Inderal)

### Ventricular Fibrillation

A. General information
  1. Rapid and disorganized rhythm caused by quivering of the ventricles
  2. No atrial activity is seen
  3. May be caused by idiopathic sudden death, electrical shock
B. Assessment findings
  1. Ventricular rate: greater than 300
  2. Ventricular rhythm irregular, without specific pattern
  3. QRS shape and duration: irregular, undulating waves without recognizable QRS pattern
C. Treatment: counter-shock (defibrillation)

## Myocardial Infarction (MI)

A. General information
  1. The death of myocardial cells from inadequate oxygenation, often caused by a sudden complete blockage of a coronary artery; characterized by localized formation of necrosis (tissue destruction) with subsequent healing by scar formation and fibrosis.
  2. Risk factors: atherosclerotic CAD, thrombus formation, hypertension, diabetes mellitus, hyperlipidemia, and genetic predisposition
B. Assessment findings (see also Angina Pectoris)
  1. Pain usually substernal with radiation to the neck, arm, jaw, or back; severe, crushing, viselike with sudden onset; *unrelieved by rest or nitrates*
  2. Nausea and vomiting
  3. Dyspnea
  4. Skin: cool, clammy, ashen
  5. Elevated temperature
  6. Initial increase in blood pressure and pulse, with gradual drop in blood pressure
  7. Restlessness
  8. Occasional findings: rales or crackles; presence of $S_4$; pericardial friction rub; split $S_1$, $S_2$
  9. Diagnostic tests
     a. Elevated WBC
     b. Elevated CPK and CPK-MB
     c. Elevated SGOT or AST
     d. Elevated LDH, $LDH_1$, and $LDH_2$
     e. Elevated troponin levels
     f. ECG changes (specific changes dependent on location of myocardial damage and phase of the MI; inverted T wave and ST segment changes seen with myocardial ischemia
     g. Increased ESR, elevated serum cholesterol

C. Nursing interventions
   1. Establish a patent IV line
   2. Provide pain relief; morphine sulfate IV (given IV because after an infarction there is poor peripheral perfusion and because serum enzymes would be affected by IM injections) as ordered.
   3. Administer oxygen as ordered to relieve dyspnea and prevent arrhythmias.
   4. Provide bed rest with semi-Fowler's position to decrease cardiac workload.
   5. Monitor ECG and hemodynamic procedures.
   6. Administer antiarrhythmias as ordered.
   7. Perform complete lung/cardiovascular assessment.
   8. Monitor urinary output and report output of less than 30 mL/hour; indicates decreased cardiac output.
   9. Maintain full liquid diet with gradual increase to soft; low sodium.
   10. Maintain quiet environment.
   11. Administer stool softeners as ordered to facilitate bowel evacuation and prevent straining.
   12. Relieve anxiety associated with coronary care unit (CCU) environment.
   13. Administer anticoagulants, as ordered.
   14. Administer thrombolytics (tissue-type plasminogen activator or t-pa and streptokinase) and monitor for side effects (bleeding).
   15. Provide client teaching and discharge planning concerning
       a. Effects of MI, healing process, and treatment regimen
       b. Medication regimen including name, purpose, schedule, dosage, side effects
       c. Risk factors, with necessary lifestyle modifications
       d. Dietary restrictions: low sodium, low cholesterol, avoidance of caffeine
       e. Importance of participation in a progressive activity program
       f. Resumption of sexual activity according to physician's orders (usually 4–6 weeks)
       g. Need to report the following symptoms: increased persistent chest pain, dyspnea, weakness, fatigue, persistent palpitations, light-headedness
       h. Enrollment of client in a cardiac rehabilitation program

## Percutaneous Transluminal Coronary Angioplasty

A. General information
   1. Percutaneous transluminal coronary angioplasty (PTCA), with or without placement of a stent, can be performed as an alternative to coronary artery bypass graft surgery (CABG).
   2. The aim of PTCA is to revascularize the myocardium, decrease angina, and increase survival.
   3. PTCA is performed in the cardiac catheterization lab and is accomplished by insertion of a balloon-tipped catheter into the stenotic, diseased coronary artery. The balloon is inflated with a controlled pressure and thereby decreases the stenosis of the vessel.
B. Nursing interventions: preoperative and postoperative care is similar to the care of the client undergoing cardiac catheterization.

## Coronary Artery Bypass Surgery (CABG)

A. General information
   1. A coronary artery bypass graft is the surgery of choice for clients with severe CAD.
   2. New supply of blood brought to diseased/occluded coronary artery by bypassing the obstruction with a graft that is attached to the aorta proximally and to the coronary artery distally.
   3. Several bypasses can be performed depending on the location and extent of the blockage.
   4. Procedure frequently requires use of extracorporeal circulation (heart-lung machine, cardiopulmonary bypass). Some clients may be candidates for off pump coronary artery bypass (OPCAB).
B. Nursing interventions: preoperative
   1. Explain anatomy of the heart, function of coronary arteries, effects of CAD.
   2. Explain events of the day of surgery: length of time in surgery, length of time until able to see family.
   3. Orient to the critical and coronary care units and introduce to staff.
   4. Explain equipment to be used (monitors, hemodynamic procedures, ventilator, endotracheal tube, drainage tubes).
   5. Demonstrate activity and exercises (turning from side to side, dangling, sitting in a chair, ROM exercises for arms and legs, effective deep breathing, and coughing).
   6. Reassure client that pain medication is available.
C. Nursing interventions: postoperative
   1. Maintain patent airway.
   2. Promote lung reexpansion.
      a. Monitor drainage from chest/mediastinal tubes, and check patency of chest drainage system.
      b. Assist client with turning, coughing, and deep breathing.
   3. Monitor cardiac status.
      a. Monitor vital signs and cardiac rhythm and report significant changes, particularly temperature elevation.
      b. Perform peripheral pulse checks.

c. Carry out hemodynamic monitoring.
d. Administer anticoagulants as ordered and monitor hematologic test results carefully.

4. Maintain fluid and electrolyte balance.
   a. Maintain accurate I&O with hourly outputs; report if less than 30 mL/hour urine.
   b. Assess color, character, and specific gravity of urine.
   c. Daily weights.
   d. Assess lab values, particularly BUN, creatinine, sodium, and potassium levels.

5. Maintain adequate cerebral circulation: frequent neuro checks.

6. Provide pain relief.
   a. Administer narcotics cautiously and monitor effects.
   b. Assist with positioning for maximum comfort.
   c. Teach relaxation techniques.

7. Prevent abdominal distension.
   a. Monitor nasogastric drainage and maintain patency of system.
   b. Assess for bowel sounds every 2–4 hours.
   c. Measure abdominal girths if necessary.

8. Monitor for and prevent the following complications.
   a. Thrombophlebitis/pulmonary embolism
   b. Cardiac tamponade
   c. Arrhythmias
      1) Maintain continuous ECG monitoring and report changes.
      2) Assess electrolyte levels daily and report significant changes, particularly potassium.
      3) Administer antiarrhythmics as ordered.
   d. Heart failure

9. Provide client teaching and discharge planning concerning
   a. Limitation with progressive increase in activities
      1) Encourage daily walking with gradual increase in distance weekly
      2) Avoid heavy lifting and activities that require continuous arm movements (vacuuming, playing golf, bowling)
      3) Avoid driving a car until physician permits
   b. Sexual intercourse: can usually be resumed by third or fourth week post-op; avoid sexual positions in which the client would be supporting weight
   c. Medical regimen: ensure client/family are aware of drugs, dosages, proper times of administration, and side effects
   d. Meal planning with prescribed modifications (decreased sodium, cholesterol, and possibly carbohydrates)

e. Wound cleansing daily with mild soap and $H_2O$ and report signs of infection
f. Symptoms to be reported: fever, dyspnea, chest pain with minimal exertion

## Heart Failure (HF)

A. General information: inability of the heart to pump an adequate supply of blood to meet the metabolic needs of the body.

B. Types
1. Left-sided heart failure
   a. Left ventricular damage causes blood to back up through the left atrium and into the pulmonary veins. Increased pressure causes transudation into the interstitial tissues of the lungs with resultant pulmonary congestion.
   b. Caused by left ventricular damage (usually due to an MI), hypertension, ischemic heart disease, aortic valve disease, mitral stenosis
   c. Assessment findings
      1) Dyspnea, orthopnea, PND, tiredness, muscle weakness, cough
      2) Tachycardia, PMI displaced laterally, possible $S_3$, bronchial wheezing, rales or crackles, cyanosis, pallor
      3) Decreased $pO_2$, increased $pCO_2$
      4) Diagnostic tests
         a) Chest X-ray: shows cardiac hypertrophy
         b) PAP and PCWP usually increased; however, this is dependent on the degree of heart failure
      5) Echocardiography: shows increased size of cardiac chambers
2. Right-sided heart failure
   a. Weakened right ventricle is unable to pump blood into the pulmonary system; systemic venous congestion occurs as pressure builds up.
   b. Caused by left-sided heart failure, right ventricular infarction, atherosclerotic heart disease, COPD, pulmonic stenosis, pulmonary embolism.
   c. Assessment findings
      1) Anorexia, nausea, weight gain
      2) Dependent pitting edema, jugular venous distension, bounding pulses, hepatomegaly, cool extremities, oliguria
      3) Elevated CVP, decreased $pO_2$, increased ALT (SGPT)
      4) Diagnostic tests
         a) Chest X-ray: reveals cardiac hypertrophy
         b) Echocardiography: indicates increased size of cardiac chambers

3. High-output failure
    a. Cardiac output is adequate but exceeded by the metabolic needs of the tissues; the exorbitant demands made on the heart eventually cause ventricular failure.
    b. Caused by hyperthyroidism, anemia, AV fistula, pregnancy
C. Medical management (all types)
    1. Determination and elimination/control of underlying cause
    2. Drug therapy: digitalis preparations, diuretics, vasodilators
    3. Sodium-restricted diet to decrease fluid retention
    4. If medical therapies unsuccessful, mechanical assist devices (intra-aortic balloon pump), cardiac transplantation, or mechanical hearts may be employed.
D. Nursing interventions
    1. Monitor respiratory status and provide adequate ventilation (when HF progresses to pulmonary edema).
        a. Administer oxygen therapy.
        b. Maintain client in semi- or high-Fowler's position.
        c. Monitor ABGs.
        d. Assess for breath sounds, noting any changes.
    2. Provide physical and emotional rest.
        a. Constantly assess level of anxiety.
        b. Maintain bed rest with limited activity.
        c. Maintain quiet, relaxed environment.
        d. Organize nursing care around rest periods.
    3. Increase cardiac output.
        a. Administer digitalis as ordered and monitor effects.
        b. Monitor ECG and hemodynamic monitoring.
        c. Administer vasodilators as ordered.
        d. Monitor vital signs.
    4. Reduce/eliminate edema.
        a. Administer diuretics as ordered.
        b. Daily weights.
        c. Maintain accurate I&O.
        d. Assess for peripheral edema.
        e. Measure abdominal girths daily.
        f. Monitor electrolyte levels.
        g. Monitor CVP and Swan-Ganz readings.
        h. Provide sodium-restricted diet as ordered.
        i. Provide meticulous skin care.
    5. Provide client teaching and discharge planning concerning
        a. Need to monitor self daily for signs and symptoms of HF (pedal edema, weight gain of 1–2 kg in a 2-day period, dyspnea, loss of appetite, cough)
        b. Medication regimen including name, purpose, dosage, frequency, and side effects (digitalis, diuretics)

c. Prescribed dietary plan (low sodium; small, frequent meals)
d. Need to avoid fatigue and plan for rest periods

## Pulmonary Edema

A. General information
    1. A medical emergency that occurs when the capillary pressure within the lungs becomes so great that fluid moves from the intravascular space into the alveoli, bronchi, and bronchioles. Death occurs by suffocation if this condition is untreated.
    2. Caused by left-sided heart failure, rapid administration of IV fluids.
B. Medical management
    1. Oxygen therapy
    2. Endotracheal/nasotracheal intubation (possible)
    3. Drug therapy
        a. Morphine sulfate to induce vasodilation and decrease anxiety; 5 mg IV, administer slowly
        b. Digitalis to improve cardiac output
        c. Diuretics (furosemide [Lasix] is drug of choice) to relieve fluid retention
        d. Aminophylline to relieve bronchospasm and increase cardiac output; 250–500 mg IV, administer slowly
        e. Vasodilators (nitroglycerin, isosorbide dinitrate) to dilate the vessels, thereby reducing amount of blood returned to the heart
    4. Rotating tourniquets or phlebotomy
C. Assessment findings
    1. Dyspnea
    2. Cough with large amounts of blood-tinged sputum
    3. Tachycardia, pallor, wheezing, rales or crackles, diaphoresis
    4. Restlessness, fear/anxiety
    5. Jugular vein distension
    6. Decreased $pO_2$, increased $pCO_2$, elevated CVP
D. Nursing interventions
    1. Assist with intubation (if necessary) and monitor mechanical ventilation.
    2. Administer oxygen by mask in high concentrations (40–60%) if not intubated.
    3. Place client in semi-Fowler's position or over bedside table to ease dyspnea.
    4. Administer medications as ordered.
    5. Assist with phlebotomy (removal of 300–500 mL of blood from a peripheral vein) if performed.
    6. CVP/hemodynamic monitoring.
    7. Provide client teaching and discharge planning concerning
        a. Prescribed medications, including name, purpose, schedule, dosage, and side effects

**b.** Dietary restrictions: low sodium, low cholesterol
  **c.** Importance of adhering to planned rest periods with gradual progressive increase in activities
  **d.** Daily weights
  **e.** Need to report the following symptoms to physician immediately: dyspnea, persistent productive cough, pedal edema, restlessness

## Pacemakers

**A.** General information
  1. A pacemaker is an electronic device that provides repetitive electrical stimulation to the cardiac musculature to control the heart rate.
  2. Artificial pacing system consists of a battery-powered generator and a pacing wire that delivers the stimulus to the heart.

**B.** Indications for use
  1. Adams-Stokes attack
  2. Acute MI with Mobitz II AV block
  3. Third-degree AV block with slow ventricular rate
  4. Right bundle branch block
  5. New left bundle branch block
  6. Symptomatic sinus bradycardia
  7. Sick sinus syndrome
  8. Arrhythmias (during or after cardiac surgery)
  9. Drug-resistant tachyarrhythmia

**C.** Modes of pacing
  1. Fixed rate: pacemaker fires electrical stimuli at preset rate, regardless of the client's rate and rhythm.
  2. Demand: pacemaker produces electrical stimuli only when the client's own heart rate drops below the preset rate per minute on the generator.

**D.** Types of pacemakers
  1. Temporary
    **a.** Used in emergency situations and performed via an endocardial (transvenous) or transthoracic approach to the myocardium.
    **b.** Performed at bedside or using fluoroscopy.
  2. Permanent
    **a.** Endocardial or transvenous procedure involves passing endocardial lead into right ventricle with subcutaneous implantation of pulse generator into right or left subclavian areas. Usually done under local anesthesia.
    **b.** Epicardial or myocardial method involves passing the electrode transthoracically to the myocardium where it is sutured in place. The pulse generator is implanted into the abdominal wall.

**E.** Nursing interventions
  1. Assess pacemaker function
    **a.** Monitor heart rate, noting deviations from the preset rate.
    **b.** Observe the presence of pacemaker spikes on ECG tracing or cardiac monitor; spike before P wave with atrial pacemaker; spike before QRS complex with ventricular pacemaker
    **c.** Assess for signs of pacemaker malfunction, such as weakness, fainting, dizziness, or hypotension.
  2. Maintain the integrity of the system
    **a.** Ensure that catheter terminals are attached securely to the pulse generator (temporary pacemaker)
    **b.** Attach pulse generator to client securely to prevent accidental dislodgment (temporary pacemaker)
  3. Provide safety and comfort
    **a.** Provide safe environment by properly grounding all equipment in the room.
    **b.** Monitor electrolyte level periodically, particularly potassium.
  4. Prevent infection
    **a.** Assess vital signs, particularly temperature changes.
    **b.** Assess catheter insertion site daily for signs of infection.
    **c.** Maintain sterile dressing over catheter insertion site.

**F.** Provide client teaching and discharge planning concerning
  1. Fundamental concepts of cardiac physiology
  2. Daily pulse check for 1 minute
  3. Need to report immediately any sudden slowing or increase in pulse rate
  4. Importance of adhering to weekly monitoring schedule during first month after implantation and when battery depletion is anticipated (depending on type of battery)
  5. Wear loose-fitting clothing around the area of the pacemaker for comfort
  6. Notify physician of any pain or redness over incision site
  7. Avoid trauma to area of pulse generator
  8. Avoid heavy contact sports
  9. Carry an identification card/bracelet that indicates physician's name, type and model number of pacemaker, manufacturer's name, pacemaker rate
  10. Display identification card and request scanning by hand scanner when going through weapons detector at airport
  11. Remember that periodic hospitalization is necessary for battery changes/pacemaker unit replacement

## Cardiac Arrest

**A.** General information: sudden, unexpected cessation of breathing and adequate circulation of blood by the heart
**B.** Medical management
  1. Cardiopulmonary resuscitation (CPR)

2. Drug therapy
  a. Lidocaine, procainamide, verapamil for ventricular tachycardia
  b. Dopamine (Intropin), isoproterenol (Isuprel), norepinephrine (Levophed): see also Drugs Used to Treat Shock, Table 4-9
  c. Epinephrine to enhance myocardial automaticity, excitability, conductivity, and contractility
  d. Atropine sulfate to reduce vagus nerve's control over the heart, thus increasing the heart rate
  e. Sodium bicarbonate to correct respiratory and metabolic acidosis
  f. Calcium chloride: calcium ions help the heart beat more effectively by enhancing the myocardium's contractile force
3. Defibrillation (electrical countershock)
C. Assessment findings: unresponsiveness, cessation of respiration, pallor, cyanosis, absence of heart sounds/blood pressure/palpable pulses, dilation of pupils, ventricular fibrillation or asystole (if client on a monitor)
D. Nursing interventions: monitored arrest caused by ventricular fibrillation
1. CPR until defibrillation possible.
2. If defibrillation unsuccessful, continue CPR and assist with administration of and monitor effects of additional emergency drugs.
3. If defibrillation successful, monitor client status.

### Cardiopulmonary Resuscitation (CPR)

A. General information: process of externally supporting the circulation and respiration of a person who has had a cardiac arrest
B. Nursing interventions: unwitnessed cardiac arrest
1. Assess LOC.
  a. Shake victim's shoulder and shout.
  b. If no response, summon help.
2. Position victim supine on a firm surface.
3. Open airway.
  a. Use head tilt, chin lift maneuver.
  b. Place ear over nose and mouth.
    1) Look to see if chest is moving.
    2) Listen for escape of air.
    3) Feel for movement of air against face.
  c. If no respiration, proceed to #4.
4. Ventilate twice, allowing for deflation between breaths.
5. Assess circulation: in adults palpate for carotid pulse; if not present, proceed to #6.
6. Initiate external cardiac compressions
  a. Proper placement of hands: lower half of the sternum
  b. Depth of compressions: 1½–2 inches for adults
  c. 30 compressions (at rate of 80–100 per minute) with 2 ventilations

7. According to the American Heart Association in March 2008, new guidelines were issued that stressed the importance of chest compressions, especially if the bystander was not trained to perform rescue breathing.

## Endocarditis

A. General information
1. Inflammation of the endocardium; platelets and fibrin deposit on the mitral and/or aortic valves causing deformity, insufficiency, or stenosis.
2. Caused by bacterial infection: commonly *S. aureus, S. viridans*, B-hemolytic streptococcus, gonococcus
3. Precipitating factors: rheumatic heart disease, open-heart surgery procedures, GU/Ob-Gyn instrumentation/surgery, dental extractions, invasive monitoring, septic thrombophlebitis
B. Medical management
1. Drug therapy
  a. Antibiotics specific to sensitivity of organism cultured
  b. Penicillin G and streptomycin if organism not known
  c. Antipyretics
2. Cardiac surgery to replace affected valve
C. Assessment findings
1. Fever, malaise, fatigue, dyspnea and cough (if extensive valvular damage), acute upper quadrant pain (if splenic involvement), joint pain
2. Petechiae, murmurs, edema (if extensive valvular damage), splenomegaly, hemiplegia and confusion (if cerebral infarction), hematuria (if renal infarction)
3. Elevated WBC and ESR, decreased Hgb and Hct
4. Diagnostic tests: positive blood culture for causative organism
D. Nursing interventions
1. Administer antibiotics as ordered to control the infectious process.
2. Control temperature elevation by administration of antipyretics.
3. Assess for vascular complications (see Thrombophlebitis and Pulmonary Embolism).
4. Provide client teaching and discharge planning concerning
  a. Types of procedures/treatments (e.g., tooth extractions, GU instrumentation) that increase the chances of recurrences
  b. Antibiotic therapy, including name, purpose, dose, frequency, side effects
  c. Signs and symptoms of recurrent endocarditis (persistent fever, fatigue, chills, anorexia, joint pain)
  d. Avoidance of individuals with known infections

## Pericarditis

A. General information
1. An inflammation of the visceral and parietal pericardium
2. Caused by a bacterial, viral, or fungal infection; collagen diseases; trauma; acute MI; neoplasms; uremia; radiation therapy; drugs (procainamide, hydralazine, doxorubicin HCl [Adriamycin])

B. Medical management
1. Determination and elimination/control of underlying cause
2. Drug therapy
   a. Medication for pain relief
   b. Corticosteroids, salicylates (aspirin), and indomethacin (Indocin) to reduce inflammation
   c. Specific antibiotic therapy against the causative organism may be indicated.

C. Assessment findings
1. Chest pain with deep inspiration (relieved by sitting up), cough, hemoptysis, malaise
2. Tachycardia, fever, pleural friction rub, cyanosis or pallor, accentuated component of $S_2$, pulsus paradoxus, jugular vein distension
3. Elevated WBC and ESR, normal or elevated AST (SGOT)
4. Diagnostic tests
   a. Chest X-ray may show increased heart size if effusion occurs
   b. ECG changes: ST elevation (precordial leads and 2- or 3-limb heads), T wave inversion

D. Nursing interventions
1. Ensure comfort: bed rest with semi- or high-Fowler's position.
2. Monitor hemodynamic parameters carefully.
3. Administer medications as ordered and monitor effects.
4. Provide client teaching and discharge planning concerning:
   a. Signs and symptoms of pericarditis indicative of a recurrence (chest pain that is intensified by inspiration and position changes, fever, cough)
   b. Medication regimen including name, purpose, dosage, frequency, side effects

## Cardiac Tamponade

A. General information
1. An accumulation of fluid/blood in the pericardium that prevents adequate ventricular filling; without emergency treatment client will die.
2. Caused by blunt or penetrating chest trauma, malignant pericardial effusion; can be a complication of cardiac surgery.

B. Medical management: emergency treatment of choice is pericardiocentesis (insertion of a needle into the pericardial sac to aspirate fluid/blood and relieve the pressure on the heart)

C. Assessment findings
1. Chest pain
2. Hypotension, distended neck veins, tachycardia, muffled or distant heart sounds, paradoxical pulse, pericardial friction rub
3. Elevated CVP, decreased Hgb and Hct if massive hemorrhage
4. Diagnostic test: chest X-ray reveals enlarged heart and widened mediastinum.

D. Nursing interventions
1. Administer oxygen therapy
2. Monitor CVP/IVs closely
3. Assist with pericardiocentesis
   a. Monitor ECG, blood pressure, and pulse.
   b. Assess aspirated fluid for color, consistency.
   c. Send specimen to lab immediately.

## Cardiogenic Shock

See Table 4-9.

# The Blood Vessels

## Hypertension

A. General information
1. According to the World Health Organization, hypertension is a persistent elevation of the systolic blood pressure above 140 mm Hg and of the diastolic above 90 mm Hg.
2. Types
   a. Essential (primary, idiopathic): marked by loss of elastic tissue and arteriosclerotic changes in the aorta and larger vessels coupled with decreased caliber of the arterioles
   b. Benign: a moderate rise in blood pressure marked by a gradual onset and prolonged course
   c. Malignant: characterized by a rapid onset and short dramatic course with a diastolic blood pressure of more than 150 mm Hg
   d. Secondary: elevation of the blood pressure as a result of another disease such as renal parenchymal disease, Cushing's disease, pheochromocytoma, primary aldosteronism, coarctation of the aorta
3. Essential hypertension usually occurs between ages 30 and 50; more common in men over 35, women over 45; African-Americans affected twice as often as white Americans
4. Risk factors for essential hypertension include positive family history, obesity, stress, cigarette smoking, hypercholesteremia, increased sodium intake

B. Medical management
1. Diet and weight reduction (restricted sodium, kcal, cholesterol)

2. Lifestyle changes: alcohol moderation, exercise regimen, cessation of smoking
3. Antihypertensive drug therapy (see Table 2-17)

C. Assessment findings
1. Pain similar to anginal pain; pain in calves of legs after ambulation or exercise (intermittent claudication); severe occipital headaches, particularly in the morning; polyuria; nocturia; fatigue; dizziness; epistaxis; dyspnea on exertion
2. Blood pressure consistently above 140/90, retinal hemorrhages and exudates, edema of extremities (indicative of right-sided heart failure)
3. Rise in systolic blood pressure from supine to standing position (indicative of essential hypertension)
4. Diagnostic tests; elevated serum uric acid, sodium, cholesterol levels

D. Nursing interventions
1. Record baseline blood pressure in three positions (lying, sitting, standing: also known as "orthostatics") and in both arms.
2. Continuously assess blood pressure and report any variables that relate to changes in blood pressure (positioning, restlessness).
3. Administer antihypertensive agents as ordered; monitor closely and assess for side effects.
4. Monitor intake and hourly outputs.
5. Provide client teaching and discharge planning concerning
   a. Risk factor identification and development/implementation of methods to modify them
   b. Restricted sodium, kcal, cholesterol diet; include family in teaching
   c. Antihypertensive drug regimen (include family); see Table 2-17
      1) Names, actions, dosages, and side effects of prescribed medications
      2) Take drugs at regular times and avoid omission of any doses
      3) Never abruptly discontinue the drug therapy
      4) Supplement diet with potassium-rich foods if taking potassium-wasting diuretics
      5) Avoid hot baths, alcohol, or strenuous exercise within 3 hours of taking medications that cause vasodilation
   d. Development of a graduated exercise program
   e. Importance of routine follow-up care

## Arteriosclerosis Obliterans

A. General information
1. A chronic occlusive arterial disease that may affect the abdominal aorta or the lower extremities. The obstruction to blood flow with resultant ischemia usually affects the femoral, popliteal, aortal, and iliac arteries.
2. Occurs most often in men ages 50–60
3. Caused by atherosclerosis
4. Risk factors: cigarette smoking, hyperlipidemia, hypertension, diabetes mellitus

B. Medical management
1. Drug therapy
   a. Vasodilators: papaverine, isoxsuprine HCl (Vasodilan), nylidrin HCl (Arlidin), nicotinyl alcohol (Roniacol), cyclandelate (Cyclospasmol), tolazoline HCl (Priscoline) to improve arterial circulation; effectiveness questionable
   b. Analgesics to relieve ischemic pain
   c. Anticoagulants to prevent thrombus formation
   d. Lipid-reducing drug: cholestyramine (Questran), colestipol HCl (Cholestid), dextrothyroxine sodium (Choloxin), clofibrate (Atromid-S), gemfibrozil (Lopid), niacin, lovastatin (Mevacor) (see Unit 2)
2. Surgery: bypass grafting, endarterectomy, balloon catheter dilation; lumbar sympathectomy (to increase blood flow), amputation may be necessary

C. Assessment findings
1. Pain, both intermittent claudication and rest pain, numbness or tingling of the toes
2. Pallor after 1–2 minutes of elevating feet, and dependent hyperemia/rubor; diminished or absent dorsalis pedis, posterior tibial and femoral pulses; trophic changes; shiny, taut skin with hair loss on lower legs
3. Diagnostic tests
   a. Oscillometry may reveal decrease in pulse volume
   b. Doppler ultrasound reveals decreased blood flow through affected vessels
   c. Angiography reveals location and extent of obstructive process
4. Elevated serum triglycerides; sodium

D. Nursing interventions
1. Encourage slow, progressive physical activity (out of bed at least 3–4 times per day, walking 2 times per day).
2. Administer medications as ordered.
3. Assist with Buerger-Allen exercises 4 times a day.
   a. Client lies with legs elevated above heart for 2–3 minutes
   b. Client sits on edge of bed with legs and feet dependent and exercises feet and toes—upward and downward, inward and outward—for 3 minutes
   c. Client lies flat with legs at heart level for 5 minutes
4. Assess for sensory function and trophic changes.
5. Protect client from injury.

6. Provide client teaching and discharge planning concerning:
   a. Restricted kcal, low-saturated-fat diet; include family
   b. Importance of continuing with established exercise program
   c. Measures to reduce stress (relaxation techniques, biofeedback)
   d. Importance of avoiding smoking, constrictive clothing, standing in any position for a long time, injury
   e. Importance of foot care, immediately taking care of cuts, wounds, injuries
7. Prepare client for surgery if necessary.

## Thromboangiitis Obliterans (Buerger's Disease)

A. General information
   1. Acute, inflammatory disorder affecting medium/smaller arteries and veins of the lower extremities. Occurs as focal, obstructive process; results in occlusion of a vessel with subsequent development of collateral circulation.
   2. Most often affects men ages 25–40.
   3. Disease is idiopathic; high incidence among smokers.
B. Medical management: see Arteriosclerosis Obliterans, only really effective treatment is cessation of smoking.
C. Assessment findings
   1. Intermittent claudication, sensitivity to cold (skin of extremity may at first be white, changing to blue, then red)
   2. Decreased or absent peripheral pulses (posterior tibial and dorsalis pedis), trophic changes, ulceration and gangrene (advanced)
   3. Diagnostic tests: same as in Arteriosclerosis Obliterans except no elevation in serum triglycerides
D. Nursing interventions
   1. Prepare client for surgery.
   2. Provide client teaching and discharge planning concerning:
      a. Drug regimen (vasodilators, anticoagulants, analgesics) to include names, dosages, frequency, and side effects
      b. Need to avoid trauma to the affected extremity
      c. Need to maintain warmth, especially in cold weather
      d. Importance of stopping smoking.

## Raynaud's Phenomenon

A. General information
   1. Intermittent episode of arterial spasms, most frequently involving the fingers
   2. Most often affects women between the teenage years and age 40
   3. Cause unknown

4. Predisposing factors: collagen diseases (systemic lupus erythematosus, rheumatoid arthritis), trauma (e.g., from typing, piano playing, operating a chain saw)
B. Medical management: vasodilators, catecholamine-depleting antihypertensive drugs (reserpine, guanethidine monosulfate [Ismelin])
C. Assessment findings
   1. Coldness, numbness, tingling in one or more digits; pain (usually precipitated by exposure to cold, emotional upsets, tobacco use)
   2. Intermittent color changes (pallor, cyanosis, rubor); small ulcerations and gangrene at tips of digits (advanced)
D. Nursing interventions
   1. Provide client teaching concerning:
      a. Importance of stopping smoking
      b. Need to maintain warmth, especially in cold weather
      c. Need to use gloves when handling cold objects/opening freezer or refrigerator door
      d. Drug regimen

## Aneurysms

An aneurysm is a sac formed by dilation of an artery secondary to weakness and stretching of the arterial wall. The dilation may involve one or all layers of the arterial wall.

### Classification

A. Fusiform: uniform spindle shape involving the entire circumference of the artery
B. Saccular: outpouching on one side only, affecting only part of the arterial circumference
C. Dissecting: separation of the arterial wall layers to form a cavity that fills with blood
D. False: the vessel wall is disrupted, blood escapes into surrounding area but is held in place by surrounding tissue

### Thoracic Aortic Aneurysm

A. General information
   1. An aneurysm, usually fusiform or dissecting, in the descending, ascending, or transverse section of the thoracic aorta
   2. Usually occurs in men ages 50–70
   3. Caused by arteriosclerosis, infection, syphilis, hypertension
B. Medical management
   1. Control of underlying hypertension
   2. Surgery: resection of the aneurysm and replacement with a Teflon/Dacron graft; clients will need extracorporeal circulation (heart-lung machine).
C. Assessment findings
   1. Often asymptomatic
   2. Deep, diffuse chest pain; hoarseness; dysphagia; dyspnea

3. Pallor, diaphoresis, distended neck veins, edema of head and arms
4. Diagnostic tests
   a. Aortography shows exact location of the aneurysm
   b. X-rays: chest film reveals abnormal widening of aorta; abdominal film may show calcification within walls of aneurysm
D. Nursing interventions: see Cardiac Surgery.

*Abdominal Aortic Aneurysm*

A. General information
   1. Most aneurysms of this type are saccular or dissecting and develop just below the renal arteries but above the iliac bifurcation
   2. Occur most often in men over age 60
   3. Caused by atherosclerosis, hypertension, trauma, syphilis, other types of infectious processes
B. Medical management: surgical resection of the lesion and replacement with a graft (extracorporeal circulation not needed)
C. Assessment findings
   1. Severe mid- to low-abdominal pain, low-back pain
   2. Mass in the periumbilical area or slightly to the left of the midline with bruits heard over the mass
   3. Pulsating abdominal mass
   4. Diminished femoral pulses
   5. Diagnostic tests: same as for thoracic aneurysms
D. Nursing interventions: preoperative
   1. Prepare client for surgery: routine pre-op care.
   2. Assess rate, rhythm, character of the peripheral pulses and mark all distal pulses.
E. Nursing interventions: postoperative
   1. Provide routine post-op care.
   2. Monitor the following parameters:
      a. Hourly circulation checks noting rate, rhythm, character of all pulses distal to the graft
      b. CVP/PAP/PCWP
      c. Hourly outputs through Foley catheter (report less than 30 mL/hour)
      d. Daily BUN/creatinine/electrolyte levels
      e. Presence of back pain (may indicate retroperitoneal hemorrhage)
      f. IV fluids
      g. Neuro status including LOC, pupil size and response to light, hand grasp, movement of extremities
      h. Heart rate and rhythm via monitor
   3. Maintain client flat in bed without sharp flexion of hip/knee (avoid pressure on femoral/popliteal arteries).
   4. Auscultate lungs and encourage turning, coughing, and deep breathing.
   5. Assess for signs and symptoms of paralytic ileus.

6. Prevent thrombophlebitis.
   a. Encourage client to dorsiflex foot while in bed.
   b. Use elastic stockings or sequential compression devices as ordered.
   c. Assess for signs and symptoms (see Thrombophlebitis).
7. Provide client teaching and discharge planning concerning
   a. Importance of changes in color/temperature of extremities
   b. Avoidance of prolonged sitting, standing, and smoking
   c. Need for a gradual progressive activity regimen
   d. Adherence to low-cholesterol, low-saturated fat diet
   e. Adherence to activity restrictions and avoid lifting heavy objects (limit 15 to 20 pounds).

*Femoral-Popliteal Bypass Surgery*

A. General information
   1. Most common type of surgery to correct arterial obstructions of the lower extremities
   2. Procedure involves bypassing the occluded vessel with a graft, such as Teflon, Dacron, or an autogenous artery or vein (saphenous).
B. Nursing interventions: preoperative
   1. Provide routine pre-op care.
   2. Monitor and correct potassium imbalances to prevent cardiac arrhythmias.
   3. Assess for focus of infection (infected tooth) or infectious processes (urinary tract infections).
   4. Mark distal peripheral pulses.
C. Nursing interventions: postoperative
   1. Provide routine post-op care.
   2. Assess the following
      a. Circulation, noting rate, rhythm, and quality of peripheral pulses distal to the graft; color; temperature; and sensation
      b. Signs and symptoms of thrombophlebitis
      c. Neuro checks
      d. Hourly outputs
      e. CVP
      f. Wound drainage, noting amount, color, and characteristics
   3. Elevate legs above the level of the heart.
   4. Encourage turning, coughing, and deep breathing while splinting incision.

## Venous Stasis Ulcers

A. General information
   1. Usually a complication of thrombophlebitis and varicose veins.
   2. Ulcers result from incompetent valves in the veins, causing high pressure with rupture of small skin veins and venules.

**B.** Medical management
  1. Antibiotic therapy (specific to organism cultured); topical bacteriocidal solutions
  2. Skin grafting
  3. Enzymatic or surgical debridement
**C.** Assessment findings
  1. Pain in the limb in dependent position or during ambulation
  2. Skin of leathery texture, brownish pigment around ankles; positive pulses but edema makes palpation difficult.
**D.** Nursing interventions
  1. Provide bed rest, elevating extremity.
  2. Provide a balanced diet with added protein and vitamin supplements.
  3. Administer antibiotics as ordered to control infection.
  4. Promote healing by cleansing ulcer with prescribed agents.
  5. Provide client teaching and discharge planning concerning
      **a.** Importance of avoiding trauma to affected limb
      **b.** Skin care regimen
      **c.** Use of elastic support stockings (after ulcer is healed)
      **d.** Need for planned rest periods with elevation of the extremities
  6. Adherence to balanced diet with vitamin supplements.

## Thrombophlebitis

**A.** General information
  1. Inflammation of the vessel wall with formation of a clot (thrombus); may affect superficial or deep veins.
  2. Most frequent veins affected are the saphenous, femoral, and popliteal.
  3. Can result in damage to the surrounding tissues, ischemia, and necrosis.
  4. Risk factors: obesity, HF, prolonged immobility, MI, pregnancy, oral contraceptives, trauma, sepsis, cigarette smoking, dehydration, severe anemias, venous cannulation, complication of surgery.
**B.** Medical management
  1. Anticoagulant therapy
      **a.** Heparin
          1) Blocks conversion of prothrombin to thrombin and reduces formation or extension of thrombus
          2) Side effects: spontaneous bleeding, injection site reactions, ecchymoses, tissue irritation and sloughing, reversible transient alopecia, cyanosis, pain in arms or legs, thrombocytopenia
      **b.** Warfarin (Coumadin)
          1) Blocks prothrombin synthesis by interfering with vitamin K synthesis

  2) Side effects
      **a)** GI: anorexia, nausea and vomiting, diarrhea, stomatitis
      **b)** Hypersensitivity: dermatitis, urticaria, pruritus, fever
      **c)** Other: transient hair loss, burning sensation of feet, bleeding complications
  2. Surgery
      **a.** Vein ligation and stripping
      **b.** Venous thrombectomy: removal of a clot in the iliofemoral region
      **c.** Plication of the inferior vena cava: insertion of an umbrella-like prosthesis into the lumen of the vena cava to filter incoming clots. (See Figure 4-10).
**C.** Assessment findings
  1. Pain in the affected extremity
  2. Superficial vein: tenderness, redness, induration along course of the vein
  3. Deep vein: swelling, venous distension of limb, tenderness over involved vein, positive Homan's sign, cyanosis

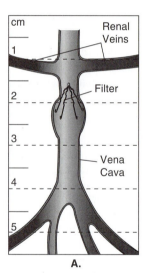

**A.**

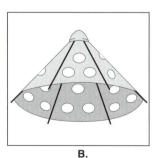

**B.**

**Figure 4-10** Vena caval filters to prevent embolus from traveling to the lungs, heart, or brain. (A) Greenfield; (B) Umbrella

4. Elevated WBC and ESR
5. Diagnostic tests
   a. Venography (phlebography): increased uptake of radioactive material
   b. Doppler ultrasonography: impairment of blood flow ahead of thrombus
   c. Venous pressure measurements: high in affected limb until collateral circulation is developed
D. Nursing interventions
   1. Provide bed rest, elevating involved extremity to increase venous return and decrease edema.
   2. Apply continuous warm, moist soaks to decrease lymphatic congestion.
   3. Administer anticoagulants as ordered
      a. Heparin
         1) Monitor PTT; dosage should be adjusted to keep PTT between 1.5–2.5 times normal control level.
         2) Use infusion pump to administer IV heparin.
         3) Ensure proper injection technique.
            a) Use 26- or 27-gauge syringe with ½–⅝-inch needle, inject into fatty layer of abdomen above iliac crest.
            b) Avoid injecting within 2 inches of umbilicus.
            c) Insert needle at 45–90° to skin.
            d) Do not withdraw plunger to assess blood return.
            e) Apply gentle pressure after removal of needle, avoid massage.
         4) Assess for increased bleeding tendencies (hematuria; hematemesis; bleeding gums; petechiae of soft palate, conjunctiva, retina; ecchymoses, epistaxis, bloody sputum, melena) and instruct client to observe for and report these.
         5) Have antidote (protamine sulfate) available.
         6) Instruct client to avoid aspirin, antihistamines, and cough preparations containing glyceryl guaiacolate, and to obtain physician's permission before using other OTC drugs.
      b. Warfarin (Coumadin)
         1) Assess PT daily; dosage should be adjusted to maintain PT at 1.5–2.5 times normal control level; INR of 2.
         2) Obtain careful medication history (there are many drug-drug interactions).
         3) Advise client to withhold dose and notify physician immediately if bleeding or signs of bleeding occur (see Heparin).
         4) Instruct client to use a soft toothbrush and to floss gently.
         5) Have antidote (vitamin K) available.
         6) Alert client to factors that may affect the anticoagulant response (high-fat diet or sudden increases in vitamin K-rich foods).
         7) Instruct client to wear Medic-Alert bracelet.
   4. Assess vital signs every 4 hours.
   5. Monitor for chest pain or shortness of breath (possible pulmonary embolism).
   6. Measure thighs, calves, ankles, and instep every morning.
   7. Provide client teaching and discharge planning concerning:
      a. Need to avoid standing, sitting for long periods; constrictive clothing; crossing legs at the knees; smoking; oral contraceptives
      b. Importance of adequate hydration to prevent hypercoagulability
      c. Use of elastic stockings when ambulatory
      d. Importance of planned rest periods with elevation of the feet
      e. Drug regimen
      f. Plan for exercise/activity
         1) Begin with dorsiflexion of the feet while sitting or lying down
         2) Swim several times weekly
         3) Gradually increase walking distance
      g. Importance of weight reduction if obese

## Pulmonary Embolism

A. General information
   1. Most pulmonary emboli arise as detached portions of venous thrombi formed in the deep veins of the legs, right side of the heart, or pelvic area.
   2. Distribution of emboli is related to blood flow; emboli involve the lower lobes of the lung because of higher blood flow.
   3. Embolic obstruction to blood flow increases venous pressure in the pulmonary artery and pulmonary hypertension.
   4. Risk factors: venous thrombosis, immobility, pre- and post-op states, trauma, pregnancy, HF, use of oral contraceptives, obesity
B. Medical management
   1. Drug therapy
      a. Anticoagulants (see Thrombophlebitis)
      b. Thrombolytics: streptokinase or urokinase
      c. Dextran 70 to decrease blood viscosity and aggregation of blood cells
      d. Narcotics for pain relief
      e. Vasopressors (in the presence of shock)
   2. Surgery: embolectomy (surgical removal of an embolus from the pulmonary arteries)
C. Assessment findings
   1. Chest pain (pleuritic), severe dyspnea, feeling of impending doom

2. Tachypnea, tachycardia, anxiety, hemoptysis, shock symptoms (if massive)
3. Decreased $pCO_2$; increased pH (due to hyperventilation)
4. Increased temperature
5. Intensified pulmonic $S_2$; rales or crackles
6. Diagnostic tests
    a. Pulmonary angiography: reveals location/extent of embolism
    b. Lung scan reveals adequacy/inadequacy of pulmonary circulation
D. Nursing interventions
1. Administer medications as ordered; monitor effects and side effects.
2. Administer oxygen therapy to correct hypoxemia.
3. Assist with turning, coughing, deep breathing, and passive ROM exercises.
4. Provide adequate hydration to prevent hypercoagulability.
5. Offer support/reassurance to client/family.
6. Elevate head of bed to relieve dyspnea.
7. Provide client teaching and discharge planning: same as for thrombophlebitis.

## Varicose Veins

A. General information
1. Dilated veins that occur most often in the lower extremities and trunk. As the vessel dilates, the valves become stretched and incompetent with resultant venous pooling/edema
2. Most common between ages 30 and 50
3. Predisposing factor: congenital weakness of the veins, thrombophlebitis, pregnancy, obesity, heart disease
B. Medical management: vein ligation (involves ligating the saphenous vein where it joins the femoral vein and stripping the saphenous vein system from groin to ankle)
C. Assessment findings
1. Pain after prolonged standing (relieved by elevation)
2. Swollen, dilated, tortuous skin veins
3. Diagnostic tests
    a. Trendelenburg test: varicose veins distend very quickly (less than 35 seconds)
    b. Doppler ultrasound: decreased or no blood flow heard after calf or thigh compression
D. Nursing interventions
1. Elevate legs above heart level.
2. Measure circumference of ankle and calf daily.
3. Apply knee-length elastic stockings.
4. Provide adequate rest.
5. Prepare client for vein ligation, if necessary.
    a. Provide routine pre-op care; usually outpatient surgery.
    b. In addition to routine post-op care:
        1) Keep affected extremity elevated above the level of the heart to prevent edema.

2) Apply elastic bandages and stockings, which should be removed every 8 hours for short periods and reapplied.
3) Assist out of bed within 24 hours, ensuring that elastic stockings are applied.
4) Assess for increased bleeding, particularly in the groin area.
6. Provide client teaching and discharge planning: same as for Thrombophlebitis.

## Amputation

A. General information
1. Surgical procedure done for peripheral vascular disease if medical management is ineffective and the symptoms become worse.
2. The level of amputation is determined by the extent of the disease process.
    a. Above knee (AKA): performed between the lower third to the middle of the thigh
    b. Below knee (BKA): usually done in middle third of leg, leaving a stump of 12.5–17.5 cm
B. Nursing interventions: preoperative
1. Provide routine pre-op care.
2. Offer support/encouragement and accept client's response of anger/grief.
3. Discuss
    a. Rehabilitation program and use of prosthesis
    b. Upper extremity exercises such as push-ups in bed
    c. Crutch walking
    d. Amputation dressings/cast
    e. Phantom limb sensation as a normal occurrence
C. Nursing interventions: postoperative
1. Provide routine post-op care.
2. Prevent hip/knee contractures.
3. Avoid letting client sit in chair with hips flexed for long periods of time.
4. Have client assume prone position several times a day and position hip in extension (unless otherwise ordered).
5. Avoid elevation of the stump after 12–24 hours.
6. Observe stump dressing for signs of hemorrhage and mark outside of dressing so rate of bleeding can be assessed.
7. Administer pain medication as ordered.
8. Ensure that stump bandages fit tightly and are applied properly to enhance prosthesis fitting.
9. Initiate active ROM exercises of all joints (when medically advised), crutch walking, and arm/shoulder exercises.
10. Provide stump care.
    a. Inspect daily for signs of skin irritation.
    b. Wash thoroughly daily with warm water and bacteriostatic soap; rinse and dry thoroughly.
    c. Avoid use of irritating substances such as lotions, alcohol, powders.

## Sample Questions

163. An adult is admitted to the coronary care unit to rule out a myocardial infarction. The client states, "I am not sure if it is just angina, and I cannot understand the difference between angina and heart attack pain." Which response is most appropriate for the nurse to make?
    1. Anginal pain usually stops after resting.
    2. Anginal pain produces clenching of the fists over the chest while acute MI pain does not.
    3. Anginal pain requires morphine for relief.
    4. Anginal pain radiates to the left arm while acute MI pain does not.

164. An adult woman is admitted to the cardiac care unit with a myocardial infarction. The morning after admission she and her husband tell the nurse that she must be home tonight to care for the children when her husband goes to work. What nursing diagnosis describes this problem?
    1. Anxiety related to physical limitations.
    2. Alteration in cardiac output.
    3. Knowledge deficit related to disease process.
    4. Impaired home maintenance.

165. The nurse is caring for an adult admitted to the coronary care unit with a myocardial infarction. During the second night in the CCU, the client develops heart failure. What is the basis for insertion of a pulmonary artery catheter?
    1. It provides information about pulmonary resistance.
    2. It measures myocardial oxygen consumption.
    3. It increases renal blood flow.
    4. It controls afterload.

166. The nurse is planning care for a client who is in heart failure. Which of the following goals are appropriate? Select all that apply.
    ____ An increase in cardiac output.
    ____ An elevation in renal blood flow.
    ____ A reduction in the heart's workload.
    ____ A decrease in myocardial contractility.

167. The nurse is caring for an adult who is being treated for a myocardial infarction. Oxygen is ordered. Administering oxygen to this client is related to which of the following client problems?
    1. Anxiety.
    2. Chest pains.
    3. Ineffective myocardial perfusion.
    4. Alteration in heart rate, rhythm, or conduction.

168. The nurse reading an ECG rhythm strip notes that there are 8 QRS complexes in a 6-second strip. What would be the heart rate?
    1. 48.
    2. 64.
    3. 80.
    4. 120.

169. A 57-year-old is being treated in the clinic for hypertension. His blood pressure is 170/92 and he is complaining of fatigue and lassitude. He has been taking propranolol (Inderal) 80 mg bid. What action by the client will assure the nurse that teaching has been successful?
    1. Checks his pulse for bradycardia.
    2. Makes an appointment as soon as he notices fatigue.
    3. Stops the drug when he experiences chest pain.
    4. Takes the drug with breakfast and dinner.

170. A 56-year-old obese man is recovering from a bowel resection for cancer of the colon. On his third post-op day he complains that the area around the calf of his leg is warm and tender. What assessment will the nurse observe that will suggest the client has a deep vein thrombosis?
    1. Absence of a pulse distal to the clot.
    2. Cyanosis distal to the clot.
    3. Pain on dorsiflexion.
    4. Reddened area around the clot.

171. A client with a history of venous insufficiency came to the medical clinic complaining of severe pain in the legs. They were swollen and covered with deep, draining, foul-smelling ulcers. What would the nurse suspect as an underlying cause of the venous insufficiency?
    1. Congestive heart failure.
    2. Hypertrophied leg muscles.
    3. Decreased hemoglobin levels.
    4. Poor blood return to the heart.

172. A 65-year-old man is admitted with venous stasis ulcers and chronic venous insufficiency. To help control the swelling, what intervention should the nurse teach the client to perform?
    1. Exercise vigorously.
    2. Restrict fluid intake.
    3. Promote gravity drainage.
    4. Eat a high-protein, low-salt diet.

173. Which are some of the common symptoms associated with cardiovascular disease?

**4**

1. Shortness of breath, chest discomfort, palpitations.
2. Dyspnea, chest discomfort, sputum production.
3. Fatigue, weight changes, mood swings.
4. Mood swings, headaches, fainting.

174. Which of the following assessment findings by the nurse is abnormal?
   1. $S_1$ heard at the fourth-fifth left intercostal space in a 35-year-old man.
   2. $S_2$ heard at the second-third left intercostal space in a 40-year-old female.
   3. $S_4$ heard at the apex in an 80-year-old male.
   4. $S_3$ heard at the apex in a 15-year-old female.

175. Which of the following instructions should the nurse give to a client prior to an exercise electrocardiogram?
   1. Avoid coffee, tea, and alcohol the day of the test.
   2. Smoking is permitted up to the time of the test.
   3. Allow only 3 hours of sleep the night prior to the test.
   4. Take all medications as prescribed prior to the test.

176. To prevent possible complication, which of the following questions should a nurse ask a client prior to a cardiac catheterization?
   1. "Have you ever had a cardiac catheterization before?"
   2. "Can you eat shellfish?"
   3. "Have you ever had general anesthesia before?"
   4. "Have you ever had a heart attack?"

177. Which of the following should the nurse include in the plan of care for a post-op coronary arteriogram client?
   1. Assess pedal pulses.
   2. Assess lung sounds.
   3. Provide early ambulation.
   4. Monitor vital signs every 8 hours.

178. A client has the following rhythm. The client has no pulse or blood pressure.

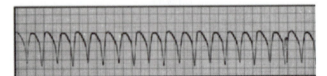

How should the nurse interpret this rhythm?
1. Ventricular tachycardia.
2. Ventricular fibrillation.
3. Sinus tachycardia.
4. Supraventricular tachycardia.

179. A client has the following rhythm. The client has no pulse or blood pressure.

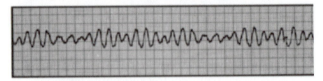

How should the nurse interpret this rhythm?
1. Ventricular tachycardia.
2. Ventricular fibrillation.
3. Sinus tachycardia.
4. Supraventricular tachycardia.

180. A client had a myocardial infarction yesterday. His cardiac monitor shows 6 to 8 PVCs per minute, with occasional couplets. What is the nurse's best action?
   1. Monitor the client for development of ventricular tachycardia.
   2. Administer the ordered prn dose of lidocaine.
   3. Perform a precordial thump.
   4. Initiate manual chest compressions.

181. A client is admitted in cardiogenic shock. What will be inserted to best evaluate the heart's hemodynamic performance?
   1. Intra-arterial line.
   2. Pulmonary artery catheter.
   3. Intra-aortic balloon pump (IABP).
   4. Triple lumen catheter.

182. Which of the following statements by a client to the nurse indicates a risk factor for coronary artery disease?
   1. "I exercise four times a week."
   2. "No one in my family has heart problems."
   3. "My cholesterol is 189."
   4. "I smoke 1½ packs of cigarettes per day."

183. An adult female has a history of coronary artery disease and angina pectoris. After walking to the bathroom, she complains of aching substernal pain that radiates to her left shoulder. What is the nurse's best action?
   1. Provide a warm shoulder massage.
   2. Administer a prn dose of nitroglycerin sublingually.

3. Use pillows to support and immobilize the left shoulder.

4. Administer a prn dose of aspirin or acetaminophen (Tylenol).

184. A nitroglycerin transdermal patch was prescribed 6 weeks ago for an adult to treat angina pectoris. How will the nurse know the patch is effective?

1. The client's serum cholesterol level has decreased.

2. The client's pressure is within normal limits.

3. The client reports no episodes of chest pain.

4. Pulse oximetry shows the client's oxygen saturation is improved.

185. An adult has developed angina pectoris secondary to coronary artery disease. A low-fat, low-cholesterol diet is prescribed for the client. The nurse should praise the client for a wise choice if which of the following was selected for an evening snack?

1. Cheese cubes and crackers.

2. Tuna salad sandwich.

3. No-added sugar ice cream.

4. Jello mold with fruit slices.

186. Lidocaine is mixed 2 g in 500 mL $D_5W$. The nurse prepared to start an infusion at 2 mg/h using a 60-drop tubing. Which of the following is the correct rate to start the infusion on a pump?

1. 15 mL.

2. 30 mL.

3. 45 mL.

4. 60 mL.

187. An adult male is transferred to the step-down unit on the third day after a myocardial infarction. Which of the following should the nurse include in his care plan at this time?

1. Enforcing complete bed rest.

2. Supervising short walks in the hallway.

3. Performing passive range of motion exercises.

4. Having him sit on the side of the bed and dangle his legs.

188. A 55-year-old man with a history of angina pectoris complains of chest pain radiating to the jaw. After taking three nitroglycerin gr 1/150 tablets he is still having the chest pain. His skin is cool and pale and he is diaphoretic and mildly short of breath. What is the nurse's priority action?

1. Auscultate heart and lung sounds.

2. Administer another nitroglycerin tablet.

3. Encourage the man to void.

4. Assist him to a supine position.

189. An adult male is being discharged from the hospital following a myocardial infarction. Knowing he will wait 4–6 weeks before having sexual activity, what statement demonstrates the client understands the guidelines taught?

1. Bedtime is the best time to have intercourse.

2. He should exercise for 10–15 minutes before intercourse, to "warm up."

3. He should take a nitroglycerin before intercourse to prevent chest pain.

4. It is best to avoid having intercourse when the stomach is empty.

190. An adult is scheduled for a percutaneous transluminal coronary angioplasty (PTCA). The adult asks the nurse, "Can you tell me again what the doctor is going to do?" What is the nurse's best response?

1. "A clot dissolving drug is administered through a catheter into the blocked section of your artery."

2. "A piece of vein from your leg is used to bypass the blocked section of your artery."

3. "A tiny rotating blade is used to scrape off the plaque that is blocking your artery."

4. "A balloon is placed next to the plaque blocking your artery, then the balloon is inflated to crush the plaque."

191. A man is being discharged following coronary artery bypass graft surgery (CABG). The nurse recognizes that he needs additional teaching if he makes which of the following statements?

1. "I'll be going to a support group to help me quit smoking."

2. "I will take a walk twice a week."

3. "I should bake or broil my chicken instead of frying it."

4. "I've learned a breathing exercise to help me calm down if I get upset."

192. Which of the following assessment findings by the nurse indicates right ventricular failure in a client?

1. Pink frothy sputum.

2. Paroxysmal nocturnal dyspnea.

3. Jugular venous distention.

4. Crackles.

193. A nurse is assessing a client with fatigue, tachycardia, crackles, and pink frothy sputum. Which nursing diagnosis is of the *most* importance?

1. Impaired skin integrity.
2. Impaired gas exchange.
3. Potential for injury.
4. Anxiety.

194. An adult is admitted with an acute exacerbation of congestive heart failure. Assessment reveals tachycardia, hypertension, and crackles in the bases of the lung fields. The medications of 0.5 mg of digoxin (Lanoxin) IV and 40 mg of furosemide (Lasix) IV are administered immediately. How would the nurse be aware that the medications are having a therapeutic effect?
    1. The client's pulse rate decreases below 100.
    2. The client has an increased urine specific gravity.
    3. The client expectorates frothy sputum.
    4. The client's lungs are clear to auscultation.

195. A client is admitted with pulmonary edema. The nurse is preparing to administer morphine sulfate. What beneficial effect does morphine have in pulmonary edema?
    1. Decreases anxiety, work of breathing, and vasodilates.
    2. Decreases respiratory rate.
    3. Provides an analgesic and sedative effect.
    4. Decreases anxiety and vasoconstricts.

196. An adult female is being discharged after having a ventricular demand pacemaker inserted. The nurse should include which of the following in the teaching plan for this client?
    1. She should not use remote control devices (e.g., TV channel selector).
    2. She must leave the room while a microwave oven is in operation.
    3. She will need to avoid air travel.
    4. She should not pass through metal detectors.

197. An adult has a ventricular demand pacemaker that is set at 72 beats per minute. The nurse knows that the client's pacemaker is functioning correctly if which of the following appears on the ECG?
    1. Pacemaker spikes instead of QRS complexes.
    2. Pacemaker spikes followed by QRS complexes.
    3. Pacemaker spikes before each P wave.
    4. Pacemaker spikes appearing only if the heart rate is over 72.

198. Which strategy by the nurse provides safety during a defibrillation attempt?

1. A verbal and visual check of "all clear."
2. No lubricant on the paddles.
3. Placing paddles lightly on the chest.
4. Standing in alignment with the bed while administering the shock.

199. An adult client has experienced a cardiac arrest and the nurse is performing CPR. What is the correct hand position on the client's chest?
    1. Over the upper half of the sternum.
    2. Two finger widths below the sternal notch.
    3. Two finger widths above the xiphoid process.
    4. Over the xiphoid process.

200. A client with a history of a myocardial infarction 2 days ago reports chest pain that is worse on inspiration but is relieved on sitting forward. Based on this finding, what does the nurse suspect the client is experiencing?
    1. Endocarditis.
    2. Angina pectoris.
    3. Pericarditis.
    4. Recurrent myocardial infarction.

201. An adult has prazocin hydrochloride (Minipress) prescribed to treat hypertension. What instructions should the nurse provide to the client?
    1. Take the medication with meals.
    2. Take the first dose at bedtime.
    3. Report a pulse rate below 50 to the physician.
    4. Check the ankles daily for edema.

202. An adult has essential hypertension. She is being treated with a thiazide diuretic and dietary and lifestyle modifications. The nurse knows that she understands the treatment if she makes which of the following statements?
    1. "I will use soy sauce or mustard instead of salt on my food."
    2. "I need to cut back to two, 4-ounce glasses of wine a day."
    3. "I will stop riding my bike because vigorous exercise will raise my blood pressure."
    4. "Smoking helped cause my hypertension, but quitting won't reverse the damage."

203. Hydrochlorothiazide is prescribed to treat high blood pressure. Which dietary modifications will the nurse instruct the client to increase?
    1. Fresh oranges.
    2. Cold cereals.
    3. Cola drinks.
    4. Cranberry juice.

204. A client reports an aching pain and cramping sensation that occurs while walking. The pain disappears after cessation of walking. What condition does the nurse suspect is occurring?
    1. Deep venous thrombosis (DVT).
    2. Raynaud's disease.
    3. Arteriosclerosis obliterans.
    4. Thrombophlebitis.

205. An adult has severe arteriosclerosis obliterans and complains of intermittent claudication after walking 20 feet. How should the nurse plan to position the client when she is in bed?
    1. Supine with legs elevated.
    2. In semi-Fowler's position with knees extended.
    3. In reverse Trendelenburg position.
    4. In Trendelenburg position.

206. An adult female experiences painful arterial spasms in her hands due to Raynaud's phenomenon. Which of the following should the nurse include in the teaching plan for her?
    1. Drink a hot beverage, such as tea or coffee, to relieve spasms.
    2. Reduce intake of high fat or high cholesterol foods.
    3. Raise the hands above the head to relieve spasms.
    4. Wear gloves when handling refrigerated foods.

207. Which assessment finding by the nurse would indicate an abdominal aortic aneurysm?
    1. Knifelike pain in the back.
    2. Pulsatile mass in the abdomen.
    3. Unequal femoral pulses.
    4. Boardlike rigid abdomen.

208. A nurse is assessing a post-op femoral popliteal bypass client. Which of the following assessment findings indicates a complication?
    1. BP 110/80, HR 86, RR 20.
    2. Small amount of dark-red blood on dressing.
    3. A decrease in pulse quality in the operated leg.
    4. Swelling of the operative leg.

209. An adult has just returned to the surgical unit after a femoral-popliteal bypass on the right leg. The nurse should place the client in what position?
    1. Fowler's position with the right leg extended.
    2. Supine with the right knee flexed 45°.
    3. Supine with the right leg extended and flat on the bed.
    4. Semi-Fowler's position with the right leg elevated on two pillows.

210. The client has a large, venous stasis ulcer on her left ankle. Wound care is performed three times a week by a home health nurse. What instruction should the nurse include in the teaching?
    1. Dangle the legs for 5–10 minutes several times a day.
    2. Wear heavy cotton or wool socks when going outdoors.
    3. Soak the feet in tepid water three or four times daily.
    4. Take frequent rest periods with her legs elevated.

211. The nurse assesses signs of bleeding in a client taking Coumadin and notifies the physician. Which of the following would the nurse expect to administer?
    1. Packed RBCs.
    2. Plasma protein.
    3. Platelets.
    4. Vitamin K.

212. A client is being discharged after treatment of deep venous thrombosis. Coumadin (warfarin) 2.5 mg daily is prescribed. The nurse recognizes that which of the following statements indicates that the client understands the effects of Coumadin?
    1. "I'll use an electric razor to shave my legs."
    2. "This will prevent me from having future DVTs."
    3. "I need to eat more salads and fresh fruits."
    4. "I will take aspirin instead of Tylenol for headaches."

213. An adult female, who was admitted 4 hours ago with thrombophlebitis in the left leg, suddenly becomes confused and dyspneic. She begins coughing up blood-streaked sputum and complains of chest pain that worsens on inspiration. What is the nurse's best response?
    1. Apply soft restraints to prevent excessive movement.
    2. Perform a Heimlich maneuver.
    3. Place her in bed in semi-Fowler's position.
    4. Place her in Trendelenburg position on her left side.

214. A client is admitted to rule out pulmonary embolism (PE) from a deep venous thrombosis. A Dextran 70 infusion is ordered for the client. What is the action of Dextran?
    1. Increase blood viscosity.
    2. Decrease platelet adhesion.
    3. Decrease plasma volume.
    4. Increase the hemoglobin.

**215.** A client reports aching, heaviness, itching, and moderate swelling of the legs. On assessment, the nurse notes dilated tortuous skin veins. What condition does the nurse suspect?

1. Thrombophlebitis.
2. Venous thrombosis.
3. Varicose veins.
4. Chronic venous insufficiency.

**216.** An adult had an above-the-knee amputation of the left leg 2 days ago. The nurse should include which of the following in the care plan?

1. Resting in a prone or supine position with the stump extended several times a day.
2. Using a rolled towel or small pillow to elevate the stump at all times.
3. Applying warm soaks to the stump to reduce phantom limb pain.
4. Avoiding turning to the left side until the stump has healed completely.

**217.** An adult male had a below-the-knee amputation of the right foot 2 days ago. He is complaining of pain in his right foot. What is the best response by the nurse?

1. Explain to him that this is a common sensation after amputation.
2. Remind him that that foot was amputated and therefore cannot have pain.
3. Apply an ice pack to the stump.
4. Show him the stump so he will realize his right foot is gone.

## Answers and Rationales

**163. 1.** Anginal pain is of short duration and is usually relieved by rest.

**164. 3.** The nurse should assess the couple's understanding of the disease process and rehabilitation, so that they can make rational decisions.

**165. 1.** The Swan-Ganz catheter measures pulmonary artery and capillary wedge pressures, which are good indicators of increase in pulmonary pressure caused by increase in left ventricular pressure.

**166.** *An increase in cardiac output* should be checked. This is an appropriate goal.

*An elevation in renal blood flow* should be checked. This is an appropriate goal. Renal blood flow will increase as cardiac output increases.

*A reduction in the heart's workload* should be checked. Reducing the venous return or the cardiac workload is an appropriate goal.

**167. 3.** With acute myocardial infarction there is ineffective myocardial perfusion, resulting in a decrease in the amount of oxygen available for tissue perfusion. Oxygen is administered to improve tissue perfusion in these clients.

**168. 3.** A regular heart rate is calculated by multiplying the number of QRS complexes in 6 seconds (8 QRS complexes) by 10 (because there are 60 seconds in 1 minute). The heart rate is 80. This method is not accurate if the client's heart rate is irregular.

**169. 1.** A common side effect of propranolol is slowed pulse rate because the drug is a beta blocker.

**170. 3.** Pain on dorsiflexion is a common manifestation of deep vein thrombosis.

**171. 4.** Venous insufficiency is stasis of venous blood flow or poor blood return to the heart. The leg muscles that normally compress the veins to force blood upward are not effective.

**172. 3.** Swelling is minimized by promoting gravity drainage. This could be accomplished by elevating the extremities.

**173. 1.** Some of the most common clinical manifestations of cardiovascular disease are shortness of breath, chest pain or discomfort, dyspnea, palpitations, fainting, and peripheral skin changes such as edema.

**174. 3.** $S_4$ is an abnormal heart sound. It is indicative of decreased ventricular compliance.

**175. 1.** Avoid any stimulants such as coffee, tea, or a depressant such as alcohol.

**176. 2.** Shellfish contains iodine, which is also in the contrast media used during a catheterization. It is *imperative* to obtain information regarding iodine allergies.

**177. 1.** Assessment of pedal pulses is imperative after a cardiac catheterization. Evaluation of presence and quality of pulses indicates blood flow to the catheterized extremity.

**178. 1.** The above rhythm is ventricular tachycardia.

**179. 2.** The above rhythm is ventricular fibrillation.

**180. 2.** Lidocaine, a class I antidysrhythmic drug, is indicated when the client has six or more PVCs per minute, multifocal PVCs, couplets or triplets, or PVCs occurring on the downslope of the T wave. Any of these situations is likely to progress to the more dangerous ventricular tachycardia or ventricular fibrillation if not treated immediately.

**181. 2.** A pulmonary artery catheter will show all right and left heart hemodynamic pressures and provide for cardiac output measurements.

**182. 4.** Smoking has been determined to increase the risk of coronary heart disease.

**183. 2.** Nitroglycerin dilates peripheral veins, reducing venous return to the heart. This immediately decreases cardiac workload, relieving ischemia and chest pain. It also dilates coronary arteries, improving oxygen supply to the heart.

**184. 3.** Nitroglycerin reduces cardiac workload and improves myocardial oxygenation. This prevents episodes of anginal pain.

**185. 4.** Most fruits and vegetables are low in fat and cholesterol-free. Jello also has no fat or cholesterol.

**186. 2.** 30 mL is 2 mg/h.
1000 mg = 1 g. 2 g is 200 mg.
2000 mg:500 mL::2 mg: x mL
2000x = 1000
      x = 0.5 mL/hr
60 drops = 1 mL 60 drops × 0.5 mL = 30 mL/hr.

**187. 2.** To improve activity tolerance, supervised walks for gradually increasing distances are encouraged when the client is transferred out of the coronary care unit.

**188. 1.** Assessment is important to identify the probable cause of the pain so that definitive intervention can be planned. Dysrhythmias are a common complication of MI. Crackles in the lungs and an $S_3$ gallop may indicate heart failure.

**189. 3.** Nitroglycerin is used prophylactically before activities that are known to cause chest pain, including sexual intercourse.

**190. 4.** PTCA is also called balloon angioplasty because a balloon-tipped catheter is used. When the balloon is inflated, the plaque is compressed, leaving the artery unobstructed.

**191. 2.** Aerobic exercise, such as walking, helps to slow formation of atherosclerotic plaques in coronary artery disease. The client needs to make the necessary lifestyle changes to prevent further progression of his disease. Riding instead of walking would not provide aerobic exercise. Therefore, this statement shows that the client needs further teaching.

**192. 3.** Jugular venous distention is seen in right ventricular failure as volume overload occurs. This overload is reflected upward into the jugulars.

**193. 2.** With left ventricular heart failure, carbon dioxide and oxygen exchange is impaired due to fluid overload and leads to hypoxia.

**194. 4.** Crackles in the lungs are a sign of pulmonary edema due to HF. Improved cardiac output due to digoxin and reduced extracellular fluid volume due to furosemide should result in reduction of pulmonary edema.

**195. 1.** This is the beneficial effect of morphine in pulmonary edema.

**196. 4.** Metal detectors generate strong magnetic fields that can alter pacemaker settings or produce interference that causes malfunction.

**197. 2.** The ventricular pacemaker stimulates the ventricle if no atrial impulse is transmitted through the AV node. The appearance of the QRS complex shows that the ventricle has responded to the stimulus.

**198. 1.** The nurse must make sure both verbally and visually that all health care providers are clear.

**199. 3.** This hand position would depress the lower half of the sternum, which would compress the heart effectively.

**200. 3.** The pain of pericarditis is exacerbated with respirations. Rotating the trunk and sitting up frequently relieves the pain.

**201. 2.** First dose syncope occurs with prazocin. To reduce the risk of fainting, the client should take the first dose at bedtime.

**202. 2.** Moderation in alcohol intake is an important lifestyle change for controlling high blood pressure. Alcohol adds empty calories to the diet and elevates arterial blood pressure.

**203. 1.** Oranges are high in potassium. Thiazide diuretics, such as hydrochlorothiazide, deplete body potassium by increasing urinary excretion, so potassium intake should be increased.

**204. 3.** Intermittent claudication is the main symptom of narrowing of the arteries (arteriosclerosis).

**205. 3.** Gravity facilitates improved arterial blood flow. The reverse Trendelenburg position, in which the feet are below heart level, is used to improve circulation to the lower extremities.

**206. 4.** Cold induces arterial spasms. When the hands will be exposed to cold, warm gloves or mittens should be worn.

**207. 2.** A pulsating abdominal mass is a common finding of an abdominal aortic aneurysm.

**208. 3.** A decrease in pulse quality signifies a decrease in the patency of the artery.

**209. 3.** The best position for the affected leg is extended and flat in the bed. Elevating the leg would allow gravity to impede circulation. Having the leg dependent would promote development of edema, which could also impair circulation.

**210. 4.** Elevating the legs improves venous drainage and reduces edema, which will promote wound healing.

**211. 4.** An injection of vitamin K will increase the synthesis of prothrombin and balance clotting time, thereby decreasing the chance of bleeding.

**212. 1.** Warfarin is an anticoagulant, which increases the risk of bleeding from any injury. Use of an electric razor reduces the risk of a cut, which might bleed excessively.

**213. 3.** Her symptoms suggest that the client has pulmonary emboli. Her activity should be limited to prevent further embolization, and her head should be elevated to promote lung expansion and ease dyspnea.

**214. 2.** Dextran coats the platelet surface to decrease adhesion. In doing so, the plasma volume expands, and viscosity is decreased.

**215. 3.** This describes varicose veins.

**216. 1.** It is essential to prevent contractures of the hip joint so that the client will be able to walk with a prosthesis. Lying supine or prone with the stump extended helps to prevent hip contractures.

**217. 1.** Phantom limb pain is common after amputation. It is a real sensation and needs to be acknowledged by the nurse.

# The Hematologic System

## OVERVIEW OF ANATOMY AND PHYSIOLOGY

The structures of the hematologic or hematopoietic system include the blood, blood vessels, and blood-forming organs (bone marrow, spleen, liver, lymph nodes, and thymus gland). The major function of blood is to carry necessary materials (oxygen, nutrients) to cells and to remove carbon dioxide and metabolic waste products. The hematologic system also plays an important role in hormone transport, the inflammatory and immune responses, temperature regulation, fluid-electrolyte balance, and acid-base balance.

### Bone Marrow

A. Contained inside all bones, occupies interior of spongy bones and center of long bones; collectively one of the largest organs of the body (4–5% of total body weight)

B. Primary function is hematopoiesis (the formation of blood cells)
C. Two kinds of bone marrow, red and yellow
   1. Red (functioning) marrow
      a. Carries out hematopoiesis; production site of erythroid, myeloid, and thrombocytic components of blood; one source of lymphocytes and macrophages
      b. Found in ribs, vertebral column, other flat bones
   2. Yellow marrow: red marrow that has changed to fat; found in long bones; does not contribute to hematopoiesis
D. All blood cells start as stem cells in the bone marrow; these mature into the different, specific types of cells, collectively referred to as formed elements of blood or blood components: erythrocytes, leukocytes, and thrombocytes.

### Blood

A. Composed of plasma (55%) and cellular components (45%); see Figure 4-11.

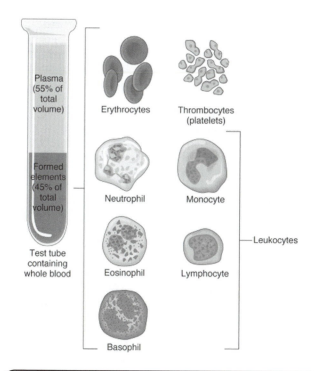

**Figure 4-11** Components of blood

**B.** Hematocrit
1. Reflects portion of blood composed of red blood cells
2. Centrifugation of blood results in separation into top layer of plasma, middle layer of leukocytes and platelets, and bottom layer of erythrocytes.
3. Majority of formed elements is erythrocytes; volume of leukocytes and platelets is negligible.

**C.** Distribution
1. 1300 mL in pulmonary circulation
   **a.** 400 mL arterial
   **b.** 60 mL capillary
   **c.** 840 mL venous
2. 3000 mL in systemic circulation
   **a.** 550 mL arterial
   **b.** 300 mL capillary
   **c.** 2150 mL venous

## Plasma

**A.** Liquid part of blood; yellow in color because of pigments
**B.** Consists of serum (liquid portion of plasma) and fibrinogen
**C.** Contains plasma proteins such as albumin, serum globulins, fibrinogen, prothrombin, plasminogen
1. Albumin: largest of plasma proteins, involved in regulation of intravascular plasma volume and maintenance of osmotic pressure

2. Serum globulins: alpha, beta, gamma
   **a.** Alpha: role in transport of steroids, lipids, bilirubin
   **b.** Beta: role in transport of iron and copper
   **c.** Gamma: role in immune response, function of antibodies
3. Fibrinogen, prothrombin, plasminogen (see Blood Coagulation)

## Cellular Components

Cellular components or formed elements of blood are erythrocytes (red blood cells [RBCs]), which are responsible for oxygen transport; leukocytes (white blood cells [WBCs]), which play a major role in defense against microorganisms; and thrombocytes (platelets), which function in hemostasis.

**A.** Erythrocytes
1. Bioconcave disc shape, no nucleus, chiefly sacs of hemoglobin
2. Cell membrane is highly diffusible to $O_2$ and $CO_2$
3. RBCs are responsible for oxygen transport via hemoglobin (Hgb)
   **a.** Two portions: iron carried on heme portion; second portion is protein
   **b.** Normal blood contains 12–18 g Hgb/ 100 mL blood; higher (14–18 g) in men than in women (12–14 g)
4. Production
   **a.** Start in bone marrow as stem cells, released as reticulocytes (immature cells), mature into erythrocytes
   **b.** Erythropoietin stimulates differentiation; produced by kidneys and stimulated by hypoxia
   **c.** Iron, vitamin $B_{12}$, folic acid, pyridoxine (vitamin $B_6$), and other factors required for erythropoiesis
5. Hemolysis (destruction)
   **a.** Average life span 120 days
   **b.** Immature RBCs destroyed in either bone marrow or other reticuloendothelial organs (blood, connective tissue, spleen, liver, lungs, and lymph nodes)
   **c.** Mature cells removed chiefly by liver and spleen
   **d.** Bilirubin: by-product of Hgb released when RBCs destroyed, excreted in bile
   **e.** Iron: freed from Hgb during bilirubin formation; transported to bone marrow via transferrin and reclaimed for new Hgb production
   **f.** Premature destruction: may be caused by RBC membrane abnormalities, Hgb abnormalities, extrinsic physical factors (such as the enzyme defects found in G6PD)
   **g.** Normal age RBCs may be destroyed by gross damage as in trauma or extravascular hemolysis (in spleen, liver, bone marrow)

**B.** Leukocytes: granulocytes and mononuclear cells: involved in protection from bacteria and other foreign substances

1. Granulocytes: eosinophils, basophils, and neutrophils
   a. Eosinophils: involved in phagocytosis and allergic reactions
   b. Basophils: involved in prevention of clotting in microcirculation and allergic reactions
   c. Eosinophils and basophils are reservoirs of histamine, serotonin, and heparin
   d. Neutrophils: involved in short-term phagocytosis
      1) mature neutrophils: polymorphonuclear leukocytes
      2) immature neutrophils: band cells (bacterial infection usually produces increased numbers of band cells)
2. Mononuclear cells: monocytes and lymphocytes: large nucleated cells
   a. Monocytes: involved in long-term phagocytosis; play a role in immune response
      1) largest leukocyte
      2) produced by bone marrow: give rise to histiocytes (Kupffer cells of liver), macrophages, and other components of reticuloendothelial system
   b. Lymphocytes: immune cells; produce substances against foreign cells; produced primarily in lymph tissue (B cells) and thymus (T cells) (see also Immune Response).

**C.** Thrombocytes (platelets)
1. Fragments of megakaryocytes formed in bone marrow
2. Production regulated by thrombopoietin
3. Essential factor in coagulation via adhesion, aggregation, and plug formation
4. Release substances involved in coagulation

## Blood Groups

**A.** Erythrocytes carry antigens, which determine the different blood groups.

**B.** Blood-typing systems are based on the many possible antigens, but the most important are the antigens of the ABO and Rh blood groups because they are most likely to be involved in transfusion reactions.

1. ABO typing
   a. Antigens of system are labelled A and B.
   b. Absence of both antigens results in type O blood.
   c. Presence of both antigens is type AB.
   d. Presence of either A or B results in type A and type B, respectively.
   e. Nearly half the population is type O, the universal donor.

   f. Antibodies are automatically formed against the ABO antigens not on person's own RBCs; transfusion with mismatched or incompatible blood results in a transfusion reaction (see Table 4-19).
2. Rh typing
   a. Identifies presence or absence of Rh antigen (Rh positive or Rh negative).
   b. Anti-Rh antibodies not automatically formed in Rh-negative person, but if Rh-positive blood is given, antibody formation starts and a second exposure to Rh antigen will trigger a transfusion reaction.
   c. Important for Rh-negative woman carrying Rh-positive baby; first pregnancy not affected, but in a subsequent pregnancy with an Rh-positive baby, mother's antibodies attack baby's RBCs (see Unit 6).

## Blood Coagulation

Conversion of fluid blood into a solid clot to reduce blood loss when blood vessels are ruptured.

**A.** Systems that initiate clotting
1. Intrinsic system: initiated by contact activation following endothelial injury ("intrinsic" to vessel itself)
   a. Factor XII initiates as contact made between damaged vessel and plasma protein
   b. Factors VIII, IX, and XI activated
2. Extrinsic system
   a. Initiated by tissue thromboplastins, released from injured vessels ("extrinsic" to vessel)
   b. Factor VII activated

**B.** Common pathway: activated by either intrinsic or extrinsic pathways
1. Platelet factor 3 (PF3) and calcium react with factors X and V.
2. Prothrombin converted to thrombin via thromboplastin.
3. Thrombin acts on fibrinogen, forming soluble fibrin.
4. Soluble fibrin polymerized by factor XIII to produce a stable, insoluble fibrin clot.

**C.** Clot resolution: takes place via fibrinolytic system by plasmin and proteolytic enzymes; clot dissolves as tissue repairs.

## Spleen

**A.** Largest lymphatic organ: functions as blood filtration system and reservoir

**B.** Vascular, bean shaped; lies beneath the diaphragm, behind and to the left of the stomach; composed of a fibrous tissue capsule surrounding a network of fiber

**C.** Contains two types of pulp

**Table 4-19** Complications of Blood Transfusion

| Type | Causes | Mechanism | Occurrence | Signs and Symptoms | Intervention |
|------|--------|-----------|------------|--------------------|--------------|
| Hemolytic | ABO incompatibility; Rh incompatibility; use of dextrose solutions; wide temperature fluctuations | Antibodies in recipient plasma react with antigen in donor cells. Agglutinated cells block capillary blood flow to organs. Hemolysis (Hgb into plasma and urine). | *Acute:* first 5 min after completion of transfusion *Delayed:* days to 2 weeks after | Headache, lumbar or sternal pain, nausea, vomiting, diarrhea, fever, chills, flushing, heat along vein, restlessness, anemia, jaundice, dyspnea, signs of shock, renal shutdown, DIC | Stop transfusion. Continue saline IV. Send blood unit and client blood sample to lab. Watch for hemoglobinuria. Treat or prevent shock, DIC, and renal shutdown. |
| Allergic | Transfer of an antigen or antibody from donor to recipient; allergic donors | Immune sensitivity to foreign serum protein | Within 30 min of start of transfusion | Urticaria, laryngeal edema, wheezing, dyspnea, bronchospasm, headache, anaphylaxis | Stop transfusion. Administer antihistamine and/or epinephrine. Treat life-threatening reactions. |
| Pyrogenic | Recipient possesses antibodies directed against WBCs; bacterial contamination; multitransfused clients; multiparous clients | Leukocyte agglutination Bacterial organisms | Within 15–90 min after initiation of transfusion | Fever, chills, flushing, palpitations, tachycardia, occasional lumbar pain | Stop transfusion. Treat temperature. Transfuse with leukocyte-poor blood or washed RBCs. Administer antibiotics prn. |
| Circulatory overload | Too rapid infusion in susceptible clients | Fluid volume overload | During and after transfusion | Dyspnea, tachycardia, orthopnea, increased blood pressure, cyanosis, anxiety | Slow infusion rate. Use packed cells instead of whole blood. Monitor CVP through a separate line. |
| Air embolism | Blood given under air pressure following severe blood loss | Bolus of air blocks pulmonary artery outflow | Anytime | Dyspnea, increased pulse, wheezing, chest pain, decreased blood pressure, apprehension | Clamp tubing. Turn client on left side. |
| Thrombo-cytopenia | Use of large amounts of banked blood | Platelets deteriorate rapidly in stored blood | When large amounts of blood given over 24 hr | Abnormal bleeding | Assess for signs of bleeding. Initiate bleeding precautions. Use fresh blood. |
| Citrate intoxication | Large amounts of citrated blood in clients with decreased liver function | Citrate binds ionic calcium | After large amounts of banked blood | Neuromuscular irritability Bleeding due to decreased calcium | Monitor/treat hypocalcemia. Avoid large amounts of citrated blood. Monitor liver function. |
| Hyperkalemia | Potassium levels increase in stored blood | Release of potassium into plasma with red cell lysis | In clients with renal insufficiency | Nausea, colic, diarrhea, muscle spasms, ECG changes (tall peaked T-wave, short Q-T segment) | Administer blood less than 5–7 days old in clients with impaired potassium excretion. |

1. Red pulp: located between the fibrous strands, composed of RBCs, WBCs, and macrophages
2. White pulp: scattered throughout the red pulp, produces lymphocytes and sequesters lymphocytes, macrophages, and antigens

D. 1–2% of red cell mass or 200 mL blood/minute stored in spleen; blood comes via the splenic artery to the pulp for cleansing, then passes into splenic venules that are lined with phagocytic cells, and finally to the splenic vein to the liver.

E. Important hematopoietic site in fetus; postnatally produces lymphocytes and monocytes

F. Important in phagocytosis; removes misshapen erythrocytes, unwanted parts of erythrocytes

G. Also involved in antibody production by plasma cells and iron metabolism (iron released from Hgb portion of destroyed erythrocytes returned to bone marrow)

H. In the adult, functions of the spleen can be taken over by the reticuloendothelial system.

## Liver

See also Gastrointestinal Tract.

A. Involved in bile production (via erythrocyte destruction and bilirubin production) and erythropoiesis (during fetal life and when bone marrow production is insufficient).

B. Kupffer cells of liver have reticuloendothelial function as histiocytes; phagocytic activity and iron storage.

C. Liver also involved in synthesis of clotting factors, synthesis of antithrombins.

# ASSESSMENT

## Health History

A. Presenting problem
1. Nonspecific symptoms may include chills, fatigue, fever, weakness, weight loss, night sweats, delayed wound healing, malaise, lethargy, depression, cold/heat intolerance
2. Note specific signs and symptoms
   a. Skin: prolonged bleeding, petechiae, jaundice, ecchymosis, pruritus, pallor
   b. Eyes: visual disturbance, yellowed sclera
   c. Ears: vertigo, tinnitus
   d. Mouth and nose: epistaxis; gingival bleeding, ulceration, pain; dysphagia, hoarseness
   e. Neck: nuchal rigidity, lymphadenopathy
   f. Respiratory: dyspnea, orthopnea, palpitations, chest discomfort or pain, cough (productive or dry), hemoptysis
   g. GI: melena, abdominal pain, change in bowel habits
   h. GU: hematuria, recurrent infection, amenorrhea, menorrhagia
   i. CNS: confusion, headache, paresthesias, syncope
   j. Musculoskeletal: joint, back, or bone pain

B. Lifestyle: exposure to chemicals, occupational exposure to radiation

C. Use of medications
1. Iron, vitamins ($B_6$, $B_{12}$, folic acid)
2. Corticosteroids
3. Anticoagulants
4. Antibiotics
5. Aspirin or aspirin-containing compounds
6. Cold or allergy preparations
7. Antiarrhythmics
8. Blood transfusions (cryoprecipitates)
9. Cancer chemotherapy drugs
10. Immunosuppressant drugs

D. Medical history
1. Surgery: splenectomy, tumor resection, cardiac valve replacement, GI tract resection
2. Allergies: multiple transfusions with whole blood or blood products, other known allergies
3. Mononucleosis; radiation therapy; recurrent infections; malabsorption syndrome; anemia; delayed wound healing; thrombophlebitis, pulmonary embolism, deep venous thrombosis (DVT); liver disease, ETOH abuse, vitamin K deficiency; angina pectoris, atrial fibrillation

E. Family history; jaundice, anemia, bleeding disorders (hemophilia, polycythemia), malignancies, congenital blood dyscrasias

## Physical Examination

A. Auscultate for heart murmurs; bruits (cerebral, cardiac, carotid); pericardial or pleural friction rubs; bowel sounds.

B. Inspect for
1. Flush or pallor of mucous membranes, nail beds, palms, soles of feet
2. Infection or pallor of sclera, conjunctiva
3. Cyanosis
4. Jaundice of skin, mucous membranes, conjunctiva
5. Signs of bleeding, petechiae, ecchymoses, oral mucosal bleeding (especially gums), epistaxis, hemorrhage from any orifice
6. Ulcerations or lesions
7. Swelling or erythema
8. Neurologic changes: pain and touch, position and vibratory sense, superficial and deep tendon reflexes

C. Palpate lymph nodes; note location, size, texture, sensation, fixation; palpate the ribs for sternal, bone tenderness.

D. Evaluate joint range of motion and tenderness.

E. Percuss for lung excursion, splenomegaly, hepatomegaly.

## Laboratory/Diagnostic Tests

A. Blood
   1. Complete blood count (CBC) with differential and peripheral smear
      a. White blood cell count (WBC) with differential
      b. Hgb and HCT
      c. Platelet and reticulocyte count
      d. Red blood cell count (RBC) with peripheral smear
   2. Coagulation studies
      a. Prothrombin time (PT)
      b. Partial thromboplastin time (PTT)
      c. Fibrin split products (FSP)
      d. Lee-White clotting time (whole blood clotting time)
   3. Blood chemistry
      a. Blood urea nitrogen (BUN)
      b. Creatinine
      c. Bilirubin: direct and indirect
      d. Uric acid
   4. Miscellaneous
      a. Erythrocyte sedimentation rate (ESR)
      b. Serum protein electrophoresis
      c. Serum iron and total iron-binding capacity
      d. Plasma protein assays
      e. Direct and indirect Coombs' tests
B. Urine and stool
   1. Urinalysis
   2. Hematest
   3. Bence-Jones protein assay (urine)
C. Radiologic
   1. Chest or other X-ray as indicated by history and physical exam
   2. Radionuclide scans (e.g., bone scan)
   3. Lymphangiography
D. Bone marrow aspiration and biopsy
   1. Puncture of iliac crest (preferred site), vertebrae body, sternum, or tibia (in infants) to collect tissue from bone marrow
   2. Purpose: study cells involved in blood production
   3. Nursing care
      a. Confirm that consent form has been signed.
      b. Allay client anxiety; prepare client for a sharp, brief pain when bone marrow is aspirated into syringe.
      c. Position client and assist physician to maintain sterile field.
      d. Immediately after the aspiration, apply pressure to the site for at least 5 minutes and longer, if necessary.
      e. Check the site frequently for signs of bleeding or infection.
      f. Send specimen to laboratory.
E. See Table 4-20

**Table 4-20** Normal Adult Values

| | |
|---|---|
| Hematocrit | |
| Male | 41.5–50.4% |
| Female | 35.9–44.6% |
| Hemoglobin | |
| Male | 14.0–17.5 g/dL |
| Female | 12.3–15.3 g/dL |
| Red cell count | 4.7–6.1 M/mL |
| White cell count | 4.8–10.8 K/mL |
| Mean corpuscular volume (MCV) | 81–99 fL |
| Mean corpuscular hemoglobin (MCH) | 27–34 pg |
| Mean corpuscular hemoglobin concentration (MCHC) | 32–36 g/dL |
| Platelet count | 150–400 K/mL |
| Neutrophils | 35–70% |
| Lymphocytes | 25–45% |
| Monocytes | 0–12% |
| Eosinophils | 0–7% |
| Basophils | 0–2% |

## ANALYSIS

Nursing diagnoses for clients with disorders of the hematologic system may include:
A. Imbalanced nutrition
B. Risk for infection
C. Ineffective tissue perfusion: cerebral, peripheral
D. Impaired gas exchange
E. Ineffective protection
F. Risk for impaired skin integrity
G. Impaired oral mucous membrane
H. Risk for activity intolerance
I. Acute pain
J. Anxiety

## PLANNING AND IMPLEMENTATION

### Goals

A. Optimal nutrition will be maintained.
B. Client will be free from infection.
C. Adequate cerebral and peripheral tissue perfusion will be maintained.
D. Client will maintain optimal respiratory function.
E. Client will maintain adequate protective mechanisms.
F. Optimal skin integrity will be maintained.
G. Client maintains optimal health of oral mucous membranes.
H. Client will have increased strength and endurance.
I. Client's pain will be relieved/controlled.
J. Client's anxiety will be relieved/reduced.

# Interventions

## Blood Transfusion and Component Therapy

A. Purpose: improve oxygen transport (RBCs); volume expansion (whole blood, plasma, albumin); provision of proteins (fresh frozen plasma, albumin, plasma protein fraction); provision of coagulation factors (cryoprecipitate, fresh frozen plasma, fresh whole blood); provision of platelets (platelet concentrate, fresh whole blood)

B. Blood and blood products
1. Whole blood; provides all components
   a. Large volume can cause difficulty: 12–24 hours for Hgb and HCT to rise
   b. Complications: volume overload, transmission of hepatitis or AIDS, transfusion reaction, infusion of excess potassium and sodium, infusion of anticoagulant (citrate) used to keep stored blood from clotting, calcium binding and depletion (citrate) in massive transfusion therapy
2. Red blood cells
   a. Provide twice the amount of Hgb as an equivalent amount of whole blood
   b. Indicated in cases of blood loss, pre- and post-op clients, and those with incipient congestive failure
   c. Complications: transfusion reaction (less common than with whole blood due to removal of plasma proteins)
3. Fresh frozen plasma
   a. Contains all coagulation factors including V and VIII
   b. Can be stored frozen for 12 months; takes 20 minutes to thaw
   c. Hang immediately upon arrival to unit (loses its coagulation factors rapidly)
4. Platelets
   a. Will raise recipient's platelet count by 10,000/mm$^3$
   b. Pooled from 4–8 units of whole blood
   c. Single-donor platelet transfusions may be necessary for clients who have developed antibodies; compatibility testing may be necessary
5. Factor VIII fractions (cryoprecipitate): contains Factors VIII, fibrinogen, and XIII
6. Granulocytes
   a. Do not increase WBC; increase marginal pool (at tissue level) rather than circulating pool
   b. Premedication with steroids, antihistamines, and acetaminophen
   c. Respiratory distress with shortness of breath, cyanosis, and chest pain may occur; requires cessation of transfusion and immediate attention
   d. Shaking chills or rigors common, require brief cessation of therapy, administration of meperidine IV until rigors are diminished, and resumption of transfusion when symptoms relieved
7. Volume expanders: albumin; percentage concentration varies (50–100 mL/unit); hyperosmolar solutions should not be used in dehydrated clients.

C. Nursing care
1. Assess client for history of previous blood transfusions and any adverse reactions.
2. Ensure that the adult client has an 18–20 gauge IV catheter in place.
3. Use 0.9% sodium chloride.
4. At least two nurses should verify the ABO group, Rh type, client and blood numbers, and expiration date.
5. Take baseline vital signs before initiating transfusion.
6. Start transfusion slowly (2 mL/minute).
7. Stay with the client during the first 15 minutes of the transfusion and take vital signs frequently.
8. Maintain the prescribed transfusion rate.
   a. Whole blood: approximately 3–4 hours
   b. RBCs: approximately 2–4 hours
   c. Fresh frozen plasma: as quickly as possible
   d. Platelets: as quickly as possible
   e. Cryoprecipitate: rapid infusion
   f. Granulocytes: usually over 2 hours
   g. Volume expanders: volume-dependent rate
9. Monitor for adverse reactions (see Table 4-19).
10. Document the following:
    a. Blood component unit number (apply sticker if available)
    b. Date infusion starts and ends
    c. Type of component and amount transfused
    d. Client reaction and vital signs
    e. Signature of transfusionist
    f. If a reaction occurs, follow facility protocol for blood packaging and assessing client.

# EVALUATION

A. Client maintains normal weight; no evidence of malnutrition.
B. Client's temperature is within normal range; no signs of infection.
C. Client neuro status is within normal limits.
D. Client demonstrates adequate peripheral capillary refill, sensation, and movement; palpable peripheral pulses; skin warm, dry, and usual color.
E. Client's respirations are of normal rate, rhythm, and depth; lungs clear to auscultation.
F. Client verbalizes signs and symptoms of infection and preventive measures; reports signs and symptoms of infection immediately.
G. Client's skin remains clear and intact.
H. Client's oral mucous membranes are healthy and intact.

I. Client experiences increased strength and endurance.
J. Client reports relief/control of pain.
K. Client expresses relief/reduction in anxiety.

# DISORDERS OF THE HEMATOLOGIC SYSTEM

## Anemias

### Iron-Deficiency Anemia

A. General information
1. Chronic microcytic, hypochromic anemia caused by either inadequate absorption or excessive loss of iron
2. Acute or chronic bleeding principal cause in adults (chiefly from trauma, dysfunctional uterine bleeding, and GI bleeding)
3. May also be caused by inadequate intake of iron-rich foods or by inadequate absorption of iron (from chronic diarrhea, malabsorption syndromes, high cereal-product intake with low animal protein ingestion, partial or complete gastrectomy, pica)
4. Incidence related to geographic location, economic class, age group, and sex
   a. More common in developing countries and tropical zones (blood-sucking parasites)
   b. Women between ages 15 and 45 and children affected more frequently, as are the poor
5. In iron-deficiency states, iron stores are depleted first, followed by a reduction in Hgb formation.

B. Assessment findings
1. Mild cases usually asymptomatic
2. Palpitations, dizziness, and cold sensitivity
3. Brittleness of hair and nails; pallor
4. Dysphagia, stomatitis, and atrophic glossitis
5. Dyspnea, weakness
6. Laboratory findings
   a. RBCs small (microcytic) and pale (hypochromic)
   b. Hgb markedly decreased
   c. HCT moderately decreased
   d. Serum iron markedly decreased
   e. Hemosiderin absent from bone marrow
   f. Serum ferritin decreased
   g. Reticulocyte count decreased

C. Nursing interventions
1. Monitor for signs and symptoms of bleeding through hematest of all elimination including stool, urine, and gastric contents.
2. Provide for adequate rest: plan activities so as not to overtire.
3. Provide a thorough explanation of all diagnostic tests used to determine sources of possible bleeding (helps allay anxiety and ensure cooperation).
4. Administer iron preparations as ordered.
   a. Oral iron preparations: route of choice
      1) Give following meals or a snack.
      2) Dilute liquid preparations well and administer using a straw to prevent staining teeth.
      3) When possible administer with orange juice as vitamin C (ascorbic acid) enhances iron absorption.
      4) Warn clients that iron preparations will change stool color and consistency (dark and tarry) and may cause constipation.
      5) Antacid ingestion will decrease oral iron effectiveness; milk products and eggs inhibit absorption.
   b. Parenteral: used in clients intolerant to oral preparations, who are noncompliant with therapy, or who have continuing blood losses.
      1) Use one needle to withdraw and another to administer iron preparations as tissue staining and irritation are a problem.
      2) Use the Z-track injection technique to prevent leakage into tissues
      3) Do not massage injection site but encourage ambulation as this will enhance absorption; advise against vigorous exercise and constricting garments.
      4) Observe for local signs of complications: pain at the injection site, development of sterile abscesses, lymphadenitis as well as fever, headache, urticaria, hypotension, or anaphylactic shock.
5. Provide dietary teaching regarding food high in iron (meats, fortified cereals, nuts, seeds, dried beans, dried fruit).
6. Encourage ingestion of roughage and increase fluid intake to prevent constipation if oral iron preparations are being taken.

### Pernicious Anemia

A. General information
1. Chronic progressive, macrocytic anemia caused by a deficiency of intrinsic factor; the result is abnormally large erythrocytes and hypochlorhydria (a deficiency of hydrochloric acid in gastric secretions)
2. Characterized by neurologic and GI symptoms; death usually results if untreated
3. Lack of intrinsic factor is caused by gastric mucosal atrophy (possibly due to heredity, prolonged iron deficiency, or an autoimmune disorder); can also result in clients who have

had a total gastrectomy if vitamin $B_{12}$ not administered

4. Usually occurs in men and women over age 50, with an increase in blue-eyed persons of Scandinavian descent

5. Pathophysiology
   a. Intrinsic factor is necessary for the absorption of vitamin $B_{12}$ into the small intestine.
   b. $B_{12}$ deficiency diminishes DNA synthesis, which results in defective maturation of cells (particularly rapidly dividing cells such as blood cells and GI tract cells).
   c. $B_{12}$ deficiency can alter structure and function of peripheral nerves, spinal cord, and the brain.

B. Medical management
   1. Drug therapy
      a. Vitamin $B_{12}$ injections: monthly maintenance
      b. Iron preparations (if Hgb level inadequate to meet increased numbers of erythrocytes)
      c. Folic acid
         1) Controversial
         2) Reverses anemia and GI symptoms but may intensify neurologic symptoms
         3) May be safe if given in small amounts in addition to vitamin $B_{12}$
   2. Transfusion therapy

C. Assessment findings
   1. Anemia, weakness, pallor, dyspnea, palpitations, fatigue
   2. GI symptoms: sore mouth; smooth, beefy, red tongue; weight loss; dyspepsia; constipation or diarrhea; jaundice
   3. CNS symptoms; tingling, paresthesias of hands and feet, paralysis, depression, psychosis
   4. Laboratory tests
      a. Erythrocyte count decreased
      b. Blood smear: oval, macrocytic erythrocytes with a proportionate amount of Hgb
      c. Bone marrow
         1) Increased megaloblasts (abnormal erythrocytes)
         2) Few normoblasts or maturing erythrocytes
         3) Defective leukocyte maturation
      d. Bilirubin (indirect): elevated unconjugated fraction
      e. Serum LDH elevated
      f. Positive Schilling test
         1) Measures absorption of radioactive vitamin $B_{12}$ both before and after parenteral administration of intrinsic factor
         2) Definitive test for pernicious anemia
         3) Used to detect lack of intrinsic factor
         4) Fasting client is given radioactive vitamin $B_{12}$ by mouth and

nonradioactive vitamin $B_{12}$ IM to saturate tissue binding sites and to permit some excretion of radioactive vitamin $B_{12}$ in the urine if it is absorbed
         5) 24–48 hour urine collection is obtained; client is encouraged to drink fluids
         6) If indicated, second stage Schilling test performed 1 week after first stage. Fasting client is given radioactive vitamin $B_{12}$ combined with human intrinsic factor and test is repeated.
      g. Gastric analysis: decreased free hydrochloric acid
      h. Large numbers of reticulocytes in the blood following parenteral vitamin $B_{12}$ administration

D. Nursing interventions
   1. Provide a nutritious diet high in iron, protein, and vitamins (fish, meat, milk/milk products, and eggs).
   2. Avoid highly seasoned, coarse, or very hot foods if client has mouth sores.
   3. Provide mouth care before and after meals using a soft toothbrush and nonirritating rinses.
   4. Bed rest may be necessary if anemia is severe.
   5. Provide safety when ambulating (especially if carrying hot items, etc.).
   6. Provide client teaching and discharge planning concerning:
      a. Dietary instruction
      b. Importance of lifelong vitamin $B_{12}$ therapy
      c. Rehabilitation and physical therapy for neurologic deficits, as well as instruction regarding safety

## Aplastic Anemia

A. General information
   1. Pancytopenia or depression of granulocyte, platelet, and erythrocyte production due to fatty replacement of the bone marrow
   2. Bone marrow destruction may be idiopathic or secondary
   3. Secondary aplastic anemia may be caused by
      a. Chemical toxins (e.g., benzene)
      b. Drugs (e.g., chloramphenicol, cytotoxic drugs)
      c. Radiation
      d. Immunologic injury

B. Medical management
   1. Blood transfusions: key to therapy until client's own marrow begins to produce blood cells
   2. Aggressive treatment of infections
   3. Bone marrow transplantation
   4. Drug therapy
      a. Corticosteroids and/or androgens to stimulate bone marrow function and to

increase capillary resistance (effective in children but usually not in adults)

   **b.** Estrogen and/or progesterone to prevent amenorrhea in female clients
   **5.** Identification and withdrawal of offending agent or drug
**C.** Assessment findings
   **1.** Fatigue, dyspnea, pallor
   **2.** Increased susceptibility to infection
   **3.** Bleeding tendencies and hemorrhage
   **4.** Laboratory findings: normocytic anemia, granulocytopenia, thrombocytopenia
   **5.** Bone marrow biopsy: marrow is fatty and contains very few developing cells
**D.** Nursing interventions
   **1.** Administer blood transfusions as ordered.
   **2.** Provide nursing care for client with bone marrow transplantation.
   **3.** Administer medications as ordered.
   **4.** Monitor for signs of infection and provide care to minimize risk.
      **a.** Maintain neutropenic precautions.
      **b.** Encourage high-protein, high-vitamin diet to help reduce incidence of infection.
      **c.** Provide mouth care before and after meals.
   **5.** Monitor for signs of bleeding and provide measures to minimize risk.
      **a.** Use a soft toothbrush and electric razor.
      **b.** Avoid intramuscular injections.
      **c.** Hematest urine and stool.
      **d.** Observe for oozing from gums, petechiae, or ecchymoses.
   **6.** Provide client teaching and discharge planning concerning
      **a.** Self-care regimen
      **b.** Identification of offending agent and importance of avoiding it (if possible) in future

## Hemolytic Anemia

**A.** General information
   **1.** A category of diseases in which there is an increased rate of RBC destruction.
   **2.** May be congenital or acquired.
      **a.** Congenital: includes hereditary spherocytosis, G6PD deficiency, sickle cell anemia, thalassemia
      **b.** Acquired: includes transfusion incompatibilities, thrombotic thrombocytopenic purpura, disseminated intravascular clotting, spur cell anemia
   **3.** Cause often unknown, but erythrocyte life span is shortened and hemolysis occurs at a rate that the bone marrow cannot compensate for.
   **4.** The degree of anemia is determined by the lag between erythrocyte hemolysis and the rate of bone marrow erythropoiesis.
   **5.** Diagnosis is based on laboratory evidence of an increased rate of erythrocyte destruction

and a corresponding compensatory effort by bone marrow to increase production.
**B.** Medical management
   **1.** Identify and eliminate (if possible) causative factors
   **2.** Drug therapy
      **a.** Corticosteroids in autoimmune types of anemia
      **b.** Folic acid supplements
   **3.** Blood transfusion therapy
   **4.** Splenectomy
**C.** Assessment findings
   **1.** Clinical manifestations vary depending on severity of anemia and the rate of onset (acute vs. chronic)
   **2.** Pallor, scleral icterus, and slight jaundice (chronic)
   **3.** Chills, fever, irritability, precordial spasm, and pain (acute)
   **4.** Abdominal pain and nausea, vomiting, diarrhea, melena
   **5.** Hematuria, marked jaundice, and dyspnea
   **6.** Splenomegaly and symptoms of cholelithiasis, hepatomegaly
   **7.** Laboratory tests
      **a.** Hgb and HCT decreased
      **b.** Reticulocyte count elevated (compensatory)
      **c.** Coombs' test (direct): positive if autoimmune features present
      **d.** Bilirubin (indirect): elevated unconjugated fraction
**D.** Nursing interventions
   **1.** Monitor for signs and symptoms of hypoxia including confusion, cyanosis, shortness of breath, tachycardia, and palpitations.
   **2.** Note that the presence of jaundice may make assessment of skin color in hypoxia unreliable.
   **3.** If jaundice and associated pruritus are present, avoid soap during bathing and use cool or tepid water.
   **4.** Frequent turning and meticulous skin care are important as skin friability is increased.
   **5.** Teach clients about the nature of the disease and identification of factors that predispose to episodes of hemolytic crisis.

## Splenectomy

**A.** General information
   **1.** Indications
      **a.** Rupture of the spleen caused by trauma, accidental tearing during surgery, diseases causing softening or damage (e.g., infectious mononucleosis)
      **b.** Hypersplenism: excessive splenic damage of cellular blood components
      **c.** As the spleen is a major source of antibody formation in children, splenectomy is not recommended during the early years of

life; if absolutely necessary, client should receive prophylactic antibiotics post-op

2. Primary hypersplenism can be alleviated with splenectomy; procedure is palliative only in secondary hypersplenism

B. Nursing interventions: postoperatively
1. Provide routine preoperative care and explain what to expect postoperatively.
2. Administer pneumococcal vaccine as ordered since client will be at increased risk for pneumococcal infections for several years after splenectomy.

C. Nursing interventions: postoperatively
1. Be aware that it is crucial to monitor carefully for hemorrhage and shock as clients with pre-op bleeding tendencies will remain at risk post-op.
2. Monitor post-op temperature elevation: fever may not be the best indicator of post-op complications such as pneumonia or urinary tract infection, as fever without concomitant infection is common following splenectomy.
3. Observe for abdominal distension and discomfort secondary to expansion of the intestines and stomach; an abdominal binder may reduce distension.
4. Know that postoperative infection in a child is considered life threatening; administer prophylactic antibiotics as ordered.
5. Ambulate early and provide chest physical therapy as location of the incision makes post-op atelectasis or pneumonia a risk.
6. Emphasize to client the need to report even minor signs or symptoms of infection immediately to the physician.

## Sickle Cell Anemia

See Unit 5

# Disorders of Platelets and Clotting Mechanism

## Disseminated Intravascular Coagulation (DIC)

A. General information
1. Diffuse fibrin deposition within arterioles and capillaries with widespread coagulation all over the body and subsequent depletion of clotting factors.
2. Hemorrhage from kidneys, brain, adrenals, heart, and other organs.
3. Cause unknown.
4. Clients are usually critically ill with an obstetric, surgical, hemolytic, or neoplastic disease.
5. May be linked with entry of thromboplastic substances into the blood.
6. Pathophysiology

a. Underlying disease (e.g., toxemia of pregnancy, cancer) causes release of thromboplastic substances that promote the deposition of fibrin throughout the microcirculation.
b. Microthrombi form in many organs, causing microinfarcts and tissue necrosis.
c. RBCs are trapped in fibrin strands and are hemolysed.
d. Platelets, prothrombin, and other clotting factors are destroyed, leading to bleeding.
e. Excessive clotting activates the fibrinolytic system, which inhibits platelet function, causing further bleeding.

7. Mortality rate is high, usually because underlying disease cannot be corrected.

B. Medical management
1. Identification and control of underlying disease is key
2. Blood transfusions: include whole blood, packed RBCs, platelets, plasma, cryoprecipitates, and volume expanders
3. Heparin administration
   a. Somewhat controversial
   b. Inhibits thrombin thus preventing further clot formation, allowing coagulation factors to accumulate

C. Assessment findings
1. Petechiae and ecchymoses on the skin, mucous membranes, heart, lungs, and other organs
2. Prolonged bleeding from breaks in the skin (e.g., IV or venipuncture sites)
3. Severe and uncontrollable hemorrhage during childbirth or surgical procedures
4. Mental status changes
5. Oliguria and acute renal failure
6. Convulsions, coma, death
7. Laboratory findings
   a. PT prolonged
   b. PTT usually prolonged
   c. Thrombin time usually prolonged
   d. Fibrinogen level usually decreased
   e. Platelet count usually depressed
   f. Fibrin split products elevated
   g. Protamine sulfate test strongly positive
   h. Factor assays (II, V, VII) depressed

D. Nursing interventions
1. Monitor blood loss and attempt to quantify.
2. Observe for signs of additional bleeding or thrombus formation.
3. Monitor appropriate laboratory data.
4. Prevent further injury.
   a. Avoid IM injections.
   b. Apply pressure to bleeding sites.
   c. Turn and position client frequently and gently.
   d. Provide frequent nontraumatic mouth care (e.g., soft toothbrush or gauze sponge).
5. Provide emotional support to client and significant others.

6. Administer blood transfusions and medications as ordered.
7. Teach client the importance of avoiding aspirin or aspirin-containing compounds.

## Hemophilia

See Unit 5.

## Idiopathic Thrombocytopenic Purpura

See Unit 5.

# Immunologic Disorders

## Acquired Immune Deficiency Syndrome (AIDS)

A. General information
1. Characterized by severe deficits in cellular immune function; manifested clinically by opportunistic infections and/or unusual neoplasms
2. Etiologic factors
   a. Results from infection with human immunodeficiency virus (HIV), a retrovirus that preferentially infects helper T-lymphocytes ($T_4$ cells)
   b. Transmissible through sexual contact, contaminated blood or blood products, and from infected woman to child in utero or possibly through breast-feeding
   c. HIV is present in an infected person's blood, semen, and other body fluids
3. Epidemiology is similar to that of hepatitis B; increased incidence in populations in which sexual promiscuity is common and in IV drug abusers
4. Proposed strategies for prevention
   a. Early detection; include HIV testing as routine part of medical care
   b. Expand opportunities for testing outside of the medical settings
   c. Behavior modification with persons diagnosed with HIV and partners
   d. Reduce viral load in pregnant woman with HIV; reduce perinatal transmission of HIV disease to newborn
B. Medical management
1. No effective cure for AIDS at present; several categories of antiretroviral drugs are available (see Table 4-21).
2. Highly active antiretroviral therapy (HAART) refers to combination of antiretroviral drugs to avoid development of viral resistance to drugs; drug therapy is initiated as early as possible to reduce HIV RNA levels in blood and to maintain or increase CD4+ levels to greater than 200 cells/μL

3. Drugs used to treat *Pneumocystis carinii* pneumonia (PCP) include:
   a. PO or IV trimethoprim-sulfamethoxazole (Bactrim, Septra); side effects include rash, leukopenia, fever
   b. IM or IV pentamidine (Pentam 300); side effects include hepatotoxicity, nephrotoxicity, blood sugar imbalances, abscess or necroses at IM injection site, hypotension
   c. Corticosteroids are also frequently used.
C. Assessment findings (see Table 4-22)
1. Fatigue, weakness, anorexia, weight loss, diarrhea, pallor, fever, night sweats
2. Shortness of breath, dyspnea, cough, chest pain, and progressive hypoxemia secondary to infection (pneumonia)
3. Progressive weight loss secondary to anorexia, nausea, vomiting, diarrhea, and a general wasting syndrome; fatigue, malaise
4. Temperature elevations (persistent or intermittent); night sweats
5. Neurologic dysfunction secondary to acute meningitis, progressive dementia, encephalopathy, encephalitis
6. Presence of opportunistic infection, for example
   a. *Pneumocystis carinii* pneumonia
   b. Herpes simplex, cytomegalovirus, and Epstein-Barr viruses

---

**Table 4-21** Antiretroviral Drug Classifications

**Nucleoside Reverse Transcriptase Inhibitors (NRTIs)**
Zidovudine (AZT, ZDV, Retrovir)—the first developed drug
Didanosine (ddl, Videx)
Stavudine (d4T, Zerit)
Lamivudine (3TC, Epivir)
Abacavir (Ziagen)

**Nucleotide Reverse Transcriptase Inhibitor**
Tenofovir DF (viread)

**Nonnucleoside Reverse Transcriptase Inhibitors (NNRTIs)**
Nevirapine (Viramune)
Delavirdne (Rescriptor)
Efavirenz (Sustival)

**Protease Inhibitors (PIs)**
Saquinavir (Fortovase)
Indinavir (Crixivan)
Ritonavir (Norvir)
Nelfinavir (Viracept)
Amprenavir (Agenerase)
Kaletra (combination of lopinavir and ritonvir)

**Fusion Inhibitor (Entry Inhibitor)**
Enfuvirtide (Fuzeon)

---

*Adapted from Broyles, B.E., Reiss, B.S., & Evans, M.E. (2007). Pharmacological aspects of nursing care (7th ed.). New York: Thomson Delmar Learning.*

**Table 4-22** Classification System for HIV Infection

| CD4 + T-cell categories | A<br>Asymptomatic, acute HIV or PGL | B<br>Symptomatic, not (A) or (C) conditions | C<br>AIDS-indicator conditions |
|---|---|---|---|
| (1) 500/uL | A1 | B1 | C1 |
| (2) 200–499/uL | A2 | B2 | C2 |
| (3) < 200/uL | A3 | B3 | C3 |

| **Clinical Category A** | **Clinical Category B** | **Clinical Category C** |
|---|---|---|
| 1 or more of the following, confirmed HIV infection, and without conditions in B and C<br>• Asymptomatic HIV infection<br>• Persistent Generalized Lymphadenopathy (PGL)<br>• Acute (primary) HIV infection with accompanying illness or history of acute HIV infection | • Candidiasis (oral or vaginal), frequent or poorly resistant to therapy<br>• Cervical dysplasia/cervical carcinoma in situ<br>• Fever or diarrhea exceeding 1 month<br>• Hairy leukoplakia, oral<br>• Herpes zoster, involving 2 episodes or more than one dermatome<br>• ITP<br>• PID<br>• Peripheral neuropathy | • Candidiasis of bronchi, trachea, or lungs<br>• Cervical cancer, invasive<br>• Coccidiomycosis<br>• Cryptosporidiosis<br>• Cytomegalovirus<br>• Encephalopathy<br>• Herpes simplex: chronic ulcer—exceeding 1 month duration<br>• Histoplasmosis<br>• Kaposi's sarcoma<br>• Lymphoma<br>• Mycobacterium–avium complex<br>• Mycobacterium tuberculosis<br>• *Pneumocystis carinii* pneumonia<br>• Salmonella<br>• Toxoplasmosis of brain<br>• Wasting syndrome due to HIV |

*NOTE:* Adapted from 1993 *Revised Classification System for HIV Infections and Expanded Surveillance Case Definition for AIDS Among Adolescents and Adults,* by Centers for Disease Control and Prevention, U.S. Department of Health and Human Services, 1993, Atlanta, GA: Author.

c. Candidiasis: oral or esophageal
        d. Mycobacterium-avium complex
    7. Neoplasms
        a. Kaposi's sarcoma
        b. CNS lymphoma
        c. Burkitt's lymphoma
        d. Diffuse undifferentiated non-Hodgkin's lymphoma
    8. Laboratory findings: diagnosis based on clinical criteria and positive HIV antibody test—ELISA (enzyme-linked immunosorbent assay) confirmed by Western blot assay. Other lab findings may include
        a. Leukopenia with profound lymphopenia
        b. Anemia
        c. Thrombocytopenia
        d. Decreased circulatory CD4 lymphocyte cells
        e. Low CD4:CD8 lymphocyte ratio
D. Nursing interventions
    1. Administer medications as ordered for concomitant disease; monitor for signs of medication toxicity.
    2. Monitor respiratory status; provide care as appropriate for respiratory problems, e.g., pneumonia.

3. Assess neurological status; reorient client as needed; provide safety measures for the confused/disoriented client.
4. Assess for signs and symptoms of fluid and electrolyte imbalances; monitor lab studies; ensure adequate hydration.
5. Monitor client's nutritional intake; provide supplements, total parenteral nutrition, etc., as ordered.
6. Assess skin daily (especially perianal area) for signs of breakdown; keep skin clean and dry; turn q4 h while in bed.
7. Inspect oral cavity daily for ulcerations, signs of infection; instruct client to rinse mouth with normal saline and hydrogen peroxide or normal saline and sodium bicarbonate rinses.
8. Observe for signs and symptoms of infection; report immediately if any occur.
9. If severe leukopenia develops, institute neutropenic precautions
    a. Prevent trauma to skin and mucous membranes, e.g., avoid enemas, rectal temperatures; minimize all parenteral infections
    b. Do not place client in a room with clients having infections

          c. Screen visitors for colds, infections, etc.
          d. Do not allow fresh fruits, vegetables, or plants in client's room.
          e. Mask client when leaving room for walks, X-rays, etc.
    10. Institute blood and body fluid precautions
    11. Provide emotional support for client/significant others; help to decrease sense of isolation
    12. Provide client teaching and discharge planning concerning
          a. Importance of observing for signs of infections and notifying physician immediately if any occur
          b. Ways to reduce chance of infection
                1) Clean kitchen and bathroom surfaces regularly with disinfectants.
                2) Avoid direct contact with pet's litter boxes or stool, bird cage droppings, and water in fish tanks.
                3) Avoid contact with people with infections, e.g., cold, flu.
                4) Importance of balancing activity with rest.
                5) Need to eat a well-balanced diet with plenty of fluids.
          c. Prevention of disease transmission
                1) Use safer sex practices, e.g., condoms for sexual intercourse.
                2) Do not donate blood, semen, organs.
                3) Do not share razors, toothbrushes, or other items that may draw blood.
                4) Inform all physicians, dentists, sexual partners of diagnosis.
          d. Resources include Public Health Service, National Gay Task Force, American Red Cross, local support groups

## Malignancies

### Multiple Myeloma

A. General information
    1. A neoplastic condition characterized by the abnormal proliferation of plasma cells in the bone marrow, causing the development of single or multiple tumors composed of abnormal plasma cells. Disease disseminates into lymph nodes, liver, spleen, and kidneys and causes bone destruction throughout the body.
    2. Cause unknown, but environmental factors thought to be involved
    3. Disease occurs after age 40; affects men twice as often as women
    4. Pathophysiology
          a. Bone demineralization and destruction with osteoporosis and a negative calcium balance
          b. Disruption of erythrocyte, leukocyte, and thrombocyte production

B. Medical management
    1. Drug therapy
          a. Analgesics for bone pain
          b. Chemotherapy (melphalan [Alkeran] and cyclophosphamide [Cytoxan]) to reduce tumor mass; may intensify the pancytopenia to which these clients are prone; requires careful monitoring of laboratory studies
          c. Antibiotics to treat infections
          d. Gammaglobulin for infection prophylaxis
          e. Corticosteroids and mithramycin for severe hypercalcemia
    2. Radiation therapy to reduce tumor mass and for palliation of bone pain
    3. Transfusion therapy

C. Assessment findings
    1. Headache and bone pain increasing with activity
    2. Pathologic fractures
    3. Skeletal deformities of sternum and ribs
    4. Loss of height (spinal column shortening)
    5. Osteoporosis
    6. Renal calculi
    7. Anemia, hemorrhagic tendencies, and increased susceptibility to infection
    8. Hypercalcemia
    9. Renal dysfunction secondary to obstruction of convoluted tubules by coagulated protein particles
    10. Neurologic dysfunction: spinal cord compression and paraplegia
    11. Laboratory tests
          a. Radiologic: diffuse bone lesions, widespread demineralization, osteoporosis, osteolytic lesions of skull
          b. Bone marrow; many immature plasma cells; depletion of other cell types
          c. CBC: reduced Hgb, WBC, and platelet counts
          d. Serum globulins elevated
          e. Bence-Jones protein: positive (abnormal globulin that appears in the urine of clients with multiple myeloma and other bone tumors)

D. Nursing interventions
    1. Provide comfort measures to help alleviate bone pain.
    2. Encourage ambulation to slow demineralization process.
    3. Promote safety as clients are prone to pathologic and other fractures.
    4. Encourage fluids: 3000–4000 mL/day to counteract calcium overload and to prevent protein from precipitating in the renal tubules.
    5. Provide nursing care for clients with bleeding tendencies and susceptibility to infection.
    6. Provide a supportive atmosphere to enhance communication and reduce anxiety.

7. Provide client teaching and discharge planning concerning
   a. Crucial importance of long-term hydration to prevent urolithiasis and renal obstruction
   b. Safety measures vital to decrease the risk of injury
   c. Avoidance of crowds or sources of infection if leukopenic

## Polycythemia Vera

A. General information
   1. An increase in both the number of circulating erythrocytes and the concentration of Hgb within the blood
   2. Three forms: polycythemia vera, secondary polycythemia, and relative polycythemia
   3. Classified as a myeloproliferative disorder (bone marrow overgrowth)
   4. Cause unknown, but thought to be a form of malignancy similar to leukemia
   5. Usually develops in middle age, common in Jewish men
   6. Pathophysiology
      a. A pronounced increase in the production of erythrocytes accompanied by an increase in the production of myelocytes (leukocytes within bone marrow) and thrombocytes.
      b. The consequences of this overproduction are an increase in blood viscosity, an increase in total blood volume (2–3 times greater than normal), and severe congestion of all tissues and organs with blood.

B. Assessment findings
   1. Ruddy complexion and duskiness of mucosa secondary to capillary congestion in the skin and mucous membranes
   2. Hypertension associated with vertigo, headache, and "fullness" in the head secondary to increased blood volume
   3. Symptoms of HF secondary to overwork of the heart
   4. Thrombus formation: CVA, MI, gangrene of the extremities, DVT, and pulmonary embolism can occur
   5. Bleeding and hemorrhage secondary to congestion and overdistension of capillaries and venules
   6. Hepatomegaly and splenomegaly
   7. Peptic ulcer secondary to increased gastric secretions
   8. Gout secondary to increased uric acid released by nucleoprotein breakdown
   9. Laboratory tests
      a. CBC: increase in all mature cell forms (erythrocytes, leukocytes, and platelets)
      b. HCT: increased
      c. Bone marrow: increase in immature cell forms

   d. Bilirubin (indirect): increase in unconjugated fraction
   e. Liver enzymes may be increased
   f. Uric acid increased
   g. Hematuria and melena possible

C. Nursing interventions
   1. Monitor for signs and symptoms of bleeding complications.
   2. Force fluids and record I&O.
   3. Prevent development of DVT.
   4. Monitor for signs and symptoms of CHF.
   5. Provide care for the client having a phlebotomy.
   6. Prevent/provide care for bleeding or infection complications.
   7. Administer medications as ordered.
      a. Radioactive phosphorus ($^{32}$P): reduction of erythrocyte production, produces a remission of 6 months to 2 years
      b. Nitrogen mustard, busulfan (Myleran), chlorambucil, cyclophosphamide to effect myelosuppression
      c. Antigout and peptic ulcer drugs as needed.
   8. Provide client teaching and discharge planning concerning
      a. Decrease in activity tolerance, need to space activity with periods of rest
      b. Phlebotomy regimens: outclient frequency is determined by HCT; importance of long-term therapy
      c. High fluid intake
      d. Avoidance of iron-rich foods to avoid counteracting the therapeutic effects of phlebotomy
      e. Recognition and reporting of bleeding
      f. Need to avoid persons with infections, especially in leukopenic clients.

## Leukemia

See Unit 5.

## Hodgkin's and Non-Hodgkin's Lymphoma

See Unit 5.

 **Sample Questions**

218. A client is admitted to the hospital with a bleeding ulcer and is to receive 4 units of packed cells. Which nursing intervention is of PRIMARY importance in the administration of blood?
   1. Checking the flow rate.
   2. Identifying the client.
   3. Monitoring the vital signs.
   4. Maintaining blood temperature.

219. Within 20 minutes of the start of transfusion, the client develops a sudden fever. What is the nurse's first action?
    1. Force fluids.
    2. Continue to monitor the vital signs.
    3. Increase the flow rate of IV fluids.
    4. Stop the transfusion.

220. A male client who is HIV positive is admitted to the hospital with a diagnosis of *Pneumocystis carinii* pneumonia. His live-in partner has accompanied him. During the history interview, the nurse is aware of feeling a negative attitude about the client's lifestyle, what action is most appropriate?
    1. Share these feelings with the client.
    2. Develop a written interview form.
    3. Avoid eye contact with the client.
    4. Discuss the negative feelings with the charge nurse.

221. What should the client at risk for developing AIDS be advised to do?
    1. Abstain from anal intercourse.
    2. Have an ELISA test for antibodies.
    3. Have a semen analysis done.
    4. Inform all sexual contacts.

222. A client who is HIV positive should have the mouth examined for which oral problem common associated with AIDS?
    1. Halitosis.
    2. Carious teeth.
    3. Creamy white patches.
    4. Swollen lips.

223. The nurse is caring for a client who is HIV positive. To prevent the spread of the HIV virus, what do the Centers for Disease Control and Prevention (CDC) recommend?
    1. Universal blood and body fluid precautions.
    2. Laminar flow rooms during active infection.
    3. Body systems isolation.
    4. Needle and syringe precautions.

224. An adult has been diagnosed with some type of anemia. The results of his blood tests showed: decreased WBC, normal RBC, decreased HCT, decreased Hgb. Based on these data, which of the following nursing diagnoses should the nurse prioritize as being the most important?
    1. Potential for infection.
    2. Alteration in nutrition.
    3. Self-care deficit.
    4. Fluid volume excess.

225. A client has the following blood lab values:
    Platelets 50,000/uL
    RBCs 3.5 ($\times 10^6$)
    Hemoglobin 10 g/dL
    Hematocrit 30%
    WBCs 10,000/uL
    Which nursing instruction should be included in the teaching plan?
    1. Bleeding precautions.
    2. Seizure precautions.
    3. Isolation to prevent infection.
    4. Control of pain with analgesics.

226. A hospitalized client has the following blood lab values:
    WBC 3,000/uL
    RBC 5.0 ($\times 10^6$)
    platelets 300,000
    What would be a priority nursing intervention?
    1. Preventing infection.
    2. Controlling blood loss.
    3. Alleviating pain.
    4. Monitoring blood transfusion reactions.

227. A man's blood type is AB and he requires a blood transfusion. To prevent complications of blood incompatibilities, which blood type(s) may the client receive?
    1. Type A or B blood only.
    2. Type AB blood only.
    3. Type O blood only.
    4. Either type A, B, AB, or O blood.

228. Which nursing intervention is appropriate for the nurse to take when setting up supplies for a client who requires a blood transfusion?
    1. Add any needed IV medication in the blood bag within one-half hour of planned infusion.
    2. Obtain blood bag from laboratory and leave at room temperature for at least one hour prior to infusion.
    3. Prime tubing of blood administration set with 0.9% NS solution, completely filling filter.
    4. Use a small-bore catheter to prevent rapid infusion of blood products that may lead to a reaction.

229. A client who is receiving a blood transfusion begins to experience chills, shortness of breath, nausea, excessive perspiration, and a vague sense of uneasiness. What is the nurse's first best action?
    1. Report the signs and symptoms to the physician.
    2. Stop the transfusion.

3. Monitor the client's vital signs.

4. Assess respiratory status.

230. A client with iron deficiency anemia is ordered parenteral iron to be given intramuscularly. Which of the following actions should the nurse take in the preparation/administration of this medication?

1. Use the same large (19–20) gauge needle for drawing up the medication and injecting it.

2. Inject medication into the upper arm muscle.

3. Use a 1-inch needle to administer the medication.

4. Use the Z-track technique to administer the medication.

231. The nurse has been teaching an adult who has iron deficiency anemia about those foods that she needs to include in her meal plans. Which of the following, if selected, would indicate to the nurse that the client understands the dietary instructions?

1. Citrus fruits and green leafy vegetables.

2. Bananas and nuts.

3. Coffee and tea.

4. Dairy products.

232. In assessing clients for pernicious anemia, the nurse should be alert for which of the following risk factors?

1. Positive family history.

2. Acute or chronic blood loss.

3. Infectious agents or toxins.

4. Inadequate dietary intake.

233. A client has been scheduled for a Schilling test. What instruction will the nurse give the client?

1. Take nothing by mouth for 12 hours prior to the test.

2. Collect his urine for 12 hours.

3. Administer a fleets enema the evening before the test.

4. Empty his bladder immediately before the test.

234. A 40-year-old woman with aplastic anemia is prescribed estrogen with progesterone. The nurse can expect that these medications are given for which of the following reasons?

1. To stimulate bone growth.

2. To regulate fluid balance.

3. To enhance sodium and potassium absorption.

4. To promote utilization and storage of fluids.

235. Which of the following lab value profiles should the nurse know to be consistent with hemolytic anemia?

1. Increased RBC, decreased bilirubin, decreased hemoglobin and hematocrit, increased reticulocytes.

2. Decreased RBC, increased bilirubin, decreased hemoglobin and hematocrit, increased reticulocytes.

3. Decreased RBC, decreased bilirubin, increased hemoglobin and hematocrit, decreased reticulocytes.

4. Increased RBC, increased bilirubin, increased hemoglobin and hematocrit, decreased reticulocytes.

236. A client is admitted for a splenectomy. What problem is the nurse aware that could develop?

1. Infection.

2. Congestive heart failure.

3. Urinary retention.

4. Viral hepatitis.

237. An adult is diagnosed with disseminated intramuscular coagulation (DIC). The nurse should identify that the client is at risk for which of the following nursing diagnoses?

1. Risk for increased cardiac output related to fluid volume excess.

2. Disturbed sensory perception related to bleeding into tissues.

3. Alteration in tissue perfusion related to bleeding and diminished blood flow.

4. Risk for aspiration related to constriction of the respiratory musculature.

238. A client diagnosed with DIC is ordered heparin. What is the reason for this medication?

1. Prevent clot formation.

2. Increase blood flow to target organs.

3. Increase clot formation.

4. Decrease blood flow to target organs.

239. A 34-year-old client is diagnosed with AIDS. His pharmacologic management includes zidovudine (AZT). During a home visit, the client states, "I don't understand how this medication works. Will it stop the infection?" What is the nurse's best response?

1. "The medication helps to slow the disease process, but it won't cure or stop it totally."

2. "The medication blocks reverse transcriptase, the enzyme required for HIV replication."

3. "Don't you know? There aren't any medications to stop or cure HIV."
4. "No, it won't stop the infection. In fact, sometimes the HIV can become immune to the drug itself."

240. Which statement, from a participant attending a class on AIDS prevention, indicates an understanding of how to reduce transmission of HIV?
1. "Mothers who are HIV-positive should still be encouraged to breastfeed their babies because breast milk is superior to cow's milk."
2. "I think a needle exchange program, where clean needles are exchanged for dirty needles, should be offered in every city."
3. "Females taking birth control pills are protected from getting HIV."
4. "It's okay to use natural skin condoms since they offer the same protection as the latex condoms."

241. What should be included in the teaching plan to young adults about the spread of AIDS?
1. Heterosexual transmission of HIV is on the rise.
2. The increase of HIV in children is primarily attributed to the rise in sexual abuse.
3. Herpes zoster is a form of the HIV virus.
4. Transmission of HIV by IV drug users is prominent even when sterile equipment is used.

242. What orders would likely be included for a client diagnosed with multiple myeloma?
1. Bed rest.
2. Corticosteroid therapy.
3. Fluid restrictions.
4. Calcium replacement therapy.

243. Which client statement would indicate to the nurse that the client with polycythemia vera is in need of further instruction?
1. "I'll be flying overseas to see my son and grandchildren for the holidays."
2. "I plan to do my leg exercises at least three times a week."
3. "I'm going to be walking in the mall every day to build up my strength."
4. "At night when I sleep, I like to use two pillows to raise my head up."

# Answers and Rationales

218. **2.** The most important consideration in transfusion therapy is to give the correct blood product to the correct client.

219. **4.** Sudden development of fever during a blood transfusion may be indicative of a pyrogenic reaction. The most appropriate nursing action is to discontinue the blood flow to prevent a more severe reaction.

220. **4.** When performing the interview, it is important to communicate an attitude of trust. If the nurse senses negative feelings with a client, it is necessary to share this information with the charge nurse, who will obtain a more accurate assessment. This strategy also provides the opportunity for the nurse to seek the counsel of others.

221. **2.** The ELISA test detects the presence of antibodies to the AIDS virus and is a useful screening tool. It is not a definitive diagnostic test but provides additional information for the high-risk individual.

222. **3.** Creamy white patches indicating an opportunistic infection (candidiasis) are often seen in the client with AIDS.

223. **1.** Universal blood and body fluid precautions, general infection control outlines, and disease-specific measures are recommended by the CDC for AIDS and AIDS-related infections.

224. **1.** These blood values are consistent with a diagnosis of aplastic anemia in which the nurse's primary goals are to prevent complications from infection and hemorrhage. Whenever WBC blood levels are low, this should cue the nurse to recognize that the client's immune system is weakened and the potential for infection is great.

225. **1.** The RBCs are decreased (normal 4.5–5.0), which is associated with either the decreased production of RBCs, increased destruction of RBCs, or blood loss. Both hemoglobin (normal 12–18) and hematocrit (normal 38–54) values are subsequently decreased. Low platelets (normal 150,000–400,000) are most frequently associated with a tendency to bleed. These factors support the need for the nurse to monitor the client closely for bleeding problems.

226. **1.** The WBC is very low (normal 4,000–11,000). This indicates that the client's immune system is deficient and the client is subject to infection.

227. **4.** Persons with type AB blood, because they are universal blood recipients, are able to receive either type A, B, AB, or O blood. People with any blood type other than AB, are restricted as to the type of blood they can receive.

228. **3.** The tubing is primed with 0.9% NS solution. If the filter is not completely primed, debris will coagulate in the filter and the transfusion will be slowed. In addition, saline is prepared to infuse in case a transfusion reaction occurs.

229. **2.** The signs and symptoms the client is experiencing are indicative of a transfusion reaction and the transfusion must first be discontinued.

230. **4.** A Z-track injection technique should be used to prevent leakage of the iron to subcutaneous tissues.

231. **1.** Dark, leafy green vegetables (as well as meats, eggs, legumes, and whole-grain or enriched breads and cereals) are rich in iron. In addition, both citrus foods and green leafy vegetables are high in vitamin C, which aids in iron absorption.

232. **1.** There is a familial predisposition for pernicious anemia, and although the disease cannot be prevented, it can be controlled if detected and treated early. Pernicious anemia occurs as a result of the lack of the protein intrinsic factor that is secreted by the gastric mucosa.

233. **1.** The client is to fast for 12 hours prior to the test. No food or drink is permitted. Following administration of the vitamin $B_{12}$ dose, food is delayed for 3 hours.

234. **1.** In aplastic anemia, the bone marrow elements (erythrocytes, leukocytes, and platelets) are suppressed. Treatments include, but are not limited to, bone marrow transplantation, transfusions to reduce symptomatology, and drugs to stimulate bone marrow function. Drugs like estrogen and progesterone work to stimulate bone growth. Estrogen and progesterone also stop menstruation so there is less blood loss.

235. **2.** Decreased RBCs are a result of the excessive destruction of the red blood cells. With this destruction, there is a subsequent decrease in both hemoglobin and hematocrit. In addition, this increased destruction causes an elevation in bilirubin levels. The reticulocyte count is high because the numbers of immature RBCs are increased when RBCs are being destroyed. This count reflects the bone marrow activity, which is active in producing RBCs to compensate for the destruction.

236. **1.** Following a splenectomy, immunologic deficiencies may develop, and vulnerability to infection is greatly increased. The postsplenectomy client is highly susceptible to infection from organisms such as *Pneumococcus*. A preventive measure is immunization with Pneumovax.

237. **3.** Cerebral, cardiopulmonary, and peripheral tissue perfusion is affected by DIC. The many clots can cause obstruction to blood flow and tissue damage can subsequently occur.

238. **1.** In DIC, the paradoxical events of hemorrhage and clotting occur. Although it may seem counterproductive to administer heparin while a client is bleeding, it is necessary to prevent the clotting that is simultaneously occurring in the microcirculation. It is critical that the client be monitored closely.

239. **1.** This statement answers the client's question in a simple, matter of fact manner that is truthful and to the point.

240. **2.** Although needle exchange programs are very controversial, it is evident the transmission of HIV can be significantly reduced when needle exchange programs are introduced.

241. **1.** Heterosexual transmission of HIV is a concern, especially in this age group. It is on the rise and this is often overlooked because the more known transmissions take place among homosexuals and IV drug abusers.

242. **2.** Corticosteroids may be added to the chemotherapy regime because of their antitumor effect. In addition, they assist in the excretion of calcium, which helps to treat the hypercalcemia that occurs in clients who have multiple myeloma.

243. **1.** With polycythemia vera, maintaining oxygenation is critical. High altitudes can precipitate hypoxia. This client needs further instruction.

# The Respiratory System

## OVERVIEW OF ANATOMY AND PHYSIOLOGY

### Upper Respiratory Tract

Structures of the respiratory system, primarily an air conduction system, include the nose, pharynx, and larynx. Air is filtered, warmed, and humidified in the upper airway before passing to lower airway (see Figure 4-12).

#### Nose

A. External nose is a framework of bone and cartilage, internally divided into two passages or nares (nasal cavities) by the septum; air enters the system through the nares.
B. The septum is covered with a mucous membrane, where the olfactory receptors are located. Turbinates, located internally, assist in warming and moistening the air.
C. The major functions of the nose are warming, moistening, and filtering the air.

#### Pharynx

A. Muscular passageway commonly called the throat.
B. Air passes through the nose to the pharynx, composed of three sections

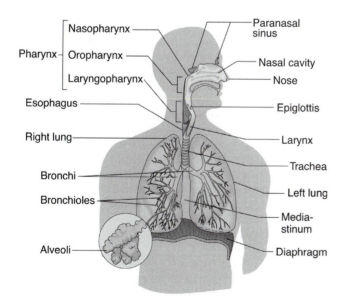

**Figure 4-12** The respiratory system

1. Nasopharynx: located above the soft palate of the mouth, contains the adenoids and openings to the eustachian tubes.
2. Oropharynx: located directly behind the mouth and tongue, contains the palatine tonsils; air and food enter body through oropharynx.
3. Laryngopharynx: extends from the epiglottis to the sixth cervical level.

#### Larynx

A. Sometimes called "voice box," connects upper and lower airways; framework is formed by the hyoid bone, epiglottis, and thyroid, cricoid, and arytenoid cartilages. The opening of the larynx is called the glottis.
B. Larynx opens to allow respiration and closes to prevent aspiration when food passes through the pharynx.
C. Vocal cords of larynx permit speech and are involved in the cough reflex.

### Lower Respiratory Tract

Consists of the trachea, bronchi and branches, and the lungs and associated structures (see Figure 4-12).

#### Trachea

A. Air moves from the pharynx to larynx to trachea (length 11–13 cm, diameter 1.5–2.5 cm in adult).
B. Extends from the larynx to the second costal cartilage, where it bifurcates and is supported by 16–20 C-shaped cartilage rings.
C. The area where the trachea divides into two branches is called the carina.

#### Bronchi

A. Formed by the division of the trachea into two branches (bronchi)
   1. Right mainstem bronchus: larger and straighter than the left; further divides into three lobar branches (upper, middle, and lower lobar bronchi) to supply the three lobes of right lung. If passed too far, endotracheal tube might enter right mainstem bronchus; only right lung is then intubated.
   2. Left mainstem bronchus: divides into the upper and lower lobar bronchi, to supply two lobes of left lung.
B. At the point a bronchus reaches about 1 mm in diameter it no longer has a connective tissue sheath and is called a bronchiole.

## Bronchioles

A. In the bronchioles, airway patency is primarily dependent upon elastic recoil formed by network of smooth muscles.
B. The tracheobronchial tree ends at the terminal bronchioles. Distal to the terminal bronchioles the major function is no longer air conduction, but gas exchange between blood and alveolar air. The *respiratory bronchioles* serve as the transition to the alveolar epithelium.

## Lungs (Right and Left)

A. Main organs of respiration, lie within the thoracic cavity on either side of the heart.
B. Broad area of lung resting on diaphragm is called the base; the narrow, superior portion is the apex.
C. Each lung is divided into lobes: three in the right lung, two in the left.
D. Pleura: serous membrane covering the lungs; continuous with the parietal pleura that lines the chest wall.
E. Lungs and associated structures are protected by the chest wall.

## Chest Wall

A. Includes the rib cage, intercostal muscles, and diaphragm.
B. Parietal pleura lines the chest wall and secretes small amounts of lubricating fluid into the intrapleural space (space between the visceral and parietal pleura). This fluid holds the lung and chest wall together as a single unit while allowing them to move separately.
C. The chest is shaped and supported by 12 pairs of ribs and costal cartilages; the ribs have several attached muscles.
   1. Contraction of the external intercostal muscles raises the rib cage during inspiration and helps increase the size of the thoracic cavity.
   2. The internal intercostal muscles tend to pull ribs down and in and play a role in forced expiration.
D. The diaphragm is the major muscle of ventilation (the exchange of air between the atmosphere and the alveoli). Contraction of muscle fibers causes the dome of the diaphragm to descend, thereby increasing the volume of the thoracic cavity. As exertion increases, additional chest muscles or even abdominal muscles may be employed in moving the thoracic cage.

## Pulmonary Circulation

A. Provides for reoxygenation of blood and release of $CO_2$; gas transfer occurs in the pulmonary capillary bed.
B. Pulmonary arteries arise from the right ventricle of the heart and continue to the bronchi and alveoli, gradually decreasing in size to capillaries.
C. The capillaries, after contact with the gas-exchange surface of the alveoli, reform to form the pulmonary veins.
D. The two pulmonary veins, superior and inferior, empty into the left atrium.

## Gas Exchange
### Alveolar Ducts and Alveoli

A. Alveolar ducts arise from the respiratory bronchioles and lead to the alveoli.
B. Alveoli are the functional cellular units of the lungs; about half arise directly from the alveolar ducts and are responsible for about 35% of alveolar gas exchange.
C. Alveoli produce surfactant, a phospholipid substance found in the fluid lining the alveolar epithelium. Surfactant reduces surface tension and increases the stability of the alveoli and prevents their collapse.
D. Alveolar sacs form the last part of the airway; functionally the same as the alveolar ducts, they are surrounded by alveoli and are responsible for 65% of the alveolar gas exchange.

## ASSESSMENT

## Health History

A. Presenting problem
   1. Nose/nasal sinuses: symptoms may include colds, discharge, epistaxis, sinus problems (swelling, pain)
   2. Throat: symptoms may include sore throat, hoarseness, difficulty swallowing, strep throat
   3. Lungs: symptoms may include
      a. Cough: note duration; frequency; type (dry, hacking, bubbly, barky, hoarse, congested); sputum (productive vs nonproductive); circumstances related to cough (time of day, positions, talking, anxiety); treatment.
      b. Dyspnea: note onset, severity, duration, efforts to treat, whether associated with radiation, if accompanied by cough or diaphoresis, time of day when it most likely occurs, interference with ADL, whether precipitated by any specific activities, whether accompanied by cyanosis.
      c. Wheezing
      d. Chest pain
      e. Hemoptysis
B. Lifestyle: smoking (note type of tobacco, duration, number per day, number of years of smoking, inhalation, related cough, desire to quit); occupation (work conditions that could irritate

respiratory system [asbestos, chemical irritants, dry-cleaning fumes] and monitoring or protection of exposure conditions); geographical location (environmental conditions that could irritate respiratory system [chemical plants/industrial pollutants]); type and frequency of exercise/recreation.

C. Nutrition/diet: fluid intake per 24-hour period; intake of vitamins
D. Past medical history: immunizations (yearly immunizations for colds/flu; frequency and results of tuberculin skin testing); allergies (foods, drugs, contact or inhalant allergens, precipitating factors, specific treatment, desensitization)

## Physical Examination

A. Inspect for configuration of the chest (kyphosis, scoliosis, barrel chest) and cyanosis.
B. Determine rate and pattern of breathing (normal rate 12–18/minute); note tachypnea, hyperventilation, or labored breathing pattern.
C. Palpate skin, subcutaneous structures, and muscles for texture, temperature, and degree of development.
D. Palpate for tracheal position, respiratory excursion (symmetric or asymmetric movement of the chest), and for fremitus.
    1. Fremitus is normally increased in intensity at second intercostal spaces at sternal border and interscapular spaces only.
    2. Increased intensity elsewhere may indicate pneumonia, pulmonary fibrosis, or tumor.
    3. Decreased intensity may indicate pneumothorax, pleural effusion, COPD.
E. Percuss lung fields (should find resonance over normal lung tissue, note hyperresonance or dullness) and for diaphragmatic excursion (normal distance between levels of dullness on full expiration and full inspiration is 6–12 cm).
F. Auscultate for normal (vesicular, bronchial, bronchovesicular) and adventitious (rales or crackles, rhonchi, pleural friction rub) breath sounds (see Figure 4-13).

## Laboratory/Diagnostic Tests

A. Arterial blood gases (ABGs)
    1. Measure base excess/deficit, blood pH, $CO_2$, total $CO_2$, $O_2$ content, $O_2$ saturation ($SaO_2$), $pCO_2$ (partial pressure of carbon dioxide), $pO_2$ (partial pressure of oxygen)
    2. Nursing care
        a. If drawn by arterial stick, place a 4 × 4 bandage over puncture site after withdrawal of needle and maintain pressure with two fingers for at least 2 minutes.
        b. Gently rotate sample in test tube to mix heparin with the blood.
        c. Place sample in ice-water container until it can be analyzed.

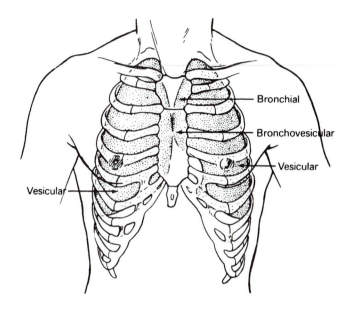

**Figure 4-13** Locations for hearing normal breath sounds

B. Pulmonary function studies
    1. Evaluation of lung volume and capacities by spirometry: tidal volume (TV), vital capacity (VC), inspiratory and expiratory reserve volume (IRV and ERV), residual volume (RV), inspiratory capacity (IC), functional residual capacity (FRC)
    2. Involves use of a spirometer to diagram movement of air as client performs various respiratory maneuvers; shows restriction or obstruction to airflow, or both
    3. Nursing care
        a. Carefully explaining procedure will help allay anxiety and ensure cooperation.
        b. Perform tests before meals.
        c. Withhold medication that may alter respiratory function unless otherwise ordered.
        d. After procedure assess pulse and provide for rest period.
C. Hematologic studies (ESR, Hgb and hct, WBC)
D. Sputum culture and sensitivity
    1. Culture: isolation and identification of specific microorganism from a specimen
    2. Sensitivity: determination of antibiotic agent effective against organism (sensitive or resistant)
    3. Nursing care
        a. Explain necessity of effective coughing.
        b. If client unable to cough, heated aerosol will assist with obtaining a specimen.
        c. Collect specimen in a sterile container that can be capped afterwards.
        d. Volume need not exceed 1–3 mL.
        e. Deliver specimen to lab rapidly.

E. Tuberculin skin test
1. Intradermal test done to detect tuberculosis infection; does not differentiate active from dormant infections
2. Purified protein derivative (PPD) tuberculin administered to determine any previous sensitization to tubercle bacillus
3. Several methods of administration
   a. Mantoux test: 0.1 mL solution containing 0.5 tuberculin units of PPD-tuberculin is injected into the forearm.
   b. Tine test: a stainless steel disc with 4 tines impregnated with PPD-tuberculin is pressed into the skin.
4. Results: read within 48–72 hours; inspect skin and circle zone of induration with a pencil; measure diameter in mm
   a. Negative: zone diameter less than 5 mm
   b. Doubtful or probable: zone diameter 5–10 mm
   c. Positive: zone diameter 10 mm or more

F. Thoracentesis
1. Insertion of a needle through the chest wall into the pleural space to obtain a specimen for diagnostic evaluation, removal of pleural fluid accumulation, or to instill medication into the pleural space
2. Nursing care: prior to procedure
   a. Confirm that a signed permit has been obtained.

   b. Explain procedure; instruct client not to cough or talk during procedure.
   c. Position client at side of bed, with upper torso supported on overbed table, feet and legs well supported. (See Figure 4-14)
   d. Assess vital signs.
3. Nursing care: following procedure
   a. Observe for signs and symptoms of pneumothorax, shock, leakage at puncture site.
   b. Auscultate chest to ascertain breath sounds.

G. Bronchoscopy
1. Insertion of a fiber-optic scope into the bronchi for diagnosis, biopsy, specimen collection, examination of structures/tissues, removal of foreign bodies
2. Nursing care: prior to procedure
   a. Confirm that a signed permit has been obtained.
   b. Explain procedure, remove dentures, and provide good oral hygiene.
   c. Keep client NPO 6–12 hours pretest.
3. Nursing care: following procedure
   a. Position client on side or in semi-Fowler's.
   b. Keep NPO until return of gag reflex.
   c. Assess for and report frank bleeding.
   d. Apply ice bags to throat for comfort; discourage talking, coughing, smoking for a few hours to decrease irritation.

## ANALYSIS

Nursing diagnoses for the client with a respiratory dysfunction may include:
A. Impaired gas exchange
B. Ineffective airway clearance
C. Ineffective breathing pattern
D. Impaired verbal communication
E. Activity intolerance
F. Anxiety
G. Imbalanced nutrition: less than body requirements
H. Risk for infection

## PLANNING AND IMPLEMENTATION

### Goals

A. Adequate ventilation will be maintained.
B. Maintenance of patent airway.
C. Effective breathing patterns will be maintained.
D. Client will communicate in an effective manner.
E. Client will demonstrate increased tolerance for activity.
F. Anxiety will be reduced.
G. Adequate nutritional status will be maintained.
H. Client remains free from infection.

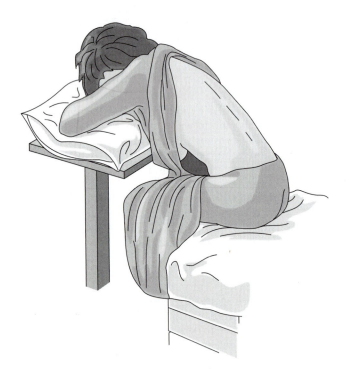

**Figure 4-14** Client position for thoracentesis

# Interventions

## Chest Drainage Systems

A. Insertion of a catheter into the intrapleural space to maintain constant negative pressure when air/fluid have accumulated.

B. Chest tube is attached to underwater drainage to allow for the escape of air/fluid and to prevent reflux of air into the chest.

C. For evacuation of air, chest tube is placed in the second or third intercostal space, anterior or midaxillary line (air rises to the upper chest).

D. For drainage of fluid, chest tube is placed in the eighth or ninth intercostal space, midaxillary line.

E. Chest tube is connected to tubing for the collection system; the distal end of the collection tubing must be placed below the water level in order to prevent atmospheric air from entering the pleural space.

F. Traditional water-seal drainage; also known as wet suction; can be set up using one, two, or three bottles. No longer used in the United States because it has been replaced by the newer technology of dry-suction water-seal drainage. For explanatory purposes it is included here. Also may be used in other countries.

   1. One-bottle system (Figure 4-15A)
      a. Operates by gravity, not suction; the bottle serves as both collection chamber and water seal.
      b. Two hollow tubes (glass rods) are inserted into the stopper of the bottle; the drainage tube is connected to the glass rod that is submerged approximately 2 cm below the water level; the second glass tube allows for the escape of air.
      c. If considerable drainage accumulates it is difficult for the client to expel air and fluid from the pleural space. If this occurs, the glass rod may be pulled up or a new drainage bottle may be set up (according to physician's orders).

   2. Two-bottle system (see Figure 4-15B,C)
      a. One bottle serves as a drainage collection chamber, the other as a water seal.
      b. The first bottle is the drainage collection chamber and has two short tubes in the rubber stopper. One of these tubes is attached to the drainage tubing coming from the client; the other is attached to the underwater tube of the second bottle (the water-seal bottle). The air vent of the water-seal bottle must be left open to atmospheric air. If suction is used, the first bottle serves as drainage collection and water-seal chamber, and the second bottle serves as the suction chamber.

   3. Three-bottle system (Figure 4-15D)
      a. This system has a drainage collection, a water-seal, and a suction-control bottle.
      b. The third bottle controls the amount of pressure in the system. The suction-control bottle has three tubes inserted in the stopper, two short and one long. One short tube is joined with the tubing to the former air vent of the water-seal bottle; the second short tube is connected to suction. The third (long) tube (or suction-control tube) is located between the short tubes and has one end open to the atmosphere and the other below the water level.
      c. The depth to which the suction-control tube is immersed controls the amount of pressure within the system. The pressure is determined by the physician.

G. Dry-suction water-seal drainage; also referred to as dry suction; has three chambers (collection chamber, water seal chamber, and wet suction control chamber) (see Figure 4-15E).

H. Dry-suction one-way valve system (also known as Heimlich Flutter Valve); allows unidirectional flow of air and fluid from pleural space, prevents reflux, sets up quickly in emergency, works when knocked over, works well for ambulatory clients.

I. Nursing care: without suction
   1. Prepare the unit for use and connect the chest catheter to the drainage tubing.
   2. Examine the entire system to ensure airtightness and absence of obstruction from kinks or dependent loops of tubing.
   3. Note oscillation of the fluid level within the water-seal tube. It will rise on inspiration and fall on expiration due to changes in the intrapleural pressure. If oscillation stops and system is intact, notify physician.
   4. Check the amount, color, and characteristics of the drainage. If drainage ceases and system is not blocked, assess for signs of respiratory distress from fluid/air accumulation.
   5. Always keep drainage system lower than the level of the client's chest.
   6. Keep Vaseline gauze at bedside at all times in case chest tube falls out.
   7. Keep clamps at bedside in case of accidental disconnection. Clamp, troubleshoot, and immediately reconnect.
   8. Encourage coughing and deep breathing to facilitate removal of air and drainage from pleural cavity.
   9. Provide ROM exercises.

J. Nursing care: with suction
   1. Attach suction tubing to suction apparatus, and chest catheter to drainage tubing.
   2. Open suction slowly until a stream of bubbles is seen in the suction chamber. There should be continuous bubbling in this chamber and intermittent bubbling in the water seal. Check for an air leak in the system if bubbling in water seal is constant; notify physician if air leak.

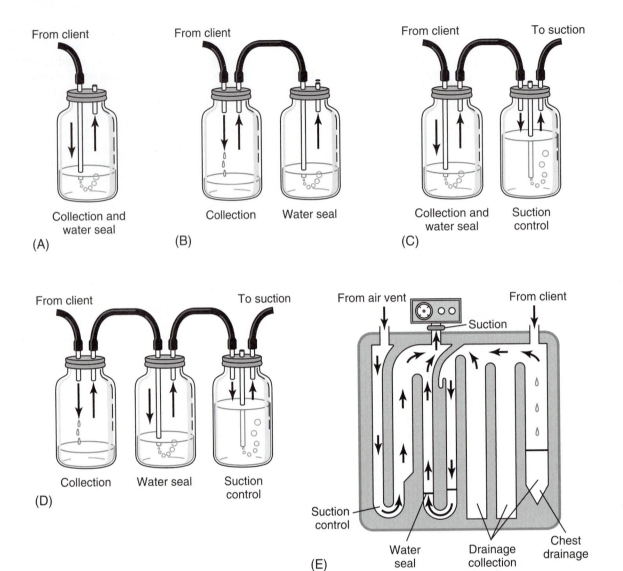

**Figure 4-15** Water-seal drainage systems: (A) one-bottle system; (B) two-bottle system; (C) two-bottle system with suction; (D) three-bottle system; (E) underwater seal chest drainage device

3. Check drainage, keep drainage system below level of client's chest, keep Vaseline gauze at bedside, encourage coughing and deep breathing, and provide ROM exercises.

**K.** General principles of chest tube management:
1. Never clamp chest tubes over an extended period of time unless a specific order is written by the physician. Clamping the chest tubes of a client with air in the pleural space will cause increased pressure buildup and possible tension pneumothorax.
2. Removal of the chest tube: instruct the client to perform Valsalva maneuver; apply a Vaseline or gauze dressing to the site (per hospital protocol).

3. If the water-seal bottle should break, immediately obtain some type of fluid-filled container to create an emergency water seal until a new unit can be obtained.

### Heimlich Flutter Valve

**A.** This disposable valve allows a unidirectional flow of air and fluid from the pleural space into a drainage bag and prevents any reflux of air or fluid. A water-seal drainage system is not necessary.
**B.** Controlled suction can be attached if ordered.
**C.** The valve is encased in clear plastic, which eliminates the possibility of kinks. Its small size, approximately 7 inches, permits greater mobility.

## Chest Physiotherapy

A. General information
   1. Used for individuals with increased production of secretions or thick, sticky secretions, and for clients with impaired removal of secretions or with ineffective cough. May also be used as a preventive measure for clients with weakness of the muscles of respiration or a predisposition to increased production or thickness of secretions.
   2. Includes the techniques of postural drainage, percussion, and vibration.
      a. Postural drainage: uses gravity and various positions to stimulate the movement of secretions.
         1) Postural drainage positions are determined by the areas of involved lung, assessed by chest X-ray and physical assessment findings.
         2) Careful positioning is required to help secretions flow from smaller airways into the segmental bronchus and larger airways where secretions can be coughed up.
      b. Percussion: involves clapping with cupped hands on the chest wall over the segment to be drained.
         1) The hand is cupped by holding the fingers together so that the shape of the hand conforms with chest wall.
         2) Clapping should be vigorous but not painful.
      c. Vibration: in this technique the hand is pressed firmly over the appropriate segment of chest wall, and muscles of upper arm and shoulder are tensed (isometric contraction); done with flattened, not cupped hand; mechanical vibration is performed by a hand-held instrument.

B. Nursing care
   1. Perform procedure before or 3 hours after meals.
   2. Administer bronchodilators about 20 minutes before procedure.
   3. Remove all tight/constricting clothing.
   4. Have all equipment available (tissues, emesis basin, towel, paper bag).
   5. Assist client to correct prescribed position for postural drainage (client to assume each postural drainage position for approximately 3–5 minutes).
   6. Place towel over area to be percussed.
   7. Instruct client to take several deep breaths.
   8. Percuss designated area for approximately 3 minutes during inspiration and expiration.
   9. Vibrate same designated area during exhalations of 4–5 deep breaths.
   10. Assist client with coughing when in postural drainage position; some clients may need to sit upright to produce a cough.
   11. Repeat the same procedure in all designated positions.
   12. After procedure, assist client to comfortable position and provide good oral hygiene.

## Mechanical Ventilation

A. General information
   1. Ventilation is performed by mechanical means in individuals who are unable to maintain normal levels of oxygen and carbon dioxide in the blood.
   2. Indicated in clients with COPD, obesity, neuromuscular disease, severe neurologic depression, thoracic trauma, ARDS; clients who have undergone thoracic or open-heart surgery are likely to be maintained on mechanical ventilation post-op.

B. Types (positive pressure ventilators)
   1. Positive pressure-cycled ventilator: pushes air into the lungs until a predetermined pressure is reached within the tracheobronchial tree; expiration occurs by passive relaxation of the diaphragm.
   2. Volume-cycled ventilator: most popular type for intubated adults and older children; delivers air into the lungs until a certain predetermined tidal volume is reached before terminating inspiration.
   3. Time-cycled ventilator: terminates inspiration after a preset time; tidal volume is regulated by adjusting length of inspiration and flow rate of pressurized gas.

C. Modes of mechanical ventilation
   1. Assist/control mode: client's inspiratory effort triggers ventilator, which then delivers breath; may be set to deliver breath automatically if client does not trigger it. The same tidal volume is delivered with each breath.
   2. Intermittent mandatory ventilation (IMV): client may breathe at own rate. IMV breaths are delivered under positive pressure; however, all other respirations taken by the client are delivered at ambient pressure and tidal volume is of client's own determination.
   3. Positive end expiratory pressure (PEEP): ventilator delivers additional positive pressure at the end of expiration, which maintains the alveoli in an expanded state.
   4. Controlled mandatory ventilation (CMV): all breaths initiated by ventilator as there is no pressure sensed by the machine. Same tidal volume is delivered with each breath.
   5. Continuous positive airway pressure (CPAP): achieves the same results as PEEP, except CPAP is used on adult clients who are on a T-piece.
   6. Pressure support (PS): client's inspiratory efforts trigger each breath; every breath ventilator assisted without dyssynchrony, which can occur with SIMV. Often used prior to extubation.

**D.** Nursing care

   **1.** Assess for decreased cardiac output and administer appropriate nursing care.

   **2.** Monitor for positive water balance. Pressure breathing may cause increase in antidiuretic hormone (ADH) and retention of water.

     **a.** Maintain accurate I&O.

     **b.** Assess daily weights.

     **c.** Take PCWP readings as ordered.

     **d.** Palpate for peripheral edema.

     **e.** Auscultate chest for altered breath sounds.

   **3.** Monitor for barotrauma (see Tension Pneumothorax).

     **a.** Assess ventilator settings every 4 hours.

     **b.** Auscultate breath sounds every 2 hours.

     **c.** Monitor ABGs.

     **d.** Perform complete pulmonary physical assessment every shift.

   **4.** Monitor for GI problems (stress ulcer).

   **5.** Administer muscle relaxants, tranquilizers, analgesics, or paralyzing agents as ordered to increase client-machine synchrony by relaxing the client.

## Oxygen Therapy

**A.** Most common therapy for clients with respiratory disease

**B.** Indications include arterial hypoxemia; COPD; ARDS; tissue, cellular, and circulatory hypoxia

**C.** Delivery systems

   **1.** Low-flow system: delivers oxygen at variable liter flows designed to add to client's inspired air.

     **a.** Nasal cannula

       **1)** Most common mode of oxygen delivery; consists of delivering 100% oxygen through two prongs inserted 1 cm into each nostril; general flow rates of 1–4 liters/minute are used with desired $FiO_2$ range of 24–40%.

       **2)** Nursing care

         **a)** Instruct client to breathe through the nose.

         **b)** Remove cannula and clean nares every 8 hours.

         **c)** Provide mouth care every 2–3 hours.

         **d)** Use gauze pads behind ears to decrease irritation.

         **e)** Assess arterial $pO_2$ frequently.

     **b.** Standard mask

       **1)** Simple face mask that covers the nose and mouth and provides an additional area for oxygen collection; ranges: 6–12 liters/minute; $FiO_2$: 40–65%.

       **2)** Nursing care

         **a)** Instruct client to breathe through the nose.

         **b)** Remove and clean mask every 2–3 hours.

         **c)** Monitor carefully in clients who are prone to develop obstructed airways.

         **d)** Replace mask with nasal cannula during meals and reposition mask immediately after eating.

     **c.** Nonrebreathing mask

       **1)** Standard mask with a reservoir bag designed to deliver 90–100% oxygen; a one-way valve between reservoir bag and mask allows the client to inhale only from the reservoir bag and exhale through separate valves on the side of the mask; ranges: 6–15 liters/minute; $FiO_2$: 60–90%.

       **2)** Nursing care

         **a)** Instruct client to breathe through the nose.

         **b)** Ensure that bag does not collapse completely with each inspiration.

         **c)** Remove and clean mask every 2–3 hours.

   **2.** High-flow system: client receives entire inspired gas from the apparatus, flow rates must exceed the volume of air required for a person's minute ventilation; Venturi mask commonly used.

     **a.** Provides precise delivery of oxygen concentrations of 24–50%.

     **b.** Nursing care

       **1)** Provide supplemental oxygen by cannula during meals and other activities where mask interferes.

       **2)** Remove and clean mask every 2–3 hours.

## Tracheobronchial Suctioning

**A.** Suction removal of secretions from the tracheobronchial tree using a sterile catheter inserted into the airway.

**B.** Catheters may be inserted through various routes: nasopharyngeal, oropharyngeal, or via an artificial airway.

**C.** Purposes

   **1.** Maintain a patent airway through removal of secretions

   **2.** Promote adequate exchange of oxygen/carbon dioxide

   **3.** Substitute for effective coughing

   **4.** Obtain a specimen for analysis

**D.** Procedure

   **1.** Gather suctioning equipment (receptacle for secretions, sterile catheter, sterile gloves, and container of sterile normal saline), or use inline device for endotracheal tube suctioning.

   **2.** Turn vacuum on and test suction system.

   **3.** Place client in semi- to high-Fowler's position.

   **4.** Apply sterile glove, fill sterile cup with solution, and attach sterile catheter to connecting tube.

5. Increase inspired oxygen concentration to highest point and hyperinflate the lungs before and after each catheter insertion by using self-inflating bag; have client deep breathe if able.
6. Use gloved hand to insert catheter.
    a. Oral route
        1) If oral airway in place, slide the catheter alongside it and back to the pharynx; if no oral airway in place, have client protrude the tongue and guide the catheter into the oropharynx.
        2) Insert during inspiration until cough is stimulated or secretion obtained.
    b. Nasal route: advance catheter along the floor of the nares or pass it through an artificial nasal airway (nasal trumpet) until cough is stimulated or secretions obtained.
    c. Artificial airway: insert the catheter into the artificial airway until cough is stimulated or secretions obtained.
7. Do not cover the thumb control and do not apply suction during insertion of the catheter.
8. During withdrawal, rotate the catheter while applying intermittent suction.
9. Whole suctioning procedure including insertion and removal of the catheter should not exceed 10 seconds.
10. If it is necessary to continue the suctioning process, hyperinflate the lungs, allow the client to rest briefly, and repeat the process.
11. Discard catheter, glove, and cup; record amount, color, characteristics of the secretions obtained; note client's tolerance of procedure.
12. Auscultate for changes in breath sounds.

## Tracheostomy Care

A. Performed to avoid bacterial contamination and obstruction of tracheostomy tube; frequency varies depending on amount of secretions
B. Procedure
    1. Explain procedure and provide reassurance to the client.
    2. If not contraindicated, place client in semi-Fowler's position to promote lung reexpansion.
    3. Disconnect ventilator or humidification device.
    4. Suction trachea to clear secretions.
    5. Reconnect ventilator or humidifier.
    6. Remove all tracheostomy dressing.
    7. Assemble equipment ("trach care kit").
    8. Set up sterile field and put on sterile glove.
        a. For a single-cannula tube
            1) With sterile gloved hand, wipe client's neck under trach tube flanges with presoaked sterile sponge.
            2) Wipe skin around tracheostomy with a second sponge until cleansed thoroughly (may use wet cotton-tipped applicators to cleanse around stoma).
            3) Use each sponge or applicator only once.
            4) Allow area to dry and apply a new sterile dressing (free of lint and fibers).
            5) Change tracheostomy ties as needed.
        b. For a double-cannula tube (nondisposable inner cannula)
            1) Disconnect ventilator or humidification device and unlock the inner cannula of trach tube using ungloved hand.
            2) Place inner cannula in basin containing $H_2O_2$ to remove encrustations.
            3) If client on a ventilator, insert another inner cannula while old one is being cleaned and reconnect client to ventilator.
            4) Cleanse stomal area and trach tube flanges with presoaked gauze sponges.
            5) Clean inner cannula.
            6) Remove excess liquid by gentle shaking.
            7) If client not on a ventilator, gently reinsert inner cannula into tracheostomy tube and lock in place.
            8) Allow area to dry, apply dressing and new tracheostomy ties as described above.
        c. For a double-cannula tube (disposable inner cannula)
            1) Disconnect ventilator tube.
            2) Remove inner cannula.
            3) Insert replacement cannula.
            4) Cleanse stomal area and trach tube flanges with presoaked gauze sponges.
            5) Allow area to dry, apply dressing and new tracheostomy ties as described above.

# EVALUATION

A. Client demonstrates ABGs or $O_2$ saturation within normal limits; absence of dyspnea and cyanosis; usual or improved breath sounds and usual mentation.
B. Client demonstrates effective coughing with expectoration of secretions; absence of dyspnea; rate and depth of ventilation within normal range; improved breath sounds.
C. ABGs or $O_2$ saturation within normal range; lungs clear to auscultation; rate and depth of respirations within client's normal range; effective use of muscles of respiration.
D. Client identifies plans for appropriate alternate speech methods.
E. Client demonstrates increased activity tolerance with absence of dyspnea and excessive fatigue and vital signs within normal limits.

F. Improved rest/sleep patterns; respiratory rate and rhythm within client's normal range; demonstrates effective problem-solving abilities.

G. Client demonstrates behaviors/lifestyle changes to regain and maintain appropriate body weight. Verbalizes importance of nutrition to general well-being. Stable weight; improved anthropometric measurements.

H. Vital signs within client's normal range; client verbalizes understanding of causative/risk factors and utilizes techniques to promote a safe environment.

# DISORDERS OF THE RESPIRATORY SYSTEM

## Chronic Obstructive Pulmonary Disease (COPD)

Refers to respiratory conditions that produce obstruction of airflow; includes emphysema, bronchitis, and bronchiectasis. Asthma is now considered a separate disorder because it is often reversible.

### Emphysema

A. General information
1. Enlargement and destruction of the alveolar, bronchial, and bronchiolar tissue with resultant loss of recoil, air trapping, thoracic overdistension, sputum accumulation, and loss of diaphragmatic muscle tone
2. These changes cause a state of carbon dioxide retention, hypoxia, and respiratory acidosis.
3. Caused by cigarette smoking, infection, inhaled irritants, heredity, allergic factors, aging

B. Assessment findings
1. Anorexia, fatigue, weight loss, clubbing (bulbous enlargement of distal fingers/nails)
2. Feeling of breathlessness, cough, sputum production, flaring of the nostrils, use of accessory muscles of respiration, increased rate and depth of breathing, dyspnea
3. Decreased respiratory excursion, resonance to hyperresonance, decreased breath sounds with prolonged expiration, normal or decreased fremitus
4. Diagnostic tests: $pCO_2$ elevated or normal; $pO_2$ normal or slightly decreased

C. Nursing interventions
1. Administer medications as ordered.
   a. Bronchiodilators: aminophylline, isoproterenol (Isuprel), terbutaline (Brethine), metaproterenol (Alupent), theophylline, isoetharine (Bronkosol); used in treatment of bronchospasm

b. Antimicrobials: tetracycline, ampicillin to treat bacterial infections
c. Corticosteroids: prednisone
2. Facilitate removal of secretions.
   a. Ensure fluid intake of at least 3 liters/day.
   b. Provide (and teach client) chest physical therapy, coughing and deep breathing, and use of hand nebulizers.
   c. Suction as needed.
   d. Provide oral hygiene after expectoration of sputum.
3. Improve ventilation.
   a. Position client in semi- or high-Fowler's.
   b. Instruct client to use diaphragmatic muscle to breathe.
   c. Encourage productive coughing after all treatments (splint abdomen to help produce more expulsive cough).
   d. Employ pursed-lip breathing techniques (prolonged, slow relaxed expiration against pursed lips).
   e. Oxygen delivery is used with caution, usually via nasal cannula keeping pulse oximetry at or above 90% (keep oxygen flow rate low to prevent suppressing respiratory drive).
4. Provide client teaching and discharge planning concerning
   a. Prevention of recurrent infections
      1) Avoid crowds and individuals with known infection.
      2) Adhere to high-protein, high-carbohydrate, increased vitamin C diet.
      3) Receive immunizations for influenza and pneumonia.
      4) Report changes in characteristics and color of sputum immediately.
      5) Report worsening of symptoms (increased tightness of chest, fatigue, increased dyspnea).
   b. Control of environment
      1) Use home humidifier at 30–50% humidity.
      2) Wear scarf over nose and mouth in cold weather to prevent bronchospasm.
      3) Avoid smoking and contact with environmental smoke.
      4) Avoid abrupt changes in temperature.
   c. Avoidance of inhaled irritants
      1) Stay indoors if pollution levels are high.
      2) Use air conditioner with high-efficiency particulate air filter to remove particles from air.
   d. Increasing activity tolerance
      1) Start with mild exercises, such as walking, and gradually increase amount and duration.
      2) Use breathing techniques (pursed lip, diaphragmatic) during

activities/exercises to control breathing.

3) Have oxygen available as needed to assist with activities.
4) Plan activities that require low amounts of energy.
5) Plan rest periods before and after activities.

## Bronchitis

A. General information
1. Excessive production of mucus in the bronchi with accompanying persistent cough.
2. Characteristic changes include hypertrophy/hyperplasia of the mucus-secreting glands in the bronchi, decreased ciliary activity, chronic inflammation, and narrowing of the small airways.
3. Caused by the same factors that cause emphysema.
B. Medical management: drug therapy includes bronchodilators, antimicrobials, expectorants (e.g., Robitussin)
C. Assessment findings
1. Productive (copious) cough, dyspnea on exertion, use of accessory muscles of respiration, scattered rales and rhonchi
2. Feeling of epigastric fullness, slight cyanosis, distended neck veins, ankle edema
3. Diagnostic tests: increased $pCO_2$, decreased $pO_2$
D. Nursing interventions: same as for emphysema

## Bronchiectasis

A. General information
1. Permanent abnormal dilation of the bronchi with destruction of muscular and elastic structure of the bronchial wall
2. Caused by bacterial infection; recurrent lower respiratory tract infections; congenital defects (altered bronchial structures); lung tumors; thick, tenacious secretions
B. Medical management: same as for emphysema
C. Assessment findings
1. Chronic cough with production of mucopurulent sputum, hemoptysis, exertional dyspnea, wheezing
2. Anorexia, fatigue, weight loss
3. Diagnostic tests
a. Bronchoscopy reveals sources and sites of secretions
b. Possible elevation of WBC
D. Nursing interventions: same as for emphysema

## Asthma

See Unit 5.

## Pulmonary Tuberculosis

A. General information
1. Bacterial infectious disease caused by *M. tuberculosis* and spread via airborne droplets when infected persons cough, sneeze, or laugh.
2. Once inhaled, the organisms implant themselves in the lung and begin dividing slowly, causing inflammation, development of the primary tubercle, and eventual caseation and fibrosis.
3. Infection spreads via the lymph and circulatory systems.
4. The CDC (2006) reports that the highest incidence is in foreign-born persons and racial/ethnic minority populations (Hispanics, African Americans, Asians). Socially and economically disadvantaged, alcoholic, and malnourished individuals are affected more often.
5. The causative agent, *M. tuberculosis*, is an acid-fast bacillus spread via droplet nuclei from infected persons.
B. Assessment findings
1. Cough (yellow mucoid sputum), dyspnea, hemoptysis, rales or crackles
2. Anorexia, malaise, weight loss, afternoon low-grade fever, pallor, pain, fatigue, night sweats
3. Diagnostic tests
a. Chest X-ray indicates presence and extent of disease process but cannot differentiate active from inactive form
b. Skin test (PPD) positive; area of induration 10 mm or more in diameter after 48 hours
c. Sputum positive for acid-fast bacillus (three samples is diagnostic for disease)
d. Culture positive
e. WBC and ESR increased
C. Nursing interventions
1. Administer medications as ordered (see Unit 2).
2. Prevent transmission.
a. Strict isolation not required if client/significant others adhere to special respiratory precautions for tuberculosis.
b. Client should be in a well-ventilated private room, with the door kept closed at all times.
c. All visitors and staff should wear masks when in contact with the client and should discard the used masks before leaving the room; client should wear a mask when leaving the room for tests.
d. All specimens should be labeled "AFB precautions."
e. Handwashing is required after direct contact with the client or contaminated articles.
3. Promote adequate nutrition.
a. Make ongoing assessments of client's appetite and do kcal counts for 3 days; consult dietitian for diet guidelines.

b. Offer small, frequent feedings and nutritional supplements; assist client with menu selection stressing balanced nutrition.

c. Weigh client at least twice a week.

d. Encourage activity as tolerated to increase appetite.

4. Prevent social isolation.

   a. Impart a comfortable, confident attitude when caring for the client.

   b. Explain the nature of the disease to the client, significant others, and visitors in simple terms.

   c. Stress that visits are important, but isolation precautions must be followed.

5. Vary the client's routine to prevent boredom.

6. Discuss the client's feelings and assess for boredom, depression, anxiety, fatigue, or apathy; provide support and encourage expression of concerns.

7. Provide client teaching and discharge planning concerning:

   a. Medication regimen: prepare a sheet with each drug name, dosage, time due, and major side effects; stress importance of following medication schedule for prescribed period of time (usually 9 months); include significant others

   b. Transmission prevention: client should cover mouth when coughing, expectorate into a tissue and place it in a paper bag; client should also wash hands after coughing or sneezing; stress importance of plenty of fresh air; include significant others

   c. Importance of notifying physician at the first sign of persistent cough, fever, or hemoptysis (may indicate recurrence)

   d. Need for follow-up care including physical exam, sputum cultures, and chest X-rays

   e. Availability of community health services

   f. Importance of high-protein, high-carbohydrate diet with inclusion of supplemental vitamins

# Histoplasmosis

A. General information: a systemic fungal disease caused by inhalation of dust contaminated by Histoplasma capsulatum; fungus has been found in poultry house litter, caves, areas harboring bats, and in bird roosts.

B. Medical management: antifungal agent Amphotericin B

   1. Very toxic: toxicity includes anorexia, chills, fever, headache, and renal failure

   2. Acetaminophen, Benadryl, and steroids given with Amphotericin B to prevent reactions

C. Assessment findings

   1. Symptoms similar to tuberculosis or pneumonia

      a. Cough
      b. Fever
      c. Joint pain
      d. Malaise

   2. Sometimes asymptomatic

   3. Diagnostic tests

      a. Chest X-ray (often appears similar to tuberculosis)

      b. Histoplasmin skin test (read the same as PPD)

D. Nursing interventions

   1. Monitor respiratory status

   2. Administer medications as ordered; observe for severe side effects of Amphotericin B: fever (acetaminophen given prophylactically), anaphylactic reaction (Benadryl and steroids given prophylactically), abnormal renal function with hypokalemia and azotemia.

# Chest Trauma

## Fractured Ribs

A. General information

   1. Common chest injury resulting from blunt trauma.

   2. Ribs 4–8 are most commonly fractured because they are least protected by chest muscles. Splintered or displaced fractured ribs may penetrate the pleura and lungs.

B. Medical management: drug therapy consists of narcotics, intercostal nerve block (injection of intercostal nerves above and below the injury with an anesthetic agent) for pain relief.

C. Assessment findings

   1. Pain, especially on inspiration

   2. Point tenderness and bruising at injury site, splinting with shallow respirations, apprehensiveness

   3. Diagnostic tests

      a. Chest X-ray reveals area and degree of fracture

      b. $pCO_2$ elevated; $pO_2$ decreased (later)

D. Nursing interventions

   1. Provide pain relief/control.

      a. Administer ordered narcotics and analgesics cautiously and monitor effects.

      b. Place client in semi- or high-Fowler's position to ease pain associated with breathing.

   2. Monitor client closely for complications.

      a. Assess for bloody sputum (indicative of lung penetration).

      b. Observe for signs and symptoms of pneumothorax or hemothorax.

## Flail Chest

A. General information

   1. Fracture of several ribs and resultant instability of the affected chest wall.

2. Chest wall is no longer able to provide the bony structure necessary to maintain adequate ventilation; consequently, the flail portion and underlying tissue move paradoxically (in opposition) to the rest of the chest cage and lungs.
   3. The flail portion is sucked in on inspiration and bulges out on expiration.
   4. Result is hypoxia, hypercarbia, and increased retained secretions.
   5. Caused by trauma (sternal rib fracture with possible costochondral separations).
B. Medical management
   1. Internal stabilization with a volume-cycled ventilator
   2. Drug therapy (narcotics, sedatives)
C. Assessment findings
   1. Severe dyspnea; rapid, shallow, grunty breathing; paradoxical chest motion
   2. Cyanosis, possible neck vein distension, tachycardia, hypotension
   3. Diagnostic tests
      a. $pO_2$ decreased
      b. $pCO_2$ elevated
      c. pH decreased
D. Nursing interventions
   1. Maintain an open airway: suction secretions/blood from nose, throat, mouth, and via endotracheal tube; note changes in amount, color, characteristics.
   2. Monitor mechanical ventilation.
   3. Encourage turning, coughing, and deep breathing.
   4. Monitor for signs of shock.

## Pneumothorax/Hemothorax

A. General information
   1. Partial or complete collapse of the lung due to an accumulation of air or fluid in the pleural space
   2. Types
      a. Spontaneous pneumothorax: the most common type of closed pneumothorax; air accumulates within the pleural space without an obvious cause. Rupture of a small bleb on the visceral pleura most frequently produces this type of pneumothorax. Occurs most often among tall, thin men between the ages of 20 and 40 years.
      b. Open pneumothorax: air enters the pleural space through an opening in the chest wall; usually caused by stabbing or gunshot wound.
      c. Tension pneumothorax: air enters the pleural space with each inspiration but cannot escape; causes increased intrathoracic pressure and shifting of the mediastinal contents to the unaffected side (mediastinal shift).

      d. Hemothorax: accumulation of blood in the pleural space; frequently found with an open pneumothorax resulting in a hemopneumothorax.
B. Assessment findings
   1. Sudden sharp pain in the chest, dyspnea, diminished or absent breath sounds on affected side, decreased respiratory excursion on affected side, hyperresonance on percussion, decreased vocal fremitus, tracheal shift to the opposite side (tension pneumothorax accompanied by mediastinal shift)
   2. Weak, rapid pulse; anxiety; diaphoresis
   3. Diagnostic tests
      a. Chest X-ray reveals area and degree of pneumothorax
      b. $pCO_2$ elevated
      c. $pO_2$, pH decreased
C. Nursing interventions
   1. Provide nursing care for the client with an endotracheal tube: suction secretions, vomitus, blood from nose, mouth, throat, or via endotracheal tube; monitor mechanical ventilation.
   2. Restore/promote adequate respiratory function.
      a. Assist with thoracentesis and provide appropriate nursing care.
      b. Assist with insertion of a chest tube to water-seal drainage and provide appropriate nursing care.
      c. Continuously evaluate respiratory patterns and report any changes.
   3. Provide relief/control of pain.
      a. Administer narcotics/analgesics/sedatives as ordered and monitor effects.
      b. Position client in high-Fowler's position.

## Atelectasis

A. General information
   1. Collapse of part or all of a lung due to bronchial obstruction
   2. May be caused by intrabronchial obstruction (secretions, tumors, bronchospasm, foreign bodies); extrabronchial compression (tumors, enlarged lymph nodes); or endobronchial disease (bronchogenic carcinoma, inflammatory structures)
B. Assessment findings
   1. Signs and symptoms may be absent depending upon degree of collapse and rapidity with which bronchial obstruction occurs
   2. Dyspnea, decreased breath sounds on affected side, decreased respiratory excursion, dullness to flatness upon percussion over affected area
   3. Cyanosis, tachycardia, tachypnea, elevated temperature, weakness, pain over affected area
   4. Diagnostic tests
      a. Bronchoscopy: may or may not reveal an obstruction

    **b.** Chest X-ray shows diminished size of affected lung and lack of radiance over atelectic area

    **c.** pO$_2$ decreased

**C.** Nursing interventions (prevention of atelectasis in hospitalized clients is an important nursing responsibility)

  **1.** Turn and reposition every 1–2 hours while client is bedridden or obtunded.

  **2.** Encourage mobility (if permitted).

  **3.** Promote liquification and removal of secretions.

  **4.** Avoid administration of large doses of sedatives and opiates that depress respiration and cough reflex.

  **5.** Prevent abdominal distension.

  **6.** Administer prophylactic antibiotics as ordered to prevent respiratory infection.

## Pleural Effusion

**A.** General information

  **1.** Collection of fluid in the pleural space

  **2.** A symptom, not a disease; may be produced by numerous conditions

  **3.** Classification

    **a.** Transudative: accumulation of protein-poor, cell-poor fluid

    **b.** Suppurative (empyema): accumulation of pus

  **4.** May be found in clients with liver/kidney disease, pneumonia, tuberculosis, lung abscess, bronchial carcinoma, leukemia, trauma, pulmonary edema, systemic infection, disseminated lupus erythematosus, polyarteritis nodosa

**B.** Medical management

  **1.** Identification and treatment of the underlying cause

  **2.** Thoracentesis

  **3.** Drug therapy

    **a.** Antibiotics: either systemic or inserted directly into pleural space

    **b.** Fibrinolytic enzymes: trypsin, streptokinase-streptodornase to decrease thickness of pus and dissolve fibrin clots

  **4.** Closed chest drainage

  **5.** Surgery: open drainage

**C.** Assessment findings

  **1.** Dyspnea, dullness over affected area upon percussion, absent or decreased breath sounds over affected area, pleural pain, dry cough, pleural friction rub

  **2.** Pallor, fatigue, fever, and night sweats (with empyema)

  **3.** Diagnostic tests

    **a.** Chest X-ray positive if greater than 250 mL pleural fluid

    **b.** Pleural biopsy may reveal bronchogenic carcinoma

    **c.** Thoracentesis may contain blood if cause is cancer, pulmonary infarction, or tuberculosis; positive for specific organism in empyema

**D.** Nursing interventions: vary depending on etiology

  **1.** Assist with repeated thoracentesis.

  **2.** Administer narcotics/sedatives as ordered to decrease pain.

  **3.** Assist with instillation of medication into pleural space (reposition client every 15 minutes to distribute the drug within the pleurae).

  **4.** Place client in high-Fowler's position to promote ventilation.

## Pneumonia

**A.** General information

  **1.** An inflammation of the alveolar spaces of the lung, resulting in consolidation of lung tissue as the alveoli fill with exudate.

  **2.** The various types of pneumonias are classified according to the offending organism.

  **3.** Bacterial pneumonia accounts for 10% of all hospital admissions; affects infants and elderly most often, and most often occurs in winter and early spring.

  **4.** Caused by various organisms: *D. pneumoniae, S. aureus, E. coli, H. influenzae.*

**B.** Assessment findings

  **1.** Cough with greenish to rust-colored sputum production; rapid, shallow respirations with an expiratory grunt; nasal flaring; intercostal rib retraction; use of accessory muscles of respiration; dullness to flatness upon percussion; possible pleural friction rub; high-pitched bronchial breath sounds; rales or crackles (early) progressing to coarse (later)

  **2.** Fever, chills, chest pain, weakness, generalized malaise

  **3.** Tachycardia, cyanosis, profuse perspiration, abdominal distension

  **4.** Diagnostic tests

    **a.** Chest X-ray shows consolidation over affected areas

    **b.** WBC increased

    **c.** pO$_2$ decreased

    **d.** Sputum specimens reveal particular causative organism

**C.** Nursing interventions

  **1.** Facilitate adequate ventilation.

    **a.** Administer oxygen as needed and assess its effectiveness.

    **b.** Place client in semi-Fowler's position.

    **c.** Turn and reposition frequently clients who are immobilized/obtunded.

    **d.** Administer analgesics as ordered to relieve pain associated with breathing (codeine is drug of choice).

    **e.** Auscultate breath sounds every 2–4 hours.

    **f.** Monitor ABGs.

2. Facilitate removal of secretions (general hydration, deep breathing and coughing, tracheobronchial suctioning as needed, expectorants as ordered, aerosol treatments via nebulizer, humidification of inhaled air, chest physical therapy).
3. Observe color, characteristics of sputum and report any changes; encourage client to perform good oral hygiene after expectoration.
4. Provide adequate rest and relief/control of pain.
   a. Provide bed rest with limited physical activity.
   b. Limit visits and minimize conversations.
   c. Plan for uninterrupted rest periods.
   d. Institute nursing care in blocks to ensure periods of rest.
   e. Maintain pleasant and restful environment.
5. Administer antibiotics as ordered, monitor effects and possible toxicity.
6. Prevent transmission (respiratory isolation may be required for clients with staphylococcal pneumonia).
7. Control fever and chills: monitor temperature and administer antipyretics as ordered, maintain increased fluid intake, provide frequent clothing and linen changes.
8. Provide client teaching and discharge planning concerning prevention of recurrence.
   a. Medication regimen/antibiotic therapy
   b. Need for adequate rest, limited activity, good nutrition with adequate fluid intake, and good ventilation
   c. Need to continue deep breathing and coughing for at least 6–8 weeks after discharge
   d. Availability of vaccines (pneumonococcal pneumonia, influenza)
   e. Techniques that prevent transmission (use of tissues when coughing, adequate disposal of secretions)
   f. Avoidance of persons with known respiratory infections
   g. Need to report signs and symptoms of respiratory infection (persistent or recurrent fever; changes in characteristics, color of sputum; chills; increased pain; difficulty breathing; weight loss; persistent fatigue)
   h. Need for follow-up medical care and evaluation

## Bronchogenic Carcinoma

A. General information
   1. The majority of primary pulmonary tumors arise from the bronchial epithelium and are therefore referred to as bronchogenic carcinomas.
   2. Characteristic pathologic changes include nonspecific inflammation with hypersecretion of mucus, desquamation of cells, hyperplasia, and obstruction.
   3. Metastasis occurs primarily by direct extension and via the circulatory or lymphatic system.
   4. Men over age 40 affected most often; 1 out of every 10 heavy smokers; affects right lung more often than left.
   5. Caused by inhaled carcinogens (primarily cigarette smoke but also asbestos, nickel, iron oxides, air silicone pollution; preexisting pulmonary disorders [TB, COPD]).
B. Medical management: depends on cell type, stage of disease, and condition of client; may include
   1. Radiation therapy
   2. Chemotherapy: usually includes cyclophosphamide, methotrexate, vincristine, doxorubicin, and procarbazine; concurrently in some combination
   3. Surgery: when entire tumor can be removed
C. Assessment findings
   1. Persistent cough (may be productive or blood tinged), chest pain, dyspnea, unilateral wheezing, friction rub, possible unilateral paralysis of the diaphragm
   2. Fatigue, anorexia, nausea, vomiting, pallor
   3. Diagnostic tests
      a. Chest X-ray may show presence of tumor or evidence of metastasis to surrounding structures
      b. Sputum for cytology reveals malignant cells
      c. Bronchoscopy: biopsy reveals malignancy
      d. Thoracentesis: pleural fluid contains malignant cells
      e. Biopsy of scalene lymph nodes may reveal metastasis
D. Nursing interventions
   1. Provide support and guidance to client as needed.
   2. Provide relief/control of pain.
   3. Administer medications as ordered and monitor effects/side effects.
   4. Control nausea: administer medications as ordered, provide good oral hygiene, provide small and more frequent feedings.
   5. Provide nursing care for a client with a thoracotomy.
   6. Provide client teaching and discharge planning concerning:
      a. Disease process, diagnostic and therapeutic interventions
      b. Side effects of radiation and chemotherapy
      c. Realistic information about prognosis

## Thoracic Surgery

A. General information
   1. Types
      a. Exploratory thoracotomy: anterior or posterolateral incision through the fourth,

fifth, sixth, or seventh intercostal spaces to expose and examine the pleura and lung

    **b.** Lobectomy: removal of one lobe of a lung; treatment for bronchiectasis, bronchogenic carcinoma, emphysematous blebs, lung abscesses

    **c.** Pneumonectomy: removal of an entire lung; most commonly done as treatment for bronchogenic carcinoma

    **d.** Segmental resection: removal of one or more segments of lung; most often done as treatment for bronchiectasis

    **e.** Wedge resection: removal of lesions that occupy only part of a segment of lung tissue; for excision of small nodules or to obtain a biopsy

  **2.** Nature and extent of disease and condition of client determine type of pulmonary resection.

**B.** Nursing interventions: preoperative

  **1.** Provide routine pre-op care.

  **2.** Perform a complete physical assessment of the lungs to obtain baseline data.

  **3.** Explain expected post-op measures: care of incision site, oxygen, suctioning, chest tubes (except if pneumonectomy performed).

  **4.** Teach client adequate splinting of incision with hands or pillow for turning, coughing, and deep breathing.

  **5.** Demonstrate ROM exercises for affected side.

  **6.** Provide chest physical therapy to help remove secretions.

**C.** Nursing interventions: postoperative

  **1.** Provide routine postoperative care.

  **2.** Promote adequate ventilation.

    **a.** Perform complete physical assessment of lungs and compare with preoperative findings.

    **b.** Auscultate lung fields every 1–2 hours.

    **c.** Encourage turning, coughing, and deep breathing every 1–2 hours after pain relief obtained.

    **d.** Perform tracheobronchial suctioning if needed.

    **e.** Assess for proper maintenance of chest drainage system (except after pneumonectomy).

    **f.** Monitor ABGs and report significant changes.

    **g.** Place client in semi-Fowler's position (if pneumonectomy performed, follow surgeon's orders about positioning, often on back or operative side, but not turned to unoperative side).

  **3.** Provide pain relief.

    **a.** Administer narcotics/analgesics prior to turning, coughing, and deep breathing.

    **b.** Assist with splinting while turning, coughing, deep breathing.

  **4.** Prevent impaired mobility of the upper extremities by doing ROM exercises; passive day of surgery, then active.

  **5.** Provide client teaching and discharge planning concerning

    **a.** Need to continue with coughing/deep breathing for 6–8 weeks post-op and to continue ROM exercises

    **b.** Importance of adequate rest with gradual increases in activity levels

    **c.** High-protein diet with inclusion of adequate fluids (at least 2 liters/day)

    **d.** Chest physical therapy

    **e.** Good oral hygiene

    **f.** Need to avoid persons with known upper respiratory infections

    **g.** Adverse signs and symptoms (recurrent fever; anorexia; weight loss; dyspnea; increased pain; difficulty swallowing; shortness of breath; changes in color, characteristics of sputum) and importance of reporting to physician

    **h.** Avoidance of crowds and poorly ventilated areas

## Acute Respiratory Distress Syndrome (ARDS)

**A.** General information

  **1.** A form of pulmonary insufficiency more commonly encountered in adults with no previous lung disorders than in those with existing lung disease.

  **2.** Initial damage to the alveolar-capillary membrane with subsequent leakage of fluid into the interstitial spaces and alveoli, resulting in pulmonary edema and impaired gas exchange.

  **3.** There is cell damage, decreased surfactant production, and atelectasis, which in turn produce hypoxemia, decreased compliance, and increased work of breathing.

  **4.** Predisposing conditions include shock, trauma, infection, fluid overload, aspiration, oxygen toxicity, smoke inhalation, pneumonia, DIC, drug allergies, drug overdoses, neurologic injuries, fat emboli.

  **5.** Has also been called shock lung.

**B.** Assessment findings

  **1.** Dyspnea, cough, tachypnea with intercostal/suprasternal retraction, scattered to diffuse rales/rhonchi

  **2.** Changes in orientation, tachycardia, cyanosis (rare)

  **3.** Diagnostic tests

    **a.** $pCO_2$ increased and $pO_2$ decreased

    **b.** Hypoxemia

    **c.** Hgb and hct possibly decreased

    **d.** $pO_2$ and $O_2$ saturation not reflective of high $O_2$ administration

**C.** Nursing interventions

  **1.** Promote optimal ventilatory status.

    **a.** Perform ongoing assessment of lungs with auscultation every 1–2 hours.

b. Elevate head and chest.
   c. Administer/monitor mechanical ventilation with PEEP.
   d. Assist with chest physical therapy as ordered.
   e. Encourage coughing and deep breathing every hour.
   f. Monitor ABGs, $O_2$ saturation, and report significant changes.
2. Promote rest by spacing activities and treatments.
3. Maintain fluid and electrolyte balance.
4. Treat cause.

# Cancer of the Larynx

A. General information
   1. Most common upper respiratory malignancy.
   2. The majority of laryngeal malignancies are squamous cell carcinomas.
   3. Types
      a. Supraglottic (also called extrinsic laryngeal cancer): involves the epiglottis and false cords and is likely to produce no symptoms until advanced stages.
      b. Glottic (also referred to as intrinsic laryngeal cancer): affects the true vocal cords; the most frequently occurring laryngeal cancer; produces early symptoms.
   4. Occurs most often in white men in middle or later life
   5. Caused by cigarette smoking, excessive alcohol consumption, chronic laryngitis, vocal abuse, family predisposition to cancer of larynx
B. Medical management
   1. Radiation therapy: may be effective in cases of localized disease, affecting only one vocal cord
   2. Chemotherapy: used as adjuvant therapy to help shrink tumor and eradicate metastases (experimental)
   3. Surgery
      a. Partial laryngectomy: a lesion on the true cord on one side is removed along with adjoining tissue. Useful in early, intrinsic lesions. Client is able to talk and has a normal airway post-op.
      b. Total laryngectomy
      c. Radical neck dissection
         1) Performed when metastasis from cancer of the larynx is suspected
         2) Includes removal of entire larynx, lymph nodes, sternocleidomastoid muscle, internal jugular vein, and spinal accessory nerve
         3) May also involve removal of the mandible, submaxillary gland, part of the thyroid and parathyroid gland
         4) Nursing care: same as for total laryngectomy, below

C. Assessment findings
   1. Supraglottic: localized throat pain; burning when drinking hot liquids or orange juice; lump in the neck; eventual dysphagia; dyspnea; weight loss; debility; cough; hemoptysis; muffled voice
   2. Glottic: progressive hoarseness (more than 2-week duration), eventual dyspnea
   3. Enlarged cervical lymph nodes
D. Nursing interventions: provide care for the client with a laryngectomy.

## Total Laryngectomy

A. General information: consists of removal of the entire larynx, hyoid bone, pre-epiglottic space, cricoid cartilage, and 3–4 rings of trachea. The pharyngeal opening to the trachea is closed and remaining trachea brought out to the neck to form a permanent tracheostomy. The result is loss of normal speech and breathing and loss of olfaction.
B. Nursing care: preoperative
   1. Provide routine pre-op care.
   2. Explain expected procedures after surgery including suctioning, humidification, coughing and deep breathing, IV fluids, nasogastric tube feedings, tracheostomy or laryngectomy tube.
   3. Reinforce physician's teaching regarding loss of normal speech, breathing patterns, and sense of smell.
   4. Encourage client/significant others to talk about fears and hopes following surgery.
   5. Introduce client to changes in modes of communication (esophageal speech, artificial larynx).
   6. Establish method of communication to be used immediately post-op (Magic Slate, gestures).
C. Nursing interventions: postoperative
   1. Promote optimum ventilatory status.
   2. Suction nose frequently because of rhinitis.
   3. Assess function of tracheostomy/laryngectomy tube and suction as needed.
   4. Promote pain relief.
      a. Elevate head of bed to decrease pressure on suture line.
      b. Administer analgesics as needed and monitor effects.
      c. Assist with moving head and turning by supporting back of neck with hands.
   5. Promote wound drainage.
      a. Elevate head of bed to promote lymphatic drainage from head.
      b. Monitor amount, characteristics of drainage.
   6. Promote nutrition.
      a. Institute and monitor tube feedings as ordered.
      b. Increase fluid intake as tolerated to improve hydration.

c. Encourage self-feeding.
   d. Advance to normal diet as soon as client able to tolerate.
7. Prevent infection.
   a. Assess WBC and report significant increases.
   b. Take temperature every 4 hours.
   c. Maintain sterile technique when suctioning and performing tracheostomy care.
   d. Observe stoma/suture lines for signs of infection.
   e. Provide frequent oral hygiene.
   f. Monitor sputum and drainage for changes in color, odor, characteristics.
8. Enhance communication.
   a. Carry out modes of communication determined pre-op.
   b. Assess nonverbal behavior.
   c. Allow client time to ask questions and do not anticipate answers.
   d. Arrange for volunteer laryngectomy client to visit client and assist with esophageal speech, artificial larynx, and living with a laryngectomy.
   e. Consult with speech therapist if needed.
   f. Progress to normal diet as soon as possible to regain muscle tone of throat and abdomen.
9. Support client during adaptation to altered physical status.
   a. Encourage client to discuss feelings about changes in appearance, body functioning, and lifestyle; be aware of nonverbal responses to the changes.
   b. Assist to identify and use coping techniques that have been helpful in past.
   c. Suggest flattering clothing styles that don't emphasize chest or neck configuration.
   d. Monitor for and support behaviors indicative of positive adaptation to changes (e.g., interest in appearance).
10. Assess for respiratory complications (dyspnea, cyanosis, tachycardia, tachypnea, restlessness).
11. Provide client teaching and discharge planning concerning
   a. Tracheostomy/laryngectomy and stomal care
   b. Proper administration of nasogastric tube feedings and maintenance of nasogastric tube
   c. Control of dryness/crusting of tongue by brushing tongue regularly with soft toothbrush and toothpaste and using mouthwashes
   d. Need for humidified air at home
   e. Importance of protecting the stoma with a shield or towel while showering, directing shower nozzle away from stoma

   f. Need to use only electric razors for 6 months after surgery as facial area will be numb
   g. Need to lean forward when expectorating secretions and to cover stoma when coughing or sneezing
   h. Snorkle devices to enable swimming (caution is advised since drowning can occur rapidly in these clients)
   i. Need to wear an identification bracelet indicating that client is a neck breather
   j. Types of stoma guards available
   k. Necessity of installing smoke detectors since sense of smell is lost
   l. Information about prosthetic devices, speech therapy, and reconstructive surgery

# Sample Questions

244. A male client is admitted following an automobile accident. He is very anxious, dyspneic, and in severe pain. The left chest wall moves in during inspiration and balloons out when he exhales. What condition are these symptoms most suggestive of?
   1. Hemothorax.
   2. Flail chest.
   3. Atelectasis.
   4. Pleural effusion.

245. A young man is admitted with a flail chest following a car accident. He is intubated with an endotracheal tube and is placed on a mechanical ventilator (control mode, positive pressure). Which physical finding alerts the nurse to an additional problem in respiratory function?
   1. Dullness to percussion in the third to fifth intercostal space, midclavicular line.
   2. Decreased paradoxical motion.
   3. Louder breath sounds on the right chest.
   4. pH of 7.36 in arterial blood gases.

246. The nurse is caring for a client who has had a chest tube inserted and connected to a portable water-seal drainage. The nurse determines the drainage system is functioning correctly when which of the following is observed?
   1. Continuous bubbling in the water-seal chamber.
   2. Fluctuation in the water-seal (U-tube) chamber.
   3. Suction tubing attached to a wall unit.
   4. Vesicular breath sounds throughout the lung fields.

247. The nurse is caring for a client who has just had a chest tube attached to a portable water-seal drainage system.
    1. Observe for intermittent bubbling in the water-seal chamber.
    2. Flush the chest tubes with 30 to 60 mL of NSS q4 to 6 hours.
    3. Maintain the client in an extreme lateral position.
    4. Strip the chest tubes in the direction of the client.

248. The nurse enters the room of a client who has a chest tube attached to a water-seal drainage system and notices the chest tube is dislodged from the chest. What is the most appropriate nursing intervention?
    1. Notify the physician.
    2. Insert a new chest tube.
    3. Cover the insertion site with petroleum gauze.
    4. Instruct the client to breathe deeply until help arrives.

249. An adult is ordered oxygen via nasal prongs. What is true of administering oxygen this way?
    1. Mixes room air with oxygen.
    2. Delivers a precise concentration of oxygen.
    3. Requires humidity during delivery.
    4. Is less traumatic to the respiratory tract.

250. An adult is receiving oxygen by nasal prongs. Which statement by the client indicates that client teaching regarding oxygen therapy has been effective?
    1. "I was feeling fine so I removed my nasal prongs."
    2. "It will be good to rest from taking deep breaths now that my oxygen is on."
    3. "Don't forget to come back quickly when you get me out of bed; I don't like to be without my oxygen for too long."
    4. "My family was angry when I told them they could not smoke in my room."

251. The client diagnosed with tuberculosis is taught prevention of disease transmission. Which correct answer will the client state is a means of transmission?
    1. Hands.
    2. Droplet nuclei.
    3. Milk products.
    4. Eating utensils.

252. The treatment plan for a client newly diagnosed with tuberculosis is likely to include which of the following medications as initial treatment?
    1. Ethambutol (Myambutol) and isoniazid (INH).
    2. Streptomycin and penicillin G (Crysticillin).
    3. Tetracycline and thioridazine (Mellaril).
    4. Pyridoxine (Beesix) and tetracycline.

253. A 64-year-old has been smoking since he was 11 years old. He has a long history of emphysema and is admitted to the hospital because of a respiratory infection that has not improved with outpatient therapy. Which finding would the nurse expect to observe during the client's nursing assessment?
    1. Electrocardiogram changes.
    2. Increased anterior-posterior chest diameter.
    3. Slow, labored respiratory pattern.
    4. Weight-height relationship indicating obesity.

254. Supplemental low-flow oxygen therapy is prescribed for a man with emphysema. Which is the most essential action for the nurse to initiate?
    1. Anticipate the need for humidification.
    2. Notify the physician that this order is contraindicated.
    3. Place the client in an upright position.
    4. Schedule frequent pulse oximeter checks.

255. When auscultating the lung fields, a sound described as a rustling, like the wind in the trees, is heard. What is the correct term for this occurrence?
    1. Crackles.
    2. Rhonchi.
    3. Wheezes.
    4. Vesicular.

256. The nurse's assessment of a client with lung cancer reveals the following: copious secretions, dyspnea, and cough. Based on these finding, what is the most appropriate nursing diagnosis?
    1. Impaired gas exchange.
    2. Ineffective airway clearance.
    3. Pain.
    4. Altered tissue perfusion.

257. A client has just had arterial blood gases drawn. What will the nurse do with the specimen collected?
    1. Gently shake the syringe.
    2. Place the sample in a syringe of warm water.
    3. Aspirate 0.5 mL of heparin into the syringe.
    4. Have the specimen analyzed immediately.

258. The nurse is to obtain a sputum specimen from a client. Select the correct set of statements instructing the client in the proper technique for obtaining a sputum specimen.
   1. "Collect the specimen right before bed. Spit carefully into the container."
   2. "Brush your teeth, then cough into the container. Do this first thing in the morning."
   3. "Right after lunch, cough and spit into the container."
   4. "Spit into the container, then add two tablespoons of water."

259. The nurse is checking tuberculin skin test results at a health clinic. One client has an area of induration measuring 12 mm in diameter. What does this finding indicate?
   1. This finding is a normal reading.
   2. This finding indicates active TB.
   3. This is a positive reaction and can indicate exposure to TB.
   4. This client needs to come back in two more days and let the nurse look at the area of induration again.

260. An adult has undergone a bronchoscopy. Which assessment findings indicate to the nurse that he is ready for discharge?
   1. Use of accessory muscles for breathing, decreased lung sounds.
   2. Stable vital signs, return of gag and cough reflex.
   3. Hemoptysis, rhonchi.
   4. Development of tachycardia with occasional PVCs, able to eat and drink.

261. An adult has a chest tube to a Pleur-evac® drainage system attached to a wall suction. An order to ambulate the client has been received. How should the nurse ambulate the client safely?
   1. Clamp the chest tube and carefully ambulate the client a short distance.
   2. Question the order to ambulate the client.
   3. Carefully ambulate the client, keeping the Pleur-evac lower than the client's chest.
   4. Disconnect the Pleur-evac from the client's chest tube, leave it attached to the bed, ambulate the client, and then reconnect the chest tube when he is returned to bed.

262. Approximately 10 minutes after a client returns from surgery with a tracheostomy tube the nurse assesses increasing noisy respiration and an increased pulse. What action should be taken immediately?

   1. Take the client's blood pressure.
   2. Suction the tracheostomy tube.
   3. Drain water from the O₂ tubing.
   4. Change the tracheostomy tube.

263. The nurse will perform chest physiotherapy (CPT) on a client every 4 hours. What is the appropriate action by the nurse?
   1. Gently slap the chest wall.
   2. Use vibration techniques to move secretions from affected lung areas during the inspiration phase.
   3. Perform CPT at least 2 hours after meals.
   4. Plan apical drainage at the beginning of the CPT session.

264. A client is on a ventilator. The ventilator alarm goes off. The nurse assesses the client and observes increased respiratory rate, use of accessory muscles, and agitation. What should be the nurse's first action?
   1. Remove the client from the ventilator and ambu bag the client, while continuing to assess to determine the cause of the client's distress.
   2. Call respiratory therapy to check the ventilator.
   3. Notify the physician.
   4. Turn off the alarm.

265. A client with respiratory failure is on a ventilator. The alarm goes off. What should be the nurse's first action?
   1. Notify the physician.
   2. Assess the client to determine the cause of the alarm.
   3. Turn off the alarm.
   4. Disconnect the client and use the ambu bag to ventilate the client.

266. A nurse is setting up oxygen for an adult male. He is to receive oxygen at 2 liters per nasal cannula. What should be included for this treatment?
   1. Adjust the flow rate to keep the reservoir bag inflated ⅔ full during inspiration.
   2. Monitor the client carefully for risk of aspiration.
   3. Make sure the valves and rubber flaps are patent, functional, and not stuck.
   4. Remind the client not to use Vaseline lip balm.

267. A long-term COPD client is receiving oxygen at 1 liter/minute. A family member decides she "doesn't look too good" and increases her

oxygen to 7 liter/minute. What should the nurse's initial action be?

1. Thank the client's cousin and continue to observe the client.
2. Immediately decrease the oxygen.
3. Notify the physician.
4. Add humidity to the oxygen.

268. An adult is receiving oxygen per face mask at 40%. The nurse should include which of the following in her plan of care?

1. Provide good skin care, making sure the mask fits well.
2. Keep all visitors out of the room.
3. Turn off the CPAP during the day.
4. Keep the bag inflated at all time.

269. An adult has a new tracheostomy in place. He has a small amount of thin, white secretions. The stoma is pink with no drainage noted. How often should the nurse perform trach care?

1. 4 hours.
2. 8 hours.
3. 24 hours.
4. Every hour.

270. A female client is admitted to the hospital. She has smoked two packs per day for 30 years. While providing her history, she becomes breathless, pauses frequently between words, and appears very anxious. She has a cough with thick white sputum production. Her chest is barrel shaped. Based on the data, on what condition will the nurse develop a plan of care?

1. Pneumonia.
2. Chronic obstructive pulmonary disease.
3. Tuberculosis.
4. Asthma.

271. A 68-year-old male is being admitted to the hospital for an exacerbation of his COPD. What will most likely be included in the plan of care?

1. Placed on 10 liters of oxygen per nasal cannula.
2. Placed in respiratory isolation.
3. Require frequent rest periods throughout the day.
4. Placed on fluid restriction.

272. A client with suspected tuberculosis will most likely relate which clinical manifestations?

1. Fatigue, weight loss, low-grade fevers, night sweats.
2. Asymmetrical chest expansion.

3. Rapid shallow breathing, prolonged labored expiration, stridor.
4. Dyspnea, hypoxemia, decreased pulmonary compliance.

273. An adult is being admitted to the nursing unit with a diagnosis of pneumonia. She has a history of arrested TB. What will be the nurse's initial action?

1. Place the client in respiratory isolation.
2. Encourage cough and deep breathing.
3. Force fluids.
4. Administer O₂.

274. An adult is being followed in the outpatient clinic for a diagnosis of active TB. She is receiving isoniazid 200 mg po daily, rifampin 500 mg po daily, and streptomycin 1500 mg IM twice weekly. Which statement by the client best indicates she understands her therapeutic regime?

1. "I'm glad I only have to take these drugs for a couple of weeks."
2. "I need to take these two drugs every day and come back to the clinic once a week for the shot."
3. "It may work best to take these pills in the evening right before bed."
4. "I'm glad my birth control pills aren't affected by these drugs—the doctor told me not to get pregnant!"

275. The nurse is counseling the family of an 18-year-old with active TB, about measures to prevent transmission of the disease. Which statement by the family best indicates understanding of these instructions?

1. "I won't let her and her sister share clothes."
2. "We will have to keep her in her room."
3. "We all need to wash our hands carefully, but especially our daughter."
4. "We cannot get TB from exposure to her sputum."

276. An elderly client has fallen and broken her eighth rib on her left side. The nurse should include which of the following when developing the plan of care?

1. Bind the client's chest with a 6-inch Ace bandage.
2. Keep the client on bed rest for 3 days.
3. Encourage the client to use her incentive spirometer and cough and deep breathe.
4. Administer large doses of narcotic analgesic so that the client will be able to more fully participate in pulmonary care.

277. A man is injured in an industrial accident. The industrial nurse assesses him and observes use of accessory muscles, severe chest pain, agitation, shortness of breath. The nurse also notices one side of his chest moving differently than the other. The nurse suspects flail chest. What will be the nurse's initial action?

1. Apply a sandbag to the flail side of his chest.
2. Prepare for intubation and mechanical ventilation.
3. Prepare for chest tube placement.
4. Administer pain medication.

278. What manifestation would the client with pleural effusion display?

1. Pain.
2. Swelling.
3. Dyspnea.
4. Increased sputum production.

279. An 86-year-old female was admitted to the hospital two days ago with pneumonia. She now has an order to be up in the chair as much as possible. How will the nurse plan the client's morning care?

1. Get her up before breakfast. Have her eat in the chair, then bathe while still up.
2. Allow her to eat breakfast in bed, rest for 30 minutes, get up in the chair, and rest for a few minutes. Allow her to wash her hands and face—nurse to complete bath.
3. Allow her to eat in bed, get her up, and provide her with a pan of water for her to bathe.
4. Get her up before breakfast, have her bathe before breakfast, eat in the chair, then a rest in the chair.

280. A client has been admitted to the hospital. Lung assessment reveals the following: bronchial breath sounds over (L) lower lobe, diminished breath sounds (L) lower lobe, tactile fremitus present, percussion dulled in this area. Based on the assessment findings, what condition does the nurse suspect?

1. Pneumonia.
2. Asthma.
3. Emphysema.
4. Early left-sided heart failure.

281. A nurse is teaching a class in a community center about lung cancer. Which statement best demonstrates the client's understanding of the risk factors for lung cancer?

1. "My husband smokes, but I don't! So, I really don't need to worry about getting lung cancer."

2. "I guess I will need to eat more green and yellow vegetables."
3. "Just because I have COPD doesn't mean that I have a higher risk."
4. "I've worked with asbestos all my life and have never had any problems."

282. An adult male was diagnosed with lung cancer 18 months ago. He is now in the terminal stages and is experiencing severe generalized pain. He has ordered morphine sulfate 10 mg IM q 4–6 h prn. What is the most appropriate action by the nurse?

1. Teach him that the pain medicine prescribed will take away all his pain and he will have no discomfort.
2. Counsel him about the addictive qualities of his prescribed narcotic.
3. Inform him that he may only ask for the pain medicine every 4 hours and there is nothing else you can offer in between medication times.
4. Encourage him to ask for the pain medicine before the pain becomes too severe.

283. A client is admitted to the nursing unit from the recovery room following a left pneumonectomy. What will the nurse expect in the plan of care?

1. Have a chest tube to water seal.
2. Have a chest tube to suction.
3. Be monitored closely for respiratory and cardiac complications.
4. Have his left arm maintained in a sling to prevent pain and discomfort.

284. An adult who has had a right thoracotomy for a wedge resection of his lung repeatedly refuses to do breathing or arm exercises because of the pain. What should the nurse include on the client's plan of care?

1. Offer the client pain medication immediately after arm exercises are completed.
2. Offer the client sips of ice water prior to a deep breathing and coughing session.
3. Schedule the client's activity 30–45 minutes after his IM injection of pain medication.
4. Have the client hold a pillow against his abdomen for support.

285. The nurse may expect a client with suspected early ARDS to exhibit which of the following?

1. $PaO_2$ of 90, $PaCO_2$ of 45, X-ray showing enlarged heart, bradycardia.
2. Thick green sputum production, $PaO_2$ of 75, pH 7.45.

3. Restlessness, suprasternal retractions, $PaO_2$ of 65.
4. Wheezes, slow deep respirations, $PaCO_2$ of 55, pH of 7.25.

286. The client had a removal of the larynx and a permanent opening made into the trachea. What is the correct name of this procedure?
   1. Total laryngectomy.
   2. Tracheostomy.
   3. Radical neck dissection.
   4. Partial laryngectomy.

287. An adult will undergo a total laryngectomy tomorrow. She is concerned about communicating post-op. The nurse should plan for her to communicate by which method the first 24–48 hours after surgery?
   1. Using the artificial larynx.
   2. Writing or pointing on a communication board.
   3. Using esophageal speech.
   4. Using a voice button.

288. An adult has had a total laryngectomy. The nurse is discussing options for verbal communication with the client. Which statement indicates the client understands the available options for verbal communication?
   1. "Because of the arthritis in my hands, I think the voice button method would be easiest to use."
   2. "By the time I leave the hospital, I will be able to talk."
   3. "If I use the esophageal speech, my voice will be high pitched and soft."
   4. "Using an artificial larynx will make me sound sort of monotone."

289. An adult is ready for discharge after undergoing a total laryngectomy. The nurse is discussing safety aspects of his home care. Which statement by the client best indicates that he understands the safety aspects of his care at home?
   1. "It is okay to swim as long as I'm careful."
   2. "I should use paper tissues to cover my stoma when I'm coughing."
   3. "I should not wear anything to cover my stoma."
   4. "I will need to use a humidifier in my home."

## Answers and Rationales

244. **2.** Paradoxical breathing movements (opposite the normal) are characteristic of flail chest. The flail portion is sucked in on inspiration and bulges out on expiration. Flail chest occurs when there are multiple rib fractures due to trauma.

245. **3.** Louder breath sounds on the right side of the chest indicate that the endotracheal tube may be misplaced and is aerating only one lung.

246. **2.** Fluctuation in the water-seal chamber demonstrates that the tubing system is patent.

247. **1.** Intermittent bubbling in the water-seal chamber indicates that air is leaving the thoracic cavity. If there is no bubbling in the water-seal chamber, it indicates either obstruction of the tubing or reexpansion of the lung. Reexpansion of the lung is unlikely, as the tube has just been inserted.

248. **3.** Covering the insertion site with petroleum gauze is a priority nursing measure that prevents air from entering the chest cavity.

249. **1.** Low-flow oxygen systems provide an oxygen concentration that is determined by the amount of air drawn into the system and the dilution of oxygen with room air.

250. **4.** Oxygen is a flammable gas and smoking is not permitted in the area.

251. **2.** The most frequent means of transmission of the tubercle bacillus is by droplet nuclei. The bacillus is present in the air as a result of coughing, sneezing, and expectorating by infected persons.

252. **1.** Ethambutol, isoniazid, streptomycin, and rifampin are first-line drugs used in the treatment of tuberculosis.

253. **2.** An increased anterior-posterior chest diameter, commonly referred to as "barrel chest," is seen in clients with emphysema as a result of chronic hyperinflation of the lungs.

254. **4.** The stimulus to breathe in a client with emphysema becomes low oxygen levels rather than rising $CO_2$ levels. Frequent pulse oximeter checks are necessary to see how the client handles low-flow oxygen administration.

255. **4.** This is a description of the normal vesicular breath sounds. They are low pitched, soft sounds heard over the peripheral lung fields where air flows through smaller bronchioles.

256. **2.** A client with lung cancer demonstrating the assessment findings provided would indicate a nursing diagnosis of ineffective airway clearance. The goal is this client will breathe without dyspnea or discomfort and maintain a patent airway.

257. **4.** The sample must be analyzed within 20 minutes, or if the client has leukocytosis immediately, to ensure accurate results.

258. **2.** Teeth are brushed to reduce contamination, then the client coughs into the container. Sputum is best collected in the morning when it is more plentiful.

259. **3.** A positive reaction is present when the induration is greater than 10 mm in diameter. The positive reaction indicates exposure to TB or the presence of inactive disease, not active disease.

260. **2.** Vital signs are taken frequently. Nothing is given by mouth until the cough and swallow reflexes have returned. Both are important criteria for discharge.

261. **3.** The Pleur-evac must not be raised above chest level because it can cause backflow of the fluid into the pleural space precipitating collapse of the lung or mediastinal shift. The Pleur-evac must remain upright and the chest tube should not have traction on it.

262. **2.** Noisy, increasing respirations and increasing pulse are signs that the client requires suctioning.

263. **3.** Chest physiotherapy should be performed at least 2 hours after meals to reduce the risk of vomiting and aspiration.

264. **1.** The nurse's best initial action should be to remove the client from the ventilator, ventilating the client with an ambu bag. Obviously, the client is experiencing respiratory distress and is not receiving adequate ventilation. The nurse should continue to closely assess to determine the cause and determine if the respiratory distress is related to ventilator malfunction or change in client status.

265. **2.** It is important for the nurse to quickly assess the client and determine the cause of the alarm. Once the cause has been determined, the nurse must intervene promptly to prevent complications.

266. **4.** Oxygen supports combustion. Smoking is not permitted in the room while $O_2$ is set up or being administered. A sign should be posted to that effect.

267. **2.** The COPD client's drive to breathe is hypoxia. In COPD the $CO_2$ level gradually rises over time and central chemoreceptors are no longer sensitive to high $CO_2$ levels. Instead, the peripheral chemoreceptors found in the carotid and aortic arch bodies become the major stimuli for breathing. When the client with COPD receives high levels of $O_2$, the hypoxic drive to breathe is eliminated. The client experiences respiratory depression that may lead to apnea.

268. **1.** The mask must fit properly, as a poor-fitting mask reduces the amount of oxygen delivered. The mask may also cause skin breakdown, so it is very important to provide skin care. Loosen the strap holding the mask frequently and assess the skin.

269. **2.** Trach care should be provided once every 8 hours.

270. **2.** These are signs and symptoms of COPD. The nurse would also need to evaluate breathing rate/pattern, use of accessory muscles for breathing, cyanosis, capillary refill, and clubbing of fingernails.

271. **3.** A major goal for the COPD client is that the client will use a breathing pattern that does not lead to tiring and to plan activities so that the client does not become overtired. Care should be spaced, allowing frequent rest periods, to prevent fatigue.

272. **1.** Typically, the client with TB will present with fatigue, lethargy, nausea, anorexia, weight loss, low-grade fever, and night sweats.

273. **1.** The client should be placed in respiratory isolation until active TB is ruled out. TB is spread by droplet infection, thus her sputum should be handled according to respiratory isolation protocol.

274. **3.** These medications frequently cause nausea. The nausea may be decreased if the medications are taken at bedtime.

275. **3.** Handwashing is the best tool for prevention of infection. The client should wash her hands very carefully after any contact with body substances, masks, or soiled tissues. The family should also use good handwashing techniques.

276. **3.** Pulmonary care is a vital part of the management of this type of client. Measures are taken to prevent stasis of secretions and promote chest expansion, preventing complications such as atelectasis and pneumonia.

277. **2.** Based on the client's symptoms the nurse suspects impending respiratory failure and should prepare for intubation and mechanical ventilation.

278. **3.** With pleural effusions, lung expansion may be restricted and the client will experience dyspnea, primarily on exertion.

279. **2.** This plan allows frequent rest periods for the client. The client should not rush through morning care activities as rushing will increase hypoxemia, dyspnea, and fatigue.

280. **1.** In a client with pneumonia, bronchial breath sounds are heard over areas of density or consolidation. Breath sounds are diminished when the airflow is decreased as is typical with pneumonia. Tactile fremitus is increased over the affected area. Percussion is dulled. In pneumonia, the alveoli fill with fluid, red cells, and white cells creating consolidation.

281. **2.** Research has shown that there may be a correlation between vitamin A deficiency in the diet and the development of lung cancer. Daily consumption of green and yellow vegetables is encouraged.

282. **4.** A preventive approach to pain control provides a more consistent level of relief and reduces client anxiety, which in turn can reduce discomfort and pain.

283. **3.** Post-op respiratory insufficiency may result from an altered level of consciousness related to anesthesia, pain medications, decreased respiratory effort secondary to pain, or inadequate airway clearance. So the client must be monitored very closely with frequent vital sign checks and respiratory assessments.

284. **3.** Thirty or 45 minutes after the administration of IM pain medication is the time when the pain medication is most effective. Thus, this is the best time to schedule coughing and deep breathing and arm exercises.

285. **3.** It is common for the client to have suprasternal and intercostal retractions as the client loses lung capacity. The nurse should anticipate restlessness, apprehension, agitation, sluggishness, disorientation, and tachycardia.

286. **1.** A total laryngectomy is the removal of the larynx and formation of the tracheostomy. The esophagus remains attached to the pharynx. No air will enter through the nose. The client will breathe through the tracheostomy. The procedure is indicated for large glottic tumors with fixation of vocal cords.

287. **2.** For the first few days after surgery, the client should communicate by writing. If the client is very tired, a communication board may be used allowing the client to point to statements.

288. **4.** An artificial larynx is an electronic device held along the neck and vibration produces mechanical speech. The speech quality is monotone and artificial.

289. **4.** To substitute for the nose and pharynx, where air is usually warmed and humidified, a humidifier, pans of water, or houseplants should be used to increase the humidity in the home.

# The Gastrointestinal System

## OVERVIEW OF ANATOMY AND PHYSIOLOGY

The organs of the digestive system are grouped into the alimentary canal (GI tract), consisting of the mouth, esophagus, stomach, and small and large intestine; and the accessory digestive organs, including the liver, pancreas, gallbladder, and ductal system (Figure 4-16). The primary functions of this system are movement of food, digestion, absorption, elimination, and provision of a continuous supply of nutrients, electrolytes, and water.

## Mouth

A. Consists of the lips and oral cavity: provides entrance and initial processing for nutrients and sensory data, such as taste, texture, and temperature.
B. Oral cavity contains the teeth, used for mastication, and the tongue, which assists in deglutition, taste sensation, and mastication.
C. The salivary glands, located in the mouth, produce secretions containing ptyalin for starch digestion and mucus for lubrication.

4

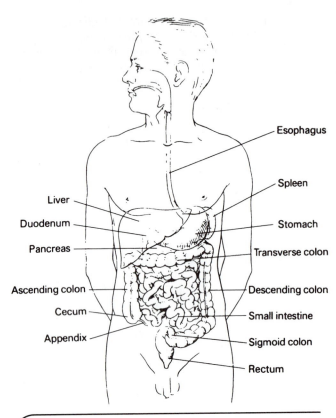

**Figure 4-16** Anterior view of the structures of the GI tract

D. The pharynx aids in swallowing and functions in ingestion by providing a route for food to pass from the mouth to the esophagus.

## Esophagus

Muscular tube that receives food from the pharynx and propels it into the stomach by peristalsis.

## Stomach

A. Located on the left side of the abdominal cavity, occupying the hypochondriac, epigastric, and umbilical regions.
B. Stores and mixes food with gastric juices and mucus, producing chemical and mechanical changes in the bolus of food.
  1. The secretion of digestive juices is stimulated by smelling, tasting, and chewing food, which is known as the cephalic phase of digestion.
  2. The gastric phase is stimulated by the presence of food in the stomach; regulated by neural stimulation via the PNS and hormonal stimulation through secretions of gastrin by the gastric mucosa.
  3. After processing in the stomach, the food bolus, called chyme, is released into the small intestine through the duodenum.

C. Two sphincters control the rate of food passage.
  1. Cardiac sphincter: located at the opening between the esophagus and stomach
  2. Pyloric sphincter: located between the stomach and duodenum
D. Three anatomic divisions: fundus, body, and antrum.
E. Gastric secretions
  1. Pepsinogen: secreted by chief cells, located in fundus, aids in protein digestion
  2. Hydrochloric acid: secreted by parietal cells, functions in protein digestion, released in response to gastrin
  3. Intrinsic factor: secreted by parietal cells, promotes absorption of vitamin $B_{12}$
  4. Mucoid secretions: coat stomach wall and prevent autodigestion

## Small Intestine

A. Composed of the duodenum, jejunum, and ileum
B. Extends from the pylorus to the ileocecal valve, which regulates flow into the large intestine and prevents reflux into the small intestine.
C. Major functions of the small intestine are digestion and absorption of the end products of digestion.
D. Structural features
  1. Villi (functional units of the small intestine): fingerlike projections located in the mucous membrane; contain goblet cells that secrete mucus and absorptive cells that absorb digested foodstuffs.
  2. Crypts of Lieberkuhn: produce secretions containing digestive enzymes.
  3. Brunner's glands: found in the submucosa of the duodenum, secrete mucus.

## Large Intestine

A. Divided into four parts: cecum (with appendix), colon (ascending, transverse, descending, sigmoid), rectum, and anus.
B. Serves as a reservoir for fecal material until defecation occurs; functions to absorb water and electrolytes.
C. Microorganisms present in the large intestine are responsible for a small amount of further breakdown and also make some vitamins.
  1. Amino acids are deaminated by bacteria, resulting in ammonia, which is converted to urea in the liver.
  2. Bacteria in the large intestine aid in the synthesis of vitamin K and some of the vitamin B groups.
D. Feces (solid waste) leave the body via the rectum and anus.
  1. Anus contains internal sphincter (under involuntary control) and external sphincter (voluntary control)

2. Fecal matter usually 75% water and 25% solid wastes (roughage, dead bacteria, fat, protein, inorganic matter)

## Liver

A. Largest internal organ; located in the right hypochondriac and epigastric regions of the abdomen.
B. Liver lobules: functional units of the liver, composed of hepatic cells.
C. Hepatic sinusoids (capillaries) are lined with Kupffer cells, which carry out the process of phagocytosis.
D. Portal circulation brings blood to the liver from the stomach, spleen, pancreas, and intestines.
E. Functions
   1. Metabolism of fats, carbohydrates, and proteins; oxidizes these nutrients for energy and produces compounds that can be stored
   2. Production of bile
   3. Conjugation and excretion (in the form of glycogen, fatty acids, minerals, fat-soluble and water-soluble vitamins) of bilirubin
   4. Storage of vitamins A, D, B$_{12}$, and iron
   5. Synthesis of coagulation factors
   6. Detoxification of many drugs and conjugation of sex hormones

## Biliary System

Consists of the gallbladder and associated ductal system (bile ducts), see Figure 4–17.
A. Gallbladder: lies on the undersurface of the liver, functions to concentrate and store bile.
B. Ductal system: provides a route for bile to reach the intestines.

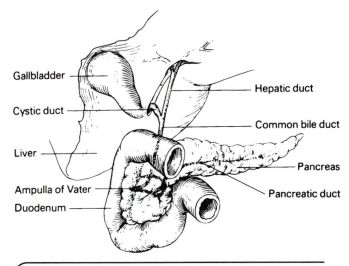

Gallbladder
Cystic duct
Liver
Ampulla of Vater
Duodenum
Hepatic duct
Common bile duct
Pancreas
Pancreatic duct

**Figure 4–17** Gallbladder and ductal system

1. Bile is formed in the liver and excreted into the hepatic duct.
2. Hepatic duct joins with the cystic duct (which drains the gallbladder) to form the common bile duct.
3. If sphincter of Oddi is relaxed, bile enters the duodenum. If contracted, bile is stored in gallbladder.

## Pancreas

A. Positioned transversely in the upper abdominal cavity.
B. Consists of a head, body, and tail along with a pancreatic duct, which extends along the gland and enters the duodenum via the common bile duct.
C. Has both exocrine and endocrine functions; function in GI system is exocrine.
   1. Exocrine cells in the pancreas secrete trypsinogen and chymotrypsin for protein digestion, amylase to break down starch to disaccharides, and lipase for fat digestion.
   2. Endocrine function is related to islets of Langerhans.

## Physiology of Digestion and Absorption

A. Digestion: physical and chemical breakdown of food into absorptive substances
   1. Initiated in the mouth where food mixes with saliva and starch is broken down.
   2. Food then passes into the esophagus where it is propelled into the stomach.
   3. In the stomach, food is processed by gastric secretions into a substance called chyme.
   4. In the small intestine, carbohydrates are hydrolyzed to monosaccharides, fats to glycerol, and fatty acids and proteins to amino acids to complete the digestive process.
      a. When chyme enters the duodenum, mucus is secreted to neutralize hydrochloric acid; in response to release of secretin, pancreas releases bicarbonate to neutralize acid chyme.
      b. Cholecystokinin and pancreozymin (CCK-PZ) are also produced by the duodenal mucosa; stimulate contraction of the gallbladder along with relaxation of the sphincter of Oddi (to allow bile to flow from the common bile duct into the duodenum), and stimulate release of pancreatic enzymes.

# ASSESSMENT

## Health History

A. Presenting problem
  1. Mouth: symptoms may include dental caries, bleeding gums, dryness or increased salivation, odors, difficulty chewing (note use of dentures)
  2. Ingestion: symptoms may include:
     a. Changes in appetite: anorexia or hyperorexia; note food preferences/dislikes.
     b. Food intolerances: allergies, fluid, fatty foods.
     c. Weight gain/loss: note symptoms/situations that might interfere with appetite (stress, deliberate weight reduction, dental problems); note average weight and percent gain/loss within past 2–9 months.
     d. Dysphagia: note level of sensation where problem occurs, whether it occurs with foods/fluids.
     e. Nausea: note onset and duration, existence of associated symptoms (weakness, headache, vomiting), occurrence before or after meals.
     f. Vomiting: note onset and duration; foods/fluids that can be maintained; associated symptoms (fever, diarrhea).
     g. Regurgitation (reflux): note whether occurs with ingestion of certain foods, any associated symptoms (vomiting), occurrence with certain positions (supine, recumbent).
  3. Digestion/absorption: symptoms may include
     a. Dyspepsia (indigestion): note location of discomfort, whether associated with certain foods, time of day/night of occurrence, associated symptoms (vomiting).
     b. Heartburn (pyrosis): note location, whether pain radiates, whether it occurs before or after meals, time of day when discomfort is most noticeable, foods that aggravate or eliminate symptoms.
     c. Pain: character, frequency, location, duration, distribution, aggravating or alleviating factors.
  4. Bowel habits: symptoms may include
     a. Constipation: note number of stools/day or week, changes in size or color of stool, alterations in food/fluid intake, presence of tenesmus, painful defecation, associated symptoms (abdominal pain, cramps)
     b. Diarrhea: note number of stools/day, consistency, quantity, odor, interference with ADL, associated symptoms (nausea, vomiting, flatus, abdominal distension)
  5. Hepatic/biliary problems: symptoms may include
     a. Jaundice: note location, duration, notable increase/decrease in degree.
     b. Pruritus: note location, distribution, onset.
     c. Urine changes: note color, onset, notable increase or decrease in color change, associated symptoms (pain).
     d. Clay-colored stools: note onset, number/day, associated symptoms (pain, problems with ingestion/digestion).
     e. Increased bleeding: note ecchymoses, purpura, bleeding gums, hematuria.
B. Lifestyle: eating behaviors (rapid ingestion, skipping meals, snacking), cultural/religious values (vegetarian, kosher foods), ingestion of alcohol, smoking
C. Use of medications: note use of antacids, antiemetics, antiflatulents, vitamin supplements; aspirin and anti-inflammatory agents
D. Past medical history: childhood, adult, psychiatric illness; surgery; bleeding disorders; menstrual history; exposure to infectious agents; allergies

## Physical Examination

A. Mouth: inspect/palpate
  1. Outer/inner lips: color, texture, moisture
  2. Buccal mucosa: color, texture, lesions, ulcerations
  3. Teeth/gums: missing teeth, cavities, tenderness, swelling
  4. Tongue: protrusion without deviation, texture, color, moisture
  5. Palates (hard and soft): color
B. Abdomen: divided into regions and quadrants (see Figure 4-18); note specific location of any abnormality.
  1. Inspect skin: color, scars, striae, pigmentation, lesions, vascularity.
  2. Inspect architecture: contour, symmetry, distension, umbilicus.
  3. Inspect movement: peristalsis, pulsations.
  4. Auscultate peristaltic sounds.
     a. Normal: bubbling, gurgling, 5–30 times/minute
     b. Increased (hyperactive): may indicate diarrhea, gastroenteritis, early intestinal obstruction
     c. Decreased (hypoactive): may indicate constipation, late intestinal obstruction, use of anticholinergics, post-op anesthesia
  5. Auscultate arterial sounds: note presence or absence of bruits in aorta/renal arteries.
  6. Percuss for tenderness/masses; determine distribution of tympany and dullness
     a. Liver span: normal 6–12 cm dullness at the midclavicular line; determine shifting dullness (ascites)
     b. Stomach: normal tympany

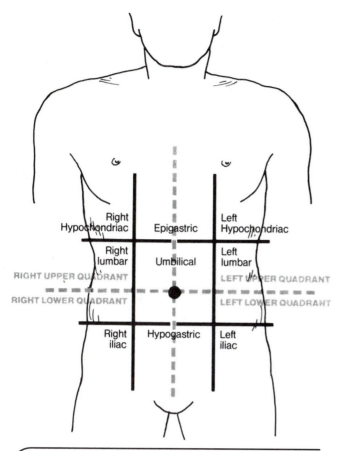

**Figure 4-18** Abdominal quadrants (broken lines) and regions (solid lines)

c. Spleen: normal tympany, dullness only if enlarged
d. Small/large intestine: normal tympany
e. Bladder: normal tympany, dullness if full

7. Palpate to depth of 1 cm (light palpation) to determine areas of tenderness, muscle guarding, and masses

8. Palpate to a depth of 4–8 cm (deep palpation) to identify rigidity, masses, ascites, tenderness, liver margins, spleen

## Laboratory/Diagnostic Tests

A. Blood chemistry and electrolyte analysis: albumin, alkaline phosphatase, ammonia, amylase, bilirubin, chloride, LDH, lipase, potassium, SGOT or AST, serum glutamic pyruvic transaminase (SGPT or ALT), sodium

B. Hematologic studies: Hgb and HCT, PT, WBC

C. Serologic studies: carcinoembryonic antigen (CEA), hepatitis-associated antigens, *Helicobacter pylori*

D. Urine studies: amylase, bilirubin

E. Fecal studies: for blood, fat, infectious organisms
   1. A freshly passed, warm stool is the best specimen.
   2. For fat or infectious organisms collect three separate specimens and label day #1, day #2, day #3.

F. Upper GI series (barium swallow)
   1. Fluoroscopic examination of upper GI tract to determine structural problems and gastric emptying time; client must swallow barium sulfate or other contrast medium; sequential films taken as it moves through the system.
   2. Nursing care: pretest
      a. Keep NPO after midnight or 6–8 hours pretest.
      b. Explain that the barium will taste chalky.
   3. Nursing care: posttest: administer laxatives to enhance elimination of barium and prevent obstruction or impaction.

G. Lower GI series (barium enema)
   1. Barium is instilled into the colon by enema; client retains the contrast medium while X-rays are taken to identify structural abnormalities of the large intestine or colon.
   2. Nursing care: pretest
      a. Keep NPO for 8 hours pretest.
      b. Give enemas until clear the morning of test.
      c. Administer laxative or suppository.
      d. Explain that cramping may be experienced during the procedure.
   3. Nursing care: posttest: administer laxatives and fluids to assist in expelling barium.

H. Endoscopy (esophagogastroduodenoscopy)
   1. Direct visualization of the esophagus, stomach, and duodenum by insertion of a lighted fiberscope
   2. Used to observe structures, ulcerations, inflammation, tumors; may include a biopsy
   3. Nursing care: pretest
      a. Keep NPO for 6–8 hours.
      b. Ensure consent form has been signed.
      c. Explain that a local anesthetic will be used to ease discomfort and that speaking during the procedure will not be possible; the client should expect hoarseness and a sore throat for several days.
   4. Nursing care: posttest
      a. Keep NPO until return of gag reflex.
      b. Assess vital signs and for pain, dysphagia, bleeding.
      c. Administer warm normal saline gargles for relief of sore throat.

I. Colonoscopy
   1. Endoscopic visualization of the large intestine: may include biopsy and removal of foreign substances.
   2. Nursing care: pretest
      a. Keep NPO for 8 hours pretest.
      b. Administer laxatives for 1–3 days before the exam, and sometimes enemas until clear the night before the test.
      c. Ensure a consent form has been signed.

d. Explain to client that when the instrument is inserted into the rectum a feeling of pressure might be experienced.
   3. Nursing care: posttest
      a. Observe for rectal bleeding and signs of perforation.
      b. Schedule planned rest periods for the client.
J. Sigmoidoscopy
   1. Endoscopic visualization of the sigmoid colon
   2. Used to identify inflammation or lesions, or remove foreign bodies.
   3. Nursing care: pretest
      a. Offer a light supper and light breakfast.
      b. Do bowel prep.
      c. Explain to client that the sensation of an urge to defecate or abdominal cramping might be experienced.
   4. Nursing care: posttest: assess for signs of bowel perforation.
K. Gastric analysis
   1. Insertion of a nasogastric tube to examine fasting gastric contents for acidity and volume
   2. Nursing care: pretest
      a. Keep NPO 6–8 hours pretest.
      b. Advise client about no smoking, anticholinergic medications, antacids for 24 hours prior to test.
      c. Inform client that tube will be inserted into the stomach via the nose, and instruct to expectorate saliva to prevent buffering of secretions.
   3. Nursing care: posttest: provide frequent mouth care.
L. Oral cholecystogram
   1. Injection of a radiopaque dye and X-ray examination to visualize the gallbladder
   2. Used to determine the gallbladder's ability to concentrate and store the dye and to assess patency of the biliary duct system
   3. Nursing care: pretest
      a. Offer a low-fat meal the evening before the test and black coffee, tea, or water the morning of the exam.
      b. Check for iodine sensitivity and administer six dye tablets (Telepaque) as ordered.
   4. Nursing care: posttest: observe for side effects of the dye (nausea, vomiting, diarrhea).
M. Liver biopsy (closed needle)
   1. Invasive procedure where a specially designed needle is inserted into the liver to remove a small piece of tissue for study
   2. Nursing care: pretest
      a. Ensure client has signed consent form.
      b. Keep NPO 6–8 hours pretest.
      c. Instruct client to hold breath during the biopsy.
   3. Nursing care: posttest
      a. Assess vital signs every hour for 8–12 hours.
      b. Place client on right side for a few hours with a pillow against the abdomen to provide pressure on the liver.
      c. Observe puncture site for hemorrhage.
      d. Assess for complications of shock and pneumothorax.
N. Endoscopic Retrograde Cholangiopancreatography (ERCP)
   1. Flexible fiber-optic endoscope permits direct visualization of biliary structures and pancreas.
   2. Consent and NPO status required.
   3. Moderate sedation used.

## ANALYSIS

Nursing diagnoses for the client with a disorder of the digestive system may include:
A. Risk for deficient fluid volume
B. Disturbed body image
C. Imbalanced nutrition: less than body requirements
D. Diarrhea
E. Constipation
F. Pain
G. Ineffective breathing pattern
H. Impaired verbal communication
I. Impaired skin integrity

## PLANNING AND IMPLEMENTATION

### Goals

A. Restoration of fluid and electrolyte balance.
B. Client will express feelings of self-worth.
C. Adequate nutritional status will be maintained.
D. Client will experience decreased frequency of regular bowel habits.
E. Client will establish regular bowel habits of appropriate amount and consistency.
F. Client will be free from pain.
G. Effective breathing patterns will be maintained.
H. Effective communication methods will be established.
I. Skin integrity will be restored/maintained.

### Interventions

#### Enemas

A. General information
   1. Instillation of fluid into the rectum, usually for the purpose of stimulating defecation. The various types include:
      a. Cleansing enema (tap water, normal saline, or soap): used to treat constipation or feces impaction, as bowel cleansing prior to

diagnostic procedures or surgery, to help establish regular bowel functions.

   b. Retention enema (mineral oil, olive oil, cottonseed oil): usually administered to lubricate or soften a hard fecal mass to facilitate defecation.

B. Nursing care for a cleansing enema
   1. Explain procedure and that breathing through the mouth relaxes abdominal musculature and helps to avoid cramps; explain the need to take adequate time to defecate.
   2. Assemble equipment: prepare solution at 105°–110° and have bedpan, commode, or nearby bathroom ready for use.
   3. Position client and drape adequately.
   4. Place waterproof pad under buttocks.
   5. Lubricate tube and allow solution to fill the tubing, displacing air.
   6. Insert rectal tube 4–5 inches without using force; request that client take several deep breaths.
   7. Administer 500–1000 mL of solution over 5–10 minutes; if cramping occurs slow the speed of instillation.
   8. After administration, have the client retain solution until the urge to defecate becomes strong.
   9. Document amount, color, characteristics of stool, and client's reaction during procedure.
   10. Assess for dizziness, light-headedness, abdominal cramps, nausea.
   11. Monitor electrolyte levels if client is to receive repeated enemas.

C. Nursing care for a retention enema: same as for a cleansing enema except:
   1. Oil is used instead of water (comes prepared in commercial kits and is given at body temperature).
   2. Administer 150–200 mL of prepared solution.
   3. Instruct client to retain oil for at least 30 minutes in order for it to take effect.

## Gastrostomy

A. General information
   1. Insertion of a catheter through an abdominal incision into the stomach where it is secured with sutures or by balloon fixation.
   2. Used as an alternative method of feeding, either temporary or permanent, for clients who have problems with swallowing, ingestion, and digestion.

B. Nursing care
   1. Maintain skin integrity: inspect and cleanse skin around stoma frequently; keep deep area dry to avoid excoriation.
   2. Maintain patency of the gastrostomy tube.
      a. Assess for residual before each feeding (check orders concerning withholding feeding).
      b. Irrigate tube before and after meals.
      c. Measure/record any drainage.

3. Promote adequate nutrition.
   a. Administer feeding with client in high-Fowler's and keep head of bed elevated for 30 minutes after meals to prevent regurgitation.
   b. Maintain feeding at room temperature.
   c. Ensure that prescribed amount of feeding be given within prescribed amount of time.
   d. Weigh client daily.
   e. Monitor I&O until feedings are well tolerated.
   f. Monitor for signs of dehydration.

## Nasogastric (NG) Tubes

A. General information
   1. Soft rubber or plastic tube inserted through a nostril and into the stomach for gastric decompression, feeding, or obtaining specimens for analysis of stomach contents
   2. Types
      a. Levin: single-lumen, nonvented
      b. Salem: a tube within a tube; vented to provide constant inflow of atmospheric air

B. Nursing care
   1. Insertion of the tube
      a. Explain the purpose of the tube and the procedure for insertion.
      b. Measure the tube: distance on the tube from the tip of the nose to the ear lobe plus the distance from the ear lobe to the tip of the xiphoid.
      c. Instruct client to bend head forward if possible during insertion.
   2. Monitor functioning of system and ensure patency of the NG tube: abdominal discomfort/distension, nausea and vomiting, and little or no drainage in collection bottle are all signs that system is not functioning properly.
      a. Assess the position: aspirate gastric contents to confirm that tube is in stomach; inject 10 mL air through tube and auscultate for rapid influx.
      b. Check that tubing is free of kinks; irrigate as per physician order.
      c. Record amount, color, and odor of drainage.
   3. Provide measures to ensure maximal comfort.
      a. Apply water-soluble lubricant to lips to prevent dryness.
      b. Keep nares free from secretions.
      c. Provide periodic warm saline gargles to prevent dryness.
      d. Provide frequent mouth care with toothbrush/toothpaste or flavored mouthwashes.
      e. If allowed, give client hard candy or gum to stimulate the flow of saliva and prevent dryness.

**f.** Elevate head and chest during and for 1–2 hours after feedings to prevent reflux (most comfortable position when suction is used).

    **4.** Monitor/maintain fluid and electrolyte balance.

        **a.** Assess for signs of metabolic alkalosis (suctioning causes excessive loss of hydrochloric acid and potassium).

        **b.** Administer IV fluids as ordered.

        **c.** If suction used, irrigate NG tube with normal saline to decrease sodium loss.

        **d.** Keep accurate I&O.

        **e.** If suction used provide ice chips sparingly (if allowed) to avoid dilution of electrolytes.

        **f.** Monitor lab values and electrolytes frequently.

### *Intestinal Tubes*

**A.** General information

    **1.** Tube is inserted via a nostril through the stomach and into the intestine for decompression proximal to an obstruction, relief of an obstruction, decompression of post-op edema at the surgical site.

    **2.** Types

        **a.** Cantor tube: single lumen

        **b.** Harris tube: single lumen

        **c.** Miller-Abbott: double lumen

**B.** Nursing care

    **1.** Facilitate placement of the tube.

        **a.** Position client in high-Fowler's while tube is being passed from the nose to the stomach; then place client on right side to aid in advancing the tube from the stomach to duodenum.

        **b.** Continuously monitor tube markings.

        **c.** Tape tube in place only after placement in duodenum is confirmed by X-ray.

    **2.** Provide measures for maximal comfort, as for NG tube.

## EVALUATION

**A.** Adequate urine output; stable vital signs; moist mucous membranes; adequate skin turgor and mobility; electrolyte levels within normal range.

**B.** Client expresses interest in personal well-being; actively participates in ADL, treatments, and care.

**C.** Stable weight; improved anthropometric measurements; laboratory values within normal limits; client verbalizes types of foods that should be included or eliminated from prescribed diet.

**D.** Client reports reduction in frequency of stools and return to more normal stool consistency; laboratory values within normal range.

**E.** Client reports increased frequency with improved consistency of stool.

**F.** Relaxed facial expression; decreased abdominal distension; healed mouth ulcers.

**G.** Improved respiratory rate, depth, and rhythm; lungs clear to auscultation; effective use of muscles of respiration.

**H.** Client effectively uses artificial means of communication (artificial larynx, sign language, or esophageal speech).

**I.** No redness, irritation, or breakdown; client demonstrates techniques to prevent skin breakdown.

## DISORDERS OF THE GASTROINTESTINAL SYSTEM

### Nausea and Vomiting

**A.** General information

    **1.** Nausea: a feeling of discomfort in the epigastrium with a conscious desire to vomit; occurs in association with and prior to vomiting.

    **2.** Vomiting: forceful ejection of stomach contents from the upper GI tract. Emetic center in medulla is stimulated (e.g., by local irritation of intestine or stomach or disturbance of equilibrium), causing the vomiting reflex.

    **3.** Nausea and vomiting are the two most common manifestations of GI disease.

    **4.** Contributing factors

        **a.** GI disease

        **b.** CNS disorders (meningitis, CNS lesions)

        **c.** Circulatory problems (HF)

        **d.** Metabolic disorders (uremia)

        **e.** Side effects of certain drugs (chemotherapy, antibiotics)

        **f.** Pain

        **g.** Psychic trauma

        **h.** Response to motion

**B.** Assessment findings

    **1.** Weakness, fatigue, pallor, possible lethargy

    **2.** Dry mucous membrane and poor skin turgor/mobility (if prolonged with dehydration)

    **3.** Serum sodium, calcium, potassium decreased

    **4.** BUN elevated (if severe vomiting and dehydration)

**C.** Nursing interventions

    **1.** Maintain NPO until client able to tolerate oral intake.

    **2.** Administer medications as ordered and monitor effects/side effects.

        **a.** Phenothiazines: chlorpromazine (Thorazine), perphenazine (Trilafon), prochlorperazine (Compazine), Promethazine (Phenergan), trifluoperazine (Stelazine)

    **b.** Antihistamines: benzquinamide (Emetecon), dimenhydrinate (Dramamine), diphenhydramine (Benadryl), hydroxyzine (Atarax, Vistaril), cyclizine (Marezine), meclizine (Antivert), promethazine (Phenergan)

    **c.** Other drugs to help control nausea and vomiting: thiethylperazine (Torecan), trimethobenzamide (Tigan), metoclopramide (Reglan)

  **3.** Notify physician if vomiting pattern changes.

  **4.** Maintain fluid and electrolyte balance.

    **a.** Administer IV fluids as ordered, keep accurate record of I&O.

    **b.** Record amount/frequency of vomitus.

    **c.** Assess skin tone/turgor for degree of hydration.

    **d.** Monitor laboratory/electrolyte values.

    **e.** Test NG tube drainage or vomitus for blood, bile; monitor pH.

  **5.** Provide measures for maximum comfort.

    **a.** Institute frequent mouth care with tepid water/saline mouthwashes.

    **b.** Remove encrustations around nares.

    **c.** Keep head of bed elevated and avoid sudden changes in position.

    **d.** Eliminate noxious stimuli from environment.

    **e.** Keep emesis basin clean.

    **f.** Maintain quiet environment and avoid unnecessary procedures.

  **6.** When vomiting subsides provide clear fluids (ginger ale, warm tea) in small amounts, gradually introduce solid foods (toast, crackers), and progress to bland foods (baked potato), in small amounts.

  **7.** Provide client teaching and discharge planning concerning:

    **a.** Avoidance of situations, foods, or liquids that precipitate nausea and vomiting

    **b.** Need for planned, uninterrupted rest periods

    **c.** Medication regimen, including side effects

    **d.** Signs of dehydration

    **e.** Need for daily weights with frequent anthropometric measurements

## Anorexia/Eating Disorders

See Unit 7.

## Diarrhea

**A.** General information

  **1.** Increase in peristaltic motility, producing watery or loosely formed stools. Diarrhea is a symptom of other pathologic processes.

  **2.** Causes

    **a.** Chronic bowel disorders

    **b.** Malabsorption problems

    **c.** Intestinal infections

    **d.** Biliary tract disorders

    **e.** Hyperthyroidism

    **f.** Saline laxatives

    **g.** Magnesium-based antacids

    **h.** Stress

    **i.** Antibiotics

    **j.** Neoplasms

    **k.** Highly seasoned foods

**B.** Assessment findings

  **1.** Abdominal cramps/distension, foul-smelling watery stools, increased peristalsis

  **2.** Anorexia, thirst, tenesmus, anxiety

  **3.** Decreased potassium and sodium if severe

**C.** Nursing interventions

  **1.** Administer antidiarrheals: diphenoxylate with atropine (Lomotil), paregoric, loperamide (Imodium), Kaopectate as ordered; monitor effects.

  **2.** Control fluid/food intake.

    **a.** Avoid milk and milk products.

    **b.** Provide liquids with gradual introduction of bland, high-protein, high-calorie, low-fat, low-bulk foods.

  **3.** Monitor and maintain fluid and electrolyte status; record number, characteristics, and amount of each stool.

  **4.** Prevent anal excoriation.

    **a.** Cleanse rectal area after each bowel movement with mild soap and water and pat dry.

    **b.** Apply A and D ointment or Desitin to promote healing.

    **c.** Use a local anesthetic as needed.

  **5.** Provide client teaching and discharge planning concerning

    **a.** Medication regimen

    **b.** Adherence to prescribed diet and avoidance of foods that are known to produce diarrhea

    **c.** Importance of perineal hygiene and care and daily assessment of skin changes

    **d.** Importance of good handwashing techniques after each stool

    **e.** Need to report worsening of symptoms (increased abdominal cramps, increased frequency or amount of stool)

    **f.** Need to assess daily weights with frequent anthropometric measurements

## Constipation

**A.** General information

  **1.** Lengthening of normal (for individual) time period between bowel movements; small volume of dry, hard stool; results from decreased motility of the colon or from retention of feces in the colon or rectum

  **2.** Causes

    **a.** Inadequate bulk/liquids in the diet

    **b.** Lack of physical activity

c. Retention of barium after radiographic exam

d. Prolonged use of constipation medications (aluminum-based antacids, anticholinergics, antihistamines, antidepressants, phenothiazines, calcium, iron)

B. Assessment findings
   1. Feeling of abdominal fullness, pressure in the rectum; abdominal distension, dyschezia; increased flatus
   2. Hardened stool upon digital examination

C. Nursing interventions
   1. Promote adequate intake of fluids/foods and dietary modification: increase fluid intake to at least 3000 mL/day; include high-fiber foods in diet.
   2. Administer medications as ordered
      a. Cathartics: milk of magnesia, castor oil, cascara sagrada, senna (Senokot), bisacodyl (Dulcolax), psyllium (Metamucil)
      b. Stool softeners: docusate calcium (Surfak), docusate sodium (Colace)
   3. Prevent accumulation of stool in the colon/rectum.
      a. Instruct client not to suppress urge to defecate.
      b. Gently massage abdomen to promote stimulation and movement of feces.
   4. Provide client teaching and discharge planning concerning:
      a. Need to establish and maintain a regular time to defecate
      b. Diet modification
      c. Medication regimen
      d. Need to assume position of comfort when sitting on toilet

# Cancer of the Mouth

A. General information
   1. Cancer of the mouth may occur on the lips or within the mouth (tongue, floor of mouth, buccal mucosa, hard/soft palate, pharynx, tonsils).
   2. Most common type of oral tumor is squamous cell carcinoma; most malignancies occur on the lower lip.
   3. More common in men.
   4. Caused by
      a. Excessive sun exposure
      b. Tobacco (cigar, pipe, cigarette, snuff)
      c. Excessive alcohol intake
      d. Constant irritation (dental caries)
   5. Early detection is very important; most discovered by dentists in routine checkups.

B. Medical management
   1. Radiation therapy: both primary lesion and affected lymph nodes; radioactive implants
   2. Chemotherapy: sometimes indicated, not used as often as radiation therapy and surgery

3. Surgery: type depends on location and extent of the tumor
   a. Mandibulectomy: removal of the mandible
   b. Hemiglossectomy: removal of half the tongue
   c. Glossectomy: removal of the entire tongue
   d. Radical neck dissection

C. Assessment findings
   1. Ulcerations (often painless) on the lip, tongue, or buccal mucosa
   2. Pain or soreness of the tongue upon eating hot or highly seasoned foods
   3. Erythroplakia, leukoplakia
   4. Difficulty chewing/speaking, dysphagia
   5. Positive oral exfoliative cytology
   6. Positive toluidine blue test

D. Nursing interventions
   1. Provide nursing care for the client receiving radiation therapy
   2. Prepare client for surgery: in addition to routine pre-op care
      a. Inform client of expected changes post-op.
      b. Provide explanation of anticipated post-op suctioning, NG tube, drains.
   3. In addition to routine post-op care
      a. Promote drainage.
         1) Place in side-lying position initially, then Fowler's.
         2) Suction mouth (except for lip surgery).
         3) Maintain patency of drainage tubes.
      b. Promote oral hygiene/comfort.
         1) Provide mouth irrigations with sterile water, diluted peroxide, normal saline, or sodium bicarbonate.
         2) Avoid use of commercial mouthwashes, lemon and glycerine swabs.
      c. Monitor/promote optimum nutritional status.
         1) Provide tube feedings following a hemiglossectomy.
         2) Place oral fluids in back of the throat with an asepto syringe.
         3) Provide foods/fluids that are nonirritating and facilitate swallowing (yogurt, puddings).
      d. Monitor for signs and symptoms of facial nerve damage (drooping, uneven smile, circumoral numbness or tingling).

# Cancer of the Esophagus

A. General information
   1. Malignant tumors of the esophagus usually appear as ulcerated lesions, most often in middle and lower portions of the esophagus.
   2. Penetration of the muscular layers with extension to the outer wall of the esophagus is commonly found. Metastases may cause eventual esophageal obstruction.

3. More common in men than in women (4:1); usually between ages 50–70.
4. Cause unknown; contributing factors include cigarette smoking, excessive alcohol intake, trauma, poor oral hygiene, achalasia, diverticula, and lye burns.

**B.** Medical management
1. Radiation therapy: used for inoperable tumors, has been found to alleviate symptoms
2. Chemotherapy: not found effective
3. Surgery
   a. Esophagectomy: removal of part or all of the esophagus using a Dacron graft to replace the resected portion
   b. Esophagogastrostomy: resection of a portion of the esophagus (usually middle third) and anastomosis of the remaining portion of the stomach
   c. Esophagoenterostomy: resection of portion of the esophagus and anastomosis of a segment of colon to the remaining portion
   d. Palliative gastrostomy: done for the purpose of feeding the client

**C.** Assessment findings
1. Substernal burning after drinking hot fluids
2. Pain located in the substernal and epigastric areas; usually intensified with swallowing
3. Weight loss
4. Barium swallow reveals narrowing of the esophagus at the area of the tumor
5. Diagnostic test: esophagoscopy with a biopsy reveals malignant cells

**D.** Nursing interventions
1. Provide nursing care for the client receiving radiation therapy.
2. Prepare client for surgery: in addition to routine pre-op care
   a. Provide meticulous oral hygiene including teeth, gums, tongue, and mouth.
   b. Explain that client may have a chest tube if thoracic approach is used.
   c. Prepare client for feedings through a gastrostomy.
3. In addition to routine post-op care
   a. Monitor NG tube: expect bloody drainage for approximately 12 hours with gradual change to green, then to yellow.
   b. Prevent gastric reflux: place client in semi-Fowler's position; maintain upright position for 2 hours after meals when client is able to take fluids/food orally.
4. Provide emotional support to client/significant others; prognosis is grave.
5. Provide client teaching and discharge planning concerning
   a. Gastrostomy and proper dietary measures
   b. Importance of cessation of smoking and elimination of alcohol consumption
   c. Maintain good oral hygiene.
   d. Maintain a high-calorie, high-protein diet

# Esophageal Varices

See Disorders of the Liver.

# Hiatal Hernia

**A.** General information
1. Sliding hiatal hernia occurs when a portion of the stomach and vagus nerve slide upward into the thorax through an enlarged hiatus in the diaphragm.
2. Result is reflux of gastric juices and inflammation of the lower portion of the esophagus.
3. Occurs more often in women ages 40–70.
4. May be caused by congenital weakening of the muscles in the diaphragm around the esophagogastric opening; increased intra-abdominal pressure (obesity, pregnancy, ascites); trauma.

**B.** Medical management
1. Drug therapy: antacids to reduce acidity and relieve discomfort, cholinergics
2. Modification of diet: elimination of spicy foods and caffeine
3. Surgery: reduction of the hiatal hernia via an abdominal or thoracic approach

**C.** Assessment findings
1. Heartburn, especially after meals, at night, or with position changes (particularly recumbent), dysphagia, regurgitation several hours after meals without vomiting
2. Barium swallow displays protrusion of the gastric mucosa through a hiatus
3. Esophagoscopy reveals an incompetent cardiac sphincter

**D.** Nursing interventions
1. Provide a bland diet with six small feedings/day, as ordered.
2. Administer medications as ordered.
3. Prepare client for surgery: in addition to routine pre-op care
   a. Inform client about chest tubes (if thoracic approach to be used).
   b. Provide information regarding NG intubation.
4. In addition to routine post-op care
   a. Decrease/avoid gastric distension.
   b. Promote pulmonary expansion: chest tubes if a thoracic approach; semi-Fowler's position.
5. Provide client teaching and discharge planning concerning:
   a. Modification of diet
   b. Sitting up for meals and for 2 hours after meals will help reduce gastric acid reflux
   c. Use of antacids
   d. Eating small, frequent meals slowly to help prevent gastric distension
   e. Need to avoid carbonated beverages and anticholinergic drugs (and OTC medications that contain them)

f. Avoidance of heavy lifting (to prevent intra-abdominal pressure); bend, kneel, or stoop instead
g. Importance of treating persistent cough
h. Adherence to weight-reduction plan if obese

## Gastritis

A. General information
1. An acute inflammatory condition that causes a breakdown of the normal gastric protective barriers with subsequent diffusion of hydrochloric acid into the gastric lumen
2. Results in hemorrhage, ulceration, and adhesions of the gastric mucosa
3. Present in some form (mild to severe) in 50% of all adults
4. Caused by excessive ingestion of certain drugs (salicylates, steroids, Butazolidin), alcohol; food poisoning; large quantities of spicy, irritating foods in diet
B. Assessment findings
1. Anorexia, nausea and vomiting, hematemesis, epigastric fullness/discomfort, epigastric tenderness
2. Decreased Hgb and HCT (if anemic)
3. Endoscopy: inflammation and ulceration of gastric mucosa
4. Gastric analysis: hydrochloric acid usually increased, except in atrophic gastritis
C. Nursing interventions
1. Monitor and maintain fluid and electrolyte balances.
2. Control nausea and vomiting (NPO until able to tolerate foods, then bland diet).
3. Administer medications as ordered: antiemetics, antacids, sedatives.
4. Maintain patency of NG tube.
5. Provide client teaching and discharge planning concerning avoidance of foods/medications such as coffee, spicy foods, alcohol, salicylates, ibuprofen, steroids.

## Peptic Ulcer Disease

### Gastric Ulcers

A. General information
1. Ulceration of the mucosal lining of the stomach; most commonly found in the antrum
2. Gastric secretions and stomach emptying rate usually normal
3. Rapid diffusion of gastric acid from the gastric lumen into gastric mucosa, however, causes an inflammatory reaction with tissue breakdown
4. Also characterized by reflux into the stomach of bile containing duodenal contents
5. Occurs more often in men, in unskilled laborers, and in lower socioeconomic groups; peak age 40–55 years

6. Predisposing factors include smoking, alcohol abuse, emotional tension, and drugs (salicylates, steroids, Butazolidin)
7. Caused by bacterial infection (*Helicobacter pylori*)
B. Medical management
1. Supportive: rest, bland diet, stress management
2. Drug therapy: antacids, histamine ($H_2$) receptor antagonists, anticholinergics, omeprazole (Prilosec), sucralfate (Carafate); also metronidazole and amoxicillin for ulcers caused by *H. pylori*
3. Surgery: various combinations of gastric resections and anastomosis
C. Assessment findings
1. Pain located in left epigastrium, with possible radiation to the back; usually occurs 1–2 hours after meals
2. Weight loss
3. Hgb and HCT decreased (if anemic)
4. Endoscopy reveals ulceration; differentiates ulcers from gastric cancer
5. Gastric analysis: normal gastric acidity in gastric ulcer, increased in duodenal ulcer
6. Upper GI series: presence of ulcer confirmed
D. Nursing interventions
1. Administer medications as ordered (see Table 4-23).
2. Provide nursing care for the client with ulcer surgery.
3. Provide client teaching and discharge planning concerning
   a. Medical regimen
      1) Take medications at prescribed times.
      2) Have antacids available at all times.
      3) Recognize situations that would increase the need for antacids.
      4) Avoid ulcerogenic drugs (salicylates, steroids).
      5) Know proper dosage, action, and side effects.
   b. Proper diet
      1) Bland diet consisting of six small meals/day.
      2) Eat meals slowly.
      3) Avoid acid-producing substances (caffeine, alcohol, highly seasoned foods).
      4) Avoid stressful situations at mealtime.
      5) Plan for rest periods after meals.
      6) Avoid late bedtime snacks.
   c. Avoidance of stress-producing situations and development of stress-reduction methods (relaxation techniques, exercises, biofeedback).

**Table 4-23** Drug Therapy for Peptic Ulcer

| Drug Type | Action | Side Effects | Nursing Implications |
|---|---|---|---|
| **TRANQUILIZERS**<br>• Combination drug (Librax); chlordiazepoxide (Librium) and clidinium bromide (Quarzan) | Decrease vagal activity and reduce anxiety | Sedation, headache, mental depression, blurred vision, nausea, vomiting, diarrhea, physical/psychological dependence | Contraindicated with other CNS depressants, antidepressants; avoid alcohol use, narcotic analgesics. |
| **ANTICHOLINERGICS**<br>• Belladonna tincture | Decreases acetylcholine, block cholinergic receptors | Dry mouth, constipation | Contraindicated in narrow-angle glaucoma, myasthenia gravis, paralytic ileus, urinary retention. |
| • Pirenzepine (Gastrozepine) | Blocks muscarinic receptors that regulate gastric acid secretion | No severe anticholinergic side effects | |
| • Propantheline bromine (Pro-Banthine) | Decreases gastric secretions; used in irritable bowel syndrome, pancreatitis, urinary bladder spasm | Standard anticholinergic effects: dry mouth, decreased secretions, tachycardia, urinary retention | |
| • Tridihexethyl chloride (Pathilon) | Decreases gastric secretions | | |
| **ANTACIDS**<br>• Aluminum hydroxide, aluminum carbonate (Amphogel, Alternagel) | Neutralize gastric acid and reduce pepsin activity | Prolonged use may cause hypophosphatemia | |
| • Magnesium hydroxide, magnesium trisilicate, magnesium phosphate (Maalox, Gaviscon) | | Hypermagnesemia | Contraindicated in impaired renal function. |
| **HISTAMINE ($H_2$) BLOCKERS**<br>• Cimetidine (Tagamet)<br>• Rantadine (Zantac)<br>• Famotidine (Pepcid)<br>• Nizatidine (Axid) | Block $H_2$ receptor sites of parietal cells of stomach | Headaches, dizziness, constipation, pruritus, skin rash, gynecomastia, decreased libido, impotence | Do not give within 1 hour of antacids. Cimetidine may enhance effects of oral anticoagulants, theophylline, caffeine, phenytoin, diazepam, propranolol, phenobarbital, calcium channel blockers; rantadine and famotidine have fewer side effects. |
| **PROTON PUMP INHIBITORS (PPIs)**<br>• Esomeprazole magnesium (Nexium)<br>• Lansoprazole (Prevacid)<br>• Omeprazole (Prilosec)<br>• Pantoprazole (Protonix)<br>• Rabeprazole (Aciphex) | Inhibit gastric secretion regardless of acetylcholine or histamine release; used in treatment of erosive esophagitis/GERD, gastric and duodenal ulcers, *H. pylori* | | |

*(continues)*

**Table 4-23** Drug Therapy for Peptic Ulcer *(continued)*

| Drug Type | Action | Side Effects | Nursing Implications |
|---|---|---|---|
| **PEPSIN INHIBITOR**<br>• Sucralfate (Carafate) | Reacts with acid to form a paste that binds to ulcerated tissue to prevent further destruction by digestive enzyme pepsin | Dizziness, nausea, constipation, dry mouth, rash, pruritus, back pain, sleepiness | Mucosal protective drug; must be given 30 minutes before meals and at bedtime. |
| **PROSTAGLANDIN E$_1$ ANALOGUE**<br>• Misoprostol (Cytotec) | Synthetic prostaglandin replacement product that blocks secretion of excess acid and protects stomach mucosa; used adjunctively with long-term NSAIDS or ASA therapy | Diarrhea, abdominal pain, flatulence, nausea, vomiting, constipation, menstrual spotting | |
| **ANTI-INFECTIVES**<br>• Metronidazole hydrochloride (Flagyl, Protostat)<br>• Amoxicillin (Amoxil)<br>• Clarithromycin (Biaxin)<br>• Tetracycline | Used in dual, triple, quadruple combination therapy for treatment of *H. pylori* | | |

## Duodenal Ulcers

A. General information
   1. Most commonly found in the first 2 cm of the duodenum
   2. Occur more frequently than gastric ulcers
   3. Characterized by gastric hyperacidity and a significant increased rate of gastric emptying
   4. Occur more often in younger men; more women affected after menopause; peak age 35–45 years
   5. Predisposing factors include smoking, alcohol abuse, psychological stress, bacterial infection (*H. pylori*)
B. Medical management: same as for gastric ulcers
C. Assessment findings
   1. Pain located in midepigastrium and described as burning, cramping; usually occurs 2–4 hours after meals and is relieved by food.
   2. Diagnostic tests: same as for gastric ulcer.
D. Nursing interventions: same as for gastric ulcer

## Gastric Surgery

A. General information
   1. Surgery is performed when peptic ulcer disease does not respond to medical management or for gastric cancer
   2. Types
      a. Vagotomy: severing of part of the vagus nerve innervating the stomach to decrease gastric acid secretion
      b. Antrectomy: removal of the antrum of the stomach to eliminate the gastric phase of digestion
      c. Pyloroplasty: enlargement of the pyloric sphincter with acceleration of gastric emptying
      d. Gastroduodenostomy (Billroth I): removal of the lower portion of the stomach with anastomosis of the remaining portion of the duodenum
      e. Gastrojejunostomy (Billroth II): removal of the antrum and distal portion of the stomach and duodenum with anastomosis of the remaining portion of the stomach to the jejunum
      f. Gastrectomy: removal of 60–80% of the stomach
      g. Esophagojejunostomy (total gastrectomy): removal of the entire stomach with a loop of jejunum anastomosed to the esophagus
   3. Dumping syndrome
      a. Abrupt emptying of stomach contents into the intestine
      b. Common complications of gastric surgery
      c. Associated with the presence of hyperosmolar chyme in the jejunum, which draws fluid by osmosis from the extracellular fluid into the bowel. Decreased plasma volume and distension

of the bowel stimulates increased intestinal motility.
   d. Signs and symptoms include weakness, faintness, palpitations, diaphoresis, feeling of fullness, or discomfort, nausea, and occasionally diarrhea; appear 15–30 minutes after meals and last for 20–60 minutes.
B. Nursing interventions: routine preoperative care
C. Nursing interventions: postoperative
   1. Provide routine post-op care.
   2. Ensure adequate function of NG tube.
      a. Measure drainage accurately to determine necessity for fluid and electrolyte replacement; notify physician if there is no drainage.
      b. Anticipate frank, red bleeding for 12–24 hours.
   3. Promote adequate pulmonary ventilation.
      a. Place client in mid- or high-Fowler's position to promote chest expansion.
      b. Teach client to splint high upper abdominal incision before turning, coughing, and deep breathing.
   4. Promote adequate nutrition.
      a. After removal of NG tube, provide clear liquids with gradual introduction of small amounts of bland food at frequent intervals.
      b. Monitor weight daily.
      c. Assess for regurgitation; if present, instruct client to eat smaller amounts of food at a slower pace.
   5. Provide client teaching and discharge planning concerning:
      a. Gradually increasing food intake until able to tolerate three meals/day
      b. Daily monitoring of weight
      c. Stress-reduction measures
      d. Need to report signs of complications to physician immediately (hematemesis, vomiting, diarrhea, pain, melena, weakness, feeling of abdominal fullness/distension)
      e. Methods of controlling symptoms associated with dumping syndrome
         1) Avoidance of concentrated sweets
         2) Adherence to six, small, dry meals/day
         3) Maintenance of modified diet
         4) Refraining from taking fluids during meals but rather 2 hours after meals
         5) Assuming a recumbent position for ½ hour after meals

## Cancer of the Stomach

A. General information
   1. Most often develops in the distal third and may spread through the walls of the stomach into adjacent tissues, lymphatics, regional lymph nodes, and other abdominal organs, or through the bloodstream to the lungs and bones.
   2. Affects men twice as often as women; more frequent in African Americans and Asians; most commonly occurs between ages 50 and 70
   3. Causes
      a. Excessive intake of highly salted or smoked foods
      b. Diet low in quantity of vegetables and fruits
      c. Atrophic gastritis
      d. Achlorhydria
      e. *Helicobacter pylori* infection
B. Medical management
   1. Chemotherapy
   2. Radiation therapy
   3. Treatment for anemia, gastric decompression, nutritional support, fluid and electrolyte maintenance
   4. Surgery: type depends on location and extent of lesion.
      a. Subtotal gastrectomy (Billroth I or II)
      b. Total gastrectomy
C. Assessment findings
   1. Fatigue, weakness, dizziness, shortness of breath, nausea and vomiting, hematemesis, weight loss, indigestion, epigastric fullness, feeling of early satiety when eating, epigastric pain (later)
   2. Pallor, lethargy, poor skin turgor and mobility, palpable epigastric mass
   3. Diagnostic tests
      a. Stool for occult blood positive
      b. CEA positive
      c. Hgb and HCT decreased
      d. SGOT (AST), SGPT (ALT), LDH, serum amylase elevated (if liver and pancreatic involvement)
      e. Gastric analysis reveals histologic changes
D. Nursing interventions
   1. Give consistent nutritional assessment and support.
   2. Provide care for the client receiving chemotherapy.
   3. Provide care for the client with gastric surgery (see Gastric Surgery).

## Hernias

A. General information
   1. Protrusion of a viscus from its normal cavity through an abnormal opening/weakened area
   2. Occurs anywhere but most often in the abdominal cavity
   3. Types
      a. Reducible: can be manually placed back into the abdominal cavity.

b. Irreducible: cannot be placed back into the abdominal cavity.
c. Inguinal: occurs when there is weakness in the abdominal wall where the spermatic cord in men and round ligament in women emerge.
d. Femoral: protrusion through the femoral ring; more common in females.
e. Incisional: occurs at the site of a previous surgical incision as a result of inadequate healing postoperatively.
f. Umbilical: most commonly found in children.
g. Strangulated: irreducible, with obstruction to intestinal flow and blood supply.

B. Medical management
1. Manual reduction, use of a truss (firm support)
2. Bowel surgery if strangulated
3. Herniorrhaphy: surgical repair of the hernia by suturing the defect

C. Assessment findings
1. Vomiting, protrusion of involved area (more obvious after coughing), and discomfort at site of protrusion
2. Crampy abdominal pain and abdominal distention (if strangulated with a bowel obstruction)

D. Nursing interventions
1. Observe client for complications such as strangulation.
2. Prepare client for herniorrhaphy, provide routine pre-op care.
3. In addition to routine post-op care
   a. Assess for possible distended bladder, particularly with inguinal hernia repair.
   b. Discourage coughing, but deep breathing and turning should be done.
   c. Assist to splint incision when coughing or sneezing.
   d. Apply ice bags to scrotal area (if inguinal repair) to decrease edema.
   e. Scrotal (athletic) or abdominal binder support may be ordered in some cases.
4. Provide client teaching and discharge planning concerning:
   a. Need to avoid strenuous physical activities (e.g., heavy lifting, pulling, pushing) for at least 6 weeks.
   b. Need to report any difficulty with urination.

## Intestinal Obstructions

A. General information
1. Mechanical intestinal obstruction: physical blockage of the passage of intestinal contents with subsequent distension by fluid and gas; caused by adhesions, hernias, volvulus, intussusception, inflammatory bowel disease, foreign bodies, strictures, neoplasms, fecal impaction

2. Paralytic ileus (neurogenic or adynamic ileus): interference with the nerve supply to the intestine resulting in decreased or absent peristalsis; caused by abdominal surgery, peritonitis, pancreatic toxic conditions, shock, spinal cord injuries, electrolyte imbalances (especially hypokalemia)
3. Vascular obstructions: interference with the blood supply to a portion of the intestine, resulting in ischemia and gangrene of the bowel; caused by an embolus, atherosclerosis

B. Assessment findings
1. Small intestine: nonfecal vomiting; colicky intermittent abdominal pain
2. Large intestine: cramplike abdominal pain, occasional fecal-type vomitus; client will be unable to pass stools or flatus
3. Abdominal distension, rigidity, high-pitched bowel sounds above the level of the obstruction, decreased or absent bowel sounds distal to obstruction
4. Diagnostic tests
   a. Flat-plate (X-ray) of the abdomen reveals the presence of gas/fluid
   b. HCT increased
   c. Serum sodium, potassium, chloride decreased
   d. BUN increased

C. Nursing interventions
1. Monitor fluid and electrolyte balance, prevent further imbalance; keep client NPO and administer IV fluids as ordered.
2. Accurately measure drainage from NG/intestinal tube.
3. Place client in Fowler's position to alleviate pressure on the diaphragm and encourage nasal breathing to minimize swallowing of air and further abdominal distension.
4. Institute comfort measures associated with NG intubation and intestinal decompression.
5. Prevent complications.
   a. Measure abdominal girth daily to assess for increasing abdominal distension.
   b. Assess for signs and symptoms of peritonitis.
   c. Monitor urinary output.

## Chronic Inflammatory Bowel Disorders
### Regional Enteritis (Crohn's Disease)

A. General information
1. Chronic inflammatory bowel disease that can affect both the large and small intestine; terminal ileum, cecum, and ascending colon most often affected
2. Characterized by granulomas that may affect all the bowel wall layers with resultant thickening, narrowing, and scarring of the intestinal wall

3. Both sexes affected equally; more common in the Jewish population; two age peaks: 20–30 years and 40–60 years
4. Cause unknown; contributing factors include food allergies, autoimmune reaction, psychologic disorders

B. Medical management
1. Diet: high calorie, high vitamin, high protein, low residue, milk free; supplementary iron preparations
2. Drug therapy: antimicrobials (especially sulfasalazine) to prevent or control infection, corticosteroids, antidiarrheals, anticholinergics
3. Supplemental parenteral nutrition
4. Surgery: resection of diseased portion of bowel and temporary or permanent ileostomy

C. Assessment findings
1. Right, lower quadrant tenderness and pain; abdominal distension
2. Nausea and vomiting, 3–4 semisoft stools/day with mucus and pus
3. Decreased skin turgor, dry mucus membranes
4. Increased peristalsis
5. Pallor
6. Diagnostic tests
   a. Hgb and HCT (if anemic) decreased
   b. Sigmoidoscopy negative or reveals scattered ulcers
   c. Barium enema shows narrowing with areas of strictures separated by segments of normal bowel

D. Nursing interventions
1. Provide appropriate nutrition while reducing bowel motility.
   a. Administer/monitor TPN.
   b. Provide high-protein, high-calorie, low-residue diet with no milk products (if able to tolerate oral foods/fluids).
   c. Weigh daily, monitor kcal counts, and take periodic anthropometric measurements.
   d. Record number and characteristics of stools daily.
   e. Administer antidiarrheals, antispasmodics, and anticholinergics as ordered.
   f. Provide tepid fluids to avoid stimulation of the bowel.
   g. Omit gas-producing foods/fluids from diet.
   h. Administer/monitor enteral tube feedings as ordered.
2. Promote comfort/rest: provide good perineal care with frequent washing and adequate drying after each bowel movement; apply analgesic or protective ointment as needed; provide sitz baths as needed.
3. Provide care for the client with bowel surgery.

## Ulcerative Colitis

A. General information
1. Inflammatory disorder of the bowel characterized by inflammation and ulceration that starts in the rectosigmoid area and spreads upward. The mucosa of the bowel becomes edematous, thickened with eventual scar formation. The colon consequently loses its elasticity and absorptive capabilities.
2. Occurs more often in women and the Jewish population, usually between ages 15 and 40.
3. Cause unknown; contributing factors include autoimmune factors, viral infection, allergies, emotional stress, insecurity.

B. Medical management
1. Mild to moderate form
   a. Low-roughage diet with no milk products
   b. Drug therapy (antimicrobials, corticosteroids, anticholinergics, antidiarrheals, immunosuppressives, hematinic agents)
2. Severe form: client kept NPO with IVs and electrolyte replacements, NG tube with suction, blood transfusions, surgery

C. Assessment findings
1. Severe diarrhea (15–20 liquid stools/day containing blood, mucus, and pus); severe tenesmus, weight loss, anorexia, weakness, crampy discomfort
2. Decreased skin turgor, dry mucous membranes
3. Low-grade fever, abdominal tenderness over the colon
4. Diagnostic tests
   a. Sigmoidoscopy reveals mucosa that bleeds easily with ulcer development
   b. Hgb and HCT decreased

D. Nursing interventions: same as for Crohn's disease

## Diverticulosis/Diverticulitis

A. General information
1. A diverticulum is an outpouching of the intestinal mucosa, most commonly found in the sigmoid colon.
2. Diverticulosis: multiple diverticula of the colon
3. Diverticulitis: inflammation of the diverticula
4. Men affected more often than women, more common in obese individuals; usually occurs between ages 40 and 45
5. Caused by stress, congenital weakening of muscular fibers of intestine, and dietary deficiency of roughage and fiber

B. Medical management
1. High-residue diet with no seeds for diverticulosis; low-residue diet for diverticulitis
2. Drug therapy: bulk laxatives, stool softeners, anticholinergics, antibiotics
3. Surgery (rare): resection of diseased portion of colon with temporary colostomy may be indicated

C. Assessment findings
1. Intermittent lower left quadrant pain and tenderness over rectosigmoid area

2. Alternating constipation and diarrhea with blood and mucus
3. Diagnostic tests
   a. Barium enema indicates an inflammatory process
   b. Hgb and HCT decreased (if anemic)
D. Nursing interventions
   1. Administer medications as ordered.
   2. Provide nursing care for the client with bowel surgery.
   3. Provide client teaching and discharge planning concerning:
      a. Importance of adhering to dietary regimen.
      b. Prevention of increased intraabdominal pressure.
      c. Signs and symptoms of peritonitis and need to notify physician immediately if they occur.

## Cancer of the Colon/Rectum

A. General information
   1. Adenocarcinoma is the most common type of colon cancer and may spread by direct extension through the walls of the intestine or through the lymphatic or circulatory system. Metastasis is most often to the liver.
   2. Second most common site for cancer in men and women; usually occurs between ages 50 and 60
   3. May be caused by diverticulosis, chronic ulcerative colitis, familial polyposis
B. Medical management: chemotherapy, radiation therapy, bowel surgery
C. Assessment findings
   1. Alternating diarrhea/constipation, lower abdominal cramps, abdominal distension
   2. Weakness, anorexia, weight loss, pallor, dyspnea
   3. Diagnostic tests
      a. Stool for occult blood positive
      b. Hgb and HCT decreased
      c. CEA positive
      d. Sigmoidoscopy reveals a mass
      e. Barium enema shows a colon mass
      f. Digital rectal exam indicates a palpable mass
D. Nursing interventions
   1. Administer chemotherapy agents as ordered, provide care for the client receiving chemotherapy.
   2. Provide care for the client receiving radiation therapy.
   3. Provide care for the client with bowel surgery.

## Bowel Surgery

A. General information: type of surgery varies depending on location and extent of lesion; may be indicated in Crohn's disease, ulcerative colitis, intestinal obstructions, colon/rectal cancer.

B. Types: see Table 4-24.
C. Nursing interventions common to all bowel surgery
   1. In addition to routine pre-op care:
      a. Ensure adherence to dietary restrictions.
         1) Offer clear liquids only on day before surgery.
         2) Provide high-calorie, low-residue diet 3–5 days before surgery.

**Table 4-24** Bowel Surgeries

| Type | Procedures |
| --- | --- |
| Abdominoperineal resection | Distal sigmoid colon, rectum, and anus are removed through a perineal incision and a permanent colostomy is created. Surgery of choice for cancer of the colon/rectum. |
| Ileostomy | Opening of the ileum onto the abdominal surface; most frequently done for treatment of ulcerative colitis, but may also be done for Crohn's disease. |
| Continent ileostomy (Kock's pouch) | An intra-abdominal reservoir with a nipple valve is formed from the distal ileum. The pouch acts as a reservoir for fecal material and is cleaned at regular intervals by insertion of a catheter. |
| Cecostomy | An opening between the cecum and the abdominal base temporarily diverts the fecal flow to rest the distal portion of the colon after some types of surgery. |
| Temporary colostomy | Usually located in the ascending or transverse colon; most often done to rest the bowel. |
| Double-barreled colostomy | The colon is resected and both ends are brought through the abdominal wall creating two stomas, a proximal and a distal; done most often for an obstruction or tumor in the descending or transverse colon. |
| Loop colostomy | Often a temporary procedure whereby a loop of bowel is brought out above the skin surface and held in place by a glass rod. There is one stoma but two openings, a proximal and a distal. |
| Permanent colostomy | Consists of a single stoma made when the distal portion of the bowel is removed; most often located in the sigmoid or descending colon. |
| Resection with anastomosis | Diseased part of the bowel is removed and remaining portions anastomosed, allowing elimination through the rectum. |

    **b.** Assist with bowel preparation.
        **1)** Administer antibiotics 3–5 days pre-op to decrease bacteria in intestine.
        **2)** Administer enemas (possibly with added antibiotics) to further cleanse the bowel.
    **c.** Administer vitamins C and K (decreased by bowel cleansing) to prevent post-op complications.
  **2.** In addition to routine post-op care:
    **a.** Promote elimination.
        **1)** Assess for signs of returning peristalsis.
        **2)** Monitor characteristics of initial stools.
    **b.** Monitor and maintain fluid and electrolyte balance.

**D.** Additional nursing interventions specific to abdominoperineal resection
  **1.** Reinforce and change perineal dressings as needed.
  **2.** Record type, amount, color of drainage.
  **3.** Irrigate with normal saline or hydrogen peroxide.
  **4.** Provide warm sitz baths 4 times per day.
  **5.** Cover wound with dry dressing.

**E.** Additional nursing interventions specific to colostomy
  **1.** Prevent skin breakdown.
    **a.** Cleanse skin around stoma with mild soap and water and pat dry.
    **b.** Use a skin barrier to protect skin around the stoma.
    **c.** Assess skin regularly for irritation.
    **d.** Avoid the use of adhesives on irritated skin.
  **2.** Control odor, maintain pleasant environment.
    **a.** Change pouch/seal whenever necessary.
    **b.** Empty or clean bag frequently, and provide ventilation afterwards; use deodorizer in bag/room if needed.
    **c.** Avoid gas-producing foods.
  **3.** Promote adequate stomal drainage.
    **a.** Assess stoma for color and intactness.
    **b.** Expect mucoid/serosanguinous drainage during the first 24 hours, then liquid type.
    **c.** Assess for flatus indicating return of intestinal function.
    **d.** Monitor for changing consistency of fecal drainage.
  **4.** Irrigate colostomy as needed.
    **a.** Position client on toilet or in high-Fowler's if client on bed rest.
    **b.** Fill irrigation bag with desired amount of water (500–1000 mL) and hang bag so the bottom is at shoulder height.
    **c.** Remove air from tubing and lubricate the tip of the catheter or cone.
    **d.** Remove old pouch and clean skin and stoma with water.

    **e.** Gently dilate stoma and insert the irrigation catheter or cone snugly.
    **f.** Open tubing and allow fluid to enter the bowel.
    **g.** Remove catheter or cone and allow fecal contents to drain.
    **h.** Observe and record amount and character of fecal return.
  **5.** Promote adequate nutrition.
    **a.** Assess return of peristalsis.
    **b.** Advance diet as tolerated, add new foods gradually.
    **c.** Avoid constipating foods.
  **6.** Provide at least 2500 mL liquid/day.
  **7.** Encourage client to discuss concerns and feelings about surgery.
  **8.** Provide client teaching and discharge planning concerning:
    **a.** Recognition of complications and need to report immediately
        **1)** Changes in odor, consistency, and color of stools
        **2)** Bleeding from the stoma
        **3)** Persistent constipation or diarrhea
        **4)** Changes in the contour of the stoma
        **5)** Persistent leakage around the stoma
        **6)** Skin irritation despite treatment
    **b.** Proper procedure for colostomy irrigation.

## Peritonitis

**A.** General information
  **1.** Local or generalized inflammation of part or all of the parietal and visceral surfaces of the abdominal cavity
  **2.** Initial response: edema, vascular congestion, hypermotility of the bowel and outpouring of plasmalike fluid from the extracellular, vascular, and interstitial compartments into the peritoneal space
  **3.** Later response: abdominal distension leading to respiratory compromise, hypovolemia results in decreased urinary output
  **4.** Intestinal motility gradually decreases and progresses to paralytic ileus
  **5.** Caused by trauma (blunt or penetrating), inflammation (ulcerative colitis, diverticulitis), volvulus, intestinal ischemia, or intestinal obstruction

**B.** Medical management
  **1.** NPO with fluid replacement
  **2.** Drug therapy: antibiotics to combat infection, analgesics for pain
  **3.** Surgery
    **a.** Laparotomy: opening made through the abdominal wall into the peritoneal cavity to determine the cause of peritonitis
    **b.** Depending on cause, bowel resection may be necessary

C. Assessment findings
1. Severe abdominal pain, rebound tenderness, muscle rigidity, absent bowel sounds, abdominal distension (particularly if large bowel obstruction)
2. Anorexia, nausea, and vomiting
3. Shallow respirations; decreased urinary output; weak, rapid pulse; elevated temperature
4. Diagnostic tests
   a. WBC elevated
   b. HCT elevated (if hemoconcentration)
D. Nursing interventions
1. Assess respiratory status for possible distress.
2. Assess characteristics of abdominal pain and changes over time.
3. Administer medications as ordered.
4. Perform frequent abdominal assessment.
5. Monitor and maintain fluid and electrolyte balance; monitor for signs of septic shock.
6. Maintain patency of NG or intestinal tubes.
7. Place client in Fowler's position to localize peritoneal contents.
8. Provide routine pre- and post-op care if surgery ordered.

# Hemorrhoids

A. General information
1. Congestion and dilation of the veins of the rectum and anus; usually result from impairment of flow of blood through the venous plexus
2. May be internal (above the anal sphincter) or external (outside anal sphincter)
3. Most commonly occur between ages 20 and 50
4. Predisposing conditions include occupations requiring long periods of standing; increased intra-abdominal pressure caused by prolonged constipation, pregnancy, heavy lifting, obesity, straining at defecation; portal hypertension
B. Medical management
1. Stool softeners, local anesthetics, or anti-inflammatory creams
2. Diet modification: high fiber, adequate liquids
3. Hemorrhoidectomy: surgical excision of hemorrhoids indicated when there is prolapse, severe pain, and excessive bleeding
C. Assessment findings
1. Bleeding with defecation, hard stools with streaks of blood
2. Pain with defecation, sitting, or walking
3. Protrusion of external hemorrhoids upon inspection
4. Diagnostic tests
   a. Proctoscopy reveals presence of internal hemorrhoids
   b. Hgb and HCT decreased if bleeding excessive, prolonged

D. Nursing interventions: preoperative
1. Prepare client for hemorrhoidectomy.
2. In addition to routine pre-op care, provide laxatives/enemas to promote cleansing of the bowel.
E. Nursing interventions: postoperative
1. Provide routine post-op care.
2. Assess for rectal bleeding: inspect rectal area/dressings every 2–3 hours and report significant increases in bloody drainage.
3. Promote comfort.
   a. Assist client to side-lying or prone position, provide flotation pad when sitting.
   b. Administer analgesics as ordered and monitor effects.
4. Promote elimination: administer stool softeners as ordered and, if possible, administer analgesic before first post-op bowel movement.
5. Provide client teaching and discharge planning concerning:
   a. Dietary modifications (high fiber and ingestion of at least 2000 mL/day)
   b. Need to defecate when urge is felt
   c. Use of stool softeners as needed until healing occurs
   d. Sitz baths after each bowel movement for at least 2 weeks after surgery
   e. Perineal care
   f. Recognition and reporting immediately to physician of the following signs and symptoms
      1) Rectal bleeding
      2) Continued pain on defecation
      3) Puslike drainage from rectal area

# DISORDERS OF THE LIVER

## Hepatitis

A. General information
1. Widespread inflammation of the liver tissue with liver cell damage due to hepatic cell degeneration and necrosis; proliferation and enlargement of the Kupffer cells; inflammation of the periportal areas (may cause interruption of bile flow)
2. Hepatitis A
   a. Incubation period: 15–45 days
   b. Transmitted by fecal/oral route: often occurs in crowded living conditions; with poor personal hygiene; or from contaminated food, milk, water, or shellfish
3. Hepatitis B
   a. Incubation period: 50–180 days
   b. Transmitted by blood and body fluids (saliva, semen, vaginal secretions): often from contaminated needles among IV drug abusers; intimate/sexual contact

4. Hepatitis C
   a. Incubation period: 7–50 days
   b. Transmitted by parenteral route: through blood and blood products, needles, syringes
5. Hepatitis D
   a. Incubation period: 14–56 days
   b. Transmitted by blood and body fluids; seen in persons who have hepatitis B
6. Hepatitis E
   a. Incubation period: 15–64 days
   b. Transmitted by fecal/oral route; usually water-borne; seen in travelers returning from underdeveloped countries

B. Assessment findings
   1. Preicteric stage
      a. Anorexia, nausea and vomiting, fatigue, constipation or diarrhea, weight loss
      b. Right upper quadrant discomfort, hepatomegaly, splenomegaly, lymphadenopathy
   2. Icteric stage
      a. Fatigue, weight loss, light-colored stools, dark urine
      b. Continued hepatomegaly with tenderness, lymphadenopathy, splenomegaly
      c. Jaundice, pruritus
   3. Posticteric stage
      a. Fatigue, but an increased sense of well-being
      b. Hepatomegaly gradually decreasing
   4. Diagnostic tests
      a. Hepatitis A, B, C
         1) SGPT (ALT), SGOT (AST), alkaline phosphatase, bilirubin, ESR: all increased (preicteric)
         2) Leukocytes, lymphocytes, neutrophils: all decreased (pericteric)
         3) Prolonged PT
      b. Hepatitis A
         1) Hepatitis A virus (HAV) in stool before onset of disease
         2) Anti-HAV (IgG) appears soon after onset of jaundice; peaks in 1–2 months and persists indefinitely
         3) Anti-HAV (IgM): positive in acute infection; lasts 4–6 weeks
      c. Hepatitis B
         1) HBsAg (surface antigen): positive, develops 4–12 weeks after infection
         2) Anti-HBsAG: negative in 80% of cases
         3) Anti-HBc: associated with infectivity, develops 2–16 weeks after infection
         4) HBeAg: associated with infectivity and disappears before jaundice
         5) Anti-HBe: present in carriers, represents low infectivity
      d. Hepatitis C
         1) Initial screening test enzyme-linked immunoabsorbent assay (ELISA) test

         2) If ELISA test is positive and ALT is normal then recombinant immunoblot assay (RIBA) done
         3) Reverse transcription polymerase chain reaction (RT-PCR) test can pick up virus 2–3 weeks after exposure
      e. Hepatitis D: rise in hepatitis D virus antibodies (anti-HDV) titer
      f. Hepatitis E: testing usually done only for symptomatic persons who have traveled to high-risk areas; hepatitis E antibodies (anti-HEV) present

C. Nursing interventions
   1. Promote adequate nutrition.
      a. Administer antiemetics as ordered, 30 minutes before meals to decrease occurrence of nausea and vomiting.
      b. Provide small, frequent meals of a high-carbohydrate, moderate- to high-protein, high-vitamin, high-calorie diet.
      c. Avoid very hot or very cold foods.
   2. Ensure rest/relaxation: plan schedule for rest and activity periods, organize nursing care to minimize interruption.
   3. Monitor/relieve pruritus (see Cirrhosis of the Liver).
   4. Administer corticosteroids as ordered.
   5. Institute isolation procedures as required; pay special attention to good hand-washing technique and adequate sanitation.
   6. In hepatitis A administer immune serum globulin (ISG) early to exposed individuals as ordered.
   7. In hepatitis B
      a. Screen blood donors for HBsAg.
      b. Use disposable needles and syringes.
      c. Instruct client/others to avoid sexual intercourse while disease is active.
      d. Administer ISG to exposed individuals as ordered.
      e. Administer hepatitis B immunoglobulin (HBIG) as ordered to provide temporary and passive immunity to exposed individuals.
      f. To produce active immunity, administer hepatitis B vaccine to those individuals at high risk.
   8. In non-A, non-B: use disposable needles and syringes; ensure adequate sanitation.
   9. In hepatitis C: Medications used are interferon combined with ribavirin. Side effects may include flu-like symptoms, nausea; hair loss; emotional changes.
   10. Provide client teaching and discharge planning concerning:
      a. Importance of avoiding alcohol
      b. Avoidance of persons with known infections
      c. Balance of activity and rest periods
      d. Importance of not donating blood

4

e. Dietary modifications
f. Recognition and reporting of signs of inadequate convalescence: anorexia, jaundice, increasing liver tenderness/discomfort
g. Techniques/importance of good personal hygiene

# Cirrhosis of the Liver

A. General information
1. Chronic, progressive disease characterized by inflammation, fibrosis, and degeneration of the liver parenchymal cells
2. Destroyed liver cells are replaced by scar tissue, resulting in architectural changes and malfunction of the liver
3. Types
   a. Laënnec's cirrhosis: associated with alcohol abuse and malnutrition; characterized by an accumulation of fat in the liver cells, progressing to widespread scar formation.
   b. Postnecrotic cirrhosis: results in severe inflammation with massive necrosis as a complication of viral hepatitis.
   c. Cardiac cirrhosis: occurs as a consequence of right-sided heart failure; manifested by hepatomegaly with some fibrosis.
   d. Biliary cirrhosis: associated with biliary obstruction, usually in the common bile duct; results in chronic impairment of bile excretion.
4. Occurs twice as often in men as in women; ages 40–60
B. Assessment findings
1. Fatigue, anorexia, nausea and vomiting, indigestion, weight loss, flatulence, irregular bowel habits
2. Early symptoms: hepatomegaly; pain in right upper quadrant. Late symptoms: hard nodular liver upon palpitation; atrophy of liver
3. Changes in mood, alertness, and mental ability; sensory deficits; gynecomastia, decreased axillary and pubic hair in males; amenorrhea in young females
4. Jaundice of the skin, sclera, and mucous membranes; pruritus
5. Easy bruising, spider angiomas, palmar erythema
6. Muscle atrophy
7. Diagnostic tests
   a. SGOT (AST), SGPT (ALT), LDH alkaline phosphatase increased
   b. Serum bilirubin increased
   c. PT prolonged
   d. Serum albumin decreased
   e. Hgb and HCT decreased
C. Nursing interventions
1. Provide sufficient rest and comfort.

a. Provide bed rest with bathroom privileges.
b. Encourage gradual, progressive, increasing activity with planned rest periods.
c. Institute measures to relieve pruritus.
   1) Do not use soaps and detergents.
   2) Bathe in tepid water followed by application of an emollient lotion.
   3) Provide cool, light, nonrestrictive clothing.
   4) Keep nails short to avoid skin excoriation from scratching.
   5) Apply cool, moist compresses to pruritic areas.
2. Promote nutritional intake.
   a. Encourage small frequent feedings.
   b. Promote a high-calorie, low- to moderate-protein, high-carbohydrate, low-fat diet, with supplemental vitamin therapy (vitamins A, B-complex, C, D, K, and folic acid).
3. Prevent infection.
   a. Prevent skin breakdown by frequent turning and skin care.
   b. Provide reverse isolation for clients with severe leukopenia; pay special attention to handwashing technique.
   c. Monitor WBC.
4. Monitor/prevent bleeding.
5. Administer diuretics as ordered.
6. Provide client teaching and discharge planning concerning:
   a. Avoidance of agents that may be hepatotoxic (sedatives, opiates, or OTC drugs detoxified by the liver)
   b. How to assess for weight gain and increased abdominal girth
   c. Avoidance of persons with upper respiratory infections
   d. Recognition and reporting of signs of recurring illness (liver tenderness, increased jaundice, increased fatigue, anorexia)
   e. Avoidance of all alcohol
   f. Avoidance of straining at stool, vigorous blowing of nose and coughing, to decrease the incidence of bleeding

# Ascites

A. General information
1. Accumulation of free fluid in the abdominal cavity
2. Most frequently caused by cirrhotic liver damage, which produces hypoalbuminemia, increased portal venous pressure, and hyperaldosteronism
3. May also be caused by HF
B. Medical management
1. Supportive: modify diet, bed rest, salt-poor albumin

2. Diuretic therapy (see Unit 2)
3. Surgery
    a. Paracentesis: insertion of a needle into the peritoneal cavity through the abdomen to remove abnormally large amounts of peritoneal fluid.
        1) Peritoneal fluid assessed for cell count, specific gravity, protein, and microorganisms.
        2) Used in clients with acute respiratory or abdominal distress secondary to ascites.
    b. LeVeen shunt (peritoneal-venous shunt): used in chronic, unmanageable ascites
        1) Permits continuous reinfusion of ascitic fluid back into the venous system through a silicone catheter with a one-way pressure-sensitive valve.
        2) One end of the catheter is implanted into the peritoneal cavity and is channeled through the subcutaneous tissue to the superior vena cava, where the other end of the catheter is implanted; the valve opens when pressure in the peritoneal cavity is 3–5 cm of water higher than in superior vena cava, thereby allowing ascitic fluid to flow into the venous system.
C. Assessment findings
    1. Anorexia, nausea and vomiting, fatigue, weakness, changes in mental functioning
    2. Positive fluid wave and shifting dullness on percussion, flat or protruding umbilicus, abdominal distension/tautness with striae and prominent veins, abdominal pain
    3. Peripheral edema, shortness of breath
    4. Diagnostic tests
        a. Potassium and serum albumin decreased
        b. PT prolonged
        c. LDH, SGOT (AST), SGPT (ALT), BUN, sodium increased
D. Nursing interventions
    1. Monitor nutritional status/provide adequate nutrition with modified diet.
        a. Restrict sodium to 200–500 mg/day.
        b. Restrict fluids to 1000–1500 mL/day.
        c. Promote high-calorie foods/snacks.
    2. Monitor/prevent increasing edema.
        a. Administer diuretics as ordered and monitor for effects.
        b. Measure I&O.
        c. Monitor peripheral pulses.
        d. Measure abdominal girth.
        e. Inspect/palpate extremities, sacrum.
        f. Administer salt-poor albumin to replace vascular volume.
    3. Monitor/promote skin integrity.
        a. Reposition frequently.
        b. Apply lotions to stretched areas.
        c. Assess for redness, breakdown.

4. Promote comfort: place client in mid- to high-Fowler's and reposition frequently.
5. Provide nursing care for the client undergoing paracentesis.
    a. Confirm that client has signed a consent form.
    b. Instruct client to empty bladder before the procedure to prevent inadvertent puncture of the bladder during insertion of trocar.
    c. Inform client that a local anesthetic will be provided to decrease pain.
    d. Place in sitting position to facilitate the flow of fluid by gravity.
    e. Measure abdominal girth and weight before and after the procedure.
    f. Record color, amount, and consistency of fluid withdrawn and client tolerance during procedure.
    g. Assess insertion site for leakage.
6. Provide routine pre- and post-op care for the client with LeVeen shunt.

# Esophageal Varices

A. General information
    1. Dilation of the veins of the esophagus, caused by portal hypertension from resistance to normal venous drainage of the liver into the portal vein
    2. Causes blood to be shunted to the esophagogastric veins, resulting in distension, hypertrophy, and increased fragility.
    3. Caused by portal hypertension, which may be secondary to cirrhosis of the liver (alcohol abuse), swallowing poorly masticated food, increased intra-abdominal pressure
B. Medical management
    1. Iced normal saline lavage
    2. Transfusions with fresh whole blood
    3. Vitamin K therapy
    4. Sengstaken-Blakemore tube: a three-lumen tube used to control bleeding by applying pressure on the cardiac portion of the stomach and against bleeding esophageal varices. One lumen serves as NG suction, a second lumen is used to inflate the gastric balloon, the third to inflate the esophageal balloon.
    5. Intra-arterial or IV vasopressin
    6. Injection sclerotherapy
    7. Surgery for portal hypertension (decompresses esophageal varices and helps to maintain optimal portal perfusion)
        a. Ligation of esophageal and gastric veins to stop acute bleeding
        b. Portacaval shunt: end-to-side or side-to-side anastomosis of the portal vein to the inferior vena cava
        c. Splenorenal shunt: end-to-side or side-to-side anastomosis of the splenic vein to the left renal vein

       d. Mesocaval shunt: end-to-side or use of a
          graft to anastomose the inferior vena cava
          to the side of the superior mesenteric vein
C. Assessment findings
   1. Anorexia, nausea and vomiting, hematemesis,
      fatigue, weakness
   2. Splenomegaly, increased splenic dullness,
      ascites, caput medusae, peripheral edema, bruits
   3. Diagnostic tests
      a. PT prolonged
      b. Hematest of vomitus positive
      c. Serum albumin, RBC, Hgb, and HCT
         decreased
      d. LDH, SGOT (AST), SGPT (ALT), BUN,
         increased
D. Nursing interventions
   1. Monitor/provide care for client with
      Sengstaken-Blakemore tube.
      a. Facilitate placement of the tube: check and
         lubricate tip and elevate head of bed.
      b. Prevent dislodgment of the tube by placing
         client in semi-Fowler's position; maintain
         traction by securing the tube to a piece of
         sponge or foam rubber placed on the nose.
      c. Keep scissors at bedside at all times.
      d. Monitor respiratory status; assess for signs
         of distress and if respiratory distress occurs
         cut the tubing to deflate the balloons and
         remove tubing immediately.
      e. Label each lumen to avoid confusion;
         maintain prescribed amount of pressure on
         esophageal balloon and deflate balloon as
         ordered to avoid necrosis.
      f. Observe nares for skin breakdown and
         provide mouth and nasal care every
         1–2 hours (encourage client to expectorate
         secretions, suction gently if unable).
   2. Promote comfort: place client in semi-Fowler's
      position (if not in shock); provide mouth care.
   3. Monitor for further bleeding and for signs and
      symptoms of shock; hematest all secretions.
   4. Administer vasopressin as ordered and
      monitor effects.
   5. Provide routine pre- and post-op care if the
      client has portasystemic or portacaval shunt.
   6. Provide client teaching and discharge
      planning concerning:
      a. Minimizing esophageal irritation
         (avoidance of salicylates, alcohol; use of
         antacids as needed; importance of chewing
         food thoroughly)
      b. Avoidance of increased abdominal,
         thoracic, and portal pressure
      c. Recognition and reporting of signs of
         hemorrhage

## Hepatic Encephalopathy

A. General information
   1. Frequent terminal complication in liver disease

   2. Diseased liver is unable to convert ammonia to
      urea, so that large quantities remain in the
      systemic circulation and cross the blood/brain
      barrier, producing neurologic toxic symptoms.
   3. Caused by cirrhosis, GI hemorrhage,
      hyperbilirubinemia, transfusions (particularly
      with stored blood), thiazide diuretics, uremia,
      dehydration
B. Assessment findings
   1. Early in course of disease: changes in mental
      functioning (irritability); insomnia, slowed
      affect; slow slurred speech; impaired
      judgment; slight tremor; Babinski's reflex,
      hyperactive reflexes
   2. Progressive disease: asterixis, disorientation,
      apraxia, tremors, fetor hepaticus, facial
      grimacing
   3. Late in disease: coma, absent reflexes
   4. Diagnostic tests
      a. Serum ammonia levels increased
         (particularly later)
      b. PT prolonged
      c. Hgb and HCT decreased
C. Nursing interventions
   1. Conduct ongoing neurologic assessment and
      report deteriorations.
   2. Restrict protein in diet; provide high
      carbohydrate intake and vitamin K
      supplements.
   3. Administer enemas, cathartics, intestinal
      antibiotics, and lactulose as ordered to reduce
      ammonia levels.
   4. Protect client from injury: keep side rails up;
      provide eye care with use of artificial tears/eye
      patch.
   5. Avoid administration of drugs detoxified in
      liver (phenothiazines, gold compounds,
      methyldopa, acetaminophen).
   6. Maintain client on bed rest to decrease
      metabolic demands on liver.

## Cancer of the Liver

A. General information
   1. Primary cancer of the liver is extremely rare,
      but it is a common site for metastasis because
      of liver's large blood supply and portal
      drainage. Primary cancers of the colon,
      rectum, stomach, pancreas, esophagus, breast,
      lung, and melanomas frequently metastasize to
      the liver.
   2. Enlargement, hemorrhage, and necrosis are
      common occurrences; primary liver tumors
      often metastasize to the lung.
   3. Higher incidence in men.
   4. Prognosis poor; disease well advanced before
      clinical signs evident.
B. Medical management
   1. Chemotherapy and radiotherapy (palliative) to
      decrease tumor size and pain

**2.** Resection of liver segment or lobe if tumor is localized

**C.** Assessment findings

   **1.** Weakness, anorexia, nausea and vomiting, weight loss, slight increase in temperature

   **2.** Right upper quadrant discomfort/tenderness, hepatomegaly, blood-tinged ascites, friction rub over liver, peripheral edema, jaundice

   **3.** Diagnostic tests: same as cirrhosis of the liver plus:

     **a.** Blood sugar decreased

     **b.** Alpha fetoprotein increased

     **c.** Abdominal X-ray, liver scan, liver biopsy all positive

**D.** Nursing interventions: same as for cirrhosis of the liver plus:

   **1.** Provide emotional support for client/significant others regarding poor prognosis.

   **2.** Provide care of the client receiving radiation therapy or chemotherapy.

   **3.** Provide care of client with abdominal surgery plus:

     **a.** Preoperative

       **1)** Perform bowel prep to decrease ammonium intoxication.

       **2)** Administer vitamin K to decrease risk of bleeding.

     **b.** Postoperative

       **1)** Administer 10% glucose for first 48 hours to avoid rapid blood sugar drop.

       **2)** Monitor for hyper/hypoglycemia.

       **3)** Assess for bleeding (hemorrhage is most threatening complication).

       **4)** Assess for signs of hepatic encephalopathy.

# DISORDERS OF THE GALLBLADDER

## Cholecystitis/Cholelithiasis

**A.** General information

   **1.** Cholecystitis: acute or chronic inflammation of the gallbladder, most commonly associated with gallstones. Inflammation occurs within the walls of the gallbladder and creates a thickening accompanied by edema. Consequently, there is impaired circulation, ischemia, and eventual necrosis.

   **2.** Cholelithiasis: formation of gallstones, cholesterol stones most common variety

   **3.** Most often occurs in women after age 40, in postmenopausal women on estrogen therapy, in women taking oral contraceptives, and in the obese; Caucasians and Native Americans are also more commonly affected.

   **4.** Stone formation may be caused by genetic defect of bile composition, gallbladder/bile stasis, infection.

   **5.** Acute cholecystitis usually follows stone impaction, adhesions; neoplasms may also be implicated.

**B.** Medical management

   **1.** Supportive treatment: NPO with NG intubation and IV fluids

   **2.** Diet modification with administration of fat-soluble vitamins

   **3.** Drug therapy

     **a.** Narcotic analgesics (Demerol is drug of choice) for pain. Morphine sulfate is contraindicated because it causes spasms of the sphincter of Oddi.

     **b.** Anticholinergics (atropine) for pain. (Anticholinergics relax smooth muscle and open bile ducts.)

     **c.** Antiemetics

   **4.** Surgery: cholecystectomy/choledochostomy

**C.** Assessment findings

   **1.** Epigastric or right upper quadrant pain, precipitated by a heavy meal or occurring at night

   **2.** Intolerance for fatty foods (nausea, vomiting, sensation of fullness)

   **3.** Pruritus, easy bruising, jaundice, dark amber urine, steatorrhea

   **4.** Diagnostic tests

     **a.** Direct bilirubin transaminase, alkaline phosphatase, WBC, amylase, lipase: all increased

     **b.** Oral cholecystogram (gallbladder series): positive for gallstone

**D.** Nursing interventions

   **1.** Administer pain medications as ordered and monitor for effects.

   **2.** Administer IV fluids as ordered.

   **3.** Provide small, frequent meals of modified diet (if oral intake allowed).

   **4.** Provide care to relieve pruritus.

   **5.** Provide care for the client with a cholecystectomy or choledochostomy.

## Cholecystectomy/Choledochostomy

**A.** General information

   **1.** Cholecystectomy: removal of the gallbladder with insertion of a T-tube into the common bile duct if common bile duct exploration is performed

   **2.** Choledochostomy: opening of common duct, removal of stone, and insertion of a T-tube

   **3.** Cholecystectomy performed via laparoscopy for uncomplicated cases when client has not had previous abdominal surgery

**B.** Nursing interventions: routine preoperative care

**C.** Nursing interventions: postoperative

   **1.** Provide routine post-op care.

   **2.** Position client in semi-Fowler's or side-lying positions; reposition frequently.

3. Splint incision when turning, coughing, and deep breathing.
4. Maintain/monitor functioning of T-tube.
   a. Ensure that T-tube is connected to closed gravity drainage.
   b. Avoid kinks, clamping, or pulling of the tube.
   c. Measure and record drainage every shift.
   d. Expect 300–500 mL bile-colored drainage first 24 hours, then 200 mL/24 hours for 3–4 days.
   e. Monitor color of urine and stools (stools will be light colored if bile is flowing through T-tube but normal color should reappear as drainage diminishes).
   f. Assess for signs of peritonitis.
   g. Assess skin around T-tube; cleanse frequently and keep dry.
5. Provide client teaching and discharge planning concerning
   a. Adherence to dietary restrictions
   b. Resumption of ADL (avoid heavy lifting for at least 6 weeks; resume sexual activity as desired unless ordered otherwise by physician); clients having laparoscopy cholecystectomy usually resume normal activity within 2 weeks.
   c. Recognition and reporting of signs of complications (fever, jaundice, pain, dark urine, pale stools, pruritus)

## Appendicitis

See Unit 5.

# DISORDERS OF THE PANCREAS

## Pancreatitis

A. General information
   1. An inflammatory process with varying degrees of pancreatic edema, fat necrosis, or hemorrhage
   2. Proteolytic and lipolytic pancreatic enzymes are activated in the pancreas rather than in the duodenum, resulting in tissue damage and autodigestion of the pancreas
   3. Occurs most often in the middle aged
   4. Caused by alcoholism, biliary tract disease, trauma, viral infection, penetrating duodenal ulcer, abscesses, drugs (steroids, thiazide diuretics, and oral contraceptives), metabolic disorders (hyperparathyroidism, hyperlipidemia)
B. Medical management
   1. Drug therapy
      a. Analgesics to relieve pain. Note: Morphine is contraindicated due to the spasmodic effects of opiates on the sphincter of Oddi,

which will cause exacerbation of symptoms.
      b. Smooth-muscle relaxants (papaverine, nitroglycerin) to relieve pain
      c. Anticholinergics (atropine, propantheline bromide [Pro-Banthine]) to decrease pancreatic stimulation
      d. Antacids to decrease pancreatic stimulation
      e. $H_2$ antagonists, vasodilators, calcium gluconate
   2. Diet modification
   3. NPO (usually)
   4. Peritoneal lavage
   5. Dialysis
C. Assessment findings
   1. Pain located in left upper quadrant with radiation to back, flank, or substernal area; may be accompanied by difficulty breathing and is aggravated by eating
   2. Vomiting, shallow respirations (with pain), tachycardia, decreased or absent bowel sounds, abdominal tenderness with muscle guarding, positive Grey Turner's spots (ecchymoses on flanks) and positive Cullen's sign (ecchymoses of periumbilical area)
   3. Diagnostic tests
      a. Serum amylase and lipase, urinary amylase, blood sugar, lipid levels: all increased
      b. Serum calcium decreased
      c. CT scan shows enlargement of the pancreas
D. Nursing interventions
   1. Administer analgesics, antacids, anticholinergics as ordered, monitor effects.
   2. Withhold food/fluid and eliminate odor and sight of food from environment to decrease pancreatic stimulations.
   3. Maintain NG tube and assess for drainage.
   4. Institute nonpharmacologic measures to decrease pain.
      a. Assist client to positions of comfort (knee-chest; fetal position).
      b. Teach relaxation techniques and provide a quiet, restful environment.
   5. Provide client teaching and discharge planning concerning
      a. Dietary regimen when oral intake permitted
         1) High-carbohydrate, high-protein, low-fat diet
         2) Eating small, frequent meals instead of three large ones
         3) Avoiding caffeine products
         4) Eliminating alcohol consumption
         5) Maintaining relaxed atmosphere after meals
      b. Recognition and reporting of signs of complications
         1) Continued nausea and vomiting
         2) Abdominal distension with increasing fullness

3) Persistent weight loss
4) Severe epigastric or back pain
5) Frothy/foul-smelling bowel movements
6) Irritability, confusion, persistent elevation of temperature (2 days)

# Cancer of the Pancreas

A. General information
   1. Most pancreatic tumors are adenocarcinomas and half occur in the head of the pancreas
   2. Tumor growth results in common bile duct obstruction with jaundice
   3. Occurs more often in men and in the African-American and Jewish populations; ages 45–65
   4. Contributing factors: chemical carcinogens, cigarette smoking, high-fat diet, diabetes mellitus
   5. Prognosis generally poor
B. Medical management
   1. Radiation therapy
   2. Whipple's procedure (pancreatoduodenectomy): resection of the proximal pancreas, adjoining duodenum, distal portion of the stomach, and distal segment of the common bile duct
   3. Drug therapy
      a. Pancreatic enzymes; oral hypoglycemic agents or insulin, bile salts necessary after surgery
      b. Chemotherapy may also be used
C. Assessment findings
   1. Anorexia; rapid, progressive weight loss; dull abdominal pain located in upper abdomen or left hypochondriacal region with radiation to the back, related to eating; jaundice
   2. Diagnostic tests
      a. Increased serum lipase (early)
      b. Increased bilirubin (conjugated)
      c. Increased serum amylase
D. Nursing interventions
   1. See Pancreatitis.
   2. Provide care for the client receiving radiation therapy or chemotherapy.
   3. Routine pre- and post-op care (for clients undergoing Whipple's procedure).
   4. Provide emotional support to client/significant others.
   5. Provide client teaching and discharge planning concerning
      a. Need to eat small frequent meals of a low-fat, high-calorie diet with vitamin supplements.
      b. Importance of adhering to medication regimen after surgery.

# Sample Questions

290. An adult client has a nasogastric tube in place to maintain gastric decompression. Which nursing action will relieve discomfort in the nostril with the NG tube?
   1. Remove any tape and loosely pin the tube to his gown.
   2. Lubricate the NG tube with viscous xylocaine.
   3. Loop the NG tube to avoid pressure on the nares.
   4. Replace the NG tube with a smaller diameter tube.

291. An adult client has just returned to his room following a bowel resection and end-to-end anastomosis. What type of drainage will the nurse expect in the early post-op period?
   1. Clear.
   2. Mucoid.
   3. Scant.
   4. Discolored.

292. A client with a long history of ulcerative colitis is experiencing an exacerbation of the disease and is admitted with severe diarrhea, electrolyte disturbances, and severe abdominal pain. He questions the nurse about his prognosis. What is the nurse's best response?
   1. "You should ask your physician about this."
   2. "Don't worry, colitis is rarely fatal."
   3. "It depends on the form of the disease."
   4. "Tell me what you know about this disease."

293. The nurse questions a client with hepatitis B. How long ago could the client have been exposed to hepatitis B?
   a. 3–7 days.
   b. 7–14 days.
   c. 40–50 days.
   d. 60–160 days.

294. A client has a history of peptic ulcer disease. He has had numerous bleeding episodes in the past and is admitted to the hospital for evaluation. His physician has prescribed cimetidine (Tagamet). What is the primary reason for the client to take Tagamet?
   1. Blocks the secretion of gastric hydrochloric acid.
   2. Coats the gastric mucosa with a protective membrane.

3. Increases the sensitivity of $H_2$ receptors.

4. Releases basal gastric acid.

295. An adult has a Billroth II procedure and does well postoperatively. The nurse knows the client understands discharge teaching when the client recognizes that symptoms of dizziness, sweating, and weakness in the weeks following the surgery are usually associated with what condition?

1. Afferent loop syndrome.

2. Dumping syndrome.

3. Pernicious anemia.

4. Marginal ulcers.

296. A client has had a significant problem with alcohol abuse for the past 15 years. His wife brings him to the emergency department because he is increasingly confused and is coughing blood. His medical diagnosis is cirrhosis of the liver. He has ascites and esophageal varices. Which symptom is the client least likely to have?

1. Bulging flanks.

2. Protruding umbilicus.

3. Abdominal distension.

4. Bluish discoloration of the umbilicus.

297. What is the major dietary treatment for ascites?

1. High protein.

2. Increased potassium.

3. Restricted fluids.

4. Restricted sodium.

298. Which laboratory value would the nurse expect to find in a client as a result of liver failure?

1. Decreased serum creatinine.

2. Decreased sodium.

3. Increased ammonia.

4. Increased calcium.

299. A man is admitted with bleeding esophageal varices. A Sengstaken-Blakemore tube is inserted in an effort to stop the bleeding. After the Sengstaken-Blakemore tube is inserted, the client has difficulty breathing. Based on this information, what is the first action the nurse should take?

1. Deflate the esophageal balloon.

2. Encourage him to take deep breaths.

3. Monitor his vital signs.

4. Notify the physician.

300. A client is scheduled for a esophagoduodenoscopy. In planning for the post-procedural care, what is the most effective nursing action to prevent respiratory complications?

1. Keep the client positioned on his left side for 8–10 hours.

2. Assess for a gag reflex before offering the client anything to eat or drink.

3. Provide throat lozenges for complaints of a sore throat.

4. Position the client in high Fowler's until he is fully awake and alert.

301. A client is being evaluated for cancer of the colon. In preparing the client for a barium enema, which intervention will be included that pertains to the procedure?

1. Placement on a low-residue diet 1 to 2 days before the study.

2. Given an oil retention enema the morning of the study.

3. Instruction to swallow six radiopaque tablets the evening before the study.

4. Positioning in a high Fowler's position immediately following the procedure.

302. A client complains of excessive weight loss and anorexia. Laboratory studies show that he is anemic. Hepatocellular carcinoma is suspected. A liver biopsy is performed at the bedside. What intervention will be expected after the procedure?

1. Encourage to ambulate to prevent the formation of venous thrombosis.

2. Ask to turn, cough, and deep breathe every 2 hours for the next 8 hours.

3. Place in a high Fowler's position to maximize thoracic expansion.

4. Position on his right side with a pillow under the costal margin, and immobile for several hours.

303. A client has a fecal impaction. The physician orders an oil-retention enema followed by a cleansing enema. What is the reason for administering an oil-retention enema to the client?

1. Lubricate the walls of the intestinal tract.

2. Soften the fecal mass and lubricate the walls of the rectum and colon.

3. Reduce bacterial content of the fecal mass.

4. Coat the walls of the intestines to prevent irritation by the hardened fecal mass.

304. A client has amyotrophic lateral sclerosis. His neurologic status has continued to deteriorate. He is receiving enteral feedings through a gastrostomy tube. What priority assessment

should be performed before administering a bolus feeding?

1. Check the expiration date of the prepared enteral feeding.
2. Confirm the presence of a gag reflex.
3. Check placement of feeding tube.
4. Review laboratory studies for indications of electrolyte imbalances.

305. An adult is 8 hours post-op a Billroth II (gastric resection) for an intractable gastric ulcer. The drainage from his nasogastric decompression tube is thickened and the volume of secretions has dramatically reduced in the last 2 hours. The client complains that he feels like he is going to vomit. What is the most appropriate nursing action?

1. Reposition the nasogastric tube by advancing it gently.
2. Notify the physician of your findings.
3. Irrigate the nasogastric tube with 50 mL of sterile normal saline.
4. Discontinue the low-intermittent suctioning.

306. A client is receiving chemotherapy for cancer of the liver. Her physician has prescribed metoclopramide for the nausea and vomiting associated with the chemotherapy. Metoclopramide has anticholinergic and extrapyramidal side effects. Due to the side effects of this mediation, which nursing diagnosis is the client at high risk for?

1. Hyperglycemia related to increased gastric emptying.
2. Injury related to decreased visual acuity and ataxia.
3. Decreased cardiac output related to reduced heart rate.
4. Fluid volume deficit related to frequent episodes of diarrhea.

307. An adult develops diarrhea secondary to hyperosmolar enteral therapy. The care plan now includes giving the client water every 4 to 6 hours and after feedings. Which of the following findings would indicate that fluid therapy was effective?

1. Dry mucous membranes.
2. Hyperactive bowel sounds.
3. Increased urinary output.
4. Hypokalemia.

308. An elderly client complains of frequent episodes of constipation. What is an effective strategy for preventing constipation?

1. Reducing fluid intake to encourage bulk formation in the intestinal lumen.
2. Use of laxatives daily to establish a regular elimination pattern.
3. A regimen of exercises directed at toning the abdominal muscles.
4. Setting a routine for bowel elimination just before bedtime.

309. A client is scheduled for a resection of the lower thoracic esophagus to remove a malignant tumor. What intervention would be included in the postoperative care?

1. Keep the client in a supine position to encourage thoracic expansion.
2. Carefully advance the nasogastric tube past the anastomosis site.
3. Frequently assess the client's breath sounds.
4. Provide a regular diet high in protein.

310. A client has been experiencing frequent episodes of "heartburn" and regurgitation of acrid, sour-tasting fluid. These episodes tend to occur especially after a heavy meal. The client is diagnosed with a hiatal hernia. Which statement by the client shows a good understanding of her treatment regimen?

1. "I will elevate my legs when sleeping."
2. "I will increase the roughage in my diet."
3. "I will drink more fluid with my meals."
4. "I will avoid caffeine, alcohol, and chocolate."

311. A client stockbroker has recently been diagnosed with peptic ulcer disease. Diagnostic studies confirm the presence of the gram-negative bacteria *Helicobacter pylori* in his gastrointestinal tract. If the client has a duodenal ulceration, how would the nurse expect the "ulcer pain" to be described by the client?

1. Located in the upper right epigastric area radiating to his right shoulder or back.
2. Relieved by vomiting.
3. Occurring 2 to 3 hours after a meal, often awakening him between 1:00 and 2:00 A.M.
4. Worsening with the ingestion of food.

312. A client has been diagnosed with peptic ulcer disease. Her medication regimen includes misoprostol. What therapeutic effect will be performed by misoprostol?

1. Neutralizing excess gastric acid.
2. Inhibiting gastric acid production.
3. Increasing mucous production and bicarbonate levels.
4. Increasing gastric emptying time.

313. A client has Billroth II (gastrojejunostomy) for intractable peptic ulcer disease. The nurse is instructing the client concerning the potential complication of dumping syndrome. What would be included in the client's dietary and activity instructions?
    1. A high-carbohydrate diet.
    2. Exercise after mealtime to promote the digestive process.
    3. Limit drinking fluids with meals.
    4. A protein-restricted diet.

314. A client underwent a total gastrectomy for gastric cancer. The nurse has been giving the client post-op instructions about his diet, activities, and medications. Which of the following statements indicates that he understands his post-op care?
    1. "I should take a walk after meals to aid my digestion."
    2. "Drinking more water with my meals will prevent indigestion."
    3. "I need more carbohydrates in my diet for an extra energy source."
    4. "The visiting nurse will come monthly to give an injection of vitamin B$_{12}$."

315. A client has a direct inguinal hernia. For what symptoms should the nurse be on alert for?
    1. Hypoactive bowel sounds.
    2. Passage of semi-liquid, brown stools.
    3. Vomiting of bile-stained gastric contents.
    4. Complaints of constant, localized abdominal pain.

316. An adult has developed peritonitis related to a perforated duodenal ulceration. What would the nurse expect to find during the assessment?
    1. Decreased or absent bowel sounds.
    2. Colicky abdominal pain.
    3. High-pitched bowel sounds.
    4. Alternating episodes of constipation and diarrhea.

317. What would be an appropriate nursing diagnosis for a client with ulcerative colitis?
    1. Abdominal pain, related to decreased peristalsis.
    2. Diarrhea related to hyperosmolar intestinal contents.
    3. Excess fluid volume related to increased water absorption by intestinal mucosa.
    4. Activity intolerance related to fatigue.

318. The nurse is caring for a client recently diagnosed with ulcerative colitis. The nurse has been giving dietary instructions to help prevent exacerbation of his inflammatory bowel disease. Which dietary choice indicates that the client understands the dietary instructions?
    1. Apple.
    2. Celery.
    3. Refined cereals.
    4. Hard cheeses.

319. When a client is diagnosed with ulcerative colitis, What complication would the nurse be on alert for?
    1. Intestinal obstruction.
    2. Toxic megacolon.
    3. Malnutrition from malabsorption.
    4. Fistula formation.

320. A client with diverticulosis is admitted to the hospital. What type of diet would be ordered for this client?
    1. A bland, low residue diet.
    2. A low protein, high carbohydrate diet.
    3. A soft, but high fiber diet.
    4. Saline cathartics to increase intestinal peristalsis.

321. An adult has been diagnosed with colon cancer. What would the nursing assessment most likely reveal?
    1. Epigastric pain that intensifies when the stomach is empty.
    2. Stools that are fatty and foul-smelling.
    3. Alternating episodes of diarrhea and constipation.
    4. A rigid, board-like abdomen.

322. The nurse has been instructing a client regarding identifying and alleviating the risk factors associated with colon cancer. Which statement by the client demonstrates a good understanding of the means to reduce the chances of colon cancer?
    1. "I will exercise daily."
    2. "I will include more red meat in my diet."
    3. "I will have an annual chest X-ray."
    4. "I will include more fresh fruits and vegetables in my diet."

323. An adult has a sigmoid colostomy. The nurse is performing peristomal skin care and changing the stoma pouch. What is the most appropriate nursing action?
    1. Empty the ostomy pouch when it is full.
    2. Pull flange and pouch off together to prevent spillage of stomach pouch contents.

3. Leave ¼ inch of skin exposed around stoma when determining size to cut new skin barrier.

4. Apply liquid deodorant to mucous membrane of protruding stoma.

324. An adult has a double-barreled, transverse colostomy. The nurse has formulated the nursing diagnosis: risk for impaired skin integrity related to irritation of the peristomal skin by the effluent. What is the most appropriate nursing action relevant to this nursing diagnosis?

1. Strict measurement and recording of I&O.

2. Assessing for bowel sounds when changing ostomy appliance.

3. Wash peristomal skin with an astringent solution to reduce bacterial contamination.

4. Apply skin barrier before applying flange and ostomy pouch.

325. An adult is brought to the emergency room with severe, constant, localized abdominal pain. Abdominal muscles are rigid and rebound tenderness is present. Peritonitis is suspected. The client is hypotensive and tachycardiac. What is the nursing diagnosis most appropriate to the signs/symptoms presented?

1. Deficient fluid volume related to depletion of intravascular volume.

2. Disturbed thought process related to toxic effects of elevated ammonia levels.

3. Abdominal pain related to increased intestinal peristalsis.

4. Imbalanced nutrition, less than body requirements, related to malabsorption.

326. A client has had a hemorrhoidectomy. Which activity by the client will demonstrate the client has good understanding of post-op discharge instruction?

1. Reduce her fluid intake for several weeks after her surgery.

2. Include more fresh fruits and vegetables in her diet.

3. Vigorously clean her perianal area with soap and water after every bowel movement.

4. Limit her activities to bed rest for at least 6 hours a day.

327. The client with hepatitis may be anicteric and symptomless. What sign/symptom is most likely present in the early presentation of hepatic inflammatory disorder?

1. Dark urine.

2. Ascites.

3. Occult blood in stools.

4. Anorexia.

328. A client visits her physician with flu-like symptoms that have persisted for nearly a month. She complains of headaches, malaise, anorexia, and fever. She is a childcare worker at a local daycare center with children ranging in ages from 6 months to 5 years. Based on the associated risk factors and mode of transmission, which condition is the client most likely experiencing?

1. Hepatitis A.

2. Hepatitis B.

3. Hepatitis C.

4. Hepatitis D.

329. A client that works in a community health clinic has been experiencing fatigue, headaches, diminished appetite, and a yellowish discoloration of sclera for the past 2 months. He is diagnosed with hepatitis B and asks the nurse how he contracted hepatitis. What is the nurse's most appropriate response?

1. Airborne droplets carry the infectious hepatitis B virus.

2. The hepatitis B virus is transmitted parenterally and through intimate contact.

3. An individual may contract hepatitis B by using contaminated eating utensils.

4. Hepatitis B may be transmitted through eating shellfish from contaminated water sources.

330. A client with hepatic cirrhosis related to 10-year history of alcohol abuse is at risk for injury related to portal hypertension. What is the most appropriate nursing action to decrease his risk of injury?

1. Keep his fingernails short.

2. Offer small, frequent feedings.

3. Observe stools for color and consistency.

4. Assess for jaundice of skin and sclera.

331. A client is diagnosed with Laënnec's cirrhosis. He has massive ascites formation. His respirations are rapid and shallow. The physician decides to perform a paracentesis. Which activity does the nurse give the highest priority to during the procedure?

1. Gathering the appropriate sterile equipment.

2. Labeling samples of abdominal fluid and sending them to the laboratory.

3. Positioning the client upright on the edge of the bed.

4. Measuring and recording blood pressure and pulse frequently during the procedure.

332. An adult who has a 7-year history of hepatic cirrhosis was brought to the emergency room

because he began vomiting large amounts of dark-red blood. A Sengstaken-Blakemore tube was inserted to tamponade the bleeding esophageal varices. While the balloon tamponade is in place, what is given the highest priority?

1. Assessing his stools for occult blood.
2. Evaluating capillary refill in extremities.
3. Performing frequent mouth care.
4. Auscultating breath sounds.

333. A client is experiencing advanced hepatic cirrhosis complicated by hepatic encephalopathy. He is confused, restless, and demonstrating asterixis. In developing a two-part nursing diagnosis for this condition, what would be the second part following *Disturbed Thought Processes*?

1. Massive ascites formation.
2. Increased serum ammonia levels.
3. Fluid volume excess.
4. Altered clotting mechanism.

334. A client has choledocholithiasis. During the nursing admission, the nurse notes that the client's sclera and skin are jaundiced. When complaining of abdominal distention and pain, how is the client most likely to describe this condition?

1. An intermittent, colicky pain in his left flank.
2. Pain which awakens him during the night, and is relieved by eating.
3. A vise-like pressure over his sternum.
4. Right upper quadrant pain that often radiates to his right shoulder.

335. A client is admitted to the hospital for acute cholecystitis. She is now 6 hours post-op abdominal cholecystectomy with a choledochostomy and has a T-tube in place. What is the proper management of the T-tube?

1. Hanging the T-tube drainage below the bed.
2. Notifying the physician if T-tube drainage is 75 mL for the first 24 hours after surgery.
3. Irrigating the T-tube with sterile normal saline q 2 h to prevent obstruction.
4. Clamping the T-tube if the client develops sudden, severe abdominal pain.

336. A client has experienced repeated episodes of acute pancreatitis. He has continued to consume alcohol. The nurse observes that he is doubled-over, rocking back-and-forth in pain. Why is morphine derivative contraindicated for the pain associated with acute pancreatitis?

1. It causes severe respiratory depression.

2. Depression of GI peristalsis may cause constipation.
3. Spasms of the sphincter of Oddi may occur.
4. It is rapidly metabolized by the liver.

337. A client has a 5-year history of alcohol abuse. He appears acutely ill. He is vomiting bile-stained emesis. What would be documented as signs of severe, hemorrhagic pancreatitis?

1. The presence of a positive fluid wave in the abdominal area.
2. A yellowish color of the sclera and skin.
3. Ecchymosis in the flank and around the umbilical area.
4. Bloody, foul-smelling stools.

338. A client with a 10-year history of alcohol abuse has recently been diagnosed with chronic pancreatitis. The physician has prescribed pancrelipase, a pancreatic enzyme replacement. Which statement by the client demonstrates understanding of his medication regimen?

1. "I will take this medication with a glass of milk."
2. "If my stools appear yellowish with a foul odor, I will call my doctor."
3. "I will take my medication with some antacid so it will not bother my stomach."
4. "I will be sure to thoroughly chew the capsule contents before swallowing the medication."

339. A client has been diagnosed with a malignant tumor of the head of the pancreas. A pancreatoduodenectomy (Whipple's procedure) was done to resect the tumor. The nurse recognizes that hemorrhage is a potentially major complication of a Whipple procedure. Which of the following assessment findings suggest this complication?

1. Jaundice of the skin and sclera.
2. Hyperglycemia.
3. Oliguria.
4. Bradycardia.

 **Answers and Rationales**

290. **3.** Looping the NG tube will prevent pressure on the nares that can cause pain and eventual necrosis.

291. **4.** The drainage following abdominal surgery is discolored as it is evacuating stomach and intestinal contents, not mucoid material.

292. **4.** The nurse should explore the client's motivation for posing the question and establish this current knowledge.

293. **4.** The onset of hepatitis B is long and insidious, lasting from 60 to 160 days.

294. **1.** Cimetidine (Tagemet) is a histamine antagonist that blocks the secretion of hydrochloric acid.

295. **2.** Signs of dumping syndrome include vertigo, pallor, sweating, palpitations, and weakness. Dumping syndrome occurs after a gastric resection because ingested foods rapidly enter the jejunum without proper mixing and without the normal duodenal processing. It subsides in 6–12 months.

296. **4.** Bluish discoloration of the umbilicus (Cullen's sign) is present in massive gastrointestinal hemorrhage resulting from free blood present in the abdomen. This is not consistent with cirrhosis of the liver.

297. **4.** Sodium restriction is most important for a client with cirrhosis because fluid retention contributes to ascites.

298. **3.** Increased ammonia levels could be seen because ammonia is a by-product of protein metabolism, and a diseased liver is unable to convert ammonia into urea to be excreted in the urine.

299. **1.** If the client's airway is obstructed by the Sengstaken-Blakemore tube, the esophageal balloon must be deflated so the client can breathe.

300. **2.** The client's throat is sprayed with a local anesthetic agent. Until the anesthetic agent wears off, the client is at high risk for aspiration.

301. **1.** A low-residue diet 1 to 2 days before the study aids in evacuating the lower intestinal tract of all fecal matter.

302. **4.** The client experiencing a liver biopsy is at risk for bleeding or hemorrhage related to penetration of the liver capsule. Positioning on the right side acts as a tamponade against the puncture site discouraging bleeding from the site.

303. **2.** Oil retention enemas are given to soften the hardened fecal mass and lubricate the walls of the rectum and colon. Cleansing enemas stimulate intestinal peristalsis, thus eliminating the softened fecal mass.

304. **3.** A client with altered central nervous system functioning is at high risk for aspiration. Checking for the placement of the feeding tube using several different methods, i.e., aspiration of gastric contents for residual volume, determining pH of aspirated gastric contents, and auscultating for gurgling sounds with injection of air bolus, is the priority nursing assessment to ensure client safety.

305. **2.** The nasogastric tube for gastric decompression after a gastric resection is never irrigated without a specific order from the physician. Irrigating the nasogastric tube may rupture the suture line and hemorrhaging may occur.

306. **2.** Metoclopramide blocks dopamine receptors in the chemoreceptor trigger zone (CTZ). This action results in the extrapyramidal and anticholinergic side effects that include sedation, dilated pupils and parkinsonian effects.

307. **3.** Increased urinary output is related to the resolved dehydration state. Adding fluid to the enteral feedings reduced the osmolarity of the gastrointestinal contents.

308. **3.** Exercises to strengthen the abdominal muscles are appropriate to aiding the defecation process.

309. **3.** Surgical resection of the esophagus has a relatively high mortality rate related to pulmonary complications.

310. **4.** These substances aggravate the episodes of heartburn (pyrosis) and gastroesophageal reflux.

311. **3.** Duodenal ulcer pain characteristically occurs 2 to 3 hours after a meal, often awakening the client in the very early morning hours.

312. **3.** Misoprostol, a synthetic prostaglandin, is a cytoprotective agent. By increasing mucous production and bicarbonate levels, the mucosal barrier better resists the erosive action of the gastric acid-pepsin complex.

313. **3.** Fluids with meals cause rapid emptying of the gastric contents. Fluids with meals should be limited.

314. **4.** A total gastrectomy results in a loss of intrinsic factor, which is necessary for the absorption of vitamin $B_{12}$.

315. **3.** A direct inguinal hernia is most likely to cause a small bowel obstruction. Therefore, the nurse must monitor closely for the

signs/symptoms of a small bowel mechanical obstruction, including vomiting of bile-stained gastric contents from reverse peristalsis.

316. **1.** A paralytic ileus is related to disturbance of the neural stimulation of the bowel. There is decreased or absence of bowel sounds.

317. **4.** Anorexia, weight loss, fever, vomiting, and blood loss are conditions that will cause the client to become easily fatigued. Activities are planned or restricted to conserve energy.

318. **3.** When grain is refined, most of the original fiber is removed, then vitamins and additives are added to compensate, thus producing a low-residue product.

319. **2.** Toxic megacolon is a serious complication of ulcerative colitis. Excessive dilation of the colon may lead to intestinal perforation and death.

320. **3.** A soft, high-fiber diet is indicated to increase the bulk of the stool, thereby promoting defecation. Fluid intake of 2 liters/day is recommended unless otherwise contraindicated. Seeds are not allowed.

321. **3.** A change in bowel habits such as alternating episodes of diarrhea and constipation is a common manifestation of colon cancer.

322. **4.** A diet low in fiber is a major risk factor for colon cancer. Fresh fruits and vegetables increase the fiber content of the diet, thereby reducing the risk of colon cancer.

323. **3.** Leaving ¼ inch of skin exposed around stoma when determining size to cut skin barrier prevents trauma to stoma.

324. **4.** A skin barrier applied helps prevent enzymatic activity, which is a risk for peristomal skin breakdown.

325. **1.** Hypovolemia occurs because massive amounts of fluid and electrolytes move from intestinal lumen into peritoneal cavity and deplete intravascular volume. Hypotension and tachycardia are manifestations of this massive fluid shift.

326. **2.** Post-hemorrhoidectomy diet is modified to include increased fluid and fiber intake. This promotes regular bowel elimination and reduces the occurrence of constipation.

327. **4.** Anorexia is often an early and severe symptom of hepatitis.

328. **1.** Hepatitis A is transmitted through the fecal-oral route. Childcare workers are in a high risk group because of potentially poor hygiene/sanitation practices.

329. **2.** Hepatitis B is transmitted parenterally or through intimate sexual contact with a carrier.

330. **3.** Portal hypertension puts the client at risk for injury related to bleeding/hemorrhaging esophageal varices. Monitoring stools permits early detection of bleeding in the GI tract.

331. **4.** A serious complication of a paracentesis is hypovolemic shock or vascular collapse. Early detection of this cardiovascular complication through monitoring blood pressure and pulse is a nursing priority intervention.

332. **4.** Airway obstruction and aspiration of gastric contents are potential serious complications of balloon tamponade. Frequent assessment of the client's respiratory status is the priority.

333. **2.** Hepatic cirrhosis leads to elevated serum ammonia levels, which have an adverse toxic effect on cerebral metabolism.

334. **4.** Pain related to gallstones in the common duct is located in the right upper quadrant and often radiates to the right shoulder or back.

335. **2.** The T-tube usually drains 200–500 mL in the first 24 hours. Decreased bile drainage may indicate an obstruction to bile flow or bile may be leaking into the peritoneum.

336. **3.** Morphine sulfate causes spasms of the sphincter of Oddi, which will exacerbate the episode of acute pancreatitis.

337. **3.** Cullen's sign and Turner's sign reveal discoloration and occur with intra-abdominal bleeding.

338. **2.** The presence of steatorrhea indicates that the dosage of pancrelipase needs to be adjusted.

339. **3.** Oliguria is a primary sign of hypovolemic shock related to hemorrhage.

# The Genitourinary System

## OVERVIEW OF ANATOMY AND PHYSIOLOGY

The genitourinary system includes the kidneys, ureters, urinary bladder, urethra, and the male and female genitalia. This section discusses only the male genitalia; the female reproductive system is covered in Unit 6.

### Urinary System

#### Kidneys

See Figure 4-19.

A. Two bean-shaped organs that lie in the retroperitoneal space on either side of the vertebral column; adrenal glands located on top of each kidney

B. Renal parenchyma
   1. Cortex: outermost layer; site of glomeruli and proximal and distal tubules of nephron
   2. Medulla: middle layer; formed by collecting tubules and ducts

C. Renal sinus and pelvis
   1. Papillae: projections of renal tissues located at the tips of the renal pyramids
   2. Calices
      a. Minor calyx: collects urine flow from collecting duct
      b. Major calyx: directs urine from renal sinus to renal pelvis
   3. Urine flows from renal pelvis to ureters

D. Nephron: the functional unit of the kidney (see Figure 4-20)
   1. Renal corpuscle (vascular system of nephron)
      a. Bowman's capsule: a portion of the proximal tubule, surrounds the glomerulus
      b. Glomerulus: a capillary network permeable to water, electrolytes, nutrients, and wastes; impermeable to large protein molecules
   2. Renal tubule: divided into proximal convoluted tubule, descending loop of Henle, ascending loop of Henle, distal convoluted tubule, and collecting duct

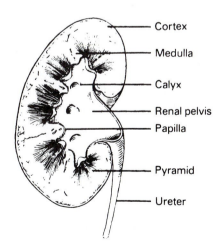

**Figure 4-19** Anatomy of the kidney

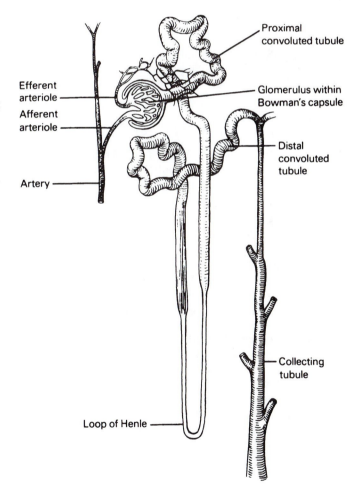

**Figure 4-20** The nephron

## Ureters

A. Two tubes approximately 25–35 cm long
B. Extend from the renal pelvis to the pelvic cavity, where they enter the bladder, convey urine from the kidneys to the bladder
C. Ureterovesical valve prevents backflow of urine into ureters

## Bladder

A. Located behind the symphysis pubis; composed of muscular, elastic tissue that makes it distensible
B. Serves as a reservoir of urine (capable of holding 1000–1800 mL; moderately full bladder usually holds about 500 mL)
C. Internal and external urethral sphincters control the flow of urine; urge to void stimulated by passage of urine past the internal sphincter (involuntary) to the upper part of the urethra. Relaxation of external sphincter (voluntary) produces emptying of the bladder (voiding, micturition).

## Urethra

A. A small tube that extends from the bladder to the exterior of the body
B. In females, located behind the symphysis pubis and anterior to the vagina; approximately 3–5 cm long
C. In males, extends the entire length of the penis; approximately 20 cm long

## Regulatory Functions of Kidney

Kidneys and urinary system play a major role in maintenance of homeostatic control of the body. Kidneys remove nitrogenous wastes and regulate fluid and electrolyte balance and acid-base balance. Urine is the end product of these mechanisms.

### Formation of Urine

A. Glomerular filtration
  1. Ultrafiltration of blood by the glomerulus; beginning of urine formation
     a. Requires hydrostatic pressure (supplied by the heart and assisted by vascular resistance [glomerular hydrostatic pressure]) and sufficient circulating volume.
     b. Pressure in Bowman's capsule opposes hydrostatic pressure and filtration; if glomerular pressure insufficient to force substances out of the blood into the tubules, filtrate formation stops.
  2. Glomerular filtration rate (GFR): amount of blood filtrated by the glomeruli in a given time; normal is 125 mL/min
  3. Filtrate formed has essentially same composition as blood plasma without the proteins; blood cells and proteins are usually too large to pass the glomerular membrane.

B. Tubular function: the tubules and collecting ducts carry out the functions of reabsorption, secretion, and excretion. Reabsorption of water and electrolytes is controlled by antidiuretic hormone (ADH), released by the pituitary, and aldosterone, secreted by the adrenal glands (see Table 4-25).
  1. Proximal convoluted tubule: reabsorption of certain constituents of the glomerular filtrate: 80% of electrolytes and $H_2O$, all glucose and amino acids, and bicarbonate; secretes organic substances and wastes.
  2. Loop of Henle: reabsorption of sodium and chloride in the ascending limb; reabsorption of water in the descending limb; concentrates/dilutes urine.
  3. Distal convoluted tubule: secretes potassium, hydrogen ions, and ammonia; reabsorbs $H_2O$ (regulated by ADH) and bicarbonate; regulates calcium and phosphate concentrations.
  4. Collecting ducts: receive urine from distal convoluted tubules and reabsorb water (regulated by ADH).
C. Normal adult produces 1 liter/day of urine.

### Blood Pressure Control

A. Kidneys regulate blood pressure partly through maintenance of volume (formation/excretion of urine).
B. The renin-angiotensin system is the other kidney-controlled mechanism that can contribute to rise in blood pressure. When blood pressure drops, the cells of the glomerulus release renin, which then activates angiotensin to cause vasoconstriction.

# Male Reproductive System

See Figure 4-21.

## Penis

A. An external structure that serves as a passageway for urine and semen
B. Capable of distension during sexual excitement
C. Distal portion, glans penis, is covered by a prepuce or foreskin that may or may not be removed (circumcised)

## Scrotum

A. Saclike structure that hangs from the root of the penis
B. Contains the testes and epididymis, and helps to regulate temperature conducive to sperm production

## Testes

A. Small oval structures suspended in the scrotum
B. Produce sperm (exocrine function) and male hormones (endocrine function, see Table 4-25).

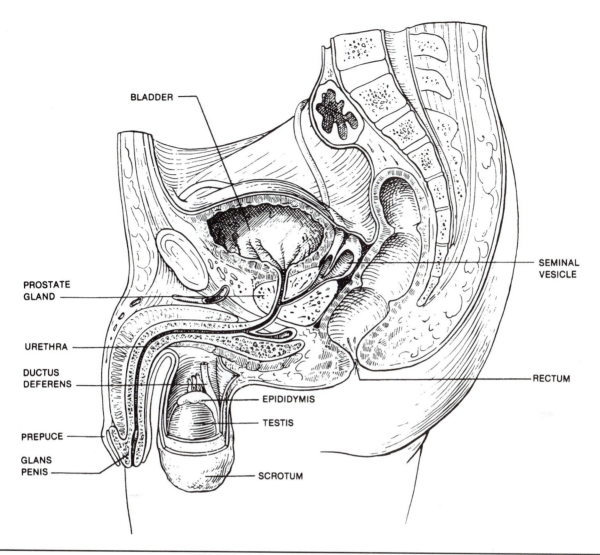

BLADDER

PROSTATE
GLAND

URETHRA

DUCTUS
DEFERENS

PREPUCE

GLANS
PENIS

SEMINAL
VESICLE

RECTUM

EPIDIDYMIS

TESTIS

SCROTUM

**Figure 4-21** The male reproductive system

## Ductal System

**A.** Epididymis: first part of ductal system
  **1.** Soft cordlike structure that lies along the posterolateral surface of each testis
  **2.** Head is attached to the top of the testis, tail is continuous with vas deferens; stores spermatozoa while they mature.
**B.** Spermatic cord: consists of vas deferens, arteries, veins, nerves, and lymphatic vessels. Vas deferens joins the duct of the seminal vesicles to become the ejaculatory duct.

## Accessory Glands

**A.** Prostate: located below the bladder and in front of the rectum; approximately 4–6 cm long
  **1.** Enclosed in firm, fibrous capsule; connected to the urethra and ejaculatory ducts

  **2.** Secretes a milky fluid that aids in the passage of spermatozoa and helps keep them viable
**B.** Cowper's glands: lie on each side of the urethra and just below the prostate; secrete a small amount of lubricating fluid.
**C.** Seminal vesicles: paired structures parallel to the bladder; secrete a portion of the ejaculate and may contribute to nutrition and activation of sperm.

## ASSESSMENT

### Health History

**A.** Presenting problem: symptoms may include:
  **1.** Pain in flank, groin; dysuria
  **2.** Changes in urination patterns: frequency, nocturia, hesitancy of stream, urgency, dribbling, incontinence, retention

3. Changes in urinary output: polyuria, oliguria, anuria
4. Changes in color/consistency of urine: dilute, concentrated, malodorous; hematuria, pyuria
B. Lifestyle: occupation (type of employment, exposure to chemicals such as carbon tetrachloride, ethylene glycol); level of activity, exercise
C. Nutrition/diet: water, calcium, dairy product intake
D. Past medical history: hypertension; diabetes mellitus; gout; cystitis; kidney infections; connective tissue diseases (systemic lupus erythematosus); infectious diseases; drug use (prescribed/OTC); previous catheterizations, hospitalizations, or surgery for renal problems
E. Family history: hypertension, diabetes mellitus, renal disease, gout, connective tissue disorders, urinary tract infections (UTIs), renal calculi

## Physical Examination

A. Inspect skin for color, turgor, and mobility; purpuric lesions; integrity.
B. Inspect mouth for color, moisture, odor, ulcerations.
C. Inspect face for edema, particularly periorbital edema.
D. Inspect abdomen and palpate bladder for distension; percuss bladder for tympany or dullness (if full).
E. Inspect extremities for edema.
F. Determine rate, rhythm, and depth of respirations.
G. Inspect muscles for tremors, atrophy.
H. Palpate right and left kidneys for tenderness, pain, enlargement; percuss costovertebral angles for tenderness/pain; fist percuss kidneys for tenderness/pain.
I. Palpate flank area for pain and prostate for size, shape, consistency.
J. Auscultate aorta and renal arteries for bruits.

## Laboratory/Diagnostic Tests

A. Urine studies
1. Urinalysis: examination to assess the nature of the urine produced
   a. Evaluates color, pH, and specific gravity.
   b. Determines presence of glucose (glycosuria), protein, blood (hematuria), ketones (ketonuria).
   c. Analyzes sediment for cells (presence of WBC called pyuria), casts, bacteria, crystals.
2. Urine culture and sensitivity: diagnoses bacterial infections of the urinary tract
3. Residual urine: amount of urine left in bladder after voiding measured via catheter (permanent or temporary) in bladder
4. Creatinine clearance: determines amount of creatinine (waste product of protein breakdown) in the urine over 24 hours, measures overall renal function

B. Urine collection methods: nursing care
1. Routine urinalysis: wash perineal area if soiled, obtain first voided morning specimen; send to lab immediately (should be examined within 1 hour of voiding).
2. Clean catch (midstream) specimen for urine culture.
   a. Cleanse perineal area.
      1) Females: spread labia and cleanse meatus front to back using antiseptic sponges.
      2) Males: retract foreskin (if uncircumsized) and cleanse glans with antiseptic sponges.
   b. Have client initiate urine stream then stop.
   c. Collect specimen in a sterile container.
   d. Have client complete urination but not in specimen container.
3. 24-hour specimen (preferred method for creatinine clearance test)
   a. Have client void and discard specimen; note time.
   b. Collect all subsequent urine specimens for 24 hours.
   c. If specimen is accidentally discarded, the test must be restarted.
   d. Record exact start and finish of collection; include date and times.
C. Blood studies
1. Bicarbonate
2. BUN: measures renal ability to excrete urea nitrogen
3. Calcium
4. Serum creatinine: specific test for renal disorders; reflects ability of kidneys to excrete creatinine
5. Phosphorus
6. Potassium
7. Sodium
8. Prostate-specific antigen (PSA)
D. KUB/plain film: an abdominal flat-plate X-ray showing the kidneys, ureters, and bladder; may identify the number and size of kidneys with tumors, malformations, and calculi
E. Intravenous pyelogram (IVP)
1. Fluoroscopic visualization of the urinary tract after injection with a radiopaque dye
2. Nursing care: pretest
   a. Assess for iodine sensitivity.
   b. Inform client he will lie on a table throughout procedure.
   c. Administer cathartic or enema the night before.
   d. Keep client NPO for 8 hours pretest.
3. Nursing care: posttest: force fluids
F. Cystoscopy
1. Use of a lighted scope (cystoscope) to inspect the bladder
   a. Inserted into the bladder via the urethra
   b. May be used to remove tumors, stones, or other foreign material (use of electrical

current to remove tumors is called fulguration); or to implant radium, place catheters in ureters

2. Nursing care: pretest
   a. Explain to client that procedure will be done under general or local anesthesia.
   b. Confirm consent form is signed.
   c. Administer sedatives 1 hour before test, as ordered.
   d. General anesthesia: keep client NPO.
   e. Local anesthesia: offer liquid breakfast.
   f. Give enemas as ordered.
3. Nursing care: posttest
   a. Provide warm sitz baths, mild analgesics to relieve discomfort after test.
   b. Monitor I&O and vital signs (especially temperature, as elevation may indicate infection).
   c. Expect mild hematuria at first; urine will be pink tinged, subsiding over 24–48 hours; monitor for large clots.
   d. Advise client that burning on urination is normal and will subside.
   e. Force fluids.

# ANALYSIS

Nursing diagnoses for the client with a disorder of the genitourinary system may include:

A. Deficient fluid volume
B. Fluid volume excess
C. Fatigue
D. Risk for injury
E. Disturbed thought processes
F. Impaired oral mucous membrane
G. Imbalanced nutrition: less than body requirements
H. Risk for infection
I. Impaired skin integrity
J. Urinary retention
K. Sexual dysfunction

# PLANNING AND IMPLEMENTATION

## Goals

A. Fluid imbalance will be resolved.
B. Client will exhibit improved sense of energy.
C. Client will not exhibit unusual bleeding.
D. Thought processes will improve.
E. Integrity of mucous membranes will be maintained.
F. Adequate nutritional status will be maintained.
G. Client will remain free from infection.
H. Adequate skin integrity will be maintained.
I. Client will demonstrate restored urinary flow.
J. Changes in sexual functioning will be accepted.

# Interventions

## Urinary Catheterization

A. General information
   1. Insertion of a catheter through the external meatus and the urethra into the bladder
   2. Purposes include relief from urinary retention, bladder decompression, prevention of bladder obstruction, instillation of medications into the bladder, splinting the bladder, and output monitoring.
B. Nursing care: insertion
   1. Explain procedure to client and collect necessary equipment (catheter set).
   2. Wash hands and position client.
   3. Use sterile technique while inserting catheter.
   4. Observe for urine return and obtain specimen.
   5. Connect drainage tubing to catheter (indwelling) and tape.
C. Nursing care: indwelling catheter
   1. Maintain catheter patency: place drainage tubing properly to avoid kinking or pinching.
   2. Observe for signs of obstruction (e.g., decreased urine in collection bag, voiding around the catheter, abdominal discomfort, bladder distension).
   3. Irrigate catheter as necessary.
   4. Ensure comfort and safety: relieve bladder spasms by administering belladonna suppositories (if ordered); ensure adequate fluid intake and provide perineal care.
   5. Prevent infection: maintain a closed drainage system and prevent backflow of urine by keeping drainage system below level of bladder.
   6. Empty collection bag at least every 8 hours.
   7. Promote acidification of the urine with acid-ash diet and ascorbic acid.
   8. Change catheter/drainage system only when necessary.

## Dialysis

A. General information
   1. Removal by artificial means of metabolic wastes, excess electrolytes, and excess fluid from clients with renal failure
   2. Principles
      a. Diffusion: movement of particles from an area of high concentration to one of low concentration across a semipermeable membrane
      b. Osmosis: movement of water through a semipermeable membrane from an area of lesser concentration of particles to one of greater concentration
B. Purposes
   1. Remove the endproducts of protein metabolism from blood
   2. Maintain safe levels of electrolytes

4

3. Correct acidosis and replenish blood bicarbonate system
4. Remove excess fluid from the blood

C. Types: hemodialysis and peritoneal dialysis

*Hemodialysis*

A. General information
1. Shunting of blood from the client's vascular system through an artificial dialyzing system, and return of dialyzed blood to the client's circulation
2. Dialysis coil acts as the semipermeable membrane; the dialysate is a specially prepared solution.
3. Access routes (see Figure 4-22)
   a. External AV shunt: one cannula inserted into an artery and the other into a vein; both are brought out to the skin surface and connected by a U-shaped shunt.
   b. AV fistula: internal anastomosis of an artery to an adjacent vein in a sideways position; fistula is accessed for hemodialysis by venipuncture; takes 4–6 weeks to be ready for use.
   c. Femoral/subclavian cannulation: insertion of a catheter into one of these large veins for easy access to circulation; procedure is similar to insertion of a CVP line; temporary, but can be used immediately; associated with more clotting problems.
   d. Graft: piece of bovine artery or vein, Gore-Tex material, or saphenous vein sutured to client's own vessel; used for clients with compromised vascular systems; provides a segment in which to place dialysis needles; ready for use in 2–3 weeks.

B. Nursing care: external AV shunt
1. Auscultate for a bruit and palpate for a thrill to ensure patency.
2. Assess for clotting (color change of blood, absence of pulsations in tubing).
3. Change sterile dressing over shunt daily.
4. Avoid performing venipuncture, administering IV infusions, giving injections, or taking a blood pressure with a cuff on the shunt arm.

C. Nursing care: AV fistula.
1. Auscultate for a bruit and palpate for a thrill to ensure patency.
2. Report bleeding, skin discoloration, drainage, and pain.
3. Avoid restrictive clothing/dressings over site.
4. Avoid administration of IV infusions, giving injections, or taking blood pressure with a cuff on the fistula extremity.

D. Nursing care: femoral/subclavian cannulation
1. Palpate peripheral pulses in cannulized extremity.
2. Observe for bleeding/hematoma formation.
3. Position catheter properly to avoid dislodgment during dialysis.

E. Nursing care: before and during hemodialysis
1. Have client void.
2. Chart client's weight.

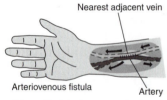

Nearest adjacent vein

Arteriovenous fistula  Artery

Edges of incision in artery and vein are sutured together to form a common opening.

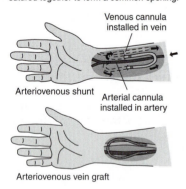

Venous cannula installed in vein

Arteriovenous shunt  Arterial cannula installed in artery

Arteriovenous vein graft

Ends of natural or synthetic graft sutured into an artery and a vein.

A.

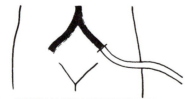

B.  FEMORAL VEIN CATHETERIZATION

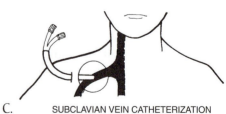

C.  SUBCLAVIAN VEIN CATHETERIZATION

**Figure 4-22** Dialysis vascular access sites. (A) Arteriovenous access; (B) femoral access; (C) subclavian access catheter

3. Assess vital signs before and every 30 minutes during procedure.
4. Withhold antihypertensives, sedatives, and vasodilators to prevent hypotensive episode (unless ordered otherwise).
5. Ensure bed rest with frequent position changes for comfort.
6. Inform client that headache and nausea may occur.
7. Monitor closely for signs of bleeding because blood has been heparinized for procedure.

F. Nursing care: postdialysis
1. Chart client's weight.
2. Assess for complications.
   a. Hypovolemic shock: may occur as a result of rapid removal or ultrafiltration of fluid from the intravascular compartment.

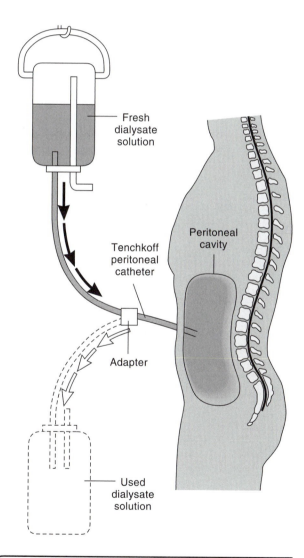

**Figure 4-23** Peritoneal dialysis removes wastes through a fluid exchange in the peritoneal cavity

Labels in figure:
- Fresh dialysate solution
- Tenchkoff peritoneal catheter
- Peritoneal cavity
- Adapter
- Used dialysate solution

b. Dialysis disequilibrium syndrome (urea is removed more rapidly from the blood than from the brain): assess for nausea, vomiting, elevated blood pressure, disorientation, leg cramps, and peripheral paresthesias.

*Peritoneal Dialysis*

A. General information: introduction of a specially prepared dialysate solution into the abdominal cavity, where the peritoneum acts as a semipermeable membrane between the dialysate and blood in the abdominal vessels (see Figure 4-23).
B. Nursing care
1. Chart client's weight.
2. Assess vital signs before, every 15 minutes during first exchange, and every hour thereafter.
3. Assemble specially prepared dialysate solution with added medications.
4. Have client void.
5. Warm dialysate solution to body temperature.
6. Assist physician with trocar insertion.
7. Inflow: allow dialysate to flow unrestricted into peritoneal cavity (10–20 minutes).
8. Dwell: allow fluid to remain in peritoneal cavity for prescribed period (30–45 minutes).
9. Drain: unclamp outflow tube and allow to flow by gravity.
10. Observe characteristics of dialysate outflow.
    a. Clear pale yellow: normal
    b. Cloudy: infection, peritonitis
    c. Brownish: bowel perforation
    d. Bloody: common during first few exchanges; abnormal if continues
11. Monitor total I&O and maintain records.
12. Assess for complications.
    a. Peritonitis resulting from contamination of solution or tubing during exchange
    b. Respiratory difficulty: may occur from upward displacement of diaphragm due to increased pressure in the peritoneal cavity; assess for signs and symptoms of atelectasis, pneumonia, and bronchitis
    c. Protein loss: most serum proteins pass through the peritoneal membrane and are lost in the dialysate fluid; monitor serum protein levels closely

## Continuous Ambulatory Peritoneal Dialysis

A. General information
1. A continuous type of peritoneal dialysis performed at home by the client or significant others.
2. Dialysate is delivered from flexible plastic containers through a permanent peritoneal catheter.
3. Following infusion of the dialysate into the peritoneal cavity, the bag is folded and tucked away during the dwell period.

**B.** Provide client teaching and discharge planning concerning:

1. Need to assess the permanent peritoneal catheter for complications
   a. Dialysate leak
   b. Exit site infection
   c. Bacterial/fungal contamination
   d. Obstruction
2. Adherence to high-protein (if indicated), well-balanced diet
3. Importance of periodic blood chemistries
4. Daily weights

## EVALUATION

**A.** Adequate urinary output with specific gravity/laboratory studies within client's normal range; stable weight; absence of edema; pulmonary congestion.

**B.** Client verbalizes increased tolerance for activities.

**C.** Skin and mucous membranes free from ecchymoses/bleeding; improved laboratory values (CBC, platelet count; clotting factors); no signs of bleeding.

**D.** Client identifies ways to compensate for cognitive impairment; demonstrates improved problem-solving skills.

**E.** Oral mucosa pink, moist, and intact; no ulcerations; saliva consistency normal; verbalizes interventions to promote/maintain healthy oral mucosa.

**F.** Stable weight gain; laboratory values within client's normal range; improved anthropometric measurements.

**G.** Vital signs within normal range; client identifies measures to prevent/reduce the risk of infection.

**H.** Skin warm and dry; absence of redness and irritation.

**I.** Voiding in adequate amounts with no palpable bladder distention; postvoid residuals less than 50 mL; absence of dribbling/overflow.

**J.** Client identifies acceptable sexual practices and explores alternate methods.

**K.** Client integrates treatment regimens into ADL; shows increased interest in appearance; actively participates in treatments.

# DISORDERS OF THE GENITOURINARY SYSTEM

## Disorders of the Urinary Tract

### Cystitis

**A.** General information
1. Inflammation of the bladder due to bacterial invasion
2. More common in women
3. Predisposing factors include stagnation of urine, obstruction, sexual intercourse, high estrogen levels

**B.** Assessment
1. Abdominal or flank pain/tenderness, frequency and urgency of urination, pain on voiding, nocturia
2. Fever
3. Diagnostic tests: urine culture and sensitivity reveals specific organism (80% *E. coli*)

**C.** Nursing interventions
1. Force fluids (3000 mL/day).
2. Provide warm sitz baths for comfort.
3. Assess urine for odor, hematuria, sediment.
4. Administer medications as ordered and monitor effects.
   a. Systemic antibiotics: ampicillin, cephalosporins, aminoglycosides
   b. Sulfonamides: sulfisoxazole (Gantrisin), sulfamethoxazole (Gantanol), trimethoprim-sulfamethoxazole (Bactrim)
   c. Antibacterials: nitrofurantoin (Macrodantin), methenamine mandelate (Mandelamine), nalidixic acid (NegGram)
   d. Urinary tract analgesic: pyridium
5. Provide client teaching and discharge planning concerning:
   a. Importance of adequate hydration
   b. Frequent voiding to avoid stagnation
   c. Proper personal hygiene; women to cleanse from front to back
   d. Voiding after sexual intercourse
   e. Acidification of the urine to decrease bacterial multiplication (acid-ash diet, vitamin C)
   f. Need for follow-up urine cultures

### Bladder Cancer

**A.** General information
1. Most common site of cancer of the urinary tract
2. Occurs in men 3 times more often than women; peak age 50–70 years
3. Predisposing factors include exposure to chemicals (especially aniline dyes), cigarette smoking, chronic bladder infections

**B.** Medical management: dependent on the staging of cell type; includes:
1. Radiation therapy, usually in combination with surgery
2. Chemotherapy: considerable research on both agents and methods of administration
   a. Methods include direct bladder instillations, intra-arterial infusions, IV infusion, oral ingestion
   b. Agents include 5-fluorouracil, methotrexate, bleomycin, mitomycin-C, hydroxyurea, doxorubicin, cyclophosphamide, cisplatin; results variable
3. Surgery: see Bladder Surgery.

**C.** Assessment findings
   1. Intermittent painless hematuria, dysuria, frequent urination
   2. Diagnostic tests
      **a.** Cytoscopy with biopsy reveals malignancy
      **b.** Cytologic exam of the urine reveals malignant cells
**D.** Nursing interventions: provide care for the client receiving radiation therapy or chemotherapy, and for the client with bladder surgery.

## Bladder Surgery

**A.** General information
   1. Cystectomy (removal of the urinary bladder) with one of the various types of urinary diversions is the surgical procedure done for bladder cancer
   2. Types of urinary diversions
      **a.** Ureterosigmoidostomy: ureters are excised from the bladder and implanted into sigmoid colon; urine flows through the colon and is excreted via the rectum
      **b.** Ileal conduit: ureters are implanted into a segment of the ileum that has been resected from the intestinal tract with formation of an abdominal stoma; most common type of urinary diversion
      **c.** Cutaneous ureterostomy: ureters are excised from the bladder and brought through abdominal wall with creation of a stoma
      **d.** Nephrostomy: insertion of a catheter into the renal pelvis via an incision into the flank or by percutaneous catheter placement into the kidney
**B.** Nursing interventions: preoperative
   1. Provide routine pre-op care.
   2. Assess client's ability to learn prior to starting a teaching program.
   3. Discuss social aspects of living with a stoma (sexuality, changes in body image).
   4. Assess understanding and emotional response of client/significant others.
   5. Perform pre-op bowel preparation for procedures involving the ileum or colon.
   6. Inform client of post-op procedures.
**C.** Nursing interventions: postoperative
   1. Provide routine post-op care.
   2. Maintain integrity of the stoma.
      **a.** Monitor for and report signs of impaired stomal healing (pale, dark red, or blue-black color; increased stomal height, edema, bleeding).
      **b.** Maintain stomal circulation by using properly fitted faceplate.
      **c.** Monitor for signs and symptoms of stomal obstruction (sudden decrease in urine output, increased abdominal tenderness and distension).
   3. Prevent skin irritation and breakdown.
      **a.** Inspect skin areas for signs of breakdown daily.
      **b.** Patch test all adhesives, sprays, and skin barriers before use.
      **c.** Change appliance only when necessary and when production of urine is slowest (early morning).
      **d.** Place wick (rolled gauze pad) on stomal opening when appliance is off.
      **e.** Cleanse peristomal skin with mild soap and water.
      **f.** Remove alkaline encrustations by applying vinegar and water solution to peristomal area.
      **g.** Implement measures to maintain urine acidity (acid-ash foods, vitamin C therapy, omission of milk/dairy products).
   4. Provide care for the client with an NG tube; will be in place until bowel motility returns.
   5. Assist client to identify strengths and qualities that have a positive effect on self-concept.
   6. Provide client teaching and discharge planning concerning
      **a.** Maintenance of stomal/peristomal skin integrity
      **b.** Proper application of appliance
      **c.** Recommended method of cleaning reusable ostomy equipment (manufacturer's recommendations)
      **d.** Information regarding prevention of UTIs (adequate fluids; empty pouch when half full; change to bedside collection bag at night)
      **e.** Control of odor (adequate fluids; avoid foods with strong odor; place small amount of vinegar or deodorizer in pouch)
      **f.** Reporting signs and symptoms of UTIs (see Cystitis).

## Nephrolithiasis/Urolithiasis

**A.** General information
   1. Presence of stones anywhere in the urinary tract; frequent composition of stones: calcium, oxalate, and uric acid
   2. Most often occurs in men age 20–55; more common in the summer
   3. Predisposing factors
      **a.** Diet: large amounts of calcium, oxalate
      **b.** Increased uric acid levels
      **c.** Sedentary lifestyle, immobility
      **d.** Family history of gout or calculi; hyperparathyroidism
**B.** Medical management
   1. Surgery
      **a.** Cystoscopic stone removal: basket extraction is invasive but effective for stones even in kidney.
      **b.** Percutaneous nephrostomy: tube is inserted through skin and underlying tissues into renal pelvis to remove calculi.
      **c.** Percutaneous nephrostolithotomy: delivers ultrasound waves through a probe placed on the calculus.

2. Extracorporeal shock-wave lithotripsy: delivers shock waves from outside the body to the stone, causing pulverization
3. Pain management and diet modification

C. Assessment findings
1. Abdominal or flank pain; renal colic; hematuria
2. Cool, moist skin
3. Diagnostic tests
   a. KUB: pinpoints location, number, and size of stones
   b. IVP: identifies site of obstruction and presence of nonradiopaque stones
   c. Urinalysis: indicates presence of bacteria, increased protein, increased WBC and RBC

D. Nursing interventions
1. Strain all urine through gauze to detect stones and crush all clots.
2. Force fluids (3000–4000 mL/day).
3. Encourage ambulation to prevent stasis.
4. Relieve pain by administration of analgesics as ordered and application of moist heat to flank area.
5. Monitor I&O.
6. Provide modified diet, depending upon stone consistency.
   a. Calcium stones: limit milk/dairy products; provide acid-ash diet to acidify urine (cranberry or prune juice, meat, eggs, poultry, fish, grapes, whole grains); take vitamin C.
   b. Oxalate stones: avoid excess intake of foods/fluids high in oxalate (tea, chocolate, rhubarb, spinach); maintain alkaline-ash diet to alkalinize urine (milk; vegetables; fruits except prunes, cranberries, and plums).
   c. Uric acid stones: reduce foods high in purine (liver, brains, kidneys, venison, shellfish, meat soups, gravies, legumes); maintain alkaline urine.
7. Administer allopurinol (Zyloprim) as ordered, to decrease uric acid production; push fluids when giving allopurinol.
8. Provide client teaching and discharge planning concerning:
   a. Prevention of urinary stasis by maintaining increased fluid intake especially in hot weather and during illness; mobility; voiding whenever the urge is felt and at least twice during the night
   b. Adherence to prescribed diet
   c. Need for routine urinalysis (at least every 3–4 months)
   d. Need to recognize and report signs/symptoms of recurrence (hematuria, flank pain)

## Pyelonephritis

A. General information
1. Inflammation of the renal pelvis; may be unilateral or bilateral, acute or chronic

2. Acute: infection usually ascends from lower urinary tract
3. Chronic: thought to be a combination of structural alterations along with infection, major cause is ureterovesical reflux, with infected urine backing up into ureters and renal pelvises; result of recurrent infections is eventual renal parenchymal deterioration and possible renal failure

B. Medical management
1. Acute: antibiotics, antispasmodics, surgical removal of any obstruction
2. Chronic: antibiotics and urinary antiseptics (sulfanomides, nitrofurantoin); surgical correction of structural abnormality if possible

C. Assessment findings
1. Acute: fever, chills, nausea and vomiting; severe flank pain or dull ache
2. Chronic: client usually unaware of disease; may have bladder irritability, chronic fatigue, or slight dull ache over kidneys; eventually develops hypertension, atrophy of kidneys

D. Nursing interventions: acute pyelonephritis
1. Provide adequate comfort and rest.
2. Monitor I&O.
3. Administer antibiotics as ordered.
4. Provide client teaching and discharge planning concerning:
   a. Medication regimen
   b. Follow-up cultures
   c. Signs and symptoms of recurrence and need to report

E. Nursing interventions: chronic pyelonephritis
1. Administer medications as ordered.
2. Provide adequate fluid intake and nutrition.
3. Support client/significant others and explain possibility of dialysis, transplant options if significant renal deterioration.

## Glomerulonephritis

See Unit 5.

## Nephrosis

See Unit 5.

## Acute Renal Failure

A. General information
1. Sudden inability of the kidneys to regulate fluid and electrolyte balance and remove toxic products from the body
2. Causes
   a. Prerenal: factors interfering with perfusion and resulting in decreased blood flow and glomerular filtrate, ischemia, and oliguria; include CHF, cardiogenic shock, acute vasoconstriction, hemorrhage, burns, septicemia, hypotension

b. Intrarenal: conditions that cause damage to the nephrons; include acute tubular necrosis (ATN), endocarditis, diabetes mellitus, malignant hypertension, acute glomerulonephritis, tumors, blood transfusion reactions, hypercalcemia, nephrotoxins (certain antibiotics, X-ray dyes, pesticides, anesthetics)

c. Postrenal: mechanical obstruction anywhere from the tubules to the urethra; include calculi, BPH, tumors, strictures, blood clots, trauma, anatomic malformation

B. Assessment findings
1. Oliguric phase (caused by reduction in glomerular filtration rate)
   a. Urine output less than 400 mL/24 hours; duration 1–2 weeks
   b. Manifested by hypernatremia, hyperkalemia, hyperphosphatemia, hypocalcemia, hypermagnesemia, and metabolic acidosis
   c. Diagnostic tests: BUN and creatinine elevated
2. Diuretic phase (slow, gradual increase in daily urine output)
   a. Diuresis may occur (output 3–5 liters/day) due to partially regenerated tubule's inability to concentrate urine
   b. Duration: 2–3 weeks; manifested by hyponatremia, hypokalemia, and hypovolemia
   c. Diagnostic tests: BUN and creatinine elevated
3. Recovery or convalescent phase: renal function stabilizes with gradual improvement over next 3–12 months

C. Nursing interventions
1. Monitor/maintain fluid and electrolyte balance.
   a. Obtain baseline data on usual appearance and amount of client's urine.
   b. Measure I&O every hour; note excessive losses.
   c. Administer IV fluids and electrolyte supplements as ordered.
   d. Weigh daily and report gains.
   e. Monitor lab values; assess/treat fluid and electrolyte and acid-base imbalances as needed.
2. Monitor alteration in fluid volume.
   a. Monitor vital signs, PAP, PCWP, CVP as needed.
   b. Weigh client daily.
   c. Maintain strict I&O records.
   d. Assess every hour for hypervolemia; provide nursing care as needed.
      1) Maintain adequate ventilation.
      2) Decrease fluid intake as ordered.
      3) Administer diuretics, cardiac glycosides, and antihypertensives as ordered; monitor effects.
   e. Assess every hour for hypovolemia; replace fluids as ordered.
   f. Monitor ECG and auscultate heart as needed.
   g. Check urine, serum osmolality/osmolarity, and urine specific gravity as ordered.
3. Promote optimal nutritional status.
   a. Weigh daily.
   b. Maintain strict I&O.
   c. Administer TPN as ordered.
   d. With enteral feedings, check for residual and notify physician if residual volume increases.
   e. Restrict protein intake.
4. Prevent complications from impaired mobility (pulmonary embolism, skin breakdown, contractures, atelectasis).
5. Prevent fever/infection.
   a. Take rectal temperature and obtain orders for cooling blanket/antipyretics as needed.
   b. Assess for signs of infection.
   c. Use strict aseptic technique for wound and catheter care.
6. Support client/significant others and reduce/relieve anxiety.
   a. Explain pathophysiology and relationship to symptoms.
   b. Explain all procedures and answer all questions in easy-to-understand terms.
   c. Refer to counseling services as needed.
7. Provide care for the client receiving dialysis if used.
8. Provide client teaching and discharge planning concerning:
   a. Adherence to prescribed dietary regime
   b. Signs and symptoms of recurrent renal disease
   c. Importance of planned rest periods
   d. Use of prescribed drugs only
   e. Signs and symptoms of UTI or respiratory infection, need to report to physician immediately

## Chronic Renal Failure

A. General information
1. Progressive, irreversible destruction of the kidneys that continues until nephrons are replaced by scar tissue; loss of renal function gradual
2. Predisposing factors: recurrent infections, exacerbations of nephritis, urinary tract obstructions, diabetes mellitus, hypertension

B. Medical management
1. Diet restrictions
2. Multivitamins
3. Hematinics
4. Aluminum hydroxide gels
5. Antihypertensives

C. Assessment findings
   1. Nausea, vomiting; diarrhea or constipation; decreased urinary output; dyspnea
   2. Stomatitis, hypotension (early), hypertension (later), lethargy, convulsions, memory impairment, pericardial friction rub, HF
   3. Diagnostic tests: urinalysis
      a. Protein, sodium, and WBC elevated
      b. Specific gravity, platelets, and calcium decreased
D. Nursing interventions
   1. Prevent neurologic complications.
      a. Assess every hour for signs of uremia (fatigue, loss of appetite, decreased urine output, apathy, confusion, elevated blood pressure, edema of face and feet, itchy skin, restlessness, seizures).
      b. Assess for changes in mental functioning.
      c. Orient confused client to time, place, date, and persons; institute safety measures to protect client from falling out of bed.
      d. Monitor serum electrolytes, BUN, and creatinine as ordered.
   2. Promote optimal GI function.
      a. Assess/provide care for stomatitis
      b. Monitor nausea, vomiting, anorexia; administer antiemetics as ordered.
      c. Assess for signs of GI bleeding.
   3. Monitor/prevent alteration in fluid and electrolyte balance.
   4. Assess for hyperphosphatemia (paresthesias, muscle cramps, seizures, abnormal reflexes), and administer aluminum hydroxide gels (Amphojel, AlternaGEL) as ordered.
   5. Promote maintenance of skin integrity.
      a. Assess/provide care for pruritus.
      b. Assess for uremic frost (urea crystallization on the skin) and bathe in plain water.
   6. Monitor for bleeding complications, prevent injury to client.
      a. Monitor Hgb, HCT, platelets, RBC.
      b. Hematest all secretions.
      c. Administer hematinics as ordered.
      d. Avoid IM injections.
   7. Promote/maintain maximal cardiovascular function.
      a. Monitor blood pressure and report significant changes.
      b. Auscultate for pericardial friction rub.
      c. Perform circulation checks routinely.
      d. Administer diuretics as ordered and monitor output.
      e. Modify digitalis dose as ordered (digitalis is excreted in kidneys).
   8. Provide care for client receiving dialysis.

## Kidney Transplantation

A. General information
   1. Transplantation of a kidney from a donor to recipient to prolong the life of person with renal failure
   2. Sources of donor selection
      a. Living relative or potential with compatible serum and tissue studies, free from systemic infection, and emotionally stable
      b. Cadavers with good serum and tissue crossmatching; free from renal disease, neoplasms, and sepsis; absence of ischemia/trauma
B. Nursing interventions: preoperative
   1. Provide routine pre-op care.
   2. Discuss the possibility of post-op dialysis/immunosuppressive drug therapy with client and significant others.
C. Nursing interventions: postoperative
   1. Provide routine post-op care.
   2. Monitor fluid and electrolyte balance carefully.
      a. Monitor I&O hourly and adjust IV fluid administration accordingly.
      b. Anticipate possible massive diuresis.
   3. Encourage frequent and early ambulation.
   4. Monitor vital signs, especially temperature; report significant changes.
   5. Provide mouth care and nystatin (Mycostatin) mouthwashes for candidiasis.
   6. Administer immunosuppressive agents as ordered.
      a. Cyclosporine (Sandimmune): does not cause significant bone marrow depression. Assess for hypertension; blood chemistry alterations (hypermagnesemia, hyperkalemia, decreased sodium bicarbonate); neurologic functioning.
      b. Azathioprine (Imuran): assess for manifestations of anemia, leukopenia, thrombocytopenia, oral lesions.
      c. Cyclophosphamide (Cytoxan): assess for alopecia, hypertension, kidney/liver toxicity, leukopenia.
      d. Antilymphocytic globulin (ALG), antithymocytic globulin (ATG): assess for fever, chills, anaphylactic shock, hypertension, rash, headache.
      e. Corticosteroids (prednisone, methylprednisolone sodium succinate [Solu-Medrol]): assess for peptic ulcer and GI bleeding, sodium/water retention, muscle weakness, delayed healing, mood alterations, hyperglycemia, acne.
   7. Assess for signs of rejection. Include decreased urinary output, fever, pain/tenderness over transplant site, edema, sudden weight gain, increasing blood pressure, generalized malaise, rise in serum creatinine, and decrease in creatinine clearance.

8. Provide client teaching and discharge planning concerning:
   a. Medication regimen: names, dosages, frequency, and side effects
   b. Signs and symptoms of rejection and the need to report immediately
   c. Dietary restrictions: restricted sodium and calories, increased protein
   d. Daily weights
   e. Daily measurement of I&O
   f. Resumption of activity and avoidance of contact sports in which the transplanted kidney may be injured

## Nephrectomy

A. General information
   1. Surgical removal of an entire kidney
   2. Indications include renal tumor, massive trauma, removal for a donor, polycystic kidneys
B. Nursing interventions: preoperative care
   1. Provide routine pre-op care.
   2. Ensure adequate fluid intake.
   3. Assess electrolyte values and correct any imbalances before surgery.
   4. Avoid nephrotoxic agents in any diagnostic tests.
   5. Advise client to expect flank pain after surgery if retroperitoneal approach (flank incision) is used.
   6. Explain that client will have chest tube if a thoracic approach is used.
C. Nursing interventions: postoperative
   1. Provide routine post-op care.
   2. Assess urine output every hour; should be 30–50 mL/hour.
   3. Observe urinary drainage on dressing and estimate amount.
   4. Weigh daily.
   5. Maintain adequate functioning of chest drainage system; ensure adequate oxygenation and prevent pulmonary complications.
   6. Administer analgesics as ordered.
   7. Encourage early ambulation.
   8. Teach client to splint incision while turning, coughing, deep breathing.
   9. Provide client teaching and discharge planning concerning:
      a. Prevention of urinary stasis
      b. Maintenance of acidic urine
      c. Avoidance of activities that might cause trauma to the remaining kidney (contact sports, horseback riding)
      d. No lifting heavy objects for at least 6 months
      e. Need to report unexplained weight gain, decreased urine output, flank pain on unoperative side, hematuria
      f. Need to notify physician if cold or other infection present for more than 3 days
      g. Medication regimen and avoidance of OTC drugs that may be nephrotoxic (except with physician approval)

# Disorders of the Male Reproductive System

## Epididymitis

A. General information
   1. Inflammation of epididymis, one of the most common intrascrotal infections
   2. May be sexually transmitted, usually caused by *N. gonorrhoeae, C. trachomatis;* also caused by GU instrumentation, urinary reflux
B. Assessment findings
   1. Sudden scrotal pain, scrotal edema, tenderness over the spermatic cord
   2. Diagnostic test: urine culture reveals specific organism
C. Nursing interventions
   1. Administer antibiotics and analgesics as ordered.
   2. Provide bed rest with elevation of the scrotum.
   3. Apply ice packs to scrotal area to decrease edema.

## Prostatitis

A. General information
   1. Inflammatory condition that affects the prostate gland
   2. Several forms: acute bacterial prostatitis, chronic bacterial prostatitis, or abacterial chronic prostatitis
   3. Acute and chronic bacterial prostatitis usually caused by *E. coli, N. gonorrhoeae, Enterobacter* or *Proteus* species, and group D streptococci
   4. Most important predisposing factor: lower UTIs
B. Assessment findings
   1. Acute: fever, chills, dysuria, urethral discharge, prostatic tenderness, copious purulent urethral discharge upon palpation
   2. Chronic: backache; perineal pain; mild dysuria; frequency; enlarged, firm, and slightly tender prostate upon palpation
   3. Diagnostic tests
      a. WBC elevated
      b. Bacteria in initial urinalysis specimens
C. Nursing interventions
   1. Administer antibiotics, analgesics, and stool softeners as ordered.
   2. Provide increased fluid intake.
   3. Provide sitz baths/rest to relieve discomfort.
   4. Provide client teaching and discharge planning concerning:
      a. Importance of maintaining adequate hydration

    **b.** Antibiotic therapy regimen (may need to remain on medication for several months)

    **c.** Activities that drain the prostate (masturbation, sexual intercourse, prostatic massage)

## Benign Prostatic Hypertrophy (BPH)

**A.** General information

    **1.** Mild to moderate glandular enlargement, hyperplasia, and overgrowth of the smooth muscles and connective tissue

    **2.** As the gland enlarges, it compresses the urethra, resulting in urinary retention.

    **3.** Most common problem of the male reproductive system; occurs in 50% of men over age 50; 75% of men over age 75

    **4.** Cause unknown; may be related to hormonal mechanism

**B.** Assessment findings

    **1.** Nocturia, frequency, decreased force and amount of urinary stream, hesitancy (more difficult to start voiding), hematuria

    **2.** Enlargement of prostate gland upon palpation by digital rectal exam

    **3.** Diagnostic tests

        **a.** Urinalysis: alkalinity increased; specific gravity normal or elevated

        **b.** BUN and creatinine elevated (if longstanding BPH)

        **c.** Prostate-specific antigen (PSA) elevated (normal is 4 ng/mL)

        **d.** Cystoscopy reveals enlargement of gland and obstruction of urine flow

**C.** Nursing interventions

    **1.** Administer antibiotics as ordered.

    **2.** Provide client teaching concerning medications

        **a.** Terazosin (Hytrin) relaxes bladder sphincter and makes it easier to urinate. May cause hypotension and dizziness.

        **b.** Finasteride (Proscar) shrinks enlarged prostate.

    **3.** Force fluids.

    **4.** Provide care for the catheterized client.

    **5.** Provide care for the client with prostatic surgery.

## Cancer of the Prostate

**A.** General information

    **1.** Second most common cause of cancer deaths in American males over age 55

    **2.** Usually an adenocarcinoma; growth related to the presence of androgens

    **3.** Spreads from the prostate to the seminal vesicles, urethral mucosa, bladder wall, external sphincter, and lymphatic system

    **4.** Highest incidence is in African-American men age 60 or over

    **5.** Cause is unknown

**B.** Medical management

    **1.** Drug therapy: estrogens, chemotherapeutic agents

    **2.** Radiation therapy

    **3.** Surgery: radical prostatectomy

    **4.** "Watchful waiting": tumor is small and slow-growing without symptoms; decide with physician to monitor condition without surgery.

**C.** Assessment findings: same as for BPH but diagnostic test results are:

    **1.** Elevated acid phosphatase (distant metastasis) and alkaline phosphatase (bone metastasis)

    **2.** Bone scan: abnormal in metastatic areas

**D.** Nursing interventions

    **1.** Administer medications as ordered and provide care for the client receiving chemotherapy.

    **2.** Provide care for the client receiving radiation therapy.

    **3.** Provide care for the client with a prostatectomy.

## Prostatic Surgery

**A.** General information

    **1.** Indicated for benign prostatic hypertrophy and prostatic cancer.

    **2.** Types

        **a.** Transurethral resection (TUR or TURP): insertion of a resectoscope into the urethra to excise prostatic tissue; good for poor surgical risks, does not require an incision; most common type of surgery or BPH

        **b.** Suprapubic prostatectomy: the prostate is approached by a low abdominal incision into the bladder to the anterior aspect of the prostate; for large tumors obstructing the urethra

        **c.** Retropubic prostatectomy: to remove a large mass high in the pelvic area; involves a low midline incision below the bladder and into the prostatic capsule

        **d.** Perineal prostatectomy: often used for prostatic cancer; the incision is made through the perineum, which facilitates radical surgery if a malignancy is found

        **e.** *da vinci* Prostatectomy: removal of prostate using robotic system with few small incisions and great precision; more benefits than traditional surgery (less pain, nerve damage, scarring, blood loss, hospital stay).

**B.** Nursing interventions: preoperative

    **1.** Provide routine pre-op care.

    **2.** Institute and maintain urinary drainage.

    **3.** Force fluids; administer antibiotics, acid-ash diet to eradicate UTI.

    **4.** Reinforce what surgeon has told client/significant others regarding effects of surgery on sexual function.

C. Nursing interventions: postoperative
1. Provide routine post-op care.
2. Ensure patency of 3-way Foley.
3. Monitor continuous bladder irrigations with sterile saline solution (removes clotted blood from bladder), and control rate to keep urine light pink changing to clear.
4. Expect hematuria for 2–3 days.
5. Irrigate catheter with normal saline as ordered.
6. Control/treat bladder spasms; encourage short, frequent walks; decrease rate of continuous bladder irrigations (if urine is not red and is without clots); administer anticholinergics (propantheline bromide [Pro-Banthine]) or antispasmodics (B&O suppositories) as ordered.
7. Prevent hemorrhage: administer stool softeners to discourage straining at stool; avoid rectal temperatures and enemas; monitor Hgb and HCT.
8. Report bright red, thick blood in the catheter; persistent clots, persistent drainage on dressings.
9. Provide for bladder retraining after Foley removal.
   a. Instruct client to perform perineal exercises (stopping and starting stream during voiding; pressing buttocks together then relaxing muscles) to improve sphincter control.
   b. Limit liquid intake in evening.
   c. Restrict caffeine-containing beverages.
   d. Withhold anticholinergics and antispasmodics (these drugs relax bladder and increase chance of incontinence) if permitted.
10. Provide client teaching and discharge planning concerning:
   a. Client and/or family education on going home with a smaller leg-bag catheter until physician office visit.
   b. Continued increased fluid intake
   c. Signs of UTI and need to report them
   d. Continued perineal exercises
   e. Avoidance of heavy lifting, straining during defecation, and prolonged travel (at least 8–12 weeks)
   f. Measures that promote urinary continence
   g. Possible impotence (more common after perineal resection)
      1) Discuss ways of expressing sexuality (massage, cuddling)
      2) Suggest alternative methods of sexual gratification and use of assistive aids
      3) Discuss possibility of penile prosthesis with physician
   h. Need for annual and self-exams

## Sample Questions

340. A client is hospitalized for bladder cancer. He is scheduled for ileal loop surgery to create a urostomy. Which information is most important for the nurse to include in a teaching plan for this client when learning to change his urostomy appliance?
    1. Change the appliance before going to bed.
    2. Cut the wafer one inch larger than the stoma.
    3. Cleanse the peristomal skin with mild soap and water.
    4. Use firm pressure to attach the wafer to the skin.

341. Which nursing intervention best prevents urinary tract infections in a person who has an ileal conduit?
    1. Allowing the bag to fill completely.
    2. Attaching a larger bag at night.
    3. Restricting fluids to less than 1000 mL daily.
    4. Changing the appliance every 8 hours.

342. An elderly client has just returned to the nursing unit after a transurethral resection. He has a 3-way indwelling urinary catheter for continuous bladder irrigation connected to straight drainage. Immediately after surgery, what color of urine does the nurse expect in the catheter bag?
    1. Clear.
    2. Light yellow.
    3. Pink or dark red.
    4. Bright red.

343. An elderly man has just returned to the nursing care unit following a transurethral resection. He has a three-way indwelling catheter with continuous bladder irrigation. He tells the nurse he has to void. What is the most appropriate nursing action?
    1. Allow him to void around the catheter.
    2. Irrigate the catheter.
    3. Notify the physician.
    4. Remove the catheter.

344. A young adult is admitted to the hospital with a diagnosis of acute renal failure. She is oliguric and has proteinuria. She asks the nurse, "How long will it be until I start to make urine again?"
    1. 1–2 days.
    2. 3–7 days.
    3. 1–2 weeks.
    4. 3–4 weeks.

345. A client who is in acute renal failure develops pulmonary edema. Nursing interventions for this person should include which of the following? Check all that apply.

____ Administering oxygen.

____ Encouraging coughing and deep breathing.

____ Placing the client in a semi-sitting position.

____ Replacing lost fluids.

346. A client is admitted to the floor from PACU with continuous bladder irrigation after undergoing a TURP. The nurse knows to increase the rate of flow of the irrigation if what condition of the urine return is present?

1. There is no return.
2. The return is slow.
3. The return is yellow and cloudy.
4. The return becomes brighter red.

347. A young man is admitted in chronic renal failure and placed on hemodialysis three times a week. Which is an attainable short-term goal for this person when he is placed on hemodialysis?

1. Understanding the treatment and its implications.
2. Independence in the care of the AV shunt.
3. Self-monitoring during dialysis.
4. Recording dialysate composition and temperature.

348. The nurse is caring for a client who is on hemodialysis and has an arteriovenous fistula. Which finding is expected when assessing the fistula?

1. Ecchymotic area.
2. Enlarged veins.
3. Pulselessness.
4. Redness.

349. A female client is to have a urine culture collected. What are the correct instructions the nurse will give the client for collecting a clean catch urine specimen?

1. Separate the labia, clean from front to back with the three wipes impregnated with the cleaning solution, and then start to void in the toilet. Stop, and finally continue to void into the sterile container.
2. Retract the foreskin, cleanse with the three cleansing sponges, and start to void. Stop, and finally continue to void into the sterile container.
3. Separate the labia, clean from back to front with the three wipes impregnated with the cleaning solution, and then start to void in

the toilet. Stop, and finally continue to void into the sterile container.
4. Retract the foreskin, clean with soap and water, and then start to void. Stop, and finally continue to void into the sterile container.

350. The nurse is to collect a urine culture specimen from a catheterized client. Which one of the following statements describes the nurse's actions for this procedure?

1. With a sterile syringe the nurse aspirates 50 mL of urine from the silicone catheter tubing.
2. With a sterile syringe, the nurse aspirates 1–3 mL from the sampling port of the catheter after first cleaning with alcohol.
3. With a sterile syringe, the nurse aspirates 1–3 mL from the distal end of the catheter after first cleaning the sampling port with soap and water.
4. The nurse disconnects the catheter from the tubing and allows a small volume of urine to drain into a sterile container.

351. The nurse is ordered to perform a urinary catheterization for post-void residual volume (PVR) on a client with urinary incontinence. Several minutes after the client voids, the nurse obtains a residual urine of 30 mL. How does the nurse interpret this result?

1. Adequate bladder emptying.
2. Inadequate bladder emptying.
3. Decreased urethral pressure.
4. Increased urethral pressure.

352. Post cystoscopy, which one of the following assessment findings would the nurse expect to find?

1. Gross hematuria and pain.
2. Pink-tinged urine and burning on voiding.
3. Colicky pain and bladder distention.
4. Flank pain and bladder distention.

353. A post-op client is unable to void and is ordered to have an indwelling catheter inserted immediately. What is the nurse's greatest concern?

1. Teaching the client deep breathing techniques to decrease post-op pain, preprocedure.
2. Maintaining strict aseptic technique.
3. Medicating the client for pain, before the procedure.
4. Teaching the client the signs and symptoms of urinary tract infection.

**354.** The nurse is assessing a client with an indwelling catheter and finds the catheter is not draining and the client's bladder is distended. What is the nurse's first best action?

1. Notify the physician.
2. Assess the catheter tubing for kinks and position so downhill flow is initiated.
3. Change the catheter.
4. Aspirate urine for culture.

**355.** The nurse is teaching a client about the concept of dialysis and how it works for the body. What statement best describes the nurse's understanding of dialysis?

1. It will move blood through a semipermeable membrane into a dialysate that is used to remove waste products as well as correct fluid and electrolyte imbalances.
2. It will add electrolytes and water to the blood when passing through a semipermeable membrane to correct electrolyte imbalances.
3. It will increase potassium to the blood when passing through a semipermeable membrane to correct electrolyte imbalances.
4. It allows the nurse to choose to use either diffusion osmosis or ultrafiltration to correct the client's fluid and electrolyte imbalance.

**356.** A client with end-stage renal disease (ESRD) receives hemodialysis three times a week. Which statement demonstrates that dialysis is effective?

1. The client does not have a large weight gain.
2. The client has no signs and symptoms of infection.
3. The client expresses he or she can catch up on rest while on dialysis.
4. The client is able to return to employment.

**357.** The nurse is caring for a client going to hemodialysis three times a week. The client receives the following medications every morning: hydrochlorothiazide (Hydrodiuril), nitroglycerin patch (Minitran), vancomycin, and allopurinol (Zyloprim). The nurse expects to withhold which of the above medications until after hemodialysis?

1. Hydrochlorothiazide (Hydrodiuril) and vancomycin.
2. Hydrochlorothiazide (Hydrodiuril) and nitroglycerin patch (Minitran).
3. Nitroglycerin (Minitran) and allopurinol (Zyloprim).
4. Vancomycin and allopurinol (Zyloprim).

**358.** The nurse is caring for a client receiving peritoneal dialysis. The nurse is completing the exchange by draining the dialysate and notices the dialysate is cloudy. What is the nurse's interpretation of this finding?

1. The normal appearance of draining dialysate.
2. A sign of infection.
3. An indication of an impending lower back problem.
4. A sign of a vascular access occlusion.

**359.** A client is on continuous ambulatory peritoneal dialysis (CAPD). Which statement by the client demonstrates understanding of the treatment?

1. "I must increase my carbohydrate intake daily."
2. "I must maintain a positive nitrogen balance by decreasing proteins."
3. "I must take prophylactic antibiotics to prevent infection."
4. "I must be aware of the signs and symptoms of peritonitis."

**360.** A woman presents to the urgent care center with dysuria and hematuria. The woman reveals that she has a history of cystitis. The nurse should also assess for which of the following clinical manifestations suggesting cystitis?

1. Frequency and urgency of urination, flank pain, nausea, and vomiting.
2. Abscess formation and flank pain.
3. Frequency and urgency of urination, suprapubic pain, and foul smelling urine.
4. Fever, nausea, vomiting, and flank pain.

**361.** A 3-day post-op client for a ureterosigmoidostomy is complaining of cramping in lower extremities and occasional dizziness. What intervention should be given the highest priority?

1. Assessing for electrolyte imbalance.
2. Assessing for cardiac dysrhythmias.
3. Observing the client's response to surgery.
4. Verifying the temperature of the client's lower extremities.

**362.** What teaching by the nurse should be given to the client with a Kock's pouch?

1. Decreasing the client's sexual encounters.
2. Adhering to catheterization schedules.
3. Decreasing food intake to avoid embarrassing situations.
4. Decreasing fluid intake to manage the urinary diversion.

**363.** A 35-year-old male presents to the ER with hematuria, flank pain, fever, nausea, and vomiting. He is admitted and passes a "stone." The stone is sent to the laboratory and is found to be composed

of uric acid. The client is placed on allopurinol (Zyloprim). What is the action for this medication?
1. Decrease the client's serum creatinine.
2. Reduce the urinary concentration of uric acid.
3. Acidify the urine.
4. Bind oxalate in the gastrointestinal tract.

364. The nurse is caring for a client who has just been given discharge instruction for kidney stones. Which statement by the client indicates a need for further instruction?
1. "I will decrease my intake of all foods on the list you gave me that are high in purine, calcium, or oxalate."
2. "I will decrease my fluid intake."
3. "I will take my medication daily."
4. "I will return to my doctor in one week for follow-up."

365. Medication will be used in the management of a client with urolithiasis. Based on knowledge of urolithiasis, the nurse should include which of the following in planning nursing care for the client?
1. Place the client in bed with upper rails up, call bell within reach, and instructions to call to get out of bed.
2. Keep the client NPO so there will be no experience of nausea with medication administration.
3. Increase intake of purine-, calcium-, and oxalate-rich food.
4. Add Probenecid to the narcotic to prevent renal tubular excretion of the narcotic.

366. The nurse is performing discharge teaching for a client who was admitted with pyelonephritis. The client asks the nurse, "What is pyelonephritis?" What is the nurse's best response?
1. "Pyelonephritis is an inflammation of the bladder."
2. "Pyelonephritis is a rupture of the bladder."
3. "Pyelonephritis is an infection of the kidney."
4. "Pyelonephritis is an infection of the lower urinary tract."

367. On a medical-surgical unit, a client is admitted with acute renal failure. What problem must the nurse assess for continually?
1. Hyponatremia and hyperkalemia.
2. Decreased BUN and creatinine.
3. Alkalosis.
4. Hypercalcemia.

368. The client with chronic renal failure complains of irritating white crystals on his skin. The nurse recognizes this finding as uremic frost and takes which of the following nursing actions?
1. Administers an antihistamine because the doctor would prescribe one to relieve itching.
2. Increases fluids to prevent crystal formation and decrease itching.
3. Provides skin care with tepid water and applies lotion on the skin to relieve itching.
4. Permits the client to soak in a bathtub to remove crystals.

369. The nurse has been working with a client with chronic renal failure. Which of the following behaviors would indicate to the nurse that the client understands his dietary regimen?
1. He reports eating two bananas for breakfast, rice and beans for lunch, and fruit salad, green beans, and an 8 oz. T-bone steak for dinner.
2. He reports eating bacon and eggs for breakfast, hot dogs and sauerkraut for lunch, and baked canned ham with green beans for dinner.
3. He reports eating an apple and oatmeal for breakfast, homemade tomato soup for lunch, and pasta with fish for dinner.
4. He reports eating half a honeydew melon and three eggs for breakfast, a baked potato with processed cheese spread and broccoli for lunch, and chicken, yams, pinto beans, squash, and 8 oz. of pecans for dinner.

370. A client who has been in intensive care, for cardiogenic shock related to a myocardial infarction, is recovering. He is transferred to the renal unit in renal failure. The client's spouse asks the nurse "Is this acute or chronic renal failure?" What is the nurse's best response?
1. "Don't worry; this is an excellent renal unit, so we can treat either acute or chronic failure."
2. "Acute renal failure always progresses to chronic renal failure."
3. "Acute renal failure is glomerular degeneration whereas chronic renal failure is the result of cardiovascular collapse."
4. "Acute renal failure generally results from decreased blood to the kidneys, nephrotoxicity, or muscle injury. The myocardial infarction caused extensive heart muscle damage decreasing blood to the kidneys."

371. What should be assessed immediately post kidney transplant?
1. Fluid and electrolyte imbalances.
2. Infection.
3. Hepatotoxicity.
4. Cardiomegaly.

372. An adult had a renal transplant, as a result of glomerulonephritis, and is at the physician's office for a follow-up visit. The client tells the office nurse "I am not worried about rejection. I am not going to come here weekly." What defense mechanism is the client expressing?

1. Projection.
2. Intellectualization.
3. Denial.
4. Regression.

373. The nurse will complete which one of the following initial assessments on the client immediately post-op nephrectomy?

1. Performing cardiovascular assessment.
2. Ordering laboratory studies monitoring renal functions and electrolytes.
3. Inspecting the incision site for bleeding.
4. Obtaining a urine culture.

374. The nurse is completing an admission assessment on a client with benign prostatic hyperplasia (BPH). What in-depth assessment should the nurse obtain?

1. Laboratory studies.
2. Urinary patterns.
3. Electrocardiograms.
4. Internal bleeding.

375. A client with BPH is at the clinic for follow-up. Which of the following statements indicates to the nurse his understanding of management of his condition?

1. "As soon as I finish this visit I won't ever have to worry about BPH again."
2. "I don't know how I am going to get used to voiding every 2 to 3 hours."
3. "I will wear an athletic supporter while I am awake."
4. "I am going to avoid fluids while at work to prevent dribbling."

376. A client who is 8 hours post-transurethral resection prostatectomy (TURP) asks the nurse "Why are there blood clots in my bag?" How does the nurse interpret this occurrence?

1. After all surgery bleeding is normal.
2. It is common for blood clots to be irrigated from the bladder for a day or so.
3. The physician needs to be called as the client is hemorrhaging.
4. The client is tugging on the catheter causing irritation to the bladder mucosa.

377. A 68-year-old client, 48 hours post-transurethral resection prostatectomy asks "How will my sex life be affected?" The nurse's best response would be,

1. "I will get the physician to determine if your sex life was affected during surgery."
2. "Only your doctor can answer that. Why don't you ask him prior to discharge."
3. "A transurethral prostatectomy does not usually result in erectile dysfunction."
4. "Don't you remember, before surgery you were told that you would not be able to engage in sexual intercourse but you can express your love for your spouse by alternate acts such as cuddling."

378. Following a prostatectomy, the client has a 3-way, indwelling catheter for continuous bladder irrigation. During evening shift, 2400 mL of irrigant was instilled. At the end of the shift, the drainage bag was drained of 2900 mL of fluid. What is the total urine output for the shift?

1. 5300 mL.
2. 2900 mL.
3. 240 mL.
4. 500 mL.

 ## Answers and Rationales

340. **3.** Cleansing the peristomal skin is critical to maintenance of skin integrity.

341. **2.** Attaching a larger bag at night helps to prevent reflux of urine into the stoma during a period when the bag is emptied less frequently.

342. **3.** The urine is expected to be pink or dark red for up to 36 hours after a transurethral resection.

343. **2.** Blood clots obstructing the catheter can produce the sensation of needing to void. Irrigating the catheter will remove any blood clots, allowing the urine to drain freely.

344. **3.** The oliguric period in acute renal failure is usually 1–2 weeks.

345. *Administered oxygen* should be checked. Oxygenation is seriously compromised in pulmonary edema.

*Encouraging coughing and deep breathing* should be checked. Coughing and deep breathing may help with oxygenation.

*Placing the client in a semi-sitting position* should be checked. This position facilitates breathing.

346. **4.** If return becomes brighter red, the solution rate should be increased to flush the irrigation tube of clots.

347. **1.** Prior to the start of dialysis the client should fully comprehend its meaning and the changes in lifestyle required.

348. **2.** Leaking of arterial blood into an AV fistula causes the veins to enlarge so they are easier to access for hemodialysis.

349. **1.** Women should separate the labia, clean from front to back, and then proceed to void into the toilet. Stop, and finally continue to void into the sterile container.

350. **2.** Several milliliters of urine for culture can be aspirated with a 21-gauge needle and 3-mL syringe after the sampling port or the distal catheter has been swabbed with alcohol or iodine swabs. The urinary catheter and drainage system should remain a closed system to prevent infection.

351. **1.** Measurement of post-void residual volume (PVR) should be performed for all clients with urinary incontinence. Catheterization is performed several minutes after the client voids. A residual of less than 50 mL signifies adequate bladder emptying.

352. **2.** Pink-tinged urine and burning on voiding for a day or two following the procedure are expected.

353. **2.** Strict aseptic technique is vital to prevent urinary tract infection. The client is positioned on the back with heels flat on the bed with legs separated. The meatus is cleansed with an iodine solution. The catheter is lubricated with a water-soluble jelly and is inserted through the urethra into the bladder until urine starts to flow. The balloon is inflated and the catheter is taped securely to the leg.

354. **2.** Possible signs of indwelling catheter obstruction can be pain, distention, and no urinary output. Possible causes of obstruction include blood clots, mineral sediment, or mucous plugs in the catheter or tubing. The most effective strategies to promote drainage are to place the tubing so downhill flow is unobstructed and to empty the collection system regularly. Irrigation and catheter changes should be performed when all other means fail as they are associated with a high potential for infection.

355. **1.** Dialysis allows substances to move from the blood through a semipermeable membrane into a dialysis solution (dialysate) to correct fluid and electrolyte imbalances as well as remove waste products that accumulate when the client is in renal failure. The principles of dialysis include diffusion, osmosis, and ultrafiltration.

356. **4.** By the client returning to employment, it helps to maintain a positive self-image and to continue to be a productive member of society. It will be an ongoing assessment of the client's fluid status and sign/symptoms of infection.

357. **2.** The morning of dialysis antihypertensives, nitrates, and sedatives are usually withheld as they may precipitate hypotensive episodes.

358. **2.** Peritonitis is usually caused by *Staphylococcus*. The first indication of peritonitis is cloudy dialysate.

359. **4.** Peritonitis is a life-threatening complication of CAPD, which is manifested by abdominal pain and distention, diarrhea, vomiting, and fever. Clients are given antibiotics orally or parenterally as necessary, not prophylactically.

360. **3.** The signs and symptoms of cystitis are frequency and urgency of urination, suprapubic pain, dysuria, foul-smelling urination, and sometimes pyuria. Some clients with cystitis may be asymptomatic.

361. **1.** In this surgical procedure, the client's ureters are anastomosed to the sigmoid colon. This results in the client having drainage from the rectum, which often leads to acidosis and electrolyte imbalance involving potassium, chloride, and magnesium.

362. **2.** The client with a Kock's pouch should be taught about living with a stoma, how to self-catheterize and irrigate the appliance, increasing fluid intake to dilute urine to prevent irritation of the stoma, and lastly, stoma care. The client will need to self-catheterize at regular intervals.

363. **2.** Allopurinol (Zyloprim) reduces the urinary concentration of uric acid to decrease the recurrence of uric acid stones.

364. **2.** A high fluid intake of at least 3000 mL/day is needed to remove minerals prior to precipitation.

365. **1.** Nursing care priorities for the client with urolithiasis include pain relief and prevention of urinary tract obstruction and recurrence of stones. The nurse can expect to administer narcotics and maintain client safety.

366. **3.** Pyelonephritis is an inflammation or infection of the kidney or kidney pelvis.

367. **1.** The most common findings in acute renal failure include elevations in BUN and creatinine, metabolic acidosis, hyponatremia, hyperkalemia, hypocalcemia, and hypophosphatemia.

368. **3.** Skin care should be provided for the client by bathing with tepid water and oils to reduce dryness and itching.

369. **3.** A client with chronic renal failure needs to adhere to a low-protein, low-sodium, and low-potassium diet. This meal plan would fall into these restrictions.

370. **4.** A myocardial infarction causes decreased cardiac output, which may cause acute renal failure. The other mechanisms responsible for acute renal failure are nephrotoxicity, trauma, burns, sepsis, and mismatched blood. Chronic renal failure results from irreversible damage to the nephrons and glomeruli. Diseases commonly responsible for chronic renal failure are diabetes, hypertension, and kidney infections.

371. **1.** The immediate assessments to be performed for a kidney recipient are fluid and electrolyte status, intake and output, and blood pressure.

372. **3.** Denial is disowning intolerable thoughts. The client is denying feelings of anxiety and the seriousness of potential rejection of the organ.

373. **3.** The renal system is highly vascular; the client is at risk for post-op bleeding.

374. **2.** Benign prostatic hyperplasia (BPH) is the growth of new cells in the prostate gland, resulting in urinary obstruction; therefore, assessment of the obstructive symptoms are: decrease in the force of the urinary stream; hesitancy in initiation of urine; dribbling; urinary retention; incomplete bladder emptying; nocturia; dysuria; and urgency.

375. **2.** Clients with BPH should void every 2 to 3 hours to flush the urinary tract.

376. **2.** Blood clots are normal after a prostatectomy for the first 36 hours. Large quantities of bright red blood may indicate hemorrhage.

377. **3.** Prior to surgery, the client should be informed that his sexual functioning will not be hampered other than retrograde ejaculation, which is not physically harmful.

378. **4.** Urine output is calculated by subtracting the amount of irrigant instilled from the total fluid removed from the drainage bag (2900 mL drainage − 2400 mL irrigant = 500 mL urine).

# The Musculoskeletal System

## OVERVIEW OF ANATOMY AND PHYSIOLOGY

The musculoskeletal system consists of the bones, muscles, joints, cartilage, tendons, ligaments, and bursae. Its major function is to provide a structural framework for the body and to provide a means for movement.

## Bones

A. Functions
   1. Provide support to skeletal framework
   2. Assist in movement by acting as levers for muscles
   3. Protect vital organs and soft tissues
   4. Manufacture RBCs in the red bone marrow (hematopoiesis)
   5. Provide site for storage of calcium and phosphorus
B. Types of bones
   1. Long: central shaft (diaphysis) made of compact bone and two ends (epiphyses) composed of cancellous bone (e.g., femur and humerus)
   2. Short: cancellous bone covered by thin layer of compact bone (e.g., carpals and tarsals)
   3. Flat: two layers of compact bones separated by a layer of cancellous bone (e.g., skull and ribs)
   4. Irregular: sizes and shapes vary (e.g., vertebrae and mandible)

## Joints

A. Articulation of bones occurs at joints; movable joints provide stabilization and permit a variety of movements
B. Classification (according to degree of movement)
   1. Synarthroses: immovable joints
   2. Amphiarthroses: partially movable joints
   3. Diarthroses (synovial): freely movable joints
      a. Have a joint cavity (synovial cavity) between the articulating bone surfaces
      b. Articular cartilage covers the ends of the bones
      c. A fibrous capsule encloses the joint
      d. Capsule is lined with synovial membrane that secretes synovial fluid to lubricate the joint and reduce friction

## Muscles

A. Functions
   1. Provide shape to the body
   2. Protect the bones
   3. Maintain posture
   4. Cause movement of body parts by contraction
B. Types of muscles
   1. Cardiac: involuntary; found only in heart
   2. Smooth: involuntary; found in walls of hollow structures (e.g., intestines)
   3. Striated (skeletal): voluntary
C. Characteristics of skeletal muscles
   1. Muscles are attached to the skeleton at the point of origin and to bones at the point of insertion.
   2. Have properties of contraction and extension, as well as elasticity, to permit isotonic (shortening and thickening of the muscle) and isometric (increased muscle tension) movement.
   3. Contraction is innervated by nerve stimulation.

## Cartilage

A. A form of connective tissue
B. Major functions are to cushion bony prominences and offer protection where resiliency is required

## Tendons and Ligaments

A. Composed of dense, fibrous connective tissue
B. Functions
   1. Ligaments attach bone to bone
   2. Tendons attach muscle to bone

## ASSESSMENT

## Health History

A. Presenting problem
   1. Muscles: symptoms may include pain, cramping, weakness
   2. Bones and joints: symptoms may include stiffness, swelling, pain, redness, heat, limitation of movement
B. Lifestyle: usual patterns of activity and exercise (limitations in ADL, use of assistive devices such as canes or walkers), nutrition (obesity) and diet, occupation (sedentary, heavy lifting, or pushing)
C. Use of medications: drugs taken for musculoskeletal problems
D. Past medical history: congenital defects, trauma, inflammations, fractures, back pain
E. Family history: arthritis, gout

## Physical Examination

A. Inspect for overall body build, posture, and gait.
B. Inspect and palpate joints for swelling, deformity, masses, movement, tenderness, crepitations.
C. Inspect and palpate muscles for size, symmetry, tone, strength.

## Laboratory/Diagnostic Tests

A. Hematologic studies
   1. Muscle enzymes: CPK, aldolase, SGOT (AST)
   2. Erythrocyte sedimentation rate (ESR)
   3. Rheumatoid factor
   4. Complement fixation
   5. Lupus erythematosus cells (LE prep)
   6. Antinuclear antibodies (ANA)
   7. Anti-DNA
   8. C-reactive protein
   9. Uric acid
B. X-rays: detect injury to or tumors of bone or soft tissue
C. Bone scan
   1. Measures radioactivity in bones 2 hours after IV injection of a radioisotope; detects bone tumors, osteomyelitis.
   2. Nursing care
      a. Have client void immediately before the procedure.
      b. Explain that client must remain still during the scan itself.
D. Arthroscopy
   1. Insertion of fiber-optic endoscope (arthroscope) into a joint to visualize it, perform biopsies, or remove loose bodies from the joint
   2. Performed in OR using aseptic technique
   3. Nursing care
      a. Maintain pressure dressing for 24 hours.
      b. Advise client to limit activity for several days.
E. Arthrocentesis: insertion of a needle into the joint to aspirate synovial fluid for diagnostic purposes or to remove excess fluid
F. Myelography
   1. Lumbar puncture used to withdraw a small amount of CSF, which is replaced with a

radiopaque dye; used to detect tumors or herniated intravertebral discs

2. Nursing care: pretest
   a. Keep NPO after liquid breakfast.
   b. Check for iodine allergy.
   c. Confirm that consent form has been signed and explain procedure to client.
3. Nursing care: posttest (see also Lumbar Puncture)
   a. If oil-based dye (e.g., iophendylate [Pantopaque]) was used, keep client flat for 12 hours.
   b. If water-based dye (e.g., metrizamide [Amipaque]) was used
      1) Elevate head of bed 30–45°; to prevent upward displacement of dye, which may cause meningeal irritation and possibly seizures.
      2) Institute seizure precautions and do not administer any phenothiazine drugs to client, e.g., prochlorperazine (Compazine).

G. Electromyography
   1. Measures and records activity of contracting muscles in response to electrical stimulation; helps differentiate muscle disease from motor neuron dysfunction
   2. Nursing care: explain procedure to the client and advise that some discomfort may occur due to needle insertion

# ANALYSIS

Nursing diagnoses for clients with disorders of the musculoskeletal system may include:
A. Risk for injury
B. Risk for disuse syndrome
C. Impaired physical mobility
D. Bathing/hygiene self-care deficit
E. Dressing/grooming self-care deficit
F. Toileting self-care deficit
G. Body-image disturbance
H. Pain

# PLANNING AND IMPLEMENTATION

## Goals

Client will:
A. Be free from injury.
B. Be free from complications of immobility.
C. Attain optimal level of mobility.
D. Perform self-care activities at optimal level.
E. Adapt to alterations in body image.
F. Achieve maximum comfort level.

## Interventions

### Preventing Complications of Immobility

*Range-of-Motion (ROM) Exercises*

A. Movement of joint through its full ROM to prevent contractures and increase or maintain muscle tone/strength
B. Types
   1. Active: carried out by client; increases and maintains muscle tone; maintains joint mobility
   2. Passive: carried out by nurse without assistance from client; maintains joint mobility only; body part not to be moved beyond its existing ROM
   3. Active assistive: client moves body part as far as possible and nurse completes remainder of movement
   4. Active resistive: contraction of muscles against an opposing force; increases muscle size and strength

*Isometric Exercises*

A. Active exercise through contraction/relaxation of muscle; no joint movement; length of muscle does not change.
B. Client increases tension in muscle for several seconds and then relaxes.
C. Maintains muscle strength and size.

*Assistive Devices for Walking*

A. Cane
   1. Types: single, straight-legged cane; tripod cane; quad cane.
   2. Nursing care: teach client to hold cane in hand opposite affected extremity and to advance cane at the same time the affected leg is moved forward.
B. Walker
   1. Mechanical device with four legs for support.
   2. Nursing care: teach client to hold upper bars of walker at each side, then to move the walker forward and step into it.
C. Crutches: teaching the client proper use of crutches is an important nursing responsibility.
   1. Ensure proper length
      a. When client assumes erect position the top of crutch is 2 inches below the axilla, and the tip of each crutch is 6 inches in front and to the side of the feet.
      b. Client's elbows should be slightly flexed when hand is on hand grip.
      c. Weight should not be borne by the axillae.
   2. Crutch gaits
      a. Four-point gait: used when weight bearing is allowed on both extremities
         1) Advance right crutch.

**2)** Step forward with left foot.

**3)** Advance left crutch.

**4)** Step forward with right foot.

  **b.** Two-point gait: typical walking pattern, an acceleration of four-point gait

    **1)** Step forward moving both right crutch and left leg simultaneously.

    **2)** Step forward moving both left crutch and right leg simultaneously.

  **c.** Three-point gait: used when weight bearing is permitted on one extremity only

    **1)** Advance both crutches and affected extremity several inches, maintaining good balance.

    **2)** Advance the unaffected leg to the crutches, supporting the weight of the body on the hands.

  **d.** Swing-to gait: used for clients with paralysis of both lower extremities who are unable to lift feet from floor

    **1)** Both crutches are placed forward.

    **2)** Client swings forward to the crutches.

  **e.** Swing-through gait: same indications as for swing-to gait

    **1)** Both crutches are placed forward.

    **2)** Client swings body through the crutches.

## Care of the Client with a Cast

**A.** Types of casts: long arm, short arm, long leg, short leg, walking cast with rubber heel, body cast, shoulder spica, hip spica

**B.** Casting materials

  **1.** Plaster of paris—traditional cast

    **a.** Takes 24–72 hours to dry.

    **b.** Precautions must be taken until cast is dry to prevent dents, which may cause pressure areas.

    **c.** Signs of a dry cast: shiny white, hard, resistant.

    **d.** Must be kept dry because water can ruin a plaster cast.

  **2.** Synthetic casts, e.g., fiberglass

    **a.** Strong, lightweight; sets in about 20 minutes.

    **b.** Can be dried using cast dryer or hair blow-dryer on cool setting; some synthetic casts need special lamp to harden.

    **c.** Water-resistant; however, if cast becomes wet, must be dried thoroughly to prevent skin problems under cast.

**C.** Cast drying—plaster cast

  **1.** Use palms of hands, not fingertips, to support cast when moving or lifting client.

  **2.** Support cast on rubber- or plastic-protected pillows with cloth pillowcase along length of cast until dry.

**3.** Turn client every 2 hours to reduce pressure and promote drying.

**4.** Do not cover the cast until it is dry (may use fan to facilitate drying).

**5.** Do not use heat lamp or hair dryer on plaster cast.

**D.** Assessment

  **1.** Perform neurovascular checks to area distal to cast.

    **a.** Report absent or diminished pulse, cyanosis or blanching, coldness, lack of sensation, inability to move fingers or toes, excessive swelling.

    **b.** Report complaints of burning, tingling, or numbness.

  **2.** Note any odor from the cast that may indicate infection.

  **3.** Note any bleeding on cast in a surgical client.

  **4.** Check for "hot spots" that may indicate inflammation under cast.

  **5.** Compartment syndrome: report of pain due to inadequate space for tissue swelling; treatment may include removing case and fasciotomy (surgical opening of the fascia); non-treatment could result in permanent nerve damage and deformity.

**E.** General care

  **1.** Instruct client to wiggle toes or fingers to improve circulation.

  **2.** Elevate affected extremity above heart level to reduce swelling.

  **3.** Apply ice bags to each side of the cast if ordered.

**F.** Provide client teaching and discharge planning concerning:

  **1.** Isometric exercises when cleared with physician

  **2.** Reinforcement of instructions given on crutch walking

  **3.** Do not get cast wet; wrap cast in plastic bag when bathing or take sponge bath

  **4.** If a cast that has already dried and hardened does become wet, may use blow-dryer on low setting over wet spot; if large area of plaster cast becomes wet, call physician

  **5.** Do not scratch or insert foreign bodies under cast; may direct cool air from blow-dryer under cast for itching

  **6.** Recognize and report signs of impaired circulation or of infection

  **7.** Cast cleaning

    **a.** Clean surface soil on plaster cast with a slightly damp cloth; mild soap may be used for synthetic cast

    **b.** To brighten a plaster cast, apply white shoe polish sparingly

## Care of the Client in Traction

**A.** A pulling force exerted on bones to reduce and/or immobilize fractures, reduce muscle spasm, correct or prevent deformities

B. Types
1. Skin traction: weights are attached to a moleskin or adhesive strip secured by elastic bandage or other special device (e.g., foam rubber boot) used to cover the affected limb.
   a. Buck's extension (See Figure 4-24).
      1) Exerts straight pull on affected extremity
      2) Generally used to temporarily immobilize the leg in a client with a fractured hip
      3) Shock blocks at the foot of the bed produce countertraction and prevent the client from sliding down in bed
   b. Russell traction (See Figure 4-24).
      1) Knee is suspended in a sling attached to a rope and pulley on a Balkan frame, creating upward pull from the knee; weights are attached to foot of bed (as in Buck's extension) creating a horizontal force exerted on the tibia and fibula

2) Generally used to stabilize fractures of the femoral shaft while client is awaiting surgery
3) Elevating foot of bed slightly provides countertraction
4) Head of bed should remain flat
5) Foot of bed usually elevated by shock blocks to provide countertraction
   c. Cervical traction (See Figure 4-24).
      1) Cervical head halter attached to weights that hang over head of bed
      2) Used for soft tissue damage or degenerative disc disease of cervical spine to reduce muscle spasm and maintain alignment
      3) Usually intermittent traction
      4) Elevate head of bed to provide countertraction

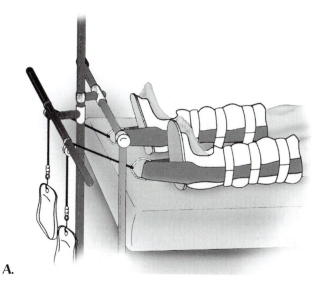

A.

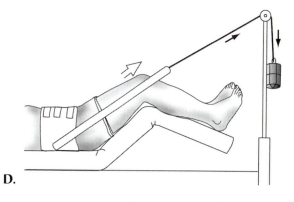

C.

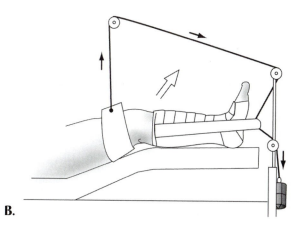

B.

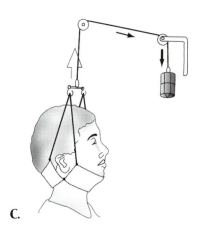

D.

**Figure 4-24** Types of traction. (**A**) Buck's extension traction; (**B**) Russell's traction; (**C**) Cervical traction; (**D**) Pelvic traction

d. Pelvic traction (See Figure 4-24).
   1) Pelvic girdle with extension straps attached to ropes and weights
   2) Used for low back pain to reduce muscle spasm and maintain alignment
   3) Usually intermittent traction
   4) Client in semi-Fowler's position with knee bent
   5) Secure pelvic girdle around iliac crests
2. Skeletal traction: traction applied directly to the bones using pins, wires, or tongs (e.g., Crutchfield tongs) that are surgically inserted; used for fractured femur, tibia, humerus, cervical spine
3. Balanced suspension traction: produced by a counterforce other than the client's weight; extremity floats or balances in the traction apparatus; client may change position without disturbing the line of traction
4. Thomas splint and Pearson attachment (usually used with skeletal traction in fractures of the femur)
   a. Hip should be flexed at 20°
   b. Use footplate to prevent foot drop
C. Nursing care
   1. Check traction apparatus frequently to ensure that:
      a. Ropes are aligned and weights are hanging freely.
      b. Bed is in proper position.
      c. Line of traction is within the long axis of the bone.
   2. Maintain client in proper alignment.
      a. Align in center of bed.
      b. Do not rest affected limb against foot of bed.
   3. Perform neurovascular checks to affected extremity.
   4. Observe for and prevent foot drop.
      a. Provide footplate.
      b. Encourage plantarflexion and dorsiflexion exercises.
   5. Observe for and prevent deep venous thrombosis (especially in Russell traction due to pressure on popliteal space).
   6. Observe for and prevent skin irritation and breakdown (especially over bony prominences and traction application sites).
      a. Russell traction: check popliteal area frequently and pad the sling with felt covered by stockinette or ABDs.
      b. Thomas splint: pad top of splint with same material as in Russell traction.
      c. Cervical traction: pad chin area and protect ears.
   7. Provide pin care for clients in skeletal traction.
      a. Usually consists of cleansing and applying antibiotic ointment, but individual agency policies may vary.
      b. Observe for any redness, drainage, odor.

8. Assist with ADL; provide overhead trapeze to facilitate moving, using bedpan, etc.
9. Prevent complications of immobility.
10. Encourage active ROM exercises to unaffected extremities.
11. Check carefully for orders about turning.
   a. Buck's extension: client may turn to unaffected side (place pillows between legs before turning).
   b. Russell traction and balanced suspension traction: client may turn slightly from side to side without turning body below the waist.
   c. May need to make bed from head to foot.

## EVALUATION

A. Client remains free from injury.
B. Client is free from complications of immobility.
   1. Maintains clear, intact skin.
   2. Has regular bowel movements.
   3. Is free from urinary tract infection/retention/calculi.
   4. Has clear breath sounds; normal rate, rhythm, and depth of respiration.
   5. Demonstrates adequate peripheral circulation.
   6. Maintains joint mobility and muscle tone.
   7. Remains oriented to time, place, and person.
   8. Is active in decision making regarding own care.
C. Optimum level of mobility is attained.
D. Client attains independence in self-care activities; uses assistive devices as necessary.
E. Client successfully adjusts to alterations in body image; exhibits increased self-esteem.
F. Pain is relieved or is more manageable.

# DISORDERS OF THE MUSCULOSKELETAL SYSTEM

## Rheumatoid Arthritis (RA)

A. General information
   1. Chronic systemic disease characterized by inflammatory changes in joints and related structures.
   2. Occurs in women more often than men (3:1); peak incidence between ages 35–45.
   3. Cause unknown, but may be an autoimmune process; genetic factors may also play a role.
   4. Predisposing factors include fatigue, cold, emotional stress, infection.
   5. Joint distribution is symmetric (bilateral); most commonly affects smaller peripheral joints of hands and also commonly involves wrists, elbows, shoulders, knees, hips, ankles, and jaw.
   6. If unarrested, affected joints progress through four stages of deterioration: synovitis, pannus formation, fibrous ankylosis, and bony ankylosis.

B. Medical management
   1. Drug therapy
      a. Aspirin: mainstay of treatment, has both analgesic and anti-inflammatory effect.
      b. Nonsteroidal anti-inflammatory drugs (NSAIDs): ibuprofen (Motrin), indomethacin (Indocin), fenoprofen (Nalfon), mefenamic acid (Ponstel), phenylbutazone (Butazolidin), piroxicam (Feldene), naproxen (Naprosyn), sulindac (Clinoril); relieve pain and inflammation by inhibiting the synthesis of prostaglandins
      c. Gold compounds (chrysotherapy)
         1) Injectable form: sodium thiomalate (Myochrysine); aurothioglucose (Solganal); given IM once a week; take 3–6 months to become effective; side effects include proteinuria, mouth ulcers, skin rash, aplastic anemia; monitor blood studies and urinalysis frequently.
         2) Oral form: auranofin (Ridaura); smaller doses are effective; take 3–6 months to become effective; diarrhea also a side effect with oral form; blood and urine studies should also be monitored.
      d. Corticosteroids
         1) Intra-articular injections temporarily suppress inflammation in specific joints.
         2) Systemic administration used only when client does not respond to less potent anti-inflammatory drugs.
      e. Methotrexate, Cytoxan given to suppress immune response; side effects include bone marrow suppression
   2. Physical therapy to minimize joint deformities
   3. Surgery to remove severely damaged joints (e.g., total hip replacement; knee replacement)
C. Assessment findings
   1. Fatigue, anorexia, malaise, weight loss, slight elevation in temperature.
   2. Joints are painful, warm, swollen, limited in motion, stiff in morning and after periods of inactivity, and may show crippling deformity in long-standing disease.
   3. Muscle weakness secondary to inactivity.
   4. History of remissions and exacerbations.
   5. Some clients have additional extra-articular manifestations: subcutaneous nodules; eye, vascular, lung, or cardiac problems.
   6. Diagnostic tests
      a. X-rays show various stages of joint disease
      b. CBC: anemia is common
      c. ESR elevated
      d. Rheumatoid factor positive
      e. ANA may be positive
      f. C-reactive protein elevated
D. Nursing interventions
   1. Assess joints for pain, swelling, tenderness, limitation of motion.

2. Promote maintenance of joint mobility and muscle strength.
   a. Perform ROM exercises several times a day; use of heat prior to exercise may decrease discomfort; stop exercise at the point of pain.
   b. Use isometric or other exercise to strengthen muscles.
3. Change position frequently; alternate sitting, standing, lying.
4. Promote comfort and relief/control of pain.
   a. Ensure balance between activity and rest.
   b. Provide 1–2 scheduled rest periods throughout day.
   c. Rest and support inflamed joints; if splints used, remove 1–2 times per day for gentle ROM exercises.
5. Ensure bed rest if ordered for acute exacerbations.
   a. Provide firm mattress.
   b. Maintain proper body alignment.
   c. Have client lie prone for ½ hour twice a day.
   d. Avoid pillows under knees.
   e. Keep joints mainly in extension, not flexion.
   f. Prevent complications of immobility.
6. Provide heat treatments (warm bath, shower, or whirlpool; warm, moist compresses; paraffin dips) as ordered.
   a. May be more effective in chronic pain.
   b. Reduce stiffness, pain, and muscle spasm.
7. Provide cold treatments as ordered; most effective during acute episodes.
8. Provide psychologic support and encourage client to express feelings.
9. Assist client in setting realistic goals; focus on client strengths.
10. Provide client teaching and discharge planning concerning
   a. Use of prescribed medications and side effects
   b. Self-help devices to assist in ADL and to increase independence
   c. Importance of maintaining a balance between activity and rest
   d. Energy conservation methods
   e. Performance of ROM, isometric, and prescribed exercises
   f. Maintenance of well-balanced diet
   g. Application of resting splints as ordered
   h. Avoidance of undue physical or emotional stress
   i. Importance of follow-up care

## Osteoarthritis

A. General information
   1. Chronic, nonsystemic disorder of joints characterized by degeneration of articular cartilage
   2. Women and men affected equally; incidence increases with age

3. Cause unknown; most important factor in development is aging (wear and tear on joints); others include obesity, joint trauma
4. Weight-bearing joints (spine, knees, hips) and terminal interphalangeal joints of fingers most commonly affected

B. Assessment findings
1. Pain (aggravated by use and relieved by rest) and stiffness of joints
2. Heberden's nodes: bony overgrowths at terminal interphalangeal joints
3. Decreased ROM, possible crepitation (grating sound when moving joint)
4. Diagnostic tests
   a. X-rays show joint deformity as disease progresses
   b. ESR may be slightly elevated when disease is inflammatory

C. Nursing interventions
1. Assess joints for pain and ROM.
2. Relieve strain and prevent further trauma to joints.
   a. Encourage rest periods throughout day.
   b. Use cane or walker when indicated.
   c. Ensure proper posture and body mechanics.
   d. Promote weight reduction if obese.
   e. Avoid excessive weight-bearing activities and continuous standing.
3. Maintain joint mobility and muscle strength.
   a. Provide ROM and isometric exercises.
   b. Ensure proper body alignment.
   c. Change client's position frequently.
4. Promote comfort/relief of pain.
   a. Administer medications as ordered: aspirin and NSAIDs most commonly used; intra-articular injections of corticosteroids relieve pain and improve mobility; calcitonin (Miacalcin) PO or nasal spray to help preservation of bone mass in lumbar spine
   b. Apply heat as ordered (e.g., warm baths, compresses, hot packs) or ice to reduce pain.
5. Prepare client for joint replacement surgery if necessary.
6. Provide client teaching and discharge planning concerning:
   a. Use of prescribed medications and side effects
   b. Importance of rest periods
   c. Measures to relieve strain on joints
   d. ROM and isometric exercises
   e. Maintenance of a well-balanced diet
   f. Use of heat/ice as ordered

## Gout

A. General information
1. A disorder of purine metabolism; causes high levels of uric acid in the blood and the precipitation of urate crystals in the joints
2. Inflammation of the joints caused by deposition of urate crystals in articular tissue
3. Occurs most often in males
4. Familial tendency

B. Medical management
1. Drug therapy
   a. Acute attack: Colchicine IV or PO (discontinue if diarrhea occurs); NSAIDs such as indomethacin (Indocin), naproxen (Naprosyn), phenylbutazone (Butazolidin)
   b. Prevention of attacks
      1) Uricosuric agents (probenecid [Benemid], sulfinpyrazone [Anturane]) increase renal excretion of uric acid
      2) Allopurinal (Zyloprim) inhibits uric acid formation
2. Low-purine diet may be recommended
3. Joint rest and protection
4. Heat or cold therapy

C. Assessment findings
1. Joint pain, redness, heat, swelling; joints of foot (especially great toe) and ankle most commonly affected (acute gouty arthritis stage)
2. Headache, malaise, anorexia
3. Tachycardia; fever; tophi in outer ear, hands, and feet (chronic tophaceous stage)
4. Diagnostic test: uric acid elevated

D. Nursing interventions
1. Assess joints for pain, motion, appearance.
2. Provide bed rest and joint immobilization as ordered.
3. Administer antigout medications as ordered.
4. Administer analgesics for pain as ordered.
5. Increase fluid intake to 2000–3000 mL/day to prevent formation of renal calculi.
6. Apply local heat or cold as ordered.
7. Apply bed cradle to keep pressure of sheets off joints.
8. Provide client teaching and discharge planning concerning:
   a. Medications and their side effects
   b. Modifications for low-purine diet: avoidance of shellfish, liver, kidney, brains, sweetbreads, sardines, anchovies
   c. Limitation of alcohol use
   d. Increase in fluid intake
   e. Weight reduction if necessary
   f. Importance of regular exercise

## Systemic Lupus Erythematosus (SLE)

A. General information
1. Chronic connective tissue disease involving multiple organ systems
2. Occurs most frequently in young women
3. Cause unknown; immune, genetic, and viral factors have all been suggested
4. Pathophysiology
   a. A defect in body's immunologic mechanisms produces autoantibodies in

the serum directed against components of the client's own cell nuclei.

   b. Affects cells throughout the body resulting in involvement of many organs, including joints, skin, kidney, CNS, and cardiopulmonary system.

B. Medical management
   1. Drug therapy
      a. Aspirin and NSAIDs to relieve mild symptoms such as fever and arthritis
      b. Corticosteroids to suppress the inflammatory response in acute exacerbations or severe disease
      c. Immunosuppressive agents such as azathioprine (Imuran), cyclophosphamide (Cytoxan) to suppress the immune response when client unresponsive to more conservative therapy
   2. Plasma exchange to provide temporary reduction in amount of circulating antibodies
   3. Supportive therapy as organ systems become involved

C. Assessment findings
   1. Fatigue, fever, anorexia, weight loss, malaise, history of remissions and exacerbations
   2. Joint pain, morning stiffness
   3. Skin lesions
      a. Erythematous rash on face, neck, or extremities may occur
      b. Butterfly rash over bridge of nose and cheeks
      c. Photosensitivity with rash in areas exposed to sun
   4. Oral or nasopharyngeal ulcerations
   5. Alopecia
   6. Renal system involvement (proteinuria, hematuria, renal failure)
   7. CNS involvement (peripheral neuritis, seizures, organic brain syndrome, psychosis)
   8. Cardiopulmonary system involvement (pericarditis, pleurisy)
   9. Increase susceptibility to infection
   10. Diagnostic tests
      a. ESR elevated
      b. CBC; anemia; WBC and platelet counts decreased
      c. ANA positive
      d. LE prep positive
      e. Anti-DNA positive
      f. Chronic false-positive test for syphilis

D. Nursing interventions
   1. Assess symptoms to determine systems involved.
   2. Monitor vital signs, I&O, daily weights.
   3. Administer medications as ordered.
   4. Institute seizure precautions and safety measures with CNS involvement.
   5. Provide psychologic support to client/significant others.
   6. Provide client teaching and discharge planning concerning:

      a. Disease process and relationship to symptoms
      b. Medication regimen and side effects
      c. Importance of adequate rest
      d. Use of daily heat and exercises as prescribed for arthritis
      e. Need to avoid physical or emotional stress
      f. Maintenance of a well-balanced diet
      g. Need to avoid direct exposure to sunlight (wear hat and other protective clothing)
      h. Need to avoid exposure to persons with infections
      i. Importance of regular medical follow-up
      j. Availability of community agencies

# Osteomyelitis

A. General information
   1. Infection of the bone and surrounding soft tissues, most commonly caused by *S. aureus*.
   2. Infection may reach bone through open wound (compound fracture or surgery), through the bloodstream, or by direct extension from infected adjacent structures.
   3. Infections can be acute or chronic; both cause bone destruction.

B. Assessment findings
   1. Malaise, fever
   2. Pain and tenderness of bone, redness and swelling over bone, difficulty with weight bearing; drainage from wound site may be present
   3. Diagnostic tests
      a. CBC: WBC elevated
      b. Blood cultures may be positive
      c. ESR may be elevated

C. Nursing interventions
   1. Administer analgesics and antibiotics as ordered.
   2. Use sterile technique during dressing changes.
   3. Maintain proper body alignment and change position frequently to prevent deformities.
   4. Provide immobilization of affected part as ordered.
   5. Provide psychologic support and diversional activities (depression may result from prolonged hospitalization).
   6. Prepare client for surgery if indicated.
      a. Incision and drainage of bone abscess
      b. Sequestrectomy: removal of dead, infected bone and cartilage
      c. Bone grafting after repeated infections
      d. Leg amputation
   7. Provide client teaching and discharge planning concerning:
      a. Use of prescribed oral antibiotic therapy and side effects
      b. Importance of recognizing and reporting signs of complications (deformity, fracture) or recurrence

# Fractures

A. General information
1. A break in the continuity of bone, usually caused by trauma
2. Pathologic fractures: spontaneous bone break, found in certain diseases or conditions (osteoporosis, osteomyelitis, multiple myeloma, bone tumors)
3. Types
   a. Complete: separation of bone into two parts
      1) Transverse
      2) Oblique
      3) Spiral
   b. Incomplete (partial): fracture does not go all the way through the bone, only part of the bone is broken.
   c. Comminuted: bone is broken or splintered into pieces.
   d. Closed or simple: bone is broken without break in skin.
   e. Open or compound: break in skin with or without protrusion of bone.
B. Medical management
1. Traction
2. Reduction
   a. Closed reduction through manual manipulation followed by application of cast
   b. Open reduction
3. Application of a cast
C. Assessment findings
1. Pain, aggravated by motion; tenderness
2. Loss of motion; edema, crepitus (grating sound), ecchymosis
3. Diagnostic test: X-ray reveals break in bone
D. Nursing interventions
1. Provide emergency care of fractures.
2. Perform neurovascular checks on affected extremity.
3. Observe for signs of compartment syndrome (swelling causes an increase within muscle compartment which causes edema and more pressure; irreversible neuromuscular damage can occur within 4 to 6 hours); signs include weak pulse, pallor followed by cyanosis, paresthesias, and severe pain.
4. Observe for signs of fat emboli (respiratory distress, mental disturbances, fever, petechiae) especially in the client with multiple long-bone fractures.
5. Encourage diet high in protein and vitamins to promote healing.
6. Encourage fluids to prevent constipation, renal calculi, and UTIs.
7. Provide care for the client in traction, with a cast, or with open reduction.
8. Provide client teaching and discharge planning concerning
   a. Cast care if indicated
   b. Crutch walking if necessary
   c. Signs of complications and need to report them

## Open Reduction and Internal Fixation (ORIF)

A. General information
1. Open reduction of fractures requires surgery to realign bones; may include internal fixation with pins, screws, wires, plates, rods, or nails
2. Indications include:
   a. Compound fractures
   b. Fractures accompanied by serious neurovascular injuries
   c. Fractures with widely separated fragments
   d. Comminuted fractures
   e. Fractures of the femur
   f. Fractures of joints
B. Nursing interventions: preoperative
1. Provide routine pre-op care.
2. Provide meticulous skin preparation to prevent infection.
C. Nursing interventions: postoperative
1. Provide routine post-op care.
2. Maintain affected limb in proper alignment.
3. Perform neurovascular checks to affected extremity.
4. Observe for post-op infection.

## Fractured Hip

A. General information
1. Fracture of the head, neck (intracapsular fracture), or trochanteric area (extracapsular fracture) of the femur
2. Occurs most often in elderly women
3. Predisposing factors include osteoporosis and degenerative changes of bone
B. Medical management
1. Buck's or Russell traction as temporary measures to maintain alignment of affected limb and reduce the pain of muscle spasm
2. Surgery
   a. Open reduction and internal fixation with pins, nails, and/or plates
   b. Hemiarthroplasty: insertion of prosthesis (e.g., Austin-Moore) to replace head of femur
C. Assessment findings
1. Pain in affected limb
2. Affected limb appears shorter, external rotation
3. Diagnostic test: X-ray reveals hip fracture
D. Nursing interventions
1. Provide general care for the client with a fracture.
2. Provide care for the client with Buck's or Russell traction.
3. Monitor for disorientation and confusion in the elderly client; reorient frequently and provide safety measures.

4. Perform neurovascular checks to affected extremity.
5. Prevent complications of immobility.
6. Encourage use of trapeze to facilitate movement.
7. Administer analgesics as ordered for pain.
8. In addition to routine post-op care for the client with open reduction and internal fixation:
   a. Check dressings for bleeding, drainage, infection: empty Hemovac and note output; keep compressed to facilitate drainage.
   b. Assess client's LOC.
   c. Reorient the confused client frequently.
   d. Avoid oversedating the elderly client.
   e. Turn client every 2 hours.
   f. Turn to unoperative side only.
   g. Place two pillows between legs while turning and when lying on side.
   h. Institute measures to prevent thrombus formation.
      1) Apply elastic stockings.
      2) Encourage plantarflexion and dorsiflexion foot exercises.
      3) Administer anticoagulants such as aspirin if ordered.
   i. Encourage quadriceps setting and gluteal setting exercises when allowed.
   j. Observe for adequate bowel and bladder function.
   k. Assist client in getting out of bed, usually on first or second post-op day.
   l. Pivot or lift into chair as ordered.
   m. Avoid weight bearing until allowed.
9. Provide care for the client with a hip prosthesis if necessary (similar to care for client with total hip replacement).

## Total Hip Replacement

A. General information
   1. Replacement of both acetabulum and head of femur with prostheses
   2. Indications
      a. Rheumatoid arthritis or osteoarthritis causing severe disability and intolerable pain
      b. Fractured hip with nonunion
B. Nursing interventions
   1. Provide routine pre-op care.
   2. In addition to routine post-op care for the client with hip surgery
      a. Maintain abduction of affected limb at all times with abductor splint or two pillows between legs.
      b. Prevent external rotation (may vary depending on type of prosthesis and method of insertion) by placing trochanter rolls along leg.
      c. Prevent hip flexion.
         1) Keep head of bed flat if ordered.
         2) May raise bed to 45° for meals if allowed.

d. Turn only to unoperative side if ordered; use abductor splint or two pillows between knees while turning and when lying on side.
e. Assist client in getting out of bed when ordered.
   1) PT usually ordered to get client out of bed day of surgery or first day post-op, and every day thereafter.
   2) Avoid weight bearing until allowed.
   3) Avoid adduction and hip flexion; do not use low chair.
3. Provide client teaching and discharge planning concerning:
   a. Prevention of adduction of affected limb and hip flexion
      1) Do not cross legs.
      2) Use raised toilet set.
      3) Do not bend down to put on shoes or socks.
      4) Do not sit in low chairs.
   b. Signs of wound infection
   c. Exercise program as ordered
   d. Partial weight bearing only until full weight bearing allowed

## Herniated Nucleus Pulposus (HNP)

A. General information
   1. Protrusion of nucleus pulposus (central part of intervertebral disc) into spinal canal causing compression of spinal nerve roots
   2. Occurs more often in men
   3. Herniation most commonly occurs at the fourth and fifth intervertebral spaces in the lumbar region
   4. Predisposing factors include heavy lifting or pulling and trauma
B. Medical management
   1. Conservative treatment
      a. Bed rest
      b. Traction
         1) Lumbosacral disc: pelvic traction
         2) Cervical disc: cervical traction
      c. Drug therapy
         1) Anti-inflammatory agents
         2) Muscle relaxants
         3) Analgesics
      d. Local application of heat and diathermy
      e. Corset for lumbosacral disc
      f. Cervical collar for cervical disc
      g. Epidural injections of corticosteroids
   2. Surgery
      a. Discectomy with or without spinal fusion
      b. Chemonucleolysis
         1) Injection of chymopapain (derivative of papaya plant) into disc to reduce size and pressure on affected nerve root
         2) Used as alternative to laminectomy in selected cases

C. Assessment findings
1. Lumbosacral disc
   a. Back pain radiating across buttock and down leg (along sciatic nerve)
   b. Weakness of leg and foot on affected side
   c. Numbness and tingling in toes and foot
   d. Positive straight-leg raise test: pain on raising leg
   e. Depressed or absent Achilles reflex
   f. Muscle spasm in lumbar region
2. Cervical disc
   a. Shoulder pain radiating down arm to hand
   b. Weakness of affected upper extremity
   c. Paresthesias and sensory disturbances
3. Diagnostic tests: myelogram localizes site of herniation
D. Nursing interventions
1. Ensure bed rest on a firm mattress with bed board.
2. Assist client in applying pelvic or cervical traction as ordered.
3. Maintain proper body alignment.
4. Administer medications as ordered.
5. Prevent complications of immobility.
6. Provide additional comfort measures to relieve pain.
7. Provide pre-op care for client receiving chemonucleolysis.
   a. Administer cimetidine (Tagamet) and diphenhydramine HCl (Benadryl) every 6 hours as ordered to reduce possibility of allergic reaction.
   b. Possibly administer corticosteroids before procedure.
8. Provide post-op care for client receiving chemonucleolysis.
   a. Observe for anaphylaxis.
   b. Observe for less serious allergic reaction (e.g., rash, itching, rhinitis, difficulty in breathing).
   c. Monitor for neurologic deficits (numbness or tingling in extremities or inability to void).
9. Provide client teaching and discharge planning concerning:
   a. Back-strengthening exercises as prescribed
   b. Maintenance of good posture
   c. Use of proper body mechanics, how to lift heavy objects correctly
      1) Maintain straight spine.
      2) Flex knees and hips while stooping.
      3) Keep load close to body.
   d. Prescribed medications and side effects
   e. Proper application of corset or cervical collar
   f. Weight reduction if needed

# Discectomy/Laminectomy

A. General information
1. Discectomy: excision of herniated fragments of intervertebral disc.
2. Laminectomy: excision of lamina to reduce pressure on the spinal cord, spinal nerves, or to provide access for removing the disc.
3. Indications
   a. Most commonly used for herniated nucleus pulposus not responsive to conservative therapy or with evidence of decreasing sensory or motor status
   b. Also indicated for spinal decompression as with spinal cord injury, to remove fragments of broken bone, or to remove spinal neoplasm or abscess
4. Spinal fusion may be done at the same time if spine is unstable
B. Nursing interventions: preoperative
1. Provide routine pre-op care.
2. Teach client log rolling (turning body as a unit while maintaining alignment of spinal column) and use of bedpan.
C. Nursing interventions: postoperative
1. Provide routine post-op care.
2. Position client as ordered.
   a. Lower spinal surgery: generally flat
   b. Cervical spinal surgery: slight elevation of head of bed to prevent edema around airway
3. Maintain proper body alignment; with cervical spinal surgery avoid neck flexion and apply cervical collar as ordered.
4. Turn client every 2 hours.
   a. Use log-rolling technique and turning sheet.
   b. Place pillows between legs while on side.
5. Assess for complications.
   a. Monitor sensory and motor status every 2–4 hours.
   b. With cervical spinal surgery client may have difficulty swallowing and coughing.
      1) Monitor for respiratory distress.
      2) Keep suction and tracheostomy set available.
6. Check dressings for hemorrhage, CSF leakage, infection.
7. Promote comfort.
   a. Administer analgesics as ordered.
   b. Provide additional comfort measures and positioning.
8. Assess for adequate bladder and bowel function.
   a. Monitor every 2–4 hours for bladder distension.
   b. Assess bowel sounds.
   c. Prevent constipation.
9. Prevent complications of immobility.
10. Assist with ambulation.
    a. Usually out of bed day after surgery.

     b. Apply brace or corset if ordered.
     c. If client allowed to sit, use straight-back chair and keep feet flat on floor.
  D. Provide client teaching and discharge planning concerning:
    1. Wound care
    2. Maintenance of good posture and proper body mechanics
    3. Activity level as ordered
    4. Recognition and reporting of signs of complications such as wound infection, sensory or motor deficits

## Spinal Fusion

A. General information
    1. Fusion of spinous processes with bone graft from iliac crest to provide stabilization of spine
    2. Performed in conjunction with laminectomy or discectomy
B. Nursing interventions
    1. Provide pre-op care as for laminectomy.
    2. In addition to post-op care for laminectomy:
      a. Position client correctly.
        1) Lumbar spinal fusion: keep bed flat for first 12 hours, then may elevate head of bed 20–30°, keep off back for first 48 hours.
        2) Cervical spinal fusion: elevate head of bed slightly.
      b. Assist with ambulation.
        1) Time varies with surgeon and extent of fusion.
        2) Usually out of bed 3–4 days post-op.
        3) Apply brace before getting client out of bed.
        4) Apply special cervical collar for cervical spinal fusion.
      c. Promote comfort: client may experience considerable pain from graft site.
    3. In addition to client teaching and discharge planning for laminectomy, advise client that:
      a. Brace will be needed for 4 months and lighter corset for 1 year after surgery.
      b. It takes 1 year until graft becomes stable.
      c. No bending, lifting, stooping, or sitting for prolonged periods for 4 months.
      d. Walking without excessive tiring is healthful exercise.
      e. Diet modification will help prevent weight gain resulting from decreased activity.

## Harrington Rod Insertion

See Unit 5.

## Amputation of a Limb

See Amputation.

## Sample Questions

379. An adult has been diagnosed with rheumatoid arthritis for the past 8 years. Her condition is deteriorating despite conservative treatment, and intramuscular gold is prescribed by the physician. When teaching about gold (chrysotherapy), what important teaching should the nurse emphasize?
  1. Cushing's syndrome is common.
  2. Improvement may not occur for 3–6 months.
  3. Side effects are rare.
  4. The need to take this drug daily.

380. A woman who has had rheumatoid arthritis for several years is admitted to the hospital. Upon physical examination of the client, what should the nurse expect to find?
  1. Asymmetric joint involvement.
  2. Heberden's nodes.
  3. Obesity.
  4. Small joint involvement.

381. An elderly client is admitted to the orthopedic unit with a diagnosis of a right intracapsular hip fracture. Buck's extension traction is employed prior to surgery. She complains of numbness in the right foot. After the nurse notes the fraction tapes are lengthwise on the opposite sides of the limb, what would be the nurse's best response?
  1. "How long has your foot been numb?"
  2. "I can adjust it for your comfort."
  3. "I'll call your doctor about it."
  4. "There is nothing wrong with the traction."

382. An elderly woman had an Austin-Moore prosthesis inserted following an intracapsular hip fracture. Which statement by the client indicates the client has understood instruction about maintaining the hip in proper position?
  1. "I shouldn't bend my knees."
  2. "Put a pillow between my legs when you turn me."
  3. "I will be sure to put my shoes on when I go for a walk."
  4. "Put the head of my bed way up so I can eat breakfast in my normal position."

383. The nurse is caring for an elderly woman who has had a fractured hip repaired. In the first few days following the surgical repair which of the following nursing measures will best facilitate the resumption of activities for this client?
  1. Arranging for a wheelchair.

2. Asking her family to visit.

3. Assisting her to sit out of bed in a chair qid.

4. Encouraging the use of an overhead trapeze.

384. A 90-year-old woman is preparing for transfer to an extended care facility to continue recovery following repair of a fractured hip. She begins to cry and says, "When you're young these things don't happen. Why did I break my hip at this age?" Which response by the nurse indicates the best understanding of risk factors for the elderly?

1. "As you age you become less aware of your surroundings and careless about safety."

2. "Nothing works as well when we are older."

3. "There are no known specific reasons why hip fractures occur more often in your age group."

4. "Your age and sex are factors in the loss of minerals from your bones, making them more likely to break."

385. An adult is admitted to the hospital. X-rays reveal a fractured tibia and a cast is applied. Of the following, which nursing action would be most important after the cast is in place?

1. Assessing for capillary refill.

2. Arranging for physical therapy.

3. Discussing cast care with the client.

4. Helping the client to ambulate.

386. A client is admitted to the floor after having a laminectomy with spinal fusion. Of the following maneuvers the client may use to avoid pain, which is unsafe?

1. Log rolling.

2. Asking for pain medication.

3. Placing pillows between her legs.

4. Sitting in semi-Fowler's.

387. A client has suffered low-back pain and sciatica for over 2 years. Why is it important for the nurse to conduct a thorough assessment of his level of discomfort from low-back pain?

1. This will provide a baseline for later comparison.

2. This is a method for identifying clients with "low back neurosis."

3. Clients who have pain localized to the back and radiating to one extremity are probably not candidates for surgery.

4. Surgery is contraindicated for clients who have had pain for less than 2 years.

388. An adult man is scheduled for a lumbar laminectomy. Preoperative teaching regarding postoperative pain management should include which of the following explanations?

1. Pain and spasm are not expected and therefore there will be minimal need for pain medication.

2. Pain and spasm are expected and pain medication will be provided as needed.

3. Pain and spasm are expected but pain medication will interfere with a neurological assessment and will therefore be given sparingly.

4. Pain and spasm are expected but pain medication will be limited as client tolerance to the medication is feared.

389. A client attends a class on osteoporosis. Which statement by the client needs further teaching about the relationship between exercise and maintenance of bone mass?

1. I will begin jogging.

2. I will begin jumping rope.

3. I will begin swimming.

4. I will begin walking.

390. In preparing a teaching plan for an adult who has had an arthroscopy, the nurse will include which of the following?

1. Client should check extremity for color, mobility, and sensation at least every 2 hours after procedure.

2. Client may return to regular activities immediately after procedure.

3. Remove compression dressing 6 to 8 hours after procedure.

4. Keep extremity in flexion for 24 hours after procedure.

391. The nursing care plan for an adult who has had a myelogram using an oil-based contrast medium should include which intervention by the nurse?

1. Give the client a light meal immediately before the myelogram, to help prevent nausea or lightheadedness.

2. Restrict fluids for 12 hours after the myelogram.

3. Keep the client in a recumbent position for 12–24 hours after the myelogram.

4. Assure the client that stiff neck or photophobia are expected side effects of the contrast medium used during the myelogram.

392. Which statement by the family tells the nurse that they understand how to perform passive range-of-motion exercises on a bed-bound family member?

1. "We should put each joint through a full series of exercises until Mother tells us she's fatigued."

2. "Every day, we should try to move all of her joints a degree or two further than they naturally go."

3. "If Mother has a muscle spasm, we should stop exercising that limb for a day or two."

4. "To exercise Mother's elbow, we would hold her upper arm still, and move her forearm."

393. An adult is learning how to use a cane. The nurse knows that the person can use the cane safely when observing which of the following?

1. The cane is held on the unaffected side; the cane and affected leg are moved forward, then the unaffected leg comes forward.

2. The cane is held on the affected side; the cane is moved forward, then the unaffected leg, then the affected leg.

3. The cane is held on the unaffected side; the cane is moved forward, then the unaffected leg, then the affected leg.

4. The cane is held on the affected side; the cane and unaffected leg are moved forward, then the affected leg comes forward.

394. An adult who has had a total hip replacement is learning how to walk with a standard (not reciprocal) walker. Which description below tells the nurse that he is using the walker correctly?

1. One side of the walker is simultaneously advanced with the opposite foot; the process is repeated on the other side.

2. Each time he steps on his nonaffected side, the client advances the walker; when moving his affected side, he steps into the walker and lifts his nonaffected foot.

3. The client balances on both feet, most weight on his nonaffected side, and lifts the walker forward; he then balances on the walker and swings both feet forward into the walker.

4. The client lifts the walker in front while balancing on both feet, then walks into the walker, supporting his body weight on his hands while advancing his affected side.

395. A man has sprained his knee and the emergency nurse is fitting him with crutches. If the man is measured while he is lying down, how does the nurse ensure the correct crutch length?

1. Measure client from anterior axillary fold to sole of foot and add 2 inches.

2. Add 6 inches to the length of the client's foot and measure the distance from that point to the client's axilla.

3. Measure from the client's axilla to his palm to get the length from the top of the crutch to

the hand piece. Measure from palm to sole to determine length of lower part of crutch.

4. Subtract 24 inches from client's height to determine length of crutch from top to tip.

396. The nurse is teaching a client with a broken left ankle how to go up stairs when using crutches. Which statement by the nurse is correct?

1. "Place both crutches on the next step, stand on the right foot and place the left foot on the step next to the crutches."

2. "Place the left crutch and right foot on the next step and push off with both arms then lift the left foot up to the step."

3. "Place the right foot on the next step, then move the crutches and the left foot onto the step."

4. "Place the right crutch and left foot on the next step; move the right crutch up onto the step, then swing the right foot up."

397. What is one major disadvantage of a fiberglass cast?

1. It is heavy.

2. It must remain dry.

3. It may cause skin irritation.

4. It must be replaced frequently.

398. Which of the following findings would alert the nurse to notify the physician of a serious complication for the client with a cast on his leg?

1. Itching under the cast.

2. Poor capillary refill of the toes.

3. Ability of client to move toes without difficulty.

4. Pain relieved by application of ice bag to cast.

399. Which intervention below would be appropriate for the nurse to teach the client with a cast on his left arm?

1. "Cover your plaster cast with plastic before taking a long bath or shower."

2. "Repair breaks in the cast with super-glue or epoxy."

3. "Remove surface dirt on your cast with a damp cloth."

4. "If your fiberglass cast gets wet, dry it with the warm setting on your blowdryer."

400. An adult is in Russell traction. It is appropriate for the nurse to make which of the following assessments because of the client's treatment modality?

1. Make sure sling under the affected knee is smooth and doesn't apply pressure in the popliteal space.

2. Ensure that both buttocks clear the mattress.

3. Check that the leg in traction is on the mattress, not elevated.

4. Assess for numbness and tingling of one or more fingers, suggesting radial, ulnar, or median nerve pressure.

401. A client's family asks why the client has been put into pelvic traction for low-back pain. What is the nurse's best response?

1. "He really needs bed rest; the traction will force him to stay in bed."

2. "By pulling on either side of the pelvis, the lower back muscles are stretched and this gives relief from the crampy back muscles."

3. "Traction helps to relieve compression of the roots of the nerves."

4. "By holding the pelvis still, the back muscles can relax and start to heal."

402. An adult's left leg is in Buck's extension traction. She complains of burning under the traction boot and the toes on that foot are cool. What is the nurse's first best action?

1. Ask, "What do you mean by 'burning'?"

2. Notify the physician at once.

3. Remove the boot, then reapply and reassess.

4. Apply an ice pack to the boot for 15 minutes.

403. A client whose left leg is in balanced suspension traction for a femur fracture needs to be moved to a new bed. What is the best way to do this safely?

1. All weights are removed from the ends of the traction ropes so the leg moves freely before the move is attempted.

2. The left leg is kept above the level of the heart.

3. Sufficient time is given to the client to move himself to the new bed at his own rate of tolerance.

4. The line of pull is maintained on the left leg.

404. Which statement best describes the nurse's assessment of the client with rheumatoid arthritis?

1. Assessment is done of the musculoskeletal, cardiac, pulmonary, and renal systems.

2. Pain is best assessed by monitoring the client's facial expression during exam and by observing limitations in the client's own movement.

3. Vital signs are an adequate assessment of the acuity of the client's level of pain.

4. The client's health history is not nearly as important as the nurse's findings on physical examination.

405. An adult is admitted to the medical unit with an acute exacerbation of rheumatoid arthritis. Which of the following will the nurse include on his nursing care plan?

1. Administer analgesics for pain when systolic blood pressure increases 20 mm Hg or more or pulse increases 20% or more.

2. Develop plan with client to meet self-care needs.

3. Instruct client to stop taking iron supplements that lead to constipation.

4. Schedule hygiene activities together in one block to provide longer rest periods before and after care.

406. An adult has rheumatoid arthritis and is taking prednisone. In creating a teaching plan, the nurse will be certain to include which of the following?

1. "You should expect to be on corticosteroids for the rest of your life."

2. "It will take 3 to 6 months for you to notice any effect from this medication."

3. "Notify your physician of any stomach upset you may have."

4. "Avoid bananas and spinach while you are taking this drug."

407. Which statement by an adult with osteoarthritis indicates to the nurse that she understands her therapeutic regimen?

1. "I will wait until my pain is very bad before I take my pain medication, or else further on in my disease, the medication won't help at all."

2. "Jogging for short distances is better for my arthritis than walking for longer distances."

3. "It would probably be a good idea for me to lose the 30 pounds my doctor recommended I lose."

4. "I should do all my house cleaning on one day, so I can rest for the remainder of the week."

408. In preparing a teaching plan for the client with osteoarthritis, the nurse would include which of the following?

1. Application of cold packs to affected joints to decrease swelling.

2. Client education regarding self-administration of medications.

3. Progressively increasing activity to point of muscle fatigue to build muscle bulk and improve rate of metabolism.

4. Teaching client that degenerative changes are progressive and that pain is a natural sequela of age.

409. The nurse, assessing a client with systemic lupus erythematosus can expect to find which of the following?
   1. Dysphagia.
   2. Decreased visual acuity or blindness.
   3. Dryness or itching of genitalia.
   4. Abnormal lung sounds.

410. A client with systemic lupus erythematosus is taking gold. Which of the following interventions would the nurse include in the teaching plan for this client?
   1. "Stop taking your anti-inflammatory medication as long as you are taking gold preparations."
   2. "You will give yourself intramuscular injections of gold preparations every day for 2 to 4 weeks, then taper down to one injection every 2 months."
   3. "You will be taking a large dose when you start taking gold capsules, and will taper down to a smaller dose as the therapy becomes effective."
   4. "Stay away from crowds during flu season and have your blood tested after every other gold injection."

411. In assessing the client with osteomyelitis, the nurse would expect to find which of the following?
   1. Pale, cool, tender skin at site.
   2. Decreased white blood cell count.
   3. Positive wound cultures.
   4. Decreased erythrocyte sedimentation rate.

412. An adult has a fractured left radius, which has been casted. While performing an assessment of this client, the nurse will correctly identify which of these findings as *emergent*?
   1. Pain at the fracture site.
   2. Swelling of fingers of left hand.
   3. Diminished capillary refill of fingers of left hand.
   4. Warm, dry fingers of left hand.

413. Which intervention by the emergency nurse is critical in caring for the client with a fractured tibia and fibula?
   1. Cutting away clothing on the injured leg.
   2. Palpation of the dorsalis pedis pulses.
   3. Administration of analgesic medications as ordered.
   4. Initiating two, large-bore IV catheters and warmed normal saline at a fast rate.

414. A 20-year-old was brought to the emergency department after an auto accident. There is a strong scent of alcohol about her, and she states she had three beers over 3 hours. Her only injury is an open fracture of the left humerus. Which assessment finding by the emergency nurse is critical?
   1. Status of client's tetanus immunization.
   2. Current blood alcohol level.
   3. Support systems available at home to assist with care.
   4. Last time client voided.

415. A firefighter fell off a roof while fighting a house fire and fractured his femur. Approximately 24 hours after the incident, the nurse finds him dyspneic, tachypneic, with scattered crackles in his lung fields; he is coughing up large amounts of thick, white sputum. What nursing diagnosis would be formulated?
   1. Respiratory compromise related to inhalation of smoke.
   2. Pneumonia related to prolonged bed rest.
   3. Fat embolism syndrome related to femur fracture.
   4. Hypovolemic shock related to multiple trauma.

416. An adult has had a total right hip replacement. Why does the operative hip need to be kept in the extension and abduction position?
   1. Reduces the risk for the development of thromboemboli.
   2. Promotes circulation to the operative site, reducing the risk of avascular necrosis.
   3. Helps to prevent dislocation of the hip prosthesis.
   4. Facilitates the drainage of blood and fluid at the operative site.

417. An adult who has had a total right hip replacement asks the nurse about "moving around in this bed." What is the nurse's best response?
   1. The client should remain supine for 48 hours after surgery, with affected leg in a slightly inward-rotation position.
   2. Although the client must remain supine, she can cross her legs to change position for comfort.
   3. A side-lying position is undesirable, but the head of the bed can be elevated 60–75° to shift weight off of back and buttocks.
   4. The client will be repositioned using an abductor pillow between the legs.

**418.** Which statement by a client who has had an open reduction/internal fixation of her fractured left hip indicates to the nurse that the client understands her care?

1. "My nephew will move my bed down to the first floor so I won't have to go upstairs when I get home."
2. "I should expect my surgical site to be swollen and red for a week or two after I get home."
3. "The night nurse will take off these thigh-high stockings at bedtime, and the day nurse will put them back on at breakfast time."
4. "I need to limit my fluid intake so I won't be getting on and off the bedpan so often; it's not good for my hip."

**419.** The nurse teaches an adult woman that because she has osteoporosis, she must take safety precautions to prevent falls, "because you could break a hip." When the client asks what one has to do with the other, what is the nurse's best response?

1. Osteoporosis yields brittle bones which break easily.
2. Osteoporosis causes changes in balance, which makes the client more susceptible to falls that could lead to hip fractures.
3. Hips are the primary sites of calcium loss in osteoporosis, making them more susceptible to fracture.
4. Both osteoporosis and hip fractures are common in elderly women.

**420.** An adult is diagnosed with a herniated nucleus pulposus at the C5-C6 interspace and a second at the C6-C7 interspace. Which of the following findings would the nurse expect to discover during the assessment?

1. Constant, throbbing headaches.
2. Numbness of the face.
3. Clonus in the lower extremities.
4. Pain in the scapular region.

**421.** An adult has undergone a cervical laminectomy. Because of the potential complications associated with this procedure, the nurse must perform which of the following assessments?

1. Assess for wheezes and stridor.
2. Check pupils for response to direct and consensual light.
3. Assess gag reflex.
4. Assess shoulder shrug and neck strength.

**422.** The nurse is caring for a person who just had a cervical laminectomy. The nurse knows that the client will most likely be maintained in what position?

1. Left lateral decubitus with neck flexed to 30°.
2. Supine, with no pillows under the head.
3. Semi-Fowler's.
4. Modified Trendelenburg, with a soft cervical collar in place.

**423.** An adult is being discharged after a lumbar laminectomy. Which statement indicates to the nurse that the client understands her discharge teaching?

1. "I can't wait to sit in my own recliner and rest while I watch my soaps!"
2. "I'll be able to man the refreshment stand at my nephew's baseball game next weekend, won't I?"
3. "My friend is getting me a footstool for in front of my sink."
4. "I have to buy a soft mattress so my spine won't be subjected to any extra pressure."

**424.** The nurse is planning post-op care for a client undergoing a laminectomy. Why does the nurse need to know whether the client will be having a spinal fusion also?

1. The contrast medium used to check the fusion site for grafting could cause an allergic reaction.
2. The client whose laminectomy is performed with a spinal fusion will be on bed rest longer than the client who does not undergo spinal fusion.
3. Clients undergoing spinal fusion will be in long torso casts for 6 to 8 weeks after surgery.
4. The client whose laminectomy is performed with a spinal fusion is at greater risk for spontaneous pneumothorax than the client who does not undergo spinal fusion.

## Answers and Rationales

**379.** **2.** Chrysotherapy often requires a 3–6 month period before effects are seen.

**380.** **4.** Small joint involvement is common in rheumatoid arthritis. All of the other symptoms are seen in osteoarthritis but not rheumatoid arthritis.

**381.** **1.** Numbness is symptomatic of circulatory or nerve impairment to the extremity. It is important to know the length of time the client has been experiencing this sensation.

382. 2. A pillow placed between the client's legs will keep the affected leg abducted and in good alignment while the client is being turned.

383. 4. Exercise is important to keep the joints and muscles functioning and to prevent secondary complications. Use of the overhead trapeze prevents hazards of immobility by permitting movement in bed and strengthening of the upper extremities in preparation for ambulation.

384. 4. Elderly females are prone to hip fractures because the cessation of estrogen production after menopause contributes to demineralization of bone.

385. 1. Good capillary refill indicates that the cast has not caused a circulatory problem in the extremity. Assessing circulation is a priority of action.

386. 4. The client returning from a lumbar spinal fusion should be kept flat in bed.

387. 1. The importance of an accurate history cannot be overemphasized in assessing the character and location of the pain. A baseline assessment of neurological signs is made so that deviation from the database can be noted. Once a pain assessment is complete a plan for pain management can be developed.

388. 2. Clients should be told that they may experience pain and spasm in the early postoperative period and that pain medication will be provided.

389. 3. Physical compression of weight-bearing joints stimulates osteoblastic deposition of calcium. Swimming does not involve weight bearing and physical compression of joints.

390. 1. Because the joint is distended with saline and the arthroscope is introduced into the joint area, the potential for neurovascular damage exists. Color (indicating adequate vascular perfusion), sensation, and mobility (indicating intact neurologic status) should be assessed, although mobility assessment will likely be limited to "wiggling the digits."

391. 3. If an oil-based contrast medium is used, the client will be kept in a recumbent position for 12–24 hours to reduce cerebrospinal fluid leakage, and thus decrease the likelihood of developing a postprocedure headache. If a water-soluble medium is used, the client will usually remain in bed, with the head elevated 15–30° (to minimize the upward migration of the medium), but some physicians may allow these clients to ambulate.

392. 4. To perform passive range of motion, the joint is supported, the bones above the joint are stabilized, and the body part distal to the joint is exercised through the range of motion. The family's description of how to maneuver the elbow illustrates this well.

393. 1. The cane, held on the unaffected side, will provide a wider base of support for the affected side while the unaffected limb is moving. The client should keep the cane close to the body to prevent leaning.

394. 4. The sequence for using a walker is balance on both feet, lift the walker and place in front of you, walk into the walker (using it for support when standing on affected limb) and then balance on both feet before repeating the sequence.

395. 1. Although measuring the client while he is lying down is not the preferred method of fitting crutches, this formula may be used successfully.

396. 3. The unaffected limb is advanced to the next step, then the crutches and the affected limb move to that step (weight stays on crutches or foot of unaffected side). A handy mnemonic for clients is, "Up with the good leg, down with the bad," meaning the "good" leg is used first when going up stairs, and the crutches and "bad" leg go to the new step first when going down stairs.

397. 3. Although fiberglass casts have other advantages, the particles of fiberglass may scratch and cause a skin reaction.

398. 2. Poor capillary refill (a "pinking up" of the toes after the nailbeds are blanched by compression, which takes more than 3 seconds) is indicative of a circulatory compromise. In this scenario, the likely cause is compartment syndrome: an increase of pressure within the cast ("compartment"). Other signs/symptoms include pain unrelieved by usual modalities, disproportional swelling, and inability to move digits.

399. 3. A damp, not wet, cloth can be used to remove superficial dirt. Stained areas can be covered with a thin layer of white shoe polish.

400. 1. Russell traction is a modification of Buck extension, used for a femur fracture that is not appropriate for internal fixation. The

modification occurs when a sling is placed under the affected knee, giving more comfort to the client, and preventing some of the rotation tendencies.

**401. 3.** Although this information may be a bit technical for the lay members of the client's family, it is the only answer that provides correct information. Increased lumbar flexion relieves compression of the lumbar nerve roots, which is why the head of the bed is elevated 30° and the knees are flexed; 15–30 lb of traction increases lumbar flexion and facilitates relief.

**402. 2.** These are signs of potential neurovascular compromise, an orthopedic emergency. Additionally, the nurse would check the capillary refill of the toes, any peripheral pulses present, and the sensation and mobility of the foot. In addition, the nurse would compare findings on the affected side with those on the nonaffected side.

**403. 4.** A vertical transfer is permitted, as long as manual traction is applied to maintain the "line of pull," that is, the direction of the traction, or "pull," which the balanced suspension device supplied.

**404. 1.** Rheumatoid arthritis is a condition with multisystem effects. The cardiopulmonary and renal systems must be assessed as well as the obvious assessment of the musculoskeletal system. Because some of the medications used in treating rheumatoid arthritis can have serious systemic effects (e.g., gold therapy, corticosteroids), this is especially true of the client on aggressive pharmacotherapy.

**405. 2.** Although this is an exacerbation of an existing problem, it is always appropriate to formulate a plan—with the client's input—as how best to meet his self-care needs. The plan will need to address protection of joints, conservation of energy, and methods to simplify work tasks. Correct use of assistive devices may also be involved in the plan.

**406. 3.** High dosage or long-term use of corticosteroids is associated with the development of gastric ulcers. Other adverse effects associated with this treatment include hypertension, hyperglycemia, infection susceptibility, and psychiatric disorders.

**407. 3.** Weight reduction can reduce stress on weight-bearing joints; because the client's physician has recommended it, we can believe that she will benefit from weight loss.

**408. 2.** Anti-inflammatory medications including salicylates and NSAIDs will be taken by the client indefinitely. The client must understand the regimen; ways to monitor for (and when possible, diminish) adverse effects must also be taught.

**409. 4.** Abnormal lung sounds are indicative of respiratory insufficiency from pleural effusions or infiltrations. Pleural effusions may occur with myocarditis, which might manifest as a pericardial friction rub assessed during the cardiovascular exam.

**410. 4.** Signs of gold toxicity include bone marrow suppression and hematuria, proteinuria, diarrhea, and stomatitis. The client receiving parenteral gold should expect to have blood and urine monitored after every other injection.

**411. 3.** Positive wound cultures are used to help determine the causative organisms and indicate which antibiotic therapy is appropriate. Blood cultures may also be positive.

**412. 3.** Diminished capillary refill suggests vascular compromise, an emergency condition.

**413. 2.** Neurovascular compromise is possible with fracture; distal pulses should be palpated to ensure circulation is adequate; the dorsalis pedis pulses in both feet should be assessed for comparison purposes. Likewise color, sensation, and mobility should be assessed. These interventions are also to be repeated at frequent intervals during the emergent phase, and especially after any intervention (i.e., splinting, casting).

**414. 1.** There is a strong risk of infection with an open fracture (a fracture with an open wound through skin surface to bone injury), and the nurse will expect the client to be given antibiotics prophylactically; in addition, tetanus immunization status must be assessed, and tetanus prophylaxis given if needed, or if the status cannot be determined.

**415. 3.** These are classic observations of the client with fat embolism syndrome, seen within 48 hours of a long-bone fracture. Onset of symptoms is rapid, and often fatal. Any respiratory difficulties, personality changes, or chest pain in clients with recent long-bone fractures must be assessed with fat embolism syndrome in mind.

**416. 3.** Positioning the client in extension and abduction helps to ensure that the femoral head part of the prosthesis remains in the acetabular cup. The use of wedge pillows or abduction splints helps in maintaining correct position.

**417. 4.** To maintain the femoral component of the prosthesis in the acetabular cup, an abductor pillow may be used to keep the legs separate; this must be maintained in all repositioning activities. The client is always encouraged to assist with repositioning, as long as the integrity of the hip position is maintained.

**418. 1.** The client will need to refrain from climbing stairs in the early recovery phase, except as guided during physical therapy sessions. Moving to the first floor is a prudent decision.

**419. 1.** Osteoporosis is a disorder in which bone formation is slower than bone resorption. The outcome of this disequilibrium is bones that are increasingly porous, brittle, and fragile. Any bone can be broken, but the trauma associated with falls frequently leads to hip fractures in clients with osteoporosis.

**420. 4.** Sometimes misinterpreted by the client as a heart attack or bursitis, pain with cervical disc herniation at this level may occur between the scapulae, in the neck or the top of the shoulders.

Stiffness, paresthesias, or numbness in upper extremities is also possible.

**421. 1.** The client is assessed for respiratory distress that would be caused by cord edema. The nurse would also look for signs of interstitial edema and/or hematoma.

**422. 2.** This position will maintain spinal alignment. Occasionally, the physician will approve the use of a pillow under the head, or the head of the bed raised 30° if a soft cervical collar is used, and if the surgical approach was posterior.

**423. 3.** When standing (for example, while washing dishes at the sink), the client should place one foot on a stool, thus alternating the weight between the feet.

**424. 2.** Because the bone graft used for fusion is taken from the iliac crest or fibula, the client will have pain and the potential for complications at those sites as well as complications from the laminectomy. Bed rest may be maintained for longer periods of time; lumbar support may be used once the client is ambulating, and pain relief must be directed at the graft site as well as the laminectomy site.

# The Endocrine System

## OVERVIEW OF ANATOMY AND PHYSIOLOGY

The endocrine system is composed of an interrelated complex of glands (pituitary, adrenals, thyroid, parathyroids, islets of Langerhans of the pancreas, ovaries, and testes) that secrete a variety of hormones directly into the bloodstream. Its major function, together with the nervous system, is to regulate body functions.

### Hormone Regulation

A. Hormones: chemical substances that act as messengers to specific cells and organs (target organs), stimulating and inhibiting various processes; two major categories
1. Local: hormones with specific effect in the area of secretion (e.g., secretin, cholecystokinin-pancreozymin [CCK-PZ])
2. General: hormones transported in the blood to distant sites where they exert their effect (e.g., cortisol)

B. Negative feedback mechanisms: major means of regulating hormone levels
1. Decreased concentration of a circulating hormone triggers production of a stimulating hormone from the pituitary gland; this hormone in turn stimulates its target organ to produce hormones.
2. Increased concentration of a hormone inhibits production of the stimulating hormone, resulting in decreased secretion of the target organ hormone.
C. Some hormones are controlled by changing blood levels of specific substances (e.g., calcium, glucose).
D. Certain hormones (e.g., cortisol or female reproductive hormones) follow rhythmic patterns of secretion.
E. Autonomic and CNS control (pituitary-hypothalamic axis): hypothalamus controls release of the hormones of the anterior pituitary gland through *releasing and inhibiting factors* that stimulate or inhibit hormone secretion.

# Structure and Function of Endocrine Glands

See Table 4-25 and Figure 4-25.

## Pituitary Gland (Hypophysis)

**A.** Located in sella turcica at the base of the brain
**B.** "Master gland" of the body, composed of three lobes

**1.** Anterior lobe (adenohypophysis)
    **a.** Secretes tropic hormones (hormones that stimulate target glands to produce their hormone): adrenocorticotropic hormone (ACTH), thyroid-stimulating hormone (TSH), follicle-stimulating hormone (FSH), luteinizing hormone (LH)
    **b.** Also secretes hormones that have direct effect on tissues: somatotropic or growth hormone, prolactin

**Table 4-25** Hormone Functions

| Endocrine Gland | Hormones | Functions |
|---|---|---|
| **Pituitary** | | |
| Anterior lobe | TSH | Stimulates thyroid gland to release thyroid hormones. |
| | ACTH | Stimulates adrenal cortex to produce and release adrenocorticoids. |
| | FSH, LH | Stimulate growth, maturation, and function of primary and secondary sex organs. |
| | GH or somatotropin | Stimulates growth of body tissues and bones. |
| Posterior lobe | Prolactin or LTH | Stimulates development of mammary glands and lactation. |
| | ADH | Regulates water metabolism; released during stress or in response to an increase in plasma osmolality to stimulate reabsorption of water and decrease urine output. |
| | Oxytocin | Stimulates uterine contractions during delivery and the release of milk in lactation. |
| Intermediate lobe | MSH | Affects skin pigmentation. |
| **Adrenal** | | |
| Adrenal cortex | Mineralocorticoids (e.g., aldosterone) | Regulate fluid and electrolyte balance; stimulate reabsorption of sodium, chloride, and water; stimulate potassium excretion. |
| | Glucocorticoids (e.g., cortisol, corticosterone) | Increase blood glucose levels by increasing rate of glyconeogenesis; increase protein catabolism, increase mobilization of fatty acids; promote sodium and water retention; anti-inflammatory effect; aid body in coping with stress. |
| | Sex hormones (androgens, estrogen, progesterone) | Influence development of secondary sex characteristics. |
| Adrenal medulla | Epinephrine, norepinephrine | Function in acute stress; increase heart rate, blood pressure; dilate bronchioles; convert glycogen to glucose when needed by muscles for energy. |
| **Thyroid** | $T_3$, $T_4$ | Regulate metabolic rate; carbohydrate, fat, and protein metabolism; aid in regulating physical and mental growth and development. |
| | Thyrocalcitonin | Lowers serum calcium by increasing bone deposition. |
| **Parathyroid** | PTH | Regulates serum calcium and phosphate levels. |
| **Pancreas (Islets of Langerhans)** | | |
| Beta cells | Insulin | Allows glucose to diffuse across cell membrane; converts glucose to glycogen. |
| Alpha cells | Glucagon | Increases blood glucose by causing glyconeogenesis and glycogenolysis in the liver; secreted in response to low blood sugar. |
| **Ovaries** | Estrogen, progesterone | Development of secondary sex characteristics in the female, maturation of sex organs, sexual functioning, maintenance of pregnancy. |
| **Testes** | Testosterone | Development of secondary sex characteristics in the male, maturation of sex organs, sexual functioning. |

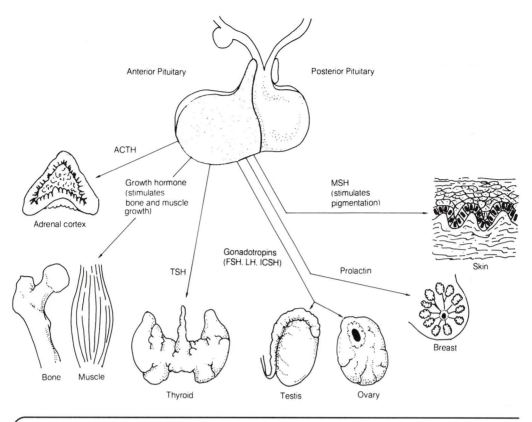

**Figure 4-25** Hormones secreted by the anterior pituitary gland

   **c.** Regulated by hypothalamic releasing and inhibiting factors and by negative feedback system
**2.** Posterior lobe (neurohypophysis): does not produce hormones; stores and releases antidiuretic hormone (ADH) and oxytocin, produced by the hypothalamus
**3.** Intermediate lobe: secretes melanocyte-stimulating hormone (MSH)

## Adrenal Glands

**A.** Two small glands, one above each kidney
**B.** Consist of two sections
   **1.** Adrenal cortex (outer portion): produces mineralocorticoids, glucocorticoids, sex hormones
   **2.** Adrenal medulla (inner portion): produces epinephrine, norepinephrine

## Thyroid Gland

**A.** Located in anterior portion of the neck
**B.** Consists of two lobes connected by a narrow isthmus
**C.** Produces thyroxine ($T_4$), triiodothyronine ($T_3$), thyrocalcitonin

## Parathyroid Glands

**A.** Four small glands located in pairs behind the thyroid gland
**B.** Produce parathormone (PTH)

## Pancreas

**A.** Located behind the stomach
**B.** Has both endocrine and exocrine functions (See Gastrointestinal System).
**C.** Islets of Langerhans (alpha and beta cells) involved in endocrine function
   **1.** Beta cells: produce insulin
   **2.** Alpha cells: produce glucagon

## Gonads

**A.** Ovaries: located in pelvic cavity, produce estrogen and progesterone
**B.** Testes: located in scrotum, produce testosterone

# ASSESSMENT

## Health History

**A.** Presenting problem: symptoms may include:
   **1.** Change in appearance: hair, nails, skin (change in texture or pigmentation); change in size, shape, or symmetry of head, neck, face, eyes, or tongue
   **2.** Change in energy level
   **3.** Temperature intolerance

4. Development of abnormal secondary sexual characteristics; change in sexual function
5. Change in emotional state, thought pattern, or intellectual functioning
6. Signs of increased activity of sympathetic nervous system (e.g., nervousness, palpitations, tremors, sweating)
7. Change in bowel habits, appetite, or weight; excessive hunger or thirst
8. Change in urinary pattern
B. Lifestyle: any increased stress
C. Past medical history: growth and development (any delayed or excessive growth); diabetes, thyroid disease, hypertension, obesity, infertility
D. Family history: endocrine diseases, growth problems, obesity, mental illness

## Physical Examination

A. Check height, weight, body stature, and body proportions.
B. Observe distribution of muscle mass, fat distribution, any muscle wasting.
C. Inspect for hair growth and distribution.
D. Check condition and pigmentation of skin; presence of striae.
E. Inspect eyes for any bulging.
F. Observe for enlargement in neck area and quality of voice.
G. Observe development of secondary sex characteristics.
H. Palpate thyroid gland (normally cannot be palpated): note size, shape, symmetry, any tenderness, presence of any lumps or nodules.

## Laboratory/Diagnostic Tests

A variety of tests may be performed to measure the amounts of hormones present in the serum or urine in assessing pituitary, adrenal, and parathyroid functions; these tests will be referred to when appropriate under specific disorders of the endocrine system.

### Thyroid Function

A. Serum studies: nonfasting blood studies (no special preparation necessary)
   1. Serum $T_4$ level: measures total serum level of thyroxine
   2. Serum $T_3$ level: measures serum triiodothyronine level
   3. TSH: measurement differentiates primary from secondary hypothyroidism
B. Radioactive iodine uptake (RAIU)
   1. Administration of $^{123}$I or $^{131}$I orally; measurement by a counter of the amount of radioactive iodine taken up by the gland after 24 hours
   2. Performed to determine thyroid function; increased uptake indicates hyperactivity; minimal uptake may indicate hypothyroidism

3. Nursing care
   a. Take thorough history; thyroid medication must be discontinued 7–10 days prior to test; medications containing iodine, cough preparations, excess intake of iodine-rich foods, and tests using iodine (e.g., IVP) can invalidate this test.
   b. Assure client that no radiation precautions are necessary.
C. Thyroid scan
   1. Administration of radioactive isotope (orally or IV) and visualization by a scanner of the distribution of radioactivity in the gland
   2. Performed to determine location, size, shape, and anatomic function of thyroid gland; identifies areas of increased or decreased uptake; valuable in evaluating thyroid nodules
   3. Nursing care: same as RAIU

### Pancreatic Function

A. Fasting blood sugar: measures serum glucose levels; client fasts from midnight before the test
B. Two-hour postprandial blood sugar: measurement of blood glucose 2 hours after a meal is ingested
   1. Fast from midnight before test
   2. Client eats a meal consisting of at least 75 g carbohydrate or ingests 100 g glucose
   3. Blood drawn 2 hours after the meal
C. Oral glucose tolerance test: most specific and sensitive test for diabetes mellitus
   1. Fast from midnight before test
   2. Fasting blood glucose and urine glucose specimens obtained
   3. Client ingests 100 g glucose; blood sugars are drawn at 30 and 60 minutes and then hourly for 3–5 hours; urine specimens may also be collected
   4. Diet for 3 days prior to test should include 200 g carbohydrate and at least 1500 kcal/day
   5. During test, assess the client for reactions such as dizziness, sweating, and weakness
D. Glycosylated hemoglobin (hemoglobin A1c) reflects the average blood sugar level for the previous 100–120 days. Glucose attaches to a minor hemoglobin (A1c). This attachment is irreversible.
   1. Fasting is not necessary.
   2. Excellent method to evaluate long-term control of blood sugar.

## ANALYSIS

Nursing diagnoses for the client with a disorder of the endocrine system may include:
A. Imbalanced nutrition: more or less than body requirements
B. Risk for infection
C. Impaired urinary elimination
D. Deficient fluid volume

E. Risk for impaired skin integrity
F. Sexual dysfunction
G. Deficient knowledge
H. Ineffective individual coping
I. Disturbed sleep pattern
J. Disturbed body image

# PLANNING AND IMPLEMENTATION

## Goals

Client will:
A. Regain optimal nutritional status.
B. Be free from infection.
C. Have adequate urinary elimination and fluid volume.
D. Maintain skin integrity.
E. Experience optimum sexual health.
F. Demonstrate and use knowledge of disease process, prescribed medications, treatments, and complications in order to maintain optimal health.
G. Use positive coping behaviors in dealing with the effects of acute and chronic illness.
H. Attain an optimal balance of rest and activity.

## Interventions

### Care of the Client on Corticosteroid Therapy

A. General information
   1. Types of preparations include cortisone, hydrocortisone, prednisone, dexamethasone (Decadron)
   2. Indications
      a. Replacement therapy in primary and secondary adrenocortical insufficiency
      b. Symptomatic treatment for anti-inflammatory effect of numerous inflammatory, allergic, or immunoreactive disorders (e.g., arthritis, SLE, bronchial asthma, skin diseases, ocular disorders, allergic diseases, inflammatory bowel disorders, cerebral edema and increased ICP, shock, nephrotic syndrome, malignancies, myasthenia gravis, multiple sclerosis)
   3. Common side effects: salt and water retention, sweating, increased appetite
   4. Adverse reactions
      a. Cardiovascular: hypertension, CHF
      b. GI: peptic ulcer, ulcerative esophagitis
      c. Integumentary: petechiae, ecchymoses, purpura, hirsutism, acne, thinning of skin, striae, redistribution of body fat in subcutaneous tissue, abnormal pigmentation, poor wound healing
      d. Endocrine: impaired glucose metabolism, hyperglycemia, menstrual dysfunction, growth retardation
      e. Musculoskeletal: muscle weakness, osteoporosis
      f. Neurologic: personality changes, headache, syncope, vertigo, irritability, insomnia, seizures
      g. Ophthalmologic: cataract formation, glaucoma
      h. Other: hypokalemia, thrombophlebitis, masking of signs of infection, increased susceptibility to infection
      i. Sudden withdrawal may precipitate acute adrenal insufficiency
B. Nursing care
   1. Administer with food or milk; instruct client to report gastric distress (antacids may be necessary).
   2. Give in a single daily dose, preferably before 9 A.M. (cortisol level is at highest peak between 6 and 8 A.M.).
   3. Instruct client to avoid infections and to report immediately if one is suspected.
   4. Instruct client never to withdraw the drug abruptly, as this may cause acute adrenal insufficiency.
   5. Observe client for any mental changes (e.g., irritability, mood swings, euphoria, depression).
   6. Alert women that menstrual irregularity may develop.
   7. Monitor blood pressure, I&O, weight, blood glucose, and serum potassium.
   8. Advise client to restrict salt intake.
   9. Encourage intake of foods high in potassium.

# EVALUATION

A. Client maintains normal weight; no evidence of malnutrition.
B. Client's temperature is within normal limits; no signs of infection.
C. Client has adequate patterns of urinary elimination.
D. Peripheral edema is reduced.
E. Blood pressure and urine output are within normal limits; no signs of dehydration.
F. Skin is intact and free from irritation.
G. Client verbalizes satisfying sexual activity/expression.
H. Client demonstrates and uses knowledge of disease process, prescribed medications, and treatments; reports any complications.
I. Client uses effective coping behaviors to successfully adapt to effects of illness, changes in body image, and loss of function.
J. Client maintains balance between activity and rest.
K. Client demonstrates increased self-esteem.

# DISORDERS OF THE ENDOCRINE SYSTEM

## Specific Disorders of the Pituitary Gland

### Hypopituitarism

A. General information
1. Hypofunction of the anterior pituitary gland resulting in deficiencies of both the hormones secreted by the anterior pituitary gland and those secreted by the target glands
2. May be caused by tumor, trauma, surgical removal, or irradiation of the gland; or may be congenital (pituitary dwarfism)

B. Medical management: specific treatment depends on cause
1. Tumor: surgical removal or irradiation of the gland
2. Regardless of cause, treatment will include replacement of deficient hormones: e.g., corticosteroids, thyroid hormone, sex hormones, gonadotropins (may be used to restore fertility).

C. Assessment findings
1. Tumor: bitemporal hemianopia, headache
2. Varying signs of hormonal disturbances depending on which hormones are being undersecreted (e.g., menstrual dysfunction, hypothyroidism, adrenal insufficiency)
3. Retardation of growth if condition occurs before epiphyseal closure
4. Diagnostic tests
   a. Skull X-ray, CT scan may reveal pituitary tumor
   b. Plasma hormone levels may be decreased depending on specific hormones undersecreted

D. Nursing interventions
1. Provide care for the client undergoing hypophysectomy or radiation therapy if indicated.
2. Provide client teaching and discharge planning concerning:
   a. Hormone replacement therapy
   b. Importance of follow-up care

### Hyperpituitarism

A. General information
1. Hyperfunction of the anterior pituitary gland resulting in oversecretion of one or more of the anterior pituitary hormones
2. Overproduction of the growth hormone produces acromegaly in adults and gigantism in children (if hypersecretion occurs before epiphyseal closure).
3. Usually caused by a benign pituitary adenoma

B. Medical management: surgical removal or irradiation of the gland

C. Assessment findings
1. Tumor: bitemporal hemianopia; headache
2. Hormonal disturbances depending on which hormones are being excreted in excess
3. Acromegaly caused by oversecretion of growth hormones: transverse enlargement of bones, especially noticeable in skull and in bones of hands and feet; features become coarse and heavy; lips become heavier; tongue enlarged
4. Diagnostic tests
   a. Skull X-ray, CT scan reveal pituitary tumor
   b. Plasma hormone levels reveal increased growth hormone, oversecretion of other hormones

D. Nursing interventions
1. Monitor for hyperglycemia and cardiovascular problems (hypertension, angina, HF) and modify care accordingly.
2. Provide psychologic support and acceptance for alterations in body image.
3. Provide care for the client undergoing hypophysectomy or radiation therapy if indicated.

### Hypophysectomy

A. General information
1. Partial or complete removal of the pituitary gland
2. Indications: pituitary tumors, diabetic retinopathy, metastatic cancer of the breast or prostate, which may be endocrine dependent
3. Surgical approaches
   a. Craniotomy: usually transfrontal
   b. Transphenoidal: incision made in inner aspect of upper lip and gingiva; sella turcica is entered through the floor of the nose and sphenoid sinuses

B. Nursing care
1. In addition to pre-op care of the craniotomy client, explain post-op expectations.
2. In addition to post-op care of the craniotomy client, observe for signs of target gland deficiencies (diabetes insipidus, adrenal insufficiency, hypothyroidism) due to total removal of the gland or to post-op edema.
   a. Perform hourly urine outputs and specific gravities; alert physician if urine output is greater than 800–900 mL/2 hours or if specific gravity is less than 1.004.
   b. Administer cortisone replacement as ordered.
3. If transphenoidal approach used:
   a. Elevate the head of the bed to 30° to decrease headache and pressure on the sella turcica.
   b. Administer mild analgesics for headache as ordered.

c. Perform frequent oral hygiene with soft swabs to cleanse the teeth and mouth rinses; no toothbrushing.
d. Observe for and prevent CSF leak from surgical site.
   1) Warn the client not to cough, sneeze, or blow nose.
   2) Observe for clear drainage from nose or postnasal drip (constant swallowing); check drainage for glucose; positive results indicate that drainage is CSF.
   3) If leakage does occur:
      a) Elevate head of bed and call the physician.
      b) Most leaks will resolve in 72 hours with bed rest and elevation.
      c) May do daily spinal taps to decrease CSF pressure.
      d) Administer antibiotics as ordered to prevent meningitis.
4. Provide client teaching and discharge planning concerning:
   a. Hormone therapy
      1) If gland is completely removed, client will have permanent diabetes insipidus
      2) Cortisone and thyroid hormone replacement
      3) Replacement of sex hormones
         a) Testosterone: may be given for impotence in men
         b) Estrogen: may be given for atropy of the vaginal mucosa in women
         c) Human pituitary gonadotropins: may restore fertility in some women
   b. Need for lifelong follow-up and hormone replacement
   c. Need to wear Medic-Alert bracelet
   d. If transphenoidal approach was used:
      1) Avoid bending and straining at stool for 2 months post-op
      2) No toothbrushing until sutures are removed and incision heals (about 10 days)

## Diabetes Insipidus

A. General information
   1. Hypofunction of the posterior pituitary gland resulting in deficiency of ADH
   2. Characterized by excessive thirst and urination
   3. Caused by tumor, trauma, inflammation, pituitary surgery
B. Assessment findings
   1. Polydipsia (excessive thirst) and severe polyuria with low specific gravity
   2. Fatigue, muscle weakness, irritability, weight loss, signs of dehydration

3. Tachycardia, eventual shock if fluids not replaced
4. Diagnostic tests
   a. Urine specific gravity less than 1.004
   b. Water deprivation test reveals inability to concentrate urine
C. Nursing interventions
   1. Maintain fluid and electrolyte balance.
      a. Keep accurate I&O.
      b. Weigh daily.
      c. Administer IV/oral fluids as ordered to replace fluid losses.
   2. Monitor vital signs and observe for signs of dehydration and hypovolemia.
   3. Administer hormone replacement as ordered.
      a. Vasopressin (Pitressin) given IV and SC; desmopressin, given PO or intranasal.
         1) Warm to body temperature before giving.
         2) Shake tannate suspension to ensure uniform dispersion.
      b. Lypressin (Diapid): nasal spray
   4. Provide client teaching and discharge planning concerning:
      a. Lifelong hormone replacement; lypressin as needed to control polyuria and polydipsia
      b. Need to wear Medic-Alert bracelet

## Syndrome of Inappropriate Antidiuretic Hormone Secretion (SIADH)

A. General information
   1. Hypersection of ADH from the posterior pituitary gland even when the client has abnormal serum osmolality.
   2. SIADH may occur in persons with bronchogenic carcinoma or other nonendocrine conditions.
B. Medical management
   1. Treat underlying cause if possible
   2. Diuretics and fluid restriction
C. Assessment findings
   1. Persons with SIADH cannot excrete a dilute urine
   2. Fluid retention and sodium deficiency.
D. Nursing interventions
   1. Administer diuretics (furosemide [Lasix]) as ordered.
   2. Restrict fluids to promote fluid loss and gradual increase in serum sodium.
   3. Monitor serum electrolytes and blood chemistries carefully.
   4. Careful intake and output, daily weight.
   5. Monitor neurologic status.

# Disorders of the Adrenal Gland
## Addison's Disease

A. General information
   1. Primary adrenocortical insufficiency; hypofunction of the adrenal cortex causes

decreased secretion of the mineralocorticoids, glucocorticoids, and sex hormones

2. Relatively rare disease caused by:
   a. Idiopathic atrophy of the adrenal cortex possibly due to an autoimmune process
   b. Destruction of the gland secondary to tuberculosis (rare, due to early TB treatment available) or fungal infection

B. Assessment findings
   1. Fatigue, muscle weakness
   2. Anorexia, nausea, vomiting, abdominal pain, weight loss
   3. History of frequent hypoglycemic reactions
   4. Hypotension, weak pulse
   5. Bronzelike pigmentation of the skin
   6. Decreased capacity to deal with stress
   7. Diagnostic tests: low cortisol levels, hyponatremia, hyperkalemia, hypoglycemia

C. Nursing interventions
   1. Administer hormone replacement therapy as ordered.
      a. Glucocorticoids (cortisone, hydrocortisone): to stimulate diurnal rhythm of cortisol release, give ⅔ of dose in early morning and ⅓ of dose in afternoon
      b. Mineralocorticoids: fludrocortisone acetate (Florinef)
   2. Monitor vital signs.
   3. Decrease stress in the environment.
   4. Prevent exposure to infection.
   5. Provide rest periods; prevent fatigue.
   6. Monitor I&O.
   7. Weigh daily.
   8. Provide small, frequent feedings of diet high in carbohydrates, sodium, and protein to prevent hypoglycemia and hyponatremia and to provide proper nutrition.
   9. Provide client teaching and discharge planning concerning:
      a. Disease process; signs of adrenal insufficiency
      b. Use of prescribed medications for lifelong replacement therapy; never omit medications
      c. Need to avoid stress, trauma, and infections, and to notify physician if these occur as medication dosage may need to be adjusted
      d. Stress management techniques
      e. Diet modification (high in protein, carbohydrates, and sodium)
      f. Use of salt tablets (if prescribed) or ingestion of salty foods (potato chips) if experiencing increased sweating
      g. Importance of alternating regular exercise with rest periods
      h. Avoidance of strenuous exercise especially in hot weather

*Addisonian Crisis*

A. General information
   1. Severe exacerbation of Addison's disease caused by acute adrenal insufficiency
   2. Precipitating factors
      a. Overexertion, infection, trauma, stess, failure to take prescribed medications
      b. Iatrogenic: surgery on pituitary or adrenal glands, rapid withdrawal of exogenous steroids in a client on long-term steroid therapy

B. Assessment findings: severe generalized muscle weakness, severe hypotension, hypovolemia, shock (vascular collapse)

C. Nursing interventions
   1. Administer IV fluids (5% dextrose in saline, plasma) as ordered to treat vascular collapse.
   2. Administer IV glucocorticoids (hydrocortisone [Solu-Cortef]) and vasopressors as ordered.
   3. If crisis precipitated by infection, administer antibiotics as ordered.
   4. Maintain strict bed rest and eliminate all forms of stressful stimuli.
   5. Monitor vital signs, I&O, daily weights.
   6. Protect client from infection.
   7. Provide client teaching and discharge planning: same as for Addison's disease.

## Cushing's Syndrome

A. General information
   1. Condition resulting from excessive secretion of corticosteroids, particularly the glucocorticoid cortisol
   2. Occurs most frequently in females between ages 30–60
   3. Primary Cushing's syndrome caused by adrenocortical tumors or hyperplasia
   4. Secondary Cushing's syndrome (also called Cushing's disease): caused by functioning pituitary or nonpituitary neoplasm secreting ACTH, causing increased secretion of glucocorticoids
   5. Iatrogenic: caused by prolonged use of corticosteroids

B. Assessment findings
   1. Muscle weakness, fatigue, obese trunk with thin arms and legs, muscle wasting
   2. Irritability, depression, frequent mood swings
   3. Moon face, buffalo hump, pendulous abdomen
   4. Purple striae on trunk, acne, thin skin
   5. Signs of masculinization in women; menstrual dysfunction, decreased libido
   6. Osteoporosis, decreased resistance to infection
   7. Hypertension, edema
   8. Diagnostic tests: cortisol levels increased, slight hypernatremia, hypokalemia, hyperglycemia

C. Nursing interventions
   1. Maintain muscle tone.
      a. Provide ROM exercises.
      b. Assist with ambulation.
   2. Prevent accidents or falls and provide adequate rest.
   3. Protect client from exposure to infection.
   4. Maintain skin integrity.
      a. Provide meticulous skin care.
      b. Prevent tearing of skin: use paper tape if necessary.
   5. Minimize stress in the environment.
   6. Monitor vital signs; observe for hypertension, edema.
   7. Measure I&O and daily weights.
   8. Provide diet low in calories and sodium and high in protein, potassium, calcium, and vitamin D.
   9. Monitor urine for glucose and acetone; administer insulin if ordered.
   10. Provide psychologic support and acceptance.
   11. Prepare client for hypophysectomy or radiation if condition is caused by a pituitary tumor.
   12. Prepare client for an adrenalectomy if condition is caused by an adrenal tumor or hyperplasia.
   13. Provide client teaching and discharge planning concerning:
      a. Diet modifications
      b. Importance of adequate rest
      c. Need to avoid stress and infection
      d. Change in medication regimen (alternate day therapy or reduced dosage) if cause of the condition is prolonged corticosteroid therapy

## Primary Aldosteronism (Conn's Syndrome)

A. General information
   1. Excessive aldosterone secretion from the adrenal cortex
   2. Seen more frequently in women, usually between ages 30–50
   3. Caused by tumor or hyperplasia of adrenal gland
B. Assessment findings
   1. Headache, hypertension
   2. Muscle weakness, polyuria, polydipsia, metabolic alkalosis, cardiac arrhythmias (due to hypokalemia)
   3. Diagnostic tests
      a. Serum potassium decreased, alkalosis
      b. Urinary aldosterone levels elevated
C. Nursing interventions
   1. Monitor vital signs, I&O, daily weights.
   2. Maintain sodium restriction as ordered.
   3. Administer spironolactone (Aldactone) and potassium supplements as ordered.
   4. Prepare the client for an adrenelectomy if indicated.

   5. Provide client teaching and discharge planning concerning
      a. Use and side effects of medication if the client is being maintained on spironolactone therapy
      b. Signs of symptoms of hypo/hyperaldosteronism
      c. Need for frequent blood pressure checks and follow-up care

## Pheochromocytoma

A. General information
   1. Functioning tumor of the adrenal medulla that secretes excessive amounts of epinephrine and norepinephrine
   2. Occurs most commonly between ages 25–50
   3. May be hereditary in some cases
B. Assessment findings
   1. Severe headache, apprehension, palpitations, profuse sweating, nausea
   2. Hypertension, tachycardia, vomiting, hyperglycemia, dilation of pupils, cold extremities
   3. Diagnostic tests
      a. Increased plasma levels of catecholamines; elevated blood sugar; glycosuria
      b. Elevated urinary catecholamines and urinary vanillylmandelic acid (VMA) levels
      c. Presence of tumor on X-ray
C. Nursing interventions
   1. Monitor vital signs, especially blood pressure.
   2. Administer medications as ordered to control hypertension.
   3. Promote rest; decrease stressful stimuli.
   4. Monitor urine tests for glucose and acetone.
   5. Provide high-calorie, well-balanced diet; avoid stimulants such as coffee, tea.
   6. Provide care for the client with an adrenalectomy as ordered; observe postadrenelectomy client carefully for shock due to drastic drop in catecholamine level.
   7. Provide client teaching and discharge planning: same as for adrenalectomy.

## Adrenalectomy

A. General information
   1. Removal of one or both adrenal glands
   2. Indications
      a. Tumors of adrenal cortex (Cushing's syndrome, hyperaldosteronism) or medulla (pheochromocytoma)
      b. Metastatic cancer of the breast or prostate
B. Nursing interventions: preoperative
   1. Provide routine pre-op care.
   2. Correct metabolic/cardiovascular problems.
      a. Pheochromocytoma: stabilize blood pressure.

b. Cushing's syndrome: treat hyperglycemia and protein deficits.
c. Primary hyperaldosteronism: treat hypertension and hypokalemia.
3. Administer glucocorticoid preparation on the morning of surgery as ordered to prevent acute adrenal insufficiency.

C. Nursing interventions: postoperative
1. Provide routine post-op care.
2. Observe for hemorrhage and shock.
a. Monitor vital signs, I&O.
b. Administer IV therapy and vasopressors as ordered.
3. Prevent infections (suppression of immune system makes clients especially susceptible).
a. Encourage coughing and deep breathing to prevent respiratory infection.
b. Use meticulous aseptic technique during dressing changes.
4. Administer cortisone or hydrocortisone as ordered to maintain cortisol levels.
5. Provide general care for the client with abdominal surgery.

D. Provide client teaching and discharge planning concerning:
1. Self-administration of replacement hormones
a. Bilateral adrenalectomy: lifelong replacement of glucocorticoids and mineralocorticoids
b. Unilateral adrenalectomy: replacement therapy for 6–12 months until the remaining adrenal gland begins to function normally
2. Signs and symptoms of adrenal insufficiency
3. Importance of follow-up care

# Specific Disorders of the Thyroid Gland
## Simple Goiter

A. General information
1. Enlargement of the thyroid gland not caused by inflammation or neoplasm
2. Types
a. Endemic: caused by nutritional iodine deficiency, most common in the "goiter belt" (midwest, northwest, and Great Lakes regions), areas where soil and water are deficient in iodine; occurs most frequently during adolescence and pregnancy
b. Sporadic: caused by:
1) Ingestion of large amounts of goitrogenic foods (contain agents that decrease thyroxine production): e.g., cabbage, soybeans, rutabagas, peanuts, peaches, peas, strawberries, spinach, radishes
2) Use of goitrogenic drugs: propylthiouracil, large doses of iodine, phenylbutazone, para-amino salicylic acid, cobalt, lithium

3) Genetic defects that prevent synthesis of thyroid hormone
3. Low levels of thyroid hormone stimulate increased secretion of TSH by pituitary; under TSH stimulation the thyroid increases in size to compensate and produces more thyroid hormone.

B. Medical management
1. Drug therapy
a. Hormone replacement with levothyroxine (Synthroid) ($T_4$), dessicated thyroid, or liothyronine (Cytomel) ($T_3$)
b. Small doses of iodine (Lugol's or potassium iodide solution) for goiter resulting from iodine deficiency
2. Avoidance of goitrogenic foods or drugs in sporadic goiter
3. Surgery: subtotal thyroidectomy (if goiter is large) to relieve pressure symptoms and for cosmetic reasons

C. Assessment findings
1. Dysphagia, enlarged thyroid, respiratory distress
2. Diagnostic tests
a. Serum $T_4$ level low-normal or normal
b. RAIU uptake normal or increased

D. Nursing interventions
1. Administer replacement therapy as ordered.
2. Provide care for client with subtotal thyroidectomy if indicated.
3. Provide client teaching and discharge planning concerning
a. Use of iodized salt in preventing and treating endemic goiter
b. Thyroid hormone replacement

## Hypothyroidism (Myxedema)

A. General information
1. Slowing of metabolic processes caused by hypofunction of the thyroid gland with decreased thyroid hormone secretion; causes myxedema in adults and cretinism in children.
2. Occurs more often in women between ages 30 and 60
3. Primary hypothyroidism: atrophy of the gland possibly caused by an autoimmune process
4. Secondary hypothyroidism: caused by decreased stimulation from pituitary TSH
5. Iatrogenic: surgical removal of the gland or overtreatment of hyperthyroidism with drugs or radioactive iodine
6. In severe or untreated cases, myxedema coma may occur
a. Characterized by intensification of signs and symptoms of hypothyroidism and neurologic impairment leading to coma
b. Mortality rate high; prompt recognition and treatment essential

    c. Precipitating factors: failure to take prescribed medications; infection; trauma, exposure to cold; use of sedatives, narcotics, or anesthetics

B. Medical management
  1. Drug therapy: levothyroxine (Synthroid), thyroglobulin (Proloid), dessicated thyroid, liothyronine (Cytomel)
  2. Myxedema coma is a medical emergency.
    a. IV thyroid hormones
    b. Correction of hypothermia
    c. Maintenance of vital functions
    d. Treatment of precipitating causes

C. Assessment findings
  1. Fatigue; lethargy; slowed mental processes; dull look; slow, clumsy movements
  2. Anorexia, weight gain, constipation
  3. Intolerance to cold; dry, scaly skin; dry, sparse hair; brittle nails
  4. Menstrual irregularities; generalized interstitial nonpitting edema
  5. Bradycardia, cardiac complications (CAD, angina pectoris, MI, CHF)
  6. Increased sensitivity to sedatives, narcotics, and anesthetics
  7. Exaggeration of these findings in myxedema coma: weakness, lethargy, syncope, bradycardia, hypotension, hypoventilation, subnormal body temperature
  8. Diagnostic tests
    a. Serum $T_3$ and $T_4$ level low
    b. Serum cholesterol level elevated
    c. RAIU decreased

D. Nursing interventions
  1. Monitor vital signs, I&O, daily weights; observe for edema and signs of cardiovascular complications.
  2. Administer thyroid hormone replacement therapy as ordered and monitor effects.
    a. Observe for signs of thyrotoxicosis (tachycardia, palpitations, nausea, vomiting, diarrhea, sweating, tremors, agitation, dyspnea).
    b. Increase dosage gradually, especially in clients with cardiac complications.
  3. Provide a comfortable, warm environment.
  4. Provide a low-calorie diet.
  5. Avoid the use of sedatives; reduce the dose of any sedative, narcotic, or anesthetic agent by half as ordered.
  6. Institute measures to prevent skin breakdown.
  7. Provide increased fluids and foods high in fiber to prevent constipation; administer stool softeners as ordered.
  8. Observe for signs of myxedema coma; provide appropriate nursing care.
    a. Administer medications as ordered.
    b. Maintain vital functions: correct hypothermia, maintain adequate ventilation.

  9. Provide client teaching and discharge planning concerning:
    a. Thyroid hormone replacement
      1) Take daily dose in the morning to prevent insomnia.
      2) Self-monitor for signs of thyrotoxicosis.
    b. Importance of regular follow-up care
    c. Need for additional protection in cold weather
    d. Measures to prevent constipation

## Hyperthyroidism (Graves' Disease)

A. General information
  1. Secretion of excessive amounts of thyroid hormone in the blood causes an increase in metabolic processes
  2. Overactivity and changes in the thyroid gland may be present
  3. Most often seen in women between ages 30–50
  4. Cause unknown, but may be an autoimmune process
  5. Symptomatic hyperthyroidism may also be called thyrotoxicosis

B. Medical management
  1. Drug therapy
    a. Antithyroid drugs (propylthiouracil and methimazole ([Tapazole]): block synthesis of thyroid hormone; toxic effects include agranulocytosis
    b. Adrenergic blocking agents (commonly propranolol [Inderal]): used to decrease sympathetic activity and alleviate symptoms such as tachycardia
  2. Radioactive iodine therapy
    a. Radioactive isotope of iodine (e.g., $^{131}$I) given to destroy the thyroid gland, thereby decreasing production of thyroid hormone
    b. Used in middle-aged or older clients who are resistant to, or develop toxicity from, drug therapy
    c. Hypothyroidism is a potential complication
  3. Surgery: thyroidectomy performed in younger clients for whom drug therapy has not been effective

C. Assessment findings
  1. Irritability, agitation, restlessness, hyperactive movements, tremor, sweating, insomnia
  2. Increased appetite, hyperphagia, weight loss, diarrhea, intolerance to heat
  3. Exophthalmos (protrusion of the eyeballs), goiter
  4. Warm, smooth skin; fine, soft hair; pliable nails
  5. Tachycardia, increased systolic blood pressure, palpitations
  6. Diagnostic tests
    a. Serum $T_3$ and $T_4$ levels elevated
    b. RAIU increased

D. Nursing interventions
  1. Monitor vital signs, daily weights.
  2. Administer antithyroid medications as ordered.
  3. Provide for periods of uninterrupted rest.
     a. Assign to a private room away from excessive activity.
     b. Administer medications to promote sleep as ordered.
  4. Provide a cool environment.
  5. Minimize stress in the environment.
  6. Encourage quiet, relaxing diversional activities.
  7. Provide a diet high in carbohydrates, protein, calories, vitamins, and minerals with supplemental feedings between meals and at bedtime; omit stimulants.
  8. Observe for and prevent complications.
     a. Exophthalmos: protect eyes with dark glasses and artificial tears as ordered.
     b. Thyroid storm: see Thyroid Storm.
  9. Provide client teaching and discharge planning concerning:
     a. Need to recognize and report signs and symptoms of agranulocytosis (fever, sore throat, skin rash) if taking antithyroid drugs
     b. Signs and symptoms of hyper/hypothyroidism

## Thyroid Storm

A. General information
  1. Uncontrolled and potentially life-threatening hyperthyroidism caused by sudden and excessive release of thyroid hormone into the bloodstream
  2. Precipitating factors: stress, infection, unprepared thyroid surgery
  3. Now quite rare
B. Assessment findings
  1. Apprehension, restlessness
  2. Extremely high temperature (up to 106°F [40.7°C]), tachycardia, HF, respiratory distress, delirium, coma
C. Nursing interventions (see also Hyperthermia)
  1. Maintain a patent airway and adequate ventilation; administer oxygen as ordered.
  2. Administer IV therapy as ordered.
  3. Administer medications as ordered: antithyroid drugs, corticosteroids, sedatives, cardiac drugs.

## Thyroidectomy

A. General information
  1. Partial or total removal of the thyroid gland
  2. Indications
     a. Subtotal thyroidectomy: hyperthyroidism
     b. Total thyroidectomy: thyroid cancer

B. Nursing interventions: preoperative
  1. Ensure that the client is adequately prepared for surgery.
     a. Cardiac status is stable.
     b. Weight and nutritional status are normal.
  2. Administer antithyroid drugs as ordered to suppress the production and secretion of thyroid hormone and to prevent thyroid storm.
  3. Administer iodine preparations (Lugol's or potassium iodide solution) to reduce the size and vascularity of the gland and prevent hemorrhage.
C. Nursing interventions: postoperative
  1. Monitor vital signs and I&O.
  2. Check dressings for signs of hemorrhage; check for wetness behind neck.
  3. Place client in semi-Fowler's position and support head with pillows.
  4. Observe for respiratory distress secondary to hemorrhage, edema of the glottis, laryngeal nerve damage, or tetany; keep tracheostomy set, oxygen, and suction nearby.
  5. Assess for signs of tetany due to hypocalcemia secondary to accidental removal of parathyroid glands; keep calcium gluconate available (see Hypoparathyroidism).
  6. Encourage the client to rest voice.
     a. Some hoarseness is common.
     b. Check every 30–60 minutes for extreme hoarseness or any accompanying respiratory distress.
  7. Observe for thyroid storm due to release of excessive amounts of thyroid hormone during surgery.
  8. Administer IV fluids as ordered until the client is tolerating fluids by mouth.
  9. Administer analgesics as ordered for incisional pain.
  10. Relieve discomfort from sore throat.
     a. Cool mist humidifier to thin secretions.
     b. Administer analgesic throat lozenges before meals and prn as ordered.
     c. Encourage fluids.
  11. Encourage coughing and deep breathing every hour.
  12. Assist the client with ambulation: instruct the client to place hands behind neck to decrease stress on suture line if added support necessary.
  13. Provide client teaching and discharge planning concerning:
     a. Signs and symptoms of hypo/hyperthyroidism
     b. Self-administration of thyroid hormones if total thyroidectomy performed
     c. Application of lubricant to the incision once sutures are removed
     d. Performance of ROM neck exercises 3–4 times a day
     e. Importance of regular follow-up care

# Specific Disorders of the Parathyroid Glands

## Hypoparathyroidism

A. General information
1. Disorder characterized by hypocalcemia resulting from a deficiency of parathormone (PTH) production
2. May be hereditary, idiopathic, or caused by accidental damage to or removal of parathyroid glands during surgery, e.g., thyroidectomy

B. Assessment findings
1. Acute hypocalcemia (tetany)
    a. Tingling of fingers and around lips, painful muscle spasms, dysphagia, laryngospasm, seizures, cardiac arrhythmias
    b. Chvostek's sign: sharp tapping over facial nerve causes twitching of mouth, nose, and eye
    c. Trousseau's sign: carpopedal spasm induced by application of blood pressure cuff for 3 minutes
2. Chronic hypocalcemia
    a. Fatigue, weakness, muscle cramps
    b. Personality changes, irritability, memory impairment
    c. Dry, scaly skin; hair loss; loss of tooth enamel
    d. Tremor, cardiac arrhythmias, cataract formation
    e. Diagnostic tests
        1) Serum calcium levels decreased
        2) Serum phosphate levels elevated
        3) Skeletal X-rays reveal increased bone density

C. Nursing interventions
1. Administer calcium gluconate by slow IV drip as ordered for acute hypocalcemia.
2. Administer medications for chronic hypocalcemia.
    a. Oral calcium preparations: calcium gluconate, lactate, carbonate (Os-Cal)
    b. Large doses of vitamin D (Calciferol) to help absorption of calcium
    c. Aluminum hydroxide gel (Amphogel) or aluminum carbonate gel, basic (Basaljel) to decrease phosphate levels
3. Institute seizure and safety precautions.
4. Provide quiet environment free from excessive stimuli.
5. Monitor for signs of hoarseness or stridor; check for Chvostek's and Trousseau's signs.
6. Keep emergency equipment (tracheostomy set, injectable calcium gluconate) at bedside.
7. For tetany or generalized muscle cramps, may use rebreathing bag to produce mild respiratory acidosis.
8. Monitor serum calcium and phosphate levels.
9. Provide high-calcium, low-phosphorus diet; milk and egg yolks are restricted because of high levels of phosphorus.
10. Provide client teaching and discharge planning concerning:
    a. Medication regimen; oral calcium preparations and vitamin D to be taken with meals to increase absorption
    b. Need to recognize and report signs and symptoms of hypo/hypercalcemia
    c. Importance of follow-up care with periodic serum calcium levels

## Hyperparathyroidism

A. General information
1. Increased secretion of PTH that results in an altered state of calcium, phosphate, and bone metabolism
2. Most commonly affects women between ages 35–65
3. Primary hyperparathyroidism: caused by tumor or hyperplasia of parathyroid glands
4. Secondary hyperparathyroidism: caused by compensatory oversecretion of PTH in response to hypocalcemia from chronic renal disease, rickets, malabsorption syndrome, osteomalacia

B. Assessment findings
1. Bone pain (especially at back), bone demineralization, pathologic fractures
2. Renal colic, kidney stones, polyuria, polydipsia
3. Anorexia, nausea, vomiting, gastric ulcers, constipation
4. Muscle weakness, fatigue
5. Irritability, personality changes, depression
6. Cardiac arrhythmias, hypertension
7. Diagnostic tests
    a. Serum calcium levels elevated
    b. Serum phosphate levels decreased
    c. Skeletal X-rays reveal bone demineralization

C. Nursing interventions
1. Administer IV infusions of normal saline solution and give diuretics as ordered; monitor I&O and observe for fluid overload and electrolyte imbalances.
2. Assist client with self-care: provide careful handling, moving, and ambulation to prevent pathologic fractures.
3. Monitor vital signs; report irregularities.
4. Force fluids; provide acid-ash juices, e.g., cranberry juice.
5. Strain urine for stones.
6. Provide low-calcium, high-phosphorus diet.
7. Provide care for the client undergoing parathyroidectomy (see Thyroidectomy).

8. Provide client teaching and discharge planning concerning
   a. Need to engage in progressive ambulatory activities
   b. Increased intake of fluids
   c. Use of calcium preparations and importance of high-calcium diet following a parathyroidectomy

# Specific Disorders of the Pancreas

## Diabetes Mellitus

A. General information
   1. Diabetes mellitus represents a heterogenous group of chronic disorders characterized by hyperglycemia.
   2. Hyperglycemia is due to total or partial insulin deficiency or insensitivity of the cells to insulin.
   3. Characterized by disorders in the metabolism of carbohydrate, fat, and protein, as well as changes in the structure and function of blood vessels.
   4. Most common endocrine problem; affects over 20 million people in the United States.
   5. Exact etiology unknown; causative factors may include:
      a. Genetics, viruses, and/or autoimmune response in Type 1
      b. Genetics and obesity in Type 2
   6. Types
      a. Type 1 (insulin-dependent diabetes mellitus [IDDM])
         1) Secondary to destruction of beta cells in the islets of Langerhans in the pancreas resulting in little or no insulin production; requires insulin injections.
         2) Usually occurs in children (see Unit 5) or in nonobese adults.
      b. Type 2 (non-insulin-dependent diabetes mellitus [NIDDM])
         1) May result from a partial deficiency of insulin production and/or an insensitivity of the cells to insulin.
         2) Usually occurs in obese adults over 40.
      c. Diabetes associated with other conditions or syndromes, e.g., pancreatic disease, Cushing's syndrome, use of certain drugs (steroids, thiazide diuretics, oral contraceptives).
   7. Pathophysiology
      a. Lack of insulin causes hyperglycemia (insulin is necessary for the transport of glucose across the cell membrane).
      b. Hyperglycemia leads to osmotic diuresis as large amounts of glucose pass through the kidney; results in polyuria and glycosuria.
      c. Diuresis leads to cellular dehydration and fluid and electrolyte depletion causing polydipsia (excessive thirst).
      d. Polyphagia (hunger and increased appetite) results from cellular starvation.
      e. The body turns to fats and protein for energy; but in the absence of glucose in the cell, fats cannot be completely metabolized and ketones (intermediate products of fat metabolism) are produced.
      f. This leads to ketonemia, ketonuria (contributes to osmotic diuresis), and metabolic acidosis (ketones are acid bodies).
      g. Ketones act as CNS depressants and can cause coma.
      h. Excess loss of fluids and electrolytes leads to hypovolemia, hypotension, renal failure, and decreased blood flow to the brain resulting in coma and death unless treated.
   8. Acute complications of diabetes include diabetic ketoacidosis (see Ketoacidosis), insulin reaction (see Insulin Reaction/Hypoglycemia), hyperglycemic hyperosmolar nonketotic coma (see Hyperglycemic Hypersmolar Coma (HHNK)).

B. Medical management
   1. Type 1: insulin, diet, exercise
   2. Type 2: ideally managed by diet and exercise; may need oral hypoglycemics or occasionally insulin if diet and exercise are not effective in controlling hyperglycemia; insulin needed for acute stresses, e.g., surgery, infection
   3. Diet Exchange (see Appendix)
      a. Type 1: consistency is imperative to avoid hypoglycemia
      b. Type 2: weight loss is important because it decreases insulin resistance
      c. High-fiber, low-fat diet also recommended
      d. Utilize Exchange list as recommended from American Diabetes Association.
   4. Drug therapy
      a. Insulin: used for Type 1 diabetes (also occasionally used in Type 2 diabetes)
         1) Types (Table 4-25)
            a) Short acting: used in treating ketoacidosis; during surgery, infection, trauma; management of poorly controlled diabetes; to supplement longer-acting insulins
            b) Intermediate: used for maintenance therapy
            c) Long acting: used for maintenance therapy in clients who experience hyperglycemia during the night with intermediate-acting insulin
         2) Various preparations of short-, intermediate-, and long-acting insulins are available (see Table 4-26)
         3) Insulin preparations can consist of a mixture of beef and pork insulin, pure beef, pure pork, or human insulin. Human insulin is the purest insulin and has the lowest antigenic effect.

**Table 4-26** Types of Insulins

| TYPE | ONSET | PEAK | DURATION |
|------|-------|------|----------|
| Humalog (Lispro) | Less than 15 minutes | 30–90 minutes | 4 hours |
| Regular | 30–60 minutes | 2–4 hours | 5–7 hours |
| NPH | 3–4 hours | 6–12 hours | 18–28 hours |
| Lente | 1–3 hours | 8–12 hours | 18–28 hours |
| Ultra Lente | 4–6 hours | 18–24 hours | 36–hours |
| 70/30 | 15–30 minutes | 2–3 hours and 8–12 hours | 18–24 hours |
| Insulin glargine | 1.1 hour | 5 hours | 24 hours |

Adapted from, Broyles, B. E. Reiss, B.S., & Evans, M.E. (2007). *Pharmacological aspects of nursing care* (7th ed.). New York: Thomson Delmar Learning.

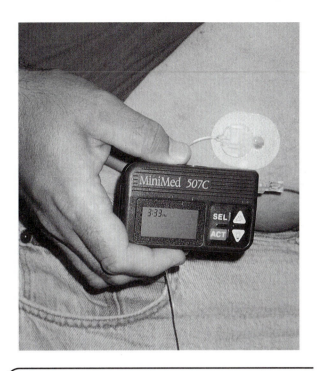

**Figure 4-26** Insulin infusion pump

4) Human insulin is recommended for all newly diagnosed Type 1 diabetics, Type 2 diabetics who need short-term insulin therapy, the pregnant client, and diabetic clients with insulin allergy or severe insulin resistance.

5) Insulin pumps are small, externally worn devices that closely mimic normal pancreatic functioning. Insulin pumps contain a 3-mL syringe attached to a long (42-inch), narrow-lumen tube with a needle or Teflon catheter at the end. The needle or Teflon catheter is inserted into the subcutaneous tissue (usually on the abdomen) and secured with tape or a transparent dressing. The needle or catheter is changed at least every 3 days. The pump is worn either on a belt or in a pocket (see Figure 4-26). The pump uses only regular insulin. Insulin can be administered via the basal rate (usually 0.5–2.0 units/hr) and by a bolus dose (which is activated by a series of button pushes) prior to each meal.

b. Oral hypoglycemic agents (Table 4-27)

1) Used for Type 2 diabetics who are not controlled by diet and exercise

2) Increase the ability of islet cells of the pancreas to secrete insulin; may have some effect on cell receptors to decrease resistance to insulin

5. Exercise: helpful adjunct to therapy as exercise decreases the body's need for insulin.

C. Assessment findings

1. All types: polyuria, polydipsia, polyphagia, fatigue, blurred vision, susceptibility to infection

2. Type 1: anorexia, nausea, vomiting, weight loss

3. Type 2: obesity; frequently no other symptoms

4. Diagnostic tests

a. Fasting blood sugar

1) A level of 126 mg/dL or greater on at least two occasions confirms diabetes mellitus

2) May be normal in Type 2 diabetes

b. Postprandial blood sugar: elevated greater than 200 mg/dL 2 hours after a meal.

c. Oral glucose tolerance test (most sensitive test): elevated greater than 200 mg/dL

d. Glycosolated hemoglobin (hemoglobin A1c) elevated; (normal range 4–6%)

D. Nursing interventions

1. Administer insulin or oral hypoglycemic agents as ordered; monitor for hypoglycemia, especially during period of drug's peak action.

2. Provide special diet as ordered.

a. Ensure that the client is eating all meals.

b. If all food is not ingested, provide appropriate substitutes according to the exchange lists or give measured amount of orange juice to substitute for leftover food; provide snack later in the day.

3. Monitor urine sugar and acetone (freshly voided specimen).

4. Perform finger sticks to monitor blood glucose levels as ordered (more accurate than urine tests).

5. Observe for signs of hypo/hyperglycemia.

6. Provide meticulous skin care and prevent injury.

7. Maintain I&O; weigh daily.

**Table 4-27** Oral Hypoglycemic Agents

| Drug | Onset of Action (hrs) | Peak Action (hrs) | Duration of Action (hrs) | Comments |
|---|---|---|---|---|
| *Oral Sulfonylureas* | | | | |
| Acetohexamide (Dymelor) | 1 | 4–6 | 12–24 | |
| Chlorpropamide (Diabinase) | 1 | 4–6 | 40–60 | |
| Glyburide (Micronase Diabeta) | 0.25–1 hr | 2–8 | 10–24 | |
| *Oral Biguanides* | | | | |
| Metformin (Glucophage) | 2–2.5 | | 10–16 | Decreases glucose production in liver; decreases intestinal absorption of glucose and improves insulin sensitivity. |
| *Oral Alpha-glucosidose Inhibitor* | | | | |
| Acarbose (Precose) | Unknown | 1 | Unknown | Delay glucose absorption and digestion of carbohydrates, lowering blood sugar. Reduces plasma glucose and insulin. Exact mechanism is unknown. Potentiates action of insulin in skeletal muscle and decreases glucose production in liver. |
| Miglitol (Glyset) | | 2–3 | | |
| Troglitazone (Rezulin) | Rapid | 2–3 | Unknown | |

8. Provide emotional support; assist client in adapting to change in lifestyle and body image.
9. Observe for chronic complications and plan care accordingly.
   a. Macrovascular: changes in large vessels
      1) Atherosclerosis: increased plaque formation (decrease lipid level)
      2) Cardiovascular, cerebral, peripheral vascular diseases (modify lifestyle-obesity, smoking, sedentary lifestyle, hypertension)
   b. Microvascular: thickening of capillaries and arterioles
      1) Diabetic retinopathy: premature cataracts (prevent/control elevated blood glucose)
      2) Diabetic nephropathy: renal disease (control blood glucose)
      3) Diabetic neuropathies: peripheral, autonomic spinal nerves affected (control blood glucose)
10. Provide client teaching and discharge planning concerning
    a. Disease process
    b. Diet
       1) Client should be able to plan meals using exchange lists before discharge
       2) Emphasize importance of regularity of meals; never skip meals
    c. Insulin
       1) How to draw up into syringe
          a) Use insulin at room temperature.

b) Gently roll vial between palms of hands.
          c) Draw up insulin using sterile technique.
          d) If mixing insulins, draw up clear insulin before cloudy insulin.
       2) Injection technique
          a) Systematically rotate sites to prevent lipodystrophy (hypertrophy or atrophy of tissue).
          b) Insert needle at a 45° or 90° angle depending on amount of adipose tissue.
       3) May store current vial of insulin at room temperature; refrigerate extra supplies.
       4) Provide many opportunities for return demonstration.
    d. Oral hypoglycemic agents
       1) Stress importance of taking the drug regularly.
       2) Avoid alcohol intake while on medication.
    e. Urine testing (not very accurate reflection of blood glucose level)
       1) May be satisfactory for Type 2 diabetics since they are more stable.
       2) Use Clinitest, Tes-Tape, Diastix for glucose testing.
       3) Perform tests before meals and at bedtime.
       4) Use freshly voided specimen.

5) Be consistent in brand of urine test used.
6) Report results in percentages.
7) Report results to physician if results are greater than 1%, especially if experiencing symptoms of hyperglycemia.
8) Urine testing for ketones should be done by Type 1 diabetics when there is persistent glycosuria, increased blood glucose levels, or if the client is not feeling well (Acetest, Ketostix).

f. Blood glucose monitoring
1) Use for Type 1 diabetics since it gives exact blood glucose level and also detects hypoglycemia.
2) Use for Type 2 diabetics to monitor effectiveness of oral and/or insulin treatment.
3) Instruct client in finger-stick technique, use of monitor device (if used), and recording and utilization of test results.

g. General care
1) Perform good oral hygiene and have regular dental exams.
2) Have regular eye exams.
3) Care for "sick days" (e.g., cold or flu)
   a) Do not omit insulin or oral hypoglycemic agents because infection causes increased blood sugar.
   b) Notify physician.
   c) Monitor urine or blood glucose levels and urine ketones frequently.
   d) If nausea and/or vomiting occurs, sip on clear liquids with simple sugars.

h. Foot care
1) Wash feet with mild soap and water and pat dry.
2) Apply lanolin to feet to prevent drying and cracking.
3) Cut toenails straight across.
4) Avoid constricting garments such as garters.
5) Wear clean, absorbent socks (cotton or wool).
6) Purchase properly fitting shoes and break new shoes in gradually.
7) Never go barefoot.
8) Inspect feet daily and notify physician if cuts, blisters, or breaks in skin occur.

i. Exercise
1) Undertake regular exercise; avoid sporadic, vigorous exercise.
2) Food intake may need to be increased before exercising.
3) Exercise is best performed after meals when the blood sugar is rising.

j. Complications
1) Learn to recognize signs and symptoms of hypo/hyperglycemia.
2) Eat candy or drink orange juice with sugar added for insulin reaction (hypoglycemia).

k. Need to wear a Medic-Alert bracelet.

*Ketoacidosis (DKA)*

A. General information
1. Acute complication of diabetes mellitus characterized by hyperglycemia and accumulation of ketones in the body; causes metabolic acidosis
2. Occurs in insulin-dependent diabetic clients
3. Precipitating factors: undiagnosed diabetes, neglect of treatment; infection, cardiovascular disorder; other physical or emotional stress
4. Onset slow, may be hours to days

B. Assessment findings
1. Polydipsia, polyphagia, polyuria
2. Nausea, vomiting, abdominal pain
3. Skin warm, dry, and flushed
4. Dry mucous membranes; soft eyeballs
5. Kussmaul's respirations or tachypnea; acetone breath
6. Alterations in LOC
7. Hypotension, tachycardia
8. Diagnostic tests
   a. Serum glucose and ketones elevated (glucose greater than 250 mg/dL)
   b. BUN, creatinine, hct elevated (due to dehydration)
   c. Serum sodium decreased, potassium (may be normal or elevated at first)
   d. ABGs: metabolic acidosis with compensatory respiratory alkalosis

C. Nursing interventions
1. Maintain a patent airway.
2. Maintain fluid and electrolyte balance.
   a. Administer IV therapy as ordered.
      1) Normal saline (0.9% NaCl), then hypotonic (0.45% NaCl) sodium chloride
      2) When blood sugar drops to 250 mg/dL, may add 5% dextrose to IV.
      3) Potassium will be added when the urine output is adequate.
   b. Observe for fluid and electrolyte imbalances, especially fluid overload, hypokalemia, and hyperkalemia.
3. Administer insulin as ordered.
   a. Regular insulin IV (drip or push) and/or subcutaneously (SC).
   b. If given IV drip, give with small amounts of albumin since insulin adheres to IV tubing.
   c. Monitor blood glucose levels frequently.
4. Check urine output every hour.
5. Monitor vital signs.

6. Assist client with self-care.
7. Provide care for the unconscious client if in a coma.
8. Discuss with client the reasons ketosis developed and provide additional diabetic teaching if indicated.

### Insulin Reaction/Hypoglycemia

A. General information
   1. Abnormally low blood sugar, usually below 50 mg/dL
   2. Usually caused by insulin overdosage, too little food, nutritional and fluid imbalances from nausea and vomiting, excessive exercise
   3. Onset rapid; may develop in minutes to hours
B. Assessment findings
   1. Headache, dizziness, difficulty with problem solving, restlessness, hunger, visual disturbances
   2. Slurred speech; alterations in gait; decreasing LOC; pallor, cold, clammy skin; diaphoresis
   3. Diagnostic test: serum glucose level 50–60 mg/dL or lower
C. Nursing interventions
   1. Administer oral sugar in the form of candy or orange juice with sugar added if the client is alert.
   2. If the client is unconscious, administer 20–50 mL 50% dextrose IV push, or 1 mg glucagon IM, IV, or SC, as ordered.
   3. Explore with client reasons for hypoglycemia and provide additional diabetic teaching as indicated.

### Hyperglycemic Hyperosmolar Nonketotic Coma (HHNK)

A. General information
   1. Complication of diabetes, characterized by hyperglycemia and a hyperosmolar state without ketosis
   2. Occurs in non-insulin-dependent diabetics or nondiabetic persons (typically elderly clients)
   3. Precipitating factors: undiagnosed diabetes; infections or other stress; certain medications (e.g., Dilantin, thiazide diuretics); dialysis; hyperalimentation; major burns; pancreatic disease
B. Assessment findings
   1. Similar to ketoacidosis but without Kussmaul respirations and acetone breath
   2. Laboratory tests
      a. Blood glucose level extremely elevated (greater than 600 mg/dL)
      b. BUN, creatine, hct elevated (due to dehydration)
      c. Urine positive for glucose
C. Nursing interventions: treatment and nursing care is similar to DKA, excluding measures to treat ketosis and metabolic acidosis.

## Sample Questions

425. A client was admitted to the hospital for uncontrolled diabetes. Lab studies reveal a fasting blood sugar of 310 mg/dL. The client is informed that Type 1 diabetes has a characteristic feature. What is it?
   1. It is associated with the destruction of beta cells.
   2. It usually causes complete fat metabolism.
   3. It often occurs in obese individuals.
   4. It is rarely controlled.

426. A diabetic client who is taking regular and NPH insulin asks why she must mix the two insulins. What would be the explanation for mixing regular and NPH insulin?
   1. Immediate onset of the regular insulin.
   2. Onset of the regular insulin within 2 hours.
   3. A peak action of the NPH insulin at 2 hours.
   4. A total duration of action of 24 hours.

427. A female client has a simple goiter. She is being seen by the community health nurse for teaching and follow-up regarding nutritional deficiencies related to her goiter. The client's problems are most likely associated with which nutritional deficiency?
   1. Calcium.
   2. Iodine.
   3. Iron.
   4. Sodium.

428. The nurse is teaching a woman who has a simple goiter. The nurse teaches the client that to enhance glandular function, she should eliminate which of the following foods?
   1. Corn.
   2. Milk.
   3. Turnips.
   4. Watermelon.

429. A client is admitted to the hospital with Addison's disease. He has a respiratory infection. When the client's vital signs are assessed, his blood pressure is 90/40. Why should the nurse notify the physician immediately?
   1. Blood gases need to be drawn.
   2. Seizure activity is imminent.
   3. Shock may be developing.
   4. The reading is atypical.

430. A client who is diagnosed with Addison's disease is admitted to the hospital. Which of the following would the nurse expect to find when assessing the client?
    1. Acne.
    2. Hyperpigmentation.
    3. Moon face.
    4. Supraclavicular fat pads.

431. A client who is diagnosed as having Addison's disease is receiving teaching about his disease from the nurse. Which statement the client makes indicates to the nurse that he understands the teaching?
    1. "I should avoid strenuous exercise during hot weather."
    2. "I should not eat salty foods."
    3. "I need to take medication only when I am having symptoms."
    4. "I should eat foods such as bananas and oranges several times daily."

432. The nurse is teaching a person who has Addison's disease about drug therapy for his condition. In evaluating the effectiveness of teaching regarding drug therapy, what should the client know and be able to verbalize?
    1. To avoid antibiotics.
    2. For lifelong therapy.
    3. To taper the steroid dose.
    4. To receive alternate-day therapy.

433. A client is newly diagnosed with Type 1 diabetes. She is hospitalized for insulin dose stabilization and is being taught insulin administration and self-monitoring of blood glucose (SMBG) levels. What is the major benefit of self-monitoring of blood glucose levels?
    1. Blood glucose is maintained at close to normal levels.
    2. Materials and laboratory expenses are cost efficient.
    3. Dependence on the health care system is reduced.
    4. Larger but fewer doses of insulin are required.

434. The nurse is teaching an adult client who has Type 1 diabetes mellitus about ketoacidosis. What is the primary cause for the development of ketoacidosis?
    1. A GI disturbance.
    2. An insulin overdosage.
    3. Omitted meals.
    4. Not taking insulin regularly.

435. A client is to have the following diagnostic procedures: serum $T_3$ and $T_4$, carotid arteriogram, and thyroid scan. In what order should the nurse schedule the tests?
    1. Arteriogram, serum $T_3$ and $T_4$, scan.
    2. Serum $T_3$ and $T_4$, scan, arteriogram.
    3. Arteriogram, scan, serum $T_3$ and $T_4$.
    4. Serum $T_3$ and $T_4$, arteriogram, scan.

436. After reading about the procedure for his upcoming thyroid scan, a client expresses concern about the dangers of being "radioactive" after the test. Which understanding about the test should guide the nurse's response?
    1. There is no danger because the thyroid scan no longer involves the use of a radioactive isotope.
    2. The radioactive isotope is only a tracer dose, which is not harmful to the client or others close to him.
    3. The client must avoid close contact with others for 5 days following the test.
    4. Wearing a lead shield during the test will protect the client from radioactivity.

437. The nurse is explaining to a client about a radioactive iodine uptake test. Which of the following OTC medications should the nurse advise the client to avoid prior to the test?
    1. Antiflatulents.
    2. Poison ivy remedies.
    3. Cough syrups.
    4. Antifungal agents.

438. Select the most accurate explanation by the nurse to a client who is to have an oral glucose tolerance test and needs to understand the procedure.
    1. "You will go to the laboratory and your blood will be drawn."
    2. "After you drink a concentrated glucose solution, you cannot eat or drink anything until your blood is drawn."
    3. "You will eat a large meal and your blood will be drawn 2 hours later."
    4. "Your blood will be drawn, you will drink a concentrated glucose solution, and your blood will be drawn again."

439. An adult is suffering from adrenocortical insufficiency and is placed on glucocorticoid therapy. The nurse plans to include which of the following administration directions?
    1. "You will need to take the large dose of the medication at bedtime and the smaller dose in the morning until the prescription is finished."

2. "You will need to take the medication at bedtime for life."

3. "You will need to take the medication in the morning until the prescription is finished."

4. "You will need to take the large dose of the medication in the morning and the smaller dose in the afternoon for life."

440. Which assessment is most important for the nurse to make when monitoring a client with a pituitary tumor that secretes ACTH?
   1. Height.
   2. Blood pressure.
   3. Pulse rate.
   4. Output.

441. The nurse is caring for a client who underwent surgical hypophysectomy. Which of the following assessments is most essential for the nurse to make immediately post-op?
   1. Blood pressure.
   2. Serum calcium levels.
   3. Patent catheter.
   4. Bowel sounds.

442. An adult has had a hypophysectomy with a complete removal of the pituitary gland. Which of the following statements represents to the nurse the most complete understanding of follow-up care?
   1. "I will need to wear a Medic-Alert bracelet."
   2. "I will need to take hormone replacements for the next 2 months."
   3. "I will need to wear a Medic-Alert bracelet and take hormone replacements for the next year."
   4. "I will need to have lifelong follow-up, to take hormone replacement therapy for the rest of my life, and to wear a Medic-Alert bracelet."

443. A client is admitted with a posterior pituitary tumor and is experiencing diabetes insipidus, a complication of that tumor. Which nursing diagnosis is most appropriate for this client?
   1. Fluid volume excess.
   2. Deficient fluid volume.
   3. Bowel incontinence.
   4. Diarrhea.

444. A client who has been taking prednisone to treat lupus erythematosus has discontinued the medication because of lack of funds to buy the drug. When the nurse becomes aware of the situation, which assessment is most important for the nurse to make first?

1. Breath sounds.
2. Capillary refill.
3. Blood pressure.
4. Skin integrity.

445. An adult is readmitted to the medical/surgical care unit in addisonian crisis. He is exhibiting signs of tachycardia, dehydration, hyponatremia, hyperkalemia, and hypoglycemia. What will the initial orders for this client include?
   1. Administration of oxygen via 100% nonrebreathing mask.
   2. Starting an IV solution of saline and dextrose.
   3. Administering potassium chloride.
   4. Preparing for an emergency tracheostomy.

446. A female client is suffering from Cushing's syndrome. She is constantly lashing out at her coworkers and family. Her husband informs the nurse of this behavior. What condition does the nurse interpret from this behavior?
   1. Mineralocorticoid excess.
   2. Glucocorticoid excess.
   3. Activity intolerance.
   4. Sensory-perceptual alterations.

447. A nurse at a weight loss center assesses a client who has a large abdomen and a rounded face. Which additional assessment finding would lead the nurse to suspect that the client has Cushing's syndrome rather than obesity from imbalance of food intake and body need?
   1. Large thighs and upper arms.
   2. Pendulous abdomen and large hips.
   3. Abdominal striae and ankle enlargement.
   4. Posterior neck fat pad and thin extremities.

448. A client has primary aldosteronism. Which assessment findings would the nurse expect to find initially?
   1. Decreased serum sodium and potassium.
   2. Decreased blood glucose and elevated temperature.
   3. Tachycardia and albuminuria.
   4. Hypertension and decreased serum potassium.

449. A client who is suspected of having a pheochromocytoma complains of sweating, palpitations, and headache. Which assessment is essential for the nurse to make first?
   1. Pupil reaction.
   2. Hand grips.
   3. Blood pressure.
   4. Blood glucose.

**450.** An adult is to have a bilateral adrenalectomy. The nurse is performing preoperative teaching. The client asks the nurse "What will I look like after surgery?" What is the nurse's best response?

1. "Don't worry about that now. You need to concentrate on the surgery."
2. "You will only have a small incision."
3. "I know you are worried, maybe we should resume the education session later."
4. "You're appearance won't change immediately after surgery."

**451.** An adult has undergone a bilateral adrenalectomy. Which of the following demonstrates to the nurse the best understanding of long-term care needs?

1. When I run out of the medication the doctor gave me, I can stop taking the hormones.
2. I can take the steroid replacement therapy once every 3 days.
3. I need to take the steroid replacement therapy every day. I should not alter the dose or stop taking it.
4. I can take the dose of the medication when I feel stressed.

**452.** An adult is admitted to the hospital for removal of a simple goiter. What is the cause of a simple goiter?

1. Low intake of fat-free foods.
2. Excessive thyroid-stimulating hormone (TSH) stimulation.
3. Excessive adrenocorticotropic hormone (ACTH) stimulation.
4. Low intake of goitrogenic foods.

**453.** An adult is currently being treated at the clinic for Graves' disease. It is essential for the nurse to assess for which of the following signs immediately?

1. Goiter.
2. Tachycardia.
3. Constipation.
4. Hypothermia.

**454.** A 35-year-old female visits her managed care physician for an annual physical examination. Routine laboratory studies reveal thyroxine ($T_4$) and triiodothyronine ($T_3$) levels are elevated, whereas the thyroid-stimulating hormone (TSH) level was undetectable. What condition would the nurse suspect?

1. Hypothyroidism.
2. Addisonian crisis.
3. Hypoparathyroidism.
4. Hyperthyroidism.

**455.** An adult who is newly diagnosed with Graves' disease asks the nurse "Why do I need to take propranolol (Inderal)?" Based on the nurse's understanding of the medication and Graves' disease, what would be the best response?

1. "The medication will limit thyroid hormone secretion."
2. "The medication will inhibit synthesis of thyroid hormones."
3. "The medication will relieve the symptoms of Graves' disease."
4. "The medication will increase the synthesis of thyroid hormones."

**456.** The nurse is preparing a room to receive a client immediately post-thyroidectomy. The nurse should be sure that which of the following equipment is available at the bedside?

1. Nasogastric tray.
2. Central venous tray set-up.
3. Tracheostomy tray.
4. Lumbar puncture tray.

**457.** An adult had a total thyroidectomy. Which statement by the client demonstrates to the nurse an adequate understanding of long-term care?

1. "I will need to take replacement hormones for the rest of my life."
2. "I should try to avoid stress and be alert for signs of recurrent hyperthyroidism."
3. "Thank goodness this is over, I will never have to worry about weight problems again!"
4. "I should increase my caloric intake to replace what I lost during the surgery."

**458.** The nurse is caring for a client who is status post-thyroidectomy. The client is exhibiting hyperreflexia, muscle twitching, and spasms. What is the first action the nurse should perform?

1. Assess for additional signs of tetany.
2. Prepare to send a blood sample to the laboratory for a calcium level.
3. Place the client in semi-Fowler's position.
4. Administer post-op pain medication.

**459.** An adult who has Graves' disease just received a dose of sodium $^{131}$I. Which of the following statements made to the nurse best demonstrates an understanding of immediate care needs?

1. "I should be able to go home after about 2 hours if I don't have any vomiting."
2. "I have my belongings with me to stay in the isolation room for the next 24 hours."

3. "My daughter is pregnant, so I told her I will not be able to see her for the next month."

4. "I brought my antithyroid drug with me so I will not miss a dose."

460. An adult has had hypoparathyroidism for 20 years. The client has come in to the center for a check-up. For what condition should the nurse assess?

1. Hypothermia.
2. Hyperthermia.
3. Tetany.
4. Hypertension.

461. A client who is newly diagnosed with Type 1 diabetes asks the nurse "Why can't I take a pill for my diabetes like my neighbor?" Select the statement that states the primary difference between Type 1 and Type 2 diabetes.

1. Type 1 diabetes and Type 2 diabetes can be controlled with injections of antibodies.
2. Type 1 diabetes is the result of autoimmune destruction of beta cell function in the pancreas, whereas Type 2 diabetes is the result of the lack of responsiveness of beta cells to insulin.
3. Type 1 diabetes insulin production is a circadian function, whereas in Type 2 diabetes, insulin production depends on serum glucose levels.
4. Type 1 diabetes has a complication known as hyperglycemic hyperosmolar nonketosis, whereas Type 2 diabetes has a complication known as diabetic ketoacidosis.

462. The nurse administers the client's morning dose of regular insulin at 0730. The nurse should anticipate to observe the client for a hypoglycemic reaction at which of the following times?

1. Immediately.
2. 1000.
3. 1300.
4. 1930.

463. The nurse is planning an education session for a client newly diagnosed with diabetes. Which concept is essential to include when developing the plan of care?

1. All diabetic teaching needs to be accomplished within 20 hours before discharge.
2. Insulin injection sites should be cleaned with iodine prior to injection.
3. Snacks should be ingested prior to physical exercise.
4. Urine sugar levels should be checked prior to insulin administration.

464. The nurse is attending a bridal shower for a friend when another guest starts to tremble and complains of dizziness. The nurse notices a medical alert bracelet for diabetes. What will be the nurse's best action?

1. Encourage the guest to eat some baked ziti.
2. Call the guest's personal physician.
3. Offer the guest a peppermint.
4. Give the guest a glass of orange juice.

465. A woman usually administers her NPH insulin at 0600. but she plans to attend a banquet and fashion show next week, at which lunch will be served at 1400. rather than noon when she usually eats lunch. Which of the following statements demonstrates to the nurse an understanding of peak action of NPH and risk for hypoglycemia?

1. "I will administer the insulin at my regular time, it is important to adhere to my schedule."
2. "I will take the insulin at 0800. that day, as the insulin peaks in 6–12 hours."
3. "I will not take any insulin until they serve the lunch at the banquet."
4. "I will take the insulin at 1000. that day as the peak action of NPH is 4 hours after administered."

466. A man is hospitalized for an infected foot ulcer. At 1100 his blood glucose is 460 mg/dL and he has been up to the bathroom seven times this morning to urinate. What will be the nurse's best action?

1. Administer regular insulin according to the physician's sliding scale order.
2. Administer NPH insulin according to the physician's sliding scale order.
3. Notify the physician.
4. Make sure the client's urinal is close to the bed so he does not have to keep getting up.

467. A client with diabetes is displaying signs of irritability and irrational behavior during an office visit. The nurse observes visible tremors in the client's hands. Based on the client's history, how are these findings interpreted?

1. Hyperglycemia.
2. Diabetic ketoacidosis (DKA).
3. Hyperglycemic hyperosmolar nonketosis (HHNK).
4. Hypoglycemia.

468. Which statement by a woman newly diagnosed with NIDDM demonstrates to the nurse an adequate understanding of dietary needs?

1. "I will increase my intake of fat and carbohydrates."
2. "Having diabetes makes it harder for my system to digest food."
3. "I met with the dietician who said to eat carbohydrates, protein, and fats together."
4. "When will I start the TPN medication to control my sugar?"

469. The client came to the diabetic clinic for follow-up teaching on the complications of diabetes. What is a correct explanation for the result of neuropathy?
    1. Microangiopathies or metabolic defects that cause by-products to accumulate in the nerve tissues.
    2. Microvascular damage to the retina.
    3. Macroangiopathy in the extremities.
    4. End-stage renal disease.

470. The nurse is teaching a client with Type 2, non-insulin-dependent diabetes about the acute metabolic complications. Why does a client with Type 2 diabetes usually not develop diabetic ketoacidosis?
    1. There is no insulin available for the state of hyperglycemia.
    2. The client with Type 2 diabetes has no protein or fat reserves.
    3. There is sufficient insulin to prevent the breakdown of protein and fatty acid for metabolic needs.
    4. There is insufficient serum glucose concentrations.

471. The primary caretaker for a man who was recently started on an oral hypoglycemic agent is his wife. The wife should know to watch for which of the following symptoms of hypoglycemia?
    1. High blood sugar readings (greater than 250 mg/dL).
    2. Presence of ketones in the urine.
    3. Significant increase in urine output.
    4. Cold sweats, weakness, and trembling.

472. Which of the following statements by a person who has diabetes mellitus shows the nurse that he has an adequate understanding of special foot care needs?
    1. "I am looking forward to the summer when I can go barefoot in my house and at the beach."
    2. "I like to use a heating pad at night as I always have cold feet."

3. "I used to take a shower every other night but now I am going to wash and examine my feet every night."
4. "I have a corn on my left foot, so I am going to go to the pharmacy to get something for it right away."

473. A client took her usual NPH insulin dose at 0600, her lunch is delayed until 1300, and she begins to feel weak. Which of the following actions by the client demonstrates an understanding of her condition?
    1. Administers an extra 4 units of regular insulin.
    2. Administers an additional 4 units of NPH insulin.
    3. Takes a nap.
    4. Drinks a cup of milk and then eats her lunch.

474. The nurse is teaching a client about diabetic management. The client asks the nurse "What is a hemoglobin A1c test?" What is the most appropriate answer by the nurse?
    1. "The hemoglobin A1c is a blood test that evaluates glycemic control over a 3-month time period by measuring the glucose attached to hemoglobin."
    2. "The hemoglobin A1c is a blood test that measures the glucose attached to hemoglobin molecule over the last 7 days."
    3. "The hemoglobin A1c test is a kidney test that measures protein to evaluate glucose control over the last 7 days."
    4. "The hemoglobin A1c test is a urine test that measures protein to evaluate glucose control over the last few months."

 **Answers and Rationales**

425. **1.** Type 1 diabetes mellitus, also know as insulin-dependent diabetes, occurs in individuals in whom the beta islet cells of the pancreas do not make insulin.

426. **4.** NPH insulin is an intermediate-acting insulin. Regular insulin is a rapid-acting insulin. Mixing the two gives insulin over a 24-hour period, requiring fewer injections for the client.

427. **2.** Lack of iodine in the diet is a primary contributor to the development of simple goiter.

428. **3.** Turnips belong to a classification of foods called exogenous goitrogens. Goitrogens are

thyroid-inhibiting substances and therefore should be avoided. Other goitrogens include rutabagas, cabbage, soybeans, peanuts, peaches, peas, strawberries, spinach, and radishes.

429. **3.** Any emotional or physical stress, such as infection, may precipitate acute adrenal crisis with vascular collapse and shock.

430. **2.** Addison's disease is characterized by bilateral hypofunction of the adrenal cortex, resulting in insufficient production of adrenal steroids including cortisol and aldosterone. There is increased production of melanocyte stimulating hormone (MSH), which stimulates production of melanin, a dark pigment. Persons with Addison's disease note that their skin is darker.

431. **1.** If the person with Addison's perspires heavily he will lose sodium and fluid and become hyponatremic and hypovolemic. He should avoid strenuous exercise during hot weather.

432. **2.** Addison's disease cannot be cured but it is controlled with lifelong hormone replacement.

433. **1.** Self-monitoring of blood glucose has become an important part of diabetes management. Maintaining good control of blood sugar reduces complications. This is the best method to keep close control.

434. **4.** In order to meet metabolic demand insulin must be taken on a regular basis. Ketoacidosis occurs when there is a lack of insulin in relation to metabolic demands.

435. **2.** The blood work can be done quickly without preparation, while the remaining tests must be scheduled in advance. The scan must precede the arteriogram, because the arteriogram dye contains iodine that will interfere with the scan.

436. **2.** The tracer dose used is much smaller than a therapeutic dose and is not harmful. The client can resume contact with others immediately following the test.

437. **3.** Many cough syrups contain iodine, which interferes with the test. Other OTC drugs to be avoided include salicylates, multivitamins, and some iodine-containing preparations found in health food stores.

438. **4.** A fasting blood glucose is drawn before Glucola is administered. The client can drink only water as blood samples are obtained at designated intervals.

439. **4.** Adrenal insufficiency requires lifelong glucocorticoid replacement therapy. Glucocorticoids are given in divided doses, two-thirds in the morning and one-third in the afternoon to reflect the body's own circadian rhythm, which decreases the side effects of therapy.

440. **2.** ACTH-secreting tumors can cause Cushing's syndrome, which can elevate the blood pressure to dangerously high levels.

441. **1.** Hypophysectomy (removal of the pituitary gland) interferes with the secretion of both glucocorticoids and antidiuretic hormone, both of which are essential to maintain fluid balance and blood pressure. Careful monitoring of blood pressure is essential to ensure that hormone replacement therapy is adequate.

442. **4.** Hormone replacement and follow-up care are needed for the rest of the client's life because the pituitary gland has been removed. This is the master gland that secretes trophic hormones that stimulate target glands to produce their hormones. A Medic-Alert bracelet is needed to alert others of the client's condition.

443. **2.** Diabetes insipidus is characterized by polydipsia and polyuria. It occurs with lesions of the hypothalamus and pituitary. Because antidiuretic hormone synthesis is affected, the client is at high risk for dehydration, which is life-threatening.

444. **3.** Withdrawal from glucocorticoid therapy can precipitate addisonian crisis, which is characterized by circulatory collapse and shock. Hypotension is a major manifestation of addisonian crisis and must be treated vigorously.

445. **2.** Management of addisonian crisis includes glucocorticoid management. Intravenous replacement of sodium and dextrose is also necessary.

446. **1.** Cushing's syndrome is caused by excessive corticosteroids. Excessive mineralocorticoid produces hypertension, acne, changes in secondary sex characteristics, and mood disturbances such as irritability, anxiety, euphoria, insomnia, irrationality, and psychosis.

447. **4.** Clients with Cushing's syndrome exhibit central obesity, with a "buffalo hump," a heavy trunk, and thin extremities. The accumulation of fat on the cheeks makes the face moon-shaped, or rounded.

448. **4.** Hypertension and hyperkalemia are the classic manifestations of primary aldosteronism, in which the adrenal cortex secretes excessive mineralocorticoid.

449. **3.** Clients with pheochromocytoma can experience episodes of life-threatening hypertension when the adrenal tumor secretes catecholamines that stimulate the sympathetic nervous system. These attacks are often accompanied by sweating, palpitations, and headache.

450. **4.** The client will have to take corticosteroids life-long, but the physical changes they may cause take time to present. Explaining all treatment and procedures can reduce the patient's stress and anxiety level for now.

451. **3.** Without adrenal glands there is a lifelong need for a constant dose for replacement therapy daily.

452. **2.** A simple goiter is an enlargement of the thyroid gland caused by excess thyroid-stimulating hormone (TSH) stimulation, growth-stimulating hormones, or excessive intake of goitrogenic foods.

453. **2.** The client with Graves' disease is at risk for tachycardia, shock, hyperthermia, weight loss, and nervousness.

454. **4.** Thyroxine and triiodothyronine levels are usually elevated and thyroid-stimulating hormone levels may be normal or undetectable in hyperthyroidism.

455. **3.** Propranolol (Inderal) is a beta-adrenergic blocker that will relieve the symptoms of Graves' disease caused by increased circulating thyroid hormone. The symptoms are heat intolerance, palpitations, nervousness, tachycardia, and tremors.

456. **3.** Oxygen, suction equipment, and a tracheostomy tray should be available in case airway obstruction occurs.

457. **1.** The administration of thyroid hormone is needed after surgery because there is no thyroid gland to perform the usual functions.

458. **2.** During a thyroidectomy it is possible for the parathyroid glands to be removed or damaged. If the parathyroid glands are disturbed, hypocalcemia may result.

459. **1.** The client remains in the outpatient department for about 2 hours to be monitored for vomiting.

460. **3.** The signs and symptoms of hypoparathyroidism are due to low serum calcium levels. A decrease in serum calcium may produce tetany. Tetany produces tingling in lips, fingers, and feet. Severe tetany is associated with muscle spasms.

461. **2.** Type 1 diabetes arises from the destruction of the beta cells, which results in little or no insulin production. Type 2 diabetes is the result of tissues being unresponsive to insulin, which eventually exhausts the production of insulin. Type 2 diabetics tend to be older than 35 years and overweight.

462. **2.** The peak action for regular insulin occurs in 2 to 4 hours after administration. If regular insulin is administered at 0730, then the client should be observed for hypoglycemia between 0930 and 1130.

463. **3.** Snacks should be eaten prior to any exercise so glucose is readily available for the body's use.

464. **4.** A conscious client experiencing hypoglycemia needs 5–20 grams of simple carbohydrates immediately. A 4–6 oz glass of orange juice would provide enough glucose to counteract hypoglycemia.

465. **2.** The peak action for NPH is 6 hours after administration; therefore, delaying the administration 2 hours in the morning will allow the client to safely eat lunch at 1400.

466. **1.** At the first sign of diabetic ketoacidosis (elevated blood glucose and frequent urination) the nurse should administer insulin per physician's order to stabilize the blood glucose level.

467. **4.** Hypoglycemia or low blood glucose occurs when there is more insulin than glucose in the serum or when blood glucose levels drop too rapidly. The signs of hypoglycemia include irritability, irrational behavior, dizziness, tremors, or loss of consciousness.

468. **3.** The client states the recommendation by the American Diabetes Association and may also use the Exchange List, knowing that eating the different groups will help keep the blood glucose from going up too quickly.

469. **1.** Neuropathy is one of the most common complications of diabetes caused by microangiopathies or metabolic defects that cause waste to build up in the nerves, resulting in demyelinization.

**470. 3.** A client with Type 2 diabetes is more likely to have hyperglycemic hyperosmolar nonketosis because there is sufficient insulin to prevent the metabolism of protein and fats for basic energy needs.

**471. 4.** The cardinal signs of hypoglycemia are cold sweats, weakness, and trembling. Additional signs include nervousness, irritability, pallor, increased heart rate, confusion, and fatigue.

**472. 3.** The client with diabetes should wash the feet daily and examine for cuts, blisters, swelling, and any red, tender spots.

**473. 4.** The client is experiencing low blood sugar or hypoglycemia; ingesting a quick-acting carbohydrate source is the best action.

**474. 1.** Glycosylated hemoglobin, also known as the hemoglobin A1c test, is used to determine glycemic control over time. Glucose attaches to hemoglobin and remains there for the life of the blood cell (120 days); therefore, the test indicates the overall glucose level of 120 days.

# The Integumentary System

## OVERVIEW OF ANATOMY AND PHYSIOLOGY

The integumentary system consists of the skin and its appendages, such as hair, nails, and various glands. The integumentary system not only provides a barrier against the external environment, it also plays a role in maintenance of the body's internal environment.

### Skin

A. Functions
  1. Protection: barrier to noxious agents (microorganisms, parasites, chemical substances) and to loss of water and electrolytes
  2. Thermoregulation: radiant cooling, evaporation
  3. Sensory perception: touch, temperature, pressure, pain
  4. Metabolism: excretion of water and sodium, production of vitamin D, wound repair
B. Layers (see Figure 4-27)
  1. Epidermis
    a. The avascular outermost layer
    b. Stratified into several layers
    c. Composed mainly of keratinocytes and melanocytes
      1) Keratinocytes produce keratin, responsible for formation of hair and nails
      2) Melanocytes produce melanin, a pigment that gives color to skin and hair
    d. Appendages (hair and nails, eccrine sweat glands, sebaceous glands, apocrine sweat glands) all derived from epidermis

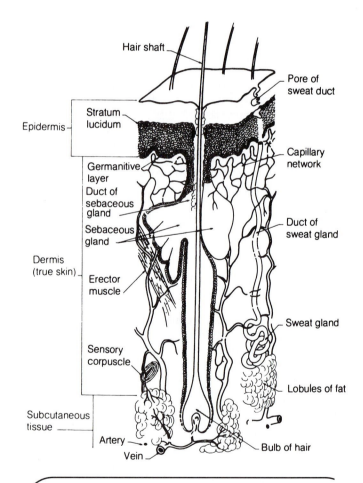

**Figure 4-27** Cross–section of skin: observe the skin layers and note the location of the glands in the dermal layer

2. Dermis: layer beneath the epidermis composed of connective tissue that contains lymphatics, nerves, and blood vessels; elasticity of skin results from presence of collagen, elastin, and reticular fibers in the dermis, which also nourish the epidermis
3. Subcutaneous layer: layer beneath the dermis composed of loose connective tissue and fat cells; stores fat; important in temperature regulation

## Hair

A. Covers most of the body surface (except palms of hands, soles of feet, lips, nipples, and parts of external genitalia).
B. Hair follicles: tube-like structures, derived from epidermis, from which hair grows.
C. Hair functions as protection from external elements and from trauma.
D. Hair growth is controlled by hormonal influences and by blood supply.
E. Loss of body hair is called alopecia.

## Nails

A. Dense layer of flat, dead cells; filled with keratin
B. Systemic illnesses may be reflected by changes in the nail or its bed; common changes include:
   1. Clubbing: enlargement of fingers and toes, nail becomes convex; caused by chronic pulmonary or cardiovascular disease
   2. Beau's line; transverse groove caused by temporary halt in nail growth because of systemic disorder

## Glands

A. Eccrine sweat glands: located all over the body; participate in heat regulation
B. Apocrine sweat glands: odiferous glands, found primarily in axillary, nipple, anal, and pubic areas; bacterial decomposition of excretions causes body odor
C. Sebaceous glands: oil glands, located all over the body except for palms of hands and soles of feet (abundant on face, scalp, upper chest, and back); produce sebum

# ASSESSMENT

## Health History

A. Presenting problem: symptoms may include changes in color or texture of skin, hair, nails; pruritus; infections; tumors; lesions; dermatitis; ecchymoses; rashes; dryness
B. Lifestyle: hygienic practices (skin-cleansing measures, use of cosmetics [type, brand names]); skin exposure (duration of exposure to sun, irritants [occupational], cold weather)
C. Nutrition/diet: intake of vitamins, essential nutrients, water; food allergies
D. Use of medications: steroids, vitamin use, hormones, antibiotics, chemotherapeutic agents
E. Past medical history: renal, hepatic, or collagen diseases; trauma or surgery; food, drug, or contact allergies
F. Family history: diabetes mellitus, allergic disorders, blood dyscrasias, specific dermatologic problems, cancer

## Physical Examination

A. Color: note areas of uniform color; pigmentation; redness, jaundice, cyanosis.
B. Vascular changes
   1. Purpuric lesions: note ecchymoses, petechiae.
   2. Vascular lesions: note angiomas, hemangiomas, venous stars.
C. Lesions: note color, type, size, distribution, location, consistency, grouping (annular, circular, linear, or clustered).
D. Edema: differentiate pitting from nonpitting.
E. Moisture content: note dryness, clamminess.
F. Temperature: note whether increased or decreased, distribution of temperature changes.
G. Texture: note smoothness, coarseness.
H. Mobility/turgor: note whether increased or decreased.

## Laboratory/Diagnostic Studies

A. Blood chemistry/electrolytes: calcium, chloride, magnesium, potassium, sodium
B. Hematologic studies: Hbg, HCT, RBC, WBC
C. Biopsy
   1. Removal of a small piece of skin for examination to determine diagnosis
   2. Nursing care: instruct client to keep biopsied area dry until healing occurs
D. Skin testing
   1. Administration of allergens or antigens on the surface of or into the dermis to determine hypersensitivity
   2. Three types: patch, scratch, and intradermal

# ANALYSIS

Nursing diagnoses for clients with a disorder of the integumentary system may include:
A. Impaired skin integrity
B. Pain
C. Disturbed body image
D. Risk for infection
E. Ineffective airway clearance
F. Ineffective peripheral tissue perfusion

# PLANNING AND IMPLEMENTATION

## Goals

A. Restoration of skin integrity.
B. Client will experience absence of pain.
C. Client will adapt to changes in appearance.
D. Client will be free from infection.
E. Maintenance of effective airway clearance.
F. Maintenance of adequate peripheral tissue perfusion.

## Interventions

### Skin Grafts

A. Replacement of damaged skin with healthy skin to provide protection of underlying structures or to reconstruct areas for cosmetic or functional purposes
B. Graft sources
   1. Autograft: client's own skin
   2. Isograft: skin from a genetically identical person (identical twin)
   3. Homograft or allograft: cadaver of same species
   4. Heterograft or xenograft: skin from another species (such as a porcine graft)
   5. Human amniotic membrane
C. Nursing care: preoperative
   1. Donor site: cleanse with antiseptic soap the night before and morning of surgery as ordered.
   2. Recipient site: apply warm compresses and topical antibiotics as ordered.
D. Nursing care: postoperative
   1. Donor site
      a. Keep area covered for 24–48 hours.
      b. Use bed cradle to prevent pressure and provide greater air circulation
      c. Outer dressing may be removed 24–72 hours postsurgery; maintain fine mesh gauze (innermost dressing) until it falls off spontaneously.
      d. Trim loose edges of gauze as it loosens with healing.
      e. Administer analgesics as ordered (more painful than recipient site).
   2. Recipient site
      a. Elevate site when possible.
      b. Protect from pressure (use bed cradle).
      c. Apply warm compresses as ordered.
      d. Assess for hematoma, fluid accumulation under graft.
      e. Monitor circulation distal to graft.
   3. Provide emotional support and monitor behavioral adjustments; refer for counseling if needed.
E. Provide client teaching and discharge planning concerning
   1. Applying lubricating lotion to maintain moisture on surfaces of healed graft for at least 6–12 months
   2. Protecting grafted skin from direct sunlight for at least 6 months
   3. Protecting graft from physical injury
   4. Need to report changes in graft (fluid accumulation, pain, hematoma)
   5. Possible alteration in pigmentation and hair growth; ability to sweat lost in most grafts
   6. Sensations may or may not return

# EVALUATION

A. Healing of burned areas; absence of drainage, edema, and pain over graft sites.
B. Relaxed facial expression/body posture; achieves effective rest patterns; participates in daily activities without pain.
C. Incorporates changes into self-concept without negating self-esteem; verbalizes about changes that occurred; demonstrates interest in physical appearance.
D. Achieves wound healing; vital signs within normal range; lungs clear; laboratory studies within normal range.
E. Lungs clear to auscultation; respiratory rate and depth within normal limits; free of dyspnea.
F. Palpable peripheral pulses of equal quality; adequate capillary refill; skin color normal in uninjured areas.

# DISORDERS OF THE INTEGUMENTARY SYSTEM

## Primary Lesions of the Skin

A. Macule: a flat, circumscribed area of color change in the skin without surface elevation, up to 2 cm in diameter
B. Papule: a circumscribed solid and elevated lesion, up to 1 cm in size
C. Nodule: a solid, elevated lesion extending deeper into the dermis, 1–2 cm in diameter
D. Wheal: a slightly irregular, transient superficial elevation of the skin with a palpable margin (e.g., hive)
E. Vesicle: circumscribed elevated lesion filled with serous fluid, less than 1 cm in diameter
F. Bulla: a vesicle larger than 1 cm in diameter
G. Pustule: a vesicle or bulla containing purulent exudate

## Contact Dermatitis

A. General information
   1. An irritation of the skin from a specific substance or from a hypersensitivity immune reaction from contact with a specific antigen

2. Caused by irritants (mechanical, chemical, biologic); allergens
B. Assessment findings
  1. Pruritus
  2. Erythema; localized edema; vesicles (oozing, crusting, and scaling [later])
  3. Diagnostic test: skin testing reveals hypersensitivity to specific antigen
C. Nursing interventions
  1. Apply wet dressings of Burrow's solution for 20 minutes 4 times a day to help clear oozing lesions.
  2. Provide relief from pruritus (see Cirrhosis of the Liver).
  3. Administer topical steroids and antibiotics as ordered.
  4. Provide client teaching and discharge planning concerning
     a. Avoidance of causative agent
     b. Preventing skin dryness
        1) Use mild soaps (Ivory).
        2) Soak in plain water for 20–30 minutes.
        3) Apply prescribed steroid cream immediately after bath.
        4) Avoid extremes of heat and cold.
     c. Allowing crusts and scales to drop off skin naturally as healing occurs
     d. Avoidance of wool, nylon, or fur fibers on sensitive skin
     e. Need to use gloves if handling irritant or allergenic substances

## Psoriasis

A. General information
  1. Chronic type of dermatitis that involves accelerated turnover rate of the epidermal cells
  2. Predisposing factors include stress, trauma, infection; changes in climate may produce exacerbations; familial predisposition to the disease
B. Medical management
  1. Topical corticosteroids
  2. Coal tar preparations
  3. Ultraviolet light
  4. Antimetabolites (methotrexate)
C. Assessment findings
  1. Mild pruritus
  2. Sharply circumscribed scaling placques that are mostly present on the scalp, elbows, and knees; yellow discoloration of nails
D. Nursing interventions
  1. Apply occlusive wraps over prescribed topical steroids.
  2. Protect areas treated with coal tar preparations from direct sunlight for 24 hours.
  3. Administer methotrexate as ordered, assess for side effects.
  4. Provide client teaching and discharge planning concerning

a. Feelings about changes in appearance of skin (encourage client to cover arms and legs with clothing if sensitive about appearance)
b. Importance of adhering to prescribed treatment and avoidance of commercially advertised products

## Acne

See Unit 5.

## Pediculosis

See Unit 5.

## Skin Cancer

A. General information
  1. Types of skin cancers
     a. Basal cell epithelioma: most common type of skin cancer; locally invasive and rarely metastasizes; most frequently located between the hairline and upper lip
     b. Squamous cell carcinoma (epidermoid): grows more rapidly than basal cell carcinoma and can metastasize; frequently seen on mucous membranes, lower lip, neck, and dorsum of the hands
     c. Malignant melanoma: least frequent of skin cancers, but most serious; capable of invasion and metastasis to other organs
  2. Precancerous lesions
     a. Leukoplakia: white, shiny patches in the mouth and on the lip
     b. Nevi (moles): junctional nevus may become malignant (signs include a color change to black, bleeding, and irritation); compound and dermal nevi unlikely to become cancerous
     c. Senile keratoses: brown, scalelike spots on older individuals
  3. Contributing factors include hereditary predisposition (fair, blue-eyed people; redheads and blondes); irritation (chemicals or ultraviolet rays)
  4. Occurs more often in those with outdoor occupations who are exposed to more sunlight
B. Medical management: varies depending on type of cancer; surgical excision with or without radiation therapy most common; chemotherapy and immunotherapy for melanoma
C. Assessment findings: characteristics depend on specific type of lesion; biopsy reveals malignant cells
D. Nursing interventions: provide client teaching concerning:
  1. Limitation of contact with chemical irritants
  2. Protection against ultraviolet radiation from sun

a. Wear thin layer of clothing.
b. Use sun block or lotion containing para-amino benzoic acid (PABA).
3. Need to report lesions that change characteristics and/or those that do not heal.

## Herpes Zoster (Shingles)

A. General information
1. Acute viral infection of the nervous system
2. The virus causes an inflammatory reaction in isolated spinal and cranial sensory ganglia and the posterior gray matter of the spinal cord
3. Contagious to anyone who has not had varicella or who is immunosuppressed
4. Caused by activation of latent varicella-zoster virus
B. Medical management
1. Analgesics
2. Corticosteroids
3. Acetic acid compresses
4. Acyclovir (Zovirax)
C. Assessment findings
1. Neuralgic pain, malaise, itching, burning
2. Cluster of skin vesicles along course of peripheral sensory nerves, usually unilateral and primarily on trunk, thorax, or face
D. Nursing interventions
1. Apply acetic acid compresses or white petrolatum to lesions.
2. Administer medications as ordered.
   a. Analgesics for pain.
   b. Systemic corticosteroids: monitor for side effects of steroid therapy.
   c. Acyclovir (Zovivax): antivalagent reduces severity when given early in illness.

## Herpes Simplex Virus, Type I

A. General information
1. Causes cold sores or fever blisters, canker sores, and herpetic whitlow
2. Common disorder, frequently seen in women
3. Primary infection occurs in children, recurrences in adults
4. Self-limiting virus
B. Assessment findings: clusters of vesicles, may ulcerate or crust; burning, itching, tingling; usually appears on lip or cheek
C. Nursing interventions: keep lesions dry; apply topical antibiotics or anesthetic as ordered; antivirals (valacyclovir) may be ordered 1–3 days.

## Burns

A. Types
1. Thermal: most common type; caused by flame, flash, scalding, and contact (hot metals, grease)
2. Smoke inhalation: occurs when smoke (particular products of a fire, gases, and superheated air) causes respiratory tissue damage
3. Chemical: caused by tissue contact, ingestion or inhalation of acids, alkalies, or vesicants
4. Electrical: injury occurs from direct damage to nerves and vessels when an electric current passes through the body.
B. Classification
1. Partial thickness
   a. Superficial partial-thickness (first degree)
      1) Depth: epidermis only
      2) Causes: sunburn, splashes of hot liquid
      3) Sensation: painful
      4) Characteristics: erythema, blanching on pressure, no vesicles
   b. Deep partial thickness (second degree)
      1) Depth: epidermis and dermis
      2) Causes: flash, scalding, or flame burn
      3) Sensation: very painful
      4) Characteristics: fluid-filled vesicles; red, shiny, wet after vesicles rupture
2. Full thickness (third and fourth degree)
   a. Depth: all skin layers and nerve endings; may involve muscles, tendons, and bones
   b. Causes: flame, chemicals, scalding, electric current
   c. Sensation: little or no pain
   d. Characteristics: wound is dry, white, leathery, or hard
C. Medical management
1. Supportive therapy: fluid management (IVs), catheterization
2. Wound care: hydrotherapy, debridement (enzymatic or surgical)
3. Drug therapy
   a. Topical antibiotics: mafenide (Sulfamylon), silver sulfadiazine (Silvadene), silver nitrate, povidone-iodine (Betadine) solution
   b. Systemic antibiotics: gentamicin
   c. Tetanus toxoid or hyperimmune human tetanus globulin (burn wound good medium for anaerobic growth)
   d. Analgesics
4. Surgery: excision and grafting
D. Assessment
1. Extent of burn injury by rule of nines: head and neck (9%); each arm (9%), each leg (18%), trunk (36%), genitalia (1%) (see Figure 4-28)
2. Lund and Browder method determines the extent of the burn injury by using client's age in proportion to relative body-part size.
3. Severity of burn
   a. Major: partial thickness greater than 25%; full thickness greater than or equal to 10%
   b. Moderate: partial thickness 15–25%, full thickness less than 10%
   c. Minor: partial thickness less than 15%; full thickness less than 2%

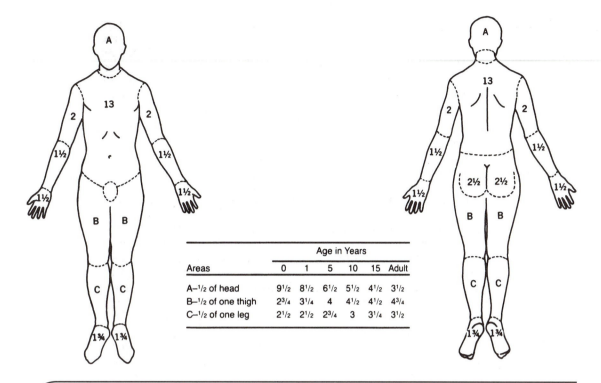

| | Age in Years | | | | | |
|---|---|---|---|---|---|---|
| Areas | 0 | 1 | 5 | 10 | 15 | Adult |
| A–1/2 of head | 9½ | 8½ | 6½ | 5½ | 4½ | 3½ |
| B–1/2 of one thigh | 2¾ | 3¼ | 4 | 4½ | 4½ | 4¾ |
| C–1/2 of one leg | 2½ | 2½ | 2¾ | 3 | 3¼ | 3½ |

**Figure 4-28** Body proportions change with growth. Shown here, in percentage, is the relationship of the body area to the whole body surface area at various ages. This method of determining the extent of the burned area is attributed to Lund and Browder

E. Stages
1. Emergent phase
   a. Remove person from source of burn.
      1) Thermal: smother burn beginning with the head.
      2) Smoke inhalation: ensure patent airway.
      3) Chemical: remove clothing that contains chemical; lavage area with copious amounts of water.
      4) Electrical: note victim position, identify entry/exit routes, maintain airway.
   b. Wrap in dry, clean sheet or blanket to prevent further contamination of wound and provide warmth.
   c. Assess how and when burn occurred.
   d. Provide IV route if possible.
   e. Transport immediately.
2. Shock phase (first 24–48 hours)
   a. Plasma to interstitial fluid shift causing hypovolemia; fluid also moves to areas that normally have little or no fluid (third-spacing).
   b. Assessment findings
      1) Dehydration, decreased blood pressure, elevated pulse, decreased urine output, thirst
      2) Diagnostic tests: hyperkalemia, hyponatremia, elevated HCT, metabolic acidosis

3. Fluid remobilization or diuretic phase (2–5 days postburn)
   a. Interstitial fluid returns to the vascular compartment.
   b. Assessment findings
      1) Elevated blood pressure, increased urine output
      2) Diagnostic tests: hypokalemia, hyponatremia, metabolic acidosis
4. Convalescent (rehabilitation) phase
   a. Starts when diuresis is completed and wound healing and coverage begin.
   b. Assessment findings
      1) Dry, waxy-white appearance of full thickness burn changing to dark brown; wet, shiny, and serous exudate in partial thickness
      2) Diagnostic test: hyponatremia
F. Nursing interventions
1. Provide relief/control of pain.
   a. Administer morphine sulfate IV and monitor vital signs closely.
   b. Administer analgesics/narcotics 30 minutes before wound care.
   c. Position burned areas in proper alignment.
2. Monitor alterations in fluid and electrolyte balance.
   a. Assess for fluid shifts and electrolyte alteration (see Table 4-5).

**Table 4-28** Guidelines and Formulas for Fluid Replacement for Burns

| Consensus Formula | Evans Formula | Brooke Army Formula | Parkland/Baxter Formula |
|---|---|---|---|
| Lactated Ringer's: 2–4 mL × wt. in kg × % body surface area (BSA) burned. Half to be given in first 8 hr after burn; remaining fluid to be given over next 16 hr. | 1. Colloids: 1 mL × wt. kg × % BSA burned<br>2. Electrolytes (saline): 1 mL × wt. kg × % BSA burned<br>3. Glucose (5% in water): 2000 mL for insensible loss<br>Day 1: Half to be given in first 8 hr; remaining half over next 16 hr.<br>Day 2: Half of previous day's colloids and electrolytes; all of insensible fluid replacement.<br>Maximum of 10,000 mL over 24 hr.<br>Second- and third-degree burns exceeding 50% BSA calculated on basis of 50% BSA. | 1. Colloids: 0.5 mL × wt. kg × % BSA burned<br>2. Electrolytes (lactated Ringer's): 1.5 mL × wt. kg × % BSA burned<br>3. Glucose (5% in water): 2000 mL for insensible loss<br>Day 1: Half to be given in first 8 hr; remaining half over next 16 hr.<br>Day 2: Half of colloids, half of electrolytes, all of insensible fluid replacement.<br>Second- and third-degree burns exceeding 50% BSA calculated on basis of 50% BSA. | Lactated Ringer's: 4 mL × wt. kg × % BSA burned.<br>Day 1: Half to be given in first 8 hr; half to be given over next 16 hr.<br>Day 2: Varies; colloid is added. |

  b. Administer IV fluids as ordered (see Table 4-28)

  c. Monitor Foley catheter output hourly (30 mL/hour desired).

  d. Weigh daily.

  e. Monitor circulation status regularly.

  f. Administer/monitor crystalloids/colloids/H$_2$O solutions.

 3. Promote maximal nutritional status.

  a. Monitor tube feedings/TPN if ordered.

  b. When oral intake permitted, provide high-calorie, high-protein, high-carbohydrate diet with vitamin and mineral supplements.

  c. Serve small portions.

  d. Schedule wound care and other treatments at least 1 hour before meals.

 4. Prevent wound infection.

  a. Place client in controlled sterile environment.

  b. Use hydrotherapy for no more than 30 minutes to prevent electrolyte loss.

  c. Observe wound for separation of eschar and cellulitis.

  d. Apply mafenide (Sulfamylon) as ordered.

   1) Administer analgesics 30 minutes before application.

   2) Monitor acid-base status and renal function studies.

   3) Provide daily tubbing for removal of previously applied cream.

  e. Apply silver sulfadiazine (Silvadene) as ordered.

   1) Administer analgesics 30 minutes before application.

   2) Observe for and report hypersensitivity reactions (rash, itching, burning sensation in unburned areas).

   3) Store drug away from heat.

  f. Apply silver nitrate as ordered.

   1) Handle carefully; solution leaves a gray or black stain on skin, clothing, and utensils.

   2) Administer analgesic before application.

   3) Keep dressings wet with solution; dryness increases the concentration and causes precipitation of silver salts in the wound.

  g. Apply povidone-iodine (Betadine) solution as ordered.

   1) Administer analgesics before application.

   2) Assess for metabolic acidosis/renal function studies.

  h. Administer gentamicin as ordered: assess vestibular/auditory and renal functions at regular intervals.

 5. Prevent GI complications.

  a. Assess for signs and symptoms of paralytic ileus.

  b. Assist with insertion of NG tube to prevent/control Curling's/stress ulcer; monitor patency/drainage.

  c. Administer prophylactic antacids through NG tube and/or IV cimetidine (Tagamet) or ranitidine (Zantac) (to prevent gastric pH of less than 5).

  d. Monitor bowel sounds.

  e. Test stools for occult blood.

6. Provide client teaching and discharge planning concerning
   a. Care of healed burn wound
      1) Assess daily for changes.
      2) Wash hands frequently during dressing change.
      3) Wash area with prescribed solution or mild soap and rinse well with $H_2O$; dry with clean towel.
      4) Apply sterile dressing.
   b. Prevention of injury to burn wound
      1) Avoid trauma to area.
      2) Avoid use of fabric softeners or harsh detergents (might cause irritation).
      3) Avoid constrictive clothing over burn wound.
   c. Adherence to prescribed diet
   d. Importance of reporting formation of blisters, opening of healed area, increased or foul-smelling drainage from wound, other signs of infection
   e. Methods of coping and resocialization

# Complementary and Alternative Medicine (CAM)

## OVERVIEW

A. Definitions
1. Alternative medicine is a holistic approach to health and focuses on balancing the body to achieve optimal wellness.
2. Alternative medical systems are built upon a complex system of theory and practice and have often evolved apart from, and earlier than, the conventional medicine that is practiced in the United States.
3. Modalities that are generally not taught widely in Western medical schools nor generally available in hospitals in the United States or other Western societies (see Table 4-29).

B. Patterns of CAM use in the United States
1. Most clients do not tell their physician they are using CAM unless specifically asked.
2. Estimates that one in three adults aged 35 to 49 years is using at least one CAM therapy.
3. Higher incidence in incomes over $50,000.
4. 42% of CAM use is for treatment of a specific disease or illness, while 58% of use is, at least in part, to prevent future illness from occurring or to maintain health and vitality.

**Table 4–29** Complementary and Alternative Modalities

| Modality | What It Is | Common Uses |
| --- | --- | --- |
| Ayurvedic Medicine | Ayurvedic tradition believes that all illnesses, physical or mental, are a state of disharmony or imbalance in the body's systems. Diagnosis is made by feeling the pulse and looking for indicators of disharmony on the tongue. Utilizes a wide variety of modalities such as medication, herbals, and massage. Nutrition and food groups play a key role in balancing the body systems. Practiced in India for more than 5000 years. | Acute and chronic illness, promotion of health and wellness |
| Aromatherapy | The use of essential oils, distilled from plants, aromatherapy treats. Oils are massaged into the skin in diluted form, inhaled, or placed in water for diffusion. Aromatherapy is often used in conjunction with massage therapy, acupuncture, reflexology, herbology, chiropractic, and other holistic treatments. | Abdominal pain, stress and anxiety, insomnia, as an antiseptic, skin conditions |
| Massage | Manipulation of muscles and other soft tissue. Improves circulation, muscle fatigue, and promotes well-being. Multiple techniques including deep tissue, vibration, effleurage, percussion. Developed in both Western and Eastern cultures. | Back and neck pain, stress, insomnia, headache, promotion of well-being |

*(continues)*

**Table 4-29** Complementary and Alternative Modalities *(continued)*

| Modality | What It Is | Common Uses |
|---|---|---|
| Chiropractic | Manipulation of the spine to promote balance and health. Misalignments of the spine thought to cause pressure on the spinal nerve roots. Pressure from trauma or poor posture leads to decreased function and wellness. Adjustment or manipulation of the spine corrects the misalignment and results in a more balanced state of health. | Back and neck pain, stress, insomnia, headache |
| Acupuncture | Based on the concept of chi, or life-force energy. Very fine needles are placed along energy lines to disperse congestion, increase energy flow, and allow the body to heal and balance. | Pain relief, smoking cessation, treatment of acute and chronic illness; also used extensively with pets |
| Biofeedback | Use of a sensor unit (TENS) allows individuals to monitor their own bodies' response to stimuli. Usually a light and sound device. A method of monitoring minute metabolic changes in one's own body with the aid of sensitive machines. Individuals use imagery, breathing techniques, and visualization to control their heart rate, breathing, and thought process. These changes are audible and visible on the biofeedback unit. | Stress-related conditions such as asthma, migraines, insomnia, and high blood pressure |
| Hypnosis | A method of focusing on the unconscious mind and accessing the subconscious to access repressed emotions, forgotten events, and memories that may assist the client to heal. Trained hypnotherapist creates a calm, safe environment for the client. Client remains aware but focused on the subconscious mind rather than the present. | Anxiety, weight loss, pain relief, phobias, chronic pain |
| Homeopathy | A healing system that uses minute amounts of natural substances, called remedies, to stimulate the individual's immune system. These substances, given in larger dose, mimic the symptoms the client is experiencing. Based on the philosophy "like cures like." | Arthritis, abdominal complaints, allergies, fatigue, menstrual irregularities |
| Herbal Medicine | The use of plant products for treatment of a wide range of chronic and acute illnesses. Plants, and their derivatives, are used in a variety of forms, including dried, distilled, tincture, pills, caplets, elixirs, and topical preparations. One of the oldest complementary therapies, it is used widely throughout the world today as the primary source of medicinal products. Not regulated by the FDA in the United States. | Acute and chronic illness including, but not limited to, asthma, arthritis, abdominal pain, menstrual irregularities, cuts and bruises; used to enhance the functioning of the body's systems |
| Reflexology | Designed to stimulate chi, or life-force energy, in the body by applying pressure to meridians, or contact points, on the feet and hands. Pressure on the reflexology points stimulates flow of chi, allowing the client to restore balance in the body and promote healing. The practitioner uses the fingers to apply pressure to the reflexology points. | Respiratory symptoms, stress, headache, fatigue, pain |
| Reiki | Use of the practitioner's hands to "channel" the universal life-force energy to the client to promote healing. Tibetan healing system. Hands may hover above the client or lightly touch. Use light hand placements to channel healing energies to the recipient. | Pain, digestive problems, stress and stress-related disorders; assist the recipient in achieving spiritual focus and clarity |
| Therapeutic Touch | Practitioner "senses" client's energy field through auditory-visual-kinetic or intuitive systems. Using the hands, the practitioner facilitates a symmetrical and rhythmical flow of energy and redirects it, allowing the individual's energy to flow freely. Treatment is complete when the practitioner senses a symmetrical state and rhythmic order. | Headache, musculoskeletal pain, emotional distress |

**475.** A client is seen in the outpatient clinic for treatment of psoriasis. The nurse should anticipate which of the following findings in this man?

1. Intense pain.
2. Discolored nails.
3. Abdominal lesions.
4. Hyperpigmented skin.

**476.** The physician prescribes coal tar preparations as part of the treatment plan for a client who has psoriasis. The nurse should include which statement in the teaching plan for this client?

1. Avoid sunlight immediately after the treatment.
2. Ingest the coal tar with liberal amounts of water.
3. Eat a high-carbohydrate diet.
4. Restrict activity for 24 hours.

**477.** An adult's shirt catches on fire and is now in flames. He panics and runs into his neighbor's yard. Which of the following interventions is appropriate? Select all that apply.

_____ Dousing the flames with water.
_____ Removing his burned clothing.
_____ Removing his jewelry.
_____ Rolling him on the ground.

**478.** The nurse is caring for a man admitted with severe burns sustained when his clothing caught fire while he was burning leaves. During the acute burn phase, which intervention will be absent from the nursing care plan?

1. Strict aseptic technique.
2. Proper alignment of all joints.
3. Maintenance of fluid and electrolyte balance.
4. Frequent and routine administration of narcotics.

**479.** The nurse is planning care for an adult man who is admitted with severe flame burns. During the first 24–48 hours of a post-burn client, which body changes can the nurse expect to occur?

1. An increase in the total volume of intravascular plasma.
2. Excessive renal perfusion with diuresis.
3. Fluid shift from interstitial spaces to plasma.
4. Fluid shift from plasma to interstitial spaces.

**480.** The nurse is caring for an adult who was admitted following severe burns sustained in a house fire.

What would an acceptable range for hourly urine output during the first 2 days post-burn?

1. 20 mL.
2. 30–50 mL.
3. 100–150 mL.
4. 150–200 mL.

**481.** The nurse is to perform a scratch test for allergy. Which statement best describes this procedure?

1. The antigen is directly applied to the skin and covered with a gauze dressing.
2. The allergen is applied superficially to a small cut of the outer layer of skin.
3. A small amount of allergen is injected into the intradermal layer of skin.
4. Suspected food allergy items are scratched from the diet, one at a time, until all allergy symptoms are no longer present.

**482.** An adult has undergone a skin graft from his left buttock to his right upper thigh. What intervention will the nurse expect to perform when caring for the recipient site?

1. Apply silver sulfadiazine to promote rapid healing.
2. Assess for bleeding and large amounts of fluid accumulation beneath the graft.
3. Encourage the client to ambulate and do leg lifts on return from the OR.
4. Encourage the client to take frequent soaking baths to relieve his soreness and discomfort.

**483.** A client with a skin graft has undergone a full-thickness skin graft from her right upper thigh to her upper chest area. What is the most appropriate nursing action in caring for the donor site?

1. Keep the fine mesh gauze dressing on her chest soaked with normal saline.
2. Completely immobilize her right upper thigh area.
3. Maintain the compression bandage on her right upper thigh for several days.
4. Remove the nylon fabric adhered to the donor site no later than 2 to 3 days after grafting has taken place.

**484.** A client has undergone a skin graft. Which finding most likely indicates that complications with the recipient site may exist?

1. Small amounts of blood beneath the graft.
2. Small amounts of serum beneath the graft.
3. A meshed pattern in the graft.
4. Continuous bleeding beneath the graft.

485. A female client has been diagnosed with atopic dermatitis. She has severe pruritis. Which interventions are most appropriate to include in the plan of care?
   1. Soak in a hot water bath at least once a day for 15–20 minutes.
   2. Avoid use of air conditioning when possible.
   3. When symptoms are worse, decrease bathing.
   4. Use a moisturizing soap.

486. The client is ordered soaks with Burrow's solution due to severe poison ivy. What is the primary reason for the soaks?
   1. To clean out the wounds.
   2. To help dry the oozing lesions.
   3. To stop the pruritus.
   4. To stop the pain from the lesions.

487. The nurse has been giving instructions to a white female about preventing skin cancer. Which statement best indicates understanding of skin cancer risk factors?
   1. "I guess because I am dark complected I will be more prone to developing skin cancer."
   2. "I used to lie in the sun all the time—now I just go to the tanning bed."
   3. "My father was treated for melanoma, but my mom says not to worry."
   4. "I really need to use sunscreen—even in winter."

488. A client presents with a diagnosis of basal cell epithelioma. What is the best description for the lesion?
   1. Dome shaped, shiny, with a well-defined border.
   2. Poorly marginated, flat red area.
   3. Red, dark blue, or purple macules.
   4. Erythema, edema, and blisters.

489. While providing a nursing history, a client with suspected malignant melanoma will most often relate which of the following?
   1. A history of intense sunlight exposure.
   2. Complaints of frequently occurring irregularly shaped, flat macules with overlying hard scale.
   3. Consistent use of sunscreen agents.
   4. Complaints of several lesions with a raised border and flattened center.

490. An adult presents with the following symptoms: clusters of vesicles on the right flank; constant, severe pain; burning; itching and discomfort in the flank area. Which of the following diagnoses would be a priority when developing a plan of care for the client?
   1. Pain, related to herpes simplex.
   2. Pain, related to herpes zoster.
   3. Pain, related to herpetic whitlow.
   4. Pain, related to staphylococcal cellulitis.

491. What should the nurse include in the plan of care for a client with herpes zoster?
   1. Teaching the client to avoid sexual contact during outbreaks.
   2. Administering analgesics and evaluating the efficacy.
   3. Informing the client that people who have not had chickenpox will not develop them from exposure to the client.
   4. Scheduling several diagnostic tests to confirm the presence of herpes zoster.

492. Which client statement best indicates the client understands how herpes simplex is transmitted?
   1. "It is okay to share towels as long as it is a family member."
   2. "I really don't need to use a condom, unless I have a sore."
   3. "Once I'm over this spell, I won't need to worry about it again."
   4. "I shouldn't have sex if some of those sores are around."

493. A client is admitted with severe flame burns resulting from smoking in bed. The nurse would expect the room environment to include which of the following?
   1. Strict isolation techniques and policies.
   2. A semi-private room.
   3. Liberal unrestricted visiting.
   4. Equipment shared between the client and the other burn client in the unit.

494. An adult client was burned severely in an industrial accident. He has second-degree burns on his right leg and arm and on his back. He has third-degree burns on his left arm. The triage nurse, using the rule of nines, estimates the extent of the client's burns as _____%.

495. An adult was burned in a house fire 16 hours ago. She suffered second- and third-degree burns over 65% of her body. She is receiving lactated Ringer's at 200 mL/h. Which intervention is a priority at this time?
   1. Monitoring hourly urine output.
   2. Assessing for signs and symptoms of infection.

3. Performing range of motion q 1–2 h.

4. Meeting the high caloric needs of the client.

496. A nurse is providing care for a severely burned client during the shock phase of the burn injury. Which assessment findings would indicate that the client is receiving adequate fluid volume replacement?
1. Urine output 20 mL/h, CVP 3, weak pulses, K⁺ level of 5.3.
2. Urine output 50 mL/h, BP 100/60, oriented to person and place.
3. Weak thready pulses, BP 70/40, pulse 130, HCT 52%.
4. Restlessness, confusion, urine output 15 mL/h, rapidly increasing weight.

497. A client with severe burns is receiving IV Zantac. Which statement best explains the reason for administration of this medication in this situation?
1. The client was treated for gastritis several years ago.
2. The medication will reduce hypoxemia in burn clients.
3. The medication is an H₂ receptor antagonist and will decrease acid secretion.
4. The medication will aid in removal of pulmonary secretions.

498. An 18-year-old was burned 6 weeks ago. She is now ready for discharge. Select the statement best reflecting understanding of discharge care.
1. "I will be so glad to get home so that I don't have to wear this pressure thing anymore."
2. "I will need to call my doctor if my temperature goes up or this burn area starts draining and oozing."
3. "I really need to stick to a low-calorie, low-protein diet."
4. "To prevent that area of new skin from feeling so tight, I can rub ice and baby oil on it."

499. A client has suffered a chemical burn. What is the nurse's best initial action?
1. Roll the client in a blanket.
2. Secure lead-lined gloves and move the client away from the chemical.
3. Flush the area with copious amounts of water or normal saline.
4. If the chemical is an acid, neutralize with a base.

500. An electrical worker has come in contact with a live power line. He is unconscious and is lying across the power line. What is the nurse's best initial action?
1. Move the person away from the power line using a wooden pole.
2. Cover the person with a blanket.
3. Grab the person and pull him away from the power lines.
4. Flush the wound with copious amounts of water.

# Answers and Rationales

475. **2.** A yellow discoloration of the nails is frequently seen in psoriasis.

476. **1.** Sunlight should be avoided after a coal tar treatment.

477. *Dousing the flames* should be selected. This is an appropriate way to smother the flames. *Removing his jewelry* should be selected. Hot metal jewelry could increase burning. Rings should be removed before edema occurs. *Rolling him on the ground* should be selected because it will smother flames.

478. **4.** Narcotics should be given only after careful assessment in this phase due to the danger of shock and respiratory depression.

479. **4.** The initial fluid alteration following a severe burn is a plasma-to-interstitial fluid and electrolyte balance, which is a nursing priority.

480. **2.** A safe range for the hourly urine output post-burn is 30–50 mL. Less than this amount would indicate severely decreased renal arterial perfusion.

481. **2.** The allergen is applied to a small superficial scratch that cuts the outer layer of the skin.

482. **2.** Bleeding and large amounts of fluid accumulation beneath the graft may prevent successful adherence of the graft.

483. **3.** Compression bandages are often applied in the operating room on top of a synthetic, semipermeable polyurethane film. This dressing allows the polyurethane film to adhere to the donor site, reducing accumulation of fluid.

484. **4.** Continuous bleeding beneath a graft may prevent adherence of the graft.

**4**

485. **4.** A moisturizing soap will help decrease the pruritus, as it will be less drying.

486. **2.** The solution helps dry up oozing lesions such as poison ivy. It does not debride wounds, prevent pain, or stop itching.

487. **4.** Almost all cases of basal and squamous cell skin cancer diagnosed each year in the United States are considered to be sun-related.

488. **1.** The most common presentation of BSE is a nodular lesion that is dome-shaped papules with well-defined borders. The lesions can have a pearly or shiny appearance because it does not keratinize.

489. **1.** The majority of malignant melanoma appears to be associated with the intensity of sunlight exposure rather than the duration.

490. **2.** Pain is a significant problem with herpes zoster. Topical solutions, cooling soaks, and use of analgesics are usually incorporated into the plan of care.

491. **2.** Pain is usually present and can be quite severe. It is important to help the client obtain relief. Cool compresses, analgesics, and topical antipruritic preparations may be used.

492. **4.** Sexual contact should be avoided during the initial and recurring infections. The client should also avoid touching the infected area, as it may be transferred to the eyes or face. Good handwashing is vital.

493. **1.** Isolation is thought by some clinicians to reduce the incidence of cross contamination significantly. However, methods vary drastically from one center to another. The single most effective technique to prevent transmission of infection is handwashing!

494. The rule of nines is a quick assessment scale used to estimate the extent of burn injury. The basis of the rule is to divide the body into areas each representing 9% or a multiple of 9% of the total body surface area. This client's injuries were assigned the following percentages: R arm 9%, L arm 9%, R leg 18%, back 18%, total 54%.

495. **1.** Urine output is the most readily available and reliable indicator for determining the adequacy of fluid resuscitation. Urine output should be monitored every hour and maintained between 30 and 50 mL/h.

496. **2.** 50 mL/h of urine is adequate, BP is stable, clear sensorium is another positive sign that adequate fluid volume replacement is occurring. Pulses should also be easily palpable.

497. **3.** Burn clients are very susceptible to development of stress ulcers. Routinely they receive Zantac to help prevent this complication.

498. **2.** This statement demonstrates that the client realizes she must be alert to the signs and symptoms of infection and notify her physician if they do occur.

499. **3.** Water will neutralize most chemicals while decreasing the heat reaction.

500. **1.** Emergency treatment starts with separating the client from the power source. It is important to use nonconductive implements such as wooden poles to prevent injury to the rescuer.

## REFERENCES AND SUGGESTED READINGS

Adams, J., & Apple, F. (2004). New blood tests for detecting heart disease. *Cardiology Patient Page*, 12–14. (Retrieved from Circulation).

*Alternative therapies in health and medicine.* Boulder, CO. InnoVision Communications, LLC. Retrieved on August 21, 2008 from http://www.alternative-therapies.com

American Association of Nurse Anesthetists. *Conscious sedation: What patients should expect.* Retrieved August 21, 2008, from http://www.aana.com/forpatients.aspx?ucNavMenu_TSMenuTargetID=68&ucNavMenu_TSMenuTargetType=4&ucNavMenu_TSMenuID=6&id=298&terms=conscious+sedation

Aschenbrenner, D., Cleveland, L., & Venable, S. (2007). *Drug therapy in nursing* (2nd ed.). Philadelphia: Lippincott Williams & Wilkins.

Barash, P., Cullen, B., Stoelting, R., Cullen, B. (2005). *Handbook of clinical anesthesia* (5th ed.). Philadelphia: Lippincott Williams & Wilkins.

Barnes, P. M., Powell-Griner, E., McFann, K., & Nahin, R. L. (2004). Complementary and alternative medicine use among adults: United States, 2002. Advance data from vital & health statistics. Hyattsville, MD: National Center for Health Statistics.

Bickley, L., & Szilagyi, P. (2005). *Bates' guide to physical examination and history taking* (9th ed.). Philadelphia: Lippincott Williams & Wilkins.

Black, J., & Hawks, J. (2008). *Medical-surgical nursing: Clinical management for positive outcomes* (8th ed.). Philadelphia: Saunders.

Board on Health Promotion and Disease Prevention and Institute of Medicine. Institute of Medicine of the National Academies. (2005). *Complementary and alternative medicine in the United States.* The National Academies Press: Washington, D.C.

Brown, K. (2003). *Emergency dysrhythmias & ECG injury patterns.* Clifton Park, NY: Thomson Delmar Learning.

Carpenito, L. (2007). *Nursing diagnosis: Application to clinical practice* (12th ed.). Philadelphia: Lippincott Williams & Wilkins.

Centers for Disease Control and Prevention. (2006). *Trends in tuberculosis incidence—United States, 2006* (March 23, 2007/56(11);245-250). Atlanta, GA.

Daniels, R., Nosek, L., & Nicoll, L. (2007). *Contemporary medical-surgical nursing.* Clifton Park, NY: Thomson Delmar Cengage Learning.

Doenges, M., & Moorehouse, M. (2008). *Application of nursing process and nursing diagnosis* (5th ed.). Philadelphia: F. A. Davis.

Eliopoulos, C. (2004). *Gerontological nursing* (6th ed.). Philadelphia: Lippincott Williams & Wilkins.

Estes, M. (2010). *Health assessment and physical examination* (4th ed.). Clifton Park, NY: Delmar Cengage Learning.

Fischbach, F. (2008). *A manual of laboratory and diagnostic tests* (8th ed.). Philadelphia: Lippincott Williams & Wilkins.

Fischbach, F., & Dunning III, M. (2005). *Nurses' quick reference to common laboratory and diagnostic tests* (4th ed.). Philadelphia: Lippincott Williams & Wilkins.

Guyton, A., & Hall, J. (2006). *Textbook of medical physiology* (11th ed.). Philadelphia: Saunders.

Hudack, C., Morton, P., & Gallo, B. (2004). *Critical care nursing: A holistic approach* (8th ed.). Philadelphia: Lippincott Williams & Wilkins.

Ignatavicius, D., & Workman, M. (2006). *Medical-surgical nursing: Critical thinking for collaborative care* (5th ed.). Philadelphia: W. B. Saunders.

Kost, M. (2002). *Administration of conscious sedation.* http://nsweb.nursingspectrum.com/ce/ce159.htm

Lemone, P., & Burke, K. (2008). *Medical-surgical nursing: Critical thinking in client care* (4th ed.). Upper Saddle River, NJ: Prentice Hall.

Lewis, S., Bucher, L., Heitkemper, M., Dirksen, S. O'Brien, P., & Bucher, L. (2007). *Medical-surgical nursing: Assessment and management of clinical problems* (7th ed.) St. Louis, MO: Elsevier, Health Science Division.

Linton, A., & Lach, H. (2006). *Matteson & McConnell's gerontological nursing: concepts and practice* (3rd ed.). St. Louis, MO: Elsevier, Health Science Division.

Mayhew, M., Edmunds, M., & Wendel, V. (2005). *Gerontological nurse practitioner: Review and resource manual.* Washington, DC: The American Nurses Credentialing Center.

Micozzi, M. S. (2005). *Fundamentals of complementary and alternative medicine.* (3rd ed.). New York: Churchill-Livingston.

Miller, C. (2003). *Nursing for wellness in older adults: Theory & practice* (4th ed.). Philadelphia: Lippincott Williams & Wilkins.

Miller, J. (2003). *Delmar's NCLEX-PN review.* Clifton Park, NY: Thomson Delmar Learning.

NANDA International. (2007). *Nursing diagnosis: Definitions & classification 2007–2008.* NANDA International, Philadelphia. Author.

Phipps, W., Long, B., Woods, N., & Cass Meyer, V. (2006). *Medical-surgical nursing concepts and clinical practice* (8th ed.). St. Louis, MO: Elsevier, Health Science Division.

Reuben, D. B., Pacala, J., & Herr, K. (2004). *Geriatrics at your fingertips* (6th ed.). Malden, MA: Blackwell.

Seeley, R., Stephens, T., & Tate, P. (2006). *Anatomy & physiology* (7th ed.). New York: McGraw Hill.

Smeltzer, S., Bare, B., & Boyer, M. (2008). *Brunner and Suddarth's textbook of medical surgical nursing* (11th ed.). Philadelphia: Lippincott Williams & Wilkins.

Spratto, G. R., & Woods, A. L. (2009). *Delmar Nurse's drug handbook 2009 Edition.* Clifton Park, NY: Delmar Cengage Learning.

# UNIT 5

# PEDIATRIC NURSING

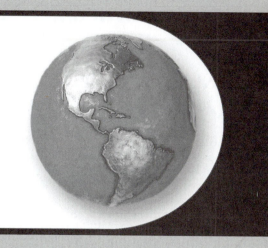

Today's pediatric nurse faces an array of challenges in providing care for children and their families. A nurse requires competent skills from a wide spectrum of both technological and psychosocial disciplines. To effectively care for children and families in a variety of settings, the nurse must have a thorough understanding of disease processes, as well as knowledge of emotional, social, cultural, and developmental needs.

To provide this essential knowledge base, this unit begins with a review of growth and development, which is basic to understanding the behavior of children and the influences of illness. The next section, multisystem stressors, emphasizes such topics as fluid, electrolyte, and acid-base imbalance, which are applicable to many pediatric health care problems.

The unit is further divided into specific body systems. For each system, there is an initial review of aspects of anatomy and physiology unique to the child. Each step of the nursing process is then reviewed, followed by discussions of the major health problems of that system.

Throughout the unit, only information specific to children is presented. In many cases, for instance, when lab tests or nursing care do not differ from those for the adult, the content is not repeated. Refer to Unit 4 for additional background information when needed.

## UNIT OUTLINE

# Growth and Development

## GENERAL PRINCIPLES

### Definition of Terms

A. *Growth:* increase in size of a structure. Human growth is orderly and predictable, but not even; it follows a cyclical pattern.

B. *Development:* increased complexity in thought, behavior, skill, or function. Development includes growth and is a process that continues over time.

C. *Maturation:* genetically determined pattern for growth and development.

D. *Gephalocaudal:* head-to-toe progression of growth and development.

E. *Proximodistal:* trunk-to-periphery (fingers and toes) progression of growth and development.

F. *Phylogeny:* development or evolution of a species or group; a pattern of development for a species.

G. *Ontogeny:* development of an individual within a species.

H. *Critical period:* specific time period during which certain environmental events or stimuli have greatest effect on a child's development.

I. *Developmental task:* skill or competency unique to a stage of development.

### Rates of Development

Growth and development are not synonymous but are closely interrelated processes directed by both genetic and environmental factors. Although changes in growth and development are more obvious in some periods than others, they are important in all periods.

A. Infancy and adolescence: fast growth periods

B. Toddler through school-age: slow growth periods

C. Fetal period and infancy: the head and neurologic tissue grow faster than other tissues.

D. Toddler and preschool periods: the trunk grows more rapidly than other tissue.

E. The limbs grow most during school-age period.

F. The trunk grows faster than other tissue during adolescence.

### Child Development Theorists

Also see Unit 7.

#### Sigmund Freud (Psychosexual Theory)

See Table 5-1.

#### Erik Erikson (Psychosocial Theory)

See Table 5-2.

#### Jean Piaget (Cognitive Theory)

See Table 5-3.

## ASSESSMENT

### Developmental Tasks

Developmental tasks are skills or competencies normally occurring at one stage and having an effect on the development of subsequent stages; fall into three categories

A. Physical tasks (e.g., learning to sit, crawl, walk; toileting)

B. Psychologic tasks (e.g., learning trust, self-esteem)

**Table 5-1** Stages of Freud's Psychosexual Development

| Stage | Age | Characteristics |
|-------|-----|-----------------|
| Oral | Birth to 1 year | Receives satisfaction from oral needs being met; attachment to mother important because she usually meets infant's needs |
| Anal | 1 to 3 years | Learns to control bodily functions, especially toileting |
| Phallic | 3 to 6 years | Fascinated with gender differences, childbirth; Oedipus or Electra complex |
| Latency | 6 to 11 years | Sexual drives submerged; appropriate gender roles adopted; learning about society |
| Genital | 12 years and older | Sexual desires directed toward opposite gender; learns how to form loving relationships and manage sexual urges in societally appropriate ways |

**Table 5-2** Stages of Erikson's Psychosocial Theory of Development

| Stage | Age | Characteristics |
|---|---|---|
| Trust versus mistrust | 1 month to 1½ years | Learns world is good and can be trusted as basic needs are met |
| Autonomy versus shame and doubt | 1½ to 3 years | Learns independent behaviors regarding toileting, bathing, feeding, dressing; exerts self; exercises choices |
| Initiative versus guilt | 3 to 6 years | Goal directed, competitive, exploratory behavior; imaginative |
| Industry versus inferiority | 6 to 11 years | Learns self-worth as gains mastery of psychosocial, physiological, and cognitive skills; becomes society or peer focused |
| Identity versus role confusion | 12 to 18 years | Develops sense of who I am; gains independence from parents; peers important |

**Table 5-3** Stages of Piaget's Theory of Cognitive Development

| Stage/Phase | Age | Characteristics |
|---|---|---|
| **Sensiomotor** | Birth to 2 years | |
| Reflexive | Birth to 1 month | Predictable, innate survival reflexes |
| Primary circular reactions | 1 to 4 months | Responds purposefully to stimuli; initiates , respects satisfying behaviors |
| Secondary circular reactions | 4 to 8 months | Learns from intentional behavior; motor skills/ vision coordinated; recognizes familiar objects |
| Coordination of secondary schemes | 8 to 12 months | Develops object permanence; anticipates others' actions; differentiates familiar/unfamiliar |
| Tertiary circular reactions | 12 to 18 months | Interested in novelty, repetition, understands causality; solicits help from others |
| Mental combinations | 18 to 24 months | Simple problem solving; imitates |
| **Preoperational** | 2 to 7 years | |
| Preconceptual | 2 to 4 years | Egocentric thought; mental imagery; increasing language |
| Intuitive | 4 to 7 years | Sophisticated language; decreasing egocentric thought; reality-based play |
| **Concrete Operations** | 7 to 11 years | Understands relationships, classification, conservation, seriation, reversibility; logical reasoning limited, less egocentric thought |
| **Formal Operation** | 11 years and older | Capable of systemic, abstract thought |

C. Cognitive tasks (e.g., acquiring concepts of time and space, abstract thought)
See Table 5-4.

## Measurement Tools

There are a number of different assessment tools for measuring the progress of growth and development.
A. Chronologic age: assessment of developmental tasks related to birth date
B. Mental age: assessment of cognitive development
 1. Measured by variety of standardized intelligence tests (IQ), such as the *Stanford Binet Intelligence Scale*
 2. Results from at least two separate testing sessions needed before determination of cognitive level is made
 3. Uses toys and language based on mental rather than chronologic age
C. *Denver II* (Revision and restandardized from *Denver Developmental Screening Test (DDST)* and its revision, the *DDST-R*).
 1. Generalized assessment tool; measures gross motor, fine motor, language, and personal-social development from newborn-6 years
 2. Does not measure intelligence

**Table 5-4** Stages, Age Ranges, and Characteristics of Human Development Related to Pediatric Nursing

| Stage | Age | Characteristics |
| --- | --- | --- |
| Infant | Birth to 1 year | Period of rapid growth and change; attachments to family members and other caregivers are formed; trust develops. |
| Toddler | 1 to 3 years | Motor ability, coordination, sensory skills developing; basic feelings, emotions, a sense of self, and being independent becomes important. |
| Preschooler | 3 to 6 years | Continued physiological, psychological, and cognitive growth; better able to care for selves; interested in playing with other children; beginning to develop a concept of who they are. |
| School age | 6 to 12 years | Interested in achievement; ability to read, write, and complete academic work advances; understanding of the world broadens. |
| Adolescent | 12 to 19 years, or later | Transition period between childhood and adulthood; physiological maturation occurs, formal operational thought begins; preparation for becoming an adult takes place. |

**D.** Growth parameters
   1. Bone age: X-ray of tarsals and carpals determines degree of ossification
   2. Growth charts: norms are expressed as percentile of height, weight, head circumference, and body mass index (BMI) for age; any child who crosses over multiple percentile lines or is above the 95th or below the 5th percentile needs further evaluation.
**E.** Correction for prematurity
   1. Subtract time premature from chronological age
   2. Use corrected age for developmental assessment until age 2

## Developmental Stages

### Infant (Birth through 12 months)

**A.** Physical tasks
   1. Neonate (Birth to 1 month)
      a. Weight: 6–8 lb (2750–3629 g); gains 5–7 oz (142–198 g) weekly for first 6 months
      b. Length: 20 inches (50 cm); grows 1 inch (2.5 cm) monthly for first 6 months
      c. Head growth
         1) Head circumference 33–35.5 cm (13–14 inches)
         2) Head circumference slightly larger than chest
         3) Increases by ½ inch (1.25 cm) monthly for first 6 months
         4) Brain growth related to myelinization of nerve fibers; increase in size of brain reflects this process, reaches ⅔ adult size at 1 year; 90% adult size at 2 years
         5) Weak neck muscles result in poor head control
      d. Vital signs
         1) Pulse: 110–160 and irregular; count for a full minute apically
         2) Respirations: 32–60 and irregular; count for full minute; neonates are abdominal breathers and obligate nose breathers
         3) Blood pressure: 75/49 mm Hg
         4) Poor development of sweating and shivering mechanisms; impaired temperature control
      e. Motor development
         1) Behavior is reflex controlled
         2) Flexed extremities
         3) Can lift head slightly off bed when prone
      f. Sensory development
         1) Hearing and touch well developed at birth
         2) Sight not fully developed until 6 years
            a) Differentiates light and dark at birth
            b) Rapidly develops clarity of vision within 1 foot
            c) Fixates on moving objects
            d) Strabismus due to lack of binocular vision
   2. 1–4 months
      a. Head growth: posterior fontanel closes
      b. Motor development
         1) Reflexes begin to fade (e.g., Moro, tonic neck)
         2) Gains head control; balances head in sitting position
         3) Rolls from back to side
         4) Begins voluntary hand-to-mouth activity

- **c.** Sensory development
  - **1)** Begins to be able to coordinate stimuli from various sense organs
  - **2)** Hearing: locates sounds by turning head and visually searching
  - **3)** Vision
    - **a)** Binocular vision developing; less strabismus
    - **b)** Beginning hand-eye coordination
    - **c)** Prefers human face
    - **d)** Follows objects 180°
    - **e)** Ability to accommodate is equal to adult

3. **5–6 months**
  - **a.** Weight: birth weight doubles; gains 3–5 oz (84–140 g) weekly for next 6 months
  - **b.** Length: gains ½ inch (1.25 cm) for next 6 months
  - **c.** Eruption of teeth begins
    - **1)** Lower incisors first
    - **2)** Causes increased saliva and drooling
    - **3)** Enzyme released with teething causes mild diarrhea, facial skin irritation
    - **4)** Slight fever may be associated with teething, but not a high fever or seizures
  - **d.** Motor development
    - **1)** Intentional rolling over
    - **2)** Supports weight on arms
    - **3)** Creeping; pushes backward with hands
    - **4)** Can grasp and let go voluntarily
    - **5)** Transfers toys from one hand to another
    - **6)** Sits with support
  - **e.** Sensory development
    - **1)** Hearing: can localize sounds above and below ear
    - **2)** Vision: smiles at own mirror image and responds to facial expressions of others
    - **3)** Taste: sucking needs have decreased and cup weaning can begin; chewing, biting, and taste preferences begin to develop

4. **7–9 months**
  - **a.** Teething continues
    - **1)** 7 months: upper central incisors
    - **2)** 9 months: upper lateral incisors
  - **b.** Motor development
    - **1)** Sits unsupported; goes from prone to sitting upright
    - **2)** Crawls; may go backwards initially
    - **3)** Pulls self to standing position
    - **4)** Develops finger-thumb opposition (pincer grasp)
    - **5)** Preference for dominant hand evident
  - **c.** Sensory development: vision
    - **1)** Can fixate on small objects
    - **2)** Beginning to develop depth perception

5. **10–12 months**
  - **a.** Weight: birth weight tripled
  - **b.** Length: 50% increase over birth length
  - **c.** Head and chest circumference equal
  - **d.** Teething
    - **1)** Lower lateral incisors erupt
    - **2)** Average of eight deciduous teeth
  - **e.** Motor development
    - **1)** Creeps with abdomen off floor
    - **2)** Walks with help or cruises
    - **3)** May attempt to stand alone
    - **4)** Can sit down from upright position
    - **5)** Weans from bottle to cup
  - **f.** Sensory development: vision
    - **1)** Able to discriminate simple geometric forms
    - **2)** Able to follow rapidly moving objects
    - **3)** Visual acuity 20/50 or better
    - **4)** Binocularity well established; if not, amblyopia may develop

**B.** Psychosocial tasks
  1. **Neonatal period**
    - **a.** Cries to express displeasure
    - **b.** Smiles indiscriminately
    - **c.** Receives gratification through sucking
    - **d.** Makes throaty sounds
  2. **1–4 months**
    - **a.** Crying becomes differentiated at 1 month
      - **1)** Decreases during awake periods
      - **2)** Ceases when parent in view
    - **b.** Vocalization distinct from crying at 1 month
      - **1)** Squeals to show pleasure at 3 months
      - **2)** Coos, babbles, laughs; vocalizes when smiling
    - **c.** Socialization
      - **1)** Stares at parents' faces when talking at 1 month
      - **2)** Smiles socially at 2 months
      - **3)** Shows excitement when happy at 4 months
      - **4)** Demands attention, enjoys social interaction with people at 4 months
  3. **5–6 months**
    - **a.** Vocalization: begins to imitate sounds
    - **b.** Socialization: recognizes parents, stranger anxiety begins to develop; comfort habits begin
  4. **7–9 months**
    - **a.** Vocalization: verbalizes all vowels and most consonants
    - **b.** Socialization
      - **1)** Shows increased stranger anxiety and anxiety over separation from parent
      - **2)** Exhibits aggressiveness by biting at times
      - **3)** Understands the word "no"
  5. **10–12 months**
    - **a.** Vocalization: imitates animal sounds, can say only 4–5 words but understands many more (ma, da)

b. Socialization
 1) Begins to explore surroundings
 2) Plays games such as pat-a-cake, peek-a-boo
 3) Shows emotions such as jealousy, affection, anger, fear (especially in new situations)
C. Cognitive tasks
 1. Neonatal period: reflexive behavior only
 2. 1–4 months
  a. Recognizes familiar faces
  b. Is interested in surroundings
  c. Discovers own body parts
 3. 5–6 months
  a. Begins to imitate
  b. Can find partially hidden objects
 4. 7–9 months
  a. Begins to understand object permanence; searches for dropped objects
  b. Reacts to adult anger; cries when scolded
  c. Imitates simple acts and noises
  d. Responds to simple commands
 5. 10–12 months
  a. Recognizes objects by name
  b. Looks at and follows pictures in book
  c. Shows more goal-directed actions
D. Nutrition
 1. Birth to 6 months
  a. Breast milk is a complete and healthful diet; supplementation may include 0.25 mg fluoride, 400 International Units vitamin D, and iron after 4 months.
  b. Commercial iron-fortified formula is acceptable alternative; supplementation may include 0.25 mg fluoride if water supply is not fluoridated.
  c. No solid foods before 5 months; too early exposure may lead to food allergies, and extrusion reflex will cause food to be pushed out of mouth.
  d. Juices may be introduced at 5–6 months, diluted 1:1 and preferably given by cup.
 2. 6–12 months
  a. Breast milk or formula continues to be primary source of nutrition.
  b. Introduction of solid foods starts with cereal (usually rice cereal), which is continued until 18 months.
  c. Introduction of other food is arbitrary; most common sequence is fruits, vegetables, meats.
   1) Introduce only one new food at a time.
   2) Separate new foods by minimum of 3–4 days.
   3) Decrease amount of formula to about 30 oz. as foods are added.
  d. Iron supplementation can be stopped.
  e. Finger foods such as cheese, meat, carrots can be started around 10 months.

f. Chopped table food or junior food can be introduced by 12 months.
g. Weaning from breast or bottle to cup should be gradual during second 6 months.
h. Breastfeeding can continue beyond 12 months.
i. No honey, nuts, egg whites until 12 months.
E. Safety
 1. Birth to 4 months
  a. Use car seat properly. Infants up to 9 kg (20 lb) and younger than 1 year should face rear.
  b. Ensure crib mattress fits snugly; do not use a pillow or comforters in the crib.
  c. Keep side rails of crib up.
  d. Position infant supine for sleep until infant is able to turn over. Prone position may increase risk for sudden infant death syndrome (SIDS).
  e. Do not leave infant unattended on bed, couch, table.
  f. Do not tie pacifier on string around infant's neck; remove bib before sleep.
  g. Remove small objects that infant could choke on.
  h. Check temperature of bath water and warmed formula or food.
  i. Use cool mist vaporizer.
 2. 5–7 months
  a. Restrain in high chair or infant seat.
  b. Do not feed hard candy, nuts, food with pits.
  c. Inspect toys for small removable parts.
  d. Be sure paint on furniture does not contain lead.
  e. Keep phone number of Poison Control Center readily available.
 3. 8–12 months
  a. Keep crib away from other furniture and windows.
  b. Keep gates across stairways.
  c. Keep safety plugs in electrical outlets.
  d. Remove hanging electrical wires and tablecloths.
  e. Use child protective caps and cabinet locks.
  f. Place cleaning solutions and medications out of reach.
  g. Do not let child use fork to self-feed.
  h. Do not leave alone in bathtub.
F. Play (Solitary)
 1. Birth to 4 months
  a. Provide variety of brightly colored objects, different sizes and textures.
  b. Hang mobiles within 8–10 inches of infant's face.
  c. Expose to various environmental sounds; use rattles, musical toys.
 2. 5–7 months
  a. Provide brightly colored toys to hold and squeeze.

b. Allow infant to splash in bath.
c. Provide crib mirror.
3. 8–12 months
a. Provide toys with movable parts and noisemakers; stack toys, blocks; pots, pans, drums to bang on; stationary activity center and push-pull toys.
b. Plays games: hide and seek, pat-a-cake.
G. Fears
1. Separation from parents
a. Searches for parents with eyes.
b. Shows preference for parents.
c. Develops stranger anxiety around 6 months.
2. Pain
a. Reacts with generalized body movement and loud crying.
b. Can be distracted with talking, sucking opportunities.

## Toddler (12 months to 3 years)

A. Physical tasks: this is a period of slow growth
1. Weight: gain of approximately 11 lb (5 kg) during this time; birth weight quadrupled by 2½ years
2. Height: grows 20.3 cm (8 inches); adult height about 2 times height at 2 years
3. Head circumference: 19½–20 inches (49–50 cm) by 2 years; anterior fontanel closes by 18 months
4. Pulse 110; respirations 26; blood pressure 99/64
5. Primary dentition (20 teeth) completed by 2½ years
6. Develops sphincter control necessary for bowel and bladder control
7. Mobility
a. Walks alone by 18 months.
b. Climbs stairs and furniture by 18 months.
c. Runs fairly well by 2 years.
d. Jumps from chair or step by 2½ years.
e. Balances on one foot momentarily by 2½ years.
f. Rides tricycle by 3 years.
B. Psychosocial tasks
1. Increases independence; better able to tolerate separation from primary caregiver.
2. Less likely to fear strangers.
3. Able to help with dressing/undressing at 18 months; dresses self at 24 months.
4. Has sustained attention span.
5. May have temper tantrums during this period; should decrease by 2½ years.
6. Vocabulary increases from about 10–20 words to over 900 words by 3 years.
7. Has beginning awareness of ownership (my, mine) at 18 months; shows proper use of pronouns (I, me, you) by 3 years.
8. Moves from hoarding and possessiveness at 18 months to sharing with peers by 3 years.

9. Toilet training usually completed by 3 years.
a. Demonstrates readiness for toilet training between 18 and 24 months
b. Indicators of readiness: walks, sits, and squats well, has voluntary control of bowel and urinary function, regular bowel movements, can communicate wetness or bowel movement, can remove clothes, wants to please caregivers, imitates
c. Daytime bladder control by 2–3 years
d. Nighttime bladder control by 3–4 years
C. Cognitive tasks
1. Follows simple directions by 2 years.
2. Begins to use short sentences at 18 months to 2 years.
3. Can remember and repeat 3 numbers by 3 years.
4. Knows own name by 12 months; refers to self, gives first name by 24 months; gives full name by 3 years.
5. Able to identify geometric forms by 18 months.
6. Achieves object permanence; is aware that objects exist even if not in view.
7. Uses "magical" thinking; believes own feelings affect events (e.g., anger causes rain).
8. Uses ritualistic behavior; repeats skills to master them and to decrease anxiety.
9. May develop dependency on "transitional object" such as blanket or stuffed animal.
D. Nutrition
1. Caloric requirement is approximately 100 calories/kg/day.
2. Increased need for calcium, iron, and phosphorus.
3. Needs 16–24 oz milk/day.
4. Appetite decreases.
5. Able to feed self.
6. Negativism may interfere with eating.
7. Initial dental examination at 3 years.
E. Safety
1. Turn pot handles toward back of stove.
2. Teach swimming and water safety; supervise near water.
3. Supervise play outdoors.
4. Avoid large chunks of meat, particularly hot dogs.
5. Do not allow child to walk around with objects such as lollipops in mouth.
6. Know when and how to use ipecac.
7. Car seat safety: children sit in forward facing car seat only after age is greater than 1 year and weight is greater than 20 lb. All car seats placed in rear seat of car. No car seats should be placed in front of the passenger side air bag.
F. Play
1. Predominantly "parallel play" period.
2. Imitation of adults often part of play.
3. Begins imaginative and make-believe play.
4. Provide toys appropriate for increased locomotive skills: push toys, rocking horse, riding toys or tricycles; swings and slide.

5. Give toys to provide outlet for aggressive feelings: work bench, toy hammer and nails, drums, pots, pans.
6. Provide toys to help develop fine motor skills, problem-solving abilities: puzzles, blocks; finger paints, crayons.
G. Fears: separation anxiety
1. Learning to tolerate and master brief periods of separation is important developmental task.
2. Increasing understanding of object permanence helps toddler overcome this fear.
3. Potential patterns of response to separation
   a. Protest: screams and cries when mother leaves; attempts to call her back.
   b. Despair: whimpers, clutches transitional object, curls up in bed, decreased activity, rocking.
   c. Denial: resumes normal activity but does not form psychosocial relationships; when mother returns, child ignores her.
4. Bedtime may represent desertion.

## Preschooler (3 to 5 years)

A. Physical tasks
1. Slower growth rate continues
   a. Weight: increases 4–6 lb (1.8–2.7 kg) a year
   b. Height: increases 2½ inches (5–6.25 cm) a year
   c. Birth length doubled by 4 years
2. Vital signs decrease slightly
   a. Pulse 90–100
   b. Respirations 24–25/minute
   c. Blood pressure: systolic 85–100 mm Hg: diastolic 60–70 mm Hg
3. Permanent teeth may appear late in preschool period; first permanent teeth are molars, behind last temporary teeth.
4. Gross motor development
   a. Walks up stairs using alternate feet by 3 years.
   b. Walks down stairs using alternate feet by 4 years.
   c. Rides tricycle by 3 years.
   d. Stands on 1 foot by 3 years.
   e. Hops on 1 foot by 4 years.
   f. Skips and hops on alternate feet by 5 years.
   g. Balances on 1 foot with eyes closed by 5 years.
   h. Throws and catches ball by 5 years.
   i. Jumps off 1 step by 3 years.
   j. Jumps rope by 5 years.
5. Fine motor development
   a. Hand dominance is established by 5 years.
   b. Builds a tower of blocks by 3 years.
   c. Ties shoes by 5 years.
   d. Ability to draw changes over this time
      1) Copies circles, may add facial features by 3 years.
      2) Copies a square, traces a diamond by 4 years.
      3) Copies a diamond and triangle, prints letters and numbers by 5 years.
   e. Handles scissors well by 5 years.
B. Psychosocial tasks
1. Becomes independent
   a. Feeds self completely.
   b. Dresses self.
   c. Takes increased responsibility for actions.
2. Aggressiveness and impatience peak at 4 years then abate; by 5 years child is eager to please and manners become more evident.
3. Gender-specific behavior is evident by 5 years.
4. Egocentricity changes to awareness of others; rules become important; understands sharing.
C. Cognitive development
1. Focuses on one idea at a time; cannot look at entire perspective.
2. Awareness of racial and sexual differences begins.
   a. Prejudice may develop based on values of parents.
   b. Manifests sexual curiosity.
   c. Sexual education begins.
   d. Beginning body awareness.
3. Has beginning concept of causality.
4. Understanding of time develops during this period.
   a. Learns sequence of daily events.
   b. Is able to understand meaning of some time-oriented words (day of week, month, etc.) by 5 years.
5. Has 2000-word vocabulary by 5 years.
6. Can name four or more colors by 5 years.
7. Is very inquisitive.
D. Nutrition
1. Caloric requirement is approximately 90 calories/kg/day.
2. May demonstrate strong taste preferences.
3. More likely to taste new foods if child can assist in the preparation.
E. Safety
1. Safety issues similar to toddler
2. Education of children concerning potential dangers important during this period
3. Car safety: children 20–40 lb and younger than age 4 should ride in car safety seat. Children over 40 lb and between ages 4 and 8 should ride in a booster seat in the rear of the car.
F. Play
1. Predominantly "associative play" period.
2. Enjoys imitative and dramatic play.
   a. Imitates same-sex role functions in play.
   b. Enjoys dressing up, dollhouses, trucks, cars, telephones, doctor and nurse kits.
3. Provide toys to help develop gross motor skills: tricycles, wagons, outdoor gym; sandbox, wading pool.
4. Provide toys to encourage fine motor skills, self-expression, and cognitive development: construction sets, blocks, carpentry tools; flash cards, illustrated books, puzzles; paints, crayons, clay, simple sewing sets.

5. Television, when supervised, can provide a quiet activity; some programs have educational content.
6. Imaginary playmates common during this period.
   a. More prevalent in bright children
   b. Help child deal with loneliness and fears
   c. Abandoned by school age

G. Fears
1. Greatest number of imagined and real fears of childhood during this period.
2. Fears concerning body integrity are common.
   a. Child is able to imagine an event without experiencing it.
   b. Observing injuries or pain in others can precipitate fear.
   c. Magical and animistic thinking allows children to develop many illogical fears (fear of inanimate objects, the dark, ghosts).
3. Exposing child to feared object in a safe situation may provide a degree of conditioning; child should progress at own rate.

## School-Age (6 to 12 years)

A. Physical tasks
1. Slow growth continues.
   a. Height: 2 inches (5 cm) per year
   b. Weight: doubles over this period
   c. At age 9, both sexes same size; age 12, girls bigger than boys
2. Dentition
   a. Loses first primary teeth at about 6 years.
   b. By 12 years, has all permanent teeth except final molars.
3. Bone growth faster than muscle and ligament development; very limber but susceptible to bone fractures during this time.
4. Vision is completely mature; hand-eye coordination develops completely.
5. Gross motor skills: predominantly involving large muscles; children are very energetic, develop greater strength, coordination, and stamina.
6. Develops smoothness and speed in fine motor control.

B. Psychosocial tasks
1. School occupies half of waking hours; has cognitive and social impact.
   a. Readiness includes emotional (attention span), physical (hearing and vision), and intellectual components.
   b. Teacher may be parent substitute, causing parents to lose some authority.
2. Morality develops
   a. Before age 9 moral realism predominates: strict superego, rule dominance; things are black or white, right or wrong.
   b. After age 9 autonomous morality develops: recognizes differing points of view, sees "gray" areas.

3. Peer relationships
   a. Child makes first real friends during this period.
   b. Is able to understand concepts of cooperation and compromise (assist in acquiring attitudes and values); learns fair play vs competition.
   c. Help child develop self-concept.
   d. Provide feeling of belonging.
4. Enjoys family activities.
5. Has some ability to evaluate own strengths and weaknesses.
6. Has increased self-direction.
7. Is aware of own body; compares self to others; modesty develops.

C. Cognitive development
1. Period of industry
   a. Is interested in exploration and adventure.
   b. Likes to accomplish or produce.
   c. Develops confidence.
2. Concept of time and space develops.
   a. Understands causality.
   b. Masters concept of conservation: permanence of mass and volume; concept of reversibility.
   c. Develops classification skills: understands relational terms; may collect things.
   d. Masters arithmetic and reading.

D. Nutrition
1. Caloric needs diminish in relation to body size: 85 kcal/kg/day.
2. "Junk" food may become a problem; excess sugar, starches, fat.
3. Obesity is a risk in this age group.
4. Nutrition education should be integrated into school program.

E. Safety
1. Incidence of accidents is decreased when compared with younger children.
2. Motor vehicle accidents most common cause of severe injury and death.
3. Other common activities associated with injuries include sports (skateboarding, rollerskating, etc.).
4. Education and supervision are key elements in prevention.
   a. Proper use of equipment
   b. Risk-taking behavior
5. Car safety: children weighing over 40 lb and younger than age 8 should ride in a booster seat placed in the rear of the car. Children over age 8 can use shoulder/lap belt combination in rear seat of the car. Children younger than age 12 should not sit in the front passenger seat or in front of an air bag.

F. Play
1. Rules and ritual dominate play; individuality not tolerated by peers; knowing rules provides sense of belonging; "cooperative play."

2. Team play: games or sports
   a. Help learn value of individual skills and team accomplishments.
   b. Help learn nature of competition.
3. Quiet games and activities: board games, collections, books, television, painting
4. Athletic activities: swimming, hiking, bicycling, skating

G. Fears: more realistic fears than younger children; include death, disease or bodily injury, punishment; school phobia may develop, resulting in psychosomatic illness.

## Adolescent (12 to 19 years)

A. Physical tasks
1. Fast period of growth
2. Vital signs approach adult norms
3. Puberty
   a. Follows same pattern for all races and cultures.
   b. Is related to hormonal changes.
   c. Results in growth spurt, change in body structure, development of secondary sex characteristics, and reproductive maturity.
   d. Girls: height increases approximately 3 inches/year; slows at menarche; stops around age 16.
   e. Boys: growth spurt starts around age 13; height increases 4 inches/year; slows in late teens.
   f. Boys double weight between 12 and 18, related to increased muscle mass.
   g. Body shape changes
      1) Boys become leaner with broader chest.
      2) Girls have fat deposited in thighs, hips, and breasts; pelvis broadens.
   h. Apocrine glands cause increased body odor.
   i. Increased production of sebum and plugging of sebaceous ducts causes acne
4. Sexual development: girls
   a. Menarche
      1) Onset about 2 years after first of pubescent changes
      2) Average age 12½ years
      3) First 1–2 years: menses irregular, infertile
   b. Menstrual cycle: controlled by complex interaction of hormones
   c. Development of secondary sex characteristics and sexual functioning under hormonal control (see Table 4-24).
   d. Breast development is first visible sign of puberty.
      1) Bud stage: areola around nipple is protuberant.
      2) Breast development is complete around the time of first menses.

5. Sexual development: boys
   a. Development of secondary sex characteristics, sex organs and function under hormonal control (see Table 4-24).
   b. Enlargement of testes is first sign of sexual maturation; occurs at approximately age 13, about 1 year before growth spurt.
   c. Scrotum and penis increase in size until age 18.
   d. Reaches reproductive maturity about age 17, with viable sperm.
   e. Nocturnal emission: a physiologic reflex to ejaculate buildup of semen; natural and normal; occurs during sleep (child should not be made to feel guilty; needs to understand that this is not enuresis).
   f. Masturbation increases (also a normal way to release semen).
   g. Pubic hair continues to grow and spread until mid 20s.
   h. Facial hair; appears first on upper lip.
   i. Voice changes due to growth of laryngeal cartilage.
   j. Gynecomastia: slight hypertrophy of breasts due to estrogen production; will pass within months but causes embarrassment.

B. Psychosocial tasks
1. Early adolescence: ages 12–14 years
   a. Starts with puberty.
   b. Physical body changes result in an altered self-concept.
   c. Tends to compare own body to others.
   d. Early and late developers have anxiety regarding fear of rejection.
   e. Fantasy life, daydreams, crushes are all normal, help in role play of varying social situations.
   f. Is prone to mood swings.
   g. Needs limits and consistent discipline.
2. Middle adolescence: ages 15–16 years
   a. Is separate from parents (except financially).
   b. Can identify own values.
   c. Can define self (self-concept, strengths and weaknesses).
   d. Involved with peer group; conforms to values/fads.
   e. Has increased heterosexual interest; communicates with opposite sex; may form "love" relationship.
   f. Sex education continues.
3. Late adolescence: ages 17–19 years
   a. Achieves greater independence.
   b. Chooses a vocation.
   c. Participates in society.
   d. Finds an identity.
   e. Finds a mate.
   f. Develops own morality.
   g. Completes physical and emotional maturity.

C. Cognitive development
1. Develops abstract thinking abilities.
2. Is often unrealistic.
3. Is capable of scientific reasoning and formal logic.
4. Enjoys intellectual abilities.
5. Is able to view problems comprehensively.
D. Nutrition
1. Nutritional requirements peak during years of maximum growth: age 10–12 in girls, 2 years later in boys.
2. Appetite increases.
3. Inadequate diet can retard growth and delay sexual maturation.
4. Food intake needs to be balanced with energy expenditure.
5. Increased needs include calcium for skeletal growth; iron for increased muscle mass and blood cell development; zinc for development of skeletal and muscle tissue and sexual maturation.
E. Safety
1. Accidents are leading cause of death: motor vehicle accidents, sports injuries, firearms accidents.
2. Safety measures include education about proper use of equipment and caution concerning risk taking.
3. Drug and alcohol use may be a serious problem during this period.
4. Adolescent characteristics of poor impulse control and recklessness make prevention complex.
F. Activities: group activities predominate (sports are important); activities involving opposite sex by middle adolescence.
G. Fears
1. Threats to body image: acne, obesity
2. Injury or death
3. The unknown

## ANALYSIS

Nursing diagnoses for problems of growth and development may include:
A. Altered family process
B. Altered health maintenance
C. Altered parenting
D. Altered thought processes
E. Delayed growth and development
F. Disturbance in self-esteem
G. Disturbed body image
H. High risk for violence
I. Impaired dentition
J. Ineffective family coping
K. Knowledge deficit (specify)
L. Risk for delayed development
M. Risk for disproportionate growth
N. Social isolation

# PLANNING AND IMPLEMENTATION

## Goals

A. Child will achieve appropriate developmental level for age.
B. Family/child will adapt successfully to developmental changes.
C. Family/child will cope successfully with crises of illness and hospitalization.
D. Family/child will cope successfully with issues related to death and dying.

## Interventions for the Ill or Hospitalized Child

### Communicating with Children

A. Speak in quiet, pleasant tones.
B. Bend down to meet child on own level.
C. Use words appropriate to age/communication ability; do not use clichès.
D. Do not explain more than is necessary.
E. Always explain what you are going to do and give the reason for it.
F. Be honest; do not lie about whether something will hurt.
G. Do not make a promise you know you cannot keep.
H. Observe nonverbal behavior for clues to level of understanding.
I. Do not threaten; and when necessary, punish the act, not the child ("I like you, but not what you did.").
J. Never shame a child by using terms like baby or sissy.
K. Allow child to show feelings (hurt and anger); provide therapeutic play, pounding or throwing toys; allow child to cry; encourage drawing and creative writing.
L. Provide time to talk; encourage a trusting environment where the child can talk without embarrassment and confide without fear.
M. Provide support to child and parents/family.
N. Teach parents to anticipate next stage of development.
O. If teaching with a child is interrupted, start over from the beginning.
P. Promote independence; allow the child to perform as many self-care activities as possible.
Q. Do not compare child's progress to that of anyone else.
R. Provide praise at every opportunity.
S. Instead of asking what something is, ask child to give it a name or tell you about it.
T. Allow choices where possible, but do not use yes/no questions unless you can accept a "no" answer ("It is time for your medication now; do you want it with milk or juice?" versus "Do you want your medication now?").
U. Involve parents in child's care.

**V.** Keep routines as much like home as possible (on admission, ask parents about routines such as toileting, eating, sleeping, and names for bowel movements and urination).

**W.** Allow parents time and opportunities to ask questions and express themselves.

**X.** If parents cannot stay with child, encourage them to bring in a favorite toy, pictures of family members, or to make a tape to be played for the child.

### Play

**A.** Play is a way to solve problems, become enculturated, express creativity, decrease stress in the environment, prepare for different situations, sublimate sensations, enhance fine and gross motor development as well as social development.

**B.** Make play appropriate for mental age and physical/disease state (e.g., appropriate for oxygen tents, isolation, hearing or vision defects).

**C.** Use multisensory stimulation.

**D.** Provide toys safe for mental age (no points, sharp edges, small parts, loud noises, propelled objects).

**E.** Offer play specific to age group.
  1. Toddler: enjoys repetition; solitary play, parallel play.
  2. Preschooler: likes to role play and make believe; associative play.
  3. School-age: likes group, organized activities (to enhance sharing); cooperative play, group goals with interaction.

### Preparation for Procedures

**A.** Allow child to play with equipment to be used.

**B.** Demonstrate procedure first on a doll.

**C.** Teach child skills that will be needed after the procedure and provide time to practice (crutches, blow bottles).

**D.** Show the child pictures of staff garb, special treatment room, special machines to be used, etc., before the procedure.

**E.** Describe sensations the child may experience during or after the procedure and what child will have to do.

**F.** Listen carefully to child to detect misconceptions or fantasies.

**G.** With younger children, the preparatory information should be simple and as close to the time of the procedure as possible.

**H.** Parents can often be helpful in preparing child for procedures, but need to be prepared as well.
  1. May need different explanation, away from child.
  2. Should have opportunity to ask questions about what will happen to child.

**I.** School-age children and adolescents may not wish parents to be present during procedure.
  1. Child's desires should be confirmed.
  2. Parents need to be assured that this is not rejection by child.

**J.** Inadequate preparation leads to heightened anxiety that may result in regressive behavior, uncooperativeness, or acting out.

## EVALUATION

**A.** Child maintains normal developmental level during hospitalization.

**B.** Parents participate in care of child during hospitalization.

## GROWTH AND DEVELOPMENT ISSUES

### Health Promotion

**A.** Immunization schedule (see Figure 5-1)

**B.** Types of immunity

**C.** Considerations concerning immunization schedule:
  1. If the immunization schedule is interrupted it is not necessary to reinstitute the entire series. Immunization should occur on the next visit as if the usual interval has elapsed.
  2. If immunization status is unknown, children should be considered susceptible and appropriate immunizations administered
  3. For children not immunized during the first year of life and who are less than 7 years old the same immunizations are given but following different time schedule.
  4. For children 7 years old and older who are not immunized, Td rather than DTaP is administered.
  5. Preterm infants are immunized according to chronological, not corrected age.
  6. Minor illnesses are not contraindications to immunization.

**D.** Contraindications for immunization
  1. Severe allergic reaction to a vaccine contraindicates further doses of that vaccine.
  2. Anaphylactic reaction to a vaccine additive contraindicates the use of vaccines containing that substance (e.g., eggs, neomycin, streptomycin).
  3. Immunocompromised persons should not receive live vaccines.
  4. Immunizations should be delayed after recent transfusion with passive immunity agents (e.g., gamma globulin).

**E.** Tuberculin testing
  1. The tuberculin skin test is the only practical tool for diagnosing tuberculosis infection.
  2. Tuberculin testing may be done at the same visit at which an immunization is being given.
  3. Routine testing is no longer recommended. Testing is always indicated for individuals with known contact with a person with tuberculosis disease.

## Recommended Immunization Schedule for Persons Aged 0 Through 6 Years—United States • 2009

*For those who fall behind or start late, see the catch-up schedule*

| Vaccine ▼  Age ► | Birth | 1 month | 2 months | 4 months | 6 months | 12 months | 15 months | 18 months | 19–23 months | 2–3 years | 4–6 years |
|---|---|---|---|---|---|---|---|---|---|---|---|
| Hepatitis B[1] | HepB | HepB | | see footnote 1 | | HepB | | | | | |
| Rotavirus[2] | | | RV | RV | RV[2] | | | | | | |
| Diphtheria, Tetanus, Pertussis[3] | | | DTaP | DTaP | DTaP | see footnote 3 | DTaP | | | | DTaP |
| Haemophilus influenzae type b[4] | | | Hib | Hib | Hib[4] | Hib | | | | | |
| Pneumococcal[5] | | | PCV | PCV | PCV | PCV | | | | | PPSV |
| Inactivated Poliovirus | | | IPV | IPV | | IPV | | | | | IPV |
| Influenza[6] | | | | | | Influenza (Yearly) | | | | | |
| Measles, Mumps, Rubella[7] | | | | | | MMR | | see footnote 7 | | | MMR |
| Varicella[8] | | | | | | Varicella | | see footnote 8 | | | Varicella |
| Hepatitis A[9] | | | | | | HepA (2 doses) | | | | HepA Series | |
| Meningococcal[10] | | | | | | | | | | MCV | |

Range of recommended ages

Certain high-risk groups

This schedule indicates the recommended ages for routine administration of currently licensed vaccines, as of December 1, 2008, for children aged 0 through 6 years. Any dose not administered at the recommended age should be administered at a subsequent visit, when indicated and feasible. Licensed combination vaccines may be used whenever any component of the combination is indicated and other components are not contraindicated and if approved by the Food and Drug Administration for that dose of the series. Providers should consult the relevant Advisory Committee on Immunization Practices statement for detailed recommendations, including high-risk conditions: http://www.cdc.gov/vaccines/pubs/acip-list.htm. Clinically significant adverse events that follow immunization should be reported to the Vaccine Adverse Event Reporting System (VAERS). Guidance about how to obtain and complete a VAERS form is available at http://www.vaers.hhs.gov or by telephone, 800-822-7967.

**1. Hepatitis B vaccine (HepB).** *(Minimum age: birth)*
**At birth:**
- Administer monovalent HepB to all newborns before hospital discharge.
- If mother is hepatitis B surface antigen (HBsAg)-positive, administer HepB and 0.5 mL of hepatitis B immune globulin (HBIG) within 12 hours of birth.
- If mother's HBsAg status is unknown, administer HepB within 12 hours of birth. Determine mother's HBsAg status as soon as possible and, if HBsAg-positive, administer HBIG (no later than age 1 week).
**After the birth dose:**
- The HepB series should be completed with either monovalent HepB or a combination vaccine containing HepB. The second dose should be administered at age 1 or 2 months. The final dose should be administered no earlier than age 24 weeks.
- Infants born to HBsAg-positive mothers should be tested for HBsAg and antibody to HBsAg (anti-HBs) after completion of at least 3 doses of the HepB series, at age 9 through 18 months (generally at the next well-child visit).
**4-month dose:**
- Administration of 4 doses of HepB to infants is permissible when combination vaccines containing HepB are administered after the birth dose.

**2. Rotavirus vaccine (RV).** *(Minimum age: 6 weeks)*
- Administer the first dose at age 6 through 14 weeks (maximum age: 14 weeks 6 days). Vaccination should not be initiated for infants aged 15 weeks or older (i.e., 15 weeks 0 days or older).
- Administer the final dose in the series by age 8 months 0 days.
- If Rotarix® is administered at ages 2 and 4 months, a dose at 6 months is not indicated.

**3. Diphtheria and tetanus toxoids and acellular pertussis vaccine (DTaP).** *(Minimum age: 6 weeks)*
- The fourth dose may be administered as early as age 12 months, provided at least 6 months have elapsed since the third dose.
- Administer the final dose in the series at age 4 through 6 years.

**4. Haemophilus influenzae type b conjugate vaccine (Hib).** *(Minimum age: 6 weeks)*
- If PRP-OMP (PedvaxHIB® or Comvax® [HepB-Hib]) is administered at ages 2 and 4 months, a dose at age 6 months is not indicated.
- TriHiBit® (DTaP/Hib) should not be used for doses at ages 2, 4, or 6 months but can be used as the final dose in children aged 12 months or older.

**5. Pneumococcal vaccine.** *(Minimum age: 6 weeks for pneumococcal conjugate vaccine [PCV]; 2 years for pneumococcal polysaccharide vaccine [PPSV])*
- PCV is recommended for all children aged younger than 5 years. Administer 1 dose of PCV to all healthy children aged 24 through 59 months who are not completely vaccinated for their age.

- Administer PPSV to children aged 2 years or older with certain underlying medical conditions (see *MMWR* 2000;49[No. RR-9]), including a cochlear implant.

**6. Influenza vaccine.** *(Minimum age: 6 months for trivalent inactivated influenza vaccine [TIV]; 2 years for live, attenuated influenza vaccine [LAIV])*
- Administer annually to children aged 6 months through 18 years.
- For healthy nonpregnant persons (i.e., those who do not have underlying medical conditions that predispose them to influenza complications) aged 2 through 49 years, either LAIV or TIV may be used.
- Children receiving TIV should receive 0.25 mL if aged 6 through 35 months or 0.5 mL if aged 3 years or older.
- Administer 2 doses (separated by at least 4 weeks) to children aged younger than 9 years who are receiving influenza vaccine for the first time or who were vaccinated for the first time during the previous influenza season but only received 1 dose.

**7. Measles, mumps, and rubella vaccine (MMR).** *(Minimum age: 12 months)*
- Administer the second dose at age 4 through 6 years. However, the second dose may be administered before age 4, provided at least 28 days have elapsed since the first dose.

**8. Varicella vaccine.** *(Minimum age: 12 months)*
- Administer the second dose at age 4 through 6 years. However, the second dose may be administered before age 4, provided at least 3 months have elapsed since the first dose.
- For children aged 12 months through 12 years the minimum interval between doses is 3 months. However, if the second dose was administered at least 28 days after the first dose, it can be accepted as valid.

**9. Hepatitis A vaccine (HepA).** *(Minimum age: 12 months)*
- Administer to all children aged 1 year (i.e., aged 12 through 23 months). Administer 2 doses at least 6 months apart.
- Children not fully vaccinated by age 2 years can be vaccinated at subsequent visits.
- HepA also is recommended for children older than 1 year who live in areas where vaccination programs target older children or who are at increased risk of infection. See *MMWR* 2006;55(No. RR-7).

**10. Meningococcal vaccine.** *(Minimum age: 2 years for meningococcal conjugate vaccine [MCV] and for meningococcal polysaccharide vaccine [MPSV])*
- Administer MCV to children aged 2 through 10 years with terminal complement component deficiency, anatomic or functional asplenia, and certain other high-risk groups. See *MMWR* 2005;54(No. RR-7).
- Persons who received MPSV 3 or more years previously and who remain at increased risk for meningococcal disease should be revaccinated with MCV.

The Recommended Immunization Schedules for Persons Aged 0 Through 18 Years are approved by the Advisory Committee on Immunization Practices (www.cdc.gov/vaccines/recs/acip), the American Academy of Pediatrics (http://www.aap.org), and the American Academy of Family Physicians (http://www.aafp.org).
DEPARTMENT OF HEALTH AND HUMAN SERVICES • CENTERS FOR DISEASE CONTROL AND PREVENTION

CS103164

**Figure 5-1** Recommended childhood immunization schedule, 2009 (Courtesy of U.S. Centers for Disease Control and Prevention. Retrieved February 24, 2009 from cdc.gov)

4. Positive reaction signifies infection with *Mycobacterium tuberculosis.*
5. Positive reaction indicates need for further evaluation.
6. Children from other countries who have received BCG vaccine against tuberculosis may show positive skin test.

F. Common childhood communicable diseases (see Table 5-5).

# Challenges of Parenting

A. Failure to thrive (FTT)
1. General information
   a. A condition in which a child fails to gain weight and is persistently less than the 5th percentile on growth charts.
   b. When related to nonorganic cause, it is usually due to a disrupted maternal-child relationship.
   c. Other pathology (especially absorption problems and hormonal dysfunction) must be ruled out before a disorder can be diagnosed as FTT.
   d. Growth and developmental delay usually improve with appropriate stimulation.
2. Assessment findings
   a. Sleep disturbances; rumination (voluntary regurgitation and reswallowing)
   b. History of parental isolation and social crisis with inadequate support systems
   c. Physical exam reveals delayed growth and development (decreased vocalization, low interest in environment) and characteristic postures (child is stiff or floppy, resists cuddling)
   d. Disturbed maternal-infant interaction may be demonstrated in feeding techniques, amount of stimulation provided by mother, ability of mother to respond to infant's cues
3. Nursing interventions
   a. Provide consistent care.
   b. Teach parents positive feeding techniques.
      1) Provide quiet environment.
      2) Follow child's rhythm of feeding.
      3) Maintain face-to-face posture with child.
      4) Talk to child encouragingly during feeding.
   c. Involve parents in care.
      1) Provide supportive environment.
      2) Give positive feedback.
      3) Demonstrate and reinforce responding to child's cues.
   d. Refer to appropriate community agencies.
B. Child abuse
1. General information
   a. Physical, emotional, or sexual abuse of children: may result from intentional and nonaccidental actions; or may be from intentional and nonaccidental acts of omission (neglect).

b. In sexual abuse, 80% of children know their abuser.
c. Problem usually related to parents' limited capacity to cope with, provide for, or relate to a child and/or to each other.
d. Adults who abuse were often themselves victims of child abuse; although abuser may care about child, pattern of response to frustration and discipline is to be abusive.
e. Occurs in all socioeconomic groups.
f. Only 10% of abusers have serious psychologic disturbances, but most have low self-esteem, little confidence, low tolerance for frustration.
g. Abuse is most common among toddlers as they exercise autonomy and parents may sense loss of power.
2. Assessment findings
   a. History may be indicative of child abuse.
      1) History inconsistent with injury
      2) Delay in seeking medical attention
      3) History changes with repetition
      4) No explanation for injury
   b. Skin injuries (bruises, lacerations, burns) are most common; may show outline of instrument used and may be in varying stages of healing.
   c. Musculoskeletal injuries, fractures (especially chip or spiral fractures), sprains, dislocations are also common; X-rays may show multiple old fractures.
   d. Signs of central nervous system (CNS) injuries include subdural hematoma, retinal hemorrhage (shaken baby syndrome).
   e. Abdominal injuries may include lacerated liver, ruptured spleen.
   f. Observation of parents and child may reveal interactional problems.
      1) Does parent respond to child's cues?
      2) Does parent comfort child?
      3) Does child respond to parent with fear?
3. Nursing interventions
   a. In emergency room: tend to physical needs of child first; determination of existence of abuse must wait until child's condition is stable.
   b. Report suspected child abuse to appropriate agency.
   c. Provide a role model for parents in terms of communication, stimulation, feeding, and daily care of child.
   d. Encourage parents to be involved in child's care.
   e. Encourage parents to express feelings concerning abuse, hospitalization, and home situation.
      1) Feelings of fear and guilt should be acknowledged.
      2) Provide reassurance.

**Table 5-5** Communicable Childhood Diseases

| Disease | Characteristics | Immunization |
|---------|----------------|--------------|
| Diphtheria | A respiratory disease caused by bacteria.<br>Bacteria forms a pseudomembrane across the trachea causing respiratory distress; also produces an exotoxin that causes myocarditis and neurologic problems. | Included in DTaP up to 6 years, then in Td, repeated every 10 years throughout life. |
| Pertussis (whooping cough) | Respiratory disease caused by bacteria; life threatening in young children.<br>Severe paroxysmal cough results in severe respiratory distress; complications include seizures, pneumonia, encephalopathy, and death. | Included in DTaP; not given after 6 years because of risk from associated side effects.<br>Do not give pertussis vaccine if child has active neurologic disorder. |
| Tetanus (lockjaw) | Neurologic disorder caused by bacterial exotoxin affects motor neurons, causing rigidity and spastic muscles; first symptom is stiffness of the jaw (trismus).<br>No immunity is conferred after having the disease; associated mortality 25–50%. | Included in DTaP up to 6 years; included in Td every 10 years throughout life.<br>May be given with a puncture wound if the wound is dirty and no immunization has been given in 5 years, or if wound is clean but more than 10 years have elapsed since previous immunization. |
| Measles (rubeola) | Viral infection producing harsh cough, maculopapular rash, photophobia, and Koplik spots; complications may include pneumonia, bacterial superinfections, and encephalitis.<br>Incubation period is 8 to 12 days.<br>Care includes keeping room darkened and providing antipruritic measures. | Maternal antibodies last for at least a year, then included in MMR given at 12 to 15 months.<br>Do not give to pregnant women or immunocompromised persons. |
| German measles (rubella) | Viral infection causing lymphadenopathy and pink maculopapular rash; very mild disease, no specific care needed; complications may include arthralgia or arthritis, especially if occurring in young adults.<br>Greatest danger is if pregnant woman contracts the disease; causes serious congenital anomalies. | Included in MMR |
| Mumps (parotitis) | Viral infection causing swelling of the salivary glands with painful swallowing.<br>Ice collar may help relieve discomfort.<br>Complications include orchitis (usually unilateral) if disease occurs after puberty, aseptic meningitis, encephalitis. | Included in MMR |
| Poliomyelitis (polio) | Viral infection, 95% of infected clients have no symptoms.<br>Virus multiplies in the GI tract and enters the bloodstream to affect the CNS, resulting in paralysis in less than 2% of infected. | IPV |
| Chickenpox (varicella) | Most common communicable childhood disease, caused by the varicella zoster virus.<br>Causes rash that starts on the trunk and spreads.<br>Rash starts as vesicles, which then erupt and crust over.<br>Highly contagious from 2 days prior to rash to 6 days after rash erupts; incubation period 21 days.<br>Once lesions have crusted or scabbed over they are no longer contagious.<br>Care is directed at comfort measures. | Short-term protection from maternal antibodies.<br>Varicella vaccine. |

f. Provide family education concerning child care, especially safety and nutrition needs, discipline, and age-appropriate stimulation.

g. Initiate referrals for long-term follow-up (community agencies, pediatric and mental health clinics, self-help groups).

C. Learning disabilities

1. General information

a. A heterogeneous group of disorders manifested by significant difficulties in acquisition and use of listening, speaking, writing, reasoning, or math skills

b. Presumed to be due to CNS dysfunction

c. Children of average or above-average IQ

d. Affects all aspects of learning, not just academics

e. Boys affected 6 times more often than girls

f. Categories include:

1) Receptive/sensory: perceptual problem (dyslexia, visual misperception)

2) Integrative: difficulty processing information (analysis, organization, sequencing, abstract thought)

3) Expressive: motor dysfunction (aphasia, writing or drawing difficulties, difficulty in sports or games)

4) Diffuse: combination of above

2. Assessment findings

a. Poor attention span

b. Poor grades, normal IQ

c. Low general information scores on standardized IQ tests

d. Decreased participation in extracurricular activities or hobbies

e. Low self-esteem due to multiple failures

f. Diagnostic tests: specific testing to confirm diagnosis and determine type of defect

3. Medical management: psychostimulants may be prescribed to reduce hyperactivity and frustration and to increase attention span and self-control; side effects include anorexia.

4. Nursing interventions

a. Environmental manipulation for behavior management

1) Limit external stimuli.

2) Maintain predictable routines.

3) Enforce limits on behavior.

b. Teaching strategies tailored for child's specific defects

1) Repeat directions often.

2) Elicit feedback from child.

3) Give time to ask questions.

4) Keep teaching sessions short.

5) Do not give nonessential information.

D. Sudden infant death syndrome (SIDS)

1. General information

a. Sudden death of any young child that is unexpected by history and in which thorough postmortem examination fails to demonstrate adequate cause of death

b. Cannot be predicted; cannot be prevented (unexpected and unexplained)

c. Peak age: 3 months; 95% by 6 months

d. Usually occurs during sleep; there is no struggle and death is silent

e. Diagnosis made at autopsy

f. Although cause of death is not known, suffocation and DTaP reactions are *not* causes of SIDS

2. Assessment findings

a. Factors associated with increased SIDS risk: prematurity, low birth weight, multiple births, siblings of SIDS victims, maternal substance abuse

b. Infants with neurologic problems and abnormal respiratory function at higher risk

c. Co-sleeping with parents, prone sleep position, soft bedding associated with higher risk

3. Nursing interventions

a. Nursing care is directed at supporting parents/family; parents usually arrive at emergency department.

b. Provide a room for the family to be alone if possible, stay with them; prepare them for how infant will look and feel (baby will be bruised and blanched due to pooling of blood until death was discovered; also will be cold).

c. Let parents say good-bye to baby (hold, rock).

d. Reinforce that death was not their fault.

e. Provide appropriate support referrals: clergy, notification of significant others, local SIDS program, visiting nurse.

f. Explain how parents can receive autopsy results.

g. Notify family physician or pediatrician.

# DEATH AND DYING

## Overview

### Parental Response to Death

A. Major life stress event

B. Initially parents experience grief in response to potential loss of child

1. Acknowledgment of terminal disease is a struggle between hope and despair with resultant awareness of inevitable death.

2. Parents will be at different stages of grief at different times and constantly changing.

C. Parental response is related to age of child, cause of death, available social support, and degree of uncertainty; response might include denial, shock, disbelief, guilt.

D. Parents often confronted with major decisions such as home care versus hospital care, use of investigational drugs, and continuation of life supports.

**E.** May have long-term disruptive effects on family system
   1. Stress may result in divorce.
   2. May contribute to behavioral problems or psychosomatic symptoms in siblings.
**F.** Bereaved parents experience intense grief of long duration.

## Child's Response to Death

**A.** Child's concept of death depends on mental age.
   1. Infants and toddlers
      a. Live only in present.
      b. Are concerned only with separation from mother and being alone and abandoned.
      c. Can sense sadness in others and may feel guilty (due to magical thinking).
      d. Do not understand life without themselves.
      e. Can sense they are getting weaker.
      f. Healthy toddlers may insist on seeing a significant other long after that person's death.
   2. Preschoolers
      a. See death as temporary; a type of sleep or separation.
      b. See life as concrete; they know the word "dead" but do not understand the finality.
      c. Fear separation from parents; want to know who will take care of them when they are dead.
      d. Dying children may regress in their behavior.
   3. School-age
      a. Have a concept of time, causality, and irreversibility (but still question it).
      b. Fear pain, mutilation, and abandonment.
      c. Will ask directly if they are dying.
      d. See death as a period of immobility.
      e. Interested in the death ceremony; may make requests for own ceremony.
      f. Feel death is punishment.
      g. May personify death (bogey man, angel of death).
      h. May know they are going to die but feel comforted by having parents and loved ones with them.
   4. Adolescents
      a. Are thinking about the future and knowing they will not participate.
      b. May express anger at impending death.
      c. May find it difficult to talk about death.
      d. Have an accurate understanding of death.
      e. May wish to write something for friends and family, make things to leave, or make a tape.
      f. May wish to plan own funeral.

## Nursing Implications

### Communicating with Dying Child

**A.** Use the child's own language.
**B.** Do not use euphemisms.
**C.** Do not expect an immediate response.
**D.** Never give up hope.

## Care Guidelines at Impending Death

**A.** Do not leave child alone.
**B.** Do not whisper in the room (increases fears).
**C.** Know that touching child is important.
**D.** Let the child and family talk and cry.
**E.** Continue to read favorite stories to child or play favorite music.
**F.** Let parents participate in care as far as they are emotionally capable.
**G.** Be aware of the needs of siblings who are in the room with the family.

## Sample Questions

1. The nurse has assessed four children of varying ages; which one requires further evaluation?
   1. A 7-month-old who is afraid of strangers.
   2. A 4-year-old who talks to an imaginary playmate.
   3. A 9-year-old with enuresis.
   4. A 16-year-old male who had nocturnal emissions.

2. The nurse is caring for a 5-year-old child who has leukemia and is now out of remission and not expected to survive. The child says to his mother, "Will you take care of me when I am dead the way you do now?" The child's mother asks the nurse how to answer her child. The nurse's response should be based on which of the following understandings of the child's behavior?
   1. The child is denying that he has a terminal illness.
   2. The child may be hallucinating.
   3. Children of this age do not understand the finality of death.
   4. Most 5-year-old children have a great fear of mutilation.

3. The nurse is talking with the mother of a 1-year-old child in well-baby clinic. Which statement the mother makes indicates a need for more instruction in keeping the child safe?
   1. "I have some syrup of ipecac at home in case my child ever needs it."
   2. "I put all the medicines on the highest shelf in the kitchen."
   3. "We have moved all the valuable vases and figurines out of the family room."
   4. "My husband put the gates up at the top and bottom of the stairs."

4. A baby was born 6 weeks prematurely and is now 2 months old, and her mother brings her to the clinic for her checkup. What will determine if the baby can receive the DTaP?
   1. The presence of sufficient muscle mass.
   2. Whether the vaccines are live or inactive.
   3. The Denver Developmental Screening results.
   4. Calculating her age by subtracting 6 weeks from the due date.

5. A 12-month-old is brought in for her well-child checkup. All of the immunizations are up to date. The child's mother asks the nurse what immunizations her child will receive today. What will be the nurse's best response?
   1. First dose of MMR.
   2. Second dose of Hib.
   3. Third dose of DtaP.
   4. Final dose of IPV.

6. The presence of what condition would necessitate a change in the standard immunization schedule for a child?
   1. Allergy to eggs.
   2. Immunosuppression.
   3. Congenital defects.
   4. Mental retardation.

7. A 2-year-old is brought to the pediatric clinic with an upper respiratory infection. After assessing the child, the nurse suspects this child may be a victim of child abuse. What physical signs usually indicate child abuse?
   1. Diaper rash.
   2. Bruises on the lower legs.
   3. Scraped and scabbed knees.
   4. Welts or bruises in various stages of healing.

8. Which action by a parent-child interaction does NOT warrant further assessment when child abuse is suspected?
   1. Appears tired and disheveled.
   2. Is hypercritical of the child.
   3. Pushes the frightened child away.
   4. Expresses far more concern than the situation warrants.

9. When child abuse is suspected, what recognizable factor will be present?
   1. Have a number of scars.
   2. Have identifiable shapes.
   3. Display an erratic pattern.
   4. Be on one side of the body.

10. The nurse is testing reflexes in a 4-month-old infant as part of the neurologic assessment. Which of the following findings would indicate an abnormal reflex pattern and an area of concern in a 4-month-old infant?
    1. Closes hand tightly when palm is touched.
    2. Begins strong sucking movements when mouth area is stimulated.
    3. Hyperextends toes in response to stroking sole of foot upward.
    4. Does not extend and abduct extremities in response to loud noise.

11. The mother of a 4-month-old infant asks the nurse when she can start feeding her baby solid food. Which of the following should the nurse include in teaching this mother about the nutritional needs of infants?
    1. Infant cereal can be introduced by spoon when the extrusion reflex fades.
    2. Solid foods should be given as soon as the infant's first tooth erupts.
    3. Pureed food can be offered when the infant has tripled his birth weight.
    4. Infant formula or breast milk provides adequate nutrients for the first year.

12. The nurse is assessing a 6-month-old infant during a well-child visit. The nurse makes all of the following observations. Which of the following assessments made by the nurse is an area of concern indicating a need for further evaluation?
    1. Absence of Moro reflex.
    2. Closed posterior fontanel.
    3. Three-pound weight gain in 2 months.
    4. Moderate head lag when pulled to sitting position.

13. The nurse is giving anticipatory guidance regarding safety and injury prevention to the parents of an 18-month-old toddler. Which of the following actions by the parents indicates understanding of the safety needs of a toddler?
    1. Supervise the child in outdoor, fenced play areas.
    2. Teach the child swimming and water safety.
    3. Use automobile booster seat with lap belt.
    4. Allow child to cross the street with 4-year-old sibling.

14. The community health nurse is making a newborn follow-up home visit. During the visit the 2-year-old sibling has a temper tantrum. The parent asks the nurse for guidance in dealing

with the toddler's temper tantrums. Which of the following is the most appropriate nursing action?

1. Help the child understand the rules.
2. Leave the child alone in his bedroom.
3. Suggest that the parent ignore the child's behavior.
4. Explain that the toddler is zealous of the new baby.

15. The parent of a 3-year-old child brings the child to the clinic for a well-child checkup. The history and assessment reveals the following findings. Which of these assessment findings made by the nurse is an area of concern and requires further investigation?

1. Unable to ride a tricycle.
2. Has ability to hop on one foot.
3. Uses gestures to indicate wants.
4. Weight gain of 4 pounds in last year.

16. The parents of a 4-year-old child tell the nurse that the child has an invisible friend named "Felix." The child blames "Felix" for any misbehavior and is often heard scolding "Felix," calling him a "bad boy." The nurse understands that the best interpretation of this behavior is which of the following?

1. A delay in moral development.
2. Impaired parent-child relationship.
3. A way for the child to assume control.
4. Inconsistent parental discipline strategies.

17. The nurse is caring for a 5-year-old child who is in the terminal stages of acute leukemia. The child refuses to go to sleep and is afraid that his parents will leave. The nurse recognizes that the child suspects he is dying and is afraid. Which of the following questions about death is most likely to be made by a 5-year-old child?

1. "What does it feel like when you die?"
2. "Who will take care of me when I die?"
3. "What will my friends do when I die?"
4. "Why do children die if they're not old?"

18. The parents of an 8-year-old child bring the child into the clinic for a school physical. The nurse makes all of the following assessments. Which assessment finding is an area of concern and needs further investigation?

1. Complains of a stomach ache on test days at school.
2. Has many evening rituals and resists going to bed at night.

3. Refers to self as being too dumb and too small during the exam.
4. Has lost three deciduous teeth and has the central and lateral incisors.

19. The nurse is performing a neurologic assessment on an 8-year-old child. As part of this neurologic assessment the nurse is assessing how the child thinks. Which of the following abilities best illustrates that the child is developing concrete operational thought?

1. Able to make change from a dollar bill.
2. Describes a ball as both red and round.
3. Tells time in terms of after breakfast and before lunch.
4. Able to substitute letters for numbers in simple problems.

20. The nurse is caring for a 10-year-old child during the acute phase of rheumatic fever. Bed rest is part of the child's plan of care. Which of the following diversional activities is developmentally appropriate and meets the health needs of this child in the acute phase of rheumatic fever?

1. Using handheld computer video games.
2. Sorting and organizing baseball cards in a notebook.
3. Playing basketball with a hoop suspended from the bed.
4. Using art supplies to make drawings about the hospital experience.

21. The nurse is caring for a 13-year-old who has been casted following spinal instrumentation surgery to correct idiopathic scoliosis. The nurse is helping the teen and family plan diversional activities while the teen is in the cast. Which of the following activities would be most appropriate to support adolescent development while the teen is casted?

1. Take the teen shopping at the mall in a wheelchair.
2. Plan family evenings playing a variety of board games.
3. Have teen regularly attend special school activities for own class.
4. Encourage siblings to spend time with teen watching television and movies.

22. A 2-month-old infant is in the clinic for a well-baby visit. Which of the following immunizations can the nurse expect to administer?

1. TD, Varicella, IPV.

2. DTaP, Varicella.

3. DTaP, MMR, Menomune.

4. DTaP, Hib, IPV, HBV.

23. An 18-month-old child with a history of falling out of his crib has been brought to the emergency room by the parents. Examination of the child reveals a skull fracture and multiple bruises on the child's body. Which of the following findings obtained by the nurse is most suggestive of child abuse?

1. Poor personal hygiene of the child.

2. Parents want to comfort child.

3. Conflicting explanations about the accident from the parents.

4. Cuts and bruises on the child's lower legs in various stages of healing.

24. The nurse is discussing the risk of sudden infant death syndrome (SIDS) in infants with the parents whose first baby died of SIDS 6 months ago. The parents express fear that other children will die from SIDS since they have already had one baby die. Which of the following statements made by the parents indicate their understanding of the relationship of future children and the risk of SIDS?

1. "Any new baby will be on home monitoring for one year to prevent SIDS."

2. "There is a 99% chance that we will not have another baby die of SIDS."

3. "Genetic testing is available to determine the likelihood of another baby dying from SIDS."

4. "There is medicine that can be used to stimulate the heart rate while the baby is sleeping."

## Answers and Rationales

1. **3.** A 9-year-old should not be wetting the bed. This child may have physiologic or psychologic problems.

2. **3.** Preschool children do not understand the finality of death. They often view it as a long sleep. It is common for preschoolers to ask who will take care of them when they die. Preschool children may know the word "dead" but do not really comprehend what it means.

3. **2.** At 1 year of age babies are, or soon will be, climbing on everything. Putting medicines on

the highest shelf is not sufficient. All medicines should be put in a locked cabinet.

4. **1.** DtaP is given intramuscularly; therefore, administration is dependent on the presence of sufficient muscle mass, which may not be present in the infant who was born prematurely.

5. **1.** Current recommendations call for measles, mumps, and rubella combined vaccine (MMR) to be given at 12-15 months.

6. **2.** Immunosuppressed clients may need alteration in immunization protection as live virus vaccines may overwhelm them.

7. **4.** Injuries at various stages of healing are symptomatic of child abuse.

8. **1.** Being tired and disheveled gives no information about the quality of the parent-child interaction. It may be a normal state for a busy parent.

9. **2.** Burns typical of child abuse have symmetrical shapes and resemble the shape of the item used to burn the child.

10. **1.** The palmar grasp is present at birth. The palmar grasp lessens by age 3 months and is no longer reflexive. The infant is able to close hand voluntarily.

11. **1.** Infant cereal is generally introduced first because of its high iron content. The infant is able to accept spoon feeding at around 4 to 5 months when the tongue thrust or extrusion reflex fades.

12. **4.** By 4 to 6 months, head control is well established. There should be no head lag when infant is pulled to a sitting position by the age of 6 months.

13. **1.** The child has great curiosity and has the mobility to explore. Toddlers need to be supervised in play areas. Play areas with soft ground cover and safe equipment need to be selected.

14. **3.** The best approach toward extinguishing attention-seeking behavior is to ignore it as long as the behavior is not inflicting injury.

15. **3.** This behavior indicates a delay in language and speech development. The child may not be able to hear. The child should have a vocabulary of about 900 words and use complete sentences of three to four words.

**16. 3.** Imaginary friends are a normal part of development for many preschool children. These imaginary friends often have many faults. The child plays the role of the parent with the imaginary friend. This becomes a way of assuming control and authority in a safe situation.

**17. 2.** The greatest fear of preschool children is being left alone and abandoned. Preschool children still think as though they are alive and need to be taken care of.

**18. 3.** The school-age years are very important in the development of a healthy self-esteem. These statements by the 8-year-old child indicate a risk for development of a sense of inferiority and need further assessment.

**19. 1.** This ability illustrates the concept of conservation, which is one of the major cognitive tasks of school-age children.

**20. 2.** The middle childhood years are times for collections. The collections of middle to late school-age children become orderly, selective, and neatly organized in scrapbooks. This quiet activity supports the development of industry and concrete operational thought as well as the physical restrictions related to the rheumatic fever.

**21. 3.** Early adolescents have a strong need to fit in and be accepted by their peers. Attending school activities helps the teen continue peer relationships and develop a sense of belonging.

**22. 4.** Healthy infants at 2 months of age receive diphtheria, tetanus, and pertussis (DTaP); hemophilus influenza (Hib); polio vaccine (IPV); and hepatitis B virus (HBV).

**23. 3.** Incompatibility between the history and the injury is probably the most important criterion on which to base the decision to report suspected abuse.

**24. 2.** Whether subsequent siblings of the SIDS infant are at risk is unclear. Even if the increased risk is correct, families have a 99% chance that their subsequent child will not die of SIDS.

# Multisystem Stressors

## GENETIC DISORDERS

A. Genes are functional units of heredity, capable of replication, mutation, and expression.
B. Teratology is the branch of embryology that deals with the study of abnormal development and congenital malformations.
   1. *Congenital disorders:* present at birth, although may not be noticeable until later; may be caused by genetic factors, nongenetic factors, or a combination.
   2. *Genetic disorders:* caused by a single aberrant gene or a deviation in chromosome structure or number.
C. In humans there are normally 46 chromosomes (23 pairs) that contain the genes.
   1. *Genotype:* the gene constitution of an individual
   2. *Phenotype:* the outward visible physical appearance/expression of a person's genes (color, size, allergies)
   3. *Karyotype:* the number and pattern of chromosomes in a cell
   4. *Allele:* one or two or more forms of a gene that controls expression of specific characteristic (e.g., genes for eye color)
      a. *Mendel's law:* for each hereditary property we receive 2 genes, 1 from each parent; 1 is dominant and expressed; 1 is recessive and not expressed.
      b. *Homozygous:* alleles for characteristic are identical; both dominant (DD) or both recessive (dd).
      c. *Heterozygous:* alleles are different (Dd).
D. Normal cell division
   1. *Meiosis:* cell division that produces gametes, each with a haploid set of chromosomes (one-half the number of the parent cell); this is reductional division, occurs in the ova and sperm.
   2. *Mitosis:* cell division that produces two cells (daughter cells), each with a full complement of chromosomes, identical to the composition of the parent cell.

## Principles of Inheritance

Traits that are controlled by genes located on autosomes are inherited according to dominant or recessive patterns. Most cases of autosomal inheritance in humans involve traits controlled by one gene.

## Autosomal Dominant

A. General information
   1. Allele responsible for the trait (or disease) is dominant.
   2. Only one parent needs to pass on the gene (child may be heterozygous for trait).
   3. Examples of inherited diseases; Huntington's chorea, myotonic muscular dystrophy, night blindness, osteogenesis imperfecta, neurofibromatosis.
B. Genetic counseling: advise parents that if one of them has a disease inherited through autosomal dominant pattern, there is a 50% chance with each pregnancy that the child will have the disease/disorder.

## Autosomal Recessive

A. General information
   1. Allele responsible for trait (or disease) will not result in expression if the other allele in the pair is dominant.
   2. Both parents must pass on the gene(s) (child is homozygous for trait).
   3. Examples of inherited diseases: cystic fibrosis, PKU, sickle cell anemia, albinism, Tay-Sachs.
B. Genetic counseling: advise parents that if both are heterozygous for the trait then:
   1. There is a 25% chance with each pregnancy of having a child with the disease/disorder.
   2. There is a 50% chance with each pregnancy of having a child who is a carrier of the disease but who will not have the symptoms.
   3. There is a 25% chance with each pregnancy of having a child who will neither have the disease nor be a carrier.

## Sex-Linked (X-Linked) Inheritance

A. General information
   1. Inheritance of characteristics located on X and Y chromosomes
   2. Only known genetic locus on the Y chromosome is associated with determination of male sex.
   3. X chromosome carries other traits in addition to determination of female sex.
   4. Sex-linked inheritance in males: even a recessive defective gene on X chromosome can manifest itself in males because there is no opposing normal gene on Y chromosome.
   5. Sex-linked inheritance in females: recessive defective gene can be masked by a normal dominant gene.
   6. Examples of sex-linked inherited disorders: color blindness, baldness, hemophilia A and B, Duchenne's muscular dystrophy.
B. Genetic counseling
   1. If a woman is a carrier for a sex-linked disorder and her partner does not have the disorder:
      a. There is a 50% chance with each pregnancy that her son will have the disorder.
      b. There is a 50% chance her daughter will become a carrier.
   2. If a man has a sex-linked disorder, all his daughters will be carriers but none will manifest the disease.
   3. For sex-linked disorders, there are no carrier states in males.

## Chromosome Alterations

A. General information: deviations from normal chromosome complement may be numeric or structural.
   1. *Mutation:* spontaneous alteration in genetic material not present in previous generation
   2. *Nondisjunction:* failure of a pair of chromosomes to separate during meiosis; results in numeric change called trisomy (47 chromosomes); can be passed on by either parent (one parent would pass 24 chromosomes)
   3. *Translocation:* the transfer of all or part of a chromosome to another location on the same chromosome or to a different chromosome after chromosome breakage
   4. *Mosaicism:* the presence in the same individual of two or more genotypically different cell lines
B. Genetic counseling: varies depending on the origin of the alteration
   1. Random risk: chromosome alterations caused by environmental agents are not likely to occur in subsequent pregnancies. Therefore, the risk of the same defect recurring is no more than for any person in the general population.
   2. High risk: at least one parent carries a chromosomal aberration or mutant gene and passes it on to the offspring (e.g., if a parent is a balanced translocation carrier, the risk of a child being affected is 1 in 4)
   3. Moderate risk: largest group; includes multifactorial disorders. Risk recurrence in these disorders is empiric, based not on genetic theory but on prior experience and observation.

# Assessment

## History

A. Careful, detailed history is the basis of genetic counseling; can help confirm diagnosis and establish recurrence risk in multifactorial disorders.
B. Family history (pattern of affected family members) is recorded in form of pedigree chart or family tree.

1. Information about affected child and immediate family: history of this pregnancy and all previous pregnancies, including stillbirths and abortions; information about siblings
2. Information about maternal relatives
   a. Mother's siblings
   b. Outcome of maternal grandmother's pregnancies
   c. Health status of maternal relatives
3. Information about paternal relatives: same as maternal

### Laboratory/Diagnostic Tests

A. Amniocentesis
   1. Examination of amniotic fluid to screen for:
      a. Some inborn errors of metabolism
      b. Chromosomal abnormalities
      c. Some CNS disorders (spina bifida)
      d. Sex of infant in sex-related disorders
   2. Indications
      a. One parent is chromosome mosaic or has balanced translocation.
      b. Mother is age 35 or older.
      c. Both parents are heterozygous for an autosomal recessive disorder.
      d. Mother is carrier of an X-linked disorder.
      e. Couple already has an affected child.
B. Karyotyping (chromosomal analysis)
   1. Confirms or refutes probable diagnosis of chromosomal abnormality.
   2. Identifies whether individual is a carrier of chromosomal abnormality.
   3. Determines infant's sex if necessary.
C. Determination of fetal status

## Analysis

Nursing diagnoses for the family/individual with a genetic disorder may include:
A. Disturbed thought processes
B. Deficient knowledge (specify)
C. Risk for altered parenting
D. Grief (anticipatory)

## Planning and Implementation

### Goals

A. Child will achieve maximum potential for cognitive and motor development.
B. Family will develop effective coping strategies.

### Interventions

A. Provide community health agency referral.
B. Support family in identification of appropriate stimulation programs for child.
C. Communicate with and provide support for parents.
D. Offer genetic counseling (see Principles of Inheritance).

## Evaluation

A. Optimum level of motor and cognitive development is attained.
B. Self-care is performed at satisfactory level.
C. Family is able to function appropriately.
D. Parents demonstrate ability to meet child's physical and developmental needs.
E. Parents derive comfort/satisfaction from parenting affected child.

## Chromosome Disorder

### Down Syndrome

A. General information
   1. One of the most common causes of mental retardation; incidence: about 1 in 600 live births
   2. Caused by an extra chromosome 21 (total 47)
      a. Most cases associated with nondisjunction; incidence increased with maternal, and to some degree paternal, age; incidence in women over age 35 markedly increased
      b. Also associated with translocation; hereditary type, incidence not increased with parental age
B. Assessment findings
   1. Head and face
      a. Small head, flat facial profile, broad flat nose
      b. Small mouth, normal-size protruding tongue
      c. Upward slanting palpebral fissure
      d. Low-set ears
   2. Extremities
      a. Short, thick fingers and hands
      b. Simian creases (single crease across palms)
      c. Muscle weakness, lax joints
   3. Associated anomalies and disorders
      a. Congenital heart defects (40% incidence)
      b. GI structural defects
      c. Increased incidence of leukemia
      d. Increased incidence of respiratory infection
      e. Visual defects: strabismus, myopia, nystagmus, cataracts
      f. Obesity in older children
   4. Retardation usually moderate, IQ 50–70
C. Nursing interventions: see also Mental Retardation.
   1. Provide parent education concerning
      a. Increased susceptibility to respiratory infection
      b. Nutritional needs, feeding techniques
      c. Medication administration if necessary
      d. Protection from injury due to hypotonia, atlanto-axial instability (weak neck)
      e. Needs of siblings
   2. Promote developmental progress
   3. Provide genetic counseling.

# FLUID AND ELECTROLYTE, ACID-BASE BALANCES

## General Principles and Variations from Adult

A. Percent body water compared to total body weight
  1. Premature infant: 90% water
  2. Infant: 75–80% water
  3. Child: 64% water
B. Infant also has a higher percentage of water in extracellular fluid compared to adults (therefore, infant has less fluid reserve).
C. Renal function
  1. Concentrating ability of kidney does not reach adult levels until approximately age 2; specific gravity of infant's urine is 1.003.
  2. Glomerular filtration rate does not reach adult levels until approximately age 2.
  3. Average urine output
    a. Infant: 5–10 mL/hour
    b. 1–10 years: 10–25 mL/hour
    c. 35 mL/hour thereafter
D. Metabolic rate in children is 2–3 times that of adults; children therefore have an increased need for nutrients and fluids, and an increased amount of waste to excrete.
E. Fluid is not conserved; there is less reserve, and children more prone to fluid volume deficit than adults; ½ of infant's extracellular fluid is exchanged each day compared with only ⅕ of adult's.
F. Children have faster respiratory rate than adults, causing more water loss through breathing.
G. Infants have a greater body surface area per kg body weight than adults, therefore fluid loss through skin (evaporation) is greater in children.

## Assessment

### Health History

A. Ascertain age, recent weight, usual feeding habits/patterns, amount and type of daily intake.
B. Determine usual voiding/stooling habits and volume of urine/stool output.
C. Identify any recent illnesses or medications taken.
D. Ascertain usual activity level.

### Physical Examination

A. Measure present weight and vital signs.
B. Observe general appearance.
  1. Muscle tone
  2. Reflex responses
  3. Activity level
C. Inspect skin and mucous membranes for turgor, color, temperature.
D. Head and face
  1. Inspect fontanels, eye orbits.
  2. Ascertain presence of tears, saliva.
E. Abdomen/genitalia
  1. Auscultate for bowel sounds, peristaltic waves.
  2. Inspect for diaper rash, urine stream.

### Laboratory/Diagnostic Tests

A. Blood studies
  1. Hbg and HCT
  2. Sodium, potassium, chloride, calcium, magnesium
  3. $pCO_2$ and $CO_2$
  4. pH
B. Urine studies: specific gravity, glucose, ketones, osmolarity, pH
C. Stool studies: culture, reducing substances, blood, sodium, potassium, pH

## Analysis

Nursing diagnoses for children with fluid/electrolyte and acid-base imbalances may include:
A. Diarrhea
B. Pain
C. Deficient fluid volume
D. Imbalanced nutrition
E. Impaired oral mucous membrane
F. Impaired skin integrity
G. Ineffective tissue perfusion
H. Impaired urinary elimination

## Planning and Implementation

### Goals

A. Child will have normal hydration status.
B. Parents will demonstrate knowledge of child's disorder, prescribed treatment, and prevention of complications.

### Interventions

A. Maintain strict I&O.
  1. Weigh diapers.
  2. Monitor urine specific gravity.
  3. Hematest stools.
B. Take daily weights.
C. Keep NPO for bowel rest.
D. Administer IV fluids.
  1. Maintenance plus replacement
  2. Generally use hypotonic solutions (0.25 NSS, 0.33 NSS, or 0.45 NSS)
E. Provide pacifier for infant.
F. Reintroduce oral fluids slowly.
  1. In children under 2 years use Pedialyte, a balanced electrolyte solution.
  2. In children over 2 use weak tea, flat soda.

3. Do not use
   a. Broth (high sodium)
   b. Milk/formula (high solute)
   c. Water, glucose water, Jell-O (no electrolytes)

## Evaluation

A. Child has adequate hydration status.
   1. Adequate I&O
   2. Normal stooling pattern
   3. Good skin turgor
   4. Normal vital signs
   5. Normal serum laboratory values
B. Parents participate in care, demonstrate understanding of signs and symptoms of disorder and treatment.

## Disorders

### Dehydration

A. The most common fluid and electrolyte disturbance in infants and children
B. Osmotic factors, particularly sodium, control the movement of fluid between extracellular and intracellular compartments and influence the types of dehydration
   1. Isotonic dehydration: most common
      a. Plasma sodium level is normal (130–150 mEq/liter).
      b. Water and electrolyte lost in proportionate amounts; net loss is isotonic.
      c. Major loss is from extracellular fluid; loss of circulating blood volume.
      d. Shock may develop if losses are severe.
   2. Hypotonic dehydration
      a. Plasma sodium level is less than 130 mEq/liter.
      b. Electrolyte deficit exceeds water deficit.
      c. May occur when fluid and electrolyte losses are replaced with plain or glucose water.
      d. Fluid lost from extracellular compartment; also moves from extracellular to intracellular compartment.
      e. Signs of decreased fluid appear sooner with smaller fluid losses than in isotonic dehydration.
      f. Shock is a frequent finding.
   3. Hypertonic dehydration
      a. Plasma sodium exceeds 150 mEq/liter.
      b. Water loss exceeds electrolyte loss; may occur when fluid and electrolyte losses are replaced with large amount of solute (hypertonic formula).
      c. Fluid shifts from the intracellular to the extracellular compartments.
      d. Physical signs of dehydration may be less apparent.
      e. Neurologic symptoms (e.g., seizures) may occur.

C. Nursing interventions
   1. Teach caregivers to watch for signs/symptoms of dehydration:
      a. A decrease in wet diapers
      b. Mouth dry inside
      c. No tears present with crying if older than 2–4 months
      d. Irritable or lethargic
      e. Sunken fontanel
      f. Pale, gray, mottled skin color
   2. Correct dehydration with oral solutions that should contain glucose, sodium, potassium, and bicarbonate (Pedialyte, Lytren, Infalyte).
   3. Administer IV fluid therapy as ordered.
   4. Assess daily weight, vital signs, I&O.
   5. Educate family on signs of dehydration and to monitor child's urine output.

### Diarrhea

A. General information
   1. A change in consistency and frequency of stool
   2. Very common in young children
   3. Caused by bacteria and viruses, parasites, poisons, inflammation, malabsorption, allergies, abnormal bowel motility, and anatomic alterations
   4. Infants can easily lose 5% of their body weight in 1 day
   5. Intestinal fluids are alkaline; large loss causes metabolic acidosis
   6. Also causes bicarbonate and potassium loss
   7. Body may use its own fat for energy, leading to ketosis
B. Assessment findings
   1. History of frequent stools; child may complain of or indicate abdominal cramping by guarding, weight loss; child may be lethargic and irritable
   2. Decreased urine output, decreased tears and saliva, dry mucous membranes, dry skin with poor tissue turgor
   3. In children less than 18 months, may find depressed anterior fontanel
   4. Soft eyeballs with sunken appearance
   5. Ashen skin color; cold extremities
   6. High-pitched cry
   7. Increased pulse rate and decreased blood pressure
   8. Diagnostic tests
      a. HCT elevated if dehydrated
      b. Serum sodium and potassium decreased
      c. BUN elevated if renal circulation is decreased
      d. CBC will show increased bands if caused by bacterial infection
      e. Low pH and positive sugar with disaccharide intolerance

**f.** Stool culture will identify specific microorganism

**g.** Leukocytes in stool if caused by enteroinvasive organisms

**C.** Nursing interventions

1. Keep NPO to rest bowel, if ordered.
2. Administer IV fluid therapy as ordered.
3. Resume oral feedings slowly; regular diet is recommended.
4. Provide skin care to prevent/treat excoriation of diaper area.
5. Test all stool and chart results.
6. Isolation may be ordered with infectious cause.

## Vomiting

**A.** General information

1. Common symptom during childhood; usually not a cause for concern
2. Differs from spitting up (dribbling of undigested formula, often with burping)
3. If prolonged may result in metabolic alkalosis or aspiration

**B.** Assessment findings: in addition to vomiting, child may have fever, abdominal pain, and distension.

**C.** Nursing interventions

1. Assist with identification and treatment of underlying cause.
   **a.** Assess for accompanying diarrhea that may indicate gastroenteritis.
   **b.** Determine whether others in family/school/etc., are also sick; may indicate food poisoning.
   **c.** Assess for history of anxiety-producing life events.
   **d.** Assess amount and force of vomitus; forceful, projectile vomiting may indicate pyloric stenosis
   **e.** Determine frequency and character of vomitus (color, whether formula or food, presence of bile or blood), relationship to feeding (new foods, overeating).
2. Prevent complications: monitor fluid/electrolyte and acid-base status
3. Administer antiemetics if ordered; trimetho-benzamide HCl (Tigan) and promethazine HCl (Phenergan) recommended for children.

# ACCIDENTS, POISONINGS, AND INGESTION

**A.** Accidents are the main cause of death in children over the age of 1 year.

**B.** 90% of accidents are preventable.

**C.** Interaction among host (the child), agent (the principal cause), and environment (⅔ of accidents occur in the home); safeguard the host while the agent and environment are made safer.

**D.** Methods of prevention

1. Childproofing the environment
2. Educating parents and child
3. Legislation (e.g., seat belts, safe toys)
4. Anticipatory guidance
5. Understanding and applying growth and development principles
   **a.** Infant: totally dependent on adults for maintenance of safe environment
   **b.** Toddler: more mobile, impatient; urge to investigate and imitate; climbing, running, jumping
   **c.** Preschooler: very curious, exploring neighborhood, running, climbing, riding bikes; can accept and respond to teaching but still needs protection
   **d.** School-age and adolescent: taking dares, sports injuries, peer pressure, learning to drive

**E.** Precipitating factors

1. Arguments or tension in the home
2. Change in routines
3. Tired child/tired parents
4. Inadequate babysitting
5. Hungry child
6. Illness in immediate family member

**F.** Potential outcomes include temporary incapacitation, permanent disfigurement, and death

## Specific Disorders

### Pediatric Poisonings

**A.** General information

1. Toddlers and suicidal adolescents most often involved
2. Deaths have declined due to continued efforts in prevention and the establishment of Poison Control Centers
3. Modes of exposure: ocular, skin, ingestion (vast majority)
4. Types of substances ingested: drugs, household products (cleaning agents), garden supplies, plants and berries
5. Most ingestions are acute in nature and accompanied by a history of invasion of the medicine chest or cabinet where household cleaners are kept
6. Chronic ingestions result in accumulation of toxic substance, such as lead

**B.** General assessment findings

1. Signs vary depending on substance ingested
2. May evidence bradycardia; tachycardia; tachypnea; slow depressed respiration; hypotension or hypertension; hypothermia or hyperpyrexia
3. Confusion, disorientation, coma, ataxia, seizures
4. Miosis, mydriasis, nystagmus
5. Jaundice, cyanosis

6. Child may have a distinctive odor: hydrocarbons, alcohol, garlic, sweat
C. General interventions
  1. Resuscitate child and stabilize condition: establish patent airway and provide measures to restore circulation as indicated.
  2. Prevent absorption.
     a. Determine what, when, and how much was ingested; will frequently not be able to identify substance.
     b. Gastric lavage; may be used to prevent absorption
        1) Use largest nasogastric (NG) or orogastric tube possible.
        2) Recommended within 1 to 2 hours after ingestion.
        3) Indicated when ingested substance is highly toxic or not absorbed by activated charcoal (i.e., lithium, iron, lead).
        4) Contraindicated in ingestion of corrosives.
        5) Complications include aspiration and perforation of esophagus.
     c. Activated charcoal: minimizes amount of toxic agent for absorption.
        1) May be given alone or following gastric lavage.
        2) Used if ingestion has occurred within 2 hours prior to treatment
        3) If liquid form, shake bottle, administer, then rinse bottle with small amount of water, shake again and administer to obtain full dose.
        4) Complications include aspiration and pneumothorax.
     d. Cathartic: may be used after emesis or lavage to speed elimination of ingested substance; recommended agents are sodium or magnesium sulfate.
  3. Provide treatment and prevention information to parents.
     a. Parents should always be instructed to save container, vomitus, spills on clothing for analysis.
     b. Teach parents about safety practices that will decrease chances of accidental poisonings; educate as to use of drugs, labeling, storage, and handling of household products, importance of child-resistant safety packaging.
     c. Advise parents to keep Poison Control Center phone number readily available (1-800-222-1222).
     d. Incorporate anticipatory guidance related to developmental stage of child.
     e. Discuss general first aid measures with parents.
     f. Syrup of ipecac is no longer recommended or sold OTC and only used by healthcare personnel.

## Salicylate Poisoning

A. General information
  1. Toxicity begins at doses of 150–200 mg/kg.
  2. Products include not only aspirin but oil of wintergreen and analgesic cold medicines.
  3. Peak effect of aspirin is 2–4 hours and effects may last 8 hours.
  4. Ingestion may be accidental or due to therapeutic overdosing.
  5. Salicylate ingestion causes
     a. Acid-base alterations
     b. Respiratory alkalosis
     c. Metabolic acidosis
     d. Impaired glucose metabolism
     e. An inhibition of prothrombin formation
B. Assessment findings
  1. Hyperventilation, confusion, loss of consciousness
  2. Hyperpnea, hyperpyrexia, dehydration
  3. CNS depression, vomiting, lethargy
  4. Coma, respiratory failure, circulatory collapse
C. Nursing interventions
  1. Assist with emergency management
  2. Administer fluid therapy
  3. Monitor vital signs, BP, urine specific gravity, I&O
  4. Monitor temperature, provide tepid sponging or cooling mattress
  5. Provide emotional support to child and family
  6. Administer vitamin K

## Acetaminophen Ingestion

A. General information
  1. Has become a commonly used analgesic-antipyretic
  2. Little associated morbidity or mortality in accidental ingestion
  3. Major risk is severe hepatic damage
B. Assessment findings
  1. Vague and nonspecific initially; nausea, vomiting, anorexia, sweating
  2. Jaundice, liver tenderness, increase in liver enzymes, abdominal pain
  3. Progression to hepatic failure
C. Nursing interventions
  1. Emesis or lavage; do *not* use activated charcoal (will bind antidote).
  2. Administer antidote (acetylcysteine [Mucomyst]): lessens hepatic damage if given within 16 hours of ingestion.

## Lead Poisoning

A. General information
  1. Increased blood lead levels resulting from ingestion and absorption of lead-containing substances
  2. Most common source: candy and spices from other countries not approved by the FDA;

found in lead-based paint (used in houses prior to 1950); toys made in China recalled in 2007 due to lead paint used

3. Toddlers and preschoolers most often affected; many have pica (tendency to eat nonfood substances)
4. Lead value of more than 10 μg/dL is considered a health hazard
5. Acute symptoms usually appear once level is 70 μg/dL
6. Lead is absorbed through the GI tract and pulmonary system; it is then deposited in bone, soft tissue, and blood; excretion occurs via urine, feces, and sweat; toxic effects are due to enzyme inhibition.
7. Low dietary iron and calcium may enhance toxic effects.
8. Widespread screening programs have diminished severe effects.

B. Assessment findings
1. Abdominal complaints including colicky pain, constipation, anorexia, vomiting, weight loss
2. Pallor, listlessness, fatigue
3. Clumsiness, irritability, loss of coordination, ataxia, seizures
4. Encephalopathy
5. Identification of lead in the blood
6. Erythrocyte protoporphyrin (EP) levels increased

C. Nursing interventions
1. Prevention
   a. Nutrition: adequate iron and calcium in diet
   b. Environment: damp mop and damp wipe floors, windowsills, cover over flaking paint, handwashing before meals, baths
2. Chelating agents
   a. Succimer (chemet)-oral
   b. Dimercaprol (BAL)-IM
   c. Disodium calcium edetate (calcium EDTA)-IV or IM
   d. IM agents-multiple injections-pain
      1) Rotate sites
      2) Warm soaks
      3) Topical analgesia (EMLA cream)
   e. All chelating agents
      1) Maintain hydration (chelation is toxic to kidneys).
      2) Measure I&O.
      3) Monitor lead levels.
3. Provide nutritional counseling.
4. Aid in eliminating environmental conditions that led to lead ingestion.

### Lyme Disease

A. General information
1. Caused by the spirochete *Borrelia burgdorferi*
2. Transmitted by a deer tick, requires 24-hour tick attachment
3. Most prevalent during summer and early fall
4. Symptoms usually involve the skin, nervous system, and joints
5. Incubation period is 3 to 32 days

B. Medical management
1. Blood tests available, but lack sensitivity and specificity, therefore diagnosis is often based on clinical and epidemiologic data.
2. Antibiotic treatment: if early infection, given for 10–21 days. If neurologic or arthritic symptoms occur, combined treatment for longer duration may be necessary.

C. Assessment findings
1. Divided into stages on the basis of chronologic relationship to the tick bite
   a. Stage I: Skin rash (erythema migrans) starting 3–32 days past tick bite and lasting about 3 weeks. Most common on thighs, buttock, axilla. Systemic symptoms of malaise, fatigue, headache, stiff neck, fever, arthralgia.
   b. Stage II: Symptoms of late disease may occur months to years after the initial disease. Includes neurologic symptoms such as facial palsies, sensory losses, focal weaknesses, cardiac rhythm abnormalities, and increased arthritis complaints involving multiple joints.

D. Nursing interventions
1. Medication administration
2. Prevention
   a. Avoid high-risk areas such as woody, grassy areas
   b. If walking in such areas, wear long pants, long-sleeved shirt, high socks, and sneakers
   c. Use insect repellents for skin and clothing
   d. After every potential exposure, check carefully for ticks
   e. Remove tick by pulling straight out with tweezers

 **Sample Questions**

25. A mother of an 8-year-old child shows the physician a "funny red circle" on the child's leg and states the child went camping last weekend. The physician draws blood to rule out Lyme disease and prescribes doxycycline for the child. The child's mother asks why an antibiotic is prescribed for a tick bite. The nurse's response is based on which of the following understandings?
   1. Lyme disease weakens the person so they are susceptible to infections.
   2. Lyme disease is caused by a spirochete that is sensitive to doxycycline.
   3. Doxycycline will kill the tick, which may still be in the child.
   4. Antibiotics are given to cure the infection at the site of the tick bite.

26. The mother of a 3-year-old child calls her nurse neighbor in a panic state, saying that the child swallowed most of a bottle of aspirin. The nurse determines that the child is still alert. What instruction should the nurse give to the mother?
    1. Induce vomiting in the child.
    2. Observe the child carefully until the ambulance arrives.
    3. Call the Poison Control Center
    4. Give the child lots of milk to drink.

27. An 8-month-old infant was admitted to the hospital with severe diarrhea and dehydration. Fluid replacement therapy was initiated. Which observation the nurse makes indicates an improvement in the infant's status?
    1. Fontanels are depressed.
    2. Infant has gained 3 oz since yesterday.
    3. Skin remains pulled together after being gently pinched and released.
    4. The infant's hematocrit is greater today than yesterday.

28. A 17-year-old has Down syndrome. He is 57 inches tall and weighs 155 pounds. In planning his care, what is the most important fact for the nurse to consider?
    1. His mental age.
    2. His chronologic age.
    3. His bone age.
    4. Growth chart percentiles.

29. What is the cause of Down syndrome?
    1. An autosomal recessive defect.
    2. An extra chromosome.
    3. A sex-linked defect.
    4. A dominant gene.

30. A 10-day-old baby is admitted with 5% dehydration. The nurse is most likely to note which of the following signs?
    1. Tachycardia.
    2. Bradycardia.
    3. Hypothermia.
    4. Hyperthermia.

31. The nurse is asked why infants are more prone to fluid imbalances than adults. What would be the nurse's best response?
    1. Adults have a greater body surface area.
    2. Adults have a greater metabolic rate.
    3. Infants have functionally immature kidneys.
    4. Infants ingest a lesser amount of fluid per kilogram.

32. A 10-month-old weighs 10 kg and has voided 100 mL in the past 4 hours. The nurse is aware that _____ is normal urine output.
    1. 1–2 mL/kg/hour.
    2. 3–5 mL/kg/hour.
    3. 7–9 mL/kg/hour.
    4. 10 mL/kg/hour.

33. A 3-month-old is NPO for surgery. What would be an appropriate method for the nurse to comfort him?
    1. Administering acetaminophen.
    2. Encouraging parents to leave so the child can rest.
    3. Offering pacifier.
    4. Giving 10 cc Pedialyte.

34. An 11-year-old is admitted for treatment of lead poisoning. The nurse includes which of the following in the plan of care?
    1. Oxygen.
    2. Strict I&O.
    3. Heme-occult stool testing.
    4. Calorie counts.

35. A 2-month-old is admitted with diarrhea. What is the best room assignment for the nurse to make?
    1. Semi-private room with no roommate.
    2. Private room with no bathroom.
    3. Semi-private room with 10-year-old who has acute lymphocytic leukemia.
    4. Open ward.

36. The nurse is discussing safety measures to prevent poisoning with the mother of a 1-year-old. Which statement by the mother demonstrates understanding of safety precautions?
    1. "I have child protection locks on my cabinet under the sink."
    2. "My child is not potty-trained, so the bathroom is safe."
    3. "I keep all poisons and cleaners above the fridge."
    4. "I don't think I have any poisons in my house."

37. The home health nurse observes a new mother providing care for her 1 month old infant. What information would the nurse give the mother to help prevent hepatitis A to herself or the infant?
    1. Avoid sexual relations for 3 months since birthing occurred.
    2. Wear gloves when changing diapers with loose stool.
    3. Clean contaminated household surfaces with a solution of ½ alcohol and ½ water.
    4. Restrict visitors from holding the infant.

38. A 16-year-old admits to her mother that she tried to commit suicide by swallowing a bottle of Tylenol (acetaminophen) 16 hours ago. Her mother brings the girl to the ER. Which is the treatment of choice for this occurrence?
    1. Ipecac syrup.
    2. Activated charcoal.
    3. Mucomyst.
    4. Milk and observation.

39. The nurse would include which of the following nursing diagnoses for a 10-year-old client with stage I Lyme disease?
    1. Decreased cardiac output.
    2. Impaired mobility.
    3. Altered cerebral tissue perfusion.
    4. Alteration in skin integrity.

## Answers and Rationales

25. **2.** Lyme disease is caused by a spirochete that is sensitive to antibiotics.

26. **3.** Because the child is still alert, the mother should call the Poison Control Center for guidance. Transport to the hospital will occur, followed by gastric lavage and activated charcoal.

27. **2.** A weight gain would suggest greater circulating volume. Blood has weight.

28. **1.** Children with Down syndrome have some degree of mental retardation and care must be geared to their mental age.

29. **2.** In Down syndrome there is an extra chromosome on the 21st pair, which is why the disease is also called trisomy 21.

30. **1.** Tachycardia is associated with dehydration.

31. **3.** Infant kidneys are unable to concentrate or dilute urine, to conserve or secrete sodium, or to acidify urine.

32. **1.** Normal urine output is 1–2 mL/kg/hour.

33. **3.** Non-nutritive sucking will help console and pacify him.

34. **2.** CaNaEDTA (treatment for lead poisoning) is nephrotoxic and strict I&O records need to be kept.

35. **2.** A bathroom is irrelevant with an infant in diapers. A private room is necessary.

36. **3.** All cleaners and poisons should be kept in high locked cabinets.

37. **2.** The mode of transmission for hepatitis A is fecal-oral route or poor hygiene. Using gloves will prevent stool on the hands, as the mother also should wash the hands afterwards. Sexual activity is related to hepatitis B, a proper cleaning solution would be with bleach and water and visitors may hold the infant after washing hands to prevent infection to the infant.

38. **3.** Mucomyst is the treatment of choice to bind with acetaminophen and help reduce levels.

39. **4.** Stage I consists of tick bite followed by small erythematous papules that may be described as burning.

# The Neurosensory System

## VARIATIONS FROM THE ADULT

### Brain and Spinal Cord

#### Size and Structure

A. Rapid head growth in early childhood: brain is 25% of adult weight at birth, 75% at 2 years, and 90% at 6 years.

B. Head growth results from development of nerve tracts within the brain and an increase in nerve fibers, not an increase in the number of neurons.

C. Infant's skull is not a rigid structure.
   1. Bones of skull are not fused until 18 months.
   2. Head circumference will increase with increase in intracranial volume in infants.
   3. Sutures may separate if there is significant gradual increase in intracranial volume up to age 12.

**D.** Fontanels ("soft spots"): areas of head not covered by skull
   1. Anterior fontanel
      **a.** Diamond-shaped opening at junction of parietal and frontal bones
      **b.** Closes between 9 and 18 months
   2. Posterior fontanel
      **a.** Triangular-shaped opening at junction of occipital and parietal bones
      **b.** Closes by 2 months
   3. Should feel flat and firm
   4. May be sunken with severe dehydration
   5. Will bulge with increased intracranial pressure (ICP)

## Function

**A.** Cortical functions (e.g., fine motor coordination) are incompletely developed at birth.
**B.** The autonomic nervous system (ANS) is intact but immature.
   1. Infant has limited ability to control body temperature
   2. Infant's heart rate very sensitive to parasympathetic stimulation
**C.** Infant's behavior primarily reflexive
   1. Neurologic exam consists of evaluating reflexes
   2. Babinski's reflex normal in infant; disappears after child begins to walk
**D.** Peripheral neurons not myelinated at birth
   1. Myelination occurs in later infancy
   2. Motor skill development depends on myelinization
**E.** Infant usually demonstrates a dominance of flexor muscles; extremities will be flexed even when infant is sleeping
**F.** Small tremors are normal findings during first few months of life: not considered seizure activity if occurring in response to environmental stimuli, if they are not accompanied by abnormal eye movements, and if movements cease with passive flexion

## Eye and Vision

**A.** Vision changes as the eye and eye muscles undergo physiologic change.
**B.** Visual function becomes more organized.
   1. Binocular vision developed by 4 months
   2. Maturation of eye muscles by 1 year
      **a.** Nystagmus common in infant
      **b.** Strabismus (eyes out of alignment when fixating on an object): due to imbalance in extraocular muscles, common up to 6 months, abnormal after 6 months
   3. Visual acuity changes
      **a.** 16 weeks: 20/50 to 20/100
      **b.** 1 year: 20/50+
      **c.** 2 years: 20/40

**d.** 3 years: 20/30
**e.** 4 years: nearly 20/20

## Ear and Hearing

**A.** Hearing is fully developed at birth.
**B.** Abnormal physical structure of ears may indicate genetic problems (low-set ears often associated with renal problems or mental retardation).

# ASSESSMENT

## History

**A.** Most important part of neurologic evaluation
**B.** Family history: seizure disorders, degenerative neurologic diseases, mental retardation, sensory defects
**C.** History of pregnancy: maternal illness, placental dysfunction, fetal movements, nuchal cord, intrapartal fetal distress, prematurity, meconium staining, Apgar scores
**D.** Child's health history: delayed motor or speech development, hypotonia, seizures, childhood illnesses
**E.** Parental concerns: development, vision, hearing

## Physical Examination

**A.** Inspect size and shape of head: note fontanels in infants, chart head circumference on growth chart.
**B.** Observe posture and activity: note flexed posture versus hypotonia or opisthotonos, symmetry of movement of extremities, excessive tremors or twitching, abnormal eye movements, ineffective suck or swallow, high-pitched cry.
**C.** Observe respiratory pattern: note apnea, ataxic breathing, asymmetric or paradoxic chest movement.
**D.** Determine developmental level with Denver II.
**E.** Vision tests
   1. Binocularity
      **a.** Corneal light reflex test: performed by shining a light at the bridge of the nose as the child looks straight ahead; light reflex should fall at the same point in both pupils; deviation indicates strabismus
      **b.** Cover/uncover test: Ask child to fix on an object. Cover one eye, assess uncovered eye movement. Uncover eye, assess that eye for movement. Repeat by covering the other eye. Normal response—no movement of either eye in response to cover/uncover maneuver.
   2. Visual acuity
      **a.** Snellen E chart or Blackbird cards for preschoolers
      **b.** Snellen alphabet chart for older children
   3. Peripheral vision
   4. Color vision

F. Auditory tests
1. Audiometry: perception of sound
2. Tympanometry: conduction of sound in middle ear
3. Crib-o-gram: neonatal motor response to sound
4. Conduction tests
5. Newborn hearing screening: auditory evoked response

## Laboratory/Diagnostic Tests

A. Same neurologic tests that are used in adults are used in children.
B. Child should be carefully prepared and informed of what to expect during the test.
C. Sedation may be necessary for tests requiring child to be immobile for extended period.
D. Positioning and immobilization is crucial to the success of lumbar puncture.

# ANALYSIS

Nursing diagnoses for the child with a disorder of the nervous system may include:
A. Impaired physical mobility
B. Disturbed thought process
C. Disturbed sensory perceptions
D. Deficient knowledge
E. Pain
F. Compromised or disabled family coping
G. Risk for injury
H. Impaired verbal communication
I. Risk for impaired skin integrity

# PLANNING AND IMPLEMENTATION

## Goals

A. Child will be protected from injury.
B. Child will be free from signs and symptoms of increased intracranial pressure.
C. Normal respiratory function will be maintained.
D. Optimum developmental level will be achieved.
E. Family will be able to care for child at home.

## Interventions

### Care of the Child with Increased Intracranial Pressure

A. General information
1. Intracranial volume and pressure can increase as a result of:
   a. Increased brain volume (cerebral edema, tumor)
   b. Increased cerebral blood volume (hematoma or hemorrhage)
   c. Increased cerebrospinal fluid (CSF) volume (hydrocephalus)
2. Herniation of brain tissue: most serious complication of increased ICP; may result in life-threatening deterioration of vital functions
B. Medical management
1. Directed toward reducing intracranial volume and controlling underlying disorder
2. Drug therapy
   a. Osmotic diuretics (mannitol, glycerol) to reduce acute brain edema; for short-term use only
   b. Corticosteroids (dexamethasone) to reduce brain swelling
      1) May be used for longer periods than osmotic diuretics
      2) Antacids may be given concomitantly to prevent gastric irritation
3. Fluid restriction, hyperventilation, temperature regulation may all be used to control increased ICP
4. Surgery: if increased ICP caused by obstruction to CSF, shunt procedures may be performed
C. Assessment findings
1. Infants
   a. Lethargy, poor feeding, anorexia, vomiting, or irritability
   b. High-pitched cry
   c. Tense, bulging fontanel; increased head circumference; separation of cranial sutures
2. Children
   a. Anorexia, nausea, vomiting, irritability, or lethargy
   b. Headache, blurred vision, papilledema
   c. Separation of cranial sutures
3. Late signs
   a. Altered level of consciousness
   b. Pupil dilation and sluggish response to light
   c. Tachycardia then bradycardia
   d. Altered respiratory rate then apnea
   e. Elevation in BP, increased pulse pressure
   f. Unstable temperature
D. Nursing interventions
1. Administer medications as ordered.
   a. With osmotic diuretics, monitor fluid and electrolyte balance carefully.
   b. With corticosteroids, monitor for signs of gastric bleeding.
2. Monitor hydration status carefully.
   a. Administer IV fluids as ordered, assess carefully for fluid overload.
   b. Assess for fluid and electrolyte imbalances.
   c. Monitor for hypovolemic shock if on strict fluid restriction.
3. Assist with hyperventilation if ordered; monitor arterial blood gases (ABGs)

4. Assist with reduction of body temperature as needed.
   a. Administer antipyretics as ordered.
   b. Use sponge baths, hypothermia pads as necessary.
5. Monitor LOC and behavioral/mental changes carefully.
6. Elevate head of bed 30–45° unless contraindicated (e.g., possible spinal injury); keep neck in neutral alignment and avoid flexion.
7. Arrange nursing care activities to minimize stimulation and keep environment as quiet as possible.
8. Prepare for shunt surgery if needed.

# EVALUATION

A. Head growth progresses normally, fontanels are flat, and seizure activity is controlled.
B. Child maintains an appropriate activity level.
C. Child is placed in an appropriate special program or school, if needed.
D. Parents demonstrate ability to perform treatments and administer appropriate medications.

# DISORDERS OF THE NERVOUS SYSTEM

## Disorders of the Brain and Spinal Cord

### Hydrocephalus

A. General information
   1. Increased amount of CSF within the ventricles of the brain
   2. May be caused by obstruction of CSF flow or by overproduction or inadequate reabsorption of CSF
   3. May result from congenital malformation or be secondary to injury, infection, or tumor
   4. Classification
      a. Noncommunicating: flow of CSF from ventricles to subarachnoid space is obstructed.
      b. Communicating: flow is not obstructed, but CSF is inadequately reabsorbed in subarachnoid space, or excess CSF is produced.
B. Assessment findings: depend on age at onset, amount of CSF in brain
   1. Infant to 2 years: enlarging head size; bulging, nonpulsating fontanels; downward rotation of eyes; separation of cranial sutures; poor feeding, vomiting, lethargy, irritability; high-pitched cry and abnormal muscle tone

2. Older children: changes in head size less common; signs of increased ICP (vomiting, ataxia, headache) common; alteration in consciousness and papilledema late signs
3. Diagnostic tests
   a. Serial transilluminations detect increases in light areas
   b. CT scan shows dilated ventricles as well as presence of mass; with dye injection shows course of CSF flow
C. Nursing interventions: provide care for the child with increased ICP and for the child undergoing shunt procedures.

### Shunts

A. General information (See Figure 5–2)
   1. Insertion of a flexible tube into the lateral ventricle of the brain
   2. Catheter is then threaded under the skin and the distal end positioned in the peritoneum (most common type) or the right atrium; a subcutaneous pump may be attached to ensure patency
   3. Shunt drains excess CSF from the lateral ventricles of the brain in communicating or noncommunicating hydrocephalus; fluid is

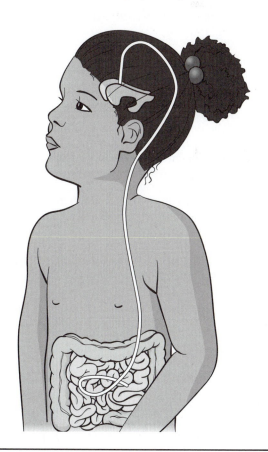

**Figure 5-2** Ventriculoperitoneal shunt

then absorbed by the peritoneum or enters the general circulation via the right atrium

B. Nursing interventions
   1. Provide routine pre-op care with special attention to monitoring neurologic status.
   2. Provide post-op care.
      a. Maintain patency of the shunt.
         1) Position child off the operative site.
         2) Pump the shunt as ordered.
         3) Observe for signs of infection of the incision.
         4) Observe for signs of increased ICP.
         5) Position the child with head slightly elevated or as ordered.
   3. Instruct parents regarding:
      a. Wound care, positioning of infant, and how to pump the shunt
      b. Signs of infection
      c. Signs of increased ICP
      d. Need for repeated shunt revisions as child grows or if shunt becomes blocked or infected
      e. Expected level of developmental functioning
      f. Availability of support groups and community agencies

## Spina Bifida (Myelodysplasia)

A. General information
   1. Failure of posterior vertebral arches to fuse during embryologic development
   2. Incidence: 2 in 1,000 infants in the United States
   3. Although actual cause is unknown, frequency of the defect is increased if a sibling has had a neural tube defect; radiation, viral, and environmental factors; and maternal folic acid deficiency have been suggested as causative.
   4. Site of the defect varies
      a. Approximately 85% of the defects in the spine involve the lower thoracic lumbar or sacral area.
      b. Defects in the upper thoracic and cervical regions make up the remaining 15%.
   5. Folic acid supplementation can decrease risk.

B. Types
   1. Spina bifida occulta
      a. Spinal cord and meninges remain in the normal anatomic position.
      b. Defect may not be visible, or may be identified by a dimple or a tuft of hair on the spine.
      c. Child is asymptomatic or may have slight neuromuscular deficit.
      d. No treatment needed if asymptomatic; otherwise treatment aimed at specific symptoms.
   2. Spina bifida cystica
      a. *Meningocele* (see Figure 5-3)

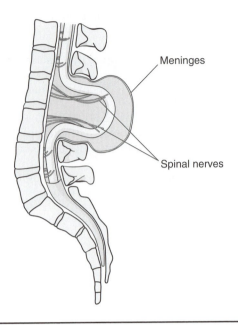

**Figure 5-3** Illustration of meningomyelocele

         1) Sac (meninges) filled with spinal fluid protrudes through opening in spinal canal; sac is covered with thin skin
         2) No nerves in sac
         3) No motor or sensory loss
         4) Good prognosis after surgery
      b. Myelomeningocele/meningomyelocele
         1) Same as meningocele except there are spinal nerves in the sac (herniation of dura and meninges).
         2) Child will have sensory/motor deficit below site of the lesion.
         3) 80% of these children have multiple handicaps.

C. Medical management
   1. Surgery
      a. Closure of the sac within 48 hours of birth to prevent infection and preserve neural tissue
      b. Shunt procedure if accompanying hydrocephalus
      c. Orthopedic procedures to correct defects of hips, knees, or feet
   2. Drug therapy
      a. Antibiotics for prevention of infections.
      b. Anticholinergic drugs to increase bladder capacity and lower intravesicular pressure.
   3. Immobilization (casts, braces, traction) for defects of the hips, knees, or feet.

D. Assessment findings
   1. Examine the defect for size, level, tissue covering, and CSF leakage.
   2. Motor/sensory involvement may include:
      a. Voluntary movement of lower extremities
      b. Withdrawal of lower extremities or crying after pinprick

    **c.** Paralysis of lower extremities

    **d.** Joint deformities

    **e.** Hydrocephalus

    **f.** Evaluate bowel and bladder function. Neurogenic bowel and bladder occur in up to 90% of the children.

  **3.** Diagnostic tests

    **a.** Prenatal

      **1)** Ultrasound image of the pregnant uterus shows fetal spinal defect and sac

      **2)** Amniocentesis: increased alphafetoprotein (AFP) level prior to 18th week of gestation

    **b.** Postbirth

      **1)** X-ray of spine shows vertebral defect; CT scan of skull may show hydrocephalus

      **2)** Myelogram shows extent of neural defect

      **3)** Encephalogram may show hydrocephalus

      **4)** Urinalysis, culture and sensitivity (C&S) may identify organism and indicate appropriate antibacterial therapy

      **5)** BUN may be increased

      **6)** Creatinine clearance rate may be decreased

**E.** Nursing interventions

  **1.** Prevent trauma to the sac.

    **a.** Cover with sterile dressing soaked with normal saline.

    **b.** Position infant prone or side-lying.

    **c.** Keep the area free from contamination by urine or feces. A protective barrier drape may be necessary.

    **d.** Inspect the sac for intactness or signs of infection.

    **e.** Administer antibiotics as ordered.

  **2.** Prevent complications.

    **a.** Observe for signs of hydrocephalus, meningitis, joint deformities.

    **b.** Clean intermittent urinary catheterization to manage neurogenic bladder.

    **c.** Administer medications to prevent urinary complications as ordered.

    **d.** Perform passive ROM exercises to lower extremities.

  **3.** Provide adequate nutrition: adapt diet and feeding techniques according to the child's position.

  **4.** Provide sensory stimulation.

    **a.** Adjust objects for visual stimulation according to child's position.

    **b.** Provide stimulation for other senses.

  **5.** Provide emotional support to parents/family.

  **6.** Provide client teaching and discharge planning to parents concerning

    **a.** Wound care

    **b.** Physical therapy, range of motion exercises

    **c.** Signs of complications

    **d.** Medication regimen: schedule, dosage, effects, and side effects

    **e.** Feeding, diapering, positioning

    **f.** Availability of appropriate support groups/community agencies/genetic counseling

## Meningitis

See Unit 4.

## Encephalitis

See Unit 4.

## Reye's Syndrome

**A.** General information

  **1.** An acute encephalopathy with fatty degeneration of the liver

  **2.** Reye's syndrome is a true pediatric emergency: cerebral complication may reach an irreversible state

  **3.** Increased ICP secondary to cerebral edema is major factor contributing to morbidity and mortality

  **4.** Early recognition and prompt management reducing mortality

  **5.** Etiology unknown; links with aspirin have been suspected but not proven

**B.** Medical management

  **1.** Proper initial staging essential.

  **2.** Treatment is supportive, based on stage of coma and level of blood ammonia.

  **3.** Treatment should take place in a pediatric intensive care unit.

**C.** Assessment findings

  **1.** Child appears to be recovering from a viral illness, such as influenza or chickenpox, during which salicylates have been administered; symptoms then appear that follow a definite pattern, which has led to clinical staging.

    **a.** Stage I: sudden onset of persistent vomiting, fatigue, listlessness

    **b.** Stage II: personality and behavior changes, disorientation, confusion, hyperreflexia

    **c.** Stage III: coma, decorticate posturing

    **d.** Stage IV: deeper coma, decerebrate rigidity

    **e.** Stage V: seizures, absent deep tendon reflexes, respiratory reflexes, flaccid paralysis

  **2.** Pathophysiologic changes include

    **a.** Increased free fatty acid level

    **b.** Hyperammonemia due to reduction of enzyme that converts ammonia to urea

    **c.** Impaired liver function

    **d.** Structural changes of mitochondria in muscle and brain tissue

    **e.** Significant swelling of the brain

**D.** Nursing interventions (depend on stage)
1. Stage I: assess hydration status: monitor skin turgor, mucous membranes, I&O, urine specific gravity; maintain IV therapy.
2. Stages I-V: assess neurologic status: monitor LOC, pupils, motor coordination, extremity movement, orientation, posturing, seizure activity.
3. Stages II-V
   **a.** Assess respiratory status: note changing rate and pattern, presence of circumoral cyanosis, restlessness, agitation.
   **b.** Assess circulatory status: frequent vital signs, note neck vein distension, skin color and temperature, abnormal heart sounds.
   **c.** Support child/family.
   1) Explain all treatments and procedures.
   2) Incorporate family members in treatment as applicable.
   3) Organize regular family and client-care conferences.
   4) Use support services as needed.
   5) Educate family on over-the-counter medications containing aspirin (i.e., Alka-Seltzer, Bufferin, Pepto-Bismol).
   **d.** Provide additional parental and community education to ensure early recognition and treatment.

## Seizure Disorders

**A.** General information
1. Seizures: recurrent sudden changes in consciousness, behavior, sensations, and/or muscular activities beyond voluntary control that are produced by excess neuronal discharge
2. Epilepsy: chronic recurrent seizures
3. Incidence higher in those with family history of idiopathic seizures
4. Cause unknown in 75% of epilepsy cases
5. Seizures may be symptomatic or acquired, caused by:
   **a.** Structural or space-occupying lesion (tumors, subdural hematomas)
   **b.** Metabolic abnormalities (hypoglycemia, hypocalcemia, hyponatremia)
   **c.** Infection (meningitis, encephalitis)
   **d.** Encephalopathy (lead poisoning, pertussis, Reye's syndrome)
   **e.** Degenerative diseases (Tay-Sachs)
   **f.** Congenital CNS defects (hydrocephalus)
   **g.** Vascular problems (intracranial hemorrhage)
6. Pathophysiology
   **a.** Normally neurons send out messages in electrical impulses periodically, and the firing of individual neurons is regulated by an inhibitory feedback loop mechanism
   **b.** With seizures, many more neurons than normal fire in a synchronous fashion in a particular area of the brain; the energy generated overcomes the inhibitory feedback mechanism
7. Classification (Table 5-6)
   **a.** Generalized: initial onset in both hemispheres, usually involves loss of consciousness and bilateral motor activity
   **b.** Partial: begins in focal area of brain and symptoms are related to a dysfunction of that area; may progress into a generalized seizure, further subdivided into simple partial or complex partial

**B.** Medical management
1. Drug therapy (refer to Anticonvulsants)
   **a.** Phenytoin (Dilantin)
   1) Often used with phenobarbital for its potentiating effect
   2) Inhibits spread of electrical discharge
   3) Side effects include gum hyperplasia, hirsutism, ataxia, gastric distress, nystagmus, anemia, sedation
   **b.** Phenobarbital: elevates the seizure threshold and inhibits the spread of electrical discharge
2. Surgery: to remove the tumor, hematoma, or epileptic focus

**C.** Assessment findings
1. Clinical picture varies with type of seizure (see Table 5-6)
2. Diagnostic tests
   **a.** Blood studies to rule out lead poisoning, hypoglycemia, infection, or electrolyte imbalances
   **b.** Lumbar puncture to rule out infection or trauma
   **c.** Skull X-rays, CT scan, or ultrasound of the head, brain scan, arteriogram, or pneumoencephalogram to detect any pathologic defects
   **d.** EEG may detect abnormal wave patterns characteristic of different types of seizures
   1) Child may be awake or asleep; sedation is ordered and child may be sleep deprived the night before the test
   2) Evocative stimulation: flashing strobe light, clicking sounds, hyperventilation

**D.** Nursing interventions
1. During seizure activity
   **a.** Protect from injury.
   1) Prevent falling, gently support head.
   2) Decrease external stimuli; do not restrain.
   3) Do not use tongue blades (they add additional stimuli).
   4) Loosen tight clothing.
   **b.** Keep airway open.
   1) Place in side-lying position.
   2) Suction excess mucus.

**Table 5-6** Types of Seizures

| Type of Seizure | Clinical Findings |
|---|---|
| *Generalized seizures* | |
| Major motor seizure (grand mal) | May be preceded by aura; tonic and clonic phases. *Tonic phase:* limbs contract or stiffen; pupils dilate and eyes roll up and to one side; glottis closes, causing noise on exhalation; may be incontinent; occurs at same time as loss of consciousness; lasts 20–40 seconds. *Clonic phase:* repetitive movements, increased mucus production; slowly tapers. Seizure ends with postictal period of confusion, drowsiness. |
| Absence seizure (petit mal) | Usually nonorganic brain damage (petit mal) present; must be differentiated from daydreaming. Sudden onset, with twitching or rolling of eyes; lasts a few seconds. |
| Myoclonic seizure | Associated with brain damage, may be precipitated by tactile or visual sensations. May be generalized or local. Brief flexor muscle spasm; may have arm extension, trunk flexion. Single group of muscles affected; involuntary muscle contractions; myoclonic jerks. |
| Akinetic seizure (tonic) | Related to organic brain damage. Sudden brief loss of postural tone, and temporary loss of consciousness. |
| Febrile seizure | Common in 5% of population under 5, familial, nonprogressive; does not generally result in brain damage. Seizure occurs only when fever is rising. EEG is normal 2 weeks after seizure. |
| *Partial seizure* | |
| Psychomotor seizure | May follow trauma, hypoxia, drug use. Purposeful but inappropriate, repetitive motor acts. Aura present; dreamlike state. |
| Simple partial seizure | Seizure confined to one hemisphere of brain. No loss of consciousness. May be motor, sensory, or autonomic symptoms. |
| Complex partial seizure | Begins in focal area but spreads to both hemispheres. Impairs consciousness. May be preceded by an aura. |
| Status epilepticus | Usually refers to generalized grand mal seizures. Seizure is prolonged (or there are repeated seizures without regaining consciousness) and unresponsive to treatment. Can result in decreased oxygen supply and possible cardiac arrest. |

c. Observe and record seizure.
  1) Note any preictal aura.
    a) Affective signs: fear, anxiety
    b) Psychosensory signs: hallucinations
    c) Cognitive signs: "déjà-vu" symptoms
  2) Note nature of the ictal phase.
    a) Symmetry of movement
    b) Response to stimuli; LOC
    c) Respiratory pattern
  3) Note postictal response: amount of time it takes child to orient to time and place; sleepiness.
2. Provide client teaching and discharge planning concerning:
  a. Care during a seizure
  b. Need to continue drug therapy
  c. Safety precautions/activity limitations
  d. Need to wear Medic-Alert identification bracelet or carry identification card
  e. Potential behavioral changes and school problems
  f. Availability of support groups/community agencies
  g. How to assist the child in explaining disorder to peers
  h. Inform parents that Ketogenic diet has had success (diet limits intake of proteins and carbohydrates)

## Cerebral Palsy (CP)

A. General information
  1. Neuromuscular disorder resulting from damage to or altered structure of the part of the brain responsible for controlling motor function
  2. Incidence: 1.5–5 in 1,000 live births
  3. May be caused by a variety of factors resulting in damage to the CNS; possible causes include:
    a. Prenatally: genetic, altered neurologic development, or infection, trauma, or anoxia to mother (toxemia, rubella, accidents, chorioamnionitis)

b. Perinatally: during the birth process (drugs at delivery, precipitate delivery, fetal distress, breech deliveries with delay)
   c. Postnatally: kernicterus or head trauma (child falls out of crib or is hit by a car)
B. Medical management
   1. Drug therapy
      a. Antianxiety agents
      b. Skeletal muscle relaxants
      c. Local nerve blocks
   2. Physical/occupational therapy
   3. Speech/audiology therapy
   4. Surgery: muscle- and tendon-releasing procedures
C. Assessment findings: disease itself does not progress once established; progressive complications, however, cause changes in signs and symptoms
   1. Spasticity: exaggerated hyperactive reflexes (increased muscle tone, increase in stretch reflex, scissoring of legs, poorly coordinated body movements for voluntary activities)
      a. Occurs with pyramidal tract lesion
      b. Found in 40% of all CP
      c. Results in contractures
      d. Also affects ability to speak: altered quality and articulation
      e. Loud noise or sudden movement causes reaction with increased spasm
      f. No parachute reflex to protect self when falling
   2. Athetosis: constant involuntary, purposeless, slow, writhing motions
      a. Occurs with extrapyramidal tract (basal ganglia) lesion
      b. Found in 40% of all CP
      c. Athetosis disappears during sleep; therefore, contractures do not develop
      d. Movements increase with increase in physical or emotional stress
      e. Also affects facial muscles
   3. Ataxia: disturbance in equilibrium; diminished righting reflex (lack of balance, poor coordination, dizziness, hypotonia)
      a. Occurs with extrapyramidal tract (cerebellar) lesion
      b. Found in 10% of all CP
      c. Muscles and reflexes are normal
   4. Tremor: repetitive rhythmic involuntary contractions of flexor and extensor muscles
      a. Occurs with extrapyramidal tract (basal ganglia) lesion
      b. Found in 5% of all CP
      c. Interferes with performance of precise movements
      d. Often a mild disability
   5. Rigidity: resistance to flexion and extension resulting from simultaneous contraction of both agonist and antagonist muscle groups

   a. Occurs with extrapyramidal tract (basal ganglia) lesion
   b. Found in 5% of all CP
   c. Diminished or absent reflexes
   d. Potential for severe contractures
6. Associated problems
   a. Mental retardation: the majority of CP clients are of normal or higher than average intelligence, but are unable to demonstrate it on standardized tests; 18–50% have some form of mental retardation
   b. Hearing loss in 13% of CP clients
   c. Defective speech in 75% of CP clients
   d. Dental anomalies (from muscle contractures)
   e. Orthopedic problems from contractures or inability to mobilize
   f. Visual disabilities in 28% due to poor muscle control
   g. Seizures
   h. Disturbances of body image, touch, perception
   i. Feelings of worthlessness
D. Nursing interventions
   1. Obtain a careful pregnancy, birth, and childhood history.
   2. Observe the child's behavior in various situations.
   3. Assist with activities of daily living (ADL), help child to learn as many self-care activities as possible; CP clients cannot do any task unless they are consciously aware of each step in the task; careful teaching and demonstration is essential.
   4. Provide a safe environment (safety helmet, padded crib).
   5. Provide physical therapy to prevent contractures and assist in mobility (braces if necessary).
   6. Provide client teaching and discharge planning concerning:
      a. Nature of disease: CP is a nonfatal, noncurable disorder
      b. Need for continued physical, occupational, and speech therapy
      c. Care of orthopedic devices
      d. Provision for child's enrollment or return to school
      e. Availability of support groups/community agencies

## Tay-Sachs Disease

A. General information
   1. Degenerative brain disease, caused by absence of hexosaminidase A from all body tissues
   2. Autosomal recessive inheritance
   3. Occurs predominantly in children of Eastern European Jewish ancestry
   4. A fatal disease; death usually occurs before age 4

**B.** Assessment findings
1. Progressive lethargy in a previously healthy 2- to 6-month-old infant
2. Loss of developmental accomplishments
3. Loss of visual acuity
4. Hyperreflexia, decerebrate posturing, dysphagia, malnutrition, seizures
5. Diagnosis confirmed by classic cherry-red spot on the macula and by enzyme measurements in serum, amniotic fluid, or white cells

**C.** Nursing interventions
1. Support parents at time of diagnosis; help them cope with feelings of anger and guilt.
2. Assist parents in planning long-term care for the child.
3. Provide genetic counseling and psychologic follow-up as needed.

# Disorders of the Eye

## Blindness

**A.** Causes
1. Genetic disorders: Tay-Sach's disease, inborn errors of metabolism
2. Maternal infections during pregnancy: TORCH syndrome
3. Perinatal: prematurity, retrolental fibroplasia
4. Postnatal: trauma, childhood infections

**B.** Medical management: treatment of causative disorders

**C.** Assessment findings
1. Vacant stare; obvious failure to look at objects
2. Rubbing eyes, tilting head, examining objects very close to the eyes
3. Does not reach for objects (over 4 months)
4. Does not smile when mother smiles (over 3 months) but does smile in response to mother's voice
5. Crawls or walks into furniture (over 12 months)
6. Does not respond to the motions of others
7. No concept of the look of an object, no concept of color or reflection of self
8. Other senses become more keenly developed to compensate
9. Unable to copy the actions of others; delayed motor milestones in accomplishing tasks but are not mentally handicapped
10. Various degrees (20/200 O.U. and worse)

**D.** Nursing interventions
1. For hospitalized child, find out parents' usual method of care.
2. Encourage infant to be active; use multisensory stimulation (rocking, water play, musical toys, touch).
3. From ages 2–5 arrange environment for maximum autonomy and safety (e.g., avoid foods with seeds and bones).
4. Speak before you touch the child, announce what you plan to do.

5. Do not rearrange furniture without first telling child.
6. For a partially sighted child
   a. Encourage child to sit in front of classroom.
   b. Speak directly to child's face; do not look down or turn back.
   c. Use large print and provide adequate nonglare lighting.
   d. Use contrasting colors to help locate areas.
7. Provide client teaching and discharge planning concerning:
   a. General child care, with adaptations for safety and developmental/functional level
   b. Availability of support groups/community agencies
   c. Special education programs
   d. Interaction with peers: assist child as necessary

## Conjunctivitis

**A.** General information: infection of membrane covering anterior surface of eye globe and inner surface of eyelid due to multiple causes (bacterial, viral, allergic)

**B.** Medical management: ophthalmic antibiotics, steroids, anesthetics

**C.** Assessment findings: weeping eye, reddened conjunctiva, sensitivity to light, eyelid stuck shut with exudate

**D.** Nursing interventions
1. Administer medications as ordered: apply ophthalmic antibiotic ointments from inner to outer canthus (do not let container touch eye).
2. Provide client teaching and discharge planning concerning measures to prevent spread of infection
   a. Very contagious if bacterial or viral; no school until antibiotics have been taken for 24–48 hours
   b. Should not share pillows, tissues, toys
   c. Good hand-washing technique
   d. Medication regimen: schedule, dosage, desired and side effects

# Disorders of the Ear

## Deafness

**A.** Causes
1. Conductive: interference in transmission from outer to middle ear from chronic otitis media, foreign bodies
2. Sensorineural: dysfunction of the inner ear; damage to cranial nerve VIII (from rubella, meningitis, drugs)

**B.** Medical management
1. Treatment of causative disorders
2. Speech/auditory therapy

**3.** Hearing aids

**4.** Surgery, depending on the cause

    **a.** Cochlear implant for neural deafness

**C.** Assessment findings

    **1.** Infant

        **a.** Fails to react to loud noises (does have a Moro reflex, but not to noise)

        **b.** Makes no attempt to locate sound

        **c.** Remains in babbling stage or ceases to babble

        **d.** Fails to develop speech

        **e.** Startled by sudden appearances

    **2.** All children

        **a.** Respond only when speaker's lips are visible

        **b.** Cannot concentrate for long on visual images; constantly scan the surroundings for change

        **c.** May have slow motor development

        **d.** Appear puzzled or withdrawn, or strain to hear

        **e.** Use high volume on TV/radio

    **3.** Audiologic testing

        **a.** Slight hearing deficit: difficulty hearing faint sounds, very little interference in school, no speech defect, benefits from favorable seating

        **b.** Mild hearing deficit: can understand conversational speech at 3–5 feet when facing the other person, decreased vocabulary, may miss half of class discussions

        **c.** Marked hearing deficit: misses most of conversation, hears loud noises, needs special education for language skills

**D.** Nursing interventions

    **1.** Speak slowly, not more loudly.

    **2.** Face child.

    **3.** Get child's attention before talking; let child see you before performing any care.

    **4.** Get feedback from child to make sure child has understood.

    **5.** Decrease outside noises that could interfere with child's ability to discern what you are saying.

    **6.** Be careful not to cover your mouth with hands.

    **7.** Teach language through visual cues, touch, and kinesthetics.

    **8.** Use body demonstrations or use doll play.

    **9.** Provide appropriate stimulation (puppets and musical toys are inappropriate).

    **10.** Provide client teaching and discharge planning concerning:

        **a.** General child care, with adaptation for safety and developmental/functional levels

        **b.** Availability of support groups/community agencies

        **c.** Special education programs

        **d.** Care and use of hearing aids, cochlear implant equipment

        **e.** Interaction with peers: assist child as needed

## *Otitis Media*

**A.** General information

    **1.** Bacterial or viral infection of the middle ear

    **2.** More common in infants and preschoolers as the ear canal is shorter and more horizontal than in older children; also found in children with cleft lip/palate

    **3.** Blockage of eustachian tube causes lymphedema and accumulation of fluid in the middle ear

**B.** Medical management

    **1.** Drug therapy

        **a.** Systemic and otic antibiotics

        **b.** Analgesics/antipyretics

    **2.** Surgery: myringotomy, with or without insertion of tubes (incision into the tympanic membrane to relieve the pressure and drain the fluid)

**C.** Assessment findings

    **1.** Dysfunction of eustachian tube

    **2.** Ear infection usually related to respiratory infection

    **3.** Increased middle ear pressure; bulging tympanic membrane

    **4.** Pain; infant pulls or touches ear frequently

    **5.** Irritability; cough; nasal congestion

    **6.** Diagnostic tests: C&S of fluid reveals causative organism

**D.** Nursing interventions

    **1.** Administer antibiotics as ordered, for a full 10-day course. When administering ear drops pull earlobe up and back for children older than 3 years and down and back if younger.

    **2.** Administer acetaminophen for fever and discomfort.

    **3.** Administer decongestants to relieve eustachian tube obstruction as ordered.

    **4.** Provide care for child with a myringotomy tube insertion (day surgery)

        **a.** Child should wear earplugs when swimming, showering, or having hair washed; do not permit diving.

        **b.** Be aware that tubes may fall out for no reason.

    **5.** Provide client teaching and discharge planning concerning:

        **a.** Medication administration

        **b.** Post-op care, depending on the type of surgery

 **Sample Questions**

**40.** An infant who was born with a myelomeningocele with accompanying hydrocephalus has had a shunt procedure to alleviate the hydrocephalus. The baby should be placed in which of the following positions?

1. Trendelenburg.
2. Supine.
3. Lithotomy.
4. Prone.

41. The nurse is caring for an infant who is born with hydrocephalus and has a shunt inserted. Which of the following signs indicates that the shunt is functioning properly?
   1. The sunset sign.
   2. A bulging anterior fontanel.
   3. Decreasing daily head circumference.
   4. Widened suture lines.

42. A 13-year-old has been diagnosed as having epilepsy. What would be a positive sign that the child is taking his Dilantin properly?
   1. Hair growth on his upper lip.
   2. Absence of seizures.
   3. Lowered hemoglobin and hematocrit.
   4. Drowsiness.

43. A 3-year-old is admitted with a diagnosis of viral meningitis. During an initial assessment, what would the nurse expect to find?
   1. Headache, fever, and petechiae.
   2. Seizures, lethargy, and hypothermia.
   3. Pallor, anorexia, and bulging fontanels.
   4. Fever, irritability, and nuchal rigidity.

44. To meet the sensory need of a child with viral meningitis, what should be included in the nursing strategies?
   1. Minimizing bright lights and noise.
   2. Promoting active range of motion.
   3. Increasing environmental stimuli.
   4. Avoiding physical contact with family members.

45. When addressing the emotional needs of the parents of a young child with meningitis, what should be the primary focus?
   1. Assuming all responsibility for physical care of the child.
   2. Providing reassurance that the symptoms will resolve within the week.
   3. Reinforcing information about the child's condition and plan of treatment.
   4. Explaining the importance of an optimistic outlook when interacting with their child.

46. A child who had meningitis is being discharged. What should be included in the discharge teaching?

1. Engaging a tutor to assist with learning problems.
2. Administering the prescribed antibiotic.
3. Notifying the physician if the child's fever or headache persists more than a few days after discharge.
4. Encouraging the child to resume normal activities immediately.

47. A 6-year-old is brought to the emergency department unconscious after being hit by a car. What information will be most helpful for the nurse performing the neurological examination of the child?
   1. Normal growth and development.
   2. The child's usual behavior and status.
   3. The child's past medical history.
   4. The child's growth and developmental progress during infancy.

48. The nurse is assessing a child who has a head injury for the occulocephalic reflex (doll's eyes). What will the nurse observe about the child's eyes if this condition is present?
   1. Move in the same direction in which his head is turned.
   2. Move in the direction opposite to which his head is turned.
   3. Remain midline when his head is turned.
   4. Move to the medial aspect of the orbit when his head is turned.

49. The pupils of a child with a head injury are dilated and react sluggishly. What occurrence is this indicative of?
   1. Barbiturate overdosage.
   2. Damage to the diencephalon.
   3. Damage to the sympathetic system.
   4. Damage to the parasympathetic system.

50. A 4-year-old female is admitted to the pediatric intensive care unit (PICU) after suffering a severe closed head injury following a car accident. An intracranial pressure (ICP) monitor is in place and reveals an ICP of 40 mm Hg. In an effort to lower the ICP, what position will the nurse know is the *best* position for the client?
   1. Supine with the head turned to the right.
   2. Supine with the head turned to the left.
   3. Supine with the head midline.
   4. Side-lying on the right with the head turned to the left.

51. A 5-year-old female is admitted to the PICU after being hit by a car while riding her bike. She

sustained a severe closed head injury and has an ICP monitor in place. Her ICP is 40 mm Hg and mannitol is ordered. What is the rationale for administering mannitol for a child with an increased ICP?

1. It will produce a rise in the intravascular osmolality, resulting in a shift of free water from the interstitial and cellular spaces to the intravascular space, thus decreasing the ICP.

2. It will produce a decrease in the intravascular osmolality, resulting in a shift of free water from the interstitial and cellular spaces to the intravascular space, thus decreasing the ICP.

3. It will produce a rise in the intravascular osmolality, resulting in a shift of free water from the intravascular space to the cellular space, thus decreasing the ICP.

4. It will produce a decrease in the intravascular osmolality, resulting in a shift of free water from the interstitial space to the cellular space, thus decreasing the ICP.

52. An infant who has a ventriculoperitoneal (VP) shunt in place for treatment of hydrocephalus is hospitalized for potential shunt malfunction. When developing the plan of care, which of the following assessment findings would the nurse list as a *positive* sign of shunt malfunction?

1. Overriding sutures.
2. Bulging, tense anterior fontanel.
3. Flat, soft anterior fontanel.
4. Consistent head circumference.

53. A male newborn was just admitted to the pediatric floor with a myelomeningocele. When developing the preoperative plan of care, the nurse lists "high risk for infection of and trauma to the nonepithelialized lesion" as the diagnosis of most concern. What would be the *most effective* strategy to prevent infection and trauma to the lesion?

1. Leave the lesion uncovered and open to the air and place the baby supine.
2. Cover the lesion with sterile, saline-soaked gauze and place the baby prone.
3. Apply lotion to the lesion and place the baby on his side.
4. Cover the lesion with dry sterile gauze and place the baby supine.

54. The nurse has been giving instructions to parents on measures to prevent Reye's syndrome. When questioning the parents on a safe medication to provide to their child during a viral illness, which choice indicates that they understand steps toward Reye's syndrome prevention?

1. Pepto-Bismol.
2. Acetaminophen (Tylenol).
3. Children's aspirin.
4. Ritalin.

55. The nurse is caring for a 5-year-old boy with a known seizure disorder. On entering his room, the nurse sees that he is experiencing a generalized, tonic-clonic seizure. What would be the nurse's first response?

1. Immediately leave the room to retrieve intravenous (IV) phenobarbital.
2. Place a metal spoon between his teeth to prevent him from biting his tongue.
3. Position him on his side to maintain a patent airway.
4. Try to hold the client down.

56. When assessing a client who is taking hydantoin (Dilantin), the nurse would recognize which of the following findings as side effects?

1. Drowsiness and irritability.
2. Slurred speech and increased salivation.
3. Hair loss and tremor.
4. Gum hyperplasia and nystagmus.

57. A 12-year-old girl with cerebral palsy has severe language deficits and poor muscle coordination. However, she can voluntarily turn her head from side to side and her mother reports that she has normal intelligence. The nurse is concerned with the child's ability to call when help is needed. Considering the child's abilities, which of the following would be the *best* way for her to call the nurse?

1. Kick the side rails of the bed.
2. Scream loudly.
3. Press the call bell with her fingers.
4. Press a large, padded call bell with her cheek.

58. The nurse is teaching a child how to prevent the spread of conjunctivitis. Which statement by the child would indicate further instruction is necessary?

1. "It is important that I wash my hands regularly."
2. "I can use a tissue to clean my eyes, but must throw it away immediately."
3. "I need to use my own washcloth and towel, not my sister's."
4. "My Dad said he would carry a handkerchief with him so I could wipe my eyes with it during the day."

59. A woman brings her daughter to the pediatric clinic because she is concerned that the child has otitis media. On examination, the nurse would recognize which of the following findings as the *most common* positive sign of otitis media?
1. Temperature of 39°C (102.2°F) and loss of appetite.
2. Pearly gray tympanic membrane and rhinorrhea.
3. Pain on pressure on the tragus and edema within the canal.
4. Feeling of "fullness" in the ear and a popping sensation during swallowing.

 **Answers and Rationales**

40. **4.** Pressure must be kept off the spinal sac.

41. **3.** With improved draining of the CSF, the head circumference should become smaller.

42. **2.** Phenytoin (Dilantin) is an antiepileptic drug that controls seizures. Absence of seizures indicates the client is taking the medication properly.

43. **4.** The clinical symptoms of viral (aseptic) meningitis include fever, irritability, and stiffness of the neck (nucchal rigidity). Other symptoms include drowsiness, photophobia, weakness, painful extremities, and sometimes seizures. Aseptic meningitis usually resolves within 2 weeks.

44. **1.** Photophobia and hypersensitivity to environmental stimuli are common clinical manifestations of meningeal irritation and infection. Comfort measures include providing an environment that is quiet and has minimal stressful stimuli.

45. **3.** Successful coping in times of anxiety and stress requires that the nurse be available to provide information that validates parental right to know and participation in their child's care.

46. **3.** Parents should be instructed to contact the physician if the child's symptoms worsen or persist. The child recovering from viral meningitis should show signs of feeling better a week after discharge.

47. **2.** The child's usual behavior and level of development is what provides critical baseline information about his pretrauma neurological condition.

48. **2.** The occulocephalic reflex occurs if, when the head of an unconscious child is turned rapidly in one direction, the eyes move in the opposite direction.

49. **4.** When dilated pupils react sluggishly to light or are nonreactive, it is an indication that there has been damage to the parasympathetic nervous system, which controls the pupillary constriction response.

50. **3.** The client's head must be kept in midline to facilitate venous return. Clients with a severe closed head injury have low intracranial compliance and turning of the head may result in an increase of ICP of 10–15 mm Hg. The head of bed (i.e., 30°) should be determined individually for each client based on the ICP and cerebral perfusion pressure (CPP) as well as the clinical appearance.

51. **1.** A shift in fluid from the interstitial and cellular space to the intravascular space will occur with a rise in intravascular osmolality, the fluid will then be diuresed resulting in a decreased ICP.

52. **2.** This is a common sign of shunt malfunction. The best way to assess an infant's fontanel is when the infant is upright and calm. In this position, a fontanel that is bulging and firm to light palpation is considered abnormal.

53. **2.** The lesion must be kept moist with sterile, saline-soaked gauze. The prone position should be maintained preoperatively to prevent tension on the lesion and minimize trauma.

54. **2.** Acetaminophen does not contain salicylates, which have been suspected as an ingredient that can lead to Reye's syndrome.

55. **3.** The first priority is to maintain a patent airway. The best position for the client during a seizure is on his side.

56. **4.** Hydantoin (Dilantin) may cause gum hyperplasia and nystagmus. Other side effects include hirsutism, ataxia, diplopia, anorexia, nausea, nervousness, and folate deficiency.

57. **4.** She is able to control her head movements voluntarily. A large padded call bell could easily be pressed when she turns her head to the side.

58. **4.** The eye should be wiped with disposable tissues after a single use and no other

individual should be exposed to items that come in contact with the infected eye.

**59.** **1.** Common signs of otitis media include fever (as high as 40°C [104°F]), postauricular and cervical lymph gland enlargement, rhinorrhea, vomiting, diarrhea, loss of appetite, and red tympanic membrane. Infants become irritable, hold their ears, and roll their head from side to side. Young children verbally complain of pain. A concurrent respiratory or pharyngeal infection may also be present.

# The Cardiovascular System

## VARIATIONS FROM THE ADULT

### Fetal Circulation

**A.** Fetal circulation differs from adult circulation in several ways and is designed to ensure a high-oxygen blood supply to the brain and myocardium.

**B.** Characteristics

1. Placenta is the source of oxygen for the fetus.
2. Fetal lungs receive less than 10% of the blood volume; lungs do not exchange gas.
3. Right atrium of fetal heart is the chamber with the highest oxygen concentration.

**C.** Pattern of altered blood flow and facilitating structures

1. Blood is carried from the placenta through the umbilical vein and enters the inferior vena cava through the ductus venosus.
2. This permits most of the highly oxygenated blood to go directly to the right atrium, bypassing the liver.
3. This right atrial blood flows directly into the left atrium through the foramen ovale, an opening between the right and left atria.
4. From the left atrium, blood flows into the left ventricle and aorta, through the subclavian arteries, to the cerebral and coronary arteries, resulting in the brain and heart receiving the most highly oxygenated blood.
5. Deoxygenated blood returns from the head and arms through the superior vena cava, enters the right atrium, and passes into the right ventricle.
6. Blood from the right ventricle flows into the pulmonary artery, but because fetal lungs are collapsed, the pressure in the pulmonary artery is very high.
7. Because pulmonary resistance is high, most of the blood passes into the distal aorta through the ductus arteriosus, which connects the pulmonary artery and the aorta distal to the origin of the subclavian arteries.
8. From the aorta, blood flows to the rest of the body.

### Normal Circulatory Changes at Birth

**A.** When the umbilical cord is clamped or severed, the blood supply from the placenta is cut off, and oxygenation must then take place in the newborn's lungs.

**B.** As the lungs expand with air, the pulmonary artery pressure decreases and circulation to lungs increases.

**C.** Structural changes

1. Ductus venosus: after the umbilical cord is severed, flow through the ductus venosus decreases and eventually ceases; it constricts within 3–7 days after birth and eventually becomes ligamentum venosum.
2. Foramen ovale
   a. Functional closure of this valvelike opening occurs when pressure in the left atrium exceeds pressure in the right.
   b. Expansion of the pulmonary artery causes a drop in pulmonary artery pressure and in right atrial and ventricular pressure.
   c. At the same time there is increased pulmonary blood flow to the left atrium and increased aortic pressure (from clamping of the umbilical cord), which in turn raises left ventricular and left atrial pressure.
   d. Anatomic closure of the foramen ovale occurs within the first weeks after birth with the deposit of fibrin.
3. Ductus arteriosus
   a. Increase in aortic blood flow increases aortic pressure and decreases right-to-left shunt through the ductus arteriosus; shunt becomes bidirectional.
   b. Increased pulmonary blood flow increases arterial oxygen, causing vasoconstriction of ductus arteriosus within hours of birth.
   c. Functional closure occurs when this constriction causes cessation of blood flow, usually 24 hours after birth.
   d. Anatomic closure occurs when there is growth of fibrous tissue in the lumen of the ductus arteriosus, by 1–3 weeks.

## Abnormal Circulatory Patterns after Birth

A. Normal blood flow in the child may be disrupted as a result of abnormal openings between the pulmonary and systemic circulations.
B. Any time there is a defect connecting systemic and pulmonary circulation, blood will go from high to low pressure (the path of least resistance).
   1. Normally pressure is higher in the systemic circulation, so blood will be shunted from systemic to pulmonary (left to right).
   2. An obstruction to pulmonary blood flow, however, may cause increased pressure proximal to the site of the obstruction.
   3. With an obstruction to pulmonary blood flow, as well as an opening between ventricles, the blood flow may be right to left (if right-sided pressure exceeds left-sided pressure).

## ASSESSMENT

### Overview

A. Approximately 40,000 babies are born with congenital heart disease (CHD) in the United States yearly.
B. One third of these babies will be seriously ill at birth, one third will have problems detected during childhood or later, and one third never have problems.
C. Etiology is multifactional.

## History

A. Family history: parental history of CHD, congenital defects in siblings, history of genetic problems in family.
B. History of pregnancy: rubella, viral infections, medications, X-ray exposure, alcohol ingestion, cigarette smoking.
C. Child's health history
   1. Presenting problem: symptoms may include:
      a. Feeding problems: fatigue, irritability, tachypnea, profuse sweating
      b. Failure to thrive
      c. Respiratory difficulties: tachypnea, difficulty breathing, frequent respiratory infections
      d. Color changes: pallor, cyanosis (persistent or intermittent)
      e. Activity intolerance
      f. All presenting symptoms must be explored within a developmental framework
   2. Past medical history: rheumatic fever; associated chromosomal abnormalities (e.g., Down syndrome)

## Physical Examination

A. Plot height and weight on growth chart; measure respiratory rate and rhythm; inspect for chest enlargement or asymmetry.
B. Inspect for presence of cyanosis: lips, mucous membranes, extremities.
C. Inspect for clubbing of fingers (thought to be caused by increased capillary formation and soft tissue fibrosis).
D. Observe for distended veins.
E. Palpate/percuss quality and symmetry of pulses, size of liver and spleen, presence of thrill over heart during expiration.
F. Auscultate for heart rate and rhythm.
G. Auscultate for abnormal heart sounds and murmurs; murmurs are caused by abnormal flow of blood between chambers or vessels; classified as:
   1. Innocent: no anatomic or physiologic abnormality
   2. Functional: no anatomic defect, but may be caused by a physiologic abnormality
   3. Organic: caused by a structural abnormality
H. Measure blood pressure in both arm and thigh.
   1. In infants under 1 year, arm and thigh blood pressure should be the same.
   2. In children over 1 year, systolic pressure in leg is usually higher by 10–40 mm Hg.
   3. A wide pulse pressure (greater than 50 mm Hg) or a narrow pulse pressure (less than 10 mm Hg) may be associated with a heart defect.
I. Select proper blood pressure cuff size.
   1. Too small a cuff can give a falsely elevated BP reading
   2. Bladder inside the cuff should be two thirds the length of the upper arm

## Laboratory/Diagnostic Tests

A. Chest X-ray
B. Cardiac fluoroscopy
C. Magnetic resonance imaging (MRI)
D. Electrocardiogram
E. Echocardiography
F. Hematologic testing: polycythemia is often associated with cyanotic heart defects
G. Cardiac catheterization
   1. Femoral vein often used for access
   2. Catheter threaded into right side of the heart since septal defects permit entry into the left side
   3. Nursing care: pretest
      a. Child's preparation should be based on developmental level, level of understanding, and past experience.
      b. Use doll play and pictures as appropriate.
      c. Describe sensations child will feel in simple terms.
      d. Administer medications as ordered.
   4. Nursing care: posttest
      a. Check extremity distal to the catheterization site for color, temperature, pulse, capillary refill.
      b. Keep extremity distal to the catheterization site extended for 6 hours.

        c. Check pressure dressing over
           catheterization site for bleeding.
        d. Monitor heart rate for signs of bradycardia,
           tachycardia, and dysrhythmia.
        e. Monitor for transient temperature elevation
           due to physiologic dehydration (NPO,
           contrast media).
        f. Monitor urine output and BP.

# ANALYSIS

Nursing diagnoses for the child with a disorder of the
cardiovascular system may include:
**A.** Delayed growth and development
**B.** Risk for injury: physiologic
**C.** Imbalanced nutrition: less than body requirements
**D.** Fear/anxiety
**E.** Risk for infection
**F.** Deficient knowledge
**G.** Decreased cardiac output
**H.** Excess fluid volume

# PLANNING AND IMPLEMENTATION

## Goals

**A.** Tissue will be adequately oxygenated.
**B.** Child will achieve normal growth and
   development milestones.
**C.** Child will be free from symptoms of complications
   of heart disease.
**D.** Parents will understand child's condition.
**E.** Parents will be able to care for child at home.

## Interventions

### Care of the Child with Heart Failure (HF)

**A.** General information
   1. Usually due to a surgically correctable
      structural abnormality of the heart that results
      in increased blood volume and pressure or
      increased pulmonary blood flow
   2. A symptom complex reflecting the heart's
      inability to meet the metabolic demands of the
      body
**B.** Medical management
   1. Directed toward improvement of cardiac
      function and energy conservation
   2. Drug therapy
      a. Digitalis to improve myocardial
         contractility and slow the heart rate
      b. ACE inhibitors to decrease cardiac
         afterload
      c. Diuretics to decrease total body water and
         to increase urine output

        d. Potassium supplement if diuretic is
           potassium depleting
   3. High-caloric formula or nasogastric feedings
      may be required to meet nutritional needs
**C.** Assessment findings
   1. Tachycardia, gallop rhythm, cardiomegaly,
      decreased peripheral pulses, and mottling of
      the extremities
   2. Tachypnea, retractions, grunting, nasal flaring,
      cough, cyanosis, orthopnea
   3. Hepatomegaly, edema, distended neck and
      peripheral veins, decreased urine output
   4. Failure to thrive, decreased exercise tolerance
**D.** Nursing interventions
   1. Decrease energy expenditure
      a. Frequent rest periods
      b. Small, frequent feedings
      c. Minimize crying
      d. Prevent cold stress
   2. Provide adequate nutrition
      a. Estimate daily caloric requirement
      b. Use soft nipple
      c. Consider gavage feeding if necessary
   3. Monitor fluid status
      a. I&O, specific gravity
      b. Daily weight
   4. Administer medications as ordered
      a. Digoxin
         1) Check dosage with another RN
         2) Give 1 hour before feeding or 2 hours
            after feeding
         3) Take apical pulse for 1 minute; if
            bradycardia is present, hold dose and
            contact physician
         4) Monitor serum potassium levels; if less
            than 3.5 mEq/liter, may be
            contraindicated
         5) Monitor therapeutic effects;
            therapeutic serum digoxin levels range
            from 0.8 to 2.0 ng/mL.
         6) Monitor for toxicity: nausea, anorexia,
            vomiting, lethargy, bradycardia
         7) Parent/child teaching
      b. ACE inhibitors—also monitor BP
      c. Diuretic (see Table 2-17)
         1) I&O
         2) Daily weight
         3) Monitor side effects: dehydration,
            electrolyte imbalance especially
            hypokalemia (potentiates digoxin and
            may lead to toxicity)
         4) Parent/child teaching
   5. Provide adequate rest
   6. Prevent infections
   7. Promote growth and development
   8. Reduce respiratory distress
      a. Position in semi- or high-Fowler's
         position
      b. Knee-chest position for children with
         tetralogy of Fallot

# EVALUATION

A. Child demonstrates optimal cardiac status.
   1. Normal color
   2. No respiratory distress
   3. Increased exercise tolerance
   4. Satisfactory growth
B. Child has no evidence of complications.
C. Parents demonstrate ability to care for child, perform necessary treatments, and administer prescribed medications.

# DISORDERS OF THE CARDIOVASCULAR SYSTEM

## Congenital Heart Defects

See Figure 5-4.

### Classification

A. Defects associated with increased pulmonary blood flow

Atrial Septal Defect

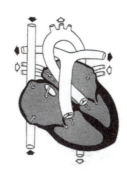

Ventricular Septal Defect

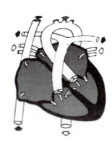

Patent Ductus Arteriosus

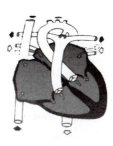

Coarctation of the Aorta

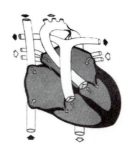

Transposition of Great Arteries

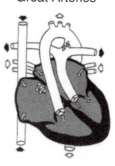

Truncus Arteriosus

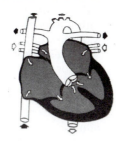

Tetralogy of Fallot

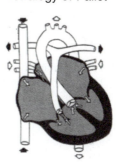

**Figure 5-4** Congenital heart abnormalities

1. Left-to-right shunting of blood across a septal defect or blood vessel (higher left side heart pressure)
2. Pulmonary overcirculation and increased work of ventricles, possible right ventricular hypertrophy
3. Risk for heart failure
4. Usually acyanotic
5. Examples: atrial septal defect, ventricular septal defect, patent ductus arteriosus, atrioventricular canal (also called endocardial cushion defect)

B. Defects associated with decreased pulmonary blood flow
1. Right-to-left shunting of blood due to presence of a defect and obstruction of pulmonary blood flow (obstructed pulmonary flow leads to higher right side heart pressure)
2. Some or most blood does not enter the pulmonary circulation and does not pick up oxygen in the lungs; instead, blood is shunted to the left side of the heart
3. Deoxygenated as well as oxygenated blood circulated to the body
4. Cyanosis and hypoxemia present
5. Example: tetralogy of Fallot

C. Defects causing obstruction to cardiac chamber outflow
1. Narrowing of outflow tract from heart to blood vessels
2. Increased work of heart as it strains to push blood out
3. Risk for heart failure and poor cardiac output
4. Examples: coarctation of the aorta, pulmonic stenosis, aortic stenosis

D. Defects associated with mixing of saturated and desaturated blood
1. Oxygenated and deoxygenated blood mixes in heart chambers
2. Increased pulmonary blood flow due to defect
3. Hypoxemia and cyanosis present, often severe
4. Risk for poor cardiac output and risk for heart failure (HF).
5. Examples: transposition of the great vessels (also called transposition of the great arteries), truncus arteriosus, hypoplastic left heart syndrome

## Increased Pulmonary Blood Flow

A. General information and medical management
1. Atrial septal defect (ASD): opening between right and left atria with left-to-right shunting of blood
   a. 15% of congenital heart defects
   b. Manifestations dependent on age and size and location of defect.
   c. Small lesions may be asymptomatic until childhood.

d. Dyspnea, tachycardia, growth failure, HF may be present. Systolic pulmonary ejection murmur present.
e. Surgical repair includes patching of defect—open heart/cardiopulmonary bypass procedure. Some defects plugged during cardiac catheterization.

2. Ventricular septal defect (VSD): opening in ventricular septum with left-to-right shunting of blood
   a. 25% of congenital heart defects.
   b. Manifestations dependent on age, size of defect, and degree of pulmonary vascular resistance. Usually found in infancy.
   c. Small lesions may be asymptomatic; may close spontaneously.
   d. With large lesions, higher pressure in ventricles results in high degree of shunting.
   e. Risk for right ventricular hypertrophy, HF, bacterial endocarditis, pulmonary problems.
   f. Dyspnea, tachycardia, growth failure, HF, frequent respiratory infections common. Harsh systolic murmur at lower left sternal border present.
   g. Surgical repair includes suturing or patching of defect using open heart/cardiopulmonary bypass procedure, usually done in infancy. Primary (complete) repair is preferred.
   h. Occasionally, surgical palliation with pulmonary artery banding for severely ill infants, with complete repair when infant is more stable. Banding decreases blood flow through pulmonary artery: decreases pressure difference between right and left ventricles to decrease left-to-right shunting of blood across defect.

3. Patent ductus arteriosus (PDA): failure of fetal ductus arteriosus to close after birth
   a. 10% of congenital heart defects in term infants, more common in preterm infants.
   b. Blood vessel connecting pulmonary artery and aorta.
   c. Higher pressure in aorta results in left-to-right shunting of blood from aorta to pulmonary circulation.
   d. Manifestations depend on size of defect. Small lesions may be asymptomatic.
   e. Risk for HF.
   f. May have bounding pulses and visible precordial pulsations (especially preterm infants). Continuous machine-like murmur at upper left sternal border.
   g. Administration of indomethacin may close defect in preterm infants.
   h. If indomethacin fails, or if not a preterm infant, surgical ligation of vessel (closed

heart procedure) or mechanical occlusion of vessel.

4. Atrioventricular canal (AV canal): combination septal defect resulting in large opening between right and left atria and ventricles and defects of valves.
   a. Most common cardiac defect in children with Down syndrome.
   b. High degree of left-to-right shunting of blood.
   c. HF commonly develops. Pulmonary flow murmurs and valvular murmurs present.
   d. Open heart/cardiopulmonary bypass surgical repair.

B. Assessment findings in conditions with increased pulmonary blood flow
   1. Poor feeding, anorexia
   2. Growth failure, poor weight gain
   3. Respiratory difficulties: tachypnea, dyspnea, orthopnea, coughing, wheezing, hoarseness, grunting, nasal flaring, retractions, frequent respiratory infections
   4. Exercise intolerance, fatigue, lethargy, excessive sweating with feeding or activity
   5. Signs/symptoms of heart failure
   6. Cardiac murmur

C. Nursing interventions
   1. Prepare child/family for diagnostic studies, surgery.
   2. Administer medications as ordered. See HF.
   3. Ensure adequate nutrition.
      a. Anticipate infant hunger to prevent crying and increased oxygen demands.
      b. Small, frequent feedings/small frequent, nutritious meals if child.
      c. Feed infants in semi-upright position.
      d. Soft nipple to decrease fatigue during infant feedings. Gavage feedings may be necessary.
      e. Burp frequently during bottle and breast feedings.
      f. Observe for tolerance of feedings if high-calorie formula or breast milk fortifier used: vomiting, diarrhea.
      g. Assist breastfeeding mothers.
      h. Monitor growth.
   4. Monitor vital signs.
   5. Provide rest.
      a. Quiet age-appropriate play if HF present.
      b. Cluster care to provide periods of undisturbed rest.
      c. Anticipate needs; prevent crying.
   6. Position semi-upright if HF or respiratory difficulty present.
   7. Prevent infections.
   8. Meet age-appropriate developmental needs.
   9. Bacterial endocarditis antibiotic prophylaxis for unrepaired ASD, VSD, PDA, and all other congenital heart defect before or after repair. Give prescribed antibiotic 1 hour before

dental, genitourinary tract, and surgical procedures. Will be required throughout life.
   10. Teach care to family.

## Decreased Pulmonary Blood Flow

A. General information and medical management
   1. Tetralogy of Fallot (TOF)
      a. Most common congenital heart defect causing cyanosis and hypoxemia; 10% of all congenital heart defect.
      b. Four associated defects: pulmonary stenosis, VSD, overriding aorta (also called dextropositioned aorta), right ventricular hypertrophy.
      c. Pulmonary stenosis creates obstruction to outflow of blood from right ventricle to pulmonary artery, causing decreased pulmonary blood flow. Increased right ventricle pressure creates right-to-left shunt. Right-shifted aorta sits over VSD so blood from both right and left ventricles flows into aorta.
      d. Aorta carries mixed oxygenated and deoxygenated blood to body.
      e. Manifestations include low oxygen saturation, cyanosis, polycythemia, activity intolerance, fatigue, poor feeding, poor growth, harsh systolic murmur along left sternal border, hypercyanotic spells (also called TET spells), also signs of chronic hypoxia.
      f. Hypercyanotic spells: occur when oxygen demand exceeds supply.
         1) Transient obstruction of pulmonary blood flow.
         2) Increasing cyanosis, tachypnea, poor muscle tone, loss of consciousness. May progress to seizures, CVA, death.
         3) Often precipitated by crying, feeding, defecation.
         4) Treat by placing in knee-chest position, give oxygen, morphine, occasionally propranolol.
      g. Surgical repair includes open heart/cardiopulmonary bypass procedure to patch VSD and relieve stenosis. Palliative surgery to increase pulmonary blood flow includes anastomosis of right or left subclavian artery to pulmonary artery (Blalock-Taussig shunt).

B. Assessment findings in conditions with decreased pulmonary blood flow
   1. Low oxygen saturation
   2. Cyanosis
   3. Polycythemia (chronic hypoxemia results in increased production of RBCs)
   4. Clubbing of digits (chronic hypoxia)
   5. Poor feeding, anorexia, fatigue, activity intolerance, growth failure, weak cry

5

6. Squatting: increases systemic vascular resistance and improves pulmonary blood flow (not seen frequently due to early repair of cardiac defects)
7. Hypercyanotic (TET) spells
8. Tachycardia, tachypnea, dyspnea
9. Cardiac murmur
10. Risk for emboli, bacterial endocarditis

C. Nursing interventions
1. Squatting: observe only. No other intervention needed unless distress develops.
2. Cluster care. Provide age-appropriate quiet activities. Promote uninterrupted rest.
3. Provide oxygen as needed.
4. Prevent crying; anticipate needs.
5. Monitor vital signs.
6. Support nutrition (see interventions for increased pulmonary blood flow).
7. Prepare child/family for diagnostic tests and surgery.
8. Administer medications as ordered.
9. Bacterial endocarditis prophylaxis as noted earlier.
10. For hypercyanotic spells, place in knee-chest position, administer oxygen, prepare to administer morphine.
11. Meet age-appropriate developmental needs.
12. Teach care to parents.

## Obstruction to Outflow

A. General information and medical management
1. Coarctation of the aorta: narrowing of a portion of aorta, usually near aortic arch beyond left subclavian artery
   a. Decreased blood flow to lower part of body, more blood shunted to arms and head.
   b. Manifestations dependent on degree of narrowing, include arm blood and pulse pressures greater than in legs, strong brachial and diminished femoral pulses, lower body cooler than upper. In older children, dizziness, headaches, fainting, epistaxis occur.
   c. Risk for heart failure, hypertension, rupture of aorta, CVA.
   d. Vascular surgery to remove narrowed portion or repair with graft.
2. Pulmonic stenosis: narrowed pulmonic valve opening
   a. Minor to moderate narrowing may be asymptomatic.
   b. Severe narrowing causes increased work of right ventricle and ventricular hypertrophy.
   c. Manifestations: cyanosis, systolic thrill, systolic ejection murmur at upper left sternal border.
   d. Repair includes balloon angioplasty to dilate stenosed area or surgical valvotomy.

3. Aortic stenosis: narrowed aortic valve
   a. Increased resistance to left ventricular blood outflow into aorta.
   b. Leads to left ventricular hypertrophy, left-sided heart failure.
   c. Manifestations include faint pulses, tachycardia, hypotension, poor feeding, exercise intolerance, aortic murmur.
   d. Repair: balloon angioplasty or valvotomy.

B. Assessment findings: HF, cardiac murmur; also see individual defects

C. Nursing interventions
1. Monitor for hypotension.
2. Monitor for HF.
3. Monitor for cyanosis and hypoxemia in children with pulmonic stenosis.
4. Prepare child and family for diagnostic/therapeutic procedures and surgery.
5. Support nutrition as noted earlier.
6. Promote rest as noted earlier.
7. Administer medications as ordered.
8. Bacterial endocarditis prophylaxis as noted earlier.
9. Meet age-appropriate developmental needs.
10. Teach care to parents.

## Lesions with Mixing of Saturated and Desaturated Blood

A. General information and medical management
1. Transposition of the great vessels (transposition of the great arteries): aorta emerges from right ventricle and pulmonary artery emerges from left ventricle.
   a. Essentially two independent circulations:
      1) Unoxygenated blood from right ventricle exits to aorta, goes to body and returns to right atrium without flowing to lungs.
      2) Oxygenated blood exits left ventricle to pulmonary arteries, goes to lungs, and returns to left atrium.
   b. Incompatible with life unless there is communication between left and right sides of heart (usually through foramen ovale or PDA).
   c. Manifestations include neonatal cyanosis, hypoxemia, systolic murmur.
   d. Treatment includes administration of Prostaglandin E to maintain patency of ductus arteriosus, balloon atrial septostomy (also called Rashkind procedure) during cardiac catheterization to improve mixing of blood in atria.
   e. Surgical repair: arterial switching procedure in newborn period or installation of atrial baffle to direct venous blood to left ventricle and oxygenated blood to right ventricle (Senning and Mustard procedures) in older children (rarely used).

2. Truncus arteriosus: failure of embryonic blood vessel to divide into aorta and pulmonary artery results in one large vessel positioned over both ventricles.
   a. Has associated large VSD.
   b. Both oxygenated and deoxygenated blood flow to systemic circulation; blood flow and pressure in pulmonary circulation are increased.
   c. Manifestations include cyanosis, growth failure, activity intolerance, HF.
   d. Treatment includes digoxin and diuretics for HF.
   e. Surgical repair includes open heart/cardiopulmonary bypass procedure to close VSD, incorporate trunk into left ventricle, grafting of right and left pulmonary arteries to right ventricle.
3. Hypoplastic left heart syndrome: poorly developed left side of heart, including hypoplastic left ventricle, aortic valve atresia or mitral valve atresia, narrowed ascending aorta and aortic arch.
   a. Some oxygenated blood flows from left atrium across foramen ovale to right atrium, enters pulmonary circulation, and flows across PDA into aorta.
   b. Clinical manifestations include progressive cyanosis, pallor, weak or absent pulses, HF, shock.
   c. Treatment includes administration of Prostaglandin E to maintain PDA, administration of medications to support blood pressure and cardiac function.
   d. Usually fatal without surgery or heart transplantation.
      1) Norwood procedure (palliative): connect pulmonary artery and aorta, create ASD, allows mixed blood to get to tissues.
      2) Repair includes intracardiac redirection of blood flow (Fontan procedure) involving open heart/cardiopulmonary bypass technique.
      3) Heart transplant may be performed.

B. Assessment findings in conditions with mixing of oxygenated and deoxygenated blood
   1. Cyanosis and hypoxemia
   2. Tachycardia, dyspnea, tachypnea
   3. Cardiac murmur
   4. Poor feeding, growth failure, activity intolerance, weak cry, lethargy
   5. Varying degrees of HF
   6. Polycythemia
   7. Clubbing of digits
   8. Risk for bacterial endocarditis, emboli, stroke

C. Nursing interventions
   1. Prepare child/family for diagnostic procedures and surgery.
   2. Assess vital signs and assess for poor cardiac output.

3. Monitor infants receiving Prostaglandin E for apnea, hypotension, hypothermia.
4. Cluster care to provide periods of uninterrupted rest.
5. Provide oxygen as ordered.
6. Prevent crying; anticipate needs.
7. Support nutrition (see interventions for increased pulmonary blood flow).
8. Bacterial endocarditis prophylaxis as noted earlier.
9. Meet age-appropriate developmental needs.
10. Teach care to parents.

## Cardiac Surgery

A. General information
   1. Surgical correction of congenital defects within the heart, or surgery of the great vessels in the immediate area surrounding the heart
   2. Open-heart surgery (uses cardiopulmonary bypass): provides a relatively blood-free operative site; heart-lung machine maintains gas exchange during surgery
   3. Closed-heart surgery does not use cardiopulmonary bypass machine; indicated for ligation of a patent ductus arteriosus or coarctation of the aorta

B. Nursing interventions: preoperative
   1. Determine the child's level of understanding; have child draw a picture, tell you a story, or use doll play.
   2. Correct misunderstandings/teach the child about the surgery using diagrams and play therapy; use terms appropriate to developmental level.
   3. Accompany the child to the operating and recovery rooms and the intensive care unit, explaining the various equipment; allow child to handle/experience it, if possible, and introduce staff and clients, depending on child's developmental/emotional levels.
   4. Have child practice post-op procedures (turning, coughing, deep breathing, etc.).
   5. Include parents in teaching sessions, but have separate sessions for the parents only.
   6. Establish pre-op baseline data for vital signs, activity/sleep patterns, I&O.

C. Nursing interventions: postoperative
   1. Prevent injury/complications.
      a. Monitor vital signs and circulatory pressure readings frequently until stable. Monitor ECG.
      b. Assess neurologic status frequently.
      c. Observe surgical site for intactness/drainage.
   2. Promote gas exchange (client may be on mechanical ventilation).
      a. Position as ordered.
      b. Administer oxygen at prescribed rate.
      c. Provide humidification.

    **d.** Suction as necessary.
    **e.** Perform postural drainage and chest percussion as ordered.
    **f.** Turn, cough, and deep breathe hourly.
    **g.** Perform routine care of chest tubes and drainage system, depending on the type of surgery.
  **3.** Monitor I&O.
  **4.** Provide nutrition as ordered.
  **5.** Provide alternative means of communication if mechanical ventilation is used, e.g., picture cards.
  **6.** Provide psychologic support of the child/family.
  **7.** Allow activity as tolerated.
  **8.** Provide client teaching and discharge planning concerning:
    **a.** Need for child/family to express feelings/fears
    **b.** Resumption of ADL
    **c.** Assisting child in dealing with peers/returning to school
    **d.** Referral for parents to support groups/community agencies

# Acquired Heart Disease

## Rheumatic Fever (RF)

**A.** General information
  **1.** An inflammatory disorder that may involve the heart, joints, connective tissue, and the CNS
  **2.** Peaks in school-age children; linked to environmental factors and family history of disorder
  **3.** Thought to be an autoimmune disorder
    **a.** Preceded by an infection of group A beta-hemolytic streptococcus (usually a strep throat); the heart itself is not infected, however.
    **b.** Antigenic markers for strep toxin closely resemble markers for heart valves; this resemblance causes antibodies made against the strep to also attack heart valves.
  **4.** Prognosis depends on degree of heart damage
**B.** Medical management
  **1.** Drug therapy
    **a.** Penicillin
      **1)** Used in the acute phase
      **2)** Used prophylactically for several years after the attack
      **3)** Erythromycin substituted if child is sensitive to penicillin
    **b.** Salicylates: for analgesic, anti-inflammatory, antipyretic effect
    **c.** Steroids: for anti-inflammatory effect
  **2.** Decrease cardiac workload: bed rest until lab studies return to normal

**C.** Assessment findings
  **1.** Major symptoms (Jones' criteria)
    **a.** Carditis
      **1)** Seen in 50% of clients
      **2)** Aschoff nodules (areas of inflammation and degeneration around heart valves, pericardium, and myocardium)
      **3)** Valvular insufficiency of mitral and aortic valves possible
      **4)** Cardiomegaly
      **5)** Shortness of breath, hepatomegaly, edema
    **b.** Polyarthritis
      **1)** Migratory, therefore no contractures develop
      **2)** Most common in large joints, which become red, swollen, painful
      **3)** Synovial fluid is sterile
      **4)** No arthralgia
    **c.** Chorea (Sydenham's chorea, St. Vitus' dance): CNS disorder characterized by abrupt, purposeless, involuntary muscular movements
      **1)** Gradual, insidious onset: starts with personality change or clumsiness
      **2)** Mostly seen in prepubertal girls
      **3)** May appear months after strep infection
      **4)** Movements increase with excitement
      **5)** Lasts 1–3 months
    **d.** Subcutaneous nodules
      **1)** Usually a sign of severe disease
      **2)** Occur with active carditis
      **3)** Firm, nontender nodes on bony prominences of joints
      **4)** Lasts for weeks
    **e.** Erythema marginatum: transient, nonpruritic rash starting with central red patches that expand; results in series of irregular patches with red, raised margins and pale centers (resemble giraffe spots)
  **2.** Minor symptoms
    **a.** Reliable history of RF, fever
    **b.** Recent history of strep infection
    **c.** Diagnostic tests: erythrocyte sedimentation rate (ESR) and antistreptolysin O (ASO) titer increased; changes on ECG
**D.** Nursing interventions
  **1.** Carditis
    **a.** Administer penicillin as ordered.
      **1)** Used prophylactically to prevent future attacks of strep and further damage to the heart
      **2)** To be taken until age 20 or for 5 years after attack, whichever is longer
    **b.** Promote bed rest until ESR returns to normal.
  **2.** Arthritis: administer aspirin as ordered, change child's position in bed frequently.

3. Chorea
    a. Decrease stimulation.
    b. Provide a safe environment: no forks with meals, assistance with mobility.
    c. Provide small, frequent meals; increased muscle activity causes increased kcal requirements.
4. Nodules and rash: none.
5. Alleviate child's anxiety about the ability of heart to continue to function.
6. Prevent recurrent infection.
7. Minimize boredom with age-appropriate sedentary play.
8. Provide client teaching and discharge planning concerning:
    a. Adaptation of home environment to promote bed rest (commode, call bell, diversional activities)
    b. Importance of prophylactic medication regimen
    c. Diet modification in relation to decreased activity/cardiac demands
    d. Avoidance of reinfections
    e. Home-bound education
    f. Availability of community agencies

 **Sample Questions**

60. A 4-year-old with tetralogy of Fallot is seen in a squatting position near his bed. What would be the nurse's response?
    1. Administer oxygen.
    2. Take no action if he looks comfortable but continue to observe him.
    3. Pick him up and place him in Trendelenburg's position in bed.
    4. Have him stand up and walk around the room.

61. A 2-month-old is suspected of having coarctation of the aorta. What is a cardinal sign of this defect?
    1. Clubbing of the digits and circumoral cyanosis.
    2. Pedal edema and portal congestion.
    3. Systolic ejection murmur.
    4. Upper extremity hypertension.

62. When assessing the apical heart rate in infants and toddlers, where is the point of maximal impulse (PMI) located?
    1. Between the third and fourth left intercostal space.
    2. Between the fourth and fifth left intercostal space.

3. At the fifth intercostal space to the right of the midclavicular line.
4. In the aortic area.

63. A 2-week-old infant has a patent ductus arteriosus. Prior to administering digoxin, which action by the nurse would be correct?
    1. Take the apical pulse for 30 seconds and multiply by 2.
    2. Give the medication if his pulse is 92, but notify the physician.
    3. Take the radial pulse for 1 full minute.
    4. Give the medication after finding that the apical pulse is 135 beats/minute.

64. The nurse is planning care for a 2-week-old infant who has a congenital heart defect. Which of the following actions are appropriate? Select all that apply.
    _____ Using a soft "preemie" nipple for feedings.
    _____ Providing passive stimulation.
    _____ Allowing him to cry to promote increased oxygenation.
    _____ Placing him in orthopneic position.

65. A 10-year-old has been hospitalized for 2 weeks with rheumatic fever. The child's mother questions whether her other children can catch the rheumatic fever. What is the nurse's best response?
    1. "The fact that you brought your child to the hospital early enough will decrease the chance of your other children getting it."
    2. "It is caused by an autoimmune reaction and is not contagious."
    3. "You appear concerned that your child's disease is contagious."
    4. "Your other children should be taking antibiotics to prevent them from catching rheumatic fever."

66. A 10-year-old child is admitted with rheumatic fever. In addition to carditis, for what other problem would the nurse assess?
    1. Arthritis.
    2. Bronchitis.
    3. Malabsorption.
    4. Oliguria.

67. An infant's blood pressure is reported to be very high. What is the most appropriate nursing action to take?
    1. Take it again in 20 minutes.
    2. Call the nursing supervisor.

3. Measure the cuff width to the infant's arm.

4. Prepare to give an antihypertensive.

68. Prior to discharge from the newborn nursery at 48 hours old, the nurse knows that murmurs are frequently assessed and are most often due to which factor?

1. A ventricular septal defect.

2. Heart disease of the newborn period.

3. Transition from fetal to pulmonic circulation.

4. Cyanotic heart disease.

69. A 10-year-old with a ventricular septal defect (VSD) is going to have a cardiac catheterization. Which of the following needs to be a high priority for the nurse to assess?

1. Capillary refill.

2. Breath sounds.

3. Arrhythmias.

4. Pedal pulses.

70. An infant with heart failure (HF) is admitted to the hospital. Which goal has the highest priority when planning nursing care?

1. The infant will maintain an adequate fluid balance.

2. The infant will have digoxin at the bedside.

3. Skin integrity will be addressed.

4. Administer medications on time.

71. An infant on the ward is receiving digoxin and diuretic therapy. The nurse knows that which of the following choices indicates no toxicity?

1. Heart rate less than 100, no dysrhythmias.

2. Heart rate of 80–100.

3. Heart rate greater than 100, no dysrhythmias.

4. Vomiting.

72. An infant with cardiac disease has been admitted to the nursery from the delivery room. Which finding helps the nurse to differentiate between a cyanotic and an acyanotic defect?

1. Infants with cyanotic heart disease feed poorly.

2. The pulse oximeter does not read above 93%.

3. Infants with cyanotic heart disease usually go directly to the operating room.

4. Cyanotic heart disease causes high fevers.

73. A child with tetralogy of Fallot has been admitted. What equipment is most important to have at the bedside?

1. Morphine.

2. A blood pressure cuff.

3. A thermometer.

4. An oxygen setup.

74. A 9-year-old boy has been transferred back to the floor after cardiac surgery. Which of the following does the nurse need to include in the plan of care to evaluate that the fluid needs are being appropriately met?

1. Call if the heart rate falls below 60 per minute.

2. Place a Foley catheter.

3. Prepare to assist with an arterial line to monitor blood pressure.

4. Calculate the daily maintenance fluid requirements and ensure correct delivery.

75. A 9-year-old girl with rheumatic fever is asking to play. Which diversional activity is the nurse likely to offer?

1. Walking to the gift store.

2. Coloring books and crayons.

3. A 300-piece puzzle.

4. A dancing contest.

76. A 10-year-old girl has been diagnosed with rheumatic fever and is now being discharged. What statement made by the parents shows an understanding of long-term care?

1. "She will need penicillin each day."

2. "She will need antibiotic prophylaxis when she has dental work."

3. "We will have yearly checkups."

4. "The murmur will always go away by adolescence."

 **Answers and Rationales**

60. **2.** Squatting is a normal response in a child who has tetralogy of Fallot. This position increases pulmonary blood flow because it changes the relationship between systemic and pulmonary vascular resistance.

61. **4.** Coarctation of the aorta is characterized by upper extremity hypertension and diminished pulses in the extremities.

62. **1.** The heartbeat is most easily counted at the point of maximum impulse. From birth through toddlerhood it is located between the third and fourth left intercostal space.

63. **4.** The apical pulse is taken for one full minute and the medication is withheld if the pulse is less than 100 beats/minute.

64. *Using a soft "preemie" nipple for feedings* should be selected. This will help to reduce energy expenditure.

*Providing passive stimulation* should be selected. This will help to reduce energy expenditure.

*Placing the child in orthopneic position* should be selected. This will help promote oxygenation.

65. **2.** Rheumatic fever is an autoimmune reaction to a streptococcal infection and is limited to the person having the reaction. It is not a contagious disease.

66. **1.** A major symptom of rheumatic fever is arthritis.

67. **3.** The cuff should be approximately two thirds the length of the humerus.

68. **3.** As the transition occurs, the murmurs may become loud, and then resolve.

69. **4.** The nurse needs to know the baseline pedal pulses.

70. **1.** This is a major priority for HF clients.

71. **3.** Infants' heart rates need to be greater than 100, with no rhythm disturbances.

72. **2.** Cyanotic heart disease is unlikely to produce a reading above 93%.

73. **4.** This is used emergently in a TET spell.

74. **4.** It is vital for pediatric nurses to know exactly how much fluid should be delivered each 24 hours to evaluate proper fluid needs.

75. **3.** This will be quiet, yet stimulating.

76. **2.** This will be necessary for many years.

# The Hematologic System

## VARIATIONS FROM THE ADULT

A. In the young child all the bone marrow is involved in blood cell formation.
B. By puberty, only the sternum, ribs, pelvis, vertebrae, skull, and proximal epiphyses of femur and humerus are involved.
C. During the first 6 months of life, fetal hemoglobin is gradually replaced by adult hemoglobin, and it is only after this that hemoglobin disorders can be diagnosed.

## ASSESSMENT

### History

A. Family history: genetic hematologic disorders, anemia, or jaundice
B. History of pregnancy: parents' blood types, anemia, infection or drug ingestion, course of labor and delivery
C. Child's health history
   1. Neonatal course: occurrence, duration, and treatment of jaundice; bleeding episodes; blood transfusions
   2. Accidents, operations, hospitalizations (any blood transfusions or unusual bleeding)
   3. Nutrition: dietary intake of iron and vitamin $B_{12}$; history of pica
   4. Ingestions: lead-based paint; drugs
   5. Ability to participate in age-appropriate activities

### Physical Examination

A. General appearance
   1. Skin: note whether cyanotic, pale, ruddy, jaundiced; note bruises or petechiae, other evidences of hemorrhage; pain, swelling around joints.
   2. Neurologic status: note listlessness or fatigue, irritability, dizziness, or lightheadedness.
B. Measure vital signs; note tachycardia or tachypnea.
C. Plot height and weight on growth chart.
D. Inspect and palpate abdomen; note enlargement of liver and spleen, pain, or tenderness on palpation.

## ANALYSIS

Nursing diagnoses for the child with a disorder of the hematologic system may include:
A. Activity intolerance
B. Pain
C. Impaired gas exchange
D. Ineffective tissue perfusion: cardiopulmonary
E. Imbalanced nutrition

## PLANNING AND IMPLEMENTATION

### Goals

A. Child will have adequate tissue oxygenation.
B. Child will be free from complications associated with hematologic diseases.
C. Child will be free from pain, or have pain controlled.
D. Optimal growth and developmental level will be achieved.
E. Parents will participate in care of child.

### Interventions

See Unit 4.

## EVALUATION

A. Serum values of hematologic components are normal.
B. Child is free from signs or symptoms of infection.
C. Child has no abnormal bleeding episodes.
D. Normal activity level is maintained without pain or fatigue.
E. Parents are able to describe symptoms of disease and complications.

F. Parents are able to administer medications and participate in child's care.

## DISORDERS OF THE HEMATOLOGIC SYSTEM

### Anemias

#### Iron Deficiency Anemia

A. General information: iron deficiency is most common cause of anemia in children; children whose diet consists mainly of cow's milk, which is low in absorbable iron, are especially vulnerable.
B. Assessment findings
   1. Pallor, fatigue, irritability
   2. History of iron-deficient diet
   3. Diagnostic tests
      a. RBC normal or slightly reduced
      b. Hgb below normal range for child
      c. HCT below normal
C. Nursing interventions
   1. Add iron to formula, food, or by vitamins by age 4–6 months.
      a. Oral iron
         1) Give iron with citrus juice and on empty stomach (iron is best absorbed in an acidic environment).

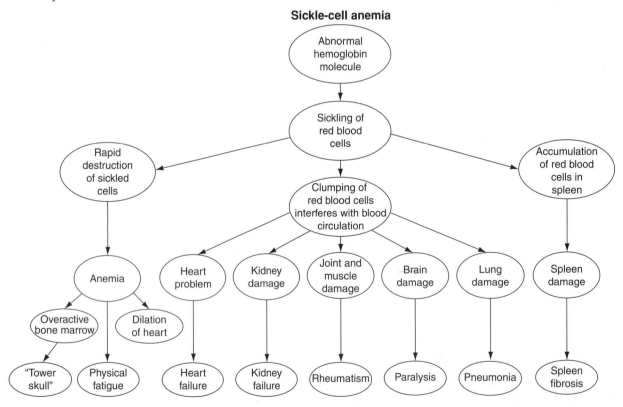

**Figure 5-5** A series of damages and effects caused by sickle-cell anemia

**2)** Have child use straw if possible, because iron stains teeth and skin.

    **b.** Administer IM iron if ordered. Use z-track method.

**2.** Provide iron-rich foods: meats, nuts, dried beans/legumes, dried fruit, dark-green leafy vegetables, whole grains, egg yolk, potatoes, shellfish.

**D.** Also see Unit 4.

## Sickle-Cell Anemia

**A.** General information (see Figure 5-5)

    **1.** Most common inherited disorder in U.S. African American population; sickle cell trait found in 10% of African Americans.

    **2.** Autosomal recessive inheritance pattern.

    **3.** Individuals who are homozygous for the sickle cell gene have the disease (more than 80% of their hemoglobin is abnormal [HgbS]).

    **4.** Those who are heterozygous for the gene have sickle cell trait (normal hemoglobin predominates, may have 25–50% HgbS). Although sickle cell trait is not a disease, carriers may exhibit symptoms under periods of severe anoxia or dehydration.

    **5.** In this disease, the structure of hemoglobin is changed; the sixth rung of the beta chain changes glutamine for valine.

    **6.** HgbS (abnormal Hgb), which has reduced oxygen-carrying capacity, replaces all or part of the hemoglobin in the RBCs.

    **7.** When oxygen is released, the shape of the RBCs changes from round and pliable to crescent-shaped, rigid, and inflexible (see Figure 5-6).

    **8.** Local hypoxia and continued sickling lead to plugging of vessels.

    **9.** Sickled RBCs live for 6–20 days instead of 120, causing hemolytic anemia.

    **10.** Usually no symptoms prior to age 6 months; presence of increased level of fetal hemoglobin tends to inhibit sickling.

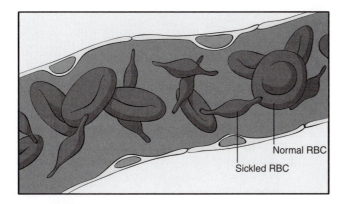

**Figure 5-6** Regular and sickled RBCs

**11.** Death often occurs in early adulthood due to occlusion or infection.

**12.** Sickle cell crisis

    **a.** Vaso-occlusive (thrombocytic) crisis: most common type

        **1)** Crescent-shaped RBCs clump together; agglutination causes blockage of small blood vessels.

        **2)** Blockage causes the blood viscosity to increase, producing sludging and resulting in further hypoxia and increased sickling.

    **b.** Splenic sequestration: often seen in toddler/preschooler

        **1)** Sickled cells block outflow tract resulting in sudden and massive collection of sickled cells in spleen.

        **2)** Blockage leads to hypovolemia and severe decrease in hemoglobin and blood pressure, leading to shock.

**B.** Medical management: sickle cell crisis

    **1.** Drug therapy

        **a.** Urea: interferes with hydrophobic bonds of the HgbS molecules

        **b.** Analgesics/narcotics to control pain

        **c.** Antibiotics to control infection

    **2.** Exchange transfusions

    **3.** Hydration: oral and IV

    **4.** Bed rest

    **5.** Surgery: splenectomy

**C.** Assessment findings

    **1.** First sign in infancy may be "colic" due to abdominal pain (abdominal infarct)

    **2.** Infants may have dactylitis (hand-foot syndrome): symmetrical painful soft tissue swelling of hands and feet in absence of trauma (aseptic, self-limiting)

    **3.** Splenomegaly: initially due to hemolysis and phagocytosis; later due to fibrosis from repeated infarct to spleen

    **4.** Weak bones or spinal defects due to hyperplasia of marrow and osteoporosis

    **5.** Frequent infections, especially with *H. influenzae* and *D. pneumoniae*

    **6.** Leg ulcers, especially in adolescents, due to blockage of blood supply to skin of legs

    **7.** Delayed growth and development, especially delay in sexual development

    **8.** CVA/infarct in the CNS

    **9.** Renal failure: difficulty concentrating urine due to infarcts; enuresis

    **10.** Heart failure due to hemosiderosis

    **11.** Priapism: may result in impotence

    **12.** Pain wherever vaso-occlusive crisis occurs

    **13.** Development of collateral circulation

    **14.** Diagnostic tests

        **a.** Hgb indicates anemia, usually 6–9 g/dL

        **b.** Sickling tests

            **1)** Sickle cell test: deoxygenation of a drop of blood on a slide with a cover slip; takes several hours for results to be read; false negatives for the trait possible.

    2) Sickledex: a drop of blood from a finger stick is mixed with a solution; mixture turns cloudy in presence of HgbS; results available within a few minutes; false negatives in anemia clients or young infants possible.

   c. Hgb electrophoresis: diagnostic for the disease and the trait; provides accurate, fast results.

D. Nursing interventions: sickle cell crisis
1. Keep child well hydrated and oxygenated.
2. Avoid tight clothing that could impair circulation.
3. Keep wounds clean and dry.
4. Provide bed rest to decrease energy expenditure and oxygen use.
5. Correct metabolic acidosis.
6. Administer medications as ordered.
   a. Analgesics: acetaminophen, Ketoralac (NSAID), morphine (avoid aspirin as it enhances acidosis, which promotes sickling).
   b. Avoid anticoagulants (sludging is not due to clotting)
   c. Antibiotics
7. Administer blood transfusions as ordered.
8. Keep arms and legs from becoming cold.
9. Decrease emotional stress.
10. Provide good skin care, especially to legs.
11. Test siblings for presence of sickle cell trait/disease.
12. Provide client teaching and discharge planning concerning:
   a. Pre-op teaching for splenectomy if needed
   b. Genetic counseling
   c. Need to avoid activities that interfere with oxygenation, such as mountain climbing, flying in unpressurized planes

# Disorders of Platelets or Clotting Mechanism

## Immune Thrombocytopenic Purpura (ITP)

A. General information
1. Formerly known as idiopathic thrombocytopenic purpura
2. Increased destruction of platelets with resultant platelet count of less than 100,000/mm$^3$ characterized by petechiae and ecchymoses of the skin
3. Autoimmune disorder; onset sudden, often preceded by a viral illness

4. The spleen is the site for destruction of platelets; spleen is not enlarged
B. Medical management
1. Drug therapy: steroids, immunosuppressive agents, anti-D antibody
2. Platelet transfusion
3. Surgery: splenectomy
C. Assessment findings
1. Petechiae: spider-web appearance of bleeding under skin due to small size of platelets
2. Ecchymosis
3. Blood in any body secretions, bleeding from mucous membranes, nosebleeds
4. Diagnostic tests: platelet count decreases, anemia
D. Nursing interventions
1. Control bleeding
   a. Administer platelet transfusions as ordered.
   b. Apply pressure to bleeding sites as needed.
   c. Position bleeding part above heart level if possible.
2. Prevent bruising.
3. Provide support to client and be sensitive to change in body image.
4. Protect from infection.
5. Measure normal circumference of extremities for baseline.
6. Administer medications orally, rectally, or IV, rather than IM; if administering immunizations, give subcutaneously (SC) and hold pressure on site for 5 minutes.
7. Administer analgesics (acetaminophen) as ordered; avoid aspirin.
8. Provide care for the client with a splenectomy.
9. Provide client teaching and discharge planning concerning:
   a. Pad crib and playpen, use rugs wherever possible.
   b. Provide soft toys.
   c. Sew pads in knees and elbows of clothing.
   d. Provide protective headgear during toddlerhood.
   e. Use soft Toothettes instead of bristle toothbrushes.
   f. Keep weight to low normal to decrease extra stress on joints.
   g. Use stool softeners to prevent straining.
   h. Avoid contact sports; suggest swimming, biking, golf, billiards.

## Hemophilia

A. General information
1. A group of bleeding disorders in which there is a deficit of one of several factors in clotting mechanism
2. Sex-linked, inherited disorder; classic form affects males only

3. Types
   a. Hemophilia A: factor VIII deficiency (75% of all hemophilia)
   b. Hemophilia B (Christmas disease): factor IX deficiency (10–12% of all hemophilia)
   c. Hemophilia C: factor XI deficiency (autosomal recessive, affects both sexes)
4. Only the intrinsic system is involved; platelets are not affected, but fibrin clot does not always form; bleeding from minor cuts may be stopped by platelets.
5. If individual has less than 20–30% of factor VIII or IX, there is an impairment of clotting and clot is jelly-like.
6. Bleeding in neck, mouth, and thorax requires immediate professional care.

B. Assessment findings
   1. Prolonged bleeding after minor injury
      a. At birth after cutting of cord
      b. Following circumcision
      c. Following IM immunizations
      d. Following loss of baby teeth
      e. Increased bruising as child learns to crawl and walk
   2. Bruising and hematomas but no petechiae
   3. Peripheral neuropathies (due to bleeding near peripheral nerves): pain, paresthesias, muscle atrophy
   4. Hemarthrosis
      a. Repeated bleeding into a joint results in a swollen and painful joint with limited mobility
      b. May result in contractures and possible degeneration of joint
      c. Knees, ankles, elbows, wrists most often affected
   5. Diagnostic tests
      a. Platelet count normal
      b. Prolonged coagulation time: PTT increased
      c. Anemia

C. Nursing interventions
   1. Control acute bleeding episode.
      a. Apply ice compress for vasoconstriction.
      b. Immobilize area to prevent clots from being dislodged.
      c. Elevate affected extremity above heart level.
      d. Provide manual pressure or pressure dressing for 15 minutes; do not keep lifting dressing to check for bleeding status.
      e. Maintain calm environment to decrease pulse.
      f. Avoid sutures, cauterization, aspirin: all exacerbate bleeding.
      g. Administer hemostatic agents as ordered.
         1) Fibrin foam
         2) Topical application of adrenalin/epinephrine to promote vasoconstriction

2. Provide care for hemarthrosis.
   a. Immobilize joint and control acute bleeding.
   b. Elevate joint in a slightly flexed position.
   c. Avoid excessive handling of joint.
   d. Administer analgesics as ordered; pain relief will minimize increases in pulse rate and blood loss.
   e. Aspirin should not be given because it inhibits platelet function.
   f. Instruct to avoid weight bearing for 48 hours after bleeding episode if bleeding is in lower extremities.
   g. Provide active or passive ROM exercises after bleeding has been controlled (48 hours), as long as exercises do not cause pain or irritate trauma site.
3. Administer factor VIII concentrate, or DDAVP as ordered
4. Provide client teaching and discharge planning concerning
   a. Prevention of trauma (see Immune Thrombocytopenic Purpura)
   b. Genetic counseling
      1) When mother is carrier: 50% chance with each pregnancy for sons to have hemophilia, 50% chance with each pregnancy for daughters to be carriers
      2) When father has hemophilia, mother is normal: no chance for children to have disease, but all daughters will be carriers
   c. Availability of support/counseling agencies

# Disorder of White Blood Cells

## Infectious Mononucleosis

A. General information
   1. Viral infection that causes hyperplasia of lymphoid tissue and a characteristic change in mononuclear cells of the blood
   2. Affects adolescents and young adults most commonly
   3. Caused by the Epstein-Barr virus, which is not highly contagious but is transmitted by saliva (the "kissing disease")
   4. Incubation period 2–6 weeks
   5. Pathophysiology: mononuclear infiltration of lymph nodes and other body tissue

B. Assessment findings
   1. Lethargy
   2. Sore throat/tonsilitis
   3. Lymphadenopathy; enlarged spleen, liver involvement
   4. Diagnostic tests
      a. Atypical WBCs increased
      b. Heterophil antibody and Monospot tests positive

**77.** The mother of a child with classic hemophilia asks the nurse what her chances are of having another child with hemophilia. What is the nurse's best response?
  1. "All of your daughters will be carriers of the disease."
  2. "If you have another son, there is almost a 100% chance he will have hemophilia."
  3. "If you have a son, there is a 50% chance he will have hemophilia but none of your daughters are likely to have it."
  4. "There is a 25% chance of having another child with hemophilia."

**78.** A 4-year-old male has been diagnosed as having iron deficiency anemia. A liquid iron preparation has been prescribed. What intervention will the nurse include in the medication administration?
  1. Ask the child if he wants to take his medicine.
  2. Mix the medication in his milk bottle and give it to him at nap time.
  3. Allow him to sip the medication through a straw.
  4. Give the medication after lunch with a sweet dessert to disguise the taste.

**79.** A 10-year-old has hemophilia A and is admitted to the hospital for hemarthrosis of the right knee. He is in a great deal of pain. Which of the following interventions would aggravate his condition?
  1. Applying an ice bag to the affected knee.
  2. Administering children's aspirin for pain relief.
  3. Elevating the right leg above the level of his heart.
  4. Keeping the right leg immobilized.

**80.** Which is a correct statement regarding a client with the sickle cell trait?
  1. The client has a chronic form of sickle cell anemia.
  2. The client has the most lethal form of the disease.
  3. The client will transmit the disease to all children.
  4. The client has some normal and some abnormal hemoglobin cells.

**81.** The mother of a child with sickle cell anemia tells the nurse that she learned that sickled blood cells do not have as long a life expectancy as normal red cells. Which answer would be correct for the nurse to tell the mother regarding how long a sickled blood cell survives?
  1. 5 days.
  2. 15 days.
  3. 30 days.
  4. 60 days.

**82.** What symptom would the child with sickle cell exhibit?
  1. Vitiligo.
  2. Hyperactivity.
  3. Mild mental retardation.
  4. Delayed physical development.

**83.** A child who has sickle cell anemia has developed stasis ulcers on her lower extremities. What is the cause of the ulcers?
  1. Poor range of motion.
  2. Ruptured blood vessels.
  3. Impaired venous circulation.
  4. Hypertrophy of muscular tissue.

**84.** Which complication is associated with sickle cell anemia?
  1. Constipation.
  2. Hypothyroidism.
  3. Addison's disease.
  4. Cerebrovascular accidents.

**85.** Both parents carry the sickle cell anemia trait. Their 8-month-old child contracted chickenpox from his brother and now is very weak, febrile, and anorexic, and cries with pain when his wrists and elbows are moved. He is admitted to the hospital with a diagnosis of sickle cell crisis. The child's mother asks the nurse why he has not been symptomatic before now. What would be the nurse's best response?
  1. High fetal hemoglobin protected him against sickling.
  2. His red blood cell levels remained normal.
  3. Maternal antibodies protected him against sickling.
  4. Sickle cell hemoglobin was not present until about 1 year of life.

**86.** In planning care for a child with newly diagnosed sickle cell anemia, what should his mother be taught to prevent vaso-occlusive crises?
  1. Prophylactic administration of acetaminophen.
  2. Eating food with a high iron content.

3. Exercising regularly.

   4. Promoting hydration.

87. How could the nurse best evaluate whether parents are giving their child with iron deficiency anemia iron as prescribed?

   1. Parents state they offer orange juice when they give the medication.

   2. Parents state the child has greenish black stools.

   3. Parents state the child experiences nausea with the iron preparation.

   4. Parents state they are giving the iron as prescribed.

88. Parents of a child who has sickle-cell anemia want to know why their child did not have the first episode until he was approximately a year old. What would be the best reply from the nurse?

   1. "Are you sure your child has sickle-cell anemia and not sickle-cell trait?"

   2. "Affected children can be asymptomatic in infancy because of high levels of fetal hemoglobin that inhibit sickling."

   3. "Have you asked your doctor about this?"

   4. "Your child probably had a crisis and you did not realize it."

89. A 5-year-old is admitted to the nursing care unit in vaso-occlusive crisis from sickle cell anemia. What is the priority nursing intervention?

   1. Teaching the family about sickle cell anemia and home care needs.

   2. Managing the child's pain.

   3. Encouraging a high-protein, high-calorie diet.

   4. Administering oxygen via nasal cannula.

90. A 3-year-old with a recent history of chickenpox is admitted to the unit with immune thrombocytopenic purpura. His platelet count is 15,000 mm$^3$/dL. His lesions are enlarging. Which of the following nursing actions best provides for the child's safety?

   1. Supervised outdoor play.

   2. Set times of rest periods.

   3. Only allowing him to have soft stuffed toys to play with.

   4. Keeping him on complete bed rest.

91. A child is admitted to the pediatric unit with hemarthrosis secondary to hemophilia. What would be the most appropriate nursing intervention?

   1. Daily bleeding times.

   2. Prophylactic antibiotic therapy.

   3. Elevating and immobilizing the affected joint.

   4. Encouraging active range of motion of affected joint.

## Answers and Rationales

77. **3.** Classic hemophilia is inherited as an X-linked recessive trait. If this family has another son, there is a 50% chance that he will have the disease. If they have a daughter she is very unlikely to have the disease but there is a 50% chance she will be a carrier.

78. **3.** Iron is given with a straw to prevent staining the teeth.

79. **2.** Aspirin is an anticoagulant. The child has a clotting disorder and has been bleeding into his knee joint. He should not receive an anticoagulant.

80. **4.** Clients with sickle cell trait inherit only one defective gene. They can synthesize both normal and abnormal hemoglobin chains.

81. **2.** The life span of a sickled cell is 6 to 20 days as opposed to 120 days for a normal red blood cell.

82. **4.** Children with sickle cell disease usually manifest growth impairment.

83. **3.** The tissues of a client with sickle cell disease are constantly vulnerable to microcirculatory interruptions.

84. **4.** The sudden appearance of a stroke in sickle cell anemia is related to the microcirculatory interruptions that are caused by the sickled cell.

85. **1.** High levels of fetal hemoglobin inhibit sickling of red cells prior to the age of 6 months.

86. **4.** Promoting good hydration is a major factor in maintaining the blood viscosity needed to maximize the circulation of red blood cells. Dehydration causes sickling of red blood cells.

87. **2.** When an adequate dosage of iron is reached, the stools usually turn a greenish black. Absence of this color stool usually gives a clue to poor compliance.

88. **2.** Children with sickle-cell anemia are often asymptomatic until at least 4 to 6 months of age.

A crisis is usually precipitated by an acute upper respiratory or gastrointestinal infection.

**89. 4.** During a vaso-occlusive crisis, tissue hypoxia and ischemia cause pain. By delivering oxygen at the prescribed rate, further tissue hypoxia can be avoided.

**90. 4.** Initially when his platelets are below 20,000 mm³/dL and he is experiencing active bleeding or progression of lesions, activity is restricted.

**91. 3.** During bleeding episodes, hemarthrosis is managed by elevating and immobilizing the joint and applying ice packs.

# The Respiratory System

## VARIATIONS FROM THE ADULT

A. Infants are obligatory nose breathers and diaphragmatic breathers.
B. Number and size of alveoli continue to increase until age 8 years.
C. Until age 5, structures of the respiratory tract have a narrower lumen and children are more susceptible to obstruction/distress from inflammation.
D. Normal respiratory rate in children is faster than in adults.
   1. Infants: 40–60/minute
   2. 1 year: 20–40/minute
   3. 2–4 years: 20–30/minute
   4. 5–10 years: 20–25/minute
   5. 10–15 years: 17–22/minute
   6. 15 and older: 15–20/minute
E. Most episodes of acute illness in young children involve the respiratory system due to frequent exposure to infection and a general lack of immunity.

## ASSESSMENT

### History

A. Presenting problem: symptoms may include cough, wheezing, dyspnea
B. Medical history: incidence of infections, respiratory allergies or asthma, prescribed and OTC medications, recent immunizations
C. Exposure to other children with respiratory infections or other communicable diseases

### Physical Examination

A. Inspect shape of chest; note:
   1. Barrel chest: occurs with chronic respiratory disease.
   2. Pectus carinatum (pigeon breast): sternum protrudes outward, producing increased A–P diameter; usually not significant.
   3. Pectus excavatum (funnel chest): lower part of sternum is depressed; usually does not produce symptoms; may impair cardiac function.
B. Note pattern of respirations.
   1. Rate
   2. Regularity
      a. Periodic respirations (periods of rapid respirations, separated by periods of slow breathing or short periods of no respirations) normal in young infants
      b. Apnea episodes (cessation of breathing for 20 seconds or more accompanied by color change or bradycardia) an abnormal finding
   3. Respiratory effort
      a. Nasal flaring: attempt to widen airway and decrease resistance
      b. Open-mouth breathing: chin drops with each inhalation
      c. Retractions: from use of accessory muscles
C. Observe skin color and temperature, particularly mucous membranes and peripheral extremities.
D. Note behavior: position of comfort, signs of irritability or lethargy, facial expression (anxiety).
E. Note speech abnormalities: hoarseness or muffled speech.
F. Observe presence and quality of cough: productive; paroxysmal, with inspiratory "whoop" characteristic of pertussis.
G. Auscultate for abnormal breath sounds (auscultation may be more difficult in infants and young children because of shallowness of respirations).
   1. Grunting on expiration
   2. Stridor: harsh inspiratory sound associated with obstruction or edema
   3. Wheezing: whistling noise during inspiration or expiration due to narrowed airways, common in asthma
   4. "Snoring": noisy breathing associated with nasal obstruction

## Laboratory/Diagnostic Tests

**A.** Pulmonary function testing is usually not done under age 6 years because children have difficulty following directions.

**B.** Chest X-rays: avoid unnecessary exposure; protect gonads and thyroid.

# ANALYSIS

Nursing diagnoses for the child with a disorder of the respiratory system may include:

**A.** Activity intolerance

**B.** Altered respiratory functions: ineffective airway clearance, ineffective breathing pattern, impaired gas exchange

**C.** Anxiety

**D.** Fatigue

**E.** Impaired oral mucous membrane

**F.** Altered nutrition

**G.** Disturbed sleep pattern

**H.** Acute pain

**I.** Deficient knowledge (caregiver) (specify)

# PLANNING AND IMPLEMENTATION

## Goals

**A.** Child will have patent airway and satisfactory oxygenation.

**B.** Child will be free from symptoms of respiratory distress.

**C.** Child will have improved ability to tolerate exercise, conserve energy.

**D.** Parents will participate in caring for child.

## Interventions

### Oxygen Tent (Croup Tent, Mist Tent, Oxygen Canopy)

**A.** General information
1. Used when desired oxygen concentration is 40% or less as oxygen concentration can be difficult to control
2. Primarily used for croup, when mist is to be delivered

**B.** Nursing care
1. Keep sides of plastic down and tucked in.
2. If tent has been opened for awhile, increase oxygen flow to raise concentration quickly.
3. If child has been out of the tent, return oxygen concentration to ordered percent before returning child to tent.
4. If tent enclosure gets too warm, add ice to cooling chamber as needed.
5. Mist is usually prescribed in addition to oxygen
   a. Keep reservoir for humidification filled.
   b. Do not allow condensation on tent walls to obstruct view of child.
   c. Keep clothes and bedding dry to avoid chilling.
6. Provide safety measures.
   a. Keep plastic away from child's face.
   b. Avoid toys that produce spark or friction, such as mechanical toys.
   c. Avoid stuffed toys because of tendency to absorb moisture.
   d. Encourage use of one or two favorite toys or transitional object in tent; other toys may be kept outside of tent in child's view.

### Vaporizers

**A.** General information
1. Same principle as oxygen tent
2. Used at home; placed at bedside; mist directed into room around child
3. Usually cool mist

**B.** Nursing responsibilities: teach parents to clean frequently because bacteria that grow in vaporizer can be dispersed into air.

### Chest Physical Therapy

**A.** Postural drainage: infants and young children do not have enough rib cage for a lower front position
1. Combine side and lower front positions
2. Five positions: upper front, upper back, lower back, right side and front, and left side and front
3. 2–5 minutes per position

**B.** Percussion
1. Do not use with clients with an acute attack of asthma or croup (dislodged mucus may cause plugging because of bronchial edema).
2. Use percussion 30 minutes before meals to clear mucus before eating, thus enhancing intake.
3. If aerosol medications are being used, administer immediately before percussion.
4. Percussion is done with cupped hand, never on bare skin, over the rib cage only
   a. Use an undershirt, gown, or diaper over skin.
   b. If infant's chest is too small for nurse's hand, a small face mask can be substituted.
   c. Be careful to avoid spine and neck during percussion.
   d. Infants can be percussed while being held on nurse's lap.
   e. If child is unable to cough during and after percussion, suction as needed.

**C.** Vibration: performed on expiration.

## Suctioning

A. Bulb syringes can be used to clear nasal stuffiness.
B. For nasotracheal and nasopharyngeal suction, use low pressure.
C. Assess response, and for improved respiratory status.

## Deep Breathing Exercises

A. Encourage deep breathing by making exercises into games (e.g., touch toes, sit-ups, jumping jacks, blowing out "flashlight," ping-pong ball games using blowing).
B. Encourage use of toys that require blowing (harmonica, bubbles).
C. Laughing and crying also stimulate coughing and deep breathing.

## Apnea Monitor

A. General information: monitors often use same three chest leads for simultaneous cardiac and respiratory rate monitoring
   1. Lead placement will differ from that usually prescribed for cardiac monitoring if apnea monitoring is also required.
   2. To monitor respiratory rate, chest leads will need to be where chest moves during inspiration.
   3. As chest wall movement rather than air entry is monitored, obstruction and dyspnea may not be recognized early.
   4. Most useful for early recognition of cessation of breathing.
B. Nursing care: when alarm sounds
   1. Note whether cardiac or respiratory rate has triggered alarm.
   2. Assess child's color, activity, and presence of respiratory effort.
   3. Auscultate cardiac and respiratory sounds.
   4. If no physical distress, check lead placement.
   5. If apneic, gently stimulate lower extremities. May need oxygen.
   6. If no improvement with stimulation and oxygen, assess need for cardiopulmonary resuscitation (CPR).

# EVALUATION

A. Child is satisfactorily oxygenated.
   1. Absence of respiratory distress
   2. Normal color and activity
   3. Decreased need for supplementary oxygen therapy
B. Parents are able to care for child at home.
   1. Identify symptoms of increased oxygen need
   2. Perform prescribed treatments
   3. Have obtained and demonstrated use of necessary equipment

# DISORDERS OF THE RESPIRATORY SYSTEM

## Tonsillitis

A. General information
   1. Inflammation of tonsils often as a result of a viral or bacterial pharyngitis
   2. 10–15% caused by group A beta-hemolytic streptococci
B. Medical management
   1. Comfort measures and symptomatic relief
   2. Antibiotics for bacterial infection, usually penicillin or erythromycin
   3. Surgery: removal of tonsils/adenoids if necessary
C. Assessment findings
   1. Enlarged, red tonsils; fever
   2. Sore throat, difficulty swallowing, mouth breathing, snoring
   3. White patches of exudate on tonsillar pillars, enlarged cervical lymph nodes
D. Nursing interventions
   1. Provide soft or liquid diet.
   2. Use cool-mist vaporizer.
   3. Administer salt water gargles, throat lozenges.
   4. Administer analgesics (acetaminophen) as ordered.
   5. Administer antibiotics as ordered; stress to parents importance of completing entire course of medication.

## Tonsillectomy

A. General information
   1. One of the most common operations performed on children
   2. Indications for tonsillectomy include recurrent tonsillitis, peritonsillar abscess, airway or esophageal obstruction
   3. Indications for adenoidectomy include nasal obstruction due to hypertrophy
B. Nursing interventions: preoperative
   1. Make pre-op preparation age-appropriate; child enters the hospital feeling well and will leave with a very sore throat.
   2. Obtain baseline bleeding and clotting times.
   3. Check for any loose teeth.
C. Nursing interventions: postoperative
   1. Position on side or abdomen to facilitate drainage of secretions.
   2. Avoid suctioning if possible; if not, be especially careful to avoid trauma to surgical site.
   3. Provide ice collar/analgesia for pain.
   4. Observe for hemorrhage; signs may include frequent swallowing, increased pulse, vomiting bright red blood (vomiting old dried blood or pink-tinged emesis is normal).

5. Offer clear, cool, noncitrus, nonred fluids when awake and alert.
6. Provide client teaching and discharge planning concerning:
   a. Need to maintain adequate fluid and food intake and to avoid spicy and irritating foods
   b. Quiet activity for a few days
   c. Need to avoid coughing, mouth gargles
   d. Chewing gum (but not Aspergum): can help relieve pain and difficulty swallowing and aids in diminishing bad breath
   e. Mild analgesics for pain
   f. Signs and symptoms of bleeding and need to report to physician

## Acute Spasmodic Laryngitis (Croup)

A. General information
   1. Respiratory distress characterized by paroxysmal attacks of laryngeal obstruction
   2. Etiology unclear but familial predisposition, allergy, viruses, psychologic factors, and anxious temperament have been implicated
   3. Common in children ages 1–3 years
   4. Attacks occur mostly at night; onset sudden and usually preceded by a mild upper respiratory infection
   5. Respiratory symptoms last several hours; may occur in a milder form on a few subsequent nights
B. Assessment findings
   1. Inspiratory stridor, hoarseness, barking cough, anxiety, retractions
   2. Afebrile, skin cool
C. Nursing interventions
   1. Instruct parents to take the child into the bathroom, close the door, turn on the hot water, and sit on floor of the steamy bathroom with child.
   2. If the laryngeal spasm does not subside the child should be taken to the emergency department.
   3. After the spasm subsides, provide cool mist with a vaporizer.
   4. Provide clear fluids.
   5. Try to keep child calm and quiet.
   6. Assure parents this is self-limiting.

## Laryngotracheobronchitis

A. General information
   1. Viral infection of the larynx that may extend into trachea and bronchi
   2. Most common cause for stridor in febrile child
   3. Parainfluenza viruses most common cause
   4. Infection causes endothelial insult, increased mucus production, edema, low-grade fever
   5. Affects children less than 5 years of age
   6. Onset more gradual than with croup, takes longer to resolve; usually develops over several days with upper respiratory infection
   7. Usually treated on outpatient basis; indications for admission include dehydration and respiratory compromise
B. Medical management
   1. Drug therapy
      a. Aerosolized racemic epinephrine
      b. Antibiotics only if secondary bacterial infection present
      c. Steroids
   2. Oxygen therapy: low concentrations to relieve mild hypoxia
   3. Oral or nasotracheal intubation for moderate hypoxia
   4. IV fluids to maintain hydration
C. Assessment findings
   1. Fever, coryza, inspiratory stridor, barking cough, tachycardia, tachypnea, retractions
   2. May have difficulty taking fluids
   3. WBC normal
D. Nursing interventions
   1. Instruct parents to take child into steamy bathroom for acute distress.
   2. Keep child calm.
   3. After distress subsides, use cool mist vaporizer in bedroom.
   4. Child may vomit large amounts of mucus after the episode; reassure parents that this is normal.
   5. For hospitalized child
      a. Monitor vital signs, I&O, skin color, and respiratory effort.
      b. Maintain hydration.
      c. Provide care for the intubated child.
      d. Plan care to disturb the child as little as possible.

## Epiglottitis

A. General information
   1. Life-threatening bacterial infection of epiglottis and surrounding structures
   2. Primary organism: *H. influenzae,* type B
   3. Often preceded by upper respiratory infection
   4. Rapid progression of swelling causes reduction in airway diameter; may lead to sudden respiratory arrest
   5. Affects children ages 3–7 years
B. Assessment findings
   1. Fever, tachycardia, inspiratory stridor (possibly), labored respirations with retractions, sore throat, dysphagia, drooling, muffled voice
   2. Irritability, restlessness, anxious-looking, quiet
   3. Position: sitting upright, head forward and jaw thrust out
   4. Diagnostic tests
      a. WBC increased
      b. Lateral neck X-ray reveals characteristic findings

C. Nursing interventions
1. Provide mist tent with oxygen.
2. Administer IV antibiotics as ordered.
3. Provide tracheostomy or endotracheal tube care; note the following:
   a. Restlessness, fatigue, dyspnea, cyanosis, pallor, tachycardia, tachypnea, diminished breath sounds, adventitious lung sounds.
   b. Need for suctioning to remove secretions; note amount, color, consistency.
4. Reassure child through touch, sound, and physically being present.
5. Involve parents in all aspects of care.
6. Avoid direct examination of the epiglottis as it may precipitate spasm and obstruction.
7. Remember this is extremely frightening experience for child and parents; explain procedures and findings; reinforce explanations of physician.

# Bronchiolitis

A. General information
1. Pulmonary viral infection characterized by wheezing
2. Usually caused by respiratory syncytial virus
3. Virus invades epithelial cells of nasopharynx and spreads to lower respiratory tract, causing increased mucus production, decreased diameter of bronchi, hyperinflation, and possible atelectasis
4. Affects infants ages 2–8 months
5. Increased incidence of asthma as child grows older

B. Medical management
1. Nebulized bronchodilators (e.g., Albuterol)
2. Steroids
3. Ribavirin—antiviral, given by aerosol (SPAG) through hood, tent, mask, or ventilator—for severe symptoms
4. Humidity, oxygen, fluids
5. Prevention: RSV antibodies
   a. RSV-IG (immune globulin)-given IV monthly
   b. Palivizumab (Synagis)-given IM monthly

C. Assessment findings
1. Difficulty feeding, fever
2. Cough, coryza
3. Wheezing, prolonged expiratory phase, tachypnea, nasal flaring, retractions (intercostal more pronounced than supraclavicular retractions)
4. Diagnostic tests
   a. WBC normal
   b. X-ray reveals hyperaeration

D. Nursing interventions
1. Provide high-humidity environment, with oxygen in some cases (instruct parents to take child into steamy bathroom if at home).
2. Offer small, frequent feedings; clear fluids if trouble with secretions.
3. Provide adequate rest.
4. Administer antipyretics as ordered to control fever.

# Asthma

A. General information (See Figure 5-7.)
1. Obstructive disease of the lower respiratory tract
2. Most common chronic respiratory disease in children, in younger children affects twice as many boys as girls; incidence equal by adolescence
3. Often caused by an allergic reaction to an environmental allergen, may be seasonal or year-round
4. Immunologic/allergic reaction results in histamine release, which produces three main airway responses
   a. Edema of mucous membranes
   b. Spasm of the smooth muscle of bronchi and bronchioles
   c. Accumulation of tenacious secretions
5. Status asthmaticus occurs when there is little response to treatment and symptoms persist

Normal

Asthma

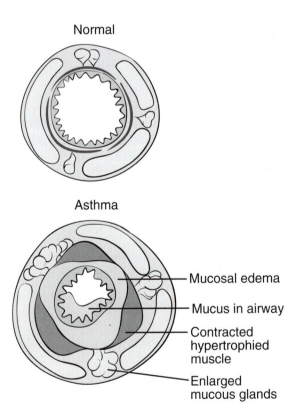

- Mucosal edema
- Mucus in airway
- Contracted hypertrophied muscle
- Enlarged mucous glands

**Figure 5-7** Pathophysiology of asthma

B. Medical management
   1. Drug therapy: Bronchodilators
      a. Beta-adrenergic agonists
         1) Metered dose inhaler (MDI)—most children will need spacers
         2) Nebulizer—infants and toddlers
         3) Rescue drugs for acute attacks
      b. Corticosteroids
         1) Inhaled by MDI or nebulizer
         2) Oral for persistent wheezing
         3) IV in hospital
      c. Nonsteroid anti-inflammatory agents
         1) Cromolyn sodium
         2) Nedocromil
         3) Leukotriene inhibitors and receptor-antagonists
         4) Used for maintenance, not rescue
      d. Xanthine-derivatives
         1) Theophylline (oral)
         2) Aminophylline (IV)
         3) Used for status asthmaticus
      e. Procedure for use of oral inhaler. See Figure 5-8.
   2. Physical therapy
   3. Hyposensitization
   4. Exercise
C. Assessment findings
   1. Family history of allergies
   2. Client history of eczema
   3. Respiratory distress: shortness of breath, expiratory wheeze, prolonged expiratory phase, air trapping (barrel chest if chronic), use of accessory muscles, irritability (from hypoxia), diaphoresis, change in sensorium if severe attack
   4. Diagnostic tests: ABGs indicate respiratory acidosis
D. Nursing interventions
   1. Place client in high-Fowler's position.
   2. Administer oxygen as ordered.
   3. Administer medications as ordered.
   4. Provide humidification/hydration to loosen secretions.
   5. Provide chest percussion and postural drainage when bronchodilation improves.
   6. Monitor for respiratory distress.
   7. Provide client teaching and discharge planning concerning:
      a. Modification of environment
         1) Ensure room is well ventilated.
         2) Stay indoors during grass cutting or when pollen count is high.
         3) Use damp dusting.
         4) Avoid rugs, draperies or curtains, stuffed animals.
         5) Avoid natural fibers (wool and feathers).
      b. Importance of moderate exercise (swimming is excellent)
      c. Purpose of breathing exercises (to increase the end expiratory pressure of each respiration)

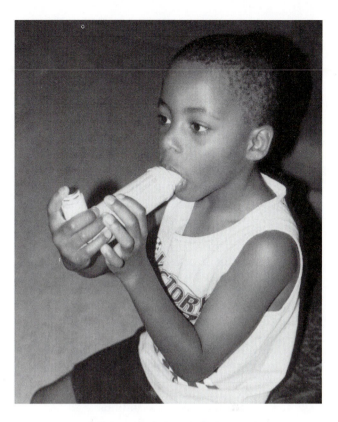

1. Attach metered dose inhaler canister to mouthpiece to spacer.
2. Shake to increase pressure in canister.
3. Blow out air.
4. Place mouthpiece in mouth and make a seal with lips.
5. Activate the canister.
6. Breathe in slowly to total lung capacity.
7. Hold breath for 5–10 seconds, then breathe normally. (For infants and small children, a mask should be used and remain in place until they have taken 5–6 breaths.)
8. Wait 60 seconds.
9. Repeat steps 2–7.
10. Rinse mouth and equipment following use to prevent fungal infections.

**Figure 5-8** Instructions for use of an oral inhaler with spacer

## Aspiration of a Foreign Object

A. General information
   1. Relatively common airway problem.
   2. Severity depends on object (e.g., pins, coins, nuts, buttons, parts of toys) aspirated and the degree of obstruction.
   3. Depending on object aspirated, symptoms will increase over hours or weeks.
   4. The curious toddler is most frequently affected.

5. If object does not pass trachea immediately, respiratory distress will be evident.
6. If object moves beyond tracheal region, it will pass into one of the main stem bronchi; symptoms will be vague, insidious.
7. Causes 400 deaths per year in children under age 4.

B. Medical management
1. Objects in upper airway require immediate removal.
2. Lower airway obstruction is less urgent (bronchoscopy or laryngoscopy).

C. Assessment findings
1. Sudden onset of coughing, dyspnea, wheezing, stridor, apnea (upper airway)
2. Persistent or recurrent pneumonia, persistent croupy cough or wheeze
3. Object not always visible on X-ray
4. Secondary infection

D. Nursing interventions
1. Perform Heimlich maneuver if indicated.
2. Reassure the scared toddler.
3. After removal, place child in high-humidity environment and treat secondary infection if applicable.
4. Counsel parents regarding age-appropriate behavior and safety precautions.

## Cystic Fibrosis (CF)

A. General information
1. Disorder characterized by dysfunction of the exocrine glands (mucus-producing glands of the respiratory tract, GI tract, pancreas, sweat glands, salivary glands)
2. Transmitted as an autosomal recessive trait
3. Incidence: According to Cystic Fibrosis Foundation: 30,000 Americans, 3000 Canadians, and 20,000 Europeans.
4. Most common lethal genetic disease among Caucasians in United States and Europe
5. Prenatal diagnosis of CF is not reliable
6. Secretions from mucous glands are thick, causing obstruction and fibrosis of tissue
7. Sweat and saliva have characteristic high levels of sodium chloride
8. Affected organs
   a. Pancreas: 85% of CF clients have pancreatic involvement
      1) Obstruction of pancreatic ducts and eventual fibrosis and atrophy of the pancreas leads to little or no release of enzymes (lipase [fats], amylase [starch], and trypsin [protein])
      2) Absence of enzymes causes malabsorption of fats and proteins
      3) Unabsorbed food fractions excreted in the stool produce steatorrhea
      4) Loss of nutrients and inability to absorb fat-soluble vitamins causes failure to thrive

   b. Respiratory tract: 99.9% of CF clients have respiratory involvement
      1) Increased production of secretions causes increased obstruction of airway, air trapping, and atelectasis
      2) Pulmonary congestion leads to cor pulmonale
      3) Eventually death occurs by drowning in own secretions
   c. Reproductive system
      1) Males are sterile
      2) Females can conceive, but increased mucus in vaginal tract makes conception more difficult
      3) Pregnancy causes increased stress on respiratory system of mother
   d. Liver: one third of clients have cirrhosis/portal hypertension
9. 95% of deaths are from abnormal mucus secretion and fibrosis in the lungs; shortened life span

B. Medical management
1. Pancreatic involvement: aimed at promoting absorption of nutrients
   a. Diet modification
      1) Infant: predigested formula
      2) Older children: may require high-calorie, high-protein, or low/limited-fat diet, but many CF clients tolerate normal diet
   b. Pancreatic enzyme supplementation: enzyme capsules, tablets, or powders (Pancrease, Cotazym, Viokase) given with meals and snacks
2. Respiratory involvement: goals are to maintain airway patency and to prevent lung infection
   a. Chest physiotherapy
   b. Antibiotics for infection

C. Assessment findings: symptoms vary greatly in severity and extent
1. Pancreatic involvement
   a. Growth failure; failure to thrive
   b. Stools are foul smelling, large, frequent, foamy, fatty (steatorrhea), contain undigested food
   c. Meconium ileus (meconium gets stuck in bowel due to lack of enzymes) in newborns
   d. Rectal prolapse is possible
   e. Voracious appetite
   f. Characteristic protruding abdomen with atrophy of extremities and buttocks
   g. Symptoms associated with deficiencies in the fat-soluble vitamins
   h. Anemia
   i. Diagnostic tests
      1) Trypsin decreased or absent in aspiration of duodenal contents
      2) Fecal fat in stool specimen increased
2. Respiratory involvement
   a. Signs of respiratory distress
   b. Barrel chest due to air trapping

c. Clubbing of digits
   d. Decreased exercise tolerance due to distress
   e. Frequent productive cough
   f. Frequent pseudomonas infections
   g. Diagnostic tests
      1) Chest X-ray reveals atelectasis, infiltrations, emphysemic changes
      2) Pulmonary function studies abnormal
      3) ABGs show respiratory acidosis
3. Electrolyte involvement
   a. Hyponatremia/heat exhaustion in hot weather
   b. Salty taste to sweat
   c. Diagnostic tests
      1) Pilocarpine iontophoresis sweat test: indicates 2–5 times normal amount of sodium and chloride in the sweat
      2) Fecal fat elevated
      3) Fecal trypsin absent or decreased
D. Nursing interventions
   1. Pancreatic involvement
      a. Administer pancreatic enzymes with meals as ordered: do not mix enzymes until ready to use them; best to mix in applesauce.
      b. Provide a high-calorie, high-carbohydrate (no empty-calorie foods), high-protein, normal-fat diet.
      c. Provide a double dose of multivitamins per day, especially fat-soluble vitamins (A, D, E, K), in water-soluble form.
      d. If low-fat diet required, MCT (medium-chain triglycerides) oil may be used.
   2. Respiratory involvement
      a. Administer antibiotics as ordered (all antibiotics for pseudomonas are given IV; doses may be above recommended levels (for virulent organisms).
      b. Administer expectorants, mucolytics (rarely used) as ordered.
      c. Avoid cough suppressants and antihistamines.
      d. Encourage breathing exercises.
      e. Provide percussion and postural drainage 4 times a day.
      f. Provide aerosol treatments as needed; handheld nebulizers, mask, intermittent positive pressure breathing (IPPB), mist tent.
   3. Electrolyte involvement
      a. Add salt to all meals, especially in summer.
      b. Give salty snacks (pretzels).
   4. Provide appropriate long-term support to child and family.
   5. Provide client teaching and discharge planning concerning:
      a. Genetic counseling

   b. Promotion of child's independence
   c. Avoidance of cigarette smoking in the house
   d. Availability of support groups/community agencies
   e. Alternative school education during extended hospitalization/home recovery

 ## Sample Questions

92. The nurse is caring for a child who had a tonsillectomy performed 4 hours ago. Which of the following is an abnormal finding and a cause for concern?
   1. An emesis of dried blood.
   2. Increased swallowing.
   3. Pink-tinged mucus.
   4. The child complains of a very sore throat.

93. A 7-year-old has been diagnosed as having cystic fibrosis. Chest physiotherapy has been ordered. When should chest percussion be performed?
   1. Before postural drainage.
   2. ½ hour before meals.
   3. Before an aerosol treatment.
   4. After suctioning.

94. The nurse is performing chest physiotherapy on a 6-year-old child who has congestion in his left lower lobe. In which position should the nurse place the child?
   1. Left side in semi-Fowler's position.
   2. Right side in semi-Fowler's position.
   3. Left side in Trendelenburg position.
   4. Right side in Trendelenburg position.

95. An infant is being evaluated for possible cystic fibrosis. The sweat test will show an elevation of which electrolyte?
   1. Chloride.
   2. Fluoride.
   3. Potassium.
   4. Calcium.

96. A 2-year-old is admitted to the hospital with cystic fibrosis. He is small for his age. What dietary suggestions can the nurse recommend to the child's mother to enhance his growth?
   1. Low-fat, low-residue, and high-potassium diet.
   2. Low-carbohydrate, soft diet with no sugar products.

3. High-carbohydrate, high-fat diet with extra water between meals.
4. High-protein, high-calorie meals with skim-milk milkshakes between meals.

97. The nurse is caring for a 2-year-old who has cystic fibrosis. His mother asks why the child developed cystic fibrosis. What explanation will the nurse provide?
   1. It develops due to meconium ileus at birth.
   2. It is an autosomal recessive genetic defect.
   3. It occurs during embryologic development.
   4. It results from chromosomal nondysjunction that occurred at conception.

98. A 2-year-old is admitted to the hospital and will need to stay for several days. The child's mother is unable to stay overnight because there is no one to care for her other children. What should the nurse recommend the mother do?
   1. Leave something of hers with the child and tell him she'll be back in the morning.
   2. Leave while he is in the playroom.
   3. Leave after he has fallen asleep.
   4. Tell him she'll be back in a few minutes after she has dinner.

99. The mother of a 2-year-old who has cystic fibrosis tells the nurse that the family is planning their first summer vacation. She wants to know if there are any special precautions needed because he has cystic fibrosis. What condition will the nurse state that children with cystic fibrosis are particularly susceptible?
   1. Severe sunburn.
   2. Infectious diarrhea.
   3. Heat exhaystion.
   4. Respiratory allergies.

100. A 4-year-old is admitted to the hospital for the treatment of an acute asthma attack. She received nebulized albuterol (Proventil) in the emergency department and was transferred to the pediatric unit with an aminophylline infusion. What significant finding will inform the nurse that the treatment is effective?
   1. A decrease in mucus production.
   2. A decrease in wheezing.
   3. An increase in blood pressure.
   4. A sleeping child.

101. A 12-month-old is hospitalized for a severe case of croup and has been placed in an oxygen tent. Today the oxygen order has been reduced from 35% to 25%. His blood gases are normal. The child refuses to stay in the oxygen tent. Attempts to placate him only cause him to become more upset. What would be an appropriate action for the nurse to perform?
   1. Restrain him in the tent and notify the physician.
   2. Take him out of the tent and notify the physician.
   3. Take him out of the tent and let him sit in the playroom.
   4. Tell him it will please his mother if he stays in the tent.

102. The nurse should recognize which of the following respiratory findings as normal in a 10-month-old infant?
   1. Respiratory rate of 60 at rest.
   2. Use of accessory muscles to assist in respiratory effort.
   3. Respiratory rate of 32 at rest.
   4. Diaphoresis with shallow respirations.

103. An 18-month-old presents with nasal flaring, intercostal and substernal retractions, and a respiratory rate of 50. What is the most appropriate nursing diagnosis?
   1. Knowledge deficit.
   2. Ineffective breathing pattern.
   3. Ineffective individual coping.
   4. High risk for altered body temperature: hyperthermia.

104. An 11-month-old is admitted to the hospital with bronchiolitis. He is currently in a croup tent with supplemental oxygen. Which toy is most appropriate for the nurse to recommend to the child's parents?
   1. A stuffed animal made from a washable fabric.
   2. A soft plastic stacking toy with multicolored rings.
   3. A set of wooden blocks.
   4. A pull toy.

105. Which of the following statements best assures the nurse that the parents understand the safety concerns related to use of a vaporizer at home?
   1. "I have a high dresser in the bedroom on which to place the vaporizer. The cord will be concealed behind the dresser."

2. "I plan to put the vaporizer on a stool next to the bed so that my child will get the most benefit from the cool mist."

3. "I purchased a warm mist vaporizer because I don't want my child to get chilled from the mist in her face."

4. "I thought I could just set the vaporizer on the floor next to the bed."

106. A 4-year-old is experiencing an acute asthma attack. Why should the nurse avoid chest percussion with this child?

1. Chest percussion may lead to increased bronchospasm and more respiratory distress.

2. Chest percussion may cause mucous plugging of the alveoli.

3. Chest percussion is useful in removing airway secretions and should be used.

4. Chest percussion will produce increased coughing and thereby enhance respiratory distress.

107. A 5-month-old has severe nasal congestion. What is the best way for the nurse to clear his nasal passages?

1. Administer saline nose drops and use a bulb syringe to clear passages.

2. Ask him to blow his nose and keep tissues handy.

3. Place him in a mist tent with 40% oxygen.

4. Administer vasoconstrictive nose drops before meals and at bedtime.

108. A 30-week gestation infant who had apnea of prematurity is ready for discharge and will be going home on apnea monitoring. What should the nurse teach the parents for proper use of the monitor?

1. The monitor is only used when the child is awake. It is not indicated at night or during naps.

2. The alarms on the monitor should be turned off when an attendant is with the infant.

3. The monitor should be kept on at all times except when the infant is being bathed. Careful attention to skin integrity and hygiene is important.

4. It is best for the parents to have 24-hour home health supervision to watch the infant while monitoring is required.

109. A 3-year-old underwent a tonsillectomy this morning. As the nurse giving discharge instructions, which comment by the child's mother suggests that she understands the care requirements?

1. "I plan to take her back to her play group tomorrow. I know she won't want to stay home."

2. "I have bought popsicles to give her later today."

3. "I will give her aspirin if she gets irritable."

4. "She is just waiting for the ice cream we promised her before she came to the hospital."

110. A 3-year-old boy presents in the ER with dysphagia, drooling, and respiratory difficulty that has increased significantly over the past 6 hours. The nurse should know that these findings are suggestive of which of the following conditions?

1. Croup.

2. Pneumonia.

3. Bronchopulmonary dysplasia.

4. Epiglottitis.

111. A 2-year-old presents to an urgent care center with respiratory distress and cyanosis. Parents report an initial episode of choking. What is the best initial action for the nurse to take?

1. Call 911 and have parents wait for an ambulance to transport the child to a pediatric hospital.

2. Administer oxygen by face mask and call the child's pediatrician.

3. Perform abdominal thrusts as described in the Heimlich maneuver.

4. Start CPR after the child loses consciousness.

 **Answers and Rationales**

**92. 2.** Increased swallowing could be a sign of hemorrhage from the surgical site.

**93. 2.** Chest percussion is done between meals to prevent vomiting, which might occur if done following meals.

**94. 4.** The affected lobe must be uppermost to be drained by gravity.

**95. 1.** There is increased excretion of chloride in the sweat of children with cystic fibrosis. A chloride level of over 60 mEq/liter is diagnostic for the disease.

96. **4.** A person with cystic fibrosis lacks pancreatic enzymes necessary for fat absorption. A diet high in protein and calories is necessary to meet the child's growth needs. Between-meal snacks, milkshakes made with skim milk may be given to provide additional protein, vitamins, and calories.

97. **2.** Cystic fibrosis is an autosomal recessive genetic disease. If both parents have the cystic fibrosis trait, each child has a 25% chance of developing the disease, a 50% chance of being a carrier, and a 25% chance of not having the disease.

98. **1.** Leaving something of his mother's with the child and telling him that she will be back in the morning is the best approach in developing trust between the mother and her child.

99. **3.** Persons with cystic fibrosis are prone to electrolyte imbalances due to increased loss of sodium and potassium in their sweat. The mother should avoid having her child become overheated and should frequently replenish body fluids with water or fruit juices.

100. **2.** Aminophylline is a bronchodilator. As it exerts its effects, wheezing will decrease.

101. **2.** The energy expended by the child in resisting the oxygen tent is causing increased respiratory effort. The child should be removed from the tent and closely monitored to be sure that he handles being in room air. The physician should be notified because the oxygen content of room air is only 20%, which is less than that ordered.

102. **3.** Rates of 20–40 breaths per minute are normal at this age.

103. **2.** The findings on assessment suggest respiratory distress. Ineffective breathing pattern is an appropriate diagnosis with the information now available.

104. **2.** Stacking toys with bright, large, colored plastic rings provide age-appropriate activity that is safe within the croup tent environment. The large rings can be held or stacked. They can be wiped down if damp. The size of the objects prevent them from creating any environmental hazards if the child is not continuously supervised.

105. **1.** It is best to keep the vaporizer out of the child's way. Concealing the cord and placing the appliance on a high surface is preferable.

106. **1.** During the course of an acute asthma attack, bronchospasm is a significant problem. Chest percussion can enhance the bronchospasm, leading to more pronounced respiratory distress.

107. **1.** Saline nose drops will help loosen secretions. The bulb syringe is necessary because the child is not old enough to effectively blow his nose.

108. **3.** Although apneic episodes are most common during sleep, they can occur at other times. Initially, it is particularly advisable to use the monitor continually except when bathing the infant.

109. **2.** Clear liquids are a good choice during the first 24 hours after surgery. Popsicles are appealing to children while providing fluids. They are less likely to irritate the surgical site than juices.

110. **4.** Epiglottitis is a medical emergency. The drooling and dysphagia are most often diagnostic of this condition.

111. **3.** The reported episode of choking and the child's condition suggest foreign body aspiration. The Heimlich maneuver should be attempted as an initial action to remove the object.

# The Gastrointestinal System

## VARIATIONS FROM THE ADULT

A. Mechanical functions of digestion are immature at birth.
1. No voluntary control over swallowing until 6 weeks
2. Stomach capacity decreased
3. Peristalsis increased, faster emptying time, more prone to diarrhea
4. Relaxed cardiac sphincter contributes to tendency to regurgitate food

B. Liver functions (glyconeogenesis and storage of vitamins) are immature throughout infancy.

C. Production of mucosal-lining antibodies is decreased.

**D.** Gastric acidity is low in infants, slowly rises until age 10, and then increases again during adolescence to reach adult levels.

**E.** Secretory cells are functional at birth, but efficiency of enzymes impaired by lower gastric pH.

**F.** Infant has decreased saliva, which causes decreased ability to digest starches.

**G.** Digestive processes are mature by toddlerhood.

**H.** Completion of myelinization of spinal cord allows voluntary control of elimination.

## ASSESSMENT

### History

**A.** Presenting problem: symptoms may include:
1. Vomiting: type, color, amount, relationship to eating or other events
2. Abnormal bowel habits: diarrhea, constipation, bleeding
3. Weight loss or growth failure
4. Pain: location; relationship to meals or other events; effect on sleep, play, appetite
5. Any other parental concerns

**B.** Diet/nutrition history: appetite, daily caloric intake, food intolerances, feeding schedule, nutritional deficits

### Physical Examination

**A.** General appearance
1. Plot height and weight on growth chart.
2. Measure midarm circumference and tricep skinfold thickness.
3. Observe color: jaundiced or pale.

**B.** Mouth
1. Note level of dentition, presence of dental caries.
2. Observe mucosal integrity.

**C.** Abdomen
1. Observe skin integrity.
2. Note abdominal distension or visible peristaltic waves (seen in pyloric stenosis).
3. Inspect for hernias (umbilical, inguinal).
4. Auscultate for bowel sounds (a sound every 10–30 seconds is normal).
5. Palpate for tenderness.
6. Palpate for liver (inferior edge normally palpated 1–2 cm below right costal margin).
7. Palpate for spleen (may be felt on inspiration 1–2 cm below left costal margin).

**D.** Vital signs: note presence of fever.

## ANALYSIS

Nursing diagnoses for the child with a disorder of the gastrointestinal system may include:

**A.** Constipation or diarrhea

**B.** Pain

**C.** Risk for deficient fluid volume

**D.** Imbalanced nutrition: less than body requirements

**E.** Impaired oral mucous membrane

**F.** Risk for impaired skin integrity

**G.** Ineffective tissue perfusion

**H.** Interrupted family processes

## PLANNING AND IMPLEMENTATION

### Goals

**A.** Child will maintain adequate nutritional intake.

**B.** Child will be free from complications of inadequate nutritional intake.

**C.** Pain will be relieved/controlled.

**D.** Child will reach optimal developmental level.

**E.** Parents will be able to care for child at home.

### Interventions

#### Nasogastric Tube Feeding

**A.** Provide continuous NG tube feedings when child needs high-calorie intake.

**B.** Use infusion pump to ensure sustained intake.

**C.** Check tube placement every 4 hours.

**D.** Check residuals and refeed every 4 hours.

#### Gastrostomy

**A.** Used for clients at high risk for aspiration.

**B.** Regulate height of tube so feeding flows in over 20–30 minutes.

#### Parenteral Nutrition

**A.** Use central venous line for high dextrose solutions (greater than 10%).

**B.** Check infusion rate and amount every 30 minutes.

**C.** Monitor urine sugar and acetone every 4 hours for 24 hours after a solution change, then every 8 hours.

**D.** Monitor for signs of hyperglycemia (nausea, vomiting, dehydration).

**E.** Provide sterile care for insertion site.
1. Change solution and tubing every 24 hours.
2. Change dressing every 1–3 days.
3. Apply restraints (if needed) to prevent dislodgment of central line.

**F.** Provide infants who are not receiving oral feedings with a pacifier to satisfy sucking needs.

## EVALUATION

**A.** Child is receiving adequate nourishment as evidenced by normal growth and development.

**B.** Skin is intact, free from signs of redness or inflammation.

C. Child is free from infection, diarrhea, or vomiting.
D. Child is free from pain.
   1. Relaxed facial expression
   2. Level of activity
   3. No guarding of abdomen
E. Parents participate in care of child.
F. Child participates in normal daily activities with family and peers.

# DISORDERS OF THE GASTROINTESTINAL SYSTEM

## Congenital Disorders

### Cleft Lip and Palate

A. General information
   1. Nonunion of the tissue and bone of the upper lip and hard/soft palate during embryologic development
   2. Familial disorder, often associated with other congenital abnormalities; incidence higher in Caucasians
      a. Cleft lip or palate: 1.5 in 1000 births
      b. Cleft lip with or without cleft palate affects more boys; cleft palate affects more girls
   3. With cleft palate, the failure of the bone and tissues to fuse results in a communication between the mouth and nose
B. Medical management: team approach for therapy
   1. Speech therapist
   2. Dentist and orthodontist
   3. Audiologist, otolaryngologist, pediatrician (these children are prone to otitis media and possible hearing loss)
   4. Surgical correction
      a. Timing varies with severity of defect; early correction helps to avoid speech defects.
      b. Cheiloplasty: correction of cleft lip
         1) Goal is to unite edges to allow lips to be both functional and cosmetically attractive.
         2) Usually performed approximately age 2 months (to prepare gums for eruption of teeth) when child is free from respiratory infection.
         3) Steri-Strips or Logan bow usually used to take tension off suture line.
      c. Cleft palate repair is usually not done until age 18 months in anticipation of speech development.
         1) Between lip and palate repair child is maintained on normal nutritional and respiratory status; also maintains normal immunization schedule.
         2) Child should be weaned and able to take liquids from a cup before palate repair.

C. Assessment findings
   1. Facial abnormality visible at birth: cleft lip or palate or both, unilateral or bilateral, partial or complete
   2. Difficulty sucking, inability to form airtight seal around nipple (size of defect may preclude breastfeeding)
   3. Formula/milk escapes through nose in infants with cleft palate
   4. Predisposition to infection because of free communication between mouth and nose
   5. Possible difficulty swallowing
   6. Abdominal distension due to swallowed air
D. Nursing interventions: preoperative cleft lip repair
   1. Feed in upright position to decrease chance of aspiration and decrease amount of air swallowed.
   2. Burp frequently; increased swallowed air causes abdominal distension and discomfort.
   3. Use a large-holed nipple; press cleft lip together with fingers to encourage sucking and to strengthen muscles needed later for speech.
   4. If infant unable to suck, use a rubber-tipped syringe and drip formula into side of mouth.
   5. Administer gavage feeding as ordered if necessary.
   6. Finish feeding with water to wash away formula in palate area.
   7. Provide small, frequent feedings.
   8. Provide emotional support for parents/family.
      a. Demonstrate benefits of surgery by showing before and after pictures.
      b. Reinforce that disorder is not their fault and that it will not affect child's life span or mental ability.
E. Nursing care: postoperative cleft lip repair
   1. Maintain patent airway (child may appear to have respiratory distress because of closure of previously open space; adaptation occurs quickly).
   2. Assess color; monitor amount of swallowing to detect hemorrhage.
   3. Do not place in prone position or with pressure on cheeks; avoid any pressure or tension on suture line.
   4. Avoid straining on suture line by anticipating child's needs.
      a. Prevent crying.
      b. Keep child comfortable and content.
   5. Use elbow restraints or pin sleeves of shirt to diaper to keep child's hands away from suture line.
   6. Resume feedings as ordered.
   7. Keep suture line clean; clean after each feeding with saline, peroxide, or water to remove crusts and prevent scarring.
   8. Provide pain control/relief.
F. Nursing interventions: preoperative cleft palate repair
   1. Prepare parents to care for child after surgery.

2. Instruct concerning feeding methods and positioning.
G. Nursing interventions: postoperative cleft palate repair
   1. Position on side for drainage of blood/mucus.
   2. Have suction available but use only in emergency.
   3. Prevent injury or trauma to suture line.
      a. Use cups only for liquids; no bottles.
      b. Avoid straws, utensils, Popsicle sticks, chewing gum.
      c. Provide soft toys.
      d. Use elbow restraints.
      e. Provide liquid diet initially, then progress to soft before returning to normal.
      f. Give water after each feeding to clean suture line.
      g. Hold and cuddle these babies to help distract them.

## Altered Connections between Trachea, Esophagus, and Stomach

A. General information
   1. Types (Figure 5-9)
      a. Esophageal atresia: esophagus ends in a blind pouch; no entry route to stomach
      b. Tracheoesophageal fistula (TEF): open connection between trachea and esophagus
      c. Esophageal atresia with TEF: esophagus ends in a blind pouch; stomach end of esophagus connects with trachea
   2. These deformities are found more often in low-birth-weight or premature infants, and are associated with polyhydramnios in the mother and multiple congenital anomalies.

B. Medical management
   1. Drug therapy: antibiotics for respiratory infections
   2. Surgery
      a. Palliative
         1) Gastrostomy for placement of a feeding tube
         2) Esophagostomy to drain secretions
      b. Corrective
         1) End-to-end anastomosis to correct the defect and restore normal anatomy
         2) Colon transplant for defects where there is insufficient tissue for an end-to-end anastomosis

C. Assessment findings
   1. Esophageal atresia
      a. History of polyhydramnios in mother (from infant's inability to swallow and excrete amniotic fluid)
      b. Inability to pass an NG tube
      c. Increased drooling and salivation
      d. Immediate regurgitation of undigested formula/milk when fed
      e. Intermittent cyanosis from choking on aspirated secretions
   2. TEF
      a. Normal swallowing but some food/mucus crosses fistula, causing choking and intermittent cyanosis
      b. Distended abdomen from inhaled air crossing fistula into stomach
      c. Aspiration pneumonia from reflux of gastric secretions into the trachea

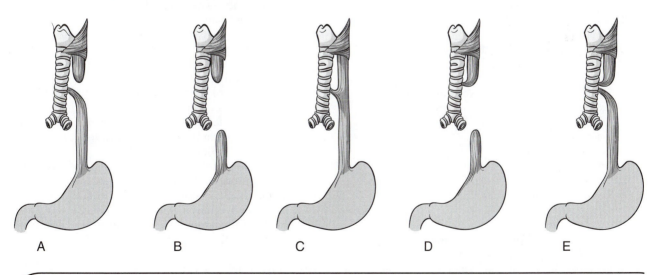

**Figure 5-9** Types of esophageal atresia and tracheoesophageal fistula. (A) Esophageal atresia with distal tracheoesophageal fistula; (B) isolated or pure esophageal atresia; (C) tracheoesophageal fistula without esophageal atresia; (D) esophageal atresia with proximal tracheoesophageal fistula; and (E) esophageal atresia with proximal and distal tracheoesophageal fistula.

3. Esophageal atresia with TEF
    a. All findings for esophageal atresia
    b. Abdominal distension and aspiration pneumonia from gas and reflux of gastric acids into trachea
4. Diagnostic tests: fluoroscopy with contrast material reveals type of defect
D. Nursing interventions: preoperative
    1. Maintain patent airway.
        a. Position according to type of defect (usually 30° head elevation).
        b. Provide continuous or prn nasal suctioning.
    2. Keep NPO.
    3. Administer IV fluids as ordered.
E. Nursing interventions: postoperative
    1. Provide nutrition.
        a. Provide gastrostomy tube feedings until the anastomosis site has healed.
        b. Start oral feedings when infant can swallow well.
        c. Progress from glucose water to small, frequent formula feedings.
    2. Promote respiratory function.
        a. Position properly.
        b. Suction as needed.
        c. Provide chest tube care.
    3. Provide client teaching and discharge planning concerning:
        a. Alternative feeding methods
        b. Signs of respiratory distress and suctioning technique

## Gastroesophageal Reflux (Chalasia)

A. General information
    1. Reversal of flow of stomach contents into lower portion of esophagus
    2. More common in premature infants due to hypotonia
    3. Caused by relaxed cardiac sphincter or overdistension of stomach by gas or overfeeding
    4. Results in local irritation of the lining of the esophagus from backflow of acidic gastric contents; sometimes causes aspiration pneumonia
B. Assessment findings
    1. Irritability
    2. "Spitting up" (versus vomiting or projectile vomiting); note relationship to feedings
    3. Diagnostic tests
        a. Muscle tone of cardiac sphincter reduced
        b. Esophageal pH: contents acidic
        c. Fluoroscopy: presence of refluxed contrast material not quickly cleared or repeated reflux
C. Nursing interventions
    1. Position with head elevated 30–45°.
    2. Give small, frequent feedings with adequate burping.

3. Provide client teaching and discharge planning: teach parents how to position and feed infant.

## Pyloric Stenosis

A. General information
    1. Hypertrophy (thickening) of the pyloric sphincter causing stenosis and obstruction
    2. Incidence: 5 in 1000 births; more common in Caucasian, firstborn, full-term boys
    3. Cause unknown; possibly familial
B. Medical management
    1. Correction of fluid electrolyte abnormalities
    2. Surgery: pyloromyotomy (Fredet-Ramstedt procedure)
C. Assessment findings
    1. Olive-size bulge under right rib cage
    2. Vomiting
        a. As obstruction increases, vomiting becomes more forceful and projectile.
        b. Vomitus does not contain bile (bile duct is distal to the pylorus).
    3. Peristaltic waves during and after feeding (look like rolling balls under abdominal wall)
    4. Failure to thrive, even though infant appears hungry after vomiting
    5. Dehydration: sunken fontanels, poor skin turgor, decreased urinary output
    6. Diagnostic tests
        a. Upper GI series reveals narrowing of the diameter of the pylorus
        b. Sodium, potassium, chloride decreased
        c. HCT increased
        d. Metabolic alkalosis
D. Nursing interventions: preoperative
    1. Administer replacement fluids and electrolytes as ordered.
    2. Prevent vomiting.
        a. May be NPO with NG tube to suction.
        b. Keep in high-Fowler's position.
        c. Place on right side after feedings.
        d. Minimize handling.
        e. Record strict I&O, daily weights, and urine specific gravity.
    3. Observe for symptoms of aspiration of vomitus.
E. Nursing interventions: postoperative
    1. Advance diet as tolerated.
    2. Place on right side after feeding. Elevate head.
    3. Monitor strict I&O, daily weights.
    4. Observe incision for signs of infection.
    5. Provide client teaching and discharge planning concerning feeding and positioning of infant.

## Intussusception

A. General information
    1. Telescoping of bowel into itself (usually at the ileocecal valve) causing edema, obstruction, and possible necrosis of the bowel

2. Most common at about age 6 months; occurs more often in boys than in girls; associated with cystic fibrosis and celiac disease
3. Cause unknown

B. Medical management
1. Barium or contrast medium enema to reduce telescoping by hydrostatic pressure
2. Surgery if barium enema unsuccessful or if signs of peritonitis

C. Assessment findings
1. Piercing cry
2. Severe abdominal pain (pulls legs up)
3. Vomiting of bile-stained fluid
4. Bloody mucus in stool
5. "Currant-jelly" stool

D. Nursing interventions
1. Provide routine pre- and post-op care for abdominal surgery.
2. Monitor for fluid and electrolyte imbalance and intervene as needed.
3. Monitor for peritonitis and intervene as needed.
4. Monitor stools. Report changes.

## Hirschsprung's Disease (Aganglionic Megacolon)

A. General information
1. Absence of autonomic parasympathetic ganglion cells in a portion of the large colon (usually occurs 4–25 cm proximally from anus), resulting in decreased motility in that portion of the colon and signs of functional obstruction
2. Usually diagnosed in infancy
3. Familial disease; more common in boys than girls; associated with Down syndrome
4. When stool enters the affected part of the colon, lack of peristalsis causes it to remain there until additional stool pushes it through; colon dilates as stool is impacted.

B. Medical management
1. Drug therapy: stool softeners
2. Isotonic enemas
3. Diet therapy: low residue
4. Surgery
   a. Palliative: loop or double-barrel colostomy
   b. Corrective: abdominal-perineal pull through; bowel containing ganglia is pulled down and anastomosed to the rectum.

C. Assessment findings
1. Failure or delay in passing meconium
2. Abdominal distension; failure to pass stool
3. Temporary relief following digital rectal exam
4. Loose stools; only liquid can get around impaction (may also be a ribbonlike stool)
5. Nausea, anorexia, lethargy
6. Possibly bile-stained or fecal vomiting
7. Loss of weight, failure to grow
8. Volvulus (bowel twists upon itself, causing obstruction and necrosis) and enterocolitis due to fecal stagnation

9. Diagnostic tests: rectal biopsy confirms presence of aganglionic cells

D. Nursing interventions
1. Administer enemas as ordered.
   a. Use mineral oil or isotonic saline.
   b. Do not use tap water or soap suds enemas in infants because of danger of water intoxication.
   c. Use volume appropriate to weight of child.
      1) Infants: 150–200 mL
      2) Children: 250–500 mL
2. Do not treat the loose stools; the child actually is constipated.
3. Administer TPN as ordered.
4. Provide a low-residue diet.
5. Provide client teaching and discharge planning concerning colostomy care and low-residue diet.

## Imperforate Anus

A. General information
1. Congenital malformation caused by abnormal fetal development
2. Many variations; anal agenesis most frequent
3. Often associated with fistula formation to rectum or vagina and other congenital anomalies
4. Surgical correction performed in stages with completion at about age 1 year
5. May need temporary colostomy

B. Medical management
1. Manual dilatation
2. Surgery: anoplasty (reconstruction of anus)
3. Prophylactic antibiotics

C. Assessment findings
1. No stool passage within 24 hours of birth
2. Meconium stool from inappropriate orifice
3. Inability to insert thermometer

D. Nursing interventions
1. If suspected, do not take rectal temperature because of risk of perforating wall and causing peritonitis.
2. Perform manual dilatation as ordered; instruct parents in proper technique.
3. After surgery prevent infection; keep anal incisional area as clean as possible.
4. After surgery use side-lying position, or have child lie prone with hips elevated.

# Acquired Gastrointestinal Disorders

## Celiac Disease

A. General information
1. Malabsorption syndrome characterized by intolerance of gluten, found in rye, oats, wheat, and barley
2. Familial disease, found more commonly in Caucasians

3. Cause unknown; thought to be an inborn error of metabolism or an immunologic disorder
4. Characterized by flat mucosal surface and atrophy of villi of the intestine; reduced absorptive surface causes marked malabsorption of fats

B. Medical management: diet therapy main intervention; gluten-free diet, TPN in children who are severely malnourished

C. Assessment findings
1. Steatorrhea: frothy, pale, bulky, foul-smelling, greasy stools
2. Chronic diarrhea during late infancy and throughout toddlerhood
3. Failure to thrive
4. Grossly distended abdomen; muscle wasting of limbs and buttocks
5. Abdominal pain, irritability, listlessness, vomiting
6. Symptoms of vitamin A, D, E, and K deficiency
7. Diagnostic tests
   a. Pancreatic enzymes and sweat chloride test normal (performed to rule out the possibility of cystic fibrosis)
   b. Jejunal and duodenal biopsies show characteristic atrophy of the mucosa

D. Nursing interventions
1. Monitor gluten-free diet (no wheat, barley, oats, and rye products)
2. Provide supplemental fat-soluble vitamins in water-soluble form
3. Provide client teaching and discharge planning concerning:
   a. Gluten-free diet; stress allowed foods and importance of reading labels carefully
   b. Avoidance of infection
   c. Assisting child to feel like a "normal" peer
   d. Importance of adhering to diet even though symptoms are controlled
   e. Importance of long-term follow-up management

## Appendicitis

A. General information
1. Inflammation of the appendix that prevents mucus from passing into the cecum; if untreated, ischemia, gangrene, rupture, and peritonitis occur
2. Most common in school-age children
3. May be caused by mechanical obstruction (fecaliths, intestinal parasites) or anatomic defect; may be related to decreased fiber in the diet

B. Assessment findings
1. Diffuse pain, localizes in lower right quadrant
2. Nausea/vomiting
3. Guarding of abdomen, rebound tenderness, walks stooped over
4. Decreased bowel sounds
5. Fever
6. Diagnostic tests
   a. WBC increased
   b. Elevated acetone in urine

C. Nursing interventions
1. Administer antibiotics/antipyretics as ordered
2. Prevent perforation of the appendix; do not give enemas or cathartics or use heating pad
3. In addition to routine pre-op care for appendectomy:
   a. Give support to parents if seeking treatment was delayed.
   b. Explain necessity of obtaining lab work prior to surgery.
4. In addition to routine post-op care:
   a. Monitor NG tube (usually with low suction).
   b. Monitor Penrose drains.
   c. Position in semi-Fowler's or lying on right side to facilitate drainage.
   d. Administer antibiotics as ordered.

## Parasitic Worms

A. General information
1. A parasite is an organism that lives in, on, or at the expense of the host.
2. Common human GI parasites are pinworms and roundworms.
3. Medication varies depending on type of parasite.

B. Assessment findings
1. Pinworms: anal irritation, itching, disturbed sleep
2. Roundworm: colic, abdominal pain, lack of appetite, weight loss

C. Nursing interventions
1. Obtain stool culture.
2. Observe for worms in all excreta (Scotch tape test for stool).
3. Instruct parents to change clothing, bed linens, towels and launder in hot water.
4. Clean toilets with disinfectant.
5. Instruct all family members to scrub hands and fingernails prior to eating and after using toilet.
6. Follow specific medication and hygiene orders given by physician.

## Giardiasis

A. General information
1. Common cause of diarrhea
2. Protozoan *Giardia lamblia*
3. Common in daycare centers
4. Cysts ingested, mature in GI tract, cysts excreted in stools, and complete maturation
5. Multiple stool cultures required as all stools don't contain cysts

6. Usually fecal-oral transmission, also contaminated water and animals
B. Assessment findings
  1. Diarrhea
  2. Vomiting, anorexia
  3. Failure to thrive
  4. Abdominal cramps
C. Medical management
  1. Metronidazole (Flagyl)
  2. Furazolidone (Furoxone)
D. Nursing interventions
  1. Hygiene, especially with diaper changes
  2. Handwashing
  3. Instructions about drug therapy

## Constipation

A. General information
  1. Decrease in number of bowel movements with large, hard stools
  2. May be caused by high fat and protein and low fluid in diet
  3. May cause bowel obstruction if severe
B. Medical management
  1. Drug therapy: stool softeners, suppositories, enemas
  2. Diet therapy: increased fluids and fiber
C. Assessment findings
  1. Less frequent stools, difficulty eliminating stool, hard consistency compared to normal pattern (children do not have to stool every day)
  2. Bleeding with stooling
  3. Abdominal pain
D. Nursing interventions
  1. Assess for other pathologic causes of constipation.
  2. Dietary modification, increase fiber and fluids.
  3. Apply lubricant around anus.
  4. Remove stool digitally if possible.
  5. Provide prune juice (1 oz); add fruits to diet.
  6. Add small amount of Karo syrup to formula.
  7. Teach parents methods to prevent further episodes.

 **Sample Questions**

112. A 9-year-old has celiac disease, which has been in good control since it was diagnosed 6 years ago. She has now been admitted to the hospital for an emergency appendectomy. Which preoperative procedure should the nurse withhold?
  1. A cleansing enema.
  2. Starting an IV.
  3. Keeping her NPO.
  4. Obtaining a blood sample for a CBC.

113. An 8-year-old has celiac disease. She had an emergency appendectomy. She is progressing well and is having her first real meal. Which food should the nurse remove from her tray?
  1. Chicken rice soup.
  2. Crackers.
  3. Hamburger patty.
  4. Fresh fruit cup.

114. A 10-month-old is brought to the clinic for a checkup and his MMR immunization. While talking to the nurse, the mother reports that her teenage babysitter has just come down with rubeola. What is the most appropriate plan of treatment for the child?
  1. Administer immune serum globulin.
  2. Administer prophylactic penicillin.
  3. Vaccinate him now with MMR.
  4. Allow him to catch measles from the babysitter in order to develop active immunity.

115. The nurse is caring for a 12-month-old child who has a cleft palate. A cleft lip was repaired when he was 2 months old. His mother asks the nurse when he will be ready for a cleft palate repair. What response would best inform the parent when the cleft palate repair can be performed?
  1. Prior to development of speech.
  2. When the child is toilet trained.
  3. When the child is completely weaned from the bottle and pacifier.
  4. When a large-holed nipple is ineffective for his feedings.

116. A 2-year-old has had a cleft palate repair. Which priority teaching fact will be included when educating the mother about the post-op period?
  1. Resume toilet training after he is up and around.
  2. Use a cup or wide bowl spoon for feeding.
  3. He will be more prone to respiratory infections now that his airway is smaller.
  4. No further treatment will be needed until his adult teeth come in at age 6.

117. What is the appropriate feeding technique for the nurse to use with an infant who has a cleft palate?
  1. Suction client prior to feeding.
  2. Feed in sitting position.
  3. Have the nurse feed the client during hospitalization.
  4. Burp client after feeding to reduce risk of aspiration.

5

118. How would you evaluate that the new nurse is using appropriate technique to feed a 3-day-old with a cleft lip?
    1. NG tube is patent.
    2. Infant is seated in upright position.
    3. The nurse uses a Nuk nipple.
    4. The nurse adds rice to formula.

119. A baby girl is born prematurely to a mother with polyhydramnios. The baby is diagnosed with esophageal atresia with tracheoesophageal fistula. What assessment finding would the nurse be likely to note?
    1. Jaundice, high bilirubin.
    2. Seedy yellow stools.
    3. Projectile emesis.
    4. Frothy saliva, drooling.

120. A 5-month-old girl is admitted with gastroesophageal reflux. Her signs and symptoms include emesis, poor weight gain, hemepositive stools, irritability, and gagging with feeds. The nurse would include which intervention?
    1. Urine dipstick each void.
    2. Appropriate feeding positioning.
    3. Biweekly weights.
    4. Monitor WBC as indicator for infection.

121. A 4-week-old is admitted for observation. Her assessment reveals projectile vomiting, visible gastric peristalsis, and an olive-shaped mass in the epigastrium. Which nursing diagnosis is of highest best priority?
    1. Altered nutrition.
    2. Self-care deficit.
    3. Impaired gas exchange.
    4. Fluid volume deficit.

122. The nurse would find which stool characteristic consistent with a diagnosis of intussusception?
    1. Yellow seedy stools.
    2. Currant jelly-like stools.
    3. Mucus-like stools.
    4. Hard black stools.

123. A 6-month-old boy is treated at home with saline enemas due to his Hirschsprung's disease. His mother asks if she can use tap water to reduce costs. Which is the best response by the nurse?
    1. "Yes, tap water is as effective as saline, just be sure to boil it first."
    2. "No, saline enemas must be used to maintain his electrolyte balance."

3. "Yes; you can use tap water after letting it run for one minute to clear any lead from the pipes."
    4. "No; tap water enemas are not allowed, but soap suds enemas are just as effective."

124. A 5-year-old boy has celiac disease. Which statement by the child informs the nurse that he is following his diet?
    1. "I had hot dogs and french fries for lunch."
    2. "I ate chicken and vegetables for dinner."
    3. "I had macaroni and cheese for lunch."
    4. "I ate soup and crackers for dinner."

125. A 14-year-old is admitted to your unit following an emergency appendectomy. What is the nurse's goal for this client?
    1. Pain related to inflamed appendix.
    2. Patient will experience minimized risk of spread of infection.
    3. Maintain NG tube decompression until bowel motility returns.
    4. Child demonstrates resolution of peritonitis.

126. A 9-year-old girl comes into the clinic with a diagnosis of pinworms. What is it essential for the nurse to teach?
    1. Check for pinworms every morning for a week with a Scotch tape test.
    2. Save the girl's next bowel movement to check for pinworms.
    3. Follow-up with local doctor in 6 months to check for recurrence.
    4. Scrub hands and fingernails thoroughly before each meal and after each use of the toilet.

 **Answers and Rationales**

112. **1.** Enemas, cathartics, and heat to the abdomen should all be avoided in appendicitis because they may cause perforation of the appendix.

113. **2.** The prescribed diet for children with celiac disease is gluten free. Crackers contain gluten.

114. **1.** Administration of immune serum globulin will provide the child with passive immunity to prevent a full-blown case of measles or reduce the severity of symptoms.

115. **1.** Cleft palate repair should be done before speech is well developed. This allows for the formation of a more normal speech pattern.

116. **2.** Care must be taken not to put anything in the mouth that could damage the suture line.

117. **2.** This position reduces the risk of aspiration.

118. **2.** This position reduces the risk of aspiration.

119. **4.** Infants with esophageal atresia (EA) with tracheoesophageal fistula (TEF) have difficulty handling their secretions.

120. **2.** It may be a challenge to find the optimum position. Best positions include upright prone and 30° head of bed elevation.

121. **4.** Infants with pyloric stenosis are at high risk for electrolyte imbalance and these need to be corrected prior to a pyloromyotomy.

122. **2.** The obstruction causes bloody mucus known as currant jelly stools.

123. **2.** Repeated water enemas cause electrolyte dilution.

124. **2.** Chicken and vegetables do not contain gluten. Gluten is in barley, rye, oats, and wheat.

125. **2.** This is an appropriate goal.

126. **4.** Handwashing prevents reinfection and/or new infections in other people.

# The Genitourinary System

## VARIATIONS FROM THE ADULT

A. Nephrons continue to develop after birth.
B. Glomerular filtration rate is 30% below adult levels at birth; reaches normal level by age 2 years.
C. Tubular functions immature at birth; tubular absorption and secretion reach adult levels by age 2 years.
D. Urethra is shorter in children and more prone to ascending infection (particularly true in girls); the urethra is also closer to anus as source of contamination.
E. Many GU conditions in children become chronic.

## ASSESSMENT

### History

A. Presenting problem: symptoms may include:
   1. Change in appearance, color, or smell of urine
   2. Change in amount, frequency, or pattern of urination
   3. Abdominal or back pain
   4. Anorexia, nausea, vomiting, weight loss
   5. Headaches, seizures
   6. Fatigue, lethargy
   7. Excessive thirst
   8. Drug use or accidental ingestions
B. Family history: kidney disease, hypertension

## Physical Examination

A. General appearance: note presence of edema.
B. Abdomen and genitalia: note abdominal distension, presence of undescended testicle, tenderness to palpation, placement of urinary meatus, urinary stream during voiding
C. Vital signs: note presence of fever; increased blood pressure (common in renal disease)

## ANALYSIS

Nursing diagnoses for the child with a disorder of the genitourinary tract may include:
A. Excess fluid volume
B. Impaired urinary elimination
C. Pain
D. Activity intolerance
E. Interrupted family process

## PLANNING AND IMPLEMENTATION

### Goals

A. Child will have normal urinary function.
B. Child's fluid and electrolyte and acid-base balances will be normal.
C. Child will be free from signs of infection.
D. Child's blood pressure will be within normal limits.
E. Parents will be able to care for child at home.

## Intervention

### Pediatric Urine Collector (PUC)

A. Used when child is not toilet trained
B. Nursing care
  1. Wash genitalia as for clean catch specimens.
  2. Apply bag directly to dry skin; do not use powder or creams.
  3. If child has not voided within 45 minutes, remove bag and repeat process.

## EVALUATION

A. Child is adequately hydrated as evidenced by normal serum electrolyte levels and normal urine output.
B. Child is free from complications such as infection, skin breakdown, or hypertension.
C. Parents demonstrate ability to administer appropriate medications and treatments.

## DISORDERS OF THE GENITOURINARY SYSTEM

### Urinary Tract Infection (UTI)

A. General information
  1. Bacterial invasion of the kidneys or bladder
  2. More common in girls, preschool, and school-age children
  3. Usually caused by *E. coli;* predisposing factors include poor hygiene, irritation from bubble baths, urinary reflux
  4. The invading organism ascends the urinary tract, irritating the mucosa and causing characteristic symptoms.
B. Assessment findings
  1. Low-grade fever
  2. Abdominal pain
  3. Enuresis, pain/burning on urination, frequency, hematuria
C. Nursing interventions
  1. Administer antibiotics as ordered; prevention of kidney infection/glomerulonephritis important. (*Note:* obtain cultures before starting antibiotics.)
  2. Provide warm baths and allow child to void in water to alleviate painful voiding.
  3. Force fluids.
  4. Encourage measures to acidify urine (cranberry juice, acid-ash diet).
  5. Provide client teaching and discharge planning concerning:
    a. Avoidance of tub baths (contamination from dirty water may allow microorganisms to travel up urethra)
    b. Avoidance of bubble baths that might irritate urethra
    c. Importance for girls to wipe perineum from front to back
    d. Increase in foods/fluids that acidify urine

## Vesicoureteral Reflux

A. General information
  1. Regurgitation of urine from the bladder via the ureters to the kidneys due to faulty valve mechanism at the vesicoureteral junction
  2. Predisposes child to:
    a. UTIs from urine stasis
    b. Pyelonephritis from chronic UTIs
    c. Hydronephrosis from increased pressure on renal pelvis
B. Assessment findings: same as for urinary tract infections
C. Nursing interventions for surgical reimplantation of ureters
  1. Assist with preoperative studies as needed (IVP, voiding cystourethrogram, cystoscopy).
  2. Provide postoperative care.
    a. Monitor drains; may have one from bladder and one from each ureter (ureteral stents).
    b. Check output from all drains (expect bloody drainage initially) and record carefully.
    c. Observe drainage from abdominal dressing; note color, amount, frequency.
    d. Administer medication for bladder spasms as ordered.

## Exstrophy of the Bladder

A. General information
  1. Congenital malformation in which nonfusion of abdominal and anterior walls of the bladder during embryologic development causes anterior surface of bladder to lie open on abdominal wall
  2. Varying degrees of defect
B. Assessment findings
  1. Associated structural changes
    a. Prolapsed rectum
    b. Inguinal hernia
    c. Widely split symphysis
    d. Rotated hips
  2. Associated anomalies
    a. Epispadias
    b. Cleft scrotum or clitoris
    c. Undescended testicles
    d. Chordee (downward deflection of the penis)
C. Medical management: two-stage reconstructive surgery, possibly with urinary diversion; usually delayed until age 3–6 months
D. Nursing interventions: preoperative
  1. Provide bladder care; prevent infection.
    a. Keep area as clean as possible; urine on skin will cause irritation and ulceration.

b. Change diaper frequently; keep diaper loose fitting.
   c. Wash with mild soap and water.
   d. Cover exposed bladder with Vaseline gauze.
E. Nursing interventions: postoperative
   1. Design play activities to foster toddler's need for autonomy (e.g., Play-Doh, talking toys, books); child will be immobilized for extended period of time.
   2. Prevent trauma; as child gets older and more mobile, trauma more likely; teach parents to avoid areas such as sandboxes.

## Undescended Testicles (Cryptorchidism)

A. General information
   1. Unilateral or bilateral absence of testes in scrotal sac
   2. Testes normally descend at 8 months of gestation, will therefore be absent in premature infants
   3. Incidence increased in children having genetically transmitted diseases
   4. Unilateral cryptorchidism most common
   5. 75% will descend spontaneously by age 1 year
B. Medical management
   1. Whether or not to treat is still controversial; if testes remain in abdomen, damage to the testes (sterility) is possible because of increased body temperature.
   2. If not descended by age 8 or 9, chorionic gonadotropin can be given.
   3. Orchipexy: surgical procedure to retrieve and secure testes placement; performed between ages 1–3 years.
C. Assessment findings: unable to palpate testes in scrotal sac (when palpating testes be careful not to elicit cremasteric reflex, which pulls testes higher in pelvic cavity)
D. Nursing interventions
   1. Advise parents of absence of testes and provide information about treatment options.
   2. Support parents if surgery is to be performed.
   3. Post-op, avoid disturbing the tension mechanism (will be in place for about 1 week).
   4. Avoid contamination of incision.

## Hypospadias

A. General information
   1. Urethral opening located anywhere along the ventral surface of penis
   2. Chordee (ventral curvature of the penis) often associated, causing constriction
   3. In extreme cases, child's sex may be uncertain
B. Medical management
   1. Minimal defects need no intervention
   2. Neonatal circumcision delayed, tissue may be needed for corrective repair
   3. Surgery performed at age 3–9 months; 2 years of age for complex repairs
C. Assessment findings
   1. Urinary meatus misplaced
   2. Inability to make straight stream of urine
D. Nursing interventions
   1. Diaper normally.
   2. Provide support for parents.
   3. Provide support for child at time of surgery.
   4. Postoperatively check pressure dressing, monitor catheter drainage, assess pain.

## Enuresis

A. General information
   1. Involuntary passage of urine after the age of control is expected (about 4 years)
   2. Types
      a. Primary: in children who have never achieved control
      b. Secondary: in children who have developed complete control and lose it
   3. May occur at any time of day but is most frequent at night
   4. More common in boys
   5. No organic cause can be identified; familial tendency
   6. Etiologic possibilities
      a. Sleep disturbances
      b. Delayed neurologic development
      c. Immature development of bladder leading to decreased capacity
      d. Psychologic problems
B. Medical management
   1. Bladder retention exercises
   2. Behavior modification, e.g., bed alarm devices
   3. Drug therapy: results are temporary; side effects may be unpleasant or even dangerous
      a. Tricyclic antidepressants: imipramine HCl (Tofranil)
      b. Anticholinergics
      c. DDAVP
C. Assessment findings
   1. Physical exam normal
   2. History of repeated involuntary urination
D. Nursing interventions
   1. Provide information/counseling to family as needed.
      a. Confirm that this is not conscious behavior and that child is not purposely misbehaving.
      b. Assure parents that they are not responsible and that this is a relatively common problem.
   2. Involve child in care; give praise and support with small accomplishments.
      a. Age 5–6 years: can strip bed of wet sheets.
      b. Age 10–12 years: can do laundry and change bed.
   3. Avoid scolding and belittling child.

# Nephrosis (Nephrotic Syndrome)

A. General information
1. Autoimmune process leading to structural alteration of glomerular membrane that results in increased permeability to plasma proteins, particularly albumin
2. Course of the disease consists of exacerbations and remissions over a period of months to years
3. Commonly affects preschoolers, boys more often than girls
4. Pathophysiology
   a. Plasma proteins enter the renal tubule and are excreted in the urine, causing proteinuria.
   b. Protein shift causes altered oncotic pressure and lowered plasma volume.
   c. Hypovolemia triggers release of renin and angiotensin, which stimulates increased secretion of aldosterone; aldosterone increases reabsorption of water and sodium in distal tubule.
   d. Lowered blood pressure also stimulates release of ADH, further increasing reabsorption of water; together with a general shift of plasma into interstitial spaces, results in edema.
5. Prognosis is good unless edema does not respond to steroids.
B. Medical management
1. Drug therapy
   a. Corticosteroids to resolve edema
   b. Antibiotics for bacterial infections
   c. Thiazide diuretics in edematous stage
2. Bed rest
3. Diet modification: high protein, low sodium
C. Assessment findings
1. Proteinuria, hypoproteinemia, hyperlipidemia
2. Dependent body edema
   a. Puffiness around eyes in morning
   b. Ascites
   c. Scrotal edema
   d. Ankle edema
3. Anorexia, vomiting and diarrhea, malnutrition
4. Pallor, lethargy
5. Hepatomegaly
D. Nursing interventions
1. Provide bed rest.
   a. Conserve energy.
   b. Find activities for quiet play.
2. Provide high-protein, low-sodium diet during edema phase only.
3. Maintain skin integrity.
   a. Do not use Band-Aids.
   b. Avoid IM injections (medication is not absorbed into edematous tissue).
   c. Turn frequently.
4. Obtain morning urine for protein studies.
5. Provide scrotal support.
6. Monitor I&O and vital signs and weigh daily.
7. Administer steroids to suppress autoimmune response as ordered.
8. Protect from known sources of infection.

# Acute Glomerulonephritis

A. General information
1. Immune complex disease resulting from an antigen-antibody reaction
2. Secondary to a beta-hemolytic streptococcal infection occurring elsewhere in the body
3. Occurs more frequently in boys, usually between ages 6–7 years
4. Usually resolves in about 14 days, self-limiting
B. Medical management
1. Antibiotics for streptococcal infection
2. Antihypertensives if blood pressure severely elevated
3. Digitalis if circulatory overload
4. Fluid restriction if renal insufficiency
5. Peritoneal dialysis if severe renal or cardiopulmonary problems develop
C. Assessment findings
1. History of a precipitating streptococcal infection, usually upper respiratory infection or impetigo
2. Edema, anorexia, lethargy
3. Hematuria or dark-colored urine, fever
4. Hypertension
5. Diagnostic tests
   a. Urinalysis reveals RBCs, WBCs, protein, cellular casts
   b. Urine specific gravity increased
   c. BUN and serum creatinine increased
   d. ESR elevated
   e. Hgb and HCT decreased
D. Nursing interventions
1. Monitor I&O, blood pressure, urine; weigh daily.
2. Provide diversional therapy.
3. Provide client teaching and discharge planning concerning:
   a. Medication administration
   b. Prevention of infection
   c. Signs of renal complications
   d. Importance of long-term follow-up

# Hydronephrosis

A. General information
1. Collection of urine in the renal pelvis due to obstruction to outflow
2. Obstruction most common at ureteral-pelvic junction (see Vesicoureteral Reflux) but may also be caused by adhesions, ureterocele, calculi, or congenital malformation
3. Obstruction causes increased intrarenal pressure, decreased circulation, and atrophy of the kidney, leading to renal insufficiency

4. May be unilateral or bilateral; occurs more often in left kidney
5. Prognosis good when treated early
B. Medical management: surgery to correct or remove obstruction
C. Assessment findings
   1. Repeated UTIs
   2. Failure to thrive
   3. Abdominal pain, fever
   4. Fluctuating mass in region of kidney
D. Nursing interventions: prepare child for multiple urologic studies (see also Vesicoureteral Reflux).

 **Sample Questions**

127. A 4-year-old has just been diagnosed as having nephrotic syndrome. What is related to his potential for impairment of skin integrity?
   1. Joint inflammation.
   2. Drug therapy.
   3. Edema.
   4. Generalized body rash.

128. A 20-month-old is admitted to the hospital with a diagnosis of cryptorchidism. What will surgical correction help to prevent?
   1. Difficulty in urinating.
   2. Sterility.
   3. Herniation.
   4. Peritonitis.

129. A 3-day-old is diagnosed with hypospadias. His parents are very upset and have been willing listeners as the nurse has explained this problem to them. In hypospadias, what primary problem will the nurse discuss with the parents?
   1. Ambiguous genitalia.
   2. Urinary incontinence.
   3. Ventral curvature of the penis.
   4. Altered location of the urethral meatus.

130. The parents of a newborn who has hypospadias ask about surgical repair. What age is the preferred time to schedule surgical repair of hypospadias?
   1. 9 months old.
   2. 5 years old.
   3. 12 years old.
   4. 17 years old.

131. The parents of a baby boy who was born with hypospadias want to know about the surgical repair. The success of hypospadias surgery will be evaluated by what occurrence?

   1. The cosmetic appearance of the penis.
   2. Maintaining stable blood pressure in the child.
   3. Observing a straight stream when he voids.
   4. His ability to void without discomfort.

132. The nurse is teaching parents about post-op care of their child who has had an orchiopexy. What instructions will the nurse give the parents?
   1. "You must tighten the rubber band around the scrotum every 4 hours to maintain the testicle."
   2. "You must increase tension on the rubber band every 4 hours."
   3. "You must check the rubber band every 4 hours to check for disconnection."
   4. "Cut the rubber band after 24 hours."

133. A baby boy is born with a hypospadias. The parents decide to wait until the child is 6 months old for the repair. The father asks the nurse why the doctor said not to have the baby circumcised. What is the nurse's best response?
   1. "It is best to wait until the baby is older and understands the surgery."
   2. "Circumcision carries a high infection rate and that may delay his hypospadias repair."
   3. "The foreskin may be used during the hypospadias repair."
   4. "He will need the foreskin to help anchor the Foley catheter after the repair."

134. The nurse is planning care for a 2-year-old who has nephrotic syndrome and is in remission. What type of diet would the nurse plan to feed this child?
   1. High protein, low calorie.
   2. High calorie, low protein.
   3. Low sodium, low fat.
   4. Regular diet, no added salt.

135. A 5-year-old girl recovered from a strep infection 2 weeks ago. She now presents with loss of appetite, dark colored urine, and orbital edema. What is the nurse's assessment?
   1. Nephrotic syndrome.
   2. Glomerulonephritis.
   3. Renal tubular acidosis.
   4. Hemolytic uremic syndrome.

136. A 4-year-old boy is admitted with glomerulonephritis. His mother asks why his eyes are so puffy. What is the nurse's best response?
   1. "This is a common finding due to circulatory congestion in the kidneys."

2. "Children cry a lot with glomerulonephritis and the puffiness should subside when he feels better."
3. "Has he been rubbing his eyes excessively?"
4. "Periorbital edema is associated with hypertension."

## Answers and Rationales

**127.** **3.** A child with nephritic syndrome will have massive edema. A child with edema is prone to skin breakdown.

**128.** **2.** If the testes remain in the abdomen beyond the age of 5, damage resulting from exposure to internal body temperature can cause sterility.

**129.** **4.** In hypospadias, the urethral opening may be anywhere along the underside of the penis.

**130.** **1.** Most surgical repairs are scheduled for the child between 6 and 18 months of age.

**131.** **3.** Observing the child void in a straight stream while standing is the expected successful outcome of hypospadias repair.

**132.** **3.** The Torek procedure attaches a rubber band from the testicle to the scrotal sac to the thigh to maintain the testicle in the pouch. The family must check the rubber band every 4 hours and call the doctor if the rubber band breaks or becomes disconnected.

**133.** **3.** The foreskin is frequently used as a flap during the repair.

**134.** **4.** The child who is in remission is allowed a regular diet; salt is restricted in the form of no added salt at the table and excluding foods with very high salt content.

**135.** **2.** Acute poststreptococcal glomerulonephritis is the most common of the noninfectious renal diseases in children.

**136.** **1.** Periorbital edema is often associated with circulatory congestion in the kidneys.

# The Musculoskeletal System

## VARIATIONS FROM THE ADULT

### Bones

A. Linear growth results from skeletal development
   1. Centers of ossification
      a. Primary centers in diaphyses
      b. Secondary centers in epiphyses
      c. Used in assessment of bone age; number of ossification centers in wrist equals age in years plus 1
      d. Centers appear earlier in girls than in boys
   2. Metaphysis
      a. Cartilaginous plate between diaphysis and epiphysis
      b. The site of active growth in long bones
      c. Disappears over time with bony fusion of diaphysis and epiphysis
      d. Linear growth ends with epiphyseal fusion
      e. Assessment of bone age includes the advancing bone edges
B. Bone circumference growth occurs as new bone tissue is formed beneath the periosteum.

C. Skeletal maturity is reached by age 17 in boys and 2 years after menarche in girls.
D. Certain characteristics of bone in children affect injury and healing, bones are more prone to injury, and injury results from relatively minor accidents.
   1. Metaphysis
      a. Absorbs shock, protects joints from injury.
      b. Traumatic injury or infection to this growth plate can cause deformity.
      c. If not injured, this growth plate participates in healing and straightening of limbs by process of remodeling.
   2. Porous bone
      a. Increases flexibility; absorbs force on impact.
      b. Allows bones to bend, buckle, and break in "greenstick" or incomplete fracture.
   3. Thicker periosteum
      a. More active osteogenic potential
      b. Healing more rapid
         1) Neonatal period: may take 2–3 weeks
         2) Early childhood: may take 4 weeks
         3) Later childhood: may take 6 weeks
         4) Adolescence: 8–10 weeks

**c.** Stiffness after immobilization is rare unless joint has been injured.

**E.** Bone growth is affected by Wolff's law: bone will grow in the direction in which stress is placed on it.

## Muscles

**A.** Muscle growth is responsible for a large part of increase in body weight.

**B.** The number of muscle fibers is constant throughout life; growth results from an increase in the size of the muscle fibers and by an increased number of nuclei per fiber.

**C.** Muscle growth most apparent in adolescence, influenced by growth hormone, adrenal androgens, and, in boys, by testosterone.

## ASSESSMENT

### History

**A.** Presenting problem: symptoms may include:
   1. Delayed motor development
   2. Injury
   3. Pain, loss of sensation, tingling
   4. Muscle weakness, loss of function of an extremity
   5. Interference with normal activity or play
   6. Other parental concerns

**B.** Family history: genetic disorders, skeletal deformities

**C.** Inadequate nutrition (e.g., vitamin D deficiency causes rickets)

### Physical Examination

**A.** General appearance: note any asymmetry, visible deformities, swelling (of joints or over bones), quality of movement (ROM, gait, guarding).

**B.** Measure muscle strength.

**C.** Identify warmth or tenderness over bones and joints.

**D.** Assess pain: note type, location, onset, relationship to activity.

**E.** Perform examination in standing, lying, and sitting positions.

## ANALYSIS

Nursing diagnoses for the child with a disorder of the musculoskeletal system may include:

**A.** Risk for activity intolerance
**B.** Pain
**C.** Deficient diversional activity
**D.** Risk for injury
**E.** Impaired physical mobility
**F.** Self-care deficit
**G.** Disturbed body image
**H.** Risk for impaired skin integrity
**I.** Ineffective tissue perfusion

## PLANNING AND IMPLEMENTATION

### Goals

**A.** Injury or deformity will be identified and treated early.
**B.** Child will achieve maximum level of mobility.
**C.** Pain will be relieved/controlled.
**D.** Child will be free from injury.
**E.** Parents will be able to care for child at home.

### Interventions

#### Care of the Child with a Cast

Also see Unit 4.
**A.** General information
   1. Initial chemical hardening reaction may cause a change in an infant's body temperature; monitor and intervene as needed.
   2. Choose toys too big to fit down cast.
   3. Do not use baby powder near cast because it clumps and provides a medium for bacterial growth.
   4. Prepare for anticipated casting by having child help apply a cast to a doll the day before.
   5. Demonstrate the use of a cast cutter on a doll before using on child to show it does not cut skin.

**B.** Care of child in hip spica cast (cast encases child from nipples to knees; legs are abducted with a bar between the thighs)
   1. Use firm mattress to allow for increased weight of plaster cast.
   2. Do not lift cast by crossbar.
   3. Protect cast from water and urine.
      **a.** Put waterproof material over petaling (Chux®, plastic diapers).
      **b.** Elevate head of bed slightly to prevent urine and stool from seeping under cast; confirm that entire body is on a slant, not just the head.
      **c.** Use Bradford frame (canvas board with opening near genitalia) and place a bedpan under opening.
   4. Use pillows to support all parts of the cast.
   5. Drape towel across top of chest part of cast during feedings to prevent crumbs from entering cast.
   6. Monitor for pain/pressure points due to growth if cast is on for a long time.

#### Care of the Child in Traction

**A.** General information
   1. Infants and young toddlers do not have enough body weight to use traditional tractions effectively.
   2. Children do not understand the necessity of maintaining proper body alignment and will need frequent repositioning.

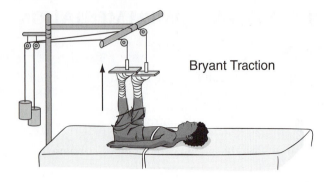

Bryant Traction

**Figure 5-10** Bryant traction

**B.** Bryant's traction: used primarily in children (See Figure 5-10.)
  1. Child is own counterweight.
  2. Both legs are at 90° angle to bed.
  3. Buttocks must be slightly off mattress in order to ensure sufficient traction on legs.
  4. Used with children under age 2 years whose weight is too low (under 30 lb [14 kg]) to counterbalance without additional gravitational force.
  5. Used for fractured femur and dislocated hip.
  6. Monitor for vascular injury to feet with frequent neurovascular checks.

### Care of the Child with a Brace

**A.** General information
  1. Orthopedic device made of metal or leather applied to the body, particularly the trunk and lower extremities, to support the weight of the body, to correct or prevent deformities, and to prevent involuntary movements in spastic conditions
  2. Types
    **a.** Milwaukee brace
      1) Steel and leather brace fitted and adapted to child individually
      2) Extends from chin cup and neck pad to pelvis
      3) Used in scoliosis to correct curvature
      4) Worn 23 hours/day, removed once daily for bathing
      5) Causes little interference with activity
    **b.** Rotowalker
      1) Used to provide upright mobility in children with lower limb paralysis
      2) Child shifts weight to achieve mobility
    **c.** Leg brace
      1) Designed to stabilize extremity and offer support during ambulation
      2) Special hinges permit hip, knee, and ankle to flex during sitting

**B.** Nursing care: provide client teaching and discharge planning concerning:
  1. Importance of meticulous skin care
  2. Need to wear protective clothing under brace
  3. Potential problems of ill-fitting braces
    **a.** Difficulty in balancing
    **b.** Muscle stress and skin breakdown
  4. Need for frequent checking and adjustment of braces with growth

## EVALUATION

**A.** Child's musculoskeletal development is normal as evidenced by normal growth and activity.
**B.** Child experiences minimal discomfort.
**C.** Injuries are prevented.
**D.** Parents demonstrate ability to identify complications and administer treatments correctly.

# DISORDERS OF THE MUSCULOSKELETAL SYSTEM

## Congenital Dislocation of the Hip (Developmental Dysplasia of the Hip)

**A.** General information
  1. Displacement of the head of the femur from the acetabulum; present at birth, although not always diagnosed immediately
  2. One of the most common congenital malformations; incidence is 2 in 1000 live births
  3. Familial disorder, more common in girls; may be associated with spina bifida
  4. Cause unknown; may be fetal position in utero (breech delivery), genetic predisposition, or laxity of ligaments
  5. The acetabulum is shallow and the head of the femur cartilaginous at birth, contributing to the dislodgment.
**B.** Medical management
  1. Goal is to enlarge and deepen socket by pressure.
  2. The earlier treatment is initiated, the shorter and less traumatic it will be.
  3. Early treatment consists of positioning the hip in abduction with the head of the femur in the acetabulum and maintaining it in position for several months.
  4. If these measures are unsuccessful, traction and casting (hip spica) or surgery may be successful.
**C.** Assessment findings
  1. May be unilateral or bilateral, partial or complete
  2. Limitation of abduction (cannot spread legs to change diaper)

3. Ortolani's click (should only be performed by an experienced practitioner)
   a. With infant in supine position (on the back), bend knees and place thumbs on bent knees, fingers at hip joint.
   b. Bring femurs 90° to hip, then abduct.
   c. With dislocation there is a palpable click where the head of the femur snaps over edge of acetabulum.
4. Barlow's test
   a. With infant on back, bend knees.
   b. Affected knee will be lower because the head of the femur dislocates toward bed by gravity (referred to as telescoping of limb).
5. Additional skin folds with knees bent, from telescoping
6. When lying on abdomen, buttocks of affected side will be flatter because head of femur falls toward bed from gravity
7. Trendelenburg test (used if child is old enough to walk)
   a. Have child stand on affected leg only.
   b. Pelvis will dip on normal side as child attempts to stay erect.
D. Nursing interventions
   1. Maintain proper positioning: keep legs abducted.
      a. Pavlik harness (place undershirt under harness and socks on legs)
      b. Frejka pillow splint (jumperlike suit to keep legs abducted)
      c. Place infant on abdomen with legs in "frog" position
      d. Other immobilization devices (splints, casts, braces)
   2. Provide adequate nutrition; adapt feeding position as needed for immobilization device.
   3. Provide sensory stimulation; adapt to immobilization device and positioning.
   4. Provide client teaching and discharge planning concerning:
      a. Application and care of immobilization devices
      b. Modification of child care using immobilization devices

## Clubfoot (Talipes)

A. General information
   1. Abnormal rotation of foot at ankle
      a. Varus (inward rotation): would walk on ankles, bottoms of feet face each other
      b. Valgus (outward rotation): would walk on inner ankles
      c. Calcaneous (upward rotation): would walk on heels
      d. Equinas (downward rotation): would walk on toes
   2. Most common deformity (95%) is talipes equinovarus.

3. Deformity almost always congenital; usually unilateral
4. Occurs more frequently in boys than in girls; may be associated with other congenital disorders but cause unknown
5. General incidence: 1 in 700–1000
B. Medical management
   1. Exercises
   2. Casting (cast is changed periodically to change angle of foot)
   3. Denis Browne splint (bar shoe): metal bar with shoes attached to the bar at specific angle
   4. Surgery and casting for several months
C. Assessment findings: foot cannot be manipulated by passive exercises into correct position (differentiate from normal clubbing of newborn's feet)
D. Nursing interventions
   1. Perform exercises as ordered.
   2. Provide cast care or care for child in a brace.
   3. Child who is learning to walk must be prevented from trying to stand; apply restraints if necessary.
   4. Provide diversional activities.
   5. Adapt care routines as needed for cast or brace.
   6. Assess toes to be sure cast it not too tight.
   7. Provide skin care.
   8. Provide client teaching and discharge planning concerning:
      a. Application/care of immobilization device
      b. Preparation for surgery if indicated
      c. Need to monitor special shoes for continued fit throughout treatment.

## Tibial Torsion

A. General information
   1. Rotational deformity of tibia (greater than that normally found in newborn)
   2. Types
      a. Internal: knee forward and foot inward
      b. External: knee forward and foot outward (rare, associated with muscle paralysis)
   3. Majority of cases resolve without treatment
B. Medical management
   1. Splinting: use of Denis Browne splint at night
   2. Surgical correction if still evident by age 3 years
C. Assessment findings: with child lying supine, assess for straight line between tibial tuberosity and 2nd toe; in tibial torsion, the line intersects the 4th or 5th toe.
D. Nursing interventions
   1. If no treatment needed, encourage parents to be patient and emphasize that condition usually resolves by itself
   2. If stretching exercises are recommended, teach parents normal ROM exercises and how to carry them out.
   3. Instruct parents on use of Denis Browne splint if needed.

## Legg–Calvè–Perthes Disease

A. General information
1. Aseptic necrosis of femoral head due to disturbance of circulation to the area
2. Primarily affects boys ages 4–10 years
3. Stages: lasting from 18 months to a few years
   a. Initial stage: may not be distinguishable from transient synovitis
   b. Avascular stage: often the first stage noticed
   c. Revascularization stage: regeneration of vascular and connective tissue
   d. Regeneration stage: formation of new bone
B. Medical management: goal is to minimize deformity until healing process is completed
1. Initial bed rest with traction and then an abduction brace
2. Possible surgery
C. Assessment findings
1. Limp, limitation of movement
2. Pain in groin, hip, and referred to knee; often difficult for child to localize pain
3. Diagnostic test: X-ray reveals opaque ossification center of head of the femur (softened in avascular stage)
D. Nursing interventions
1. Provide care for a child with a cast or brace.
2. Provide diversional activities.

## Slipped Femoral Capital Epiphysis

A. General information
1. Spontaneous displacement of proximal femoral epiphysis in a posterior and inferior direction
2. Onset insidious; usually occurs during fast growth period of adolescence (growth hormones weaken epiphyseal plate)
3. Occurs most often in very tall and very obese adolescents; boys affected more frequently
B. Medical management
1. Skeletal traction
2. Surgical stabilization with pinning
C. Assessment findings
1. Limp and referred pain to groin, hip, or knee
2. Limited internal rotation and abduction of hip
D. Nursing interventions
1. Suggest weight reduction program for obese children to decrease stress on bones.
2. Provide care for the child with a cast or traction.

## Osteogenesis Imperfecta

A. General information
1. An inherited disorder affecting collagen formation and resulting in pathologic fractures

2. Types
   a. Osteogenesis imperfecta congenita: autosomal recessive, prognosis poor
   b. Osteogenesis imperfecta tarda: autosomal dominant, less severe form, involvement of varying degrees
3. Classic picture includes soft, fragile bones; blue sclera; otosclerosis
4. Severity of symptoms decreases at puberty due to hormone production and child's ability to prevent injury
B. Medical management
1. Magnesium oxide supplements
2. Reduction and immobilization of fractures
C. Assessment findings
1. Osteogenesis imperfecta congenita
   a. Multiple fractures at birth
   b. Possible skeletal deformity due to intrauterine fracture
   c. Bones of skull are soft
   d. Occasional intracranial hemorrhage
2. Osteogenesis imperfecta tarda
   a. Delayed walking, fractures, structural scoliosis as child grows
   b. Lower limbs more frequently affected
   c. Hypermobility of joints
   d. Prone to dental caries
D. Nursing interventions
1. Support limbs, do not stretch.
2. Position with care; use blankets to aid in mobility and provide support.
3. Instruct parents in bathing, dressing, diapering.
4. Support parents; encourage expression of feelings of anger or guilt (parents may have been unjustly suspected of child abuse).

## Scoliosis

A. General information
1. Lateral curvature of the spine
2. Most commonly occurs in adolescent girls
3. Disorder has a familial pattern; associated with other neuromuscular disorders
4. Majority of the time (75% of cases) disorder is idiopathic; others causes include congenital abnormality of vertebrae, neuromuscular disorders, and trauma
5. May be functional or structural
   a. Nonstructural/functional: "C" curve of spine
      1) Due to posture, can be corrected voluntarily and disappears when child lies down
      2) Not progressive
      3) Treated with posture exercises
   b. Structural/progressive: "S" curve of spine
      1) Usually idiopathic
      2) Structural change in spine, does not disappear with position changes
      3) More aggressive intervention needed

**B.** Medical management
   **1.** Stretching exercises of the spine for nonstructural changes
   **2.** Bracing
      **a.** Milwaukee brace
      **b.** TSLO-custom molded plastic orthotic brace
      **c.** Braces worn 16–23 hours/day; off only for hygiene
   **3.** Surgical correction
      **a.** Spinal alignment
      **b.** Fusion with bone chips

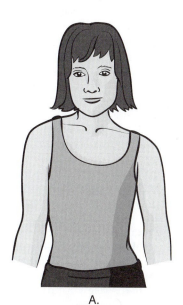

A.

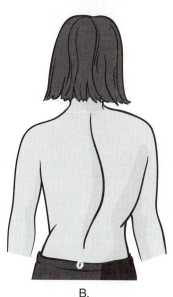

B.

**Figure 5-11** Adolescent girl with scoliosis. (A) Frontal view; (B) posterior view

   **c.** Instrumentation to stabilize position
      **1)** Harrington rod
      **2)** Luque instrumentation: wires and hooks
**C.** Assessment findings (structural scoliosis) (See Figure 5-11.)
   **1.** Failure of curve to straighten when child bends forward with knees straight and arms hanging down to feet (curve disappears with functional scoliosis)
   **2.** Uneven bra strap marks
   **3.** Uneven hips
   **4.** Uneven shoulders
   **5.** Asymmetry of rib cage
   **6.** Diagnostic test: X-ray reveals curvature
**D.** Nursing interventions
   **1.** Teach/encourage exercises as ordered.
   **2.** Provide care for child with Milwaukee brace
      **a.** Child wears brace 23 hours/day; is removed once a day for bathing.
      **b.** Monitor pressure points, adjustments may be needed to accommodate increase in height or weight.
      **c.** Promote positive body image with brace.
   **3.** Provide cast/traction care.
   **4.** Assist with modifying clothing for immobilization devices.
   **5.** Adjust diet for decreased activity.
   **6.** Provide diversional activities.
   **7.** Provide care for child with Harrington rod insertion.
   **8.** Provide client teaching and discharge planning concerning:
      **a.** Exercises
      **b.** Brace/traction/cast care
      **c.** Correct body mechanics
      **d.** Alternative education for long-term hospitalization/home care
      **e.** Availability of community agencies

## Surgical Correction for Scoliosis

**A.** General information
   **1.** Spinal fusion and installation of supports along spine
   **2.** Used for moderate to severe curvatures
   **3.** Usually results in increase in height; positive body image changes
**B.** Nursing interventions (see also Discectomy)
   **1.** Provide general pre-op teaching and care.
   **2.** In addition to routine post-op care.
      **a.** Log roll.
      **b.** Do not raise head of bed.
      **c.** Usually out of bed to chair after 48 hours with Luque procedure.
      **d.** Discuss adapting home environment to allow for privacy yet interaction with family during recovery.
      **e.** Discuss alternate methods of education during recovery period.

## Muscular Dystrophy

A. General information
1. A group of muscular diseases in children characterized by progressive muscle weakness and deformity
2. Genetic in origin; biochemical defect is suspected
3. Types
   a. Pseudohypertrophic (Duchenne type): most frequent type
      1) X-linked recessive
      2) Affects only boys
      3) Usually manifests in first 4 years
   b. Facioscapulohumeral
      1) Autosomal dominant
      2) Mild form, with weakness of facial and shoulder girdle muscles
      3) Onset usually in adolescence
   c. Limb girdle
      1) Autosomal recessive
      2) Affects boys and girls
      3) Onset usually in adolescence
   d. Congenital
      1) Autosomal recessive
      2) Onset in utero
   e. Myotonic
      1) Autosomal dominant
      2) More common in boys
      3) Onset in infancy or childhood, or adult onset
      4) Prognosis in childhood form is guarded
4. Disease causes progressive disability throughout childhood; most children with Duchenne's muscular dystrophy are confined to a wheelchair by age 8–10 years.
5. Death occurs by age 20 in 75% of clients with Duchenne's muscular dystrophy.

B. Assessment findings (Duchenne type)
1. Pelvic girdle weakness is early sign (child waddles and falls)
2. Gower's sign (child uses hands to push up from the floor)
3. Scoliosis (from weakness of shoulder girdle)
4. Contractures and hypertrophy of muscles
5. Diagnostic tests
   a. Muscle biopsy reveals histologic changes: degeneration of muscle fibers and replacement of fibers with fat.
   b. EMG shows decrease in amplitude and duration of potentials.
6. Serum enzymes increased, especially CPK

C. Nursing interventions
1. Prepare child for EMG and muscle biopsy.
2. Maintain function at optimal level; keep child as active and independent as possible.
3. Plan diet to prevent obesity.
4. Continually evaluate capabilities.

5. Support child and parents and provide information about availability of community agencies and support groups.

## Juvenile Rheumatoid Arthritis

A. General information
1. Systemic, chronic disorder of connective tissue, resulting from an autoimmune reaction
2. Results in eventual joint destruction
3. Affected by stress, climate, and genetics
4. More common in girls; peak ages 2–5 and 9–12 years
5. Types
   a. Mono/pauciarticular JRA
      1) Fewer than four joints involved (usually in legs)
      2) Asymmetric; rarely systemic
      3) Generally mild signs of arthritis
      4) Symptoms may decrease as child enters adulthood
      5) Prognosis good
   b. Polyarticular JRA
      1) Multiple joints affected
      2) Symmetrical symptoms of arthritis, disability may be mild to severe
      3) Involvement of temporomandibular joint may cause earaches
      4) Characterized by periods of remissions and exacerbations
      5) Prognosis poorer
      6) Treatment symptomatic for arthritis: physical therapy, ROM exercises, aspirin
   c. Systemic disease with polyarthritis (Still's disease)
      1) Explosive course with remissions and exacerbations lasting for months
      2) Begins with fever, rash, lymphadenopathy, anorexia, and weight loss

B. Medical management, assessment findings, and nursing interventions: see Rheumatoid Arthritis

 **Sample Questions**

137. An 18-month-old has a fractured femur and is in Bryant's traction. In evaluating the correct application of the traction, what will the nurse note?
   1. The child is being continuously and gradually pulled toward bottom of bed.
   2. The child's buttocks are raised slightly.
   3. The child's leg is at a 45° angle to the bed.
   4. The child can move the unaffected leg freely.

**138.** A 14-year-old is in a hip spica cast. Which is the correct method to turn the adolescent?

1. Use the cross bar.
2. Turn her upper body first, then turn the lower body.
3. Log-roll her.
4. Tell her to pull on the trapeze and sit up to help in turning.

**139.** A routine physical examination on a 2-day-old uncovered evidence of congenital dislocation, or dysplasia, of the right hip. When assessing the infant, what would be a sign of one-sided hip displacement?

1. An unusually narrow perineum
2. Pain where her leg is abducted.
3. Symmetrical skin folds near her buttocks and thigh.
4. Asymmetrical skin folds over the buttocks and thigh.

**140.** An infant is being treated for congenital hip dysplasia with a Pavlik harness. The baby's mother asks if she can remove the harness if it becomes soiled. What would be the nurse's best response?

1. No, the harness may not be removed.
2. No, she will only be wearing it a few days.
3. Yes, just long enough to clean the area.
4. Yes, just overnight while she is sleeping.

**141.** A 10-year-old takes aspirin QID for Still's disease (juvenile rheumatoid arthritis). What symptoms would her mother observe that would be indicative of aspirin toxicity?

1. Hypothermia.
2. Hypoventilation.
3. Decreased hearing acuity.
4. Increased urinary output.

**142.** Which of the following would the nurse include in a plan of care for a toddler with a newly applied hip spica cast?

1. Petal the cast around the perineum area with waterproof tape.
2. Teach the parents care of the child just before discharge.
3. Give the child small blocks and beads to promote eye-hand coordination.
4. Check neurovascular status every shift.

**143.** The mother of a 6-year-old asks why she was told not to use powder under her child's long leg cast. Which of the following is the most accurate basis for the nurse's response?

1. Promoting adequate circulation is a top priority.
2. Drying the cast is very important.
3. Assessing the smell of a cast is a top priority.
4. Preserving skin integrity is of the utmost importance.

**144.** In examining a newborn, the nurse notes the following: asymmetric gluteal folds, shortened right leg, and limited abduction of the right thigh. The nurse would correctly interpret these observations as which of the following?

1. Right congenital dislocated hip.
2. Spastic cerebral palsy.
3. Left hip dysplasia.
4. Myelodysplasia.

**145.** An infant with congenital hip dysplasia is placed in a Pavlik harness. In the nurse's teaching plan for the mother, which of the following would be important to include?

1. Adjustment of daily care routines as the harness is worn 24 hours a day.
2. Clothing should not be worn under the harness.
3. The harness should be removed for bathing and diapering only.
4. The infant should be confined to the crib.

**146.** In assessing a newborn for talipes equinovarus, the nurse would note which of the following?

1. The feet turn inward when the infant lies still, but they are flexible.
2. The feet are rigid and cannot be manipulated to a neutral position.
3. Uneven knee length occurs when both knees are flexed.
4. Limited abduction is observed when performing the Ortolani maneuver.

**147.** The nurse would evaluate that the parents correctly understand the care of their infant being treated for talipes equinovarus if the parents said which of the following?

1. "We will unwrap the cast every night and massage his feet with lotion to prevent skin breakdown."
2. "We'll petal the cast around the baby's groin to protect it from urine and bowel movements."
3. "Every day we'll check the baby's toes for movement and color after we squeeze them."
4. "We're so glad that the casts will cure his club feet."

**148.** Which of the following comments by the school nurse would be most appropriate in screening for scoliosis of a 13-year-old?

1. "You may leave your shirt on, but stand erect and turn to the side."
2. "Do you have any back pain?"
3. "Remove your clothes from the waist up and bend over at your waist."
4. "Have you noticed that your skirts don't hang evenly?"

149. A child is admitted to the hospital for a spinal fusion and Harrington rod insertion. What would be a nursing priority in the first 8 hours postoperatively?
1. Give fluids and fiber to promote bowel elimination.
2. Check neurovascular function in extremities.
3. Log roll every 4 hours.
4. Monitor hourly urine output.

150. The nurse would evaluate that a child understood the effective use of her Milwaukee brace for her scoliosis if she said which of the following?
1. "I'm so glad that I don't have to sleep in this brace."
2. "I've toughened my skin so I can wear the brace right next to my skin."
3. "I can't believe that I'm not allowed to chew gum anymore."
4. "I'm going to look forward to my bath time each day without this brace."

151. A 4-year-old has recently been diagnosed with Duchenne's muscular dystrophy. His parents ask if their 2-year-old daughter will get the disease. The nurse's best response would be which of the following?
1. "Every child you have has a 25% chance of developing the disease and a 50% chance of being a carrier."
2. "Sons are affected 50% of the time, whereas 50% of the time daughters will become carriers who have no symptoms."
3. "Only your sons have a 25% chance of developing the disease."
4. "Every child has a 50% chance of developing the disease."

## Answers and Rationales

137. **2.** In Bryant's traction both legs are in traction at a 90° angle and the buttocks are raised slightly off the bed.

138. **3.** The client in a hip spica cast should be turned as a unit.

139. **4.** Displacement of the hip on one side causes asymmetry of skin folds.

140. **1.** The harness is not to be removed until the hip is stable with 90° of flexion and X-ray confirmation. This usually occurs after about 3 weeks in a Pavlik harness.

141. **3.** Tinnitus or ringing in the ears is a side effect of aspirin therapy. In salicylate poisoning the child will have hypothermia, hyperventilation to compensate for metabolic acidosis, and may develop renal failure.

142. **1.** It is important to protect the cast from urine and stool to prevent skin and cast breakdown.

143. **4.** Powder may irritate the skin, leading to skin breakdown and infection.

144. **1.** These are all signs of right congenital dislocated hip in a newborn.

145. **1.** The harness is worn 24 hours a day so that parents must learn how to manage daily care (sponging and dressing the baby) with the harness on.

146. **2.** Talipes equinovarus is a rigid deformity with forefoot adduction, inversion of the heel, and plantar flexion of the feet.

147. **3.** Parents should be taught to assess neurovascular status of the toes because babies grow quickly and may outgrow the casts.

148. **3.** This is part of the screening process for scoliosis. The nurse is checking for rib hump and flank asymmetry. Also included is visual inspection of frontal and dorsal posture, observation for uneven hip and shoulder levels as well as for muscular disproportion.

149. **2.** One of the greatest risks of spinal surgery is of paralysis if the spinal cord is injured or compressed by swelling. Monitoring for sensation and movement is the top priority.

150. **4.** For best results in correction, the brace should be worn for 20–23 hours a day and only removed for hygiene and skin care.

151. **2.** Duchenne's muscular dystrophy is an X-linked recessive disorder. The defective gene is transmitted through carrier females to affected sons 50% of the time depending on which X is transmitted. Daughters have a 50% chance of becoming carriers.

# The Endocrine System

## VARIATIONS FROM THE ADULT

A. Adenohypophysis (anterior lobe of pituitary gland)
   1. Growth hormone
      a. Does not affect prenatal growth.
      b. Main effect on linear growth is through increase of cells in skeletal bones.
      c. Maintains rate of synthesis of body protein.
   2. Thyroid-stimulating hormone (TSH)
      a. Important for normal development of bones, teeth, and brain.
      b. Secretion decreases throughout childhood, then increases at puberty.
   3. Adrenocorticotropic hormone (ACTH)
      a. Little is produced throughout childhood.
      b. Becomes active in adolescence.
      c. Stimulates adrenals to secrete sex hormones.
      d. Influences production of gonadotropic hormone by hypothalamus.
         1) Gonadotropic hormones activate gonads.
         2) Gonads secrete estrogen or testosterone, which stimulate development of secondary sex characteristics.
   4. Estrogen has an inhibitory effect on epiphyseal growth.

## ANALYSIS

Nursing diagnoses for the child with a disorder of the endocrine system may include:
A. Ineffective health maintenance
B. Impaired home maintenance
C. Noncompliance
D. Disturbed body image
E. Low self-esteem

## PLANNING AND IMPLEMENTATION

### Goals

A. Any endocrine imbalance in childhood will be identified and treated.
B. Child will achieve a normal metabolic state.
C. Child will develop successful coping mechanisms for manifestations of disease.
D. Child will have no signs of complications of the disease.

## EVALUATION

A. Child receives appropriate medication, and nutritional requirements are met; symptoms of endocrine disease are controlled.
B. Child is free from complications of disease.
C. Child is achieving growth and developmental tasks on as normal a timetable as possible.
D. Child discusses feelings about body image and uses coping mechanisms that promote a positive self-image.

## DISORDERS OF THE ENDOCRINE SYSTEM

### Diabetes Mellitus

Also see Unit 4.
A. General information
   1. Most common endocrine disease of children; onset may be at any age
   2. Children typically develop Type 1: insulin-dependent diabetes mellitus
   3. Possible genetic predisposition to disease
   4. Treatments vary based on rapid growth rate in children, increased incidence of infections, and dietary fads of peers; all include insulin administration.
   5. Risk of complications is high; most commonly retinopathy, neuropathy, nephropathy, skin changes, predisposition to infection
   6. Children sometimes have one honeymoon period that occurs shortly after a child is regulated on insulin for the first time
      a. Lasts from 1 month to 1 year.
      b. Represents final effort of pancreas to provide insulin until beta cells are completely destroyed.
      c. Parents may distrust the diagnosis of diabetes and need to be reminded that symptoms will reappear and child will need insulin for life.
B. Medical management
   1. Insulin
   2. Diet therapy
   3. Exercise
   4. Prevention of complications
C. Assessment findings
   1. Rapid onset
   2. Polyuria, polydipsia, polyphagia, fatigue
   3. Weight loss

4. Ketoacidosis
5. Dry, flushed skin with hyperglycemia
D. Nursing interventions
1. Administer insulin (regular and NPH) as ordered.
2. Force fluids without sugar.
3. Monitor blood glucose levels daily.
4. Observe for hypoglycemia (insulin shock): behavior changes, sweating.
5. Provide client teaching and discharge planning concerning:
    a. Daily regimen for home care
    b. Urine and blood glucose monitoring
    c. Nutrition management
    d. Effects of infection and exercise on carbohydrate metabolism
    e. Prevention of acute and chronic complications

# Congenital Hypothyroidism (Cretinism)

A. General information
1. Disorder related to absent or nonfunctioning thyroid
2. Newborns are supplied with maternal thyroid hormones that last up to 3 months
B. Medical management
1. Prevention: neonatal screening blood test (mandatory in many states)
2. Drug therapy: thyroid hormone replacement
3. Without treatment mental retardation and developmental delay will occur after age 3 months
C. Assessment findings
1. Altered body proportions; short stature with legs shorter than they should be in proportion to trunk
2. Tongue is enlarged and protrudes from mouth; may result in breathing and feeding difficulties
3. Hypothermia with cool extremities
4. Short, thick neck; delayed dentition
5. Hypotonia
6. Low levels of $T_3$ and $T_4$
D. Nursing interventions
1. Administer oral thyroxine and vitamin D as ordered to prevent mental retardation.
2. Provide client teaching and discharge planning concerning:
    a. Medication administration and side effects
    b. Importance of continued therapy

# Hypopituitarism (Pituitary Dwarfism)

A. General information
1. Hyposecretion of growth hormone by the anterior lobe of the pituitary gland
2. Cause may be unknown or it may be due to craniopharyngioma

B. Medical management: administration of growth hormone (limited in supply since it is rendered from human cadavers)
C. Assessment findings
1. Newborn is of normal size, but child falls below the third percentile by age 1.
2. Child is well proportioned, but may be overweight for height.
3. Underdeveloped jaw, abnormal position of teeth, high voice, delayed puberty
4. Diagnostic tests
    a. X-rays reveal delayed closing of epiphyseal plates of long bones
    b. Normal IQ
D. Nursing interventions
1. Interact with child according to chronologic age/developmental level, and not according to physical appearance.
2. Administer growth hormone as ordered (because of delay in bone development, these children can still grow even when their peers have stopped).
3. Monitor for signs and symptoms of additional neurologic disorders.
4. Keep careful records of height and weight.
5. Encourage child/parents to express feelings.
6. Assist child in learning to interact normally with peers.

# Hyperpituitarism (Gigantism)

A. General information
1. Hypersecretion of growth hormone (usually related to a tumor of the anterior pituitary) resulting in enlargement of bones of head, hands, and feet, and overgrowth of long bones
2. Especially noticeable at puberty
B. Medical management
1. Surgery to remove tumor
2. Radiation therapy if there is no tumor
C. Assessment findings
1. Height beyond maximum upper percentile
2. Proportional weight and muscle growth
3. Coarse facial features
4. Signs of increased ICP if caused by a tumor
D. Nursing interventions
1. Record height and head circumference.
2. Provide nursing care for a client receiving radiation therapy.
3. Provide care for the child with a brain tumor.
4. Assist child in interacting normally with peers.

## Sample Questions

**152.** An 8-year-old is newly diagnosed with diabetes mellitus. Which of the following symptoms is different from what you would expect to find in maturity-onset (Type 2) diabetes?

1. Increased appetite.
2. Increased thirst.
3. Increased urination.
4. Weight loss.

**153.** A 7-year-old is newly diagnosed with diabetes mellitus. She had an injection of regular and NPH insulin at 0730. At 1510 she complains that she does not feel well. She is pale, perspiring, and trembling. What instructions should the nurse give the child?

1. Tell her to lie down and wait for the dinner trays to arrive.
2. Ask her to give a urine specimen and test it for sugar and acetone.
3. Give her a carbohydrate snack.
4. Administer the afternoon dose of regular insulin.

**154.** A 10-year-old with diabetes mellitus is learning how to administer her insulin. She asks the nurse why she cannot take pills like her grandmother who also has diabetes. Which would be a correct response from the nurse?

1. How long has your grandmother been taking oral medication?
2. You'll be able to stop taking insulin once you stop growing.
3. You have a different kind of diabetes and you will need to take insulin throughout your life.
4. You'll be able to switch to pills when you reach your grandmother's age.

## Answers and Rationales

**152. 4.** Weight loss is associated with juvenile diabetes, whereas weight gain develops in maturity-onset diabetes.

**153. 3.** The symptoms suggest she is having a hypoglycemic reaction from the NPH insulin and needs an afternoon snack.

**154. 3.** Juvenile or Type 1 diabetics need lifetime insulin because they no longer produce their own.

# The Integumentary System

## VARIATIONS FROM THE ADULT

**A.** Skin is only 1 mm thick at birth; approximately twice as thick at maturity.
**B.** Evaporative water loss is greater in infants and small children.
**C.** Skin is more susceptible to bacterial infection in children.
**D.** Children are more prone to toxic erythema as a result of drug reactions and skin eruptions.
**E.** Children's skin is more susceptible to sweat retention and maceration.

## ASSESSMENT

### History

**A.** Medical history: previous skin disease, allergic conditions
**B.** History of present condition: onset, relationship to eating or other activities, medication usage

### Physical Examination

**A.** Lesion type: note petechiae, erythema, ecchymosis; note secondary symptoms from rubbing, scratching, or healing.
**B.** Observe distribution pattern.
**C.** Note presence of pain or altered sensation.
**D.** Check scalp for signs of lice or nits.

## ANALYSIS

Nursing diagnoses for the child with a disorder of the integumentary system may include:
**A.** Pain
**B.** Disturbed body image
**C.** Disturbed sensory perception

D. Risk for impaired skin integrity
E. Low self-esteem

# PLANNING AND IMPLEMENTATION

## Goals

A. Child will be free from discomfort.
B. Skin integrity will be restored.
C. Spread of infection and secondary infection will be prevented.

# EVALUATION

A. Child is free from discomfort.
   1. Minimal scratching or rubbing
   2. Relaxed facial expression
   3. Minimal restlessness
B. Child's skin is clean, dry, and free from redness or signs of irritation.
C. Child is free from complications such as spread of infection.
D. Parents demonstrate satisfactory hygiene measures when caring for child with disorder of skin or scalp.

# DISORDERS OF THE INTEGUMENTARY SYSTEM

## Burns

Also see Unit 4.
A. For children, the rule of nines is modified; the head of a small child is 18–19%, the trunk 32%, each leg 15%, each arm 9½%.
B. Burns in infants and toddlers are frequently due to spills (pulling hot fluids on them or falling into hot baths); for older children, flame burns are more frequent.

## Impetigo

A. General information
   1. Superficial bacterial infection of the outer layers of skin (usually staphylococcus or streptococcus)
   2. Common in toddlers and preschoolers
   3. Related to poor sanitation
   4. Very contagious
B. Medical management: topical and systemic antibiotics
C. Assessment findings
   1. Well-demarcated lesions
   2. Macules, papules, vesicles that rupture, causing a superficial moist erosion
   3. Moist area dries, leaving a honey-colored crust

   4. Spreads peripherally
   5. Most commonly found on face, axillae, and extremities
   6. Pruritus
D. Nursing interventions
   1. Implement skin isolation techniques.
   2. Soften the skin and crusts with Burrow's solution compresses.
   3. Remove crusts gently.
   4. Cover draining lesions to prevent spread of infection.
   5. Administer antibiotics as ordered, both orally and as bacteriocidal ointments.
   6. Prevent secondary infection.
   7. Provide client teaching and discharge planning concerning:
      a. Medication administration
      b. Proper hygiene techniques

## Ringworm

A. General information
   1. Dermatomycosis due to various species of fungus
   2. Infected sites include:
      a. Scalp (tinea capitis)
      b. Body (tinea corporis)
      c. Feet (tinea pedis or athlete's foot)
   3. May be transmitted from person to person or acquired from animals or soil
B. Assessment findings
   1. Scalp
      a. Scaly circumscribed patches on the scalp
      b. Base of hair shafts are invaded by spores of the fungus; causes hair to break off, resulting in alopecia
      c. Spreads in a circular pattern
      d. Detected by Wood's lamp (fluoresces green at base of the affected hair shafts)
   2. Skin: red-ringed patches of vesicles; pain, scaling, itching
C. Nursing interventions
   1. Prevention: isolate from known infected persons.
   2. Apply antifungal ointment as ordered.
   3. Administer oral griseofulvin as ordered.

## Pediculosis (Head Lice)

A. General information
   1. Parasitic infestation
   2. Adult lice are spread by close physical contact (sharing combs, hats, etc.)
   3. Occurs in school-age children, particularly those with long hair
B. Medical management: special shampoos followed by use of fine-tooth comb to remove nits
C. Assessment findings
   1. White eggs (nits) firmly attached to base of hair shafts
   2. Pruritus of scalp

**D.** Nursing interventions
1. Institute skin isolation precautions (especially head coverings and gloves to prevent spread to self, other staff, and clients)
2. Use special shampoo and comb the hair
3. Provide client teaching and discharge planning concerning:
   a. How to check self and other family members and how to treat them
   b. Washing of clothes, bed linens, etc.; discouraging sharing of brushes, combs, and hats

# Allergies

## Diaper Rash

**A.** General information
1. Contact dermatitis
2. Plastic/rubber pants and linings of disposable diapers exacerbate the condition by prolonging contact with moist, warm environment; skin is further irritated by acidic urine
3. May also be caused by sensitivity to laundry soaps used

**B.** Medical management: exposure of skin to air/heat lamp

**C.** Assessment findings
1. Erythema/excoriation in the perineal area
2. Irritability

**D.** Nursing interventions
1. Keep area clean and dry; clean with mild soap and water after each stool and as soon as child urinates.
2. Take off diaper and expose area to air during the day.
3. Use heat lamp as ordered.
4. Provide client teaching and discharge planning concerning:
   a. Proper hygiene/infant care
   b. Diaper laundering methods
   c. Avoiding use of plastic pants or disposable diapers with a plastic lining
   d. Avoiding use of cornstarch (a good medium for bacteria once it becomes wet)
   e. Need to avoid use of commercially prepared diaper wipes because they contain chemicals and alcohol, which may be irritating

## Poison Ivy

**A.** General information
1. Contact dermatitis; mediated by T-cell response so rash is not seen for 24–48 hours after contact.
2. Poison ivy is not spread by the fluid in the vesicles; can be spread by clothes and animals that retain the plant resin.

**B.** Assessment findings: very pruritic impetigo-like lesions

**C.** Nursing interventions
1. Administer antihistamines and cortisone as ordered.
2. Provide client teaching and discharge planning concerning:
   a. Plant identification
   b. Need to wash with soap and water after contact with plant
   c. Importance of washing clothes to get the resin out

## Eczema

**A.** General information
1. Atopic dermatitis, often the first sign of an allergic predisposition in a child; many later develop respiratory allergies
2. Usually manifests during infancy

**B.** Medical management
1. Drug therapy
   a. Topical steroids
   b. Antihistamines
   c. Emollients
   d. Cautious administration of immunizations
   e. Medicated or colloid baths
2. Diet therapy: elimination diet to detect offending foods

**C.** Assessment findings
1. Erythema, weeping vesicles that rupture and crust over
2. Usually evident on cheeks, scalp, behind ears, and on flexor surfaces of extremities (rarely on diaper area)
3. Severe pruritus; scratching causes thickening and darkening of skin
4. Dry skin, sometimes urticaria

**D.** Nursing interventions
1. Avoid heat and prevent sweating; keep skin dry (moisture aggravates condition).
2. Monitor elimination diet to detect food cause.
   a. Remove all solid foods from diet (formula only).
   b. If symptoms disappear after 3 days, start one new food group every 3 days to see if symptoms reappear.
   c. The food that is suspected of causing the rash is withdrawn again to make sure symptoms go away in 3 days and is then introduced a second time (challenge test).
3. Check materials in contact with child's skin (sheets, lotions, soaps).
4. Tepid baths, mild soaps.
   a. Provide lubricant immediately after bath.
   b. Pat dry gently with soft towel (do not rub) and pat in lubricant.
   c. Avoid the use of harsh soaps (dry skin).
5. Administer topical steroids as ordered (penetrate better if applied within 3 minutes after bath). Thin layer of topical steroid.
6. Use cotton instead of wool clothing.

7. Keep child's nails short to prevent scratching and secondary infection; use gloves or elbow restraints if needed.
8. Apply wet saline or Burrow's solution compresses.
9. Double-rinse laundry.
10. Assess skin for infection.

## Acne

A. General information
   1. Skin condition associated with increased production of sebum from sebaceous glands at puberty.
   2. Lesions include pustules, papules, and comedones.
   3. Majority of adolescents experience some degree of acne, mild to severe.
   4. Lesions occur most frequently on face, neck, shoulders, and back.
   5. Caused by a variety of interrelated factors including increased activity of sebaceous glands, emotional stress, certain medications, menstrual cycle.
   6. Secondary infection can complicate healing of lesions.
   7. There is no evidence to support the value of eliminating any foods from the diet; if cause and effect can be established, however, a particular food should be eliminated.
B. Assessment findings
   1. Appearance of lesions is variable and fluctuating
   2. Systemic symptoms absent
   3. Psychologic problems such as social withdrawal, low self-esteem, feelings of being "ugly"
C. Nursing interventions
   1. Discuss OTC products and their effects.
   2. Instruct child in proper hygiene (handwashing, care of face, not to pick or squeeze any lesions).
   3. Demonstrate proper administration of topical ointments and antibiotics if indicated.

## Sample Questions

155. A 2-year-old was recently found to have impetigo. What measures should be given the highest priority to prevent its spread while in the hospital?
   1. Keeping it covered.
   2. Good handwashing.
   3. Applying A&D ointment.
   4. Placing the child in isolation.

156. A 7-year-old boy has a loss of scalp hair and is diagnosed with ringworm. What question will the nurse most likely ask?
   1. Whether the family owns any pets.
   2. From what economic background is the family.
   3. Whether other children in his classroom have ringworm.
   4. Whether the child can read the medicine directions.

157. Three school children have pediculosis capitus. The school nurse has been instructing the parents of all three students on prevention. Which statement made by one mother indicates an understanding of prevention?
   1. "I will put all of the stuffed animals in plastic bags for 2 weeks."
   2. "Since the sheets are now clean, the kids can share beds, too."
   3. "Once I cut her hair, all the nits should be gone."
   4. "I will now bathe my child every day to prevent reinfection."

158. Prior to discharge home with their new baby, which of the following will demonstrate to the nurse that the parents understand diaper rash prevention?
   1. They articulate that the baby should be checked for wet diapers every half an hour.
   2. They are observed wiping with soap and water at diaper changes.
   3. The mother discusses needs to use tight rubber pants to keep diapers from leaking.
   4. The father wipes carefully and uses a mild ointment to protect the skin.

159. A 3-year-old girl has had eczema since 4 months of age. Which statement made by her father indicates to the nurse that he understands the management of eczema?
   1. "Benadryl should be given every night before bedtime."
   2. "It's beneficial to keep her in the bubble bath for as long as possible each day."
   3. "Typical eruption areas that need to be treated include flexor surfaces of joints."
   4. "Hot water is better in which to bathe."

**155. 2.** Good handwashing is of paramount importance in preventing its spread.

**156. 1.** Pets are known to be carriers of ringworm.

**157. 1.** Stuffed animals can harbor eggs and cause reinfection.

**158. 4.** Careful cleansing on delicate skin and use of ointments helps to preserve the skin's integrity.

**159. 3.** These are the joint areas typically affected in the childhood years.

# Pediatric Oncology

## OVERVIEW

A. Cancer is the leading cause of death from disease in children from 1–14 years.
B. Incidence
   1. 6000 children develop cancer per year.
   2. 3000 children die from cancer annually.
   3. Boys are affected more frequently.
C. Leukemia is the most frequent type of childhood cancer, followed by tumors of the CNS.
D. Etiologic factors include environmental agents, viruses, familial/genetic factors, and host factors.

## Major Stressful Events

Five events have been identified as major stressors:
A. Diagnosis: child is initially hospitalized to determine extent of disease, plan course of treatment, and to educate child and family.
B. Treatment: multimodal
   1. May include surgery, radiation, chemotherapy
   2. Side effects are serious and unpleasant; child/family may complain that the "treatment is worse than the disease."
C. Remission: child is without evidence of disease, treatment continues; goals for this period include:
   1. Maintenance of normal family patterns: discipline and usual household chores
   2. Maintenance of relationships among family and friends
      a. Parents' marriage may be strained
      b. Siblings may feel neglected or jealous
   3. Attendance at school
      a. Child may fear rejection by peers due to change in appearance or not being able to keep up
      b. Teacher may be unsure as to what to say or how to treat the child
      c. Classmates need to be prepared for child's return; may have fears/concerns about whether the disease is catching and whether their friend will die
D. Recurrence
   1. An event of enormous magnitude and a cause of severe disappointment
   2. May occur while still on treatment or after treatment has been completed
E. Death

## ASSESSMENT

### History

A. Family history: some cancers suggest patterns of inheritance
B. Prenatal exposure
C. Children with chromosomal disorders have a higher-than-average incidence of cancer
D. History may elicit symptoms that have been present for a period of time
E. Presenting problems: symptoms may include:
   1. Fever, pain, bleeding
   2. Abdominal mass
   3. Night sweats, weight loss
   4. Hematuria, hypertension

### Physical Examination

A. General appearance
   1. Skin: note color, bruises, or petechiae
   2. Neurologic status: note fatigue, activity level, behavior, headache, dizziness, gait disturbances
   3. Pain: guarding of any body part, changes in range of motion
B. Measure vital signs including BP
C. Plot height and weight on growth chart
D. Inspect and palpate abdomen; note enlargement of liver and spleen
E. Palpate for enlarged lymph nodes
F. Inspect eyes for nystagmus

## Laboratory/Diagnostic Test

A. Blood studies, e.g., CBC
B. X-rays, bone scans, CT scans, MRI, ultrasound
C. Lumbar puncture
D. Bone marrow aspiration

## ANALYSIS

Nursing diagnoses for the child with cancer may include:
A. Risk for infection
B. Risk for injury
C. Fear/anxiety
D. Disturbed body image
E. Deficient knowledge

## PLANNING AND IMPLEMENTATION

### Goals

A. Child will be free from infection
B. Child will be free from pain
C. Optimum developmental level will be achieved
D. Family will develop effective coping strategies

## Interventions

### Surgery

A. May be performed for tumor removal, to obtain a biopsy, to determine extent of disease, or for palliation
B. Often used in conjunction with radiation or chemotherapy

### Radiation Therapy

A. Primarily used in children to improve prognosis
B. Goal is to achieve maximum effect on tumor while sparing normal tissue
   1. May be used for palliative relief from pain, disfigurement
   2. May be curative, destroys cancer cells/reduces size of tumor
   3. Frequently used as an adjunct to chemotherapy and surgery
   4. Must weigh gain versus risks of permanent damage to normal tissue
   5. Infants particularly susceptible to developing skeletal deformities in later years as a result of radiation
   6. Complications to growing child include scoliosis, arrested skeletal development, and pulmonary fibrosis (depends on site radiated)
   7. Dosage range varies; may be as low as 1000 rad to relieve bone pain in a specific area, to as high as 7000 rad to achieve a cure in Ewing's sarcoma
   8. Usually performed 5 days a week for 2–6 weeks

### Chemotherapy

Almost all pediatric cancer clients receive some form of drug therapy.
A. Childhood cancers are more sensitive and responsive to drugs than are adult cancers.
B. Childhood cancers tend to metastasize early and systemic treatment is needed in addition to localized treatment.

### Hematopoietic Stem Cell Transplantation (HSCT) [Previously known as Bone Marrow Transplantation]

A. General information
   1. Treatment alternative for a variety of childhood diseases including:
      a. Definite: acute lymphoblastic leukemia, acute nonlymphocytic leukemia, severe aplastic anemia, immunodeficiencies, and malignant infantile osteopetrosis
      b. Possible: chronic myelogenous leukemia, solid tumors, some hematologic disorders, and some inherited metabolic disorders
   2. Types
      a. Autologous: client transplanted with own harvested marrow
      b. Syngeneic: transplant between identical twins
      c. Allogeneic: transplant from a genetically nonidentical donor
         1) Most common transplant type
         2) Sibling most common donor
   3. Procedure
      a. Donor suitability determined through tissue antigen typing; includes human leukocyte antigen (HLA) and mixed leukocyte culture (MLC) typing.
      b. Donor bone marrow is aspirated from multiple sites along the iliac crests under general anesthesia.
      c. Donor marrow is infused IV into the recipient.
   4. Early evidence of engraftment seen during the second week posttransplant; hematologic reconstitution takes 4–6 weeks; immunologic reconstitution takes months.
   5. Hospitalization of 2 or 3 months required.
   6. Prognosis is highly variable depending on indication for use.
B. Complications
   1. Failure of engraftment
   2. Infection: highest risk in first 3–4 weeks
   3. Pneumonia: nonbacterial or interstitial pneumonias are principal cause of death during first 3 months posttransplant

4. Graft vs host disease (GVHD): principal complication; caused by an immunologic reaction of engrafted lymphoid cells against the tissues of the recipient
   a. Acute GVHD: develops within first 100 days posttransplant and affects skin, gut, liver, marrow, and lymphoid tissue
   b. Chronic GVHD: develops 100–400 days posttransplant; manifested by multiorgan involvement
5. Recurrent malignancy
6. Late complications such as cataracts, endocrine abnormalities

C. Nursing care: pretransplant
1. Extensive time must be spent with child/parents in preparing for this procedure.
2. Recipient immunosuppression attained with total body irradiation (TBI) and chemotherapy to eradicate existing disease and create space in host marrow to allow transplanted cells to grow.
3. Provide protected environment.
   a. Child should be in a laminar air flow room or on strict reverse isolation; surveillance cultures done twice a week.
   b. Encourage use of toys and familiar objects; they must be sterilized before being brought into the room.
   c. Encourage frequent contact with schoolteacher/play therapist.
   d. Introduce new people where they can be seen, but outside child's room so child can see what they look like without isolation garb.
4. Monitor central lines frequently; check patency and observe for signs of infection (fever, redness around site).
5. Provide care for the child receiving chemotherapy and radiation therapy to induce immunosuppression.
   a. Administer chemotherapy as ordered, assist with radiation therapy if required.
   b. Monitor side effects and keep child as comfortable as possible.
   c. Monitor carefully for potential infection.
   d. Child will become very ill; prepare parents.

D. Nursing care: posttransplant
1. Prevent infection.
   a. Maintain protective environment.
   b. Administer antibiotics as ordered.
   c. Assess all mucous membranes, wounds, catheter sites for swelling, redness, tenderness, pain.
   d. Monitor vital signs frequently (every 1–4 hours as needed).
   e. Collect specimens for cultures as needed and twice a week.
   f. Change IV set-ups every 24 hours.

2. Provide mouth care for stomatitis and mucositis (severe mucositis develops about 5 days after irradiation).
   a. Note tissue sloughing, bleeding, changes in color.
   b. Provide mouth rinses, viscous lidocaine, and antibiotic rinses.
   c. Do not use lemon and glycerin swabs.
   d. Administer parenteral narcotics as ordered if necessary to control pain.
   e. Provide care every 2 hours or as needed.
3. Provide skin care: skin breakdown may result from profuse diarrhea from the TBI.
4. Monitor carefully for bleeding.
   a. Check for occult blood in emesis and stools.
   b. Observe for easy bruising, petechiae on skin, mucous membranes.
   c. Monitor changes in vital signs.
   d. Check platelet count daily.
   e. Replace blood products as ordered (all blood products should be irradiated).
5. Maintain fluid and electrolyte balance and promote nutrition.
   a. Measure I&O carefully.
   b. Provide adequate fluid, protein, and caloric intake.
   c. Weigh daily.
   d. Administer fluid replacement as ordered.
   e. Monitor hydration status: check skin turgor, moisture of mucous membranes, urine output.
   f. Check electrolytes daily.
   g. Check urine for glucose, ketones, protein.
   h. Administer antidiarrheal agents as needed.
6. Provide client teaching and discharge planning concerning:
   a. Home environment (e.g., cleaning, pets, visitors)
   b. Diet modifications
   c. Medication regimen: schedule, dosages, effects, and side effects
   d. Communicable diseases and immunizations
   e. Daily hygiene and skin care
   f. Fever
   g. Activity

## STAGES OF CANCER TREATMENT

A. Induction
1. Goal: to remove bulk of tumor
2. Methods: surgery, radiation/chemotherapy, bone marrow transplant
3. Effects: often the most intensive phase; side effects of treatment are potentially life threatening

B. Consolidation
1. Goal: to eliminate any remaining malignant cells

2. Methods: often chemotherapy/radiation therapy
3. Effects: side effects will still be evident
C. Maintenance
  1. Goal: to keep child disease free
  2. Method: chemotherapy (this phase may last for several years)
D. Observation
  1. Goal: to monitor the child at intervals for evidence of recurrent disease and complications of treatment
  2. Method: treatment is complete; child may continue in this stage indefinitely
E. Late effects of treatment
  1. Impaired growth and development, usually related to radiation of growth centers
  2. CNS damage resulting in intellectual, psychologic, or neurologic sequelae
  3. Impaired pubertal development including hormonal or reproductive problems
  4. Development of secondary malignancy
  5. Psychologic problems (poor self-esteem, depression, anxiety) related to living with a life-threatening disease and complex treatment regimen

## Side Effects

A. From combined effects of treatment: nausea, vomiting, diarrhea, alopecia, anemia (low RBCs), increased susceptibility to infection (low WBCs), bleeding (low platelets), stomatitis, mucositis, pain, learning problems
B. From radiation (findings differ according to site radiated): sleepiness, reddened skin
C. From chemotherapy: drug toxicity specific to agents used; liver and renal toxicity
D. Developmental: behavior problems, avoidance of school and friends, low self-esteem or poor self-image

## Nursing Interventions

A. Help child cope with intrusive procedures.
  1. Provide information geared to developmental level and emotional readiness.
  2. Explain what is going to happen, why it is necessary, and how it will feel.
  3. Allow child to handle and manipulate equipment.
  4. Use needle play as indicated.
  5. Allow child some control in situations (e.g., positioning, selecting injection site).
B. Support child and parents.
  1. Maintain frequent clinical conferences to keep all informed.
  2. Always tell the truth.
  3. Acknowledge feelings and encourage child/family to express them, assure them that feelings are normal.

4. Provide contact with another parent or an organized support group such as Candlelighters.
5. Try to keep daily life as normal as possible.
C. Minimize side effects of treatment.
  1. Skin breakdown
    a. Keep clean and dry; wash with warm water, no soaps or creams.
    b. Do not wash off radiation markings.
    c. Avoid exposure to sunlight.
    d. Avoid all topical agents with alcohol (perfumes and powders).
    e. Do not use electric heating pads or hot water bottles.
  2. Bone marrow suppression
    a. Decreased RBCs
      1) Allow child to determine activities.
      2) Provide frequent rest periods.
    b. Decreased WBCs
      1) Avoid crowds, isolate from children with known communicable disease.
      2) Evaluate any potential site of infection.
      3) Monitor temperature elevations.
    c. Decreased platelets
      1) Make environment safe.
      2) Select activities that are physically safe.
      3) Avoid use of salicylates.
    d. Administer transfusions as ordered.
    e. Interpret peripheral blood counts to guide specific interventions and precautions.
  3. Nausea and vomiting
    a. Administer antiemetic at least half an hour before chemotherapy; repeat as necessary.
    b. Encourage relaxation techniques.
    c. Eat light meal prior to administration of therapy.
    d. Ensure adequate oral intake or administer IV fluids as necessary.
  4. Alopecia
    a. Reduce trauma of hair loss (especially in children over age 5 years).
    b. Buy wig before hair falls out.
    c. Discuss various head coverings with boys and girls.
    d. Avoid exposing head to sunlight.
    e. Discuss feelings.
  5. Stomatitis, mucositis (see Bone Marrow Transplant).
  6. Nutrition deficits
    a. Establish baseline prior to start of treatment.
    b. Measure height and weight regularly.
    c. Provide small, frequent meals.
    d. Consult dietitian as needed.
    e. Provide high-calorie, high-protein supplements.
  7. Developmental delays
    a. Discuss limit setting, discipline.
    b. Some behavior problems might be side effects of drug therapy.
    c. Facilitate return to school as soon as able.
    d. Realize changing needs of child.

# CANCERS

## Leukemia

A. General information
1. Most common form of childhood cancer
2. Peak incidence is between 2 and 3 years of age
3. Proliferation of abnormal white blood cells that do not mature beyond the blast phase
4. In the bone marrow, blast cells crowd out healthy white blood cells, red blood cells, and platelets, leading to bone marrow depression
5. Blast cells also infiltrate other organs, most commonly the liver, spleen, kidneys, and lymph tissue
6. Symptoms reflect bone marrow failure and associated involvement of other organs
7. Types of leukemia, based on course of disease and cell morphology
   a. Acute lymphocytic leukemia (ALL)
      1) 75% of childhood leukemia
      2) Malignant change in the lymphocyte or its precursors
      3) Acute onset
      4) 95% chance of obtaining remission with treatment
      5) 75% chance of surviving 5 years or more
      6) Prognostic indicators include: initial white blood count (less than 10,000/mm$^3$), child's age (2–9 years), histologic type, sex
   b. Acute nonlymphocytic leukemia (ANLL)
      1) Includes granulocytic and monocytic types
      2) 60–80% will obtain remission with treatment
      3) 30–40% cure rate
      4) Prognostic indicators less clearly defined
B. Medical management
1. Diagnosis: blood studies, bone marrow biopsy
2. Treatment stages
   a. Induction: intense and potentially life threatening
   b. CNS prophylaxis: to prevent central nervous system disease. Combination of radiation and intrathecal chemotherapy.
   c. Maintenance: chemotherapy for 2 to 3 years.
C. Assessment findings
1. Anemia (due to decreased production of RBCs), weakness, pallor, dyspnea
2. Bleeding (due to decreased platelet production), petechiae, spontaneous bleeding, ecchymoses
3. Infection (due to decreased WBC production), fever, malaise
4. Enlarged lymph nodes
5. Enlarged spleen and liver
6. Abdominal pain with weight loss and anorexia
7. Bone pain due to expansion of marrow
D. Nursing interventions
1. Monitor for signs of bleeding, anemia, thrombocytopenia, DIC.
2. Provide care for the child receiving chemotherapy and radiation therapy.
3. Provide support for child/family; needs will change as treatment progresses.
4. Support child during painful procedures (frequent bone marrow aspirations, lumbar punctures, venipunctures needed).
   a. Use distraction, guided imagery.
   b. Allow child to retain as much control as possible.
   c. Administer sedation prior to procedure as ordered.

## Brain Tumors

A. General information
1. A space-occupying mass in the brain tissue; may be benign or malignant
2. Males affected more often; peak age 3–7 years
3. Second most prevalent type of cancer in children
4. Cause unknown; genetic and environmental factors may play a role; familial tendency for brain tumors, which are found with preexisting neurocutaneous disorders.
5. Two thirds of all pediatric brain tumors are beneath the tentorium cerebelli (in the posterior fossa), often involving the cerebellum or brain stem.
6. Three fourths of brain tumors in children are gliomas (medulloblastoma and astrocytoma).
B. Types (See Figure 5–12.)
1. Medulloblastoma: highly malignant tumor usually found in cerebellum; runs a rapid course
   a. Findings include increased ICP plus unsteady walk, ataxia, anorexia, early morning vomiting
   b. Treated with radiation because complete removal is impossible
2. Astrocytoma: a benign, cystic, slow-growing tumor usually found in cerebellum
   a. Onset of symptoms is insidious.
   b. Findings include focal disturbances, papilledema, optic nerve atrophy, blindness.
3. Ependymoma: a usually benign tumor that arises in the ventricles of the brain, causing noncommunicating hydrocephalus and damage (by pressure) to other vital tissues of the brain
4. Craniopharyngioma: tumor that arises from remnants of embryonic tissue near the

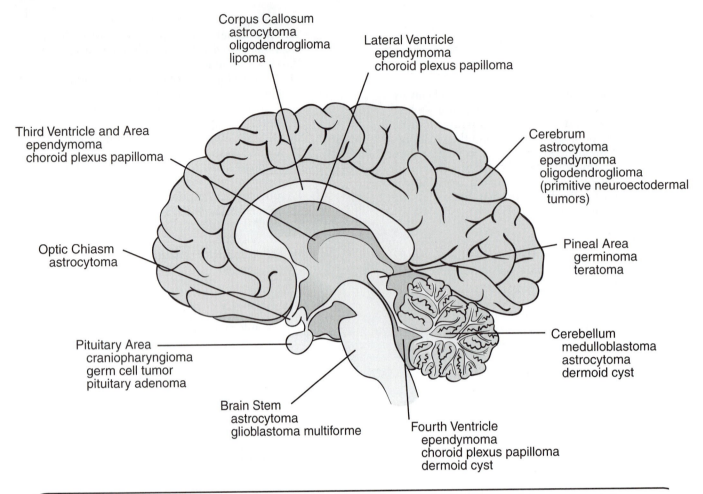

**Figure 5-12** Location of common childhood brain tumors. Source: From American Brain Tumor Association. *A primer of brain tumors: A patient's reference manual.* (2004). Des Plaines, IL: American Brain Tumor Association. Used with permission.

pituitary gland in the sella turcica, causes pressure on the third ventricle
  a. Decreased secretion of ADH causes diabetes insipidus (these children may need Pitressin).
  b. Additional symptoms include altered growth pattern, visual difficulties, difficulty regulating body temperature.
  5. Brain stem glioma: slow-growing tumor, indicated by cranial nerve palsies, ataxia
C. Medical management
  1. Surgery: some tumors entirely or partially resected; others are not amenable to surgery because of proximity to vital brain parts
  2. Radiation therapy: often used to shrink tumors
  3. Chemotherapy: vincristine, lomustine, procarbazine, intrathecal methotrexate; not as effective with brain tumors as with other childhood cancers
D. Assessment findings
  1. Symptoms dependent on location and type of tumor.

  2. A definite diagnosis is difficult in children because of the elasticity of child's skull and generally poor coordination of the young child.
  3. A decrease in school performance may be the first sign.
  4. Increased ICP
    a. Morning headache
    b. Morning vomiting without nausea; vomiting without relation to feeding schedule; projectile vomiting
    c. Personality changes
    d. Diplopia
      1) Difficult to assess in young children
      2) Observe child for tilting of head, closing or covering one eye, rubbing the eyes, or impaired eye-hand coordination
    e. Papilledema: a late sign
    f. Increased blood pressure with decreased pulse: also a late sign

g. Cranial enlargement
   1) More readily noticeable prior to 18 months when suture lines are still open
   2) Bulging, tense, pulsating fontanels
   3) Widened suture lines
   4) 90% or more on head circumference chart
5. Focal signs and symptoms
   a. Ataxia
      1) In cerebellar tumors
      2) May not be readily identified because of uncoordinated movements of young children
   b. Muscle strength
      1) Weakness with cerebellar tumors
      2) Weakness, spasticity, and paralysis of lower extremities with cerebral or brain stem tumors
      3) Change in handedness, posture, or manual coordination: may be early signs
   c. Head tilt
      1) In posterior fossa tumors
      2) Early sign of visual impairment
      3) Associated with nuchal rigidity
      4) Due to traction on the dura
   d. Ocular signs
      1) Nystagmus: corresponds to the same side as the infratentorial lesion
      2) Diplopia/strabismus: from palsy of cranial nerve VI with brain stem glioma or increased ICP
      3) Visual field deficit (child does not react to activity on periphery of vision): with craniopharyngiomas
   e. Seizures: with cerebral tumors
6. Diagnostic tests
   a. Skull X-ray reveals presence and location of tumor
   b. CT scan (with or without contrast dye) reveals position, consistency, size of tumor, and effect on surrounding tissue
   c. EEG may show seizure activity
E. Nursing interventions
   1. Obtain baseline vital signs and perform thorough neurologic assessment; monitor vital signs and neurologic status frequently.
   2. Prevent injury/complications.
      a. Institute seizure precautions.
      b. Monitor for fluid and electrolyte imbalance from vomiting.
      c. Observe for increased ICP.
      d. Provide safety measures (bed rails up).
   3. Promote comfort/relief of headache.
      a. Decrease environmental stimuli.
      b. Administer analgesics as ordered.
   4. Prevent constipation (straining increases ICP).
      a. Provide appropriate foods and fluids as ordered.
      b. Provide stool softeners as ordered.
      c. Avoid enemas, which increase ICP.
   5. Provide care for the child undergoing brain surgery.
   6. Provide care for the child undergoing radiation or chemotherapy.
   7. Provide client teaching and discharge planning concerning:
      a. Diagnostic tests (instruction needs to be appropriate to the child's developmental level)
         1) Machines will make clicking sounds
         2) Wires attached to the head for an EEG will not electrocute child
         3) Head is immobilized for a CT scan
         4) The use of contrast dye and expected sensations if used
         5) Need to lie still with the technician out of the room for most tests (younger children will be sedated for fuller cooperation)
      b. Importance of family discussion of fears/anxiety about surgery and prognosis
      c. Need to assist in implementing child's interaction with peers
      d. Available support groups and community agencies

## Brain Surgery

A. General information
   1. Indications
      a. Removal of a tumor
      b. Evacuation of a hematoma
      c. Removal of a foreign body or skull fragments resulting from trauma
      d. Aspiration of an abscess
      e. Insertion of a shunt
B. Nursing interventions: preoperative
   1. Assess the child's understanding of the procedure; have the child draw a picture, tell a story; observe doll play.
   2. Explain the procedure in terms according to the child's developmental level.
   3. Allow the child to visit the operating room/intensive care unit, if permitted, depending on the child's emotional and developmental levels.
   4. Explain that pre-op symptoms such as headache and ataxia may be temporarily aggravated.
   5. Advise child/parents that blindness may result, depending on the location of the tumor.
   6. Inform the child/parents that the head will be shaved; long hair may be saved; hats or scarves may be used to cover the head once the dressings are removed.
   7. Support the child/family if a tumor cannot be totally removed.

5

8. Provide instruction about radiation and chemotherapy (may need to be delayed because detail may be overwhelming).
9. Explain to the child/parents about the post-op dressing, monitoring devices, and possibility of facial edema.

C. Nursing interventions: postoperative
   1. Prevent injury/complications.
      a. Monitor vital signs and neuro status frequently until stable.
      b. Apply hypothermia blanket as ordered.
      c. Assess respiratory status/signs of infection.
      d. Observe the dressing for discharge/hemorrhage.
      e. Close or cover eyes, apply ice, instill saline drops or artificial tears.
      f. Position as ordered according to the location of the tumor and type of surgery.
      g. Assess for increased ICP.
      h. Institute seizure precautions.
   2. Promote comfort.
      a. Decrease environmental stimuli.
      b. Administer analgesics as ordered, first assessing LOC.
   3. Promote adequate nutrition.
      a. Administer fluids as ordered.
      b. Monitor I&O.
      c. Provide diet as ordered.
   4. Provide emotional support and encourage child/family to discuss prognosis.
   5. Provide client teaching and discharge planning concerning:
      a. Wound care
      b. Signs of increased ICP
      c. Activity level
      d. Sensation and time period of hair growth
      e. Peer acceptance
      f. Radiation/chemotherapy, if indicated
      g. Availability of support groups/community agencies

# Hodgkin's Lymphoma

A. General information
   1. Malignant neoplasm of lymphoid tissue, usually originating in localized group of lymph nodes; a proliferation of lymphocytes
   2. Metastasizes first to adjacent lymph nodes
   3. Cause unknown
   4. Most prevalent in adolescents; accounts for 5% of all malignancies
   5. Prognosis now greatly improved for these children; influenced by stage of disease and histologic type
   6. Long-term treatment effects include increased incidence of second malignancies, especially leukemia and infertility

B. Medical management
   1. Diagnosis: extensive testing to determine stage, which dictates treatment modality

   a. Lymphangiogram determines involvement of all lymph nodes (reliable in 90% of clients); is helpful in determining radiation fields
   b. Staging via laparotomy and biopsy
      1) Stage I: single lymph node involved; usually in neck; 90–98% survival
      2) Stage II: involvement of 2 or more lymph nodes on same side of diaphragm; 70–80% survival
      3) Stage III: involvement of nodes on both sides of diaphragm; 50% survival
      4) Stage IV: metastasis to other organs
   c. Laparotomy and splenectomy
   d. Lymph node biopsy to identify presence of Reed-Sternberg cells and for histologic classification
   2. Radiation: used alone for localized disease
   3. Chemotherapy: used in conjunction with radiation therapy for advanced disease

C. Assessment findings
   1. Major presenting symptom is enlarged nodes in lower cervical region; nodes are nontender, firm, and movable
   2. Recurrent, intermittent fever
   3. Night sweats
   4. Weight loss, malaise, lethargy
   5. Pruritus
   6. Diagnostic test: presence of Reed-Sternberg cells

D. Nursing interventions
   1. Provide care for child receiving radiation therapy.
   2. Administer chemotherapy as ordered and monitor/alleviate side effects.
   3. Protect client from infection, especially if splenectomy performed.
   4. Provide support for child/parents; specific needs of adolescent client must be considered.

# Non-Hodgkin's Lymphoma

A. General information
   1. Tumor originating in lymphatic tissue
   2. Significantly different from Hodgkin's lymphoma
      a. Control of primary tumor is difficult
      b. Disease is diffuse, cell type undifferentiated
      c. Tumor disseminates early
      d. Includes wide range of disease entities: lymphosarcoma, reticulum cell sarcoma, Burkitt's lymphoma
   3. Primary sites include GI tract, ovaries, testes, bone, CNS, liver, breast, subcutaneous tissues
   4. Affects all age groups.

B. Medical management
   1. Chemotherapy: multiagent regimens including cyclophosphamide (Cytoxan), vincristine,

prednisone, procarbazine, doxorubicin, bleomycin

  **2.** Radiation therapy: primary treatment in localized disease

  **3.** Surgery for diagnosis and clinical staging

**C.** Assessment findings

  **1.** Depend on anatomic site and extent of involvement

  **2.** Rapid onset and progression

  **3.** Many have advanced disease at diagnosis

**D.** Nursing interventions: provide care for child receiving chemotherapy, radiation therapy, and surgery.

## Wilms' Tumor (Nephroblastoma)

**A.** General information

  **1.** Large, encapsulated tumor that develops in the renal parenchyma, more frequently in left kidney (usually unilateral)

  **2.** Originates during fetal life from undifferentiated embryonic tissues

  **3.** Peak age of occurrence: 1–3 years

  **4.** Prognosis good if there are no metastases.

**B.** Medical management

  **1.** Nephrectomy, with total removal of tumor

  **2.** Postsurgical radiation in treatment of stages II, III, and IV; stage I disease does not usually require radiation, but it may be used if the tumor histology is unfavorable.

  **3.** Postsurgical chemotherapy: vincristine and daunorubicin, doxorubicin

**C.** Assessment findings

  **1.** Staging

    **a.** Stage I: limited to kidney

    **b.** Stage II: tumor extends beyond kidney, but is completely encapsulated

    **c.** Stage III: tumor confined to abdomen

    **d.** Stage IV: tumor has metastasized to lung, liver, bone, or brain

    **e.** Stage V: bilateral renal involvement at diagnosis

  **2.** Usually mother notices mass while bathing or dressing child; nontender, usually midline near liver

  **3.** Hypertension and possible hematuria, anemia, and signs of metastasis

  **4.** Diagnostic test: IVP reveals mass

**D.** Nursing interventions

  **1.** Do not palpate abdomen to avoid possible dissemination of cancer cells.

  **2.** Handle child carefully when bathing and giving care.

  **3.** Provide care for the client with a nephrectomy; usually performed within 24–48 hours of diagnosis.

  **4.** Provide care for the child receiving chemotherapy and radiation therapy.

## Neuroblastoma

**A.** General information

  **1.** A highly malignant tumor that develops from embryonic neural crest tissue; arises anywhere along the craniospinal axis, usually from the adrenal gland

  **2.** Incidence

    **a.** One in 10,000

    **b.** Males slightly more affected

    **c.** From infancy to age 4

  **3.** Staging

    **a.** Stage I: tumor confined to the organ of origin

    **b.** Stage II: tumor extends beyond primary site but not across midline

    **c.** Stage III: tumor extends beyond midline

    **d.** Stage IV: tumor metastasizes to skeleton (bone marrow), soft tissue (liver), and lymph nodes

**B.** Medical management: depends on the staging of tumor and age of child; includes surgery, radiation therapy, chemotherapy

**C.** Assessment findings vary, depending on the tumor site and stage

  **1.** If in the abdomen, may initially resemble Wilms' tumor

  **2.** Local signs and symptoms caused by pressure of the tumor on surrounding tissue

  **3.** Metastatic manifestations

    **a.** Ocular: supraorbital ecchymosis, periorbital edema, exophthalmos

    **b.** Cervical or supraclavicular lymphadenopathy

    **c.** Bone pain: may or may not occur with bone metastasis

    **d.** Nonspecific complaints; pallor, anorexia, weight loss, irritability, weakness

  **4.** Diagnosis usually made after metastasis has occurred

  **5.** Diagnostic tests

    **a.** X-rays of the head, chest, or abdomen reveal presence of primary tumor or metastases

    **b.** IVP: if tumor is adrenal, shows a downward displacement of the kidney on the affected side

    **c.** Bone marrow aspiration: to rule out metastasis; neuroblasts have a clumping pattern

    **d.** CBC: RBCs and platelets decreased

    **e.** Coagulation studies: abnormal due to thrombocytopenia

    **f.** Catecholamine excretion: VMA levels in urine increased

      **1)** Child must not ingest vanilla, chocolate, bananas, or nuts for 3 days prior to the test

      **2)** 24-hour urine specimen needed

**D.** Nursing interventions: same as for leukemia and brain tumors.

# Bone Tumors

## Osteogenic Sarcoma

A. General information
1. Primary bone tumor arising from the mesenchymal cells and characterized by formation of osteoid (immature bone)
2. Invades ends of long bones, most frequently distal end of femur or proximal end of tibia
3. Occurs more often in boys, usually between ages 10 and 20 years
4. Lungs most frequent site of metastasis
5. 5-year survival rate is 10–20%
B. Medical management
1. Surgery: treatment of choice
   a. Amputation: temporary prosthesis used immediately after surgery; permanent one usually fitted a few weeks later
   b. Limb salvage procedures
   c. Lung surgery if there are metastases
2. Radiation: only in areas where tumor is not accessible to surgery
3. Chemotherapy: adjuvant therapy being studied
C. Assessment findings
1. Insidious pain, increasing with activity, gradually becoming more severe
2. Tender mass, warm to touch; limitation of movement
3. Pathologic fractures
D. Nursing interventions
1. Prepare child for amputation: discuss fears, concerns, and facts of procedure; answer questions regarding prosthetic devices, limited activity
2. Assure child that phantom limb pain will subside

## Ewing's Sarcoma

A. General information
1. Primary tumor arising from cells in bone marrow
2. Invades bone longitudinally, destroying bone tissue; no new bone formation
3. Femur most frequently affected site
4. More common in males, between ages 5 and 15 years
5. Lungs most frequent site of metastasis
B. Medical management
1. High-dose radiation is primary treatment
2. Chemotherapy
3. Value of surgery presently being reassessed
C. Assessment findings
1. Pain and swelling
2. Palpable mass, may be tender, warm to touch
3. 10–30% of clients have metastatic disease at time of diagnosis

D. Nursing interventions
1. Promote exercise of affected limb to maintain function.
2. Avoid activities that may cause added stress to affected limb.

 **Sample Questions**

160. A 10-year-old is being prepared for a bone marrow transplant. Which statement by the boy will demonstrate to the nurse that he understands this treatment?
1. "I'll be much better after this blood goes to my bones."
2. "I won't feel too good until my body makes healthy cells."
3. "This will help all of the medicine they give me to work better."
4. "You won't have to wear a mask and gown after my transplant."

161. A 4-year-old has leukemia. Her mother understands the white count involvement in this disease but doesn't understand why her child has bruises and anemia. Which statement will be the best explanation for the bruises and anemia?
1. All blood cells are made in the bone marrow and therefore all types will be affected.
2. The anemia is because her child hasn't been eating well; the bruises are from the multiple needle sticks.
3. They are related to inactivity.
4. This is indicative that the end is near.

162. A 14-year-old has had an exacerbation of acute lymphocytic leukemia. What is the primary effect of leukemia on the bone marrow?
1. Crowding out of normal bone marrow cells.
2. Proliferation of cells producing blood components.
3. A selective reduction in the number of neutrophils.
4. Leukopenia, thrombocytopenia, and anemia.

163. A 14-year-old girl has acute lymphocytic leukemia and is admitted. She is terminally ill. What would be an appropriate nursing action?
1. Leave her alone as much as possible and whisper when in her room in order not to disturb her.
2. Assist her in giving away her possessions to friends and family.

3. Encourage her parents to explain to her 5-year-old sister that she will be asleep for a long time.
4. Reduce emotional stress by not having the child's parents/family participate in her care.

164. A 10-year-old is receiving cranial irradiation for a brain tumor. He has developed alopecia. Which of the following is an appropriate nursing intervention?
    1. Have the child identify famous movie stars and sports heroes who are bald.
    2. Assure the child that his hair will grow in before he leaves the hospital.
    3. Wrap a bandage around his head.
    4. Help him select a variety of hats.

165. A 6-year-old girl is newly diagnosed with acute lymphoid leukemia (ALL). During your assessment, which of the following signs and symptoms would you expect?
    1. Fever, pallor, bone and joint pain.
    2. Fever, ruddy complexion, petechiae.
    3. Abdominal pain, cystitis, swollen joints.
    4. Enlarged lymph nodes, low grade fever, night sweats.

166. A 12-year-old girl with ALL is receiving induction therapy with vincristine, prednisone, and L-asparaginase. She presents with paresthesia, alopecia, and moon face. Which of the following nursing diagnoses would be most appropriate for this child?
    1. High risk for injury.
    2. Impaired physical mobility.
    3. Body image disturbance.
    4. Altered nutrition: less than body requirements.

167. You are caring for a 10-year-old with ALL who underwent a bone marrow transplant. To provide a safe, effective care environment, what would be included in a plan of care?
    1. Rectal temperature every 4 hours to monitor for infection.
    2. Encouraging the child to go to the playroom to limit isolation.
    3. Use of a pressure-reducing mattress.
    4. Inserting a Foley catheter to monitor output.

168. A 15-year-old girl with ALL has been on maintenance therapy for 6 months. She is receiving chemotherapy of L-asparaginase, methotrexate, and cytarabine. Her absolute neutrophil count is 500/mm³. In planning for her care, which of the following would be included in a nursing care plan?
    1. Good handwashing by visitors and staff.
    2. Daily CBCs drawn.
    3. Daily physical therapy.
    4. Restriction of activity.

169. A 5-year-old boy is newly diagnosed with an astrocytoma brain tumor. His symptoms include headache, nausea, and seizures. Based on this information, which nursing diagnosis would be most appropriate for him?
    1. High risk for infection.
    2. High risk for injury.
    3. Anticipated grief.
    4. Impaired physical mobility.

170. Which of the following statements made by parents of an 8-year-old boy who just had surgery for a brain tumor reflect understanding of safety needs?
    1. "We will obtain a tutor to teach him at home."
    2. "We will not allow him to participate in sports anymore."
    3. "We will tell our other children to let him have his way and not upset him."
    4. "He will wear a helmet for sports."

171. A 16-year-old boy is admitted with Hodgkin's lymphoma. Which assessment finding would you expect?
    1. Small, tender lymph nodes in the groin.
    2. Enlarged, firm nontender nodes in the supraclavicular area.
    3. Enlarged, tender nodes all over the body.
    4. Small, nontender, nonmoveable nodes in the cervical area.

172. A 3-year-old with a Wilms' tumor is returning to the unit after surgery to remove the tumor. Which of the following actions have the highest priority in caring for this child?
    1. Maintaining NPO.
    2. Frequent blood pressure.
    3. Turning every 4 hours.
    4. Administering pain medication every 4 hours.

173. A child is to receive radiation therapy following surgery for Wilms' tumor. Which of the following measures would be important to include in the care plan prior to radiation therapy?
    1. Give compazine every 6 hours for nausea.
    2. Place a sign over the bed that reads "no needle punctures."

3. Practice lying in the required position.

4. Encourage play appropriate to age.

174. A 6-year-old boy with Ewing's sarcoma has just finished his course of chemotherapy. Which of the following statements by his parents indicate they understand the signs of complications from the chemotherapy?

1. "He will be playing football next week."

2. "We will keep him on a liquid diet until he feels better."

3. "We understand he is more susceptible to infections; we will keep him away from any sick family members."

4. "He will wear a baseball hat to bed."

 **Answers and Rationales**

160. **2.** The goal of a bone marrow transplant is to have the donor cells produce functioning blood cells for the client.

161. **1.** In leukemia, bone marrow is replaced by blast cells, resulting in decreased white cells, red cells, and platelets. The bruises are due to the child's decreased platelet count.

162. **1.** Leukemia cells are capable of an increased rate of production and a long cell life, causing crowding out of the normal bone marrow cells. Cells producing normal blood components are then unable to reproduce.

163. **2.** Adolescents who know they are dying frequently want to give away their belongings.

164. **4.** Selecting hats to cover his head will help the child deal with the change in body image.

165. **1.** The signs and symptoms of leukemia are a result of infiltration of the bone marrow. These include fever, pallor, fatigue, anorexia, petechiae, and bone and joint pain.

166. **3.** This may be especially true for this child as she is entering adolescence. Her loss of hair and "fat face" will make her different from her friends. Adolescents need to belong and be accepted by a group of peers.

167. **3.** Skin breakdown and impaired healing are common with bone marrow transplant. This is a preventive measure for the integrity of the skin.

168. **1.** Because of the maintenance therapy and neutrophil count, this client may have bone marrow suppression, which increases her risk for infection. Good handwashing is essential to help prevent infection.

169. **2.** Seizure precautions should be instituted to prevent an injury.

170. **4.** To protect the skull while it is healing, a child may need to wear a padded helmet for active sports.

171. **2.** The most common symptom of Hodgkin's disease is enlarged, firm, nontender moveable nodes in the supraclavicular area.

172. **2.** Frequent blood pressure measurements are needed to watch for signs of shock and as an indication of the functioning of the remaining kidney.

173. **3.** The child may stay in a fixed position during each therapy session, which may last 10–20 minutes. Having the child practice the required position prior to beginning radiation therapy can be helpful.

174. **3.** This client is likely to have bone marrow suppression, which increases his risk for infection and bleeding.

## REFERENCES AND SUGGESTED READINGS

American Academy of Pediatrics, Committee on Infectious Diseases. (2003). *The red book: Report of the committee on infectious diseases.* Elk Grove, IL: Author.

Axton, S., & Fugate, T. (2008). *Pediatric nursing care plans for the hospitalized child* (3rd ed.). Upper Saddle River, NJ: Pearson Education.

Ball, J. W., & Bindler, R. C. (2007). *Pediatric nursing: Caring for children* (4th ed.). Upper Saddle River, NJ: Prentice-Hall.

Centers for Disease Control and Prevention. (2004). Most recent childhood immunization schedule can be found at: Retrieved on Sep. 7, 2008, from http://www.cdc.gov/nip/recs/child-schedule.htm

*Child passenger safety.* Retrieved on Sep. 7, 2008, from www.nhtsa.dot.gov

Hockenberry, M. J., Wilson, D., Wilkenstein, M. L., & Kline, N. E. (2006). *Wong's nursing care of infants and children* (8th ed.). St. Louis, MO: Mosby.

Potts, N. & Mandleco, B. (2007). *Pediatric nursing: Caring for children and their families* (2nd ed.). Clifton Park, NY: Delmar Learning.

Zitelli, B. J., & Davis, H. (2007). *Atlas of pediatric physical diagnosis.* (5th ed.). St. Louis, MO: Mosby.

# MATERNITY AND FEMALE REPRODUCTIVE NURSING

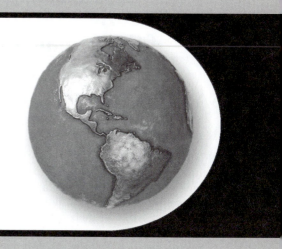

This section covers the health care needs of females from adolescence through late adulthood. Emphasis is placed on the childbearing cycle and the normal neonate, and frequently encountered health care problems. Cultural differences are addressed.

The unit begins with a review of the anatomy and physiology of the female reproductive system as a basis for understanding the entire childbearing process. Nursing process is emphasized throughout, and nursing diagnoses are used to identify the client's health care needs and to select nursing interventions.

Nursing process always must be implemented with an awareness of the interrelationship, during childbearing, of the maternal and fetal needs and their manifestations. The nurse needs to keep in mind that interventions for the mother may have an impact on the developing fetus, and vice versa. Medications for maternal conditions may affect the fetus, and fetal distress may require that the mother undergo surgery.

In this unit, a major assertion is that childbearing, for most women, is a normal, healthy life event. Discomforts and complications of childbearing also are covered, and these conditions are presented after the content that reviews the natural progression of events in pregnancy and childbearing. In this manner, the factors that alter pregnancy from a normal life event to a life crisis can be clearly identified.

In addition to childbearing, the unit includes a review of frequently encountered health care conditions of women. These conditions usually involve the reproductive system or its accessory organs and include normally occurring states, such as menopause, as well as pathologic conditions, such as gynecologic cancer.

## UNIT OUTLINE

# Overview of Anatomy and Physiology of the Female Reproductive System

## ANATOMY

### External Structures

See Figure 6-1.

A. Mons veneris: rounded, soft, fatty, and loose connective tissue over the symphysis pubis. Dark, curly pubic hair growth in typical triangular shape begins here 1 to 2 years before the onset of menstruation.

B. Labia majora: lengthwise fatty folds of skin extending from the mons to the perineum that protect the labia minora, the urinary meatus, and the vaginal introitus.

C. Labia minora: thinner, lengthwise folds of hairless skin, extending from the clitoris to the fourchette.

1. Glands in the labia minora lubricate the vulva.
2. The labia minora are very sensitive because of their rich nerve supply.
3. The space between the labia minora is called the vestibule.

D. Clitoris: small erectile organ located beneath the arch of the pubis, containing more nerve endings than the glans penis; sensitive to temperature and touch; secretes a fatty substance called smegma.

E. Vestibule: area formed by the labia minora, clitoris, and fourchette, enclosing the openings to the urethra and vagina, Skene's and Bartholin's glands; easily irritated by chemicals, discharges, or friction.

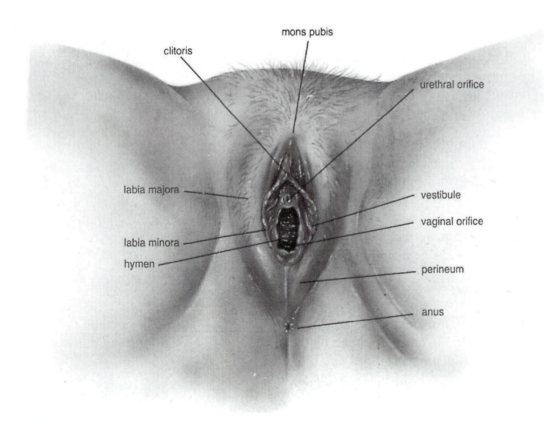

**Figure 6-1** External structures of the female reproductive system

1. Urethra: external opening to the urinary bladder
2. Skene's glands (also called *paraurethral glands*): secrete a small amount of mucus; especially susceptible to infections
3. Bartholin's glands: located on either side of the vaginal orifice; secrete clear mucus during sexual arousal; susceptible to infection, as well as cyst and abscess formation
4. Vaginal orifice and hymen: elastic, partial fold of tissue surrounding opening to the vagina

F. Fourchette: thin fold of tissue formed by the merging of the labia majora and labia minora, below the vaginal orifice.

G. Perineum: muscular, skin-covered area between vaginal opening and anus.

1. Underlying the perineum are the paired muscle groups that form the supportive "sling" for the pelvic organs, capable of great distension during the birth process.
2. An episiotomy can be made in the perineum if necessary during the birth process.

## Internal Structures

See Figure 6-2.

A. Fallopian tubes: paired tubules extending from the cornu of the uterus to the ovaries that serve as the passageway for the ova. Mucosal lining of tubes resembles that of vagina and uterus; therefore, infection may extend from lower organs.

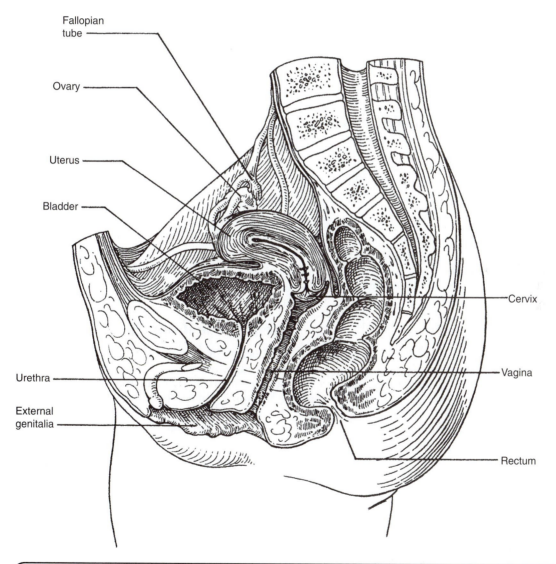

**Figure 6-2** Internal structures of the female reproductive system

B. Uterus: hollow, pear-shaped muscular organ, freely movable in pelvic cavity, comprised of *fundus, corpus, isthmus,* and *cervix.* Cervix has internal and external os, separated by the cervical canal. Wall of uterus has three layers.
  1. Endometrium: inner layer, highly vascular, shed during menstruation and following delivery
  2. Myometrium: middle layer, composed of smooth muscle fibers running in three directions; expels fetus during birth process, then contracts around blood vessels to prevent hemorrhage
  3. Parietal peritoneum: serous outer layer
C. Ovaries: oval, almond-sized organs on either side of the uterus that produce ova and hormones.
D. Vagina: muscular, distensible tube connecting perineum and cervix; the birth canal.

## The Pelvis

Right and left innominate bones, sacrum, and coccyx form the bony passage through which the baby passes during birth. Relationship between pelvic size/shape and baby may affect labor or make vaginal delivery impossible.
A. Pelvic measurements
  1. True conjugate: from upper margin of symphysis pubis to sacral promontory, should be at least 11 cm; may be obtained by X-ray or ultrasound.
  2. Diagonal conjugate: from lower border of symphysis pubis to sacral promontory; should be 12.5–13 cm; may be obtained by vaginal examination.
  3. Obstetric conjugate: from inner surface of symphysis pubis, slightly below upper border, to sacral promontory, it is the *most important pelvic measurement;* can be estimated by subtracting 1.5–2 cm from diagonal conjugate.
  4. Intertuberous diameter: measures the outlet between the inner borders of the ischial tuberosities; should be at least 8 cm.
B. Pelvic shapes
  1. Android: narrow, heart shaped; male-type pelvis
  2. Anthropoid: narrow, oval shaped; resembles ape pelvis
  3. Gynecoid: classic female pelvis; wide and well rounded in all directions
  4. Platypelloid: wide but flat; may still allow vaginal delivery
C. Pelvic divisions
  1. False pelvis: shallow upper basin of the pelvis; supports the enlarging uterus, but not important obstetrically
  2. Linea terminalis: plane dividing upper or false pelvis from lower or true pelvis
  3. True pelvis: consists of the pelvic inlet, pelvic cavity, and pelvic outlet. Measurements of true pelvis influence the conduct and progress of labor and delivery.

## The Breasts

A. Paired mammary glands on the anterior chest wall, between the second and sixth ribs, composed of glandular tissue, fat, and connective tissue.
B. Nipple and areola are darker in color than breasts.
C. Responsible for lactation after delivery.

# PHYSIOLOGY

## Menarche

Onset of the menstrual cycle; puberty.

## Menstrual Cycle

See Figure 6-3.
A. Complex pituitary/ovarian/uterine interaction.
B. Controls ripening and release of an ovum on a regular basis, and preparation for its fertilization and implantation in a thickened uterine lining (endometrium).
C. When fertilization/implantation do not occur, the endometrium is shed (menstruation), and the cycle begins again, due to follicle-stimulating hormone (FSH) and luteinizing hormone (LH) from the anterior pituitary.
D. Stages of cycle
  1. Menstruation: first days of cycle when endometrium is shed.
  2. Proliferative phase: major hormone involved is estrogen, which influences build-up of endometrium; also called *follicular phase.*
  3. Ovulation: release of ovum, usually 14 days (plus or minus 2) before end of cycle.
  4. Secretory phase: major hormone is progesterone, which influences myometrium (decreased irritability); also called *luteal phase.*

## Menopause (Climacteric)

A. Decline in ovarian function and hormone production.
B. Characterized by menstrual cycle irregularity and, in some women, by vasomotor instability and loss of bone density.
See also Menopause.

## Sexual Response in the Female: Four Phases

A. Excitement phase: vaginal lubrication and vasocongestion of external genitals.
B. Plateau phase: formation of orgasmic platform in vagina.
C. Orgasmic phase: strong rhythmic contractions of vagina and uterus.
D. Resolution phase: cervix dips into seminal pool in vagina; all organs return to previous condition.

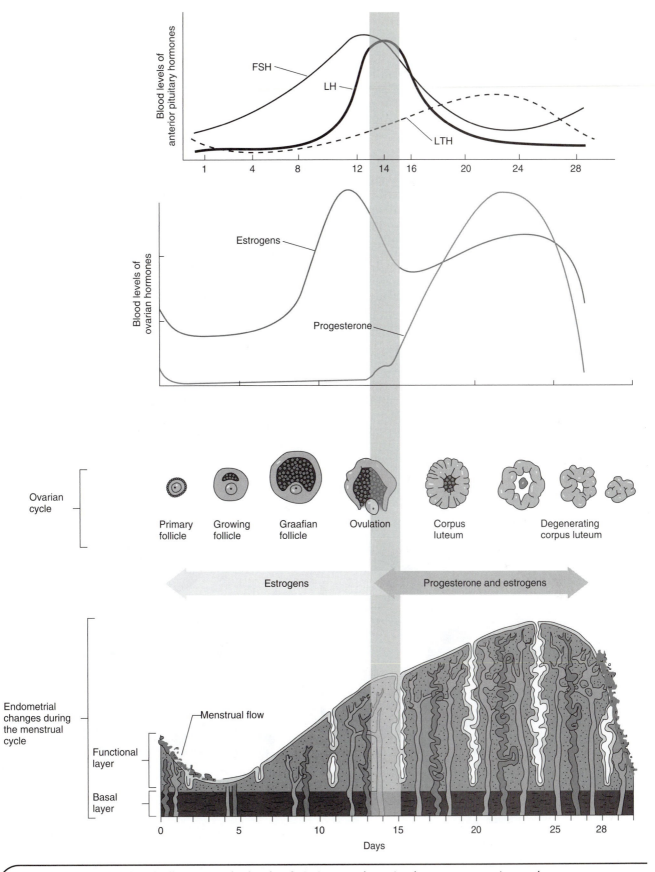

**Figure 6-3** Menstrual cycle illustrating the levels of pituitary and ovarian hormones, ovarian cycle, and endometrial changes

## CONCEPTION

See Figure 6-4.
A. The penetration of one ovum (female gamete) by one sperm (male gamete), resulting in a fertilized ovum (zygote). Each gamete has haploid number of chromosomes (23). Zygote has diploid number (46) with one of each pair from each parent.
B. Sex of child is determined at moment of conception by male gamete. If X-bearing male gamete unites with ovum, result is a female child (X + X). If Y-bearing male gamete unites with ovum, result is a male child (X + Y).
C. Usually occurs in the outer third of the fallopian tube.
D. Multiple pregnancies result from:
  1. Two or more fertilized ova (fraternal or dizygotic)
  2. Single fertilized ovum that divides—always same sex, only 1 chorion (identical or monozygotic)

## NIDATION (IMPLANTATION)

A. Burrowing of developing zygote into endometrial lining of uterus.
B. May take place 7–10 days after fertilization, while zygote develops to trophoblastic stage.
C. Chorionic villi appear on surface of trophoblast and secrete human chorionic gonadotropin (HCG), which inhibits ovulation during pregnancy by stimulating continuous production of estrogen and progesterone. This secretion of HCG forms the basis of the various tests for pregnancy.

## DEVELOPMENTAL STAGES

### Fertilized Ovum

A. From conception through first 2 weeks of pregnancy.
B. Nidation complete by the end of this period.

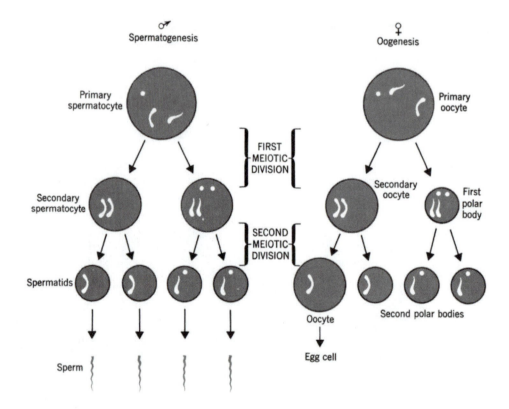

**Figure 6-4** Spermatogenesis and oogenesis. A primary spermatocyte produces four sperm, but only one egg results from meiosis of a primary oocyte. The polar bodies are functionless.

## Embryo

A. From end of second week through end of eighth week (also called period of organogenesis).
B. Critical time in development; embryo most vulnerable to teratogens (harmful substances or conditions), which can result in congenital anomalies.

## Fetus

A. From end of eighth week to termination of pregnancy.
B. Continued maturation of already-formed organ systems.

# SPECIAL STRUCTURES OF PREGNANCY

## Fetal Membranes

A. Arise from the zygote.
B. Inner (amnion) and outer (chorion).
C. Hold the developing fetus as well as the amniotic fluid.

## Amniotic Fluid

A. Clear, yellowish fluid surrounding the developing fetus.
B. Average amount 1000 mL.
C. Protects fetus.
   1. Allows free movement.
   2. Maintains temperature.
   3. Provides oral fluid.
D. Can be aspirated and tested for various diseases and abnormalities during pregnancy.
E. Alkaline pH: can be tested when membranes rupture to distinguish from urine.

## Umbilical Cord

A. Connecting link between fetus and placenta.
B. Contains two arteries and one vein supported by mucoid material (Wharton's jelly) to prevent kinking and knotting.
C. There are no pain receptors in the umbilical cord.

## Placenta

See Figure 6-5.
A. Transient organ allowing passage of nutrients and waste materials between mother and fetus.
B. Also acts as an endocrine organ and as a sieve that allows smaller particles through and holds back larger molecules. Passage of materials in either direction is effected by:
   1. Diffusion: gases, water, electrolytes.
   2. Facilitated transfer: glucose, amino acids, minerals.
   3. Pinocytosis: movement of minute particles (e.g., fats).

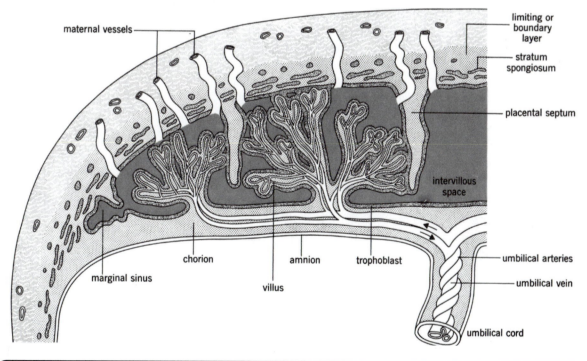

**Figure 6-5** Placental circulation. Through the placenta the fetus gets nourishment and excretes waste.

**4.** Leakage: caused by membrane defect; may allow maternal and fetal blood mixing.

**C.** Mother also transmits immunoglobulin G (IgG) to fetus through placenta, providing limited passive immunity.

**D.** Hormones produced by the placenta include:
1. HCG: early in pregnancy, responsible for continued action of corpus luteum, is basis of pregnancy tests.
2. Human chorionic somato-mammotropin/ human placental lactogen (HCS/HPL): similar to growth hormone; affects maternal insulin production; prepares breasts for lactation.
3. Estrogen and progesterone: necessary for continuation of pregnancy.

## Fetal Circulation

**A.** Arteries in cord and fetal body carry deoxygenated blood.

**B.** Vein in cord and those in fetal body carry oxygenated blood.

**C.** Ductus venosus connects umbilical vein and inferior vena cava; bypassing portal circulation; closes after birth.

**D.** Foramen ovale allows blood to flow from right atrium to left atrium, bypassing lungs. Closes functionally at birth because of increased pressure in left atrium; anatomic closure may take several weeks to several months.

**E.** Ductus arteriosus allows blood flow from pulmonary artery to aorta, bypassing fetal lungs; closes after delivery.

## Fetal Growth and Development

**A.** Organ systems develop from three primary germ layers.
1. Ectoderm: outer layer, produces skin, nails, nervous system, and tooth enamel.
2. Mesoderm: middle layer, produces connective tissue, muscles, blood, and circulatory system.
3. Endoderm: inner layer, produces linings of gastrointestinal and respiratory tracts, endocrine glands, and auditory canal.

**B.** Timetable (Figure 6-6 and Table 6-1).

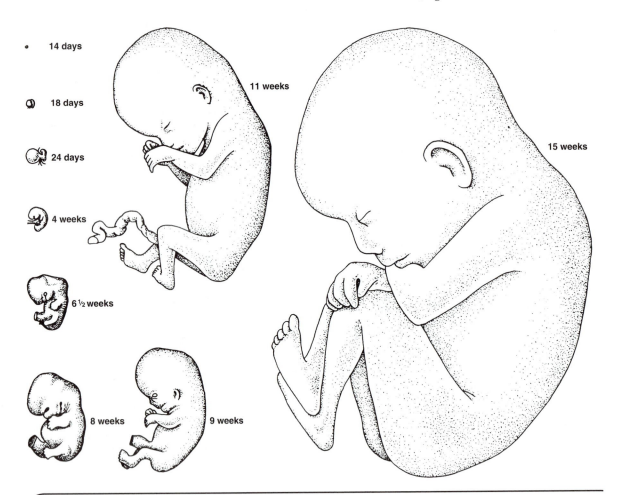

14 days

18 days

24 days

4 weeks

6 ½ weeks

8 weeks

9 weeks

11 weeks

15 weeks

**Figure 6-6** Changes in the body size of the embryo and fetus during development in the uterus (all figures are natural size)

## Table 6-1 Markers in Fetal Development

| Date* | Development |
|-------|-------------|
| 4 weeks | All systems in rudimentary form; heart chambers formed and heart is beating. Embryo length about 0.4 cm; weight about 0.4 (grams). |
| 8 weeks | Some distinct features in face; head large in proportion to rest of body; some movement. Length about 2.5 cm, weight 2 (grams). |
| 12 weeks | Sex distinguishable; ossification in most bones; kidneys secrete urine; able to suck and swallow. Length 6–8 cm, weight 19 (grams). |
| 16 weeks | More human appearance; earliest movement likely to be felt by mother; meconium in bowel; scalp hair develops. Length 11.5–13.5 cm, weight 100 (grams). |
| 20 weeks | Vernix caseosa and lanugo appear; movement usually felt by mother; heart rate audible; bones hardening. Length 16–18.5 cm, weight 300 (grams). |
| 24 weeks | Body well proportioned; skin red and wrinkled; hearing established. Length 23 cm, weight 600 (grams). |
| 28 weeks | Infant viable, but immature if born at this time. Body less wrinkled; appearance of nails. Length 27 cm, weight 1100 (grams). |
| 32 weeks | Subcutaneous fat beginning to deposit; L/S ratio in lungs now 1.2:1; skin smooth and pink. Length 31 cm, weight 1800–2100 (grams). |
| 36 weeks | Lanugo disappearing; body usually plump; L/S ratio usually 2:1; definite sleep/wake cycle. Length 35 cm, weight 2200–2900 (grams). |
| 40 weeks | Full-term pregnancy. Baby is active, with good muscle tone; strong suck reflex; if male, testes in scrotum; little lanugo. Length 40 cm, weight 3200 (grams) or more. |

*Dates are approximate, but developmental level should have been reached by the end of the time period specified.

C. Measurements of length of pregnancy
1. Days: 267–280
2. Weeks: 40, plus or minus 2
3. Months (lunar): 10
4. Months (calendar): 9
5. Trimesters: 3

D. Estimated due date/estimated date of confinement (*Nägele's rule*); see Figure 6-7. This calculation is an estimation only. Most women deliver: due date + or − 2 weeks. Sonogram dating used to confirm dates.

- Add 7 days to the first day of the last normal menstrual period
- Subtract 3 months
- Add 1 year

*Example:*

```
1st day of LNMP = September 16, 2009
     Add 7 days = September 23
Subtract 3 months = June 23
      Add 1 year = June 23, 2010, will be
                   estimated due date
```

**Figure 6-7** Nägele's rule

# PHYSICAL AND PSYCHOLOGIC CHANGES OF PREGNANCY

## Reproductive System

A. External structures: enlarged due to increased vascularity.
B. Ovaries
  1. No ovulation during pregnancy
  2. Corpus luteum persists in early pregnancy until development of placenta is complete
C. Fallopian tubes: elongate as uterus rises in pelvic and abdominal cavities.
D. Vagina
  1. Increased vascularity (*Chadwick's sign*)
  2. Estrogen-induced leukorrhea
  3. Change in pH (less acidic) may favor overgrowth of yeastlike organisms
  4. Connective tissue loosens in preparation for distention of labor and delivery
E. Cervix
  1. Softens and loosens in preparation for labor and delivery (*Goodell's sign*).
  2. Mucous production increases, and plug (operculum) is formed as bacterial barricade.
F. Uterus
  1. Hypertrophy and hyperplasia of muscle cells
  2. Development of fibroelastic tissue that increases ability to contract
  3. Shape changes from pearlike to ovoid
  4. Rises out of pelvic cavity by 16th week of pregnancy
  5. Increased vascularity and softening of isthmus (*Hegar's sign*)
  6. Mild contractions (*Braxton Hicks' sign*) beginning in the fourth month through end of pregnancy
G. Breasts
  1. Increased vascularity, sensitivity, and fullness
  2. Nipples and areola darken
  3. Nipples become more erectile

4. Proliferation of ducts and alveolar tissue evidenced by increased breast size
5. Production of colostrum by the second trimester

## Cardiovascular System

A. Blood volume expands as much as 50% to meet demands of new tissue and increased needs of all systems.
B. Progesterone relaxes smooth muscle, resulting in vasodilation and accommodation of increased volume.
C. RBC volume increases as much as 30%; may be slight decline in hematocrit as pregnancy progresses because of this relative imbalance (physiologic anemia).
D. Stroke volume and cardiac output increase.
E. WBCs increase.
F. Greater tendency to coagulation.
G. Blood pressure may drop in early pregnancy; should not rise during last half of pregnancy.
H. Heart rate increases; palpitations possible.
I. Blood flow to uterus and placenta is maximized by side-lying position.
J. Varicosities may occur in vulva and rectum as well as lower extremities.

## Respiratory System

A. Increased vascularity of mucous membranes of this system gives rise to symptoms of nasal and pharyngeal congestion and fullness in the ears.
B. Shape of thorax shortens and widens to accommodate the growing fetus.
C. Slight increase in respiratory rate.
D. Dyspnea may occur at end of third trimester before engagement or "lightening."
E. Increased respiratory volume by 40–50%.
F. Oxygen consumption increases by 15%.

## Renal System

A. Kidney filtration rate increases as much as 50%.
B. Glucose threshold drops; sodium threshold rises.
C. Water retention increases as pregnancy progresses.
D. Enlarging uterus causes pressure on bladder resulting in frequency of urination, especially during first trimester; later in pregnancy relaxed ureters are displaced laterally, increasing possibility of stasis and infection.
E. Presence of protein (not an expected component of maternal urine) indicates possible renal disease or pregnancy-induced hypertension.

## Integumentary System

A. Increased pigmentation of nipples and areolas.
B. Possible appearance of *chloasma* (mask of pregnancy): darkening of areas on forehead and cheekbones.
C. Appearance of *linea nigra,* darkened line bisecting abdomen from symphysis pubis to top of fundus.
D. Striae (stretch marks): separation of underlying connective tissue in breasts, abdomen, thighs, and buttocks; fade after delivery.
E. Greater sweat and sebaceous gland activity.

## Musculoskeletal System

A. Alterations in posture and walking gait caused by change in center of gravity as pregnancy progresses.
B. Increased joint mobility as a result of action of ovarian hormone (relaxin) on connective tissue.
C. Possible backache.
D. Occasional cramps in calf may occur with hypocalcemia.

## Neurologic System

A. Few changes with a typical pregnancy.
B. Pressure on sciatic nerve may occur later in pregnancy due to fetal position.

## Gastrointestinal System

A. Bleeding gums and hypersalivation may occur.
B. Tooth loss due to demineralization should *not* occur.
C. Nausea and vomiting in first trimester due to rising levels of HCG.
D. Appetite usually improves.
E. Cravings or desires for strange food combinations may occur.
F. Progesterone-induced relaxation of muscle tone leads to slow movement of food through GI tract; may result in heartburn.
G. Constipation may occur as water is reabsorbed in large intestine.
H. Emptying time for gallbladder may be prolonged; increased incidence of gallstones.

## Endocrine System

A. Pituitary: FSH and LH greatly decreased; oxytocin secreted during labor and after delivery; prolactin responsible for initiation and continuation of lactation.
B. Progesterone secreted by corpus luteum until formation of placenta.
C. Principal source of estrogen is placenta, synthesized from fetal precursors.
D. HCS/HPL produced by placenta; similar to growth hormone, it prepares breasts for lactation; also affects insulin/glucose metabolism. May overstress maternal pancreas.
E. Ovaries secrete relaxin during pregnancy.
F. Slight increase in thyroid activity and basal metabolic rate (BMR).
G. Pancreas may be stressed due to complex interaction of glucose metabolism, HCS/HPL, and cortisol, resulting in diminished effectiveness of insulin, and demand for increased production.

## Psychosocial Changes

A. First trimester
   1. Mother needs accurate diagnosis of pregnancy.
   2. Works through characteristic ambivalence of early pregnancy.
   3. Mother is self-centered, baby is "part" of her.
   4. Grandparents are usually the first relatives to be told of the pregnancy.
B. Second trimester
   1. Mother demonstrates growing realization of baby as separate and needing person.
   2. Fantasizes about unborn child.
C. Third trimester
   1. "Nesting" activity appears as due date approaches.
   2. Desire to be finished with pregnancy.
D. Anxiety over "safe passage" for self and baby through labor and delivery.
E. Reactions of father-to-be may parallel those of mother (e.g., ambivalence, anxiety). Additionally, as mother's pregnancy progresses he may experience similar physical changes.
F. Preparation of siblings varies according to their age and experience.

## Transcultural Concerns in Pregnancy

A. Dominant philosophy concerning pregnancy and birth may differ in non-U.S. cultures. May view this as "healthy" time, with little or no insight concerning potential complications.
B. Biological variations may occur, e.g., higher rate of complications in women with sickle cell trait or gene; diabetes mellitus seen with more frequency in pregnant American Indians; increase in parasitic infections and hepatitis in women from Southeast Asia.
C. Behaviors during pregnancy (eating, sleeping, bathing, sexual activity, etc.) will differ from culture to culture.
D. Superstition, taboos, and "old wives' tales" may play an important role.
E. Most cultures consider childbirth to be the province of women; men's roles may be limited or excluded. This may include caregivers.
F. Perception of discomfort/pain will vary; may be influenced by cultural expectations as well as mother's own experiences.
G. Despite culture, many women prefer upright position for labor and birth, rather than lying down. Additionally, many women prefer to have the freedom to move around during labor, whenever possible.
H. After delivery, cultural rituals may refer to rest, seclusion, and purification. The postpartum women may be considered vulnerable. Applications of heat or cold, in air or water, need to be specially assessed.
I. Other areas of culturally related practices may be: nutrition, clothing, activity, resumption of contact with the community, resumption of sexual activities, and return to work.
J. Infant care (feeding, cord care, circumcision, clothing, sleeping arrangements) will vary among differing cultures.
K. Control of future fertility may vary from natural methods such as breastfeeding to the use of any available means.

# The Antepartal Period

## ASSESSMENT

### Classification of Pregnancy

A. Gravida: number of times pregnant, regardless of duration, including the present pregnancy.
   1. Primagravida: pregnant for the first time
   2. Multigravida: pregnant for second or subsequent time
B. Para: number of pregnancies that lasted more than 20 weeks, regardless of outcome.
   1. Nullipara: a woman who has not given birth to a baby beyond 20 weeks' gestation.
   2. Primipara: a woman who has given birth to one baby more than 20 weeks' gestation.
   3. Multipara: Woman who has had two or more births at more than 20 weeks' gestation. . . twins or triplets count as 1 para.
   4. TPAL: Para subdivided to reflect births that went to **T**erm, **P**remature births, **A**bortions, and **L**iving children.

### Determination of Pregnancy

Diagnosis of pregnancy is based on pregnancy-related physical and hormonal changes and are classified as presumptive, probable, or positive.

## Presumptive Signs and Symptoms (Subjective)

These changes may be noticed by the mother/health care provider but are *not* conclusive for pregnancy.
A. Amenorrhea (cessation of menstruation)
B. Nausea and vomiting
C. Urinary frequency
D. Fatigue
E. Breast changes
F. Weight change
G. Skin changes
H. Vaginal changes including leukorrhea
I. Quickening

## Probable Signs and Symptoms (Objective)

These changes are usually noted by the health care provider but are *still not conclusive* for pregnancy.
A. Uterine enlargement
B. Changes in the uterus and cervix from increased vascularity
C. Ballottement: fetus rebounds against the examiner's hand when pushed gently upwards.
D. Braxton Hicks' contractions: occur early in pregnancy, although not usually sensed by the mother until the third trimester.
E. Laboratory tests for pregnancy
   1. Most tests rely on the presence of HCG in the blood or urine of the woman.
   2. Easy, inexpensive, but may give false readings with any handling error, medications, or detergent residue in laboratory equipment.
   3. Exception is the radioimmunoassay (RIA), which tests for the beta subunit of HCG and is considered to be so accurate as to be diagnostic for pregnancy.
F. Changes in skin pigmentation.

## Positive Signs and Symptoms

These signs emanate from the fetus, are noted by the health care provider, and *are conclusive* for pregnancy.
A. Fetal heartbeat: detected as early as eighth week with an electronic device; after 16th week with a more conventional auscultory device.
B. Palpation of fetal outline.
C. Palpation of fetal movements.
D. Demonstration of fetal outline by either ultrasound (after sixth week) or X-ray (after 12th week).

## ANALYSIS

Nursing diagnoses for the antepartal period *may* include:
A. Deficient knowledge: information on the following topics needs to be given and reinforced
   1. Danger signals of pregnancy to be reported
   2. Dangerous behaviors during pregnancy (e.g., smoking, using drugs [especially alcohol], use of nonprescription medications)
B. In nutrition potential: individualized nutritional information will be needed
C. Activity intolerance: need for additional rest and benefits of a moderate exercise program
D. Anxiety
E. Risk for constipation
F. Disturbed body image
G. Ineffective coping
H. Powerlessness
I. Noncompliance
J. Risk for deficient fluid volume
K. Health-seeking behaviors

# PLANNING AND IMPLEMENTATION

## Goals

A. Establish a diagnosis of pregnancy.
B. Gather initial data to form the basis for comparison with data collected as pregnancy progresses.
C. Identify high-risk factors.
D. Propose realistic and necessary interventions.
E. Promote optimal health for mother and baby, providing any needed information.
F. Provide needed information for prepared childbirth.

## Interventions

### Prenatal Care

A. Time frame
   1. First visit: may be made as soon as woman suspects she is pregnant; frequently after first missed period.
   2. Subsequent visits: Every month until the 7th or 8th month, every 2 weeks during the 8th month, and weekly during the 9th month; more frequent visits are scheduled if problems arise.
B. Conduct of initial visit
   1. Extensive collection of data about client in all pertinent areas in order to form basis for comparison with data collected on subsequent visits and to screen for any high-risk factors
      a. Menstrual history: menarche, regularity, frequency and duration of flow, last period
      b. Obstetrical history: all pregnancies, complications, outcomes, contraceptive use, sexual history
      c. Medical history: include past illnesses, surgeries; current use of medications
      d. Family history/psychosocial data
      e. Information about the father-to-be may also be significant
      f. Current concerns

2. Complete physical examination, including internal gynecologic exam and bimanual exam
3. Laboratory work, including CBC, urinalysis, Pap test, blood type and Rh, rubella titer, testing for sexually transmitted diseases (STDs), other tests as indicated (e.g., TB test, hepatitis viral studies, ECG, etc.)
C. Conduct of subsequent visits
   1. Continue collection of data, especially weight, blood pressure, urine screening for glucose and protein, evaluation of fetal development through auscultation of fetal heart rate (FHR) and palpation of fetal outline, measurement of fundal height as correlation for appropriate progress of pregnancy. Fundus palpable above symphysis at 12 weeks, at the level of umbilicus at 20 weeks, then approximately 1 cm per week until 36–38 weeks when head often descends and fundal measurement may drop somewhat.
   2. Additional tests
      a. Hemoglobin and hematocrit 26–28 weeks
      b. Glucose screen 24–28 weeks
      c. Antibody screen at 28 weeks
      d. Beginning of 9th month, test for STDs, strep, other infections
   3. Prepare for any necessary testing.
      a. Have client void (clean catch).
      b. Collect baseline data on vital signs.
      c. Collect specimen.
      d. Monitor client and fetus after procedure.
      e. Provide support to client.
      f. Document as needed.

## Nutrition during Pregnancy

A. Weight gain
   1. Variable, but 25 lb usually appropriate for average woman with single pregnancy.
   2. Woman should have consistent, predictable pattern of weight gain, with only 2–3 lb in first trimester, then average 12 oz gain every week in second and third trimesters.
   3. Gains mostly reflect maternal tissue in first half of pregnancy, and fetal tissue in second half of pregnancy.
B. Specific nutrient needs
   1. Calories: usual addition is 300 kcal/day, but there will be specific guidelines for those beginning pregnancy either over- or underweight (never less than 1800 kcal/day).
   2. Protein: additional 30 grams/day to ensure intake of 74–76 grams/day; very young pregnant adolescents and those with multiple pregnancies will need more protein.
   3. Carbohydrates: intake must be sufficient for energy needs, using fresh fruits and vegetables as much as possible to derive additional fiber benefit; teach to avoid "empty" calories.
   4. Fats: high-energy foods, which are needed to carry the fat-soluble vitamins.

5. Iron: needed by mother as well as fetus; reserves usually sufficient for first trimester, supplementation recommended after this time; iron preparations should be taken with source of vitamin C to promote absorption.
6. Calcium: 1200 mg per day needed; dairy products most frequent source, with supplementation for those with lactose intolerance.
7. Sodium: contained in most foods; needed in pregnancy; should not be restricted without serious indication.
8. Vitamins: both fat- and water-soluble are needed in pregnancy; essential for tissue growth and development, as well as regulation of metabolism. Generally not synthesized by body, nor stored in large amounts (folic acid special concern as deficiency may cause fetal anomalies and bleeding complications).
C. Dietary supplements: many health care providers supplement the pregnant woman's diet with an iron-fortified multivitamin to ensure essential levels.
D. Special concerns
   1. Religious, ethnic, and cultural practices that influence selection and preparation of foods
   2. Pica (ingestion of nonedible or non-nutritive substances)
   3. Vegan vegetarians: no meat products, may need $B_{12}$ supplement
   4. Adolescence
   5. Economic deprivation
   6. Heavy smoking, alcohol consumption, drugs
   7. Previous reproductive problems

## Education for Parenthood

A. Provision of information about pregnancy, labor and delivery, the postpartum period, and lactation.
B. Usually taught in small groups, may be individualized.
C. Topics can be grouped into early and late pregnancy, labor and delivery, and postdelivery/newborn care.
D. Emphasis placed on both physical and psychosocial changes seen in childbearing cycle.
E. Preparation for childbirth: intended to provide knowledge and alternative coping behaviors in order to diminish anxiety and discomfort, and promote cooperation with the birth process; see Table 6-2 for specific methodologies.

## Determination of Fetal Status and Risk Factors

A. Fetal diagnostic tests
   1. Used to:
      a. Identify or confirm the existence of risk factor(s)
      b. Validate pregnancy
      c. Observe progress of pregnancy

6

**Table 6-2** Methods of Childbirth

| | |
|---|---|
| Read method | The so-called natural childbirth method. Underlying concept: knowledge diminishes the fear that is key to pain. Classes include information as well as practice in relaxation and abdominal breathing techniques for labor. |
| Lamaze method | Psychoprophylactic method based on utilization of Pavlovian conditioned response theory. Classes teach replacement of usual response to pain with new, learned responses (breathing, effleurage, relaxation) in order to block recognition of pain and promote positive sense of control in labor. |
| Bradley method | Husband-coached childbirth. A modification of the Read method emphasizing working in harmony with the body. |
| Other methods | Hypnosis, yoga. |

    d. Identify optimum time for induction of labor if indicated

    e. Identify genetic abnormalities

  2. Types

    a. Chorionic villi sampling (CVS): earliest test possible on fetal cells (9–12 weeks); sample obtained by slender catheter passed through cervix to implantation site.

    b. Ultrasound: use of sound and returning echo patterns to identify intrabody structures. Useful early in pregnancy to identify gestational sac(s) and to assist in pregnancy dating. Later uses include assessment of fetal viability, growth patterns, anomalies, fluid volume, uterine anomalies, and adnexal masses. Used as an adjunct to amniocentesis; safe for fetus (no ionizing radiation).

    c. Amniocentesis: location and aspiration of amniotic fluid for examination; possible after the 14th week when sufficient amounts are present. Used to identify chromosomal aberrations, sex of fetus, levels of alpha-fetoprotein and other chemicals indicative of neural tube defects and inborn errors of metabolism, gestational age, Rh factor.

    d. X-ray: can be used late in pregnancy (after ossification of fetal bones) to confirm position and presentation; not used in early pregnancy to avoid possibility of causing damage to fetus and mother.

    e. Alpha-fetoprotein screening: Maternal serum screens. Alpha-fetoprotein is glucoprotein produced by fetal yolk sac, GI tract, and liver. Test done between 15 and 18 weeks' gestation. Elevated AFP may be associated with neural tube defects, renal anomalies. Low AFP seen with chromosomal trisomies.

    f. L/S ratio: uses amniotic fluid to ascertain fetal lung maturity through measurement of presence and amounts of the lung surfactants lecithin and sphingomyelin. At 35–36 weeks, ratio is 2:1, indicative of mature levels; once ratio of 2:1 is achieved, newborn less likely to develop respiratory distress syndrome. Phosphatidylglycerol (PG) is found in amniotic fluid after 35 weeks. In conjunction with the L/S ratio, it contributes to increased reliability of fetal lung maturity testing. May be done in laboratory or by "shake" test.

    g. Fetal movement count: teach mother to count 2–3 times daily, 30–60 minutes each time, should feel 5–6 movements per counting time. Mother should notify care giver immediately of abrupt change or no movement.

    h. PUBS (percutaneous umbilical blood sampling): uses ultrasound to locate umbilical cord. Cord blood aspirated and tested. Used in second and third trimesters.

    i. Biophysical profile: a collection of data on fetal breathing movements, body movements, muscle tone, reactive heart rate, and amniotic fluid volume. A score of 0 to 2 is given in each category, and the summative number interpreted by the physician. Primary suggested use is to identify fetuses at risk for asphyxia.

B. Electronic monitoring

  1. Nonstress test (NST) (see Table 6-3)

    a. Accelerations in heart rate accompany normal fetal movement

    b. In high-risk pregnancies, NST may be used to assess FHR on a frequent basis in order to ascertain fetal well-being.

    c. Noninvasive

  2. Contraction stress test (CST) (see Table 6-4)

    a. Based on principle that healthy fetus can withstand decreased oxygen during contraction, but compromised fetus cannot.

    b. Types

      1) Nipple-stimulated CST: massage or rolling of one or both nipples to stimulate uterine activity and check effect on FHR.

      2) Oxytocin challenge test (OCT): infusion of calibrated dose of IV oxytocin "piggybacked" to main IV line; controlled by infusion pump; amount infused increased every 15–20 minutes until three good uterine contractions are observed within 10-minute period.

      3) CST never done unless willing to deliver fetus.

**Table 6-3** Nonstress Test (NST)

| Result | Interpretation | Significance |
|---|---|---|
| Reactive | 2 or more accelerations of 15 beats/min lasting 15 sec or more in 20-min period (associated with each fetal movement) | High-risk pregnancy allowed to continue if twice weekly NSTs are reactive. |
| Nonreactive | No FHR acceleration, or accelerations less than 15 beats/min or lasting less than 15 sec through fetal movement | Need to attempt to clarify FHR pattern; implement CST and continue external monitoring. |
| Unsatisfactory | FHR pattern not able to be interpreted | Repeat NST or do CST. |

**Table 6-4** Contraction Stress Test (CST)

| Result | Interpretation | Significance |
|---|---|---|
| Negative | 3 contractions, 40–60 sec long, within 10-min period, no late decelerations | Fetus should tolerate labor if it occurs within 1 week. |
| Positive | Persistent/consistent late decelerations with more than 50% of contractions | Fetus at increased risk. May need additional testing, may try induction or cesarean birth. |
| Suspicious | Late decelerations in less than 50% of contractions | Repeat CST in 24 hr, or other fetal assessment tests. |
| Unsatisfactory | Inadequate pattern or poor tracing | Same as for suspicious. |

# EVALUATION

A. Maternal/fetal assessment data remain within acceptable limits; fetus maintains growth and development pattern appropriate to gestational age (evidenced by maternal weight gain, normal increments in fundal height, fetal activity level, other antepartal tests).
B. No complications of pregnancy are evident.
   1. Pregnant woman receives prenatal care (initial and subsequent visits).
   2. Maternal blood pressure, weight gain, and other lab test findings are within normal range.
C. Pregnant woman/family have received adequate educational instruction.
   1. Pregnant woman/family express understanding of childbirth experience and begin transition to role of parenting.
   2. Any necessary testing procedures carried out completely and correctly; client/fetus in stable condition.

# COMPLICATIONS OF PREGNANCY

Pregnancy can be complicated by situations unique to childbearing (e.g., placental bleeding), or by long-standing conditions predating pregnancy and continuing into the childbearing process (e.g., age, socioeconomic status, cardiac problems); for common discomforts of pregnancy, see Table 6-5.

## General Nursing Responsibilities

A. Teach danger signals of pregnancy early in prenatal period so that client is aware of what needs to be reported to health care provider on an immediate basis (see Table 6-6).
B. Be aware that early teaching allows the client to participate in the identification and reporting of symptoms that can indicate a problem in her pregnancy.
C. Early recognition and reporting of danger signals usually results in diminishing the risk and controlling the severity of maternal/fetal complications.
D. Interventions are specific for the individual risks.
E. Evaluation centers around whether or not the risk was controlled or eliminated, and how the maternal/fetal reaction was controlled.

## First Trimester Bleeding Complications
### Abortion

A. General information
   1. Loss of pregnancy before viability of fetus; may be spontaneous, therapeutic, or elective (for additional information on therapeutic and elective abortions see Control of Fertility). (Clients may use term "miscarriage" for spontaneous abortion.)
   2. Types
      a. Threatened abortion
         1) Cervix closed
         2) Some bleeding and contractions
         3) Fetus not expelled
      b. Inevitable
         1) Cervix open
         2) Heavier bleeding and stronger contractions
         3) Loss of fetus usually not avoidable

**Table 6-5** Common Discomforts during Pregnancy

| Discomfort | Trimester | Intervention |
|---|---|---|
| Morning sickness | First | Eat dry carbohydrate in AM; avoid fried, odorous, and greasy foods; small meals rather than large. |
| Fatigue | First | Rest frequently, as needed. |
| Urinary frequency | First, end of third | Kegel exercises, perineal pad for leakage. |
| Heartburn | Second, third | Small meals, bland foods, antacids if ordered. |
| Constipation | Second, third | Sufficient fluids, foods high in roughage, regular bowel habits. No laxatives unless ordered, including mineral oil. |
| Hemorrhoids | Third | Avoid constipation; promote regular bowel habits. |
| Varicosities | Third | Avoid crossing legs and long periods of sitting or standing; rest with feet and hips elevated; avoid elastic garters and other constrictive clothing. |
| Backache | Third | Use good posture and body mechanics; low-heeled shoes; exercises to strengthen back muscles. |
| Insomnia | Third | Conscious relaxation; supportive pillows as needed; warm shower before retiring. |
| Leg cramps | Third | Flex toes toward knees for relief; ensure adequate calcium in diet. |
| Supine hypotensive syndrome | Third | Left side–lying position. |
| Vaginal discharge | Second | Correct personal hygiene, refer to physician. Do not douche. |
| Skin changes, dryness, itching | All | Interventions are symptomatic; cool baths, lotions, oils as indicated. |

**Table 6-6** Danger Signals of Pregnancy

- Any bleeding from vagina
- Gush of fluid from vagina (clear, not urine)
- Regular contractions occurring before due date
- Severe headaches or changes in vision
- Epigastric pain
- Vomiting that persists and is severe
- Change in fetal activity patterns
- Temperature elevation, chills, or "sick" feeling indicative of infection
- Swelling in upper body, especially face and fingers

    c. Incomplete
       1) Expulsion of fetus incomplete
       2) Membranes or placenta retained
    d. Complete: all products of conception expelled
    e. Missed: fetus dies in uterus but is not expelled
    f. Habitual
       1) Three pregnancies in a row culminating in spontaneous abortion
       2) May indicate need for investigation into underlying causes

**B.** Assessment findings
  **1.** Vaginal bleeding (observing carefully for accurate determination of amount, saving all perineal pads)
  **2.** Contractions, pelvic cramping, backache
  **3.** Lowered hemoglobin if blood loss significant
  **4.** Passage of fetus/tissue

**C.** Nursing interventions
  **1.** Save all tissue passed.
  **2.** Keep client at rest and teach reason for bed rest.
  **3.** Increase fluids PO or IV.
  **4.** Prepare client for surgical intervention (D&C or suction evacuation) if needed (see also Termination of Pregnancy).
  **5.** Provide discharge teaching about limited activities and coitus after bleeding ceases.
  **6.** Observe reaction of mother and others, provide emotional support, and give opportunity to express feelings of grief and loss.
  **7.** Administer RhoGAM if mother Rh negative.

## Incompetent Cervical Os (Premature Dilation of Cervix)

**A.** General information: painless condition in which the cervix dilates without uterine contractions and allows passage of the fetus; usually the result of prior cervical trauma.
**B.** Medical management: may be treated surgically by cerclage (placement of fascia or artificial material to constrict the cervix in a "purse-string" manner).

When client goes into labor, choice of removal of suture and vaginal delivery, or cesarean birth.

C. Assessment findings
  1. History of repeated, relatively painless abortions
  2. Early and progressive effacement and dilation of cervix, usually second trimester
  3. Bulging of membranes through cervical os
D. Nursing interventions
  1. Continue observation for contractions, rupture of membranes, and monitor fetal heart tones.
  2. Position client to minimize pressure on cervix.

## Ectopic Pregnancy

A. General information
  1. Any gestation outside the uterine cavity
  2. Most frequent in the fallopian tubes, where the tissue is incapable of the growth needed to accommodate pregnancy, so rupture of the site usually occurs before 12 weeks.
  3. Any condition that diminishes the tubal lumen may predispose a woman to ectopic pregnancy
B. Assessment findings
  1. History of missed periods and symptoms of early pregnancy
  2. Abdominal pain, may be localized to one side
  3. Rigid, tender abdomen; sometimes abnormal pelvic mass
  4. Bleeding; if severe may lead to shock
  5. Low hemoglobin and hematocrit, rising WBC count
  6. HCG titers usually lower than in intrauterine pregnancy
C. Nursing interventions
  1. Prepare client for surgery.
  2. Institute measures to control/treat shock if hemorrhage severe; continue to monitor postoperatively.
  3. Allow client to express feelings about loss of pregnancy and concerns about future pregnancies.

## Hydatidiform Mole (Gestational Trophoblastic Disease)

A. General information
  1. Proliferation of trophoblasts; embryo dies. Unusual chromosomal patterns seen (either no genetic material in ovum, or 69 chromosomes). The chorionic villi change into a mass of clear, fluid-filled grapelike vessels.
  2. More common in women over 40.
  3. Cause essentially unknown.
B. Assessment findings
  1. Increased size of uterus disproportionate to length of pregnancy
  2. High levels of HCG with excessive nausea and vomiting

  3. Dark red to brownish vaginal bleeding after 12th week
  4. Anemia often accompanies bleeding
  5. Symptoms of preeclampsia before usual time of onset
  6. No fetal heart sounds or palpation of fetal parts
  7. Ultrasound shows no fetal skeleton
C. Nursing interventions
  1. Provide pre- and postoperative care for evacuation of uterus (usually suction curettage).
  2. Teach contraceptive use so that pregnancy is delayed for at least one year.
  3. Teach client need for follow-up lab work to detect rising HCG levels indicative of choriocarcinoma.
  4. Provide emotional support for loss of pregnancy.
  5. Teach about risk for future pregnancies, if indicated.

# Second Trimester Bleeding Complications

There are few unique causes of bleeding in the second trimester. Bleeding may be a late manifestation of condition usually seen in first trimester, such as spontaneous abortion or incompetent cervical os.

# Third Trimester Bleeding Complications

Placental problems are the most frequent cause of bleeding in the third trimester.

## Placenta Previa

A. General information
  1. Low implantation of the placenta so that it overlays some or all of the internal cervical os. Complete previa requires cesarean delivery. Partial may deliver vaginally if fetus in vertex presentation.
  2. Cause uncertain, but uterine factors (poor vascularity, fibroid tumors, multiple pregnancies) may be involved.
  3. Amount of cervical os involved classifies placenta previa as marginal, partial, or complete.
  4. Often diagnosed prior to 30 weeks by sonogram. Many resolve or migrate before labor.
B. Assessment findings
  1. Bright red, painless vaginal bleeding after seventh month of pregnancy is cardinal indicator. Bleeding may be intermittent, in gushes, or continuous.
  2. Uterus remains soft.
  3. FHR usually stable unless maternal shock present.

4. No vaginal exam by nurse, may result in severe bleed, if done by physician, double set-up used.
5. Diagnosis by sonography.

C. Nursing interventions
1. Ensure complete bed rest.
2. Maintain sterile conditions for any invasive procedures (including vaginal examination).
3. Make provision for emergency cesarean birth (*double set-up procedure*).
4. Continue to monitor maternal/fetal vital signs.
5. Measure blood loss carefully.
6. Assess uterine tone regularly.

## Abruptio Placentae

A. General information
1. Separation of placenta from part or all of normal implantation site, usually accompanied by pain
2. Usually occurs after 20th week of pregnancy
3. Increased risk of abruption with maternal hypertension, previous abruption, cigarette smoking, multiparity, history of abortions, cocaine use, abdominal trauma

B. Assessment findings
1. Painful vaginal bleeding
2. Tender, boardlike uterus (especially if concealed hemorrhage, then no vaginal bleeding)
3. Fetal bradycardia and late decelerations, absent FHT in complete abruption
4. Additional signs of shock

C. Nursing interventions
1. Ensure bed rest.
2. Check maternal/fetal vital signs frequently.
3. Prepare for IV infusions of fluids/blood as indicated.
4. Monitor urinary output.
5. Anticipate coagulation problems (DIC).
6. Provide support to parents as outlook for fetus is poor.
7. Prepare for emergency surgery as indicated.

## Hyperemesis Gravidarum

A. General information
1. Excess nausea and vomiting of early pregnancy leads to dehydration and electrolyte disturbances, especially acidosis.
2. Causes: possible severe reaction to HCG, not psychological, greater risk in conditions where HCG levels increased. HCG levels peak around 6 weeks after conception, plateau, then begin to decline after the 12th week. Symptoms often improve later in pregnancy but may last entire time.

B. Assessment findings
1. Nausea and vomiting, progressing to retching between meals
2. Weight loss

C. Nursing interventions
1. Begin NPO and IV fluid and electrolyte replacement. (Correction of F&E balance will decrease nausea, NPO will rest the stomach.)
2. Monitor I&O.
3. Gradually reintroduce PO intake, monitor amounts taken and retained.
4. Monitor TPN and central line placement if unable to eat.
5. Provide mouth care.
6. Offer emotional support—very demoralizing and depressing to client.
7. Refer to home health as appropriate for continued IV or TPN therapy.

## Pregnancy-Induced Hypertension

### General Information

A. Refers to condition unique to pregnancy where vasospastic hypertension is accompanied by proteinuria and edema; maternal or fetal condition may be compromised.
1. Probable cause: gradual loss of normal pregnancy-related response to angiotensin II
2. May also be related to decreased production of some vasodilating prostaglandins

B. Onset after 20th week of pregnancy, may appear in labor or up to 48 hours postpartum.

C. Characterized by widespread vasospasm.

D. Cause essentially unknown, but incidence is high in primigravidas, multiple pregnancies, maternal age under 17 or over 35, hydatidiform mole, poor nutrition, essential hypertension; familial tendency.

E. Occurs in 5–7% of all pregnant women.

F. Clinical classification of hypertensive disorders in pregnancy.
1. Pregnancy-induced hypertension (PIH)
   a. Preeclampsia—mild or severe
   b. Eclampsia
2. Chronic hypertension
3. Chronic hypertension with superimposed PIH

G. Classic triad of symptoms includes edema/weight gain, hypertension, and proteinuria. Eclampsia includes convulsions and coma.

H. Possible life-threatening complication: HELLP syndrome (hemolysis, elevated liver enzymes, lowered platelets).

I. Only known cure is delivery. Delivery may be initiated early to reduce risks and further complications.

### Mild Preeclampsia

A. Assessment findings
1. Appearance of symptoms between 20th and 24th week of pregnancy
2. Blood pressure of 140/90 or +30 systolic/+15 mm Hg diastolic on two consecutive occasions at least 6 hours apart

3. Sudden weight gain (+3 lb/month in second trimester; +1 lb/week in third trimester; or +4.5 lb/week at any time)
4. Slight generalized edema, especially of hands and face
5. Proteinuria of 300 mg/liter in a 24-hour specimen (+1 in 1 specimen)
B. Nursing interventions
1. Promote bed rest as long as signs of edema or proteinuria are minimal, preferably side-lying.
2. Provide well-balanced diet with adequate protein and roughage, no Na$^+$ restriction.
3. Explain need for close follow-up, weekly or twice-weekly visits to physician.

## Severe Preeclampsia

A. Assessment findings
1. Headaches, epigastric pain, nausea and vomiting, visual disturbances, irritability
2. Blood pressure of 150–160/100–110 mm Hg
3. Increased edema and weight gain
4. Proteinuria (5 g/24 hours) (4+) oliguria
5. Hyperreflexia of 4+, possibly with clonus
B. Medical management: magnesium sulfate
1. Magnesium sulfate acts upon the myoneural junction, diminishing neuromuscular transmission.
2. It promotes maternal vasodilation, better tissue perfusion, and has anticonvulsant effect.
3. Nursing responsibilities
a. Monitor client's respirations, blood pressure, and reflexes, as well as urinary output frequently.
b. Administer medications either IV or IM.
4. Antidote for excess levels of magnesium sulfate is calcium gluconate or calcium chloride.
C. Nursing interventions
1. Promote complete bed rest, side-lying.
2. Carefully monitor maternal/fetal vital signs.
3. Monitor I&O, results of laboratory tests.
4. Take daily weights.
5. Do daily fundoscopic examination.
6. Institute seizure precautions.
a. Restrict visitors.
b. Minimize all stimuli.
c. Monitor for hyperreflexia.
d. Administer sedatives as ordered.
7. Instruct client about appropriate diet.
8. Continue to monitor 24–48 hours postdelivery.
9. Administer medications as ordered; vasodilator of choice usually hydralazine (Apresoline).

## Eclampsia

A. Medical management (see Severe Preeclampsia).
B. Assessment findings
1. Increased hypertension precedes convulsion followed by hypotension and collapse.
2. Coma may ensue.
3. Labor may begin, putting fetus in great jeopardy.
4. Convulsion may recur.
C. Nursing interventions
1. Minimize all stimuli.
a. Darken room.
b. Limit visitors.
c. Use padded bedsides and bed rails.
2. Check vital signs and lab values frequently.
3. Seizure precautions: airway, oxygen, and suction equipment should be available at bedside.
4. Administer medications as ordered.
5. Prepare for cesarean delivery when seizures stabilized.
6. Continue observations 24–48 hours postpartum.

# PRE- AND COEXISTING DISEASES OF PREGNANCY

## Cardiac Conditions

### General Information

A. May be the result of congenital heart disease or the sequelae of rheumatic fever/heart disease.
B. May affect pregnancy, but are definitely affected by pregnancy.
C. Classification
1. Class 1: no limitation of activity
2. Class 2: slight limitation of activity
3. Class 3: considerable limitation of activity
4. Class 4: symptoms present even at rest

### Prenatal Period

A. Assessment findings
1. Evidence of cardiac decompensation especially when blood volume peaks (weeks 28–32)
2. Cough and dyspnea
3. Edema
4. Heart murmurs
5. Palpitations
6. Rales
B. Nursing interventions
1. Promote frequent rest periods and adequate sleep, decreased stress.
2. Teach client to recognize and report signs of infection, importance of prophylactic antibiotics.
3. Compare vital signs to baseline and normal values expected during pregnancy.
4. Instruct in diet to limit weight gain to 15 lb., low Na$^+$.
5. Explain rationale for anticoagulant therapy (heparin used in pregnancy) if ordered.
6. Teach danger signals for individual client.

## Intrapartal Period

**A.** Labor increases risk of congestive heart failure: milking effect of contractions and delivery increases blood volume to heart.

**B.** Nursing interventions
  1. Monitor maternal ECG and FHT continuously.
  2. Explain to client that vaginal delivery is preferred over cesarean delivery.
  3. Monitor client's response to stress of labor and watch for signs of decompensation.
  4. Administer oxygen and pain medication as ordered, epidural preferable.
  5. Position client in side-lying/low semi-Fowler's position.
  6. Provide calm atmosphere.
  7. Encourage "open-glottal" pushing during second stage of labor, forceps or vacuum extractor used to minimize pushing.

## Postpartal Period

**A.** Nursing interventions
  1. Monitor vital signs, any bleeding, strict I&O, lab test values, daily weight, rest and diet.
  2. Promote bed rest in appropriate position (see Intrapartal Period).
  3. Assist with activities of daily living (ADL) as needed.
  4. Prevent infection.
  5. Facilitate nonstressful mother/baby interactions.
  6. Help mother plan for rest and activity patterns at home, as well as household help if indicated.

# Endocrine Conditions

## Diabetes Mellitus

**A.** General information
  1. Chronic disease caused by improper metabolic interaction of carbohydrates, fats, proteins, and insulin.
  2. Interaction of pregnancy and diabetes may cause serious complications of pregnancy.
  3. Classifications of diabetes mellitus (see also Unit 4)
      **a.** Type 1, insulin-dependent diabetes mellitus, usually appears before age 30
      **b.** Type 2, noninsulin-dependent, onset usually after age 30
      **c.** Gestational diabetes, onset occurs during pregnancy
  4. Significance of diabetes in pregnancy
      **a.** Interaction of estrogen, progesterone, HCS/HPL, and cortisol raise maternal resistance to insulin (ability to use glucose at the cellular level).
      **b.** If the pancreas cannot respond by producing additional insulin, excess glucose moves across placenta to fetus, where fetal insulin metabolizes it, and acts as growth hormone, promoting macrosomia.
      **c.** Maternal insulin levels need to be carefully monitored during pregnancy to avoid widely fluctuating levels of blood glucose.
      **d.** Dose may drop during first trimester, then rise during second and third trimesters.
      **e.** Higher incidence of fetal anomalies and neonatal hypoglycemia (good control minimizes).

**B.** Assessment findings: signs of hyperglycemia
  1. Polyuria
  2. Polydipsia
  3. Weight loss
  4. Polyphagia
  5. Elevated glucose levels in blood and urine. Urine tests for elevated blood glucose less reliable in pregnancy. Blood tests (more accurate) used as follows:
      **a.** 1-hour glucose tolerance test: usually done for screening on all pregnant women 24–28 weeks' pregnant.
      **b.** 3-hour glucose tolerance test: used when results from 1 hour GTT > 140 mg/dL.
      **c.** HbA1c: reflects past 4–12-week blood levels of serum glucose.

**C.** Nursing interventions
  1. Teach client the effects and interactions of diabetes and pregnancy and signs of hyper- and hypoglycemia.
  2. Teach client how to control diabetes in pregnancy, advise of changes that need to be made in nutrition and activity patterns to promote normal glucose levels and prevent complications.
  3. Advise client of increased risk of infection and how to avoid it.
  4. Observe and report any signs of preeclampsia.
  5. Monitor fetal status throughout pregnancy.
  6. Assess status of mother and baby frequently
      **a.** Monitor carefully fluids, calories, glucose, and insulin during labor and delivery.
      **b.** Continue careful observation in postdelivery period.

# Renal Conditions

## Urinary Tract Infections (UTI)

**A.** General information
  1. Affect 10% of all pregnant women.
  2. Dilated, flaccid, and displaced ureters are a frequent site.
  3. *E. coli* is the usual cause.
  4. May cause premature labor if severe, untreated, or pyelonephritis develops.

**B.** Assessment findings
    1. Frequency and urgency of urination
    2. Suprapubic pain
    3. Flank pain (if kidney involved)
    4. Hematuria
    5. Pyuria
    6. Fever and chills
**C.** Nursing interventions
    1. Encourage high fluid intake.
    2. Provide warm baths to relieve discomfort and promote perineal hygiene.
    3. Administer and monitor intake of prescribed medications (antibiotics, urinary analgesics).
    4. Stress good bladder-emptying schedule.
    5. Monitor for signs of premature labor from severe or untreated infection.

## Other Infections

**A.** General information
    1. Pregnancy is not a prevention against pre- or coexisting infections.
    2. *Toxoplasmosis, other infections, rubella, cytomegalovirus, and herpes (TORCH infections)* are especially devastating to the fetus, causing abortions, malformations, and even fetal death.
    3. Rubella titer is assessed during early prenatal visit. If mother is deficient in rubella antibodies (titer less than 1.0), rubella virus vaccine is recommended in immediate postpartum period.
**B.** General nursing interventions
    1. Instruct the pregnant woman in signs and symptoms that indicate infection, especially fever, chills, sore throat, localized pain, or rash.
    2. Caution pregnant women to avoid obviously infected persons and other sources of infection, as danger exists for the fetus in all maternal infections.
    3. May affect delivery options.

## AIDS and Pregnancy

**A.** General information
    1. Transmission of the human immunodeficiency virus authenticated through blood, semen, vaginal secretions, and breast milk.
    2. Can be transmitted from mother to fetus during pregnancy.
    3. Cesarean delivery will not avert mother-to-fetus transmission.
    4. Breastfeeding not currently recommended for seropositive mothers.
    5. Increase in prematurity, premature rupture of membranes, low birth weight, and coexistent STDs.
    6. Pregnancy-altered immune states may result in the acceleration of opportunistic diseases,

such as *Candida albicans,* herpes, and toxoplasmosis.
    7. Treatment of the mother with AZT during pregnancy decreases the risk of transmission of the virus to the fetus.
**B.** Nursing implications
    1. Thorough review of history and any physical symptoms.
    2. Close attention to lab studies, especially CBC, leukocyte count, T-cell count, and urinalysis indicated.
    3. Strict attention to universal precautions as appropriate.
    4. Protective coverings in delivery room.
    5. Wear gloves to handle all infants until they are bathed.
    6. Suction newborn with bulb or wall suction devices only.
    7. Special assessments: respiratory, neurologic, psychosocial.

## Other Conditions of Risk in Pregnancy

### Adolescence

**A.** General information
    1. Pregnancy is a condition of both physical and psychologic risk.
    2. Adolescent is frequently undernourished and not yet completely matured either physically or psychosocially.
    3. Adolescent is uniquely unsuited for the stresses of pregnancy.
    4. Frequency of serious complications increases in adolescent pregnancy, particularly toxemia and low-birth-weight infants.
**B.** Nursing interventions
    1. Encourage adequate prenatal care.
    2. Provide health teaching to prepare for pregnancy, labor and delivery, and motherhood.
    3. Provide nutritional counseling.
    4. Teach coping skills for labor and delivery.
    5. Teach child care skills.
    6. Refer adolescent to Crisis Pregnancy Center.

### Disseminated Intravascular Coagulation (DIC)

**A.** General information
    1. Also known as *consumptive coagulopathy*
    2. A diffuse, pathologic form of clotting, secondary to underlying disease/pathology.
    3. Occurs in critical maternity problems such as abruptio placenta, dead fetus syndrome, amniotic fluid embolism, preeclampsia/eclampsia, hydatidiform mole, and hemorrhagic shock
    4. Mechanism
        a. Precoagulant substances released in the blood trigger microthrombosis in

peripheral vessels and paradoxical consumption of circulating clotting factors.
   b. Fibrin-split products accumulate, further interfering with the clotting process.
   c. Platelet and fibrinogen levels drop.
B. Assessment findings
   1. Bleeding may range from massive, unanticipated blood loss to localized bleeding (purpura and petechiae)
   2. Presence of special maternity problems
   3. Prolonged prothrombin and partial thromboplastin times
C. Nursing interventions
   1. Assist with medical management of underlying condition.
   2. Administer blood component therapy (WBCs, packed cells, fresh frozen plasma, cryoprecipitate) as ordered.
   3. Observe for signs of insidious bleeding (oozing IV site, petechiae, lowered hematocrit).
   4. Institute nursing measures for severe bleeding/shock if needed.
   5. Provide emotional support to client and family as needed.

## Anemia

A. General information
   1. Low RBC may be underlying condition
   2. May or may not be exacerbated by physiologic hemodilution of pregnancy
   3. Most common medical disorder of pregnancy
B. Assessment findings
   1. Client is pale, tired, short of breath, dizzy.
   2. Hgb is less than 11 gram/dL; hct less than 37%.
C. Nursing interventions
   1. Encourage intake of foods with high iron content.
   2. Monitor iron supplementation.
   3. Teach sequelae of iron ingestion.
   4. Assess need for parenteral iron.

## Prenatal Substance Abuse

A. General information
   1. Incidence: probably underestimated in our society.
   2. Morbidity/mortality: related to chemical used, timing, and route of administration.
B. Assessment findings
   1. Alcohol
      a. Elevates the mood, depresses the central nervous system
      b. Affects every other system in the body of the mother
      c. Displaces other nutritional food intake
      d. Greatest risk from high blood alcohol levels
      e. No safe level of maternal alcohol use in pregnancy has been established
      f. Fetus may display IUGR (intrauterine growth retardation), CNS dysfunction, and craniofacial abnormalities (fetal alcohol syndrome).
   2. Cocaine
      a. Powerful stimulant; very addictive
      b. Causes vasoconstriction, elevated BP, tachycardia
      c. May precipitate seizures
      d. Affects ability to transport $O_2$ into the blood
      e. May cause spontaneous abortion, fetal malformation, placenta abruptio, neural tube defects
      f. Newborn may display irritability, hypertonicity, poor feeding patterns, increased risk of SIDS
   3. Opiates
      a. Produce analgesia, euphoria, respiratory depression
      b. If used IV, foreign substance contamination may cause pulmonary emboli or infections
      c. If used IV, places mother at greater risk of contracting HIV, then passing it on to fetus
      d. Newborns experience withdrawal within 24–72 hours after delivery
      e. High-pitched cry, restlessness, poor feeding seen in the newborn
   4. Other chemicals
      a. May include tranquilizers, prescription medications, paint thinners, other aerosols, etc.
      b. Major danger is overdose, with accompanying cardiac/respiratory arrest
C. Nursing interventions
   1. Treatment during pregnancy may include in- or outpatient care. Alcoholics Anonymous-based programs are widely utilized.
   2. Treatment may include family therapy.
   3. Efforts to treat the chemical abuse/dependency should be maximized during pregnancy. Withdrawal is best accomplished with competent, professional help.

 **Sample Questions**

1. A 22-year-old woman has missed two of her regular menstrual periods. Her doctor confirms an early, intrauterine pregnancy. This is her first pregnancy. To determine her expected due date, which of the following assessments is most important?
   1. Date of first menstrual period.
   2. Date of last intercourse.
   3. Date of last normal menstrual period.
   4. Age at menarche.

2. A 24-year-old woman is pregnant with her first baby. During her seventh month, she complains of backache. What teaching can the nurse provide to help with comfort?
   1. Sleep on a soft mattress.
   2. Walk barefoot at least once/day.
   3. Perform Kegel exercises once/day.
   4. Wear low-heeled shoes.

3. A woman is hospitalized for the treatment of severe preeclampsia. Which of the following represents an unusual finding for this condition?
   1. Convulsions.
   2. Blood pressure 160/100.
   3. Proteinuria 4+.
   4. Generalized edema.

4. A woman is admitted with severe preeclampsia. What type of room should the nurse select for this woman?
   1. A room next to the elevator.
   2. The room farthest from the nursing station.
   3. The quietest room on the floor.
   4. The labor suite.

5. How does the action of hormones during pregnancy affect the body?
   1. Raises resistance to insulin.
   2. Blocks the release of insulin from the pancreas.
   3. Prevents the liver from metabolizing glycogen.
   4. Enhances the conversion of food to glucose.

6. A 28-year-old woman has had diabetes mellitus since she was an adolescent. She is 8 weeks pregnant. Hyperglycemia during her first trimester will have what effect on the fetus?
   1. Hyperinsulinemia.
   2. Excessive fetal size.
   3. Malformed organs.
   4. Abnormal positioning.

7. The nurse is caring for a young diabetic woman who is in her first trimester of pregnancy. As the pregnancy continues the nurse should anticipate which change in her medication needs?
   1. A decrease in the need for short-acting insulins.
   2. A steady increase in insulin requirements.
   3. Oral hypoglycemic drugs will be given several times daily.
   4. The variable pattern of insulin absorption throughout the pregnancy requires constant close adjustment.

8. A woman is pregnant and diabetic. Why would a glycosylated hemoglobin level be ordered?
   1. It is the most accurate method of determining present insulin levels.
   2. It will predict how well the pancreas can respond to the stress of pregnancy.
   3. It indicates mean glucose level over a 1- to 3-month period.
   4. It gives diagnostic information related to the peripheral effects of diabetes.

9. A 25-year-old woman is 5 months pregnant and has been suffering from morning sickness since early in her pregnancy. She is now admitted for hyperemesis gravidarum and parenteral fluid therapy is started. She has vomited twice within the last hour. What would be the priority nursing intervention to perform?
   1. Assist her with mouth care.
   2. Notify the physician.
   3. Change the IV infusion to Ringer's lactate.
   4. Warm her tray and serve it to her again.

10. A woman in her seventh month of pregnancy has a hemoglobin of 10.5 g. The nurse teaches the woman about proper nutrition during pregnancy. Which statement made by the client indicates to the nurse that teaching was effective?
    1. "I eat liver once a week."
    2. "I have an orange for breakfast."
    3. "I eat six small meals a day."
    4. "I have a green leafy vegetable occasionally."

11. A couple recently arrived in the United States from East Asia. The man brings his wife to the hospital in late labor; his mother and the woman's sister are also present. As the nurse directs the man to the dressing room to change into a scrub suit, his wife anxiously states, "No, he can't come with me. Get my sister and mother-in-law!" What would be the nurse's best response?
    1. "I'm sorry, but our hospital only allows the father into the delivery."
    2. "I'll ask the doctor if that's OK."
    3. "When I talk to your husband, I'm sure he'll want to be with you."
    4. "That's fine. I'll show your husband to the waiting area."

12. During an initial prenatal visit, a woman states that her last menstrual period began on November 21; she also reports some vaginal

bleeding about December 19. What would be the calculated expected date of birth (EDB)?

1. July 21.
2. August 28.
3. September 26.
4. October 1.

13. A 24-year-old woman comes to the clinic because she thinks she is pregnant. Which of the following is a probable sign of pregnancy that the nurse would expect this client to have?

    1. Fetal heart tones.
    2. Nausea and vomiting.
    3. Amenorrhea.
    4. Chadwick's sign.

14. A married 25-year-old housewife is 6 weeks' gestation and is being seen for her first prenatal visit. In relation to normal maternal acceptance of pregnancy, what would the nurse expect that the client feels?

    1. Some ambivalence now that the pregnancy is confirmed.
    2. Overwhelmed by the thought of future changes.
    3. Much happiness and enjoyment in the event.
    4. Detached from the event until physical changes occur.

15. A woman is entering the 20th week of pregnancy. Which normal change would the nurse expect to find on assessment?

    1. Fundus just below diaphragm.
    2. Pigment changes in skin.
    3. Complaints of frequent urination.
    4. Blood pressure returning to prepregnancy level.

16. A primigravida in the first trimester is blood type A+, rubella negative, hemoglobin 12 g, hematocrit 36%. During her second prenatal visit she complains of being very tired, experiencing frequent urination, and a white vaginal discharge; she also states that her nausea and occasional vomiting persist. Based on these findings, the nurse would select which of the following nursing diagnoses?

    1. Activity intolerance related to nutritional deprivation.
    2. Impaired urinary elimination related to a possible infection.
    3. Risk for injury related to hematologic incompatibility.
    4. Alteration in physiologic responses related to pregnancy.

17. A young woman had her pregnancy confirmed and has completed her first prenatal visit. Considering that all data were found to be within normal limits, how soon will the nurse plan the next visit?

    1. One week.
    2. Two weeks.
    3. One month.
    4. Two months.

18. Which statement by a pregnant client would indicate to the nurse that diet teaching has been effective?

    1. "The most important time to take my iron pills is during the early weeks when the baby is forming."
    2. "I don't like milk, but I'll increase my intake of cheese and yogurt."
    3. "I'll be very careful about using salt while I'm pregnant."
    4. "Because I'm overweight to begin with, I can continue my weight loss diet."

19. A woman, age 40, gravida 3 para 2, is 8 weeks pregnant. She is a full-time office manager and states she "usually unwinds with a few glasses of wine" with dinner, smokes about five cigarettes a day, and was "surprised" by this pregnancy. After the assessment, which of the following would the nurse select as the priority nursing diagnosis?

    1. Risk for an impaired bonding related to an unplanned pregnancy.
    2. Risk for injury to the fetus related to advanced age.
    3. Ineffective individual coping related to low self-esteem.
    4. Deficient knowledge related to effects of substance abuse.

20. A young couple has just completed a preconception visit in the maternity clinic. Before leaving, the woman asks the nurse why she was instructed not to take any over-the-counter medications. What would be the nurse's correct reply?

    1. "Research has found that many of these drugs have been linked to problems with getting pregnant."
    2. "At conception, and in the first trimester, these drugs can be as dangerous to the fetus as prescription drugs."
    3. "You should only take drugs that the physician has ordered during pregnancy."
    4. "Any drug is dangerous at this time; later on in pregnancy it won't matter."

21. The pregnant couple asks the nurse what is the purpose of prepared childbirth classes. What would be the nurse's best response?
    1. "The main goal of most types of childbirth classes is to provide information that will help eliminate fear and anxiety."
    2. "The desired goal is childbirth without the use of analgesics."
    3. "These classes help to eliminate the pain of childbirth by exercise and relaxation methods."
    4. "The primary aim is to keep you and your baby healthy during pregnancy and after!"

22. A woman in her 38th week of pregnancy is to have an amniocentesis to evaluate fetal maturity. The L/S (lecithin/sphingomyelin) ratio is 2:1. What is the indication of this finding?
    1. Fetal lung maturity.
    2. That labor can be induced.
    3. The fetus is not viable.
    4. A nonstress test is indicated.

23. A woman is having a contraction stress test (CST) in her last month of pregnancy. When assessing the fetal monitor strip, the nurse notices that with most of the contractions, the fetal heart rate uniformly slows at mid-contraction and then returns to baseline about 20 seconds after the contraction is over. How would the nurse interpret this test result?
    1. Negative: normal.
    2. Reactive: negative.
    3. Positive: abnormal.
    4. Unsatisfactory.

24. A woman, 36 weeks' gestation, is having a CST with an oxytocin IV infusion pump. After two contractions, the uterus stays contracted. What would be the best initial action of the nurse?
    1. Help the client turn on her left side.
    2. Turn off the infusion pump.
    3. Wait 3 minutes for the uterus to relax.
    4. Administer prn terbutaline sulfate (Brethine).

25. A pregnant woman, in the first trimester, is to have a transabdominal ultrasound. The nurse would include which of the following instructions?
    1. Nothing by mouth (NPO) from 6:00 A.M. the morning of the test.
    2. Drink one to two quarts of water and do not urinate before the test.
    3. Come to the clinic first for injection of the contrast dye.
    4. No special instructions are needed for this test.

26. A woman who is pregnant for the first time calls the clinic to say she is bleeding. To obtain important information, what question should be asked by the nurse?
    1. "When did you last feel the baby move?"
    2. "How long have you been pregnant?"
    3. "When was your pregnancy test done?"
    4. "Are you having any uterine cramping?"

27. A woman is hospitalized with a possible ectopic pregnancy. In addition to the classic symptoms of abdominal pain, amenorrhea, and abnormal vaginal bleeding, the nurse knows that which of the following factors in the woman's history may be associated with this condition?
    1. Multiparity.
    2. Age under 20.
    3. Pelvic inflammatory disease (PID).
    4. Habitual spontaneous abortions.

28. A woman is being discharged after treatment for a hydatidiform mole. The nurse should include which of the following in the discharge teaching plan?
    1. Do not become pregnant for at least one year.
    2. Have blood pressure checked weekly for 6 months.
    3. RhoGAM must be received with next pregnancy and delivery.
    4. An amniocentesis can detect a recurrence of this disorder in the future.

29. A woman, 40 weeks' gestation, is admitted to the labor and delivery unit with possible placenta previa. On the admission assessment, what would the nurse expect to find?
    1. Signs of a Couvelaire uterus.
    2. Severe lower abdominal pain.
    3. Painless vaginal bleeding.
    4. A board-like abdomen.

30. A woman, 30 weeks' gestation, is being discharged to home care with a diagnosis of placenta previa. What statement by the client indicates she understands her care at home?
    1. "As I get closer to my due date I will have to remain in bed."
    2. "I can continue with my office job because it's mostly sitting."
    3. "My husband won't be too happy with this 'no sex' order."
    4. "I'm disappointed that I will need a cesarean section."

31. A teenage client, 38 weeks' gestation, is admitted with a diagnosis of pregnancy-induced hypertension (PIH). Data include: blood pressure 160/100, generalized edema, weight gain of 10 pounds in last 2 weeks, and proteinuria of +3; the client is also complaining of a headache and nausea. In planning care for this client, which priority goal would the nurse establish?
   1. Demonstrate a decreased blood pressure within 48 hours.
   2. Not experience a seizure prior to delivery.
   3. Maintain a strict diet prior to delivery.
   4. Comply with medical and nutritional regimen.

32. A woman, 32 weeks' gestation, has developed mild PIH. What statement by the client would indicate understanding of her treatment regimen?
   1. "It is most important not to miss any of my blood pressure medication."
   2. "I will watch my diet restrictions very carefully."
   3. "I will spend most of my time in bed, on my left side."
   4. "I'm happy that this only happens during a first pregnancy."

33. A pregnant client with class 3 cardiac disease is seen during an initial prenatal visit. The nurse selects which of the following priority nursing diagnoses?
   1. Knowledge deficit related to self-care during pregnancy.
   2. Fear; client and family, related to pregnancy outcome.
   3. Alteration in nutrition related to sodium-restricted diet.
   4. Activity intolerance related to compromised cardiac status.

34. The nurse includes the importance of self-monitoring of glucose in the care plan for a diabetic client planning a pregnancy. What does the goal of this monitoring prevent?
   1. Congenital malformations in the fetus.
   2. Maternal vasculopathy.
   3. Accelerated growth of the fetus.
   4. Delayed maturation of fetal lungs.

35. What question will the nurse ask to assess a female's highest risk for developing toxoplasmosis during pregnancy?
   1. "Do you have any pets?"
   2. "Do you consume any alcohol beverages?"
   3. "Are you depressed?"
   4. "Has your blood pressure been elevated?"

## Answers and Rationales

1. **3.** The dates of the last menstrual period, especially the first day of that period, will be used in applying Nägele's rule to determine the estimated date of delivery.

2. **4.** A frequent cause of backache in the third trimester of pregnancy is the combined effect of relaxation of the sacroiliac joints and the change in the center of gravity of the pregnant woman due to the enlarging uterus. Wearing low-heeled shoes, especially when on her feet for extended periods of time, will help to minimize this discomfort.

3. **1.** Convulsions are associated with an eclamptic condition when blood pressure is increased above 160/110 mm Hg.

4. **3.** A quiet room in which stimuli are minimized and controlled is essential to the nursing care of the severely preeclamptic client.

5. **1.** Hormonal influences during pregnancy cause a resistance to insulin utilization at the cellular level. It allows sufficient glucose for placental transport to the fetus, and also prevents the blood sugar in the nondiabetic client from falling to dangerous levels. In the diabetic client, it requires increases in her insulin doses.

6. **3.** Major congenital malformations are noted in the insulin-dependent diabetic mother with poor metabolic control.

7. **2.** During the first trimester of pregnancy, there is little change in insulin requirements. In the second trimester, gradually increasing amounts of insulin are needed, with the insulin dose doubling by the end of pregnancy.

8. **3.** Glycosylated hemoglobin measurements can be used to assess prior glycemic control, giving the average over the past 1 to 3 months.

9. **1.** Frequent vomiting irritates the oral mucosa and leaves the mouth very dry and foul tasting. The first nursing action should be aimed at relieving irritation and drying of the mouth by providing mouth care.

10. **1.** Liver contains more iron than any other food source.

11. **4.** Within the traditional East Asian family, roles are clearly defined. One consideration is the East

Asian husband's lack of involvement during pregnancy and birth; this is a mutually agreeable separation of men's and women's roles.

12. **2.** If a woman has a menstrual period every 28 days and was not taking oral contraceptives, Nägele's rule may be a fairly accurate determiner of her predicted birth date. To use this method, begin with the first day of the last menstrual period, subtract 3 months, and add 7 days.

13. **4.** Probable signs of pregnancy are the result of physiologic changes in the pelvic organs and hormonal influences; for example, the mucous membranes of the vulva, vagina, and cervix become bluish (Chadwick's sign) as a result of hyperemia and proliferation of cells.

14. **1.** During the first trimester of pregnancy, women normally experience ambivalence about being pregnant. It is estimated that around 80% of women initially reject the idea of pregnancy; even women who planned pregnancy may respond at first with surprise and shock.

15. **2.** From 20–24 weeks' gestation, pigment changes in skin may occur from actions of hormones. These include the linea nigra, melasma on the face, and striae gravidarum (stretch marks).

16. **4.** All of the data stated are within the normal expected range for a first trimester pregnancy. These factors are related to hormonal changes and the growing uterus.

17. **3.** In a low-risk pregnancy, the recommended frequency of prenatal visits is: once very month until the 7th or 8th month, every 2 weeks during the 8th month, then every week until birth.

18. **2.** To meet increased calcium needs, pregnant women need to increase their intake of dairy products or consider a calcium supplement that provides 600 mg of calcium per day; it is not necessary to drink milk.

19. **4.** Evidence exists that smoking, consuming alcohol, or using social drugs during pregnancy may be harmful to the fetus.

20. **2.** It is best to avoid any medication when planning a pregnancy and during the first trimester; the greatest potential for gross abnormalities in the fetus occurs during the first trimester, when fetal organs are first developing. The greatest danger extends from day 31 after the last menstrual period to day 71.

21. **1.** All programs in prepared childbirth have some similarities; all have an educational component to help eliminate fear.

22. **1.** Lecithin and sphingomyelin are phospholipids produced by the type II alveolar cells. The L/S ratio increases with gestation and a ratio of 2:1 indicates lung maturity.

23. **3.** The CST subjects the fetus to uterine contractions that compress the arteries supplying the placenta, thus reducing placental blood flow and the flow of oxygen to the fetus; the fetus with minimal metabolic reserve will have late decelerations where the fetal heart rate does not return to the baseline until the contraction ends. Fetal compromise is therefore suggested.

24. **2.** When IV oxytocin is being used to stimulate uterine contractions in a contraction stress test, the oxytocin infusion is stopped if contractions occur more often than every 2 minutes or last longer than 60 seconds, if uterine tetany (remains contracted) takes place, or if continued fetal heart rate decelerations are noted.

25. **2.** To obtain clearer images during the first trimester, women are required to drink 1 to 2 quarts of clear fluid to fill the urinary bladder and thereby push the uterus higher into the abdomen where it can be more accurately scanned.

26. **2.** When a pregnant woman is bleeding vaginally, the nurse should first ask her how many weeks or months pregnant she is; management of bleeding differs in an early pregnancy contrasted with bleeding in late pregnancy. Additional information would include if tissue amniotic fluid was discharged and what other symptoms, such as cramps or pain, are present.

27. **3.** The incidence of ectopic pregnancy in the United States has increased by a factor of 4.9 during recent years. This is attributed primarily to the growing number of women of childbearing age who experience PID and endometriosis, who use intrauterine devices, or who have had tubal surgery.

28. **1.** The follow-up protocol of critical importance after a molar pregnancy is the assessment of serum chorionic gonadotropin (HCG); HCG is considered a highly specific tumor marker for gestational trophoblastic disease (GTD). The HCG levels are assayed at intervals for 1 year; a rise or plateau necessitates further diagnostic assessment and usually treatment. Pregnancy

would obscure the evidence of choriocarcinoma by the normal secretion of HCG.

**29. 3.** Placenta previa, when the placenta is implanted in the lower uterine segment, often is characterized by the sudden onset of bright red bleeding in the third trimester. Usually this bleeding is painless and may or may not be accompanied by contractions.

**30. 3.** In placenta previa, any sexual arousal is contraindicated because it can cause the release of oxytocin, which can cause the cervix to pull away from the low-lying placenta; this results in bleeding and potential jeopardy to the fetus.

**31. 2.** Preeclampsia may progress to eclampsia, the convulsive phase of PIH. Symptoms that herald the progression include headache, visual disturbances, epigastric pain, nausea or vomiting, hyperreflexia, and oliguria; classical signs of PIH also intensify.

**32. 3.** Modified bed rest in the left lateral position may be advised for the client with mild PIH. This position improves venous return and placental

and renal perfusion; urine output increases, and blood pressure may stabilize or decrease.

**33. 4.** Once pregnancy is established, the focus of management is on minimizing any extra cardiac demands on the pregnant woman. In class 3 cardiac disease, the client experiences fatigue, palpitation, dyspnea, or angina when she undertakes less than ordinary activity. Physical activity is markedly restricted; this includes bed rest throughout the pregnancy.

**34. 1.** There is increasing evidence that the degree of control for an insulin-dependent diabetic woman prior to conception greatly affects the fetal outcome. Studies find that poor maternal glucose control underlies the incidence of congenital malformations in the infants of diabetic mothers.

**35. 1.** Cats are intermediate hosts for toxoplasmosis. As transmission of the toxic parasite is via the cat's feces, have someone else change the litter box daily.

# Labor and Delivery

## OVERVIEW

### Five Factors of Labor (Five Ps)

#### *Passenger*

The size, presentation, and position of the fetus.
A. Fetal head (Figure 6-8)
   1. Usually the largest part of the baby; it has profound effect on birthing process.
   2. Bones of skull are joined by membranous sutures, which allow for overlapping or "molding" of cranial bones during birth process.
   3. *Anterior* and *posterior fontanels* are the points of intersection for the sutures and are important landmarks.
      a. Anterior fontanel is larger, diamond-shaped, and closes about 18 months of age.
      b. Posterior fontanel is smaller, triangular, and usually closes about 3 months of age.
   4. Fontanels are used as landmarks for internal examinations during labor to determine position of fetus.

B. Fetal shoulders: may be manipulated during delivery to allow passage of one shoulder at a time.
C. Presentation: that part of the fetus which enters the pelvis in the birth process (Figure 6-9). Types of presentation are:
   1. Cephalic: head is presenting part; usually vertex (*occiput*), which is most favorable for birth. Head is flexed with chin on chest.
   2. Breech: buttocks or lower extremities present first. Types are:
      a. Frank: thighs flexed, legs extended on anterior body surface, buttocks presenting
      b. Full or complete: thighs and legs flexed, buttocks and feet presenting (baby in squatting position)
      c. Footling: one or both feet are presenting
   3. Shoulder: presenting part is the scapula, and baby is in horizontal or transverse position. Cesarean birth indicated.
D. Position: relationship of reference point on fetal presenting part to maternal bony pelvis (Figure 6-10).
   1. Maternal bony pelvis divided into four quadrants (right and left anterior; right and left

**6**

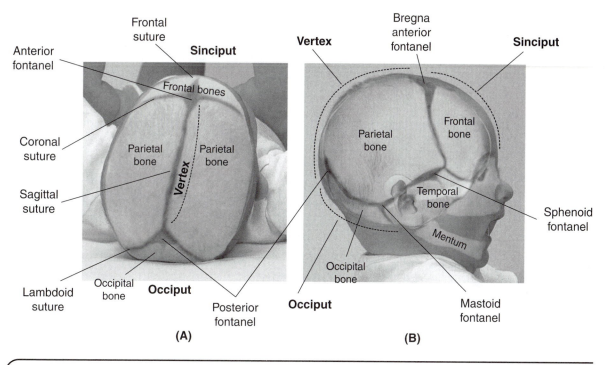

**Figure 6-8** Fetal skull–sutures and fontanels. (A) Superior view; (B) Lateral view

posterior). Relationship is expressed in a three-letter abbreviation: first the maternal side (R or L), next the fetal presentation, and last the maternal quadrant (A or P). Most common positions are:

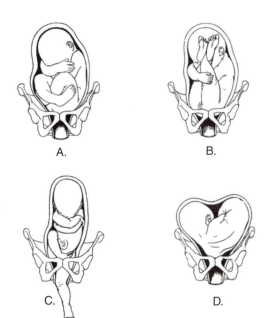

**Figure 6-9** Breech presentations. (A) Complete; (B) Frank; (C) Footling; (D) Shoulder

 a. LOA (left occiput anterior): fetal occiput is on maternal left side and toward front, face is down. This is a favorable delivery position.

 b. ROA (right occiput anterior): fetal occiput on maternal right side toward front, face is down. This is a favorable delivery position.

 c. LOP (left occiput posterior): fetal occiput is on maternal left side and toward back, face is up. Mother experiences much back discomfort during labor; labor may be slowed; rotation usually occurs before labor to anterior position, or health care provider may rotate at time of delivery.

 d. ROP (right occiput posterior): fetal occiput is on maternal right side and toward back, face is up. Presents problems similar to LOP.

2. Assessment of fetal position can be made by:

 a. Leopold's maneuvers: external palpation (4 steps) of maternal abdomen to determine fetal contours or outlines. Maternal obesity, excess amniotic fluid, or uterine tumors may make palpation less accurate.

 b. Vaginal examination: location of sutures and fontanels and determination of relationship to maternal bony pelvis.

 c. Rectal examination: now virtually completely replaced by vaginal examination.

 d. Auscultation of fetal heart tones and determination of quadrant of maternal abdomen where best heard. (Correlate with Leopold maneuvers.)

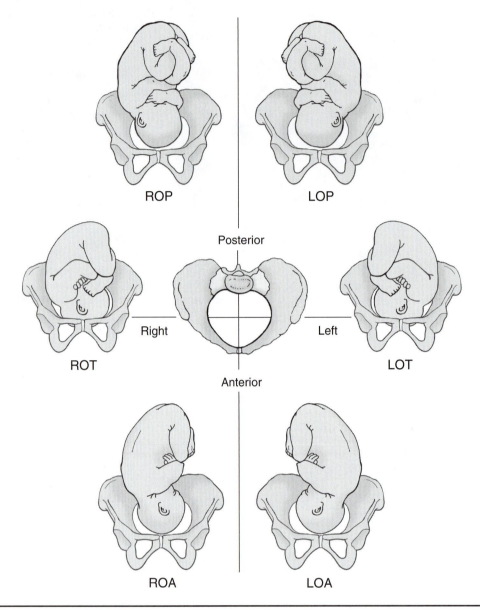

**Figure 6-10** Positions of a vertex presentation

## Passageway

Shape and measurement of maternal pelvis and distensibility of birth canal (see also Overview of Anatomy and Physiology).

A. Engagement: fetal presenting part enters true pelvis (inlet). May occur 2 weeks before labor in primipara; usually occurs at beginning of labor for multipara.

B. Station: measurement of how far the presenting part has descended into the pelvis. Referrant is ischial spines, palpated through lateral vaginal walls.
  1. When presenting part is at ischial spines, station is 0, "engaged."

  2. If presenting part is above ischial spines, station expressed as a negative number (e.g., −1, −2).
  3. If presenting part is below ischial spines, station expressed as a positive number (e.g., +1, +2).
  4. "High" or "floating" terms used to denote unengaged presenting part.

C. Soft tissue (cervix, vagina): stretches and dilates under the force of contractions to accommodate the passage of the fetus.

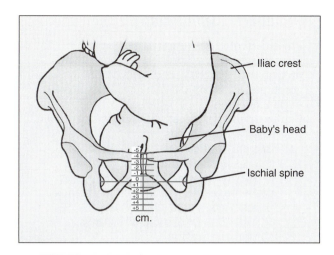

Iliac crest

Baby's head

Ischial spine

cm.

**Figure 6-11** Station, or relationship of the fetal presenting part to the ischial spines. The station illustrated is +2.

## Powers

Forces of labor, acting in concert, to expel fetus and placenta. Major forces are:
A. Uterine contractions (involuntary)
  1. Frequency: timed from the beginning of one contraction to the beginning of the next
  2. Regularity: discernible pattern; better established as labor progresses
  3. Intensity: strength of contraction; a relative assessment without the use of a monitor. May be determined by the "depressability" of the uterus during a contraction. Described as mild, moderate, or strong.
  4. Duration: length of contraction. Contractions lasting more than 90 seconds without a subsequent period of uterine relaxation may have severe implications for the fetus and should be reported.
B. Voluntary bearing-down efforts
  1. After full dilation of the cervix, the mother can use her abdominal muscles to help expel the fetus.
  2. These efforts are similar to those for defecation, but the mother is pushing out the fetus from the birth canal.
  3. Contraction of levator ani muscles.

## Position

A maternal position during the labor process.
A. Several positions possible:
  1. Not confined to lying supine in bed
  2. Lateral recumbent (usually most comfortable)
  3. Sitting in rocking chair
  4. Semi-reclined in bed

B. Position will depend on whether client has had an epidural; consider maternal needs as well as fetal well-being.

## Psychologic Response

Factors that influence labor as a positive/negative experience
A. Culture: how society views childbirth
B. Expectations/goals realistic or unattainable
C. Feedback from others involved in labor and delivery process

# The Labor Process

## Causes

Actual cause unknown. Factors involved include
A. Progressive uterine distension
B. Increasing intrauterine pressure
C. Aging of the placenta
D. Changes in levels of estrogen, progesterone, and prostaglandins
E. Increasing myometrial irritability

## Mechanisms (Vertex Presentation)

A. Engagement
  1. The biparietal diameter of the head passes the pelvic inlet.
  2. The head is fixed in the pelvis.
B. Descent: progress of the presenting part through the pelvis
C. Flexion: chin flexed more firmly onto chest by pressure on fetal head from maternal soft tissues (cervix, vaginal walls, pelvic floor)
D. Internal rotation
  1. Fetal skull rotates along axis from transverse to anteroposterior at pelvic outlet.
  2. Head passes the midpelvis.
E. Extension: head passes under the symphysis pubis and is delivered, occiput first, followed by face and chin.
F. External rotation: head rotates to full alignment with back and shoulders for shoulder delivery mechanisms.
G. *When entire body of baby has emerged from mother's body, birth is complete. This time is recorded as the time of birth.*

## Stages of Labor

A. Definitions
  1. Stage 1: from onset of labor until full dilation of cervix
    a. Latent phase: from 0–4 cm
    b. Active phase: 4–8 cm
    c. Transition phase: 8–10 cm

2. Stage 2: from full dilation of cervix to birth of baby
3. Stage 3: from birth of baby to expulsion of placenta
4. Stage 4: time after birth (usually 1–2 hours) of immediate recovery

B. Cervical changes in first stage of labor
  1. Effacement
     a. Shortening and thinning of cervix.
     b. In primipara, effacement is usually well advanced before dilation begins; in a multipara, effacement and dilation progress together.
  2. Dilation
     a. Enlargement or widening of the cervical os and canal.
     b. Full dilation is considered 10 cm.

## Duration of Labor

A. Depends on:
  1. Regular, progressive uterine contractions
  2. Progressive effacement and dilation of cervix
  3. Progressive descent of presenting part
B. Average length
  1. Primipara
     a. Stage 1: 12–13 hours
     b. Stage 2: 1 hour
     c. Stage 3: 3–4 minutes
     d. Stage 4: 1–2 hours
  2. Multipara
     a. Stage 1: 8 hours
     b. Stage 2: 20 minutes
     c. Stage 3: 4–5 minutes
     d. Stage 4: 1–2 hours

# ASSESSMENT DURING LABOR

## Fetal Assessment

### Auscultation

Auscultate FHR at least every 15–30 minutes during first stage and every 5–15 minutes during second stage (depends on risk status of client).
A. Normal range 120–160 beats/minute
B. Best recorded during the 30 seconds immediately following a contraction

### Palpation

Assess intensity of contraction by manual palpation of uterine fundus.
A. Mild: tense fundus, but can be indented with fingertips.
B. Moderate: firm fundus, difficult to indent with fingertips.
C. Strong: very firm fundus, cannot indent with fingertips.

## Electronic Fetal Monitoring

A. Placement of ultrasound transducer and tocotransducer to record fetal heartbeat and uterine contractions and display them on special graph paper for comparison and identification of normal and abnormal patterns.
B. Can be applied externally to mother's abdomen, or internally, within uterus.
  1. External application
     a. Less precise information collected
     b. May be affected by maternal movements
     c. Noninvasive: rupture of membranes not required, can be widely used
     d. Little danger associated with use
  2. Internal application
     a. More precise information collected
     b. Cervix must be dilated and membranes ruptured to be utilized
     c. Physician applies scalp electrode and uterine catheter
     d. Sterile technique must be maintained during application to reduce risk of intrauterine infection
     e. Can yield specific short-term variability
C. Pattern recognition
  1. Nurse is responsible for assessing FHR patterns, implementing appropriate nursing interventions, and reporting suspicious patterns to physician.
  2. Baseline FHR: 120–160, when uterus is not contracting.
  3. Variability is normal, indicative of intact fetal nervous system. Variability is result of interaction of sympathetic and parasympathetic nervous systems. Two types of variability are:
     a. Short-term (beat-to-beat): assessed as present/absent.
     b. Long-term (rhythmic fluctuations): classified according to number of cycles/minute. Average is 6/minute.
  4. Tachycardia
     a. FHR more than 160 beats/minute, lasting longer than 10 minutes.
     b. May have multiple causes.
     c. Oxygen may be administered.
  5. Bradycardia
     a. FHR less than 120 beats/minute lasting longer than 10 minutes.
     b. May have multiple causes.
     c. Oxygen may be administered.
  6. Early deceleration
     a. Deceleration of FHR begins early in contraction, stays within normal range, returns to baseline by end of contraction.
     b. Believed to be the result of compression of fetal head against cervix.
     c. Not an ominous pattern, no nursing interventions required.

7. Late deceleration
   a. Deceleration of FHR begins late in contraction; depth varies with strength of contraction; does not return to baseline by end of contraction.
   b. May be occasional or consistent. Gradual increase in number is always suspicious and MUST be reported/charted.
   c. Believed to be the result of uteroplacental insufficiency.
   d. An ominous pattern.
   e. Nurse should place client in side-lying position, or change maternal position, administer oxygen, discontinue any oxytocin infusion, assess variability, prepare for immediate delivery if pattern remains uncorrected.
8. Variable deceleration
   a. Onset of deceleration not related to uterine contraction.
   b. Swings in FHR abrupt and dramatic, return to baseline frequently rapid.
   c. Believed to be the result of compression of the umbilical cord.
   d. Although not an ominous pattern, continued nursing assessment required.
   e. Nurse should change maternal position to relieve pressure on cord; if no improvement seen, administer oxygen, discontinue oxytocin if infusing, prepare client for vaginal exam to assess for prolapsed cord (see also Prolapsed Umbilical Cord).
   f. If cord is prolapsed, relieve pressure on cord; do not attempt to replace cord.
   g. Cesarean delivery will be needed.

## Maternal Assessment

### Premonitory Assessment

Physiologic changes preceding labor
A. Lightening (engagement): occurs up to two weeks before labor in primipara; at beginning of labor for multipara
B. Braxton Hicks' contractions: may become more noticeable; may play a part in ripening of cervix
C. Easier respirations from decreased pressure on diaphragm
D. Frequent urination, from increased pressure on bladder
E. Restlessness/poor sleeping patterns, "nesting" behaviors

### True vs False Labor

A. True labor
   1. Contractions increased in frequency, intensity, and duration
   2. Progressive cervical changes
   3. Bloody show
   4. Progressive fetal descent
   5. Walking intensifies contractions
   6. Discomfort begins in back then radiates to abdomen
B. False labor
   1. Irregular, inefficient contractions not causing the progressive changes associated with true labor
   2. No bloody show
   3. Discomfort primarily in abdomen, may be relieved by walking
   4. Need to assess client over period of time to differentiate from true labor

## FIRST STAGE OF LABOR

### Latent Phase (0–4 cm)

#### Assessment

A. Contractions: frequency, intensity, duration
B. Membranes: intact or ruptured, color of fluid
C. Bloody show
D. Time of onset
E. Cervical changes
F. Time of last ingestion of food
G. FHR every 15 minutes; immediately after rupture of membranes
H. Maternal vital signs
   1. Temperature every 2 hours if membranes ruptured, every 4 hours if intact
   2. Pulse and respirations every hour or prn as indicated
   3. Blood pressure every half hour or prn as indicated
I. Progress of descent (station)
J. Client's knowledge of labor process
K. Client's affect
L. Client's birth plan

#### Analysis

Nursing diagnoses for the latent phase of first stage of labor may include:
A. Anxiety
B. Ineffective breathing pattern
C. Pain
D. Deficient knowledge

#### Planning and Implementation

A. Goals
   1. Complete all admission procedures.
   2. Labor will progress normally.
   3. Mother/fetus will tolerate latent phase successfully.
B. Interventions
   1. Administer perineal prep/enema if ordered/appropriate.

2. Assess vital signs, blood pressure, fetal heart, contractions, bloody show, cervical changes, descent of fetus as scheduled.
3. Maintain bed rest if indicated or required.
4. Reinforce/teach breathing techniques as needed.
5. Support laboring woman/couple based on their needs.
6. Have client attempt to void every 1–2 hours.
7. Apply external fetal monitoring if indicated or ordered.

## Evaluation

A. Admission procedures complete
B. Progress through latent stage normal, cervix dilated
C. Mother/fetus tolerate latent phase well, mother as comfortable as possible, vital signs normal; FHR maintained in response to contractions

## Active Phase (4–8 cm)

### Assessment

A. Cervical changes
B. Bloody show
C. Membranes
D. Progress of descent
E. Maternal/fetal vital signs
F. Client's affect

### Analysis

Nursing diagnoses for the active phase of first stage of labor may include:
A. Ineffective coping
B. Impaired oral mucous membranes
C. Deficient knowledge
D. Pain
E. Ineffective tissue perfusion
F. Risk for injury

### Planning and Implementation

A. Goals
   1. Progress will be normal through active phase.
   2. Mother/fetus will successfully complete active phase.
B. Interventions
   1. Continue to observe labor progress.
   2. Reinforce/teach breathing techniques as needed.
   3. Position client for maximum comfort.
   4. Support client/couple as mother becomes more involved in labor.
   5. Administer analgesia if ordered or indicated.
   6. Assist with anesthesia if given and monitor maternal/fetal vital signs.
   7. Provide ice chips or clear fluids for mother to drink if allowed/desired.

8. Keep client/couple informed as labor progresses.
9. With posterior position, apply sacral counterpressure, or have father do so.

## Evaluation

A. Labor progressing through active phase, dilation progressing
B. Mother/fetus tolerating labor appropriately
C. No complications observed

## Transition Phase (8–10 cm)

### Assessment

A. Progress of labor
B. Cervical changes
C. Maternal mood changes: if irritable or aggressive may be tiring or unable to cope
D. Signs of nausea, vomiting, trembling, crying, irritability
E. Maternal/fetal vital signs
F. Breathing patterns, may be hyperventilating
G. Urge to bear down with contractions

### Analysis

Nursing diagnoses for the transition phase of first stage of labor may include:
A. Ineffective breathing pattern
B. Powerlessness
C. Ineffective coping

### Planning and Implementation

A. Goals
   1. Labor will continue to progress through transition.
   2. Mother/fetus will tolerate process well.
   3. Complications will be avoided.
B. Interventions
   1. Continue observation of labor progress, maternal/fetal vital signs.
   2. Give mother positive support if tired or discouraged.
   3. Accept behavioral changes of mother.
   4. Promote appropriate breathing patterns to prevent hyperventilation.
   5. If hyperventilation present, have mother rebreathe expelled carbon dioxide to reverse respiratory alkalosis.
   6. Discourage pushing efforts until cervix is completely dilated, then assist with pushing.
   7. Observe for signs of delivery.

### Evaluation

A. Mother/fetus progressed through transition
B. No complications observed
C. Mother/fetus ready for second stage of labor

# SECOND STAGE OF LABOR

(See Figure 6-12)

## Assessment

A. Signs of imminent delivery
B. Progress of descent
C. Maternal/fetal vital signs
D. Maternal pushing efforts
E. Vaginal distension
F. Bulging of perineum
G. Crowning
H. Birth of baby

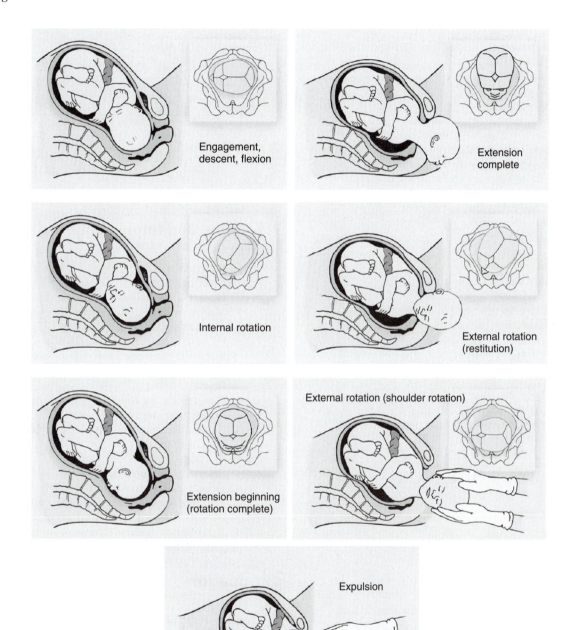

**Figure 6-12** Mechanisms of second stage labor

## Analysis

Nursing diagnoses for the second stage of labor may include:
A. Risk for injury
B. Noncompliance related to exhaustion
C. Deficient knowledge

## Planning and Implementation

A. Goals
    1. Safe delivery of living, uninjured fetus.
    2. Mother will be comfortable after tolerating delivery.
B. Interventions
    1. If necessary, transfer mother carefully to delivery table or birthing chair; support legs equally to prevent/minimize strain on ligaments.
    2. Carefully position mother on delivery table, in delivery chair, or birthing bed to prevent popliteal vein pressure.
    3. Help mother use handles or legs to pull on as she bears down with contractions.
    4. Clean vulva and perineum to prepare for delivery.
    5. Continue observation of maternal/fetal vital signs.
    6. Encourage mother in sustained (5–7 seconds) pushes with each contraction.
    7. Support father's participation if in delivery area.
    8. Catheterize mother's bladder if indicated.
    9. Keep mother informed of delivery progress.
    10. Note time of delivery of baby.

## Evaluation

A. Delivery of healthy viable fetus
B. Mother comfortable after procedure
C. No complications during procedure

## THIRD STAGE OF LABOR

### Assessment

A. Signs of placental separation
    1. Gush of blood
    2. Lengthening of cord
    3. Change in shape of uterus (discoid to globular)
B. Completeness of placenta
C. Status of mother/baby contact for first critical 1–2 hours
    1. Baby's Apgar scores (see Table 6-7)
    2. Blood pressure, pulse, respirations, lochia, fundal status of mother

### Analysis

Nursing diagnoses for the third stage of labor may include:

**Table 6-7** Apgar Scoring

| Category | 0 | 1 | 2 | Score |
|---|---|---|---|---|
| Heart Rate | Absent | <100 | >100 | _____ |
| Respiratory Effort | Absent | Slow, Irregular | Good cry | _____ |
| Muscle tone | Absent/ limp | Some flexion | Active motion | _____ |
| Reflex irritability | No response | Grimace | Cry | _____ |
| Color | Blue, pale | Body pink, extremities blue | All pink | _____ |
| | | | Total Score | _____ |

A. Pain
B. Risk for deficient fluid volume

## Planning and Implementation

A. Goals
    1. Placenta will be delivered without complications.
    2. Maternal blood loss will be minimized.
    3. Mother will tolerate procedures well.
B. Interventions
    1. Palpate fundus immediately after delivery of placenta; massage gently if not firm.
    2. Palpate fundus at least every 15 minutes for first 1–2 hours.
    3. Observe lochia for color and amount.
    4. Inspect perineum.
    5. Assist with maternal hygiene as needed.
      a. Clean gown.
      b. Warm blanket.
      c. Clean perineal pads.
    6. Offer fluids as indicated.
    7. Promote beginning relationship with baby and parents through touch and privacy.
    8. Administer medications as ordered/needed (pitocin added to IV if present).

## Evaluation

A. Placenta delivered without complications
B. Minimal maternal blood loss
C. Mother tolerated procedure well

## FOURTH STAGE OF LABOR

### Assessment

A. Fundal firmness, position
B. Lochia: color, amount

C. Perineum
D. Vital signs
E. IV if running
F. Infant's heart rate, airway, color, muscle tone, reflexes, warmth, activity state
G. Bonding/family integration

## Analysis

Nursing diagnoses for the fourth stage of labor may include:
A. Pain
B. Risk for deficient fluid volume
C. Interrupted family processes

## Planning and Implementation

A. Goal: critical first hour(s) after delivery will pass without complications for mother/baby.
B. Interventions
   1. Palpate fundus every 15 minutes for first 1–2 hours; massage gently if not firm.
   2. Check mother's blood pressure, pulse, respirations every 15 minutes for first 1–2 hours or until stable.
   3. Check lochia for color and amount every 15 minutes for first 1–2 hours.
   4. Inspect perineum every 15 minutes for first 1–2 hours.
   5. Apply ice to perineum if swollen or if episiotomy was performed (see Episiotomy).
   6. Encourage mother to void, particularly if fundus not firm or displaced.
      a. Use nursing techniques to encourage voiding.
      b. If client unable to void, get order for catheterization.
      c. Measure first voiding.
   7. Encourage early bonding; through breastfeeding if desired.

## Evaluation

A. Mother's vital signs stable, fundus and lochia within normal limits
B. Evidence of bonding; parents cuddle, touch, talk to baby
C. No complications observed for mother or baby during crucial time

## COMPLICATIONS OF LABOR AND DELIVERY

## Premature/Preterm Labor

A. General information
   1. Labor that occurs before the end of the 37th week of pregnancy.
   2. Cause is frequently unknown, but the following conditions are associated with premature labor:
      a. Cervical incompetence
      b. Preeclampsia/eclampsia
      c. Maternal injury
      d. Infection (urinary tract infection)
      e. Multiple gestation, polyhydramnios
      f. Placental disorders
   3. Preterm labor: prevention
      a. Minimize or stop smoking: a major factor in preterm labor and birth.
      b. Minimize or stop substance abuse/chemical dependency.
      c. Early and consistent prenatal care.
      d. Appropriate diet/weight gain.
      e. Minimize psychological stressors.
      f. Minimize/prevent exposure to infections.
      g. Learn to recognize signs and symptoms of preterm labor.
   4. Incidence of preterm labor is between 5% and 10% in all pregnancies and is a major cause of perinatal mortality.
B. Medical management
   1. Unless labor is irreversible, or a condition exists in which the mother or fetus would be jeopardized by the continuation of the pregnancy, or the membranes have ruptured, the usual medical intervention is to attempt to arrest the premature labor (tocolysis).
   2. Medications used in the treatment of premature labor
      a. Magnesium sulfate
         1) Stops uterine contractions with fewer side effects than beta-adrenergic drugs.
         2) Interferes with muscle contractility.
         3) Administered IV for 12 to 24 hours, PO form of magnesium may be used for maintenance.
            a) Loading dose of 4–6 g IV over 20 to 30 minutes
            b) Maintenance dose IV 1–3 g/hr (IV piggyback)
            c) Must monitor client for magnesium toxicity
         4) Few serious side effects; initially client feels hot, flushed, sweats, may complain of headache, nausea, diarrhea, dizziness, nystagmus, and lethargy.
         5) Most serious side effect: respiratory depression.
         6) Most common fetal side effect is hypotonia.
      b. Beta-adrenergic drugs—terbutaline and ritodrine.
         1) Decreases effect of calcium on muscle activation to slow or stop uterine contractions.
         2) Initially given IV, then PO brethine (terbutaline) for maintenance.

**3)** Terbutaline:
  **a)** 1–8 mg/min 3 8–12 hr
  **b)** 2.5 to 5 mg PO q 4–8 hr
**4)** Ritodrine
  **a)** 0.05–0.1 mg/min increased to 0.35 mg/min until contractions stop
  **b)** 10–20 mg q 2 hr for 24 hours
**5)** Side effects: increased heart rate, nervousness, tremors, nausea and vomiting, decrease in serum K+ level, cardiac arrhythmias, pulmonary edema.
  **c.** Nifedipine
    **1)** Calcium channel blocker
    **2)** 10–30 mg loading dose, oral or sublingual; second dose may be given in 30 min if contractions persist; 10–20 mg orally q 4–6 hr for maintenance
    **3)** Side effects: facial flushing, mild hypotension, reflex tachycardia, headache, nausea
  **d.** Indomethacin
    **1)** Prostaglandin synthetase inhibitor
    **2)** Loading dose: 50–100 mg PO or rectally: 25 mg q 4–6 hr for 24–48 hr maintenance
    **3)** Side effects: nausea, vomiting, dyspepsia
  **3.** When premature labor cannot or should not be arrested and fetal lung maturity needs to be improved, the use of betamethasone (Celestone) can improve the L/S ratio of lung surfactants. It is administered IM to the mother, usually every 12 hr × 2, then weekly until 34 weeks' gestation.
**C.** Nursing interventions
  **1.** Keep client at rest, side-lying position.
  **2.** Hydrate the client and maintain with IV or PO fluids.
  **3.** Maintain continuous maternal/fetal monitoring.
    **a.** Maternal/fetal vital signs every 10 minutes; be alert for abrupt changes.
    **b.** Monitor maternal I&O.
    **c.** Monitor urine for glucose and ketones.
    **d.** Watch cardiac and respiratory status carefully.
    **e.** Evaluate lab test results carefully.
  **4.** Administer drugs as ordered/indicated.
    **a.** Terbutaline
      **1)** Position client on side as much as possible.
      **2)** Apply external fetal monitor.
      **3)** Complete maternal/fetal assessment before each increase in dosage rate.
      **4)** Special maternal assessment includes respiratory status, blood pressure, pulse, I&O, lab values.
      **5)** Notify physician of significant changes.

  **6)** Support client through stressful period of treatment and uncertainty.
  **7)** Teach client necessity of continuing oral medication at home if discharged.
  **b.** Magnesium sulfate: carefully monitor respirations, reflexes, and urinary output (see also Severe Preeclampsia)
**5.** Keep client informed of all progress/changes.
**6.** Identify side effects/complications as early as possible.
**7.** Carry out activities designed to keep client comfortable.

# Postmature/Prolonged Pregnancy

**A.** General information
  **1.** Defined as those pregnancies lasting beyond the end of the 42nd week.
  **2.** Fetus at risk due to placental degeneration and loss of amniotic fluid (cord accidents).
  **3.** Decreased amounts of vernix also allow the drying of the fetal skin, resulting in a dry, parchmentlike skin condition.
**B.** Medical management
  **1.** Directed toward ascertaining precise fetal gestational age and condition, and determining fetal ability to tolerate labor
  **2.** Induction of labor and possibly cesarean birth
**C.** Assessment findings
  **1.** Measurements of fetal gestational age for fetal maturity
  **2.** Biophysical profile
**D.** Nursing interventions
  **1.** Perform continual monitoring of maternal/fetal vital signs.
  **2.** Support mother through all testing and labor
  **3.** Assist with amnio-infusion if ordered to increase cushion for cord.

# Prolapsed Umbilical Cord

**A.** General information
  **1.** Displacement of cord in a downward direction, near or ahead of the presenting part, or into the vagina
  **2.** May occur when membranes rupture, or with ensuing contractions
  **3.** Associated with breech presentations, unengaged presentations, and premature labors
  **4.** Obstetric emergency: if compression of the cord occurs, fetal hypoxia may result in CNS damage or death.
**B.** Assessment findings: vaginal exam identifies cord prolapse into vagina
**C.** Nursing interventions
  **1.** Check fetal heart tones immediately when membranes rupture, and again after next contraction, or within 5 minutes; report decelerations.

**2.** If fetal bradycardia, perform vaginal examination and check for prolapsed cord.

**3.** If cord prolapsed into vagina, exert upward pressure against presenting part to lift part off cord, reducing pressure on cord.

**4.** Get help to move mother into a position where gravity assists in getting presenting part off cord (knee-chest position or severe Trendelenburg's).

**5.** Administer oxygen, and prepare for immediate cesarean birth.

**6.** If cord protrudes outside vagina, cover with sterile gauze moistened with sterile saline while carrying out above tasks. Do not attempt to replace cord.

**7.** Notify physician.

## Premature Rupture of Membranes

**A.** General information
  **1.** Loss of amniotic fluid, prior to term, unconnected with labor.
  **2.** Dangers associated with this event are prolapsed cord, infection, and the potential need for premature delivery.

**B.** Assessment findings
  **1.** Report from mother/family of discharge of fluid.
  **2.** pH of vaginal fluid will differentiate between amniotic fluid (alkaline) and urine or purulent discharge (acidic).

**C.** Nursing interventions
  **1.** Monitor maternal/fetal vital signs on continuous basis, especially maternal temperature.
  **2.** Calculate gestational age.
  **3.** Observe for signs of infection and for signs of onset of labor.
    **a.** If signs of infection present, administer antibiotics as ordered and prepare for immediate delivery.
    **b.** If no maternal infection, induction of labor may be delayed.
  **4.** Observe and record color, odor, amount of amniotic fluid.
  **5.** Examine mother for signs of prolapsed cord.
  **6.** Provide explanations of procedures and findings, and support mother/family.
  **7.** Prepare mother/family for early birth if indicated.

## Fetal Distress

**A.** General information: common contributing factors are:
  **1.** Cord compression.
  **2.** Placental abnormalities.
  **3.** Preexisting maternal disease.

**B.** Assessment findings
  **1.** Decelerations in FHR

**2.** Meconium-stained amniotic fluid with a vertex presentation

**3.** Fetal scalp sampling (may be needed for a definitive diagnosis)

**C.** Nursing interventions
  **1.** Check FHR on appropriate basis, institute fetal monitoring if not already in use.
  **2.** Conduct vaginal exam for presentation and position.
  **3.** Place mother on left side, administer oxygen, check for prolapsed cord, notify physician.
  **4.** Support mother and family.
  **5.** Prepare for emergency birth if indicated.

## Dystocia

**A.** General information
  **1.** Any labor/delivery that is prolonged or difficult
  **2.** Usually results from a change in the interrelationships among the 5 Ps (factors in labor/delivery): *p*assenger, *p*assage, *p*owers, *p*osition, and *p*syche of mother.
  **3.** Frequently seen causes include
    **a.** Disproportion between fetal presentation (usually the head) and maternal pelvis (cephalopelvic disproportion [CPD]).
      **1)** If disproportion is minimal, vaginal birth may be attempted if fetal injuries can be minimized or eliminated.
      **2)** Cesarean birth needed if disproportion is great.
    **b.** Problems with presentation
      **1)** Any presentation unfavorable for delivery (e.g., breech, shoulder, face, transverse lie)
      **2)** Posterior presentation that does not rotate, or cannot be rotated with ease.
      **3)** Cesarean birth is the usual intervention.
    **c.** Problems with maternal soft tissue
      **1)** A full bladder may impede the progress of labor, as can myomata uteri, cervical edema, scar tissue, and congenital anomalies.
      **2)** Emptying the bladder may allow labor to continue; the other conditions may necessitate cesarean birth.
    **d.** Dysfunctional uterine contractions
      **1)** Contractions may be too weak, too short, too far apart, ineffectual.
      **2)** Progress of labor is affected; progressive dilation, effacement, and descent do not occur in the expected pattern.
      **3)** Classification
        **a)** Primary: inefficient pattern present from beginning of labor; usually a prolonged latent phase.

b) Secondary: efficient pattern that changes to inefficient or stops; may occur in any stage.

B. Assessment findings
1. Progress of labor slower than expected rate of dilation, effacement, descent for specific client
2. Length of labor prolonged
3. Maternal exhaustion/distress
4. Fetal distress

C. Nursing interventions
1. Individualized as to cause.
2. Provide comfort measures for client.
3. Provide clear, supportive descriptions of all actions taken.
4. Administer analgesia if ordered/indicated.
5. Prepare oxytocin infusion for induction of labor if ordered.
6. Monitor mother/fetus continuously.
7. Prepare for cesarean birth if needed.

## Precipitous Labor and Delivery

A. General information
1. Labor of less than 3 hours
2. Emergency delivery without client's physician or midwife

B. Assessment findings
1. As labor is progressing quickly, assessment may need to be done rapidly.
2. Client may have history of previous precipitous labor and delivery.
3. Desire to push.
4. Observe status of membranes, perineal area for bulging, and for signs of bleeding.

C. Nursing interventions (see Table 6-8)

## Amniotic Fluid Embolism

A. General information
1. Escape of amniotic fluid into the maternal circulation, usually in conjunction with a pattern of hypertonic, intense uterine contractions, either naturally or oxytocin induced.
2. Obstetric emergency: may be fatal to the mother and to the baby.

B. Assessment findings
1. Sudden onset of respiratory distress, hypotension, chest pain, signs of shock
2. Bleeding (DIC)
3. Cyanosis
4. Pulmonary edema

C. Nursing interventions
1. Initiate emergency life support activities for mother.
   a. Administer oxygen.
   b. Utilize CPR in case of cardiac arrest.
2. Establish IV line for blood transfusion and monitoring of CVP.

**Table 6-8** Emergency Delivery of an Infant

*If you have to deliver the baby yourself*

- Assess the client's affect and ability to understand directions, as well as other resources available (other physicians, nurses, auxiliary personnel).
- Stay with client at all times; mother must not be left alone if delivery is imminent.
- Do not prevent birth of baby.
- Maintain sterile environment if possible.
- Rupture membranes if necessary.
- Support baby's head as it emerges, preventing too-rapid delivery with gentle pressure.
- Check for nuchal cord, slip over head if possible.
- Use gentle aspiration with bulb syringe to remove blood and mucus from nose and mouth.
- Deliver shoulders after external rotation, asking mother to push gently if needed.
- Provide support for baby's body as it is delivered.
- Hold baby in head-down position to facilitate drainage of secretions.
- Promote cry by gently rubbing over back and soles of feet.
- Dry to prevent heat loss.
- Place baby on mother's abdomen.
- Check for signs of placental separation.
- Check mother for excess bleeding; massage uterus prn.
- Hold placenta as it is delivered.
- Cut cord when pulsations cease, if cord clamp is available; if no clamps, leave intact.
- Wrap baby in dry blanket, give to mother; put to breast if possible.
- Check mother for fundal firmness and excess bleeding.
- Record all pertinent data.
- Comfort mother and family as needed.

3. Administer medications to control bleeding as ordered.
4. Prepare for emergency birth of baby.
5. Keep client/family informed as possible.

## Induction of Labor

A. General information: deliberate stimulation of uterine contractions before the normal occurrence of labor.

B. Medical management: may be accomplished by
1. Amniotomy (the deliberate rupture of membranes)
2. Oxytocins, usually Pitocin
3. Prostaglandin ($PGE_2$) in gel/suppository form to improve cervical readiness

C. Assessment findings
1. Indications for use
   a. Postmature pregnancy
   b. Preeclampsia/eclampsia
   c. Diabetes
   d. Premature rupture of membranes

2. Condition of fetus: mature, engaged vertex fetus in no distress
3. Condition of mother: cervix "ripe" for induction, no CPD

D. Nursing interventions
1. Explain all procedures to client.
2. Prepare appropriate equipment and medications.
   a. Amniotomy: a small tear made in amniotic membrane as part of sterile vaginal exam
      1) Explain sensations to client.
      2) Check FHR immediately before and after procedure; marked changes may indicate prolapsed cord.
      3) Additional care as for woman with premature rupture of membranes.
   b. Oxytocin (Pitocin): IV administration, "piggybacked" to main IV
      1) Usual dilution 10 milliunit/1000 mL fluid, delivered via infusion pump for greatest accuracy in controlling dosage.
      2) Usual administration rate is 0.5–1.0 milliunit/min, increased no more than 1–2 milliunit/min at 40–60-minute intervals until regular pattern of appropriate contractions is established (every 2–3 minutes, lasting less than 90 seconds, with 30–45 second rest period between contractions).
3. Know that continuous monitoring and accurate assessments are essential.
   a. Apply external continuous fetal monitoring equipment.
   b. Monitor maternal condition on a continuous basis: blood pressure, pulse, progress of labor.
4. Discontinue oxytocin infusion when:
   a. Fetal distress is noted.
   b. Hypertonic contractions occur.
   c. Signs of other obstetric complications (hemorrhage/shock, abruptio placenta, amniotic fluid embolism) appear.
5. Notify physician of any untoward reactions.

# ANALGESIA AND ANESTHESIA

## Analgesia for Labor

### General Information

A. Definition: the easing of pain or discomfort by the administration of medication that blocks pain recognition or the raising of the pain recognition threshold.
B. Sources of pain/discomfort
1. First stage of labor: stretching of cervix and uterine contractions
2. Second stage of labor: stretching of birth canal and perineum

C. Examples of medications used systemically for labor analgesia
1. Sedatives: help to relieve anxiety; may use secobarbital (Seconal), sodium pentobarbital (Nembutal), phenobarbital.
2. Narcotic analgesics: help to relieve pain; may use morphine, meperidine (Demerol), butorphanol (Stadol), fentanyl (Sublimaze), nalbuphine hydrochloride (Nubain).
3. Narcotic antagonists: given to reverse narcotic depression of mother or baby; may use naloxone (Narcan), levallorphan (Lorfan).
4. Analgesic potentiating drugs: given to raise desired effect of analgesic without raising dose of analgesic drug; may use promethazine (Phenergan), promazine (Sparine), propiomazine (Largon), hydroxyzine (Vistaril).

D. Medication administration
1. IV: the preferred route; allows for smaller doses, better control of administration, better prediction of action.
2. IM: still widely used; needs larger dose, absorption may be delayed or erratic.
3. SC: used occasionally for small doses of nonirritating drugs.

### Assessment

A. Client's perception of pain/discomfort
B. Baseline vital signs for later comparison
C. Known allergies
D. Current status of labor: medications best given in active phase of first stage of labor
E. Time of previous doses of medications

### Analysis

Nursing diagnoses for labor analgesia may include:
A. Pain
B. Ineffective coping
C. Deficient knowledge

### Planning and Implementation

A. Goals
1. Medication will relieve maternal discomfort.
2. Maternal comfort will be achieved with least effect of medication on fetus.
B. Interventions
1. Administer medications on schedule to maximize maternal effect and minimize fetal effect.
2. Continue to observe maternal/fetal vital signs for side effects.
3. Explain to client that she must remain in bed with side rails up.
4. Record accurately drug used, time, amount, route, site, and client response.

## Evaluation

A. Medication exerts intended effect.
B. Mother reports positive response to medication.
C. Fetus shows no ill effects from medication.
D. Labor is not affected by medication.

# Anesthesia for Labor and Delivery

## General Information

A. Removal of pain perception by the administration of medication to interrupt the transmission of nerve impulses to the brain.
B. May be administered by inhalation, IV, or regional routes.
C. All methods of labor and delivery anesthesia have their drawbacks; no one method is perfect.
D. Types of labor and delivery anesthesia
   1. Inhalation: mother inhales controlled concentration of gaseous medication.
      a. Administered by trained personnel only
      b. Methoxyflurane (Penthrane) and nitrous oxide commonly used
      c. Dangers include regurgitation and aspiration, uterine relaxation, and hemorrhage postdelivery.
   2. IV: rarely used in uncomplicated vaginal deliveries; may be used for cesarean birth (as induction anesthesia).
      a. Administered by trained personnel only
      b. Sodium pentothal commonly used
   3. Regional: medication introduced to specific areas to block pain impulses
      a. Always administered by skilled personnel
      b. Medications used include tetracaine (Pontocaine), lidocaine, bupivacaine (Marcaine), mepivacaine (Carbocaine)
      c. May block nerve at the root or in a peripheral area
         1) Nerve root blocks
            a) Lumbar epidural: may be given continuously or intermittently during labor, or at time of delivery; medication is injected over dura through lumbar interspace; absorption of drug is slower, with less hypotension; client should have no postspinal headache
            b) Caudal: may be given intermittently through labor, or at time of delivery; medication is injected through sacral hiatus into peridural space; client should have no postspinal headache
            c) Subarachnoid (low spinal, saddle block): given when delivery is imminent; medication is injected into spinal fluid; mother may experience postdelivery headache; keep flat for at least 6–8 hours postspinal and encourage oral fluids postdelivery to facilitate reversal of headache.
         2) Peripheral nerve blocks
            a) Paracervical: instillation of medication into cervix; rarely used during labor because of effect on fetus; useful only in first stage of labor.
            b) Pudendal: medication injected transvaginally to affect pudendal nerve as it passes behind ischial spines on either side of vagina; useful for delivery and episiotomy if needed.
            c) Perineal (local): injected into the perineum at the time of delivery in order to perform an episiotomy

## Assessment

A. Status of labor progress
B. Maternal/fetal vital signs
C. Allergies
D. Effects of medication on client (she may need help pushing)
E. Level of anesthesia
F. Return of sensation after anesthesia

## Analysis

Nursing diagnoses for anesthesia during labor and delivery may include:
A. Impaired mobility
B. Ineffective tissue perfusion
C. Deficient knowledge
D. Impaired urinary elimination

## Planning and Implementation

A. Goals
   1. Pain relief will be obtained.
   2. Healthy maternal/fetal status will be maintained.
B. Interventions
   1. Assist client to empty bladder.
   2. Assist client to assume appropriate position.
      a. Inhalation anesthesia: supine with wedge under right hip to displace gravid uterus off inferior vena cava
      b. Pudendal and perineal: on back or left side
      c. Other regional types: on left side or sitting up
   3. Check maternal blood pressure and fetal heart rate every 3–5 minutes until stable, then every 15 minutes or prn.
   4. If blood pressure drops, turn client on left side, administer oxygen, and notify physician.

## Evaluation

A. Client experiences expected pain relief.
B. Fetus exhibits no untoward effects, FHR remains relatively stable.
C. Labor and delivery carried out as expected.
D. Client's vital signs remain within normal limits.

# OPERATIVE OBSTETRICAL PROCEDURES

## Episiotomy

A. General information
  1. Incision made in the perineum to enlarge the vaginal opening for delivery
  2. Client usually anesthetized in some manner
  3. Types
    a. Midline or median: from posterior vaginal opening through center of perineum toward anal sphincter.
      1) Most frequently used
      2) Easily done, least discomfort for client
      3) Danger of extension into anal sphincter
    b. Mediolateral: begins at posterior vaginal opening but angles off to left or right at 45° angle (rarely in the United States).
      1) Done when need for additional enlargement of vaginal opening is a possibility
      2) Mediolateral episiotomy usually more uncomfortable than median
  4. Advantages of episiotomy are:
    a. Enlarging of vaginal opening
    b. Second stage of labor shortened
    c. Stretching of perineal muscles minimized
    d. Tearing of perineum may be prevented
  5. Those opposed to episiotomies argue:
    a. Kegel exercises can prepare the perineum to stretch for delivery.
    b. Lacerations may occur anyway.
  6. Side-lying delivery minimizes the strain on the perineum and may, if used, reduce incidence of episiotomies.
B. Nursing interventions
  1. Apply ice packs to perineal area in first 12 hours to help alleviate pain and swelling.
  2. Help promote healing with warm sitz baths after first 12 hours.
  3. Observe episiotomy site for signs of infection or hematoma.
  4. Instruct client about perineal hygiene.

## Assisted Delivery: Vacuum or Forceps

A. General information
  1. Used when there is a need to shorten the second stage or the second stage has stopped.

Reasons include maternal fatigue, medical conditions, fetal distress, poor pushing, and excessive infant size.
  2. Prerequisites include: head is engaged, no CPD, membranes ruptured, cervix completely dilated, empty bladder.
B. Types of assisted deliveries
  1. Low outlet forceps used when the head is visible at the perineum.
  2. Mid and high forceps no longer used.
  3. Vacuum extraction used when head is visible—silastic suction cup applied to presenting part and gentle traction exerted while mother pushes.
C. Nursing interventions
  1. Anticipate request for forceps if possible.
  2. Monitor FHTs continuously.
  3. Explain procedure to client if awake, advise mother/family about possible presence of bruising that will go away but may contribute to jaundice, also risk of perineal or vaginal tearing.
  4. Newborn assessment should include careful examination for bruising and facial nerve damage with forceps and cephalhematoma with vacuum.
  5. Ongoing newborn assessment includes careful checking for jaundice.

## Cesarean Birth

### General Information

A. Delivery of the baby through an incision into the abdominal and uterine walls
B. Indications
  1. Fetal distress, disease, or anomaly
  2. Breech or other malpresentation, cephalopelvic disproportion, macrosomia
  3. Placenta previa or abruptio
  4. Prolapsed cord and other obstetric emergencies
  5. Failure to progress in labor
  6. Multiple gestation
  7. Maternal disease
  8. Previous uterine surgery
  9. Active herpes
C. Types
  1. Classical: vertical incisions made into both abdomen and uterus
    a. Used when rapid delivery is important, as in fetal distress, prolapsed cord, placenta abruptio
    b. Maternal bleeding greater with this method; client may have increased risk of uterine rupture of scar tissue with future pregnancies; not usually a candidate for vaginal birth in future pregnancies.
  2. Low cervical/low segment: transverse incisions made in abdomen (above pubic hairline) and in uterus
    a. Most common method used

b. Procedure may take longer than classic because of need to deflect bladder, but blood loss is lessened and adhesions are fewer.

c. Vaginal birth after this type of cesarean birth (VBAC) is a possibility.

## Preoperative

A. Assessment
   1. Maternal/fetal responses to labor
   2. Indications for cesarean birth
   3. Blood and urine test results
B. Analysis: nursing diagnoses for the preoperative phase of cesarean birth may include:
   1. Fear
   2. Knowledge deficit
   3. Powerlessness
   4. Disturbance in self-concept
C. Planning and implementation
   1. Goals
      a. Client prepared for surgery carefully and competently.
      b. Client will have procedures explained to her.
   2. Interventions
      a. Shave/prep abdomen and pubic area.
      b. Insert retention catheter into bladder.
      c. Administer preoperative medications as ordered.
      d. Explain all procedures to client.
      e. Provide emotional support to client/family as needed.
      f. Complete all preoperative charting responsibilities.
D. Evaluation
   1. Client adequately prepared for surgery
   2. Client understands all procedures

## Postoperative

A. Assessment
   1. Maternal vital signs
   2. Observation of incision for signs of infection
   3. I&O
   4. Level of consciousness/return of sensation
   5. Fundal firmness and location
   6. Lochia: color, amount, clots, odor
B. Analysis: nursing diagnoses postoperatively for cesarean birth may include:
   1. Alteration in comfort: pain
   2. High risk for fluid volume deficit
   3. High risk for alteration in parenting
   4. Altered family processes
C. Planning and implementation
   1. Goals
      a. Healing will be promoted.
      b. Bonding between mother/couple and baby will be promoted.
      c. No complications will ensue.
   2. Interventions

a. Implement general postsurgical care and general postpartum care.
b. Assist client with self-care as needed.
c. Assist mother with baby care and handling as needed.
d. Encourage client to verbalize reaction to all events.
e. Reinforce any special discharge instructions from physician.
D. Evaluation
   1. Mother and baby tolerated procedures well
   2. No postoperative complications or infection
   3. Maternal/newborn bonding occurring

 **Sample Questions**

36. The nurse is caring for a woman who is admitted to the hospital in active labor. What information is most important for the nurse to assess to avoid respiratory complications during labor and delivery?
   1. Family history of lung disease.
   2. Food or drug allergies.
   3. Number of cigarettes smoked daily.
   4. When the client last ate.

37. A woman who is gravida 1 is in the active phase of stage 1 labor. The fetal position is LOA. What should the nurse expect to see when the membranes rupture?
   1. A large amount of bloody fluid.
   2. A moderate amount of clear to straw-colored fluid.
   3. A small amount of greenish fluid.
   4. A small segment of the umbilical cord.

38. The nurse is caring for a woman in stage 1 labor. The fetal position is LOA. When the membranes rupture, what should be the nurse's first action?
   1. Notify the physician.
   2. Measure the amount of fluid.
   3. Count the fetal heart rate.
   4. Perform a vaginal examination.

39. A woman has just delivered a 9 lb 10 oz baby. After the delivery, the nurse notices that the mother is chilly and that her fundus has relaxed. The nurse administers the oxytocin that the physician orders. What occurrence will alert the nurse that the oxytocin has had the expected effect?
   1. The mother states that she feels warmer now.
   2. The mother falls asleep.

**6**

3. The baby cries.

4. The uterus becomes firm.

40. A woman had a midline episiotomy performed at delivery. What is the primary purpose of the episiotomy?

    1. Allow forceps to be applied.

    2. Enlarge the vaginal opening.

    3. Eliminate the possibility of lacerations.

    4. Eliminate the need for cesarean birth.

41. A woman is admitted to the hospital in labor. Vaginal examination reveals that she is 8 cm dilated. At this point in her labor, which of the following statements would the nurse expect her to make?

    1. "I can't decide what to name my baby."

    2. "It feels good to push with each contraction."

    3. "Take your hand off my stomach when I have a contraction."

    4. "This isn't as bad as I expected."

42. The nurse is caring for a woman who is in labor. She is 8 cm dilated. How will the nurse best support the woman during this phase of her labor?

    1. Leave her alone most of the time.

    2. Offer her a back rub during contractions.

    3. Offer her sips of oral fluids.

    4. Provide her with warm blankets.

43. A woman in labor is placed on an external fetal monitor. The nurse notices that the fetal heart rate is erratic during contractions but returns to baseline at the end of each contraction. How will this occurrence be recorded?

    1. Early decelerations.

    2. Variable decelerations.

    3. Late decelerations.

    4. Fetal distress.

44. During labor, the nurse observes variable decelerations on the external fetal monitor. What is the best action for the nurse to take at this time?

    1. Apply an oxygen mask.

    2. Change the woman's position to left side-lying.

    3. Get the woman out of bed and walk her around.

    4. Move the woman to the delivery room.

45. During delivery, a mediolateral episiotomy is performed and a 7 lb 8 oz baby delivered. Which of the following nursing assessments indicate a postpartum complication and are not normal? Check all that apply.

    _____ A foul lochial odor.

    _____ Discomfort while sitting.

    _____ Ecchymosis and edema of the perineum.

    _____ Separation of the episiotomy wound edges.

46. The nurse is talking with a woman who is 36 weeks' gestation during a prenatal visit. Which statement indicates that the woman understands the onset of labor?

    1. "I need to go to the hospital as soon as the contractions become painful."

    2. "If I experience bright red vaginal bleeding I know that I am about to deliver."

    3. "I need to go to the hospital when I am having regular contractions and bloody show."

    4. "My labor will not start until after my membranes rupture and I gush fluid."

47. Using Leopold's maneuvers to determine fetal position, the nurse finds that the fetus is in a vertex position with the back on the left side. Where is the best place for the nurse to listen for fetal heart tones?

    1. In the right upper quadrant of the mother's abdomen.

    2. In the left upper quadrant of the mother's abdomen.

    3. In the right lower quadrant of the mother's abdomen.

    4. In the left lower quadrant of the mother's abdomen.

48. Which of the following is the best way for the nurse to assess contractions in a client presenting to the labor and delivery area?

    1. Place the client on the electronic fetal monitor with the labor toco at the fundus.

    2. Ask the client to describe the frequency, duration, and strength of her contractions.

    3. Use Leopold's maneuvers to determine the quality of the uterine contractions.

    4. Place the fingertips of one hand on the fundus to determine frequency, duration, and strength of contractions.

49. As the nurse assigned to a laboring woman, you are observing the fetal heart rate. Which of the following findings would you consider abnormal for a client in active labor?

    1. A rate of 160 with no significant changes through a contraction.

2. A rate of 130 with accelerations to 150 with fetal movement.

3. A rate that varies between 120 and 130.

4. A rate of 170 with a drop to 140 during a contraction.

50. A woman arrives at the birthing center in active labor. On examination, the cervix is 5 cm dilated, membranes intact and bulging, and the presenting part at −1 station. The woman asks if she can go for a walk. What is the best response for the nurse to give?

1. "I think it would be best for you to remain in bed at this time because of the risk of cord prolapse."

2. "It's fine for you to walk, but please stay nearby. If you feel a gush of fluid, I will need to check you and your baby."

3. "It will be fine for you to walk because that will assist the natural body forces to bring the baby down the birth canal."

4. "I would be glad to get you a bean bag chair or rocker instead."

51. A primigravida presents to the labor room with rupture of membranes at 40 weeks' gestation. Her cervix is 2 cm dilated and 100% effaced. Contractions are every 10 minutes. What should the nurse include in the plan of care?

1. Allow her to ambulate as desired as long as the presenting part is engaged.

2. Assess fetal heart tones and maternal status every five minutes.

3. Place her on an electronic fetal monitor for continuous assessment of labor.

4. Send her home with instructions to return when contractions are every 5 minutes.

52. A woman who is in active labor at 4 cm dilated, 100% effaced, and 0 station is ambulating and experiences a gush of fluid. What is the most appropriate initial action for the nurse to take?

1. Send a specimen of the amniotic fluid to the laboratory for analysis.

2. Have the woman return to her room and place her in Trendelenburg position to prevent cord prolapse.

3. Have the woman return to her room so that you can assess fetal status, including auscultation of fetal heart tones for one full minute.

4. Call the woman's physician because a cesarean delivery will be required.

53. The nurse is providing care to a woman. During the most recent vaginal examination the nurse feels the cervix 6 cm dilated, 100% effaced, with the vertex at −1 station. Based on this information, the nurse is aware the woman is in which phase of labor?

1. Active labor with the head as presenting part not yet engaged.

2. Transition with the backside as presenting part fully engaged.

3. Latent phase labor with the backside as presenting part fully engaged.

4. Active labor with the head as presenting part fully engaged.

54. A woman is completely dilated and at +2 station. Her contractions are strong and last 50–70 seconds. Based on this information, the nurse should know that the client is in which stage of labor?

1. First stage.

2. Second stage.

3. Third stage.

4. Fourth stage.

55. A 28-year-old primigravida is admitted to the labor room. She is 2 cm dilated, 90% effaced, and the head is at 0 station. Contractions are every 10 minutes lasting 20–30 seconds. Membranes are intact. Admitting vital signs are: blood pressure 110/70, pulse 78, respirations 16, temperature 98.8° F, and fetal heart rate 144. What should the nurse monitor?

1. Blood pressure and contractions hourly and fetal heart rate every 15 minutes.

2. Temperature, blood pressure, and contractions every 4 hours and fetal heart rate hourly.

3. Contractions, effacement, and dilation of cervix, and fetal heart rate every hour.

4. Contractions, blood pressure, and fetal heart rate every 15 minutes.

56. A woman's cervix is completely dilated with the head at −2 station. The head has not descended in the past hour. What is the most appropriate initial assessment for the nurse to make?

1. Assess to determine if the client's bladder is distended.

2. Send the client for X-rays to determine fetal size.

3. Notify the surgical team so that an operative delivery can be planned.

4. Assess fetal status, including fetal heart tones, and scalp pH.

57. A woman who has been in labor for 6 hours is now 9 cm dilated and has intense contractions every 1 to 2 minutes. She is anxious and feels the need to bear down with her contractions. What is the best action for the nurse to take?
    1. Allow her to push so that delivery can be expedited.
    2. Encourage panting breathing through contractions to prevent pushing.
    3. Reposition her in a squatting position to make her more comfortable.
    4. Provide back rubs during contractions to distract her.

58. A newborn, at 1 minute after vaginal delivery, is pink with blue hands and feet, has a lusty cry, heart rate 140, prompt response to stimulation with crying, and maintains minimal flexion, with sluggish movement. What will the nurse record as the Apgar score?
    1. 10.
    2. 9.
    3. 8.
    4. 7.

59. A woman delivered a 7 lb boy by spontaneous vaginal delivery 30 minutes ago. Her fundus is firm at the umbilicus and she has moderate lochia rubra. Which nursing diagnosis is highest priority as the nurse plans care?
    1. Risk for infection related to episiotomy.
    2. Constipation related to fear of pain.
    3. Potential for impaired urinary elimination related to perineal edema.
    4. Deficient knowledge related to lack of knowledge regarding newborn care.

60. A woman is in the fourth stage of labor. She and her new daughter are together in the room. What assessments are essential for the nurse to make during this time?
    1. Assess the pattern and frequency of contractions and the infant's vital signs.
    2. Assess the woman's vital signs, fundus, bladder, perineal condition, and lochia. Assess the infant's vital signs.
    3. Assess the woman's vital signs, fundus, bladder, perineal condition, and lochia. Return the infant to the nursery.
    4. Assess the infant for obvious abnormalities. Assess the woman for blood loss and firm uterine contraction.

61. A woman, G3 P2, was admitted at 32 weeks' gestation contracting every 7–10 minutes. Her cervix is 2 cm dilated and 70% effaced. What should the nurse include in the plan of care for this client?
    1. Discuss with the client the need to stop working after her discharge from the hospital.
    2. Monitor the client and her fetus for response to impending delivery.
    3. Assess the client's past pregnancy history to determine if she has experienced preterm labor in the past.
    4. Start oral terbutaline to stop the contractions.

62. A woman was admitted in premature labor contracting every 5 minutes. Her cervix is 3 cm dilated and 100% effaced, IV magnesium sulfate at 1 g per hour is infusing. How will the nurse know the drug is having the desired effect?
    1. The contractions will increase in frequency to every 3 minutes, although there will be no further cervical changes.
    2. The woman will be able to sleep through her contractions due to the sedative effect of the magnesium sulfate.
    3. The contractions will diminish in frequency and finally disappear.
    4. The woman will have diminished deep tendon reflexes and her blood pressure will decrease.

63. A woman has just received an epidural for anesthesia during her labor. What should the nurse include in the plan of care because of the anesthesia?
    1. Assist the client in position changes and observe for signs of labor progress.
    2. Administer 500–1000 mL of a sugar-free crystalloid solution.
    3. Place a Foley catheter as soon as the anesthesia has been administered.
    4. Offer the client a back rub to reduce the discomfort of her contractions.

64. A woman delivered her infant son 3 hours ago. She had an episiotomy to facilitate delivery. As the nurse assigned to care for her, which of the following would be the most appropriate action?
    1. Place an ice pack on the perineum.
    2. Apply a heat lamp to the perineum.
    3. Take her for a sitz bath.
    4. Administer analgesic medication as ordered.

65. A woman is scheduled for a cesarean section delivery due to a transverse fetal lie. What is the best way for the nurse to evaluate that she understands the procedure?

1. Ask her about the help she will have at home after her delivery.
2. Give her a diagram of the body and ask her to draw the procedure for you.
3. Ask her to tell you what she knows about the scheduled surgery.
4. Provide her with a booklet explaining cesarean deliveries when she arrives at the hospital.

## Answers and Rationales

**36. 4.** Gastric motility is decreased during pregnancy. Food eaten several hours prior to the onset of labor may still be in the stomach undigested. This will influence the type of anesthesia the client may receive.

**37. 2.** With the baby in a vertex, LOA presentation and no other indicators of distress, amniotic fluid should be clear to straw-colored.

**38. 3.** Immediately after the rupture of membranes, the fetal heart tones are checked, then checked again after the next contraction or after 5–10 minutes.

**39. 4.** Oxytoxic medications such as Pitocin, Methergine, and Ergotrate are administered to stimulate uterine contractility and reverse fundal relaxation in the postdelivery client.

**40. 2.** An episiotomy is an incision made in the perineum to enlarge the vaginal opening, allowing additional room for the birth of the baby.

**41. 3.** At 8 cm dilated the client is in the transition stage of her labor. Many women experience hyperesthesia of the skin at this time and would not want to be touched during a contraction.

**42. 2.** The counterpressure of a back rub during a contraction may relieve discomfort.

**43. 2.** Variable decelerations are frequently caused by transient fetal pressure on the cord and are not a sign of fetal distress. A change in the mother's position will usually relieve the problem.

**44. 2.** Changing the position of the mother will relieve transient pressure on the umbilical cord.

**45.** *A foul lochial odor* should be checked. This is a sign of infection.

*Ecchymosis and edema of the perineum* should be checked. This could be caused by a number of things but indicates recovery will be prolonged.

*Separation of the episiotomy wound edges* should be checked. This might be due to infection or trauma. In this case the episiotomy wound would have to heal by second intention (wound left open to heal) or third intention (wound resutured).

**46. 3.** Regular contractions coupled with bloody show suggest that cervical changes are occurring as a result of contractions.

**47. 4.** The left lower quadrant is the correct location since the back is on the left and the vertex is in the pelvis.

**48. 4.** The fingertips of one hand allow the nurse to feel when the contraction begins and ends and to determine the strength of the construction by the firmness of the uterus.

**49. 4.** A rate of 170 is suggestive of fetal tachycardia. A drop to 140 during a contraction represents some periodic change, which is not a normal finding.

**50. 2.** Although there is always some risk of complications when membranes rupture, it is safe for this woman to ambulate as long as she is rechecked if rupture of membranes occurs.

**51. 1.** Ambulation will help contractions more effectively dilate the cervix. As long as the presenting part is engaged, there is no increased risk of cord prolapse.

**52. 3.** The most important nursing action after rupture of the membranes is careful fetal assessment, including fetal heart tones counted for 1 minute.

**53. 1.** At 6 cm dilation and complete effacement, active labor is occurring. A station of – 1 indicates that the vertex is above the ischial spines and not fully engaged.

**54. 2.** The second stage of labor extends from complete cervical dilation to delivery of the infant.

**55. 1.** During early labor, blood pressure and contractions should be monitored hourly and fetal heart rate every 15 minutes.

**56. 1.** A full bladder may prevent the head from moving down into the pelvic inlet. Often clients do not have the sensation of a full bladder late in labor, despite significant distention.

57. **2.** Because the client is still in transition and not ready to deliver, encouraging her to pant will diminish the urge to push.

58. **3.** This infant has 2 points for heart rate, respiratory effort, and reflex irritability. One point is awarded for color and muscle tone for a total of 8.

59. **3.** Perineal edema may affect urinary elimination. If allowed to continue, it may also lead to excessive postpartum bleeding because the uterus cannot stay firmly contracted when the bladder is excessively full.

60. **2.** Assessment of the mother during fourth stage includes elements related to her recovery from childbirth. Infant assessment focuses on stability and transition to extrauterine life.

61. **3.** As a G3 P2, the client's past pregnancy history may provide some important information that may shape the care rendered at this time.

62. **3.** If the magnesium sulfate is effective, you would expect the contractions to decrease and then disappear. You would not continue to perform vaginal exams if the desired result is occurring.

63. **1.** Epidural anesthesia may diminish the client's sensation of painful stimuli and movement. Assistance and frequent assessment are therefore essential.

64. **1.** Ice during the first 12 hours after delivery causes vasoconstriction and thereby prevents edema. Ice also provides pain relief through numbing of the area.

65. **3.** Asking for clarification of what she knows is the best way to evaluate what she understands of the procedure. If the client has additional questions, the nurse can then clarify or amplify the information.

# The Postpartum Period

## OVERVIEW

### Physical Changes of the Postpartum Period

A. The postpartum period is defined as that period of time, usually 6 weeks, in which the mother's body experiences anatomic and physiologic changes that reverse the body's adaptation to pregnancy; may also be called *involution.*
B. Begins with the delivery of the placenta and ends when all body systems are returned to, or nearly to, their prepregnant state.
C. May or may not include the return of the ovulatory/menstrual cycle.

### Specific Body System Changes
#### Reproductive System

A. Uterus undergoes involution—return to prepregnant size and position in pelvis.
  1. Fundus palpated at the umbilicus in midline at 1-hour postpartum.
  2. Fundus may rise up to 1 cm above umbilicus within 12 hours then begin descent of 1 cm per day until no longer palpable by day 10.

  3. The endometrial surface is sloughed off as *lochia,* in three stages:
     a. *Lochia rubra:* red color, days 1–3 after delivery; consists of blood and cellular debris from decidua.
     b. *Lochia serosa:* pinkish brown, days 4–10; mostly serum, some blood, tissue debris.
     c. *Lochia alba:* yellowish white, days 11–21 up to 6 weeks; mostly leukocytes, with decidua, epithelial cells, mucus.
  4. Lochia has a particular, musty odor. Foul-smelling lochia, however, may indicate infection. Some small dark clots may be normal immediately after delivery; large clots and bright red clots signify the need for close investigation.
  5. The placental site heals by means of exfoliative shedding, a process that allows the upward growth of the new endometrium and the prevention of scar tissue at the old placental site. This process may take 6 weeks.
B. Cervix
  1. Flabby immediately after delivery; closes slowly.
  2. Admits one fingertip by the end of 1 week after delivery.
  3. Shape of external os changed by delivery from round to slitlike opening.

**C.** Vagina
   1. Edematous after delivery
   2. May have small lacerations
   3. Smooth-walled for 3–4 weeks, then rugae reappear
   4. Hypoestrogenic until ovulation and menstruation resume
**D.** Ovulation/menstruation
   1. First cycle is usually anovulatory.
   2. If not lactating, menses may resume in 6–8 weeks.
   3. If lactating, menses less predictable; may resume in 12–24 weeks.
**E.** Breasts
   1. Nonlactating woman
      a. Prolactin levels fall rapidly.
      b. May still secrete colostrum for 2–3 days.
      c. Engorgement of breast tissue resulting from temporary congestion of veins and lymphatic circulation occurs on third day, lasts 24–36 hours, usually resolves spontaneously.
      d. Client should wear tight bra to compress ducts and use cold applications to reduce swelling.
   2. Lactating woman
      a. High level of prolactin immediately after delivery of placenta continued by frequent contact with nursing baby.
      b. Initial secretion is colostrum, with increasing amounts of true breast milk appearing between 48–96 hours.
      c. Milk "let-down" reflex caused by oxytocin from posterior pituitary released by sucking.
      d. Successful lactation results from the complex interaction of infant sucking reflexes and the maternal production and let-down of milk.

## Abdominal Wall/Skin

**A.** Muscles relaxed, separation of the rectus muscle (diastasis recti) from 2 to 4 cm, usually resolves by 6 weeks with exercise.
**B.** Stretch marks gradually fade to silvery-white appearance.

## Cardiovascular System

**A.** Normal blood loss in delivery of single infant is less than 500 mL (up to 1000 mL normal blood loss for a cesarean delivery).
**B.** Hematocrit usually returns to prepregnancy value within 4–6 weeks.
**C.** WBC count increases up to 20,000.
**D.** Increased clotting factors remain for several weeks leaving woman at risk for problems with thrombi.
**E.** Varicosities regress.

## Urinary System

**A.** May have difficulty voiding in immediate postpartum period as a result of urethral edema and lack of sensation.
**B.** Marked diuresis begins within 12 hours of delivery; increases volume of urinary output as well as perspiration loss.
**C.** Lactosuria may be seen in nursing mothers.
**D.** Many women will show slight proteinuria during first 1–2 days of involution.

## Gastrointestinal System

**A.** Mother usually hungry after delivery; good appetite is expected.
**B.** May still experience constipation from lack of muscle tone in abdomen and intestinal tract, and perineal soreness.
**C.** If hemorrhoids present, recommend sitz bath and foods to prevent constipation.

## Other

All other systems experience normal and rapid regression to prepregnancy status.

# POSTPARTAL PSYCHOSOCIAL CHANGES

## Adaptation to Parenthood

### Motor Skills

New parents must learn new physical skills to care for infant (e.g., feeding, holding, burping, changing diapers, skin care).

### Attachment Skills

**A.** *Bonding:* the development of a caring relationship with the baby. Behaviors include:
   1. Claiming: identifying the ways in which the baby looks or acts like members of the family.
   2. Identification: establishing the baby's unique nature (assigning the baby his or her own name).
   3. Attachment is facilitated by positive feedback between baby and caregivers.
**B.** Sensual responses enhance adaptation to parenthood.
   1. Touch: from fingertip, to open palm, to enfolding; touch is an important communication with the baby.
   2. Eye-to-eye contact: a cultural activity that helps to form a trusting relationship.
   3. Voice: parents await the baby's first cry; babies respond to the higher-pitched voice that parents use in talking to the baby.

4. Odor: babies quickly identify their own mother's breast milk by odor.
5. Entrainment: babies move in rhythm to patterns of adult speech.
6. Biorhythm: babies respond to maternal heartbeats.

## Maternal Adjustment

Takes place in three phases.

### Dependent/"Taking In"

A. 1–2 days after delivery.
B. Mother's needs predominate; mother passive and dependent.
C. Mother needs to talk about labor and delivery experiences to integrate them into the fabric of her life.
D. Mother may need help with everyday activities, as well as child care.
E. Food/sleep important.

### Dependent/Independent/"Taking Hold"

A. By third day mother begins to reassert herself.
B. Identifies own needs, especially for teaching and help with her own and baby's needs.
C. Some emotional lability, may cry "for no reason."
D. Mother requires reassurance that she can perform tasks of motherhood.

### Independent/"Letting Go"

A. Usually evident by fifth or sixth week.
B. Shows pattern of lifestyle that includes new baby but still focuses on entire family as unit.
C. Reestablishment of father-mother bond seen in this period.
D. Mother may still feel tired and overwhelmed by responsibility and conflicting demands on her time and energies.

## ASSESSMENT

## Physical

A. Vital signs
   1. Individual protocol until stable, then at least once every 8 hours.
   2. Temperature over 37.8°C (100.4°F) after first 24 hours, lasting more than 48 hours, indicative of infection.
B. Fundus
   1. Assessment done with empty bladder, one hand supporting base of uterus and one on fundus
   2. Assess for firmness and position

C. Lochia: color, amount, clots, odor
D. Perineum
   1. Healing of episiotomy if applicable
   2. Hematoma formation
   3. Development of hemorrhoids
E. Breasts: firmness, condition of nipples
F. Elimination patterns: voiding, flatus, bowels
G. Legs: pain, warmth, tenderness indicating thrombosis
H. Perform foot dorsiflexion (Homan's sign)

## Psychosocial Adjustment

A. Overall emotional status of parents
B. Parents' knowledge of infant needs
C. Previous experience of parents
D. Physical condition of infant
E. Ethnocultural background and financial status of parents
F. Additional family support available to parents

## ANALYSIS

Nursing diagnoses for the postpartum period may include:
A. Risk for constipation
B. Deficient knowledge
C. Self-care deficit
D. Impaired urinary elimination
E. Interrupted family process
F. Risk for impaired parenting
G. Ineffective role performance
H. Pain

## PLANNING AND IMPLEMENTATION

### Goals

A. Involution and return to prepregnancy state will be accomplished without complication.
B. Parental role(s) will be successfully assumed.
C. New baby will be successfully integrated into family structure.
D. Successful infant feeding patterns (bottle- or breastfeeding) will be established

### Interventions

#### Physical Care

A. Assess mother according to individual needs during first critical hours after delivery; implement nursing interventions as needed.
B. Implement routine postpartum care after first hours.

1. Administer medications as ordered (e.g., oxytocins, analgesics).
2. Teach perineal care.
3. Perform other care as needed (e.g., heat, cold applications).
4. Measure first voiding for sufficiency, observe I&O for first 24 hours.
5. Assist with breastfeeding as needed.
6. Instruct in breast care for bottle-feeding mother—good bra, limiting nipple stimulation.

C. Encourage measures to promote bowel function: roughage in diet, ambulation, sufficient fluids, attention to urge to defecate. Reassure about integrity of episiotomy.

## Adjustment to Parenthood

A. Provide time for parents to be alone with baby in crucial early time after delivery.
B. Identify learning needs of parents.
C. Plan teaching to include both parents when possible.
D. Help parents realize that fatigue is normal at this time.
E. Help parents identify and strengthen their own coping mechanisms.
F. Help parents identify resources available to them.
G. Promote positive self-esteem on part of parents as they learn new role(s).
H. Provide anticipatory guidance for after discharge.
I. Provide information about contraception if requested.
J. Prepare for discharge: reinforce physician's instructions about activities, rest, diet, drugs, exercise, resumption of sexual intercourse, return for postpartum examination.

## Infant Feeding

A. General information
1. Infancy is a time of rapid growth and development; infant doubles birth weight in 4–6 months, triples birth weight by 1 year.
2. Newborns lose up to 8% of their birth weight, then gain 4–7 ounces per week.
B. Choices in newborn nutrition
1. Breastfeeding: optimal infant nutrition, easily digested, contains antibodies to bolster the immune system as well as all nutrients needed by the infant.
   a. Helps mother's body return to prepregnant state faster.
   b. Provides some child-spacing but should not be relied on.
   c. Prolactin, stimulated by the infant's sucking, stimulates milk production.
   d. Oxytocin causes "let-down" or delivery of milk to nursing baby.

2. Formula-feeding (bottle-feeding): utilizes modified cow's milk or soy formulas as basis for provision of 20 kcal/oz.
   a. Formulas are widely available in ready-to-feed, concentrated, and powdered forms.
   b. They have supplemental vitamins; may also contain added iron.
   c. Concentrated and powdered forms require addition of prescribed amounts of water for appropriate reconstitution.
   d. Bottles and nipples should be carefully cleaned daily by hand and rinsed with boiling water or by electric dishwasher.
   e. Powdered or concentrated formulas should be mixed with tap water, bottled water or boiled water that has cooled.

C. Nursing measures to promote successful infant feeding
1. Assess previous experience and knowledge of process of infant feeding.
2. Demonstrate how to hold baby for breastfeeding and for feeding with formula.
3. Show how to burp baby.
4. Allow time for practice with selected feeding method.
5. Provide positive reinforcement for successful actions.
6. Give written instructions for at-home reference.
7. Help parents identify progress and pleasure in feeding infant.
8. If bottle-feeding, demonstrate how to prepare formula using appropriate method.
9. If breastfeeding, assess breasts for tenderness or discomfort, and examine nipples for cracks, bleeding, soreness, and erectility.
10. Assist mother with preparation: clean hands, comfortable position, support as needed (extra pillows). Demonstrate alternate infant positioning, e.g., "football hold."
11. Bring infant to nurse as soon as possible after delivery.
12. Demonstrate positioning of baby at breast, initiate rooting reflex, place entire nipple and as much of areola as possible into baby's mouth, depress fleshy part of breast away from baby's nose if needed.
13. Allow baby to nurse in short frequent periods, lengthening gradually in later days. Alternate breast offered first.
14. Help mother release baby from nipple by breaking suction of baby on nipple. Check for nipple trauma.
15. Help mother move baby to alternate breast if needed.
16. Remain with mother at each feeding until she feels confident: see also Table 6-9 for additional information on breastfeeding.

**Table 6-9** Tips for successful breastfeeding

| | |
|---|---|
| Breast care | Do not use soap on nipples or areola. Expose nipples to air to toughen them. Know how to pump breast milk if necessary and how to store expressed breast milk. |
| Nutrition | Need for good maternal nutrition while nursing.<br>• Additional 300–600 kcal/day<br>• 2–3 liters fluid/day<br>Know that certain foods may make the baby fussy and will need to be avoided temporarily. |
| Comfort | Wear well-fitting bra; use absorbent pads without plastic coating if leaking occurs. Uterine cramping during nursing normal at first. |
| Medications | Avoid medications excreted in breast milk (mother should check with physician before taking any drug while nursing). Birth control pills should not be taken while nursing (decreases milk production). |
| Sources of help | Inform mother of community support groups available for nursing mothers. |

17. Assist bottle-feeding mother with suppression of lactation, accomplished primarily by mechanical inhibition.
    a. Mechanical inhibition: usually takes 48–72 hours
       1) Snug breast binder for 2–3 days postdelivery
       2) Applications of cold (ice packs) and analgesia to relieve discomfort
       3) Avoidance of heat or other stimuli to breasts that increase milk production (including breast pumps)
       4) A well-fitting bra until lactation is suppressed
    b. No approved medications to suppress lactation.

# EVALUATION

A. Involution successfully initiated and progressing without complication
B. Parents begin to assume new role behaviors and identities
C. Beginning integration of newborn into family structure; bonding established
D. Infant feeding techniques mastered; infant growing and developing appropriately
E. Parents comfortable about infant care techniques and can demonstrate knowledge

## Teaching: Postpartum/Discharge

A. Postpartum
   1. Normal events of postpartum period: physical, psychosocial
   2. Information about feeding her infant
   3. Basic infant care, including cord care, bathing, circumcision care, dressing, handling, signs of illness
   4. Safety needs of infant
   5. Recommendations concerning activities
   6. Specific teaching about any medications
B. Discharge
   1. Reinforcement of all postpartum teaching, allowing parent(s) time to ask questions.
   2. Referrals to professional assistance (MD, CNM, hospital's maternity unit, etc.).
   3. Referrals to appropriate community assistance groups (Nursing Mothers, Mothers of Twins, etc.) that meet individual needs.
   4. Scheduled appointments for postpartal examination/newborn's first well-baby examination.
   5. Literature to reinforce all teaching. Excitement and anxiety of discharge may interfere with learning; literature will be available for quick reference.

# COMPLICATIONS OF THE POSTPARTUM PERIOD

## Postpartum Hemorrhage

A. General information
   1. Major cause of maternal death
   2. Loss of more than 500-mL blood at the time of delivery or immediately thereafter is considered postpartum hemorrhage.
   3. Major causes include:
      a. Uterine atony: loss of muscle tone in the uterus; may be the result of overdistension (large baby, multiple pregnancy, polyhydramnios), overmassage, maternal exhaustion, inhalation anesthesia
      b. Laceration of the birth canal (cervix, vagina, labia, perineum)
      c. Retained placental fragments or incomplete expulsion of placenta (usually the cause of late postpartum hemorrhage)
      d. Placenta accreta: penetration of the myometrium by the trophoblast, resulting in abnormal adherence of the placenta to the uterine wall. Rare; requires manual removal of the placenta
B. Assessment findings
   1. "Boggy" uterus, relaxed state indicating atony
   2. If uterus is firm with excess bleeding, may indicate lacerations.

3. Bright red blood, with clots
   a. Large amounts with atony
   b. Steady trickle with lacerations
4. Hemorrhage immediately after delivery with atony or lacerations
5. With retained placental fragments, delay of up to 2 weeks
6. With severe blood loss, signs and symptoms of shock
7. Full bladder may displace uterus and prevent it from contracting firmly.

C. Nursing interventions
1. Identify clients at risk for bleeding.
2. Monitor fundus frequently if bleeding occurs; when stable, every 15 minutes for 1–2 hours, then at appropriate intervals.
3. Monitor maternal vital signs for indications of shock.
4. Administer medications, IV fluids as ordered.
5. Measure I&O.
6. Remain with client for support and explanation of procedures.
7. Keep client warm.
8. Prepare for client's transfer to surgery if needed for repair of laceration or removal of placental fragment.
9. Monitor for signs of DIC.

## Thrombophlebitis

A. General information
1. Formation of a thrombus when a vein wall is inflamed
2. May be seen in the veins of the legs or pelvis
3. May result from injury, infection, or the normal increase in circulating clotting factors in the pregnant and newly delivered woman.

B. Assessment findings
1. Pain/discomfort in area of thrombus (legs, pelvis, abdomen)
2. If in the leg, pain, edema, redness over affected area
3. Elevated temperature and chills
4. Peripheral pulses may be decreased
5. Positive Homan's sign
6. If in a deep vein, leg may be cool and pale

C. Nursing interventions
1. Maintain bed rest with leg elevated on pillow. Never raise knee gatch on bed.
2. Apply moist heat as ordered.
3. Administer analgesics as ordered.
4. Provide bed cradle to keep sheets off leg.
5. Administer anticoagulant therapy as ordered (usually heparin), and observe client for signs of bleeding.
6. Apply elastic support hose if ordered, with daily inspection of legs with hose removed.
7. Teach client *not* to massage legs.
8. Allow client to express fears and reactions to condition.

9. Observe client for signs of pulmonary embolism.
10. Continue to bring baby to mother for feeding and interaction.

## Subinvolution

A. General information
1. Failure of the uterus to revert to prepregnant state through gradual reduction in size and placement
2. May be caused by infection, retained placental fragments, or tumors in the uterus

B. Assessment findings
1. Uterus remains enlarged
2. Fundus higher in the abdomen than anticipated
3. Lochia does not progress from rubra to serosa to alba
4. If caused by infection, possible leukorrhea and backache

C. Nursing interventions
1. Teach client to recognize unusual bleeding patterns.
2. Teach client usual pattern of uterine involution.
3. Instruct client to report abnormal bleeding to physician.
4. Administer oxytoxic medications if ordered.

## Postpartum Infection

A. General information
1. Any infection of the reproductive tract, associated with giving birth, usually occurring within 10 days of the birth
2. Predisposing factors include:
   a. Prolonged rupture of membranes
   b. Cesarean birth
   c. Trauma during birth process
   d. Maternal anemia
   e. Retained placental fragments
3. Infection may be localized or systemic

B. Assessment findings
1. Temperature of 37.8°C (100.4°F) or more for 2 consecutive days, excluding the first 24 hours
2. Abdominal, perineal, or pelvic pain
3. Foul-smelling vaginal discharge
4. Burning sensation with urination
5. Chills, malaise
6. Rapid pulse and respirations
7. Elevated WBC count (may be normal for postpartum initially), positive culture/sensitivity report for causative organism

C. Nursing interventions
1. Force fluids: client may need more than 3 liters/day.
2. Administer antibiotics and other medications as ordered.

3. Treat symptoms as they arise (e.g., warm sitz bath for infection in episiotomy).
4. Encourage high-calorie, high-protein diet to promote tissue healing.
5. Position client in semi- to high-Fowler's to promote drainage and prevent reflux higher into reproductive tract.
6. Support mother if isolated from baby.

## Mastitis

A. General information
   1. Infection of the breast, usually unilateral
   2. Frequently caused by cracked nipples in the nursing mother
   3. Causative organism usually hemolytic *S. aureus*
   4. If untreated, may result in breast abscess.
B. Assessment findings
   1. Redness, tenderness, or hardened area in the breast
   2. Maternal chills, malaise
   3. Elevated vital signs, especially temperature and pulse
C. Nursing interventions
   1. Teach/stress importance of hand washing to nursing mother, and wash own hands before touching client's breast.
   2. Administer antibiotics as ordered.
   3. Apply ice if ordered between feedings.
   4. Empty breast regularly: baby may continue to nurse or have mother use hospital-grade pump.

## Urinary Tract Infection

A. General information: may be caused postpartally by coliform bacteria, coupled with bladder trauma during the delivery, or a break in technique during catheterization.
B. Assessment findings
   1. Pain in the suprapubic area or at the costovertebral angle
   2. Fever
   3. Burning, urgency, frequency on urination
   4. Increased WBC count and hematuria
   5. Urine culture positive for causative organism
C. Nursing interventions
   1. Check status of bladder frequently in postpartum client.
   2. Use nursing measures to encourage client to void.
   3. Force fluids: may need minimum of 3 liters/day.
   4. Catheterize client if ordered, using sterile technique.
   5. Administer medications as ordered.
   6. Monitor status of progress through continuing lab tests.
   7. Support mother with explanations of interventions.
   8. No need for baby to be separated from mother.

 **Sample Questions**

66. On the second day postpartum, the nurse asks the new mother to describe her vaginal bleeding. What description does the nurse expect the client to say?
   1. Red and moderate.
   2. Red with clots.
   3. Scant and brown.
   4. Thin and white.

67. A woman delivers a 6 lb 4 oz (2835 g) baby boy. Which of the following statements would indicate to the nurse that the mother has begun to integrate her new baby into the family structure?
   1. "All this baby does is cry. He's not like my other child."
   2. "I wish he had curly hair like my husband."
   3. "My parents wanted a granddaughter."
   4. "When he yawns, he looks just like his brother."

68. A diabetic woman plans to breastfeed her baby. Because the woman is hyperglycemic, what explanation will the nurse give her?
   1. The glucose content of her breast milk may be high.
   2. The production of milk may be impaired.
   3. Her baby will receive insulin in the milk.
   4. Her baby will not grow well.

69. A woman and her hospital roommate each delivered a child 2 days ago. One is breastfeeding; one is using formula. Which of the following instructions can the nurse give to both mothers?
   1. Wear a good, well-supporting bra.
   2. Apply warm compresses to breast if too full.
   3. Apply cold compresses to breast if too full.
   4. Do not apply any soap to your nipples.

70. What complaint would be a common occurrence for a woman after delivery her third child?
   1. Chest pain.
   2. Afterbirth cramps.
   3. Burning on urination.
   4. Chills.

71. A woman delivered a male infant yesterday. While caring for her on her first postpartum day, which of the following behaviors would you expect?

1. Asking specific questions about home care of the infant.
2. Concern about when her bowels will move.
3. Frequent crying spells for unexplained reasons.
4. Acceptance of the nurse's suggestions about personal care.

72. A woman delivered this morning. Because this is her first child, which of the following goals is most appropriate?
    1. Early discharge for mother and baby.
    2. Rapid adaptation to role of parent.
    3. Effective education of both parents.
    4. Minimal need for expression of negative feelings.

73. A new mother is going to breastfeed her baby. What is the best indication that the let-down reflex has been achieved in a nursing mother?
    1. Increased prolactin levels.
    2. Milk dripping from the opposite breast.
    3. Progressive weight gain in the infant.
    4. Relief of breast engorgement.

74. To prevent cracked nipples while she is breastfeeding, what should the mother be taught?
    1. Apply a soothing cream prior to feeding.
    2. Nurse at least 20 minutes on each breast each feeding.
    3. Use plastic bra liners.
    4. Wash the nipples with water only.

75. What is the best indication that the breastfed baby is digesting the breast milk properly?
    1. The baby does not experience colic.
    2. The baby passes dark green, pasty stools.
    3. The baby passes soft, golden-yellow stools.
    4. The baby sleeps for several hours after each feeding.

76. Which of the following observations in the postpartum period would be of most concern to the nurse?
    1. After delivery, the mother touches the newborn with her fingertips.
    2. The new parents asked the nurse to recommend a good baby care book.
    3. A new father holds his son in the en face position while visiting.
    4. A new mother sits in bed while her newborn lies awake in the crib.

77. A woman has just delivered her first baby who will be breastfed. The nurse should include which of the following instructions in the teaching plan?
    1. Try to schedule feedings at least every three to four hours.
    2. Wash nipples with soap and water before each feeding.
    3. Avoid nursing bras with plastic lining.
    4. Supplement with water between feedings when necessary.

78. A woman's prenatal antibody titer shows that she is not immune to rubella and will receive the immunization after delivery. The nurse would include which of the following instructions in the teaching plan?
    1. Pregnancy must be avoided for the next 3 months.
    2. Another immunization should be administered in the next pregnancy.
    3. Breastfeeding should be postponed for 5 days after the injection.
    4. An injection will be needed after each succeeding pregnancy.

79. A woman had a normal vaginal delivery 12 hours ago and is to be discharged from the birthing center. Which statement by the client demonstrates understanding about the teaching related to the episiotomy and perineal area?
    1. "I know the stitches will be removed at my postpartum clinic visit."
    2. "The ice pack should be removed for 10 minutes before replacing it."
    3. "The anesthetic spray, then the heat lamp, will help a lot."
    4. "The water for the Sitz bath should be warm, about 102–105° F."

80. A new mother is bottle-feeding her newborn. Which statement by the client demonstrates understanding how to safely manage formula?
    1. "Prepared formula should be used within 48 hours."
    2. "I should mix the formula with water until it is a thin consistency."
    3. "A dishwasher is not sufficient for proper cleaning."
    4. "Prepared formula must be refrigerated until used."

81. A woman delivered her baby 12 hours ago. During the postpartum assessment, the uterus is

found to be boggy with a heavy lochia flow. What should be the initial action of the nurse?

1. Notify the physician or nurse midwife.
2. Administer prn oxytocin.
3. Encourage the woman to increase ambulation.
4. Massage the uterus until firm.

82. A breastfeeding mother is visited by the home health nurse 2 weeks after delivery. The woman is febrile with flulike symptoms; on assessment the nurse notes a warm, reddened, painful area of the right breast. What is the best initial action of the nurse?

1. Contact the physician for an order for antibiotics.
2. Advise the mother to stop breastfeeding and pumping.
3. Assess the mother's feeding technique and knowledge of breast care.
4. Obtain a sample of breast milk for culture.

83. A woman had a vaginal delivery of her second child 2 days ago. She is breastfeeding the baby without difficulty. During a postpartum assessment, what normal finding would the nurse expect?

1. Complaints of afterpains.
2. Pinkish to brownish vaginal discharge.
3. Voiding frequently, 50–75 mL per void.
4. Fundus 1 cm above the umbilicus.

84. A mother who had a vaginal delivery of her first baby 6 weeks ago is seen for her postpartum visit. She is feeling well and is bottle-feeding her infant successfully. During the physical assessment, what normal finding would the nurse expect?

1. Fundus palpated 6 cm below the umbilicus.
2. Breasts tender, some milk expressed.
3. Striae pink but beginning to fade.
4. Creamy, yellow vaginal discharge.

85. A nurse collects the following data on a woman 26 hours after a long labor and a vaginal delivery: temperature 38.3°C (101°F) blood pressure 110/70, pulse 90, some diaphoresis, output 1000 mL per 8 hours, ankle edema, lochia moderate rubra, fundus 1 cm above umbilicus and tender on palpation. The client also asks that the infant be brought back to the nursery. In the analysis of this data, the nurse would select which of the following priority nursing diagnoses?

1. Alteration in parenting related to material discomfort.
2. High risk for injury related to spread of infection.
3. Fluid volume excess related to urinary retention.
4. Knowledge deficit related to uterine subinvolution.

## Answers and Rationales

66. **1.** Lochia rubra is moderate red discharge and is present for the first 2–3 days postpartum.

67. **4.** Family identification of the newborn is an important part of attachment. The first step in identification is defined in terms of likeness to family members.

68. **1.** Glucose can be transferred from the serum to the breast, and hyperglycemia may be reflected in the breast milk.

69. **1.** A well-fitting, supportive bra with wide straps can be recommended for both the nursing and the non-nursing mother for the support of the breasts and for comfort. The nursing mother's bra should have front flaps over each breast for easy access during nursing.

70. **2.** Afterbirth cramps are most common in nursing mothers and multiparas. This mother is both. The release of oxytocin from the posterior pituitary for the "let-down" reflex of lactation causes the afterbirth cramping of the uterus.

71. **4.** During the first few days after delivery, the mother is in a dependent phase, initiating little activity by herself, and is usually content to be directed in her activities by a health care provider.

72. **3.** Both parents will need education about the new baby—how to care for the baby, information about the baby, and how to be a parent.

73. **2.** The nursing infant will stimulate let-down, resulting in milk dripping from the other breast.

74. **4.** Nipples should be washed with water only (no soap) to prevent drying.

75. **3.** Breastfed babies will pass 6–10 small, loose, yellow stools per day.

**76. 4.** During the early postpartum period, evidence of maladaptive mothering may include limited handling or smiling at the infant; studies have shown that a predictable group of reciprocal interactions, between mother and baby, should take place with each encounter to foster and reinforce attachment.

**77. 3.** Although plastic linings protect clothing from leaking milk, the nipples may become sore and prone to infection from trapped moisture; disposable nursing pads can be used to protect clothing.

**78. 1.** To prevent intrauterine infection, which can result in miscarriage, stillbirth, and congenital rubella syndrome in the fetus, women who are immunized should be advised not to become pregnant for 3 months.

**79. 2.** To attain the maximum effect of reducing edema and providing numbness of the tissues, the ice pack should remain in place approximately 20 minutes and then be removed for about 10 minutes before replacing it.

**80. 4.** Extra bottles of prepared formula are stored in the refrigerator and should be warmed slightly before feeding.

**81. 4.** A soft, boggy uterus should be massaged until firm; clots may be expressed during massage and this often tends to contract the uterus more effectively.

**82. 1.** These symptoms are signs of infectious mastitis, usually caused by *Staphylococcus aureus*; a 10-day course of antibiotics is indicated.

**83. 1.** Afterpains occur more commonly in multiparas than in primiparas and are caused by intermittent uterine contractions. Because oxytocin is released when the infant suckles, breastfeeding also increases the severity of the afterpains.

**84. 3.** At 2 weeks' postpartum, striae (stretch marks) are pink and obvious; by 6 weeks they are beginning to fade but may not achieve a silvery appearance for several more weeks.

**85. 2.** The classic definition of puerperal morbidity resulting from infection is a temperature of 38.0°C (100.4°F) or higher on any of the first 10 days postpartum exclusive of the first 24 hours; additional signs are increased pulse rate, uterine tenderness, foul-smelling lochia, and subinvolution (uterus remains enlarged).

# The Newborn

## PHYSIOLOGIC STATUS OF THE NEWBORN

### Circulatory

A. Umbilical vein and ductus venosus constrict after cord is clamped; these will become ligaments (2–3 months).
B. Foramen ovale closes functionally as respirations are established, but anatomic or permanent closure may take several months.
C. Ductus arteriosus constricts with establishment of respiratory function; later becomes ligament (2–3 months).
D. Heart rate ranges from 120–160 beats/minute at birth, with changes noted during sleep and activity.
E. Heart murmurs may be heard; usually have little clinical significance.
F. Average blood pressure is 78/42 mm Hg.
G. Peripheral circulation established slowly; may have mottled (blue/white) appearance for 24 hours (acrocyanosis).
H. RBC count high immediately after birth, then falls after first week; possible physiologic anemia of infancy.
I. Absence of normal flora in intestine of newborn results in low levels of vitamin K; prophylactic dose of vitamin K given IM on first day of life.

### Respiratory

A. "Thoracic squeeze" in vaginal delivery helps drain fluids from respiratory tract; remainder of fluid absorbed across alveolar membranes into capillaries.
B. Adequate levels of surfactants (lecithin and sphingomyelin) ensure mature lung function; prevent alveolar collapse and respiratory distress syndrome.

C. Normal respiratory rate is 30–60 breaths/minute with short periods of apnea (<15 seconds); change noted during sleep or activity.

D. Newborns are obligate nose breathers.

E. Chest and abdomen rise simultaneously; no seesaw breathing.

## Renal

A. Urine present in bladder at birth, but newborn may not void for first 12–24 hours; later pattern is 6–10 voidings/day, indicative of sufficient fluid intake.

B. Urine is pale and straw colored; initial voidings may leave brick-red spots on diaper from passage of uric acid crystals in urine.

C. Infant unable to concentrate urine for first 3 months of life.

## Digestive

A. Newborn has full cheeks due to well-developed sucking pads.

B. Little saliva is produced.

C. Hard palate should be intact; small raised white areas on palate (*Epstein's pearls*) are normal.

D. Newborn cannot move food from lips to pharynx; nipple needs to be inserted well into mouth.

E. Circumoral pallor may appear while sucking.

F. Newborn is capable of digesting simple carbohydrates and protein but has difficulty with fats in formulas.

G. Immature cardiac (esophageal) sphincter may allow reflux of food when burped; may elevate crib after feeding.

H. Stomach capacity varies; approximately 15–30 mL.

I. First stool is meconium (black, tarry residue from lower intestine); usually passed within 12–24 hours after birth.

J. Transitional stools are thin and brownish green in color; after 3 days, milk stools are usually passed—loose and golden yellow for the breastfed infant, formed and pale yellow for the formula-fed infant. Stools may vary in number from 1 every feeding to 1–2/day.

K. Feeding patterns vary; newborn may nurse vigorously immediately after birth, or may need as long as several days to learn to suck effectively. Provide support and encouragement to new mothers during this time as infant feeding is a very emotional area for new mothers.

## Hepatic

A. Liver responsible for changing hemoglobin (from breakdown of RBC) into unconjugated bilirubin, which is further changed into conjugated (water-soluble) bilirubin that can be excreted.

B. Excess unconjugated bilirubin can permeate the sclera and the skin, giving a jaundiced or yellow appearance to these tissues.

C. The liver of a mature infant can maintain the level of unconjugated bilirubin at less than 12 mg/dL. Higher levels indicate a possible dysfunction and the need for intervention.

D. This physiologic jaundice is considered normal in early newborns. It begins to appear after 24 hours, usually between 48–72 hours.

## Temperature

A. Heat production in newborn accomplished by:
   1. Metabolism of "brown fat," a special structure in newborn that is source of heat.
   2. Increased metabolic rate and activity.

B. Newborn cannot shiver as an adult does to release heat.

C. Newborn's body temperature drops quickly after birth; cold stress occurs easily.

D. Body stabilizes temperature in 8–10 hours if unstressed.

E. Cold stress increases oxygen consumption; may lead to metabolic acidosis and respiratory distress.

## Immunologic

A. Newborn has passive acquired immunity from IgG from mother during pregnancy and passage of additional antibodies in colostrum and breast milk.

B. Newborn develops own antibodies during first 3 months, but is at risk for infection during first 6 weeks.

C. Some immunizations are given before the infant is discharged. A complete list of immunizations is listed in Table 5-1.

## Neurologic/Sensory

### Six States of Consciousness

A. Deep sleep

B. Light sleep: some body movements

C. Drowsy: occasional startle; eyes glazed

D. Quiet alert: few movements, but eyes open and bright

E. Active alert: active, occasionally fussy with much facial movement

F. Crying: much activity, eyes open or closed

### Periods of Reactivity

A. First (birth through first 1–2 hours): newborn alert with good sucking reflex, irregular R/HR.

B. Second (4–8 hours after birth): may regurgitate mucus, pass meconium, and suck well

C. Equilibrium usually achieved by 8 hours of age.

### Sleep Cycle

Newborn sleeps an average of 17 hours/day.

## Hunger Cycle

Varies, depending on mode of feeding.
A. Breastfed infant may nurse every 2–3 hours.
B. Bottle-fed infant may be fed every 3–4 hours.

## Special Senses

A. Sight: eyes are sensitive to light; newborn will fix and gaze at objects, especially those with black and white, regular patterns, but eye movements are uncoordinated.
B. Hearing: can hear before birth (24 weeks); newborn seems best attuned to human speech and its cadences.
C. Taste: sense of taste established; prefers sweet-tasting fluids; derives satisfaction as well as nourishment from sucking.
D. Smell: sense is developed at birth; newborn can identify own mother's breast milk by odor.
E. Touch: newborn is well prepared to receive tactile messages; mother demonstrates touch progression in initial bonding activities.

# ASSESSMENT

## Physical Examination

A. Weight
   1. Average between 2750 and 3629 g (6–8 lb) at term
   2. Initial loss of 5–8% of body weight normal during first few days; should be regained in 1–2 weeks
B. Length: average 45.7–55.9 cm (18–22 in)
C. Head circumference: average 33–35.5 cm (13–14 in); remeasure after several days if significant molding or caput succedaneum present
D. Chest circumference: average 1.9 cm (0.75 in) less than head
E. Abdominal girth may be measured if indicated. Consistent placement of tape is important for comparison, identification of abnormalities. Measurement is best done before feeding, as abdomen relaxes after a feeding.
F. Skin
   1. Color in Caucasian infants usually pink; varies with other ethnic backgrounds.
   2. Pigmentation increases after birth.
   3. Skin may be dry.
   4. Acrocyanosis of hands and feet normal for 24 hours; may develop "newborn rash" (erythema toxicum neonatorum).
   5. Small amounts of lanugo and vernix caseosa still seen.
G. Fontanels
   1. Anterior: diamond shaped
   2. Posterior: triangular
   3. Should be flat and open

H. Ears
   1. Should be even with canthi of eyes.
   2. Cartilage should be present and firm.
I. Eyes
   1. May be irritated by medication instillation, some edema/discharge present.
   2. Color is slate blue.
J. Nodule of tissue present in breasts.
K. Female genitalia
   1. Vernix seen between labia.
   2. Blood-tinged mucoid vaginal discharge (pseudomenstruation) from high levels of circulating maternal hormones.
L. Male genitalia
   1. Testes descended or in inguinal canal
   2. Rugae cover scrotum
   3. Meatus at tip of penis
M. Legs
   1. Bowed
   2. No click or displacement of head of femur observed when hips flexed and abducted
N. Feet
   1. Flat
   2. Soles covered with creases in fully mature infant
O. Muscle tone
   1. Predominantly flexed
   2. Occasional transient tremors of mouth and chin
   3. Newborn can turn head from side to side in prone position
   4. Needs head supported when held erect or lifted
P. Reflexes present at birth
   1. Rooting, sucking, and swallowing.
   2. Tonic neck, "fencing" attitude.
   3. Grasp: newborn's fingers curl around anything placed in palm.
   4. *Moro reflex:* symmetric and bilateral abduction and extension of arms and hands; thumb and forefinger form a C; the "embrace" reflex.
   5. *Startle reflex:* similar to Moro, but with hands clenched.
   6. *Babinski's sign:* flare of toes when foot stroked from base of heel along lateral edge to great toe.
Q. Cry
   1. Loud and vigorous.
   2. Heard when infant is hungry, disturbed, or uncomfortable.

## Apgar Scoring

A. Used to evaluate the newborn in five specific categories at 1 and 5 minutes after birth (see Table 6-7).
B. The 1-minute score reflects transitional values.
C. The composite score at 5 minutes provides the best direction for the planning of newborn care.
D. Composite score interpretations
   1. 0–4: prognosis for newborn is grave.
   2. 5–7: infant needs specialized, intensive care.
   3. 7 or above: infant should do well in normal newborn nursery.

## Gestational Age Assessment

After birth, direct examination of the infant leads to an accurate assessment of maturity. This is important, as complications may vary with maturity level: pre- and postmature infants, in general, have greater difficulty adapting to extrauterine life.

A. Physical examination
   1. Skin: thickens with gestational age; may be dry/peeling if postmature.
   2. Lanugo: disappears as pregnancy progresses.
   3. Sole (plantar) creases: increase with gestational age (both depth and number).
   4. Areola of breast: at term, 5–10 mm in diameter.
   5. Ear: cartilage stiffens, recoil increases, and curvature of pinna increases with advancing gestational age.
   6. Genitalia: in the male, check for descended testicles and scrotal rugae; in the female, look for the labia majora to cover the labia minora and clitoris.

B. Neuromuscular assessment (best done after 24 hours)
   1. Resting posture: relaxed posture (extension) seen in the premature; flexion increases with maturity.
   2. Square window angle: flex hand onto underside of forearm, identify angle at which you feel resistance. Angle decreases with increasing gestational age.
   3. Arm recoil: flex infant's arms, extend for 5 seconds, then release. Note angle formed as arms recoil. Decreases with increasing gestational age.
   4. Popliteal angle: place infant on back, extend one leg, and measure angle at point of resistance. Angle becomes more acute as gestation progresses.
   5. Scarf sign: draw one arm across chest until resistance is felt; note relation of elbow to midline of chest. Resistance increases with advancing gestational age.
   6. Heel to ear: attempt to raise foot to ear, noting point at which foot slips from your grasp. Resistance increases with gestational age.

In performing gestational age assessments, the use of a specific form usually facilitates the ease and accuracy of the process.

## ANALYSIS

Nursing diagnoses for the normal newborn are related to the potential for dysfunction in transition period and first few days of life.

## PLANNING AND IMPLEMENTATION

### Goals

A. Newborn will adapt to extrauterine life.
   1. Body temperature will be maintained.
   2. Normal breathing and adequate oxygenation will be established.
   3. Cardiovascular function will be stable.
   4. Nutrition and promotion of growth will be established.
B. Positive parent-infant relationship will be established.
C. Potential dysfunctions will be identified early.
D. Needed interventions will be implemented early.

### Interventions

#### Delivery Room

A. Perform Apgar scoring at 1 and 5 minutes after birth.
B. Perform rapid, overall physical and neurologic exam.
   1. Identify obvious congenital anomalies.
   2. Count vessels in cord.
   3. Identify injuries from birth trauma.
C. Prevent heat loss.
   1. Dry infant immediately after birth.
   2. Wrap newborn warmly, cover head, or place in specially warmed area.
   3. Place newborn on warm surfaces (mother's body) or cover cool surfaces (e.g., scale).
   4. Minimize placement of newborn near cooler areas (windows, outside walls).
D. Maintain established respirations and heartbeat.
E. Identify mother and infant with matching bands.
F. Perform cord clamping if physician has not done so.
G. Allow parents to hold infant, or place in warmed unit.
H. Suction gently prn with bulb syringe.
I. Administer oxygen prn.
J. Promote bonding through early nursing if mother so desires, or by having parents hold newborn.

#### Nursery

A. Continue actions to prevent heat loss (temperature done rectally on admission then axillary; tympanic not accurate on infants).
B. When temperature stabilizes, perform complete physical and neurologic exam.
C. Administer medications as ordered.
   1. To prevent ophthalmia neonatorum, administration of 0.5% erythromycin or 1% tetracycline into conjunctival sac(s).

2. Vitamin K: prophylactic dose to prevent hemorrhage.
3. Hepatitis B vaccine in first 12 hours.
D. Measure and weigh newborn.
E. After temperature has stabilized, bathe and dress newborn, place in open crib.
F. Institute daily care routine.
   1. Take weight.
   2. Monitor temperature, apical pulse, respirations at least every shift.
   3. Suction prn.
   4. Bathe daily if ordered.
   5. Give diaper area care after each change.
   6. Continue assessment for anomalies.
   7. Allow umbilical cord to air dry by folding diaper below cord. Some institutions still use alcohol wipes.
   8. Institute feeding schedule as ordered.
   9. Note voidings and stools on daily basis.
G. Assess for physiologic jaundice (see also Hyperbilirubinemia).
   1. First manifests in the head area (test by depressing skin over bridge of nose) then progresses to chest (depress skin over sternum).
   2. Early feedings promote excretion of bilirubin in stool, diminishing incidence of jaundice.
   3. Prevention of cold stress in newborn diminishes incidence of jaundice.
   4. Loose, greenish stools and green-tinged urine are normal for these infants; advise mother.
   5. These infants need extra fluids to prevent dehydration and replace fluids being excreted.
   6. Advise parents that breast-fed infants may have increased jaundice.
      a. May not feed frequently enough in first 2 days and become dehydrated
      b. Breastmilk jaundice not a confirmed problem, usually an underfed baby.
H. Provide phototherapy if ordered, not usually required in physiologic jaundice unless levels rise rapidly or reach the high teens.
I. Monitor for pathologic jaundice.
   1. Appears at birth or in the first 24 hours.
   2. Bilirubin levels over 12 mg/dL (see Hyperbilirubinemia).
J. Male infants may need circumcision care.
   1. Observe for bleeding.
   2. Note first voiding after circumcision.
   3. Clean area appropriately.
   4. Vaseline to penis to prevent sticking to diaper.
K. Perform screening tests before discharge (PKU, hypothyroidism, galactasemia, etc.).
L. Provide teaching and demonstrations as indicated for parents (e.g., feeding, burping, holding, diapering, bathing, positioning, safety).

# EVALUATION

A. Newborn progress continually observed, normal vital signs for newborn maintained
B. No dysfunctional patterns discerned
C. No congenital anomalies identified
D. Parents comfortable with infant, have initiated bonding
E. Parents comfortable with newborn care
F. All necessary tests carried out at correct time
G. Evidence for continued growth and development at home is positive

# VARIATIONS FROM NORMAL NEWBORN ASSESSMENT FINDINGS

Some variations from the normal assessment findings in the newborn are not indicative of any disorders; others, however, provide information about likely gestational age or the possibility of the existence of a more serious disorder.

## Weight

A. Under 2500 g (5½ lb): small for gestational age (SGA)
B. Over 4100 g (9 lb): large for gestational age (LGA)

## Length

A. Under 45.7 cm (18 in): SGA
B. Over 55.9 cm (22 in): LGA

## Head Circumference

A. Under 31.7 cm (12½ in): microcephaly/SGA
B. Over 36.8 cm (14½ in): hydrocephaly/LGA

## Blood Pressure

A. Variation with activity: normal
B. Major difference between upper and lower extremities: possible aortic coarctation

## Pulse

A. Persistently under 120: possible heart block
B. Persistently over 170: possible respiratory distress syndrome

## Temperature

A. Elevated: possible dehydration or infection
B. Temperature falls with low environmental temperature, late in cold stress, sepsis, cardiac disease.

## Respirations

A. Under 25/minute: possibly result of maternal analgesia
B. Over 60/minute: possible respiratory distress

## Skin

A. Milia (blocked sebaceous glands, usually on nose and chin) are essentially normal.
B. "Stork bites"
   1. Capillary hemangiomas above eyebrows and at base of neck under hairline are essentially normal.
   2. Raised capillary hemangiomas on areas other than face or neck are *not* normal findings.
C. Newborn rash (erythema toxicum neonatorum) is normal.
D. Mongolian spots (darkened areas of pigmentation over sacral area and buttocks) are normal and fade in early childhood. (Seen in Asian and African-American babies.)
E. Fingernail scratches are normal.
F. Excess lanugo: possible prematurity.
G. Vernix
   1. Decreases after 38 weeks, full-term usually has only in creases
   2. Excess: prematurity

## Head

A. Fontanels
   1. Depressed: dehydration
   2. Bulging: increased intracranial pressure
B. Hair: coarse or brittle, possible endocrine disorder
C. Scalp: edema present at birth (*caput succedaneum*) from pressure of cervix against presenting part; crosses suture lines; disappears in 3–4 days without intervention.
D. Skull: collection of blood between a skull bone and its periosteum (*cephalhematoma*) from pressure during delivery; does not cross suture line; appears 12–24 hours after delivery; regresses in 3–6 weeks.
E. Eyes
   1. Edema from medications not uncommon
   2. Strabismus (occasional crossing of eyes) is normal
   3. Wide space between eyes is seen in fetal alcohol syndrome
F. Ears
   1. Lack of cartilage: possible prematurity
   2. Low placement: possible kidney disorder or Down's syndrome
G. Nose: copious drainage associated with syphilis
H. Mouth
   1. Thrush: appears as white patches in mouth; candida infection passed from mother during passage through birth canal.
   2. Tongue movement and excess salivation: possible esophageal atresia

## Neck

Webbing; masses in muscle

## Chest

Breast enlargement and milky secretion from breasts (witch's milk) is result of maternal hormones; self-limiting.

## Cord

Fewer than three vessels may indicate congenital anomalies.

## Female Genitalia

Pseudomenstruation is normal.

## Male Genitalia

Misplaced urinary meatus
A. Epispadias: on upper surface of penis
B. Hypospadias: on under surface of penis

## Upper Extremities

A. Extra fingers
B. Webbed fingers
C. Asymmetric movement: possible trauma or fracture

## Lower Extremities

A. Extra toes
B. Webbed toes
C. Congenital hip dysplasia
D. Few creases on soles of feet: prematurity

## Spine

Tuft of hair: possible occult spina bifida; assess pilonidal area for fistula.

## Anus

Lack of meconium after 24 hours may indicate obstruction, disease.

 **Sample Questions**

86. Which nursing action should be included in the care of the infant with a caput succedaneum?
   1. Aspiration of the trapped blood under the periosteum.
   2. Explanation to the parents about the cause/prognosis.

3. Gentle rubbing in a circular motion to decrease size.

4. Application of cold to reduce size.

87. A baby girl was born at 0915. At 0920 her heart rate was 132 beats/minute, she was crying vigorously, moving all extremities, and only her hands and feet were still slightly blue. What will the nurse record for the Apgar score?

   1. 7.
   2. 8.
   3. 9.
   4. 10.

88. Which of the following findings in a newborn baby girl is normal?

   1. Passage of meconium within the first 24 hours.
   2. Respiratory rate of 70/minute at rest.
   3. Yellow skin tones at 12 hours of age.
   4. Bleeding from umbilicus.

89. The nursery nurse carries a newborn baby into his mother's room. The mother states, "I think my baby's afraid of me. Every time I make a loud noise, he jumps." What should be the nurse's initial action?

   1. Encourage her not to be so nervous with her baby.
   2. Reassure her that this is a normal reflexive reaction for her baby.
   3. Take the baby back to the nursery for a neurologic evaluation.
   4. Wrap the baby more tightly in warm blankets.

90. A new mother asks how much weight her newborn will lose. What will be the nurse's reply?

   1. None.
   2. 2–3%.
   3. 5–8%.
   4. 10–15%.

91. Which of the following findings in a 3-hour-old full-term newborn would cause the nurse concern?

   1. Two "soft spots" between the cranial bones.
   2. Asymmetry of the head with overriding bones.
   3. Head circumference 32 cm, chest 34 cm.
   4. A sharply outlined, spongy area of edema.

92. The nurse collects the following data while assessing the skin of a 6-hour-old newborn: color pink with bluish hands and feet, some pale yellow papules with red base over trunk, small white spots on the nose, and a red area at the nape of the neck. What would be the nurse's next action?

   1. Document findings as within normal range.
   2. Isolate infant pending diagnosis.
   3. Request a dermatology consultation.
   4. Document as indicators of malnutrition.

93. While performing the discharge assessment on a 2-day-old newborn, the nurse finds that after blanching the skin on the forehead, the color turns yellow. What does this indicate?

   1. A normal biologic response.
   2. An infectious liver condition.
   3. An Rh incompatibility problem.
   4. Jaundice related to breastfeeding.

94. A newborn is 2 days old and is being breastfed. The nurse finds that yesterday her stool was thick and tarry, today it's thinner and greenish brown; she voided twice since birth with some pink stains noted on the diaper. What do these findings indicate to the nurse?

   1. Marked dehydration.
   2. Inadequate initial nutrition.
   3. Normal newborn elimination.
   4. A need for medical consultation.

95. The nurse notes the following behaviors in a 6-hour-old, full-term newborn: occasional tremors of extremities, straightens arms and hands outward and flexes knees when disturbed, toes fan out when heel is stroked, and tries to walk when held upright. What do these findings indicate to the nurse?

   1. Signs of drug withdrawal.
   2. Abnormal uncoordinated movements.
   3. Asymmetric muscle tone.
   4. Expected neurologic development.

96. While assessing a newborn, the nurse notes that the areola is flat with less than 0.5 cm of breast tissue. What does this finding indicate?

   1. That infant is male.
   2. Maternal hormonal depletion.
   3. Intrauterine growth retardation.
   4. Preterm gestational age.

97. The nurse's initial care plan for a full-term newborn includes the nursing diagnosis "risk of fluid volume depletion related to absence of intestinal flora." What would be a related nursing intervention?

   1. Administer glucose water or put to breast.
   2. Assess first void and passing of meconium.

3. Administer vitamin K injection.

4. Send cord blood to lab for Coombs' test.

98. In the time immediately following birth, why might the nurse delay instillation of eye medication to the newborn?

1. Check prenatal record to determine whether prophylactic treatment is needed.

2. Ensure that initial eye saline irrigation is completed.

3. Enable mother to breast feed the infant in the first hour of life.

4. Facilitate eye contact and bonding between parents and newborn.

99. The nurses should include which of the following instructions in the care plan for a new mother who is breastfeeding her full-term newborn?

1. Put to breast when infant shows readiness to feed.

2. Breastfeed infant every 3 to 4 hours until discharge.

3. Offer water feedings between breastfeedings.

4. Feed infant when he shows hunger by crying.

100. In the delivery area, after ensuring that the newborn has established respirations, what is the next priority of the nurse?

1. Perform the Apgar score.

2. Place plastic clamp on cord.

3. Dry infant and provide warmth.

4. Ensure correct identification.

101. During the bath demonstration, a woman asks the nurse if it is OK to use baby powder because warm weather is coming. How should the nurse respond?

1. "Just dust in on the diaper area only."

2. "It's best not to use powder on infants."

3. "First use baby oil, then the powder."

4. "If the baby is just in a diaper he'll be cool."

102. Which of the following muscles would the nurse choose as the preferred site for a newborn's vitamin K injection?

1. Gluteus medius.

2. Mid-deltoid.

3. Vastus lateralis.

4. Rectus femoris.

103. What action by the mother of the newborn will assure the nurse that she understands proper cord care for the newborn?

1. Views a videotape on newborn hygiene care.

2. Reads a booklet on care of the newborn's cord stump.

3. Says she will apply Bacitracin ointment three times per day.

4. Cleans the cord and surrounding skin with an alcohol pad.

104. What statement by a new mother demonstrates more instruction on care of the circumcised infant is needed?

1. "I know to gently retract the foreskin after the area is healed."

2. "At each diaper change I will squeeze water over the penis and pat dry."

3. "I know not to disturb the yellow exudate that will form."

4. "For the first day or so I'll apply a little A&D ointment."

105. Which statement by a new mother demonstrates proper understanding of bottle feeding her infant?

1. "I know not to prop the bottle until my baby is older."

2. "With these little bottles, he should be able to finish them."

3. "When I hold the bottle upside down, drops of milk should fall."

4. "I should burp the baby at the end of the feeding."

 **Answers and Rationales**

86. **2.** Caput succedaneum (scalp edema) will regress in a few days without interventions and without residual damage.

87. **3.** Acrocyanosis, where hands and feet are still slightly blue for the first 24 hours, is a normal variant in the newborn, but it rates a 1 on the Apgar scale. All the other descriptors are rated 2 on the Apgar scale, giving this newborn a total of 9.

88. **1.** Meconium is usually passed during the first 24 hours of life.

89. **2.** The startle reflex, normally present in neonates, is characterized by symmetric extension and abduction of the arms with fingers extended. The parent perceives this response as jumping.

90. **3.** Within 3–4 days of birth, a weight loss of 5–8% is normal.

91. **3.** The circumference of the newborn's head should be approximately 2 cm greater than the

circumference of the chest at birth and will remain in this proportion for the next few months. Any differences in head size may indicate microcephaly (abnormal smallness of head) or hydrocephalus (increased cerebrospinal fluid within the ventricles of the brain).

92. **1.** These findings of acrocyanosis (bluish discoloration of the hands and feet), erythema toxicum (newborn rash), milia, and a nevus flammeus (port wine stain) are all within the normal range for a full-term newborn.

93. **1.** Physiologic jaundice occurs after the first 24 hours of life and is caused by accelerated destruction of fetal RBCs, impaired conjugation of bilirubin, and increased bilirubin reabsorption from the intestinal tract; there is no pathologic basis.

94. **3.** Normal term newborns pass meconium within 8–24 hours of life; meconium is formed in utero and is thick, tarry, black (or dark green) in appearance. Transitional stool is a thinner brown to green. Normal voiding is 2 to 6 times daily; there may be innocuous pink stains ("brick dust spots") on the diaper from urates.

95. **4.** Tremors are common in the full-term newborn; when a newborn is startled she will exhibit the Moro reflex, that is, she will straighten arms and hands outward while the knees flex; in a newborn the Babinski reflex is displayed by a fanning and extension of the toes (in adults the toes flex); and when held upright with feet lightly touching a surface, the newborn will put one foot in front of the other and "walk."

96. **4.** At term gestation, the breast bud tissue will measure between 0.5 and 1 cm (5–10 mm).

97. **3.** The newborn is at a high risk for hemorrhage due to an absence of intestinal flora (bacteria). Vitamin K, needed for the formation of prothrombin and proconvertin for blood coagulation, is usually synthesized by these bacteria in the colon; however, they are absent in the newborn's sterile gut. This problem is prevented by the administration of vitamin K following birth.

98. **4.** The initial parental-newborn attachment period can be enhanced if the care providers keep routine investigations to a minimum, delay instillation of ophthalmic antibiotic for 1 hour, keep the room dim, and provide privacy; eye prophylaxis medication can cause chemical conjunctivitis, which may interfere with the baby's ability to focus on the parents' faces.

99. **1.** It is important for the new mother to learn and respond to her infant's early feeding cues. Early cues that indicate a newborn is interested in feeding include hand-to-hand or hand-passing-mouth motion, whimpering, sucking, and rooting.

100. **3.** After birth, the first priority is to maintain respirations, the second priority is to provide and maintain warmth; the newborn's temperature may fall 2–3°C (3.6–5°F) after birth due mainly to evaporative losses; this triggers cold-induced metabolic responses and heat production.

101. **2.** Powders and oils are not recommended for the neonate's skin; oils may clog the pores, and the small particles of powders may be inhaled by the neonate.

102. **3.** The middle third of the vastus lateralis muscle in the thigh is the preferred site for an intramuscular injection in the newborn.

103. **4.** Before discharge, parents should demonstrate proper cleaning of the cord stump by wiping it with an alcohol pad; they should know to do this 2 to 3 times a day until the cord falls off in 7–14 days.

104. **1.** A circumcision is the surgical removal of the prepuce or foreskin from the tip of the penis; any foreskin that remains should not be retracted.

105. **3.** The nipple should have a hole big enough to allow milk to flow in drops when the bottle is inverted; too large an opening may cause regurgitation, too small an opening can exhaust and upset the infant.

# The High-Risk Infant

## OVERVIEW

High-risk infants are those whose incidence of illness or death is increased because of prematurity, dysmaturity, postmaturity, physical problems, or birth complications. They are frequently the result of a high-risk pregnancy.

## ASSESSMENT

A. History of high-risk pregnancy or other factor possibly affecting fetal development
B. Apgar scores in the delivery room
C. Head-to-toe assessment of the infant (see Assessment of the Newborn)
D. Determination of gestational age

## ANALYSIS

A. Alteration in respiratory function
B. Imbalanced nutrition: less than body requirements
C. Risk for impaired skin integrity
D. Ineffective tissue perfusion
E. Risk for injury
F. Impaired gas exchange
G. Ineffective thermoregulation
H. For parents of high-risk infants
    1. Ineffective coping
    2. Deficient knowledge
    3. Anticipatory grieving
    4. Powerlessness
    5. Social isolation

## PLANNING AND IMPLEMENTATION

### Goals

A. Needs of infant for physical care will be met.
    1. Oxygen: respiratory functioning will be maintained.
    2. Humidity and warmth: temperature will be regulated and cold stress prevented.
    3. Adequate nutrition will be provided.
    4. Tender handling: newborn will receive proper skin care and positioning.
B. Infection or other complications will be prevented.
C. Normal growth and development will be promoted.
D. Needs of parents for closeness with infant will be met; attachment/bonding will be promoted.

### Interventions

A. Constantly monitor infant for subtle changes in condition and intervene promptly when necessary.
B. Conserve infant's energy and decrease physiologic stress.
C. Provide appropriate stimulation for infant growth and development.
D. Allow parents to express their reactions and feelings and assist them in attachment behaviors.
E. Teach parents care of infant in preparation for discharge.

## EVALUATION

A. Infant's physical condition stabilized and improved on a steady basis
B. Infant's growth and development steady and appropriate
C. Parents demonstrated acceptance of and comfort with infant's condition
D. Parents demonstrated comfort and confidence with infant care at discharge

## HIGH-RISK DISORDERS

### The Premature Infant

A. General information
    1. Any infant born before the end of the 37th week of pregnancy
    2. Weight usually less than 2500 grams (5½ lb)
    3. Causes include:
        a. Maternal factors: age, smoking, poor nutrition, placental problems, preeclampsia/eclampsia
        b. Fetal factors: multiple pregnancy, infection, intrauterine growth retardation (IUGR)
        c. Other: socioeconomic status, environmental exposure to harmful substance
    4. Severity of problems related to level of maturity: the earlier the infant is born, the greater the chance of complications.
    5. Major complicating conditions
        a. Respiratory distress syndrome
        b. Thermoregulatory problems

c. Conservation of energy

d. Infection

e. Hemorrhage

B. Assessment findings

1. Respiratory system

a. Insufficient surfactant

b. Apneic episodes

c. Retractions, nasal flaring, grunting, seesaw pattern of breathing, cyanosis

d. Increased respiratory rate

2. Thermoregulation: body temperature fluctuates easily (premature newborn has less subcutaneous fat and muscle mass)

3. Nutritional status

a. Poor sucking and swallowing reflexes

b. Poor gag and cough reflexes

4. Skin: lack of subcutaneous fat; reddened; translucent

5. Drainage from umbilicus/eyes

6. Cardiovascular

a. Petechiae caused by fragile capillaries and prolonged prothrombin time

b. Increased bleeding at injection sites

7. Neuromuscular

a. Poor muscle tone

b. Weak reflexes

c. Weak, feeble cry

C. Nursing interventions

1. Maintain respirations at less than 60/minute, check every 1–2 hours.

2. Administer oxygen as ordered; check concentration every 2 hours to avoid retrolental fibroplasia while providing adequate oxygenation.

3. Auscultate breath sounds to assess lung expansion.

4. Encourage breathing with gentle rubbing of back and feet.

5. Suction as needed.

6. Reposition every 1–2 hours for maximum lung expansion and prevention of exhaustion.

7. Monitor blood gases and electrolytes.

8. Maintain thermoneutral body temperature; prevent cold stress.

9. Maintain appropriate humidity level.

10. Monitor for signs of infection; these infants have little antibody production and decreased resistance.

11. Feed according to abilities.

12. Monitor sucking reflex; if poor, gavage feeding indicated. Most preterm infants require at least some gavage feeding as it diminishes the effort required for sucking while improving the caloric intake.

13. Use "preemie" nipple if bottle-feeding.

14. Monitor I&O, weight gain or loss; these infants are easily dehydrated, with poor electrolyte balance.

15. Monitor for hypoglycemia and hyperbilirubinemia.

16. Handle carefully; organize care to minimize disturbances.

17. Provide skin care with special attention to cleanliness and careful positioning to prevent breakdown.

18. Monitor heart rate and pattern at least every 1–2 hours; listen apically for 1 full minute.

19. Monitor potential bleeding sites (umbilicus, injection sites, skin); these infants have lowered clotting factors.

20. Monitor overall growth and development of infant; check weight, length, head circumference.

21. Provide tactile stimulation when caring for or feeding infant.

22. Provide complete explanations for parents.

23. Encourage parental involvement in infant's care.

24. Provide support for parents; refer to self-help group or other parents if necessary.

25. Promote parental confidence with infant care before discharge.

## The Dysmature Infant (SGA)

A. General information

1. Birth weight in the lowest 10th percentile at term

2. Causes: discounting heredity, possibly intrauterine growth retardation, infections, malformations

B. Assessment findings

1. Skin: loose and dry, little fat, little muscle mass

2. Small body makes skull look larger than normal

3. Sunken abdomen

4. Thin, dry umbilical cord

5. Little scalp hair

6. Wide skull sutures

7. Respiratory distress; may have had hypoxic episodes in utero

8. Hypoglycemia

9. Tremors

10. Weak cry

11. Lethargic

12. Cool to touch

C. Nursing interventions

1. Care of SGA infant is similar in many instances to care of preterm infant.

2. Tailor high-level nursing care to meet specific needs of infant with regard to functioning of all body systems, psychologic growth and development, parental support and teaching, and prevention of complications.

## The Postmature Infant

A. General information

1. Born after the completion of 42 weeks of pregnancy

**2.** Problems caused by progressively less efficient actions of placenta

**B.** Assessment findings

  **1.** Skin

    **a.** Vernix and lanugo completely disappeared

    **b.** Dry, cracked, parchmentlike appearance of skin

    **c.** Color: yellow to green from meconium staining

  **2.** Depleted subcutaneous fat; old looking

  **3.** Hard nails extending beyond fingertips

  **4.** Signs of birth injury or poor tolerance of birth process

**C.** Nursing interventions

  **1.** Nursing care of the postmature infant has many characteristics in common with the care given to the premature infant.

  **2.** Design high-level nursing care to identify the infant's specific physical and psychologic needs; monitor functioning of all body systems, growth and development, parental support and teaching, and prevention of complications.

# SPECIAL CONDITIONS IN THE NEONATE

## Hyperbilirubinemia

**A.** General information

  **1.** Elevated serum level of bilirubin in the newborn results in jaundice or yellow color of body tissues.

  **2.** In physiologic jaundice, average increase from 2 mg/dL in cord blood to 6 mg/dL by 72 hours; not exceeding 12 mg/dL.

  **3.** Level at which a newborn will sustain damage to body cells (especially brain cells) from high concentrations of bilirubin is termed pathologic.

  **4.** May result from immaturity of liver, Rh or ABO incompatibility, infection, birth trauma with subsequent bleeding (cephalhematoma), maternal diabetes, hypothermia, medications.

  **5.** Major complication is *kernicterus* (brain damage caused by high levels of unconjugated bilirubin).

**B.** Assessment findings

  **1.** Pathologic jaundice usually appears early, up to 24 hours after birth; represents a process ongoing before birth

  **2.** Usual pattern of progression is from head to feet. Blanch skin over bony area or look at conjunctiva and buccal membranes in dark-skinned infants

  **3.** Pallor

  **4.** Dark, concentrated urine (often dehydrated)

  **5.** Behavior changes (irritability, lethargy)

  **6.** Polycythemia

  **7.** Increased serum bilirubin (direct, indirect, and total)

**C.** Nursing interventions

  **1.** Identify conditions predisposing to hyperbilirubinemia, especially positive coombs test (test on cord blood for presence of maternal antibodies).

  **2.** Prevent progression or complications of jaundice.

  **3.** Assess jaundice levels (visually, lab tests) as needed.

  **4.** Prevent conditions that contribute to development of hyperbilirubinemia (i.e., cold stress, hypoxia, acidosis, hypoglycemia, dehydration, infection).

  **5.** Provide adequate hydration.

  **6.** Implement phototherapy if ordered; use of blue lights overhead, blanket-device wrapped around infant (Wallaby), or bili-bed.

    **a.** Overhead unit

      **1)** Unclothe infant for maximum skin exposure; minimal diaper

      **2)** Cover eyes to prevent retinal damage

      **3)** Carefully monitor temperature

      **4)** Remove baby from warmer and uncover eyes for feedings

      **5)** Ensure feedings every 3 hours

    **b.** Wallaby blanket

      **1)** Baby at bedside—explain care of unit to mother

      **2)** Keep unit on for feedings, eyes remain uncovered

      **3)** Other care as above

  **7.** Explain all tests and procedures to parents.

  **8.** Support parents with information on procedures.

## Hemolytic Disease of the Newborn (Erythroblastosis Fetalis)

**A.** General information

  **1.** Characterized by RBC destruction in the newborn, with resultant anemia and hyperbilirubinemia

  **2.** Possibly caused by Rh or ABO incompatibility between the mother and the fetus (antigen/antibody reaction)

  **3.** Mechanisms of Rh incompatibility

    **a.** Sensitization of Rh-negative woman by transfusion of Rh-positive blood

    **b.** Sensitization of Rh-negative woman by presence of Rh-positive RBCs from her fetus conceived with Rh-positive man

    **c.** Approximately 65% of infants conceived by this combination of parents will be Rh positive.

    **d.** Mother is sensitized by passage of fetal Rh-positive RBCs through placenta, either during pregnancy (break/leak in membrane) or at the time of separation of the placenta after delivery.

e. This stimulates the mother's immune response system to produce anti-Rh-positive antibodies that attack fetal RBCs and cause hemolysis.

f. If this sensitization occurs during pregnancy, the fetus is affected in utero; if sensitization occurs at the time of delivery, subsequent pregnancies may be affected.

4. ABO incompatibility

a. Same underlying mechanism

b. Mother is blood type O; infant is A, B, or AB.

c. Reaction in ABO incompatibility is less severe.

B. Rh incompatibility

1. First pregnancy: mother may become sensitized, baby rarely affected

2. Indirect Coombs' test (tests for anti-Rh-positive antibodies in mother's circulation) performed during pregnancy at first visit and again about 28 weeks' gestation. If indirect Coombs' test is negative at 28 weeks, a small dose (MicRho GAM) is given prophylactically to prevent sensitization in the third trimester. RhoGAM may also be given after second trimester amniocentesis.

3. If positive, levels are titrated to determine extent of maternal sensitization and potential effect on fetus.

4. Direct Coombs' test done on cord blood at delivery to determine presence of anti-Rh-positive antibodies on fetal RBCs.

5. If both indirect and direct Coombs' tests are negative (no formation of anti-Rh-positive antibodies) and infant is Rh positive, then Rh-negative mother can be given RhoGAM (Rho[D] human immune globulin) to prevent development of anti-Rh-positive antibodies as the result of sensitization from present (just-terminated) pregnancy.

6. In each pregnancy, an Rh-negative mother who carries an Rh-positive fetus can receive RhoGAM to protect future pregnancies if the mother has had negative indirect Coombs' tests and the infant has had a negative direct Coombs' test.

7. If mother has been sensitized (produced anti-Rh-positive antibodies), RhoGAM is not indicated.

8. RhoGAM must be injected into unsensitized mother's system within first 24 hours if possible, by 72 hours at latest.

C. ABO incompatibility

1. Reaction less severe than with Rh incompatibility

2. Firstborn may be affected because type O mother may have anti-A and anti-B antibodies even before pregnancy.

3. Fetal RBCs with A, B, or AB antigens evoke less severe reaction on part of mother, thus

fewer anti-A, anti-B, or anti-AB antibodies are produced.

4. Clinical manifestations of ABO incompatibility are milder and of shorter duration than those of Rh incompatibility.

5. Care must be taken to observe for hemolysis and jaundice.

D. Assessment findings

1. Jaundice and pallor within first 24–36 hours

2. Anemia

3. Erythropoiesis

4. Enlarged placenta

5. Edema and ascites

E. Nursing interventions

1. Determine blood type and Rh early in pregnancy.

2. Determine results of indirect Coombs' test early in pregnancy and again at 28–32 weeks.

3. Determine results of direct Coombs' test on cord blood (type and Rh, hemoglobin and hematocrit).

4. Administer RhoGAM IM to mother as ordered.

5. Monitor carefully infants of Rh-negative and Type O mothers for jaundice.

6. Set up phototherapy as ordered by physician and monitor infant during therapy.

7. Instruct parents if home device will be used.

8. Support parents with explanations and information.

# Neonatal Sepsis

A. General information

1. Associated with the presence of pathogenic microorganisms in the blood, especially gram-negative organisms (*E. coli, Aerobacter, Proteus,* and *Klebsiella*), and gram-positive group B beta-hemolytic streptococci.

2. Contributing factors

a. Prolonged rupture of membranes (more than 24 hours)

b. Prolonged or difficult labor

c. Maternal infection

d. Infection in hospital personnel

e. Aspiration at birth or later

f. Poor handwashing techniques among staff

B. Assessment findings

1. Behavioral changes: lethargy, irritability, poor feeding

2. Frequent periods of apnea

3. Jaundice

4. Hypothermia or low-grade fever

5. Vomiting, diarrhea

C. Nursing interventions

1. Perform cultures as indicated/ordered.

2. Administer antibiotics for 3 days until 72-hour cultures back—if negative, discontinue; if positive, continue with full course of specific antibiotics

3. Prevent heat loss.
4. Administer oxygen as indicated.
5. Maintain hydration.
6. Monitor vital signs (temperature, pulse, respirations) frequently.
7. Weigh daily.
8. Stroke back and feet gently to stimulate breathing if infant is apneic.
9. Promote parental attachment and involvement in newborn care.

# Hypoglycemia

A. General information
   1. Less-than-normal amount of glucose in the blood of the neonate:
   2. Common in infants of diabetic mothers (IDM), especially type III: these infants usually LGA (macrosomic) due to high maternal glucose levels that have crossed placenta, stimulating the fetal pancreas to secrete more insulin, which then acts as growth hormone.
   3. At birth, with loss of supply of maternal glucose, newborn may become hypoglycemic.
   4. Large size may have caused traumatic vaginal birth, or may have necessitated cesarean birth.
   5. Hypoglycemia can also occur in infants who are full term, SGA, postterm, septic, or with any condition that subjects the infant to stress.

B. Assessment findings
   1. May be born prematurely due to complications
   2. Although LGA, IDMs may be immature/dysmature
   3. Higher incidence of congenital anomalies in IDMs
   4. General appearance
      a. Puffy body
      b. Enlarged organs
   5. Tremors, feeding difficulty, irregular respirations, lethargy, hypothermia
   6. Hypocalcemia and hyperbilirubinemia
   7. Respiratory distress
   8. Blood glucose levels below 40 mg/dL (20 mg/dL in premature infant) using Dextristix

C. Nursing interventions
   1. Provide high-level nursing care similar to that for premature/dysmature infant.
   2. Assess blood glucose level at frequent intervals, beginning ½–1 hour after birth in at-risk infants.
   3. Feed hypoglycemic infant according to nursery protocol (formula or breast preferred) if suck/swallow reflex present and coordinated.
   4. Poor suck-swallow or lack of serum response to PO feeding, administer IV glucose.

# Infant Born to Addicted Mother

A. General information
   1. Substance may be alcohol, heroin, morphine, or any other addictive drug.
   2. Mother usually seeks prenatal care only when labor begins and has frequently taken a dose of addictive substance before seeking help, delaying withdrawal symptoms 12–24 hours.
   3. Withdrawal symptoms in the neonate may be noticed within 24 hours.

B. Assessment findings
   1. Infants born to alcohol-abusing mothers may have facial anomalies, fine-motor dysfunction, genital abnormalities (especially females), and cardiac defects; may be SGA (also called the fetal alcohol syndrome)
   2. Hyperirritability and hyperactivity
   3. High-pitched cry common
   4. Respiratory distress, tachypnea, excessive secretions
   5. Vomiting and diarrhea
   6. Elevated temperature
   7. Other signs of withdrawal: sneezing; sweating; yawning; short, nonquiet sleep; frantic sucking

C. Nursing interventions
   1. Reduce external stimuli.
   2. Handle minimally.
   3. Swaddle infant and hold close when handling.
   4. Monitor infant's vital signs.
   5. Suction/resuscitate as required.
   6. Feed frequently, with small amounts.
   7. Measure I&O.
   8. Provide careful skin care.
   9. Administer medications if ordered (may use phenobarbital or paragoric).
   10. Involve parents in care if possible.
   11. Inform parents of infant's condition/progress.

# Respiratory Distress Syndrome (RDS)

A. General information
   1. Symptoms found almost exclusively in the preterm infant.
   2. Deficiency of surfactant increases surface tension, which causes alveolar collapse.
   3. When women are likely to deliver prematurely, betamethasone is given IM in two doses, 12 hours apart.
   4. Additional factors: hypoxia, hypothermia, acidosis
   5. Sequelae of RDS may include
      a. Patent ductus arteriosus
      b. Hyperbilirubinemia
      c. Retrolental fibroplasia: retinal changes, visual impairment and eventually blindness, resulting from too-high oxygen levels during treatment
      d. Bronchopulmonary dysplasia (BPD): damage to the alveolar epithelium of the

lungs related to high oxygen concentrations and positive pressure ventilation. May be difficult to wean infant from ventilator, but most recover and have normal X-rays at 6 months to 2 years.
  e. Necrotizing enterocolitis.
B. Assessment findings
  1. Respiratory rate of over 60/minute
  2. Retractions, grunting, cyanosis, nasal flaring, chin lag
  3. Increased apical pulse
  4. Hypothermia
  5. Decreased activity level
  6. Elevated levels of carbon dioxide
  7. Metabolic acidosis
  8. X-rays show atelectasis and density in alveoli.
C. Nursing interventions
  1. Maintain infant's body temperature at 36.4°C (97.6°F).
  2. Provide sufficient caloric intake for size, age, and prevention of catabolism (usually IV glucose with gradual increase in feedings); nasogastric tube may be used.
  3. Organize care for minimal handling of infant.
  4. Administer oxygen therapy as ordered.
    a. Monitor oxygen concentration every 2–4 hours; maintain less than 40% concentration if possible.
    b. Oxygen may be administered by hood, nasal prongs, intubation, or mask.
    c. Oxygen may be at atmospheric or increased pressure.
    d. Continuous positive air pressure (CPAP) or positive end-expiratory pressure (PEEP) may be used.
    e. Oxygen should be warmed and humidified.
  5. Monitor infant's blood gases.
  6. If intubated, suction (for less than 5 seconds) prn using sterile catheter.
  7. Auscultate breath sounds.
  8. Provide chest physiotherapy, postural drainage, and percussion if ordered.
  9. Encourage parental involvement in care (visiting, stroking infant, talking).
  10. Administer surfactant via endotracheal tube and other medications as ordered.

# Necrotizing Enterocolitis (NEC)

A. General information
  1. An ischemic attack to the intestine resulting in thrombosis and infarction of affected bowel, mucosal ulcerations, pseudomembrane formation, and inflammation.
  2. Bacterial action (*E. coli*, *Klebsiella*) complicates the process, producing sepsis.
  3. May be precipitated by any event in which blood is shunted away from the intestine to the heart and brain (e.g., fetal distress, low

Apgar score, RDS, prematurity, neonatal shock, and asphyxia).
  4. Average age at onset is 4 days.
  5. Now that severely ill infants are surviving, NEC is encountered more frequently.
  6. May ultimately cause bowel perforation and death.
  7. Less common in breastfed premature infants.
B. Medical management
  1. Parenteral antibiotics
  2. Gastric decompression
  3. Correction of acidosis and fluid electrolyte imbalances
  4. Surgical removal of the diseased intestine
C. Assessment findings
  1. History indicating high-risk group
  2. Findings related to sepsis
    a. Temperature instability
    b. Apnea, labored respirations
    c. Cardiovascular collapse
    d. Lethargy or irritability
  3. Gastrointestinal symptoms
    a. Abdominal distension and tenderness
    b. Vomiting or increased gastric residual
    c. Poor feeding
    d. Hematest positive stools
    e. X-rays showing air in the bowel wall, adynamic ileus, and bowel wall thickening
D. Nursing interventions
  1. Carefully assess infants at risk for early recognition of symptoms.
  2. Discontinue oral feedings, insert nasogastric tube.
  3. Prevent trauma to abdomen by avoiding diapers and planning care for minimal handling.
  4. Maintain acid-base balance by administering fluids and electrolytes as ordered.
  5. Administer antibiotics as ordered.
  6. Stroke infant's hands and head and talk to infant as much as possible.
  7. Provide visual and auditory stimulation.
  8. Inform parents of progress and support them in expressing their fears and concerns.

# Phenylketonuria (PKU)

A. General information
  1. Inability to metabolize phenylalanine to tyrosine because of an autosomal recessive inherited disorder causing an inborn error of metabolism
  2. Phenylalanine is a composite of almost all proteins: the danger to the infant is immediate.
  3. High levels of phenylketones affect brain cells, causing mental retardation.
  4. Initial screening for diagnosis of PKU is made via the Guthrie test, done after the infant has ingested protein for a minimum of 24 hours.

5. Secondary screening
   a. Done when the infant is about 6 weeks' old.
   b. Test fresh urine with a Phenistix, which changes color.
   c. Parents send in a prepared sheet marking the color.
6. These tests, mandatory in many states, allow the early diagnosis of the disorder, and dietary interventions to minimize or prevent complications.

B. Assessment findings
   1. Phenylalanine levels greater than 8 mg/dL are diagnostic for PKU.
   2. Newborn appears normal; may be fair with decreased pigmentation.
   3. Untreated PKU can result in failure to thrive, vomiting, and eczema; by about 6 months, signs of brain involvement appear.
C. Nursing interventions
   1. Restrict protein intake.
   2. Substitute a low-phenylalanine formula (Lofenalac) for either mother's milk or formula.
   3. Provide special food lists for parents.

 **Sample Questions**

106. In differentiating physiologic jaundice from pathologic jaundice, which of the following facts is most important?
   1. Mother is 37 years of age.
   2. Infant is a term newborn.
   3. Unconjugated bilirubin level is 6 mg/dL on third day.
   4. Appears at 12 hours after birth.

107. A newborn is receiving phototherapy. What will be included during the phototherapy to meet safety needs?
   1. Limit fluid intake.
   2. Cover the infant's eyes while he is under the light.
   3. Keep him clothed to prevent skin burns.
   4. Make sure the light is not closer than 24 inches.

108. The morning temperature on a newborn is 36.4°C (97.6°F). In order to prevent cold stress, which action will be included in the plan of care?
   1. Keep the baby's head covered.
   2. Keep the baby unwrapped.
   3. Turn up the thermostat in the nursery.
   4. Use warm water for the bath.

109. A diabetic woman has a problem-free prenatal course and delivers a full-term 9 lb 2 oz girl. At 1 hour after birth, the baby exhibits tremors. The nurse performs a heel stick and a Dextrostix test. The result is 40 mg/dL. The nurse is aware these symptoms are most likely caused by what condition?
   1. Hypoglycemia.
   2. Hypokalemia.
   3. Hypothermia.
   4. Hypercalcemia.

110. A newborn weighs 1450 g, has weak muscle tone, with extremities in an extended position while at rest. The pinna is flat and does not readily recoil. Very little breast tissue is palpable. The soles have deep indentations over the upper one-third. Based on these data, what should the nurse know about the baby's gestational age?
   1. Full-term infant, 38–42 weeks' gestation.
   2. Premature infant, less than 24 weeks' gestation.
   3. Premature infant, 29–33 weeks' gestation.
   4. Postterm infant greater than 42 weeks' gestation.

111. A premature infant at 6 hours old, has respirations of 64, mild nasal flaring, and expiratory grunting. She is pink in room air, temperature is 36.5°C. The baby's mother ruptured membranes 36 hours prior to delivery. Which measures should the nurse include in the plan of care?
   1. Have respiratory therapy set up a respirator because respiratory failure is imminent. Get blood gases every hour.
   2. Encourage mother/infant interaction. Rooming in as soon as stable. Monitor vital signs every 8 hours.
   3. Observe for signs of sepsis. Cultures if ordered. Monitor vital signs at least every 2 hours for the first 24 hours. Encourage family interaction with infant.
   4. Radiant warmer for first 48 hours. Vital signs every hour. Restrict visitation due to risk of infection.

112. During the assessment of a 2-day-old infant with bruising and a cephalhematoma, the nurse notes jaundice of the face and trunk. The baby is also being breastfed. Bilirubin level is 10 mg/dL. What is the most likely interpretation of these findings?
   1. Hyperbilirubinemia due to the bruising and cephalhematoma.
   2. Pathologic jaundice requiring exchange transfusion.
   3. Breast milk jaundice.
   4. Hyperbilirubinemia due to blood group incompatibility.

113. A 6-hour-old newborn has been diagnosed with erythroblastosis fetalis. What is the cause of this condition?
    1. ABO blood group incompatibility between the father and infant.
    2. Rh incompatibility between the mother and infant.
    3. ABO blood group incompatibility between the mother and infant.
    4. Rh incompatibility between father and infant.

114. An Rh-negative mother has just given birth to an Rh-positive infant. She had a negative indirect Coombs' test at 38 weeks' gestation and her infant had a negative direct Coombs' test. What should the nurse know about these tests?
    1. Although her infant is Rh positive, she has no antibodies to the Rh factor. RhoGAM should be given.
    2. She has demonstrated antibodies to the Rh factor. She should not have any more children.
    3. She has formed antigens against the Rh factor. RhoGAM must be given to the infant.
    4. Because her infant is Rh positive, the Coombs' tests are meaningless.

115. An infant was born at 38 weeks' gestation to a heroin-addicted mother. At birth, the baby had Apgar scores of 5 at 1 minute and 6 at 5 minutes. Birth weight was at the 10th percentile for gestational age. What should the nurse include in the baby's plan of care?
    1. Administer methadone to diminish symptoms of heroin withdrawal.
    2. Promote parent-infant attachment by encouraging rooming-in.
    3. Observe for signs of jaundice because this is a common complication.
    4. Place in a quiet area of the nursery and swaddle close to promote more organized behavioral state.

116. A 36-week-gestation infant had tachypnea, nasal flaring, and intercostal retractions that increased over the first 6 hours of life. The baby was treated with IV fluids and oxygen. Which of the following assessments suggests to the nurse that the baby is improving?
    1. The baby has see-saw respirations with coarse breath sounds.
    2. The baby's respiratory rate is 50 and pulse is 136, no nasal flaring is observed.
    3. The baby has a pH of 6.97 and pO$_2$ of 61 on 40% oxygen.
    4. The baby has gained 150 grams in the 12 hours since birth.

117. You are caring for an infant. During your assessment you note a flattened philtrum, short palpebral fissures, and birth weight and head circumference below the fifth percentile for gestational age. The infant has a poor suck. Which of the following is the best interpretation of this data?
    1. Down's syndrome.
    2. Fetal alcohol syndrome.
    3. Turner's syndrome.
    4. Congenital syphilis.

118. A 2-week-old premature infant with abdominal distention, significant gastric aspirate prior to feeding, and bloody stools has also had episodes of apnea and bradycardia and temperature instability. What should the nurse include in the plan of care for this infant?
    1. Increase feeding frequency to every 2 hours.
    2. Place the infant on seizure precautions.
    3. Place the infant in strict isolation to prevent infection of other infants.
    4. Monitor infant carefully including blood pressure readings and measurements of abdominal girth.

119. A mother is taking her newborn home from the hospital at 18 hours after birth. As the nurse is giving discharge instructions, which response best validates her understanding of PKU testing?
    1. "I know you stuck my baby's heel today for that PKU test and that my doctor will recheck the test when I bring her for her 1 month appointment."
    2. "After I start my baby on cereal, I will return for a follow-up blood test."
    3. "I will have a visiting nurse come to the house each day for the first week to check the PKU test."
    4. "I will bring my baby back to the hospital or doctor's office to have a repeat PKU no later than 1 week from today."

## Answers and Rationales

106. **4.** Time is one of the most important criteria in differentiating physiologic from pathologic jaundice. Physiologic jaundice appears after 24 hours. When jaundice appears earlier, it may be pathologic.

107. **2.** The infant receiving phototherapy should have a covering put over his eyes to protect them from light.

**108. 1.** The baby's head should be kept covered. The head is the greatest source of heat loss.

**109. 1.** Tremors are symptoms of the neonatal hypoglycemia. The baby of a diabetic mother is at high risk for hypoglycemia because the infant's insulin levels are high before birth and continue to be high even though the infant has suddenly lost the influx of glucose. Immediate administration of IV glucose will be ordered for the infant.

**110. 3.** A birth weight of 1450 grams is the mean weight for an infant at 30 weeks' gestation, but falls within the 10–90th percentiles for infants between 29 and 33 weeks' gestation. The diminished muscle tone and extension of extremities at rest are also characteristic of this gestational age. The sole creases described are actually most characteristic of an infant between 32 and 34 weeks' gestation.

**111. 3.** Prolonged rupture of membranes places this premature infant at risk for sepsis. Frequent monitoring of vital signs, color, activity level, and overall behavior is particularly important because changes may provide early cues to a developing infection. Family interaction with the infant should always be a part of the nursing plan.

**112. 1.** Although hyperbilirubinemia is common in newborns, certain factors increase the likelihood of early appearance of visible jaundice. Cold stress, bruising at delivery, cephalhematoma, asphyxiation, prematurity, breastfeeding, and poor feeding are all factors that may lead to hyperbilirubinemia in otherwise normal infants.

**113. 2.** Erythroblastosis fetalis results when an Rh-negative woman makes antibodies against her Rh-positive fetus. The antibodies attack fetal red cells.

**114. 1.** Because the indirect and direct Coombs' tests were negative, antibodies to Rh have not developed. She should have RhoGAM to prevent antibody formation.

**115. 4.** Neonatal withdrawal is a common occurrence in heroin addiction. Placing the baby in a quiet area and swaddling may promote state organization and minimize some symptoms. Medication may be needed to control hyperirritability.

**116. 2.** The baby's respiratory rate and pulse are within normal limits and the nasal flaring is no longer present.

**117. 2.** Although a medical diagnosis cannot be made from the assessment data, all of the findings noted are commonly seen in infants with fetal alcohol syndrome.

**118. 4.** The infant's prematurity is the major risk factor for necrotizing enterocolitis, which affects 1–15% of all infants in NICU. Usual nonsurgical treatment includes antibiotic therapy, making the infant NPO, frequent monitoring, and respiratory and circulatory support as needed.

**119. 4.** One additional PKU test within the first week of life will validate whether PKU disease is present. The infant should have been on breast milk or formula for 48 hours prior to the test.

# Conditions of the Female Reproductive System

## INFERTILITY AND FERTILITY

### Infertility

#### General Information

A. Inability to conceive after at least 1 year of unprotected sexual relations

B. Inability to deliver a live infant after three consecutive pregnancies

C. For the male, inability to impregnate a female partner within the same conditions

D. May be primary (never been pregnant/never impregnated) or secondary (pregnant once, then unable to conceive or carry again)

E. Affects approximately 10–15% of all couples

F. Tests for infertility can include:
  1. For the female
     a. Examination of basal body temperature and cervical mucus and identification of time of ovulation
     b. Plasma progesterone level: assesses corpus luteum
     c. Hormone analysis: endocrine function

d. Endometrial biopsy: receptivity of endometrium
   e. Postcoital test: sperm placement and cervical mucus
   f. Hysterosalpingography: tubal patency/uterine cavity
   g. Rubin's test: tubal patency (uses carbon dioxide)
   h. Pelvic ultrasound: visualization of pelvic tissues
   i. Laparoscopy: visual assessment of pelvic/abdominal organs; performance of minor surgeries
2. For the male
   a. Sperm analysis: assesses composition, volume, motility, agglutination.
   b. There are fewer assessment tests as well as interventions and successes for male infertility.

## Medical Management

A. Infertility of female partner, causes and therapy
   1. Congenital anomalies (absence of organs, improperly formed or abnormal organs): surgical treatment may help in some situations but cannot replace absent structures.
   2. Irregular/absent ovulation (ovum released irregularly or not at all): endocrine therapy with clomiphene citrate (Clomid)/menotropins (Pergonal) may induce ovulation; risk of ovarian hyperstimulation and release of multiple ova.
   3. Tubal factors (fallopian tubes blocked or scarred from infection, surgery, endometriosis, neoplasms): treatment may include antibiotic therapy, surgery, hysterosalpingogram.
   4. Uterine conditions (endometrium unreceptive, infected): removal of an IUD, antibiotic therapy, or surgery may be helpful.
   5. Vaginal/cervical factors (hostile mucus, sperm allergies, altered pH due to infection): treatment with antibiotics, proper vaginal hygiene, or artificial insemination may be utilized.
B. Infertility of male partner, causes and therapy
   1. Impotence: may be helped by psychologic counseling/penile implants, medication.
   2. Low/abnormal sperm count (fewer than 20 million/mL semen, low motility, more than 40% abnormal forms): there is no good therapy, use of hormone replacement therapy has had little success.
   3. Varicocele (varicosity within spermatic cord): ligation may be successful.
   4. Infection in any area of the male reproductive system (may affect ability to impregnate): appropriate antibiotic therapy is advised.
   5. Social habits (use of nicotine, alcohol, other drugs; clothes that keep scrotal sac too close to warmth of body): changing these habits may reverse low/absent fertility.
C. Alternatives for infertile couples include
   1. Artificial insemination by husband or donor
   2. In vitro fertilization
   3. Adoption
   4. Surrogate parenting
   5. Embryo transfers
D. Accepting childlessness as a lifestyle may also be necessary; support groups (e.g., Resolve) may be helpful.

## Nursing Interventions

A. Assist with assessment including a complete history, physical exam, lab work, and tests for both partners.
B. Monitor psychologic reaction to infertility.
C. Support couple through procedures and tests.
D. Identify any existing abnormalities and provide couple with information about their condition(s).
E. Help couple acknowledge and express their feelings both separately and together.

# Control of Fertility

Voluntary prevention of conception through various means, some of which employ devices or medications.

## Methods of Conception Control

A. Natural methods
   1. Natural family planning
      a. Periodic abstinence from intercourse when ovulating
      b. Uses calculations intended to identify those days of the menstrual cycle when coitus is avoided.
         1) Basal body temperature: identification of temperature drop before ovulation, then rise past ovulation; identifies days on which coitus is avoided to avoid conception.
         2) Cervical mucus method: identification of changes in cervical mucus; when affected by estrogen and most conducive to penetration by sperm, cervical mucus is clear, stretchy, and slippery; when influenced by progesterone, cervical mucus is thick, cloudy, and sticky and does not allow sperm passage; coitus is avoided during days of estrogen-influenced mucus.
         3) Sympto-thermal: combination of basal body temperature and cervical mucus method to increase effectiveness.
   2. Coitus interruptus
      a. Withdrawal of the penis from the vagina before ejaculation.

    **b.** Not very safe; pre-ejaculatory fluids from Cowper's glands may contain live, motile sperm.

    **c.** Demands precise male control.

**B.** Chemical barriers

  **1.** Use of foams, creams, jellies, and vaginal suppositories designed to destroy the sperm or limit their motility

  **2.** Available without a prescription, widely used, especially in conjunction with the diaphragm and the condom

  **3.** Need to be placed in the vagina immediately before each act of intercourse; messy

  **4.** Some people may have allergic reaction to the chemicals

**C.** Mechanical barriers: diaphragm, condom, cervical cap, contraceptive sponge

  **1.** Diaphragm: shallow rubber dome fits over cervix, blocking passage of sperm through cervix

    **a.** Efficiency increased by use of chemical barrier as lubricant

    **b.** Woman needs to be measured for diaphragm, and refitted after childbirth or weight gain/loss of 10 lb

    **c.** Device needs to be left in place 6–8 hours after intercourse.

    **d.** Woman needs to practice insertion and removal, and to be taught how to check for holes in diaphragm, store in cool place.

  **2.** Condom: thin stretchable rubber sheath worn over penis during intercourse

    **a.** Widely available without prescription

    **b.** Applied with room at tip to accommodate ejaculate

    **c.** Applied to erect penis before vaginal penetration

    **d.** Man is instructed to hold on to rim of condom as he withdraws from female to prevent spilling semen.

  **3.** Cervical cap: cup-shaped device that is placed over cervical os and held in place by suction.

    **a.** Four sizes; client needs to be fitted

    **b.** Women need to practice insertion and removal

    **c.** Spermicidals increase effectiveness

    **d.** May be left in place for up to 24 hours

  **4.** Contraceptive sponge: small, soft insert, with indentation on one side to fit over cervix; contains spermicide

    **a.** Moistened with water and inserted with indentation snugly against cervix

    **b.** May be left in place up to 24 hours

    **c.** No professional fitting required

    **d.** May also protect against STDs

    **e.** Should not be used by women with history of toxic shock syndrome

    **f.** Problems include cost, difficulty in removal, and irritation

**D.** Hormone therapy (oral contraceptives, birth control pills)

  **1.** Ingestion of estrogen and progesterone on a specific schedule to prevent the release of FSH and LH, thus preventing ovulation and pregnancy.

  **2.** Causes additional tubal, endometrial, and cervical mucus changes.

  **3.** Available in combined or sequential types.

  **4.** Usually taken beginning on day 5 of the menstrual cycle through day 25, then discontinued.

  **5.** Withdrawal bleeding occurs within 2–3 days.

  **6.** Contraindications

    **a.** History of hypertension or vascular disorders

    **b.** Age over 35

    **c.** Cigarette smoking (heavy)

  **7.** Women using oral contraceptives need to be sure to get sufficient amounts of vitamin B as metabolism of this vitamin is affected.

  **8.** Minor side effects may include

    **a.** Weight gain

    **b.** Breast changes

    **c.** Headaches

    **d.** Vaginal spotting

  **9.** Report vision changes/disorders immediately.

**E.** Intrauterine devices (IUD)

  **1.** Placement of plastic or nonreactive device into uterine cavity

  **2.** Mode of action thought to be the creation of a sterile endometrial inflammation, discourages implantation (nidation).

  **3.** Does not affect ovulation.

  **4.** Device is inserted during or just after menstruation, while cervix is slightly open.

  **5.** May cause cramping and heavy bleeding during menses for several months after insertion.

  **6.** Tail of IUD hangs into vagina through cervix; woman taught to feel for it before intercourse and after each menses.

  **7.** A distinct disadvantage is the increased risk of pelvic infection (PID) with use of the IUD.

**F.** Surgical sterilization

  **1.** Bilateral tubal ligation in the female to prevent the passage of ova.

  **2.** Bilateral vasectomy in the male to prevent the passage of sperm.

  **3.** Both of these operations should be considered permanent.

  **4.** Female will still menstruate but will not conceive.

  **5.** Male will be incapable of fertilizing his partner after all viable sperm ejaculated from vas deferens (6 weeks or 10 ejaculations).

  **6.** There should be no effect on male capacity for erection or penetration.

  **7.** Hysterectomy also causes permanent sterility in the female.

**G.** Steroid implants: approved in 1990 by FDA; biodegradable rods containing sustained-release, low-dose progesterone. Inhibits LH (luteinizing hormone) release necessary for ovulation. Effective over 5-year time frame. Need minor surgical procedure for insertion and removal. Removal causes total reversibility of effect.

H. Injectable progestin–same action as G; lasts 3 months

## Nursing Responsibilities in Control of Fertility

A. Assess previous experience of couple or individual.
B. Obtain health history and perform physical examination.
C. Identify present needs for contraception.
D. Determine motivation regarding contraception.
E. Assist the client/couple in receiving information desired; advise about the various methods available.
F. Ensure that client/couple selects method best suited to their needs.
   1. Support choice of client/couple as right for them.
   2. Provide time for practice with method chosen, if applicable.
   3. Instruct in side effects/potential complications.
G. Encourage expression of feelings about contraception.

# Termination of Pregnancy

## General Information

A. Deliberate interruption of a pregnancy in a previable time. Legal in all states since Supreme Court ruling of January 1973, as follows
   1. First trimester: determined by pregnant woman and her physician.
   2. Second trimester: determined by pregnant woman and her physician; state can regulate the circumstances to ensure safety.
   3. Third trimester: conditions determined by state law.
B. Indications may be physical or psychologic, socioeconomic or genetic.
C. Techniques vary according to trimester.
   1. First trimester: vacuum extraction or dilation and curettage (D&C)
      a. Cervix dilated
      b. Products of conception either aspirated or scraped out
      c. Procedure is short, usually well tolerated by client, and has few complications.
   2. Second trimester
      a. Saline abortion
         1) Amniotic fluid aspirated from uterus, replaced with same amount 20% saline solution.
         2) Contractions begin in 12–24 hours; may be induced by oxytocin (Pitocin)
         3) Client is hospitalized; infection or hypernatremia possible complications

      b. Prostaglandins
         1) Injection of prostaglandin into uterus
         2) Contractions initiated in under 1 hour
         3) Side effects may include nausea and vomiting
      c. Hysterotomy
         1) Incision into uterus to remove fetus.
         2) May also be used for sterilization.
         3) Client is hospitalized.
         4) Care is similar to that for cesarean birth.
   3. Third trimester: same as second trimester, if permitted by state law.

## Assessment

A. Vaginal bleeding
B. Vital signs
C. Excessive cramping

## Analysis

A. Risk for deficient fluid volume
B. Risk for injury
C. Deficient knowledge

## Planning and Implementation

A. Goals
   1. Recovery from procedure will be free from complications.
   2. Client will be supported in her decision.
B. Interventions
   1. Explain procedure to client.
   2. Administer medications as ordered.
   3. Assist with procedure as needed.
   4. Monitor client carefully during procedure.
   5. Monitor client postprocedure.
   6. Administer postprocedure medications as ordered (analgesics, antibiotics, oxytocins, RhoGAM if mother Rh negative).
   7. Provide contraceptive information as appropriate.
   8. May need post-abortion counseling/therapy (also available at Crisis Pregnancy Centers).

## Evaluation

A. Procedure tolerated without complications; vital signs stable, no hemorrhage, products of conception evacuated, no infection
B. Client supported through procedure; emotionally stable

# MENSTRUAL DISORDERS

Menstruation is the periodic shedding of the endometrium when there has been no conception. Onset is menarche (age 11–14); cessation is menopause (average age 50).

## Assessment

A. Menstrual cycle for symptoms and pattern
B. Client discomfort with cycles
C. Knowledge base about menses

## Analysis

A. Deficient knowledge
B. Ineffective health maintenance

## Planning and Implementation

A. Goals
   1. Client will receive necessary information.
   2. Client will choose treatment/options best suited to her needs.
B. Interventions
   1. Explain menstrual physiology to client.
   2. Explain options for treatment to client.
   3. Provide time for questions.
   4. Reinforce good menstrual hygiene.
   5. Administer medications if ordered.

## Evaluation

Client demonstrates knowledge of condition and treatment options.

## Specific Disorders

### Dysmenorrhea

A. Pain associated with menstruation.
B. Usually associated with ovulatory cycles; absent when ovulation suppressed.
C. Intensified by stress, cultural factors, and presence of an IUD.
D. High levels of prostaglandins found in menstrual flow of women with dysmenorrhea.
E. Treatment my include rest, application of heat, distraction, exercise, analgesia (especially anti-prostaglandins: NSAIDs).

### Amenorrhea

A. Absence of menstruation.
B. Possibly caused by underlying abnormality of endocrine system, rapid weight loss, or strenuous exercise.
C. Treatment is individualized by cause.

### Menorrhagia

A. Excessive menstrual flow
B. Possibly caused by endocrine imbalance, uterine tumors, infection
C. Treatment individualized by cause

### Metrorrhagia

A. Intercyclic bleeding
B. Frequently the result of a disease process
C. Treatment individualized by cause

### Endometriosis

See Figure 6-13.
A. Endometrial tissue is found outside the uterus, attached to the ovaries, colon, round ligaments, etc.
B. This tissue reacts to the endocrine stimulation cycle as does the intrauterine endometrium, resulting in inflammation of the extrauterine sites, with pain and fibrosis/scar tissue formation as the eventual result.
C. Actual cause is unknown.
D. May cause dysmenorrhea, dyspareunia, and infertility.
E. Treatment may include the use of oral contraceptives to minimize endometrial buildup or medications to suppress menstruation (Danocrine, Synarel).
F. Pregnancy and lactation may also be recommended as means to suppress menstruation.
G. Surgical intervention (removal of endometrial implants) may be helpful.
H. Hysterectomy and salpingo-oophorectomy are curative.

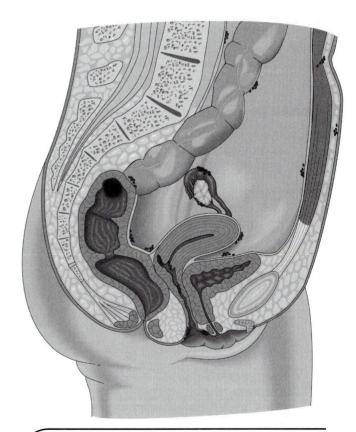

**Figure 6-13** Endometriosis can be found outside the uterus, attached to the ovaries, colon, and round ligaments

# INFECTIOUS DISORDERS

## Sexually Transmitted Diseases (STD)

Infections occurring predominantly in the genital area and spread by sexual relations.

### Assessment

A. Sexual history/social practices
B. Physical examination for signs and symptoms of specific disorder

### Analysis

A. Deficient knowledge
B. Risk for injury
C. Ineffective health maintenance

### Planning and Implementation

A. Goals
   1. Disease process will be identified and treated.
   2. Affected others will be identified and treated.
   3. Complications will be prevented.
B. Interventions
   1. Collect specimens for tests.
   2. Implement isolation technique if indicated.
   3. Teach transmission/prevention techniques.
   4. Assist in case finding.
   5. Administer medications as ordered.
   6. Inform client of any necessary lifestyle changes.

### Evaluation

A. Client receiving treatment appropriate to specific disorder, understands treatment regimen.
B. Client demonstrates knowledge of disease process and transmission.
C. Affected others have been identified and treated.

## Specific Disorders

### Herpes

A. Genital herpes is caused by herpes simplex virus type 2 ($HSV_2$).
B. Causes painful vesicles on genitalia, both external and internal.
C. There is no cure.
D. Treatment is symptomatic.
E. If active infection at the end of pregnancy, cesarean birth may be indicated, because virus may be lethal to neonate who cannot localize infection.
F. Recurrences of the condition may be caused by infection, stress, menses.
G. Acyclovir (Zovirax) reduces severity and duration of exacerbation.

### Chlamydia

A. Currently most common STD
B. Symptoms similar to gonorrhea (cervical/vaginal discharge) or may be asymptomatic
C. Can be transmitted to fetus at birth, causes neonatal ophthalmia
D. Treated with erythromycin, prophylactic treatment of neonate's eyes
E. If untreated, can lead to pelvic inflammatory disease (PID)
F. Receive regular PAP smears.

### Gonorrhea

A. Caused by *Neisseria gonorrhoeae*.
B. Symptoms may include heavy, purulent vaginal discharge, but often asymptomatic in female.
C. May be passed to fetus at time of birth, causing ophthalmia neonatorum and sepsis.
D. Treatment is penicillin; allergic clients may be treated with erythromycin or (if not pregnant) the cephalosporins.
E. All sexual contacts must be treated as well, to prevent "ping-pong" recurrence.

### Syphilis

A. Caused by *Treponema pallidum* (spirochete)
B. Crosses placenta after 16th week of pregnancy to infect fetus.
C. Initial symptoms are chancre and lymph-adenopathy and may disappear without treatment in 4–6 weeks.
D. Secondary symptoms are rash, malaise, and alopecia; these too may disappear in several weeks without treatment.
E. Tertiary syphilis may recur later in life and affect any organ system, especially cardiovascular and neurologic systems.
F. Diagnosis is made by dark-field exam and serologic tests (VDRL).
G. Treatment is penicillin, or erythromycin if penicillin allergy exists.

## Other Genital Infections

Cervical and vaginal infections may be caused by agents other than those associated with STDs. For all female clients with a vaginal infection, nursing actions should include teaching good perineal hygiene.

### Trichomonas vaginalis

A. Caused by a protozoan
B. Major symptom is profuse foamy white to greenish discharge that is irritating to genitalia.
C. Treatment is metronidazole (Flagyl) for woman and all sexual partners.

**D.** Treatment lasts 7 days, during which time a condom should be used for intercourse.

**E.** Alcohol ingestion with Flagyl causes severe gastrointestinal upset.

## *Candida albicans*

**A.** Caused by a yeast transmitted from GI tract to vagina.

**B.** Overgrowth may occur in pregnancy, with diabetes, and with steroid or antibiotic therapy.

**C.** Vaginal examination reveals thick, white, cheesy patches on vaginal walls.

**D.** Treatment is topical application of clotrimazole (Gyne-Lotrimin), nystatin (Mycostatin), or gentian violet.

**E.** *Candida albicans* causes thrush in the newborn by direct contact in the birth canal.

## *Bacterial Vaginitis*

**A.** Caused by other bacteria invading the vagina

**B.** Foul or fishy-smelling discharge

**C.** Treatment is specific to causative agent, and usually includes sexual partners for best results

## *AIDS (see Unit 4)*

## Female Reproductive System Neoplasia

The nursing diagnoses, general goals and interventions, and evaluation for the client with cancer of the reproductive system are similar to those for any client with a diagnosis of cancer. Only nursing care specific to the disorder will be discussed here.

## Fibrocystic Breast Disease

**A.** Most common benign breast lesion.

**B.** Cyst(s) may be palpated; surgical biopsy indicated for differential diagnosis.

**C.** Treatment includes surgical removal of cysts, decreasing or removing caffeine from diet, and medication to suppress menses.

## Procedure for Breast Self-Examination (BSE)

**A.** Age: routine BSE should begin as early in a woman's life as possible. Adolescence is not too early.

**B.** Timing: regularly, on a monthly basis, 3 to 7 days after the end of the menses, when breasts are least likely to be swollen or tender. After menopause, BSE should be done on one particular day/date every month.

**C.** Procedure
   1. Inspection: stand before mirror and visually inspect with arms at sides; raised over head; hands on hips with muscles tightened; then leaning forward. Assessment should include size, symmetry, shape, direction, color, skin texture and thickness, nipple size and shape, rashes or discharges. Unusual findings should be reported to health care provider.
   2. Palpation: to examine left breast, woman should be lying down, with left hand behind head and small folded towel or pillow under left shoulder. Using flattened fingertips of right hand and a rotary motion, palpate along lines of concentric circles from outer edges of breast to nipple area, or from outer edge to nipple area following wedge or wheel-spoke lines. Also palpate in the left axillary area where multiple lymph nodes are present, as well as a "tail" of breast tissue. The nipple should be gently squeezed to assess for discharges.
       **a.** To examine right breast, positions are reversed.
       **b.** Palpation activities are repeated for each breast with the woman in the sitting position.
       **c.** Unusual findings are reported to the health care provider.
       **d.** Breast self-examination (BSE) and mammograms as indicated by age and risk are primary screening tools.

## Breast Cancer

**A.** General information
   1. Most common neoplasm in women
   2. Leading cause of death in women age 40–44

**B.** Medical management
   1. Usually surgical excision; options are simple lumpectomy, simple mastectomy, modified radical mastectomy, and radical mastectomy.
   2. Adjuvant treatment with chemotherapy, radiation, and hormone therapy.

**C.** Assessment findings
   1. Palpation of lump (upper outer quadrant most frequent site) usually first symptom
   2. Skin of breast dimpled
   3. Nipple discharge
   4. Asymmetry of breasts
   5. Surgical biopsy provides definitive diagnosis

**D.** Nursing interventions
   1. Assess breasts for early identification and treatment.
   2. Support client through recommended/chosen treatment.
   3. Prepare client for mastectomy if necessary.

## Mastectomy

**A.** General information
   1. Lumpectomy: removal of lump and surrounding breast tissue; lymph nodes biopsied.
   2. Simple mastectomy: removal of breast only, lymph nodes biopsied.

3. Radical mastectomy: removal of breast, muscle layer down to chest wall, and axillary lymph nodes.

B. Nursing interventions
   1. Provide routine pre- and post-op care.
   2. Elevate client's arm on operative side on pillows to minimize edema.
   3. Do not use arm on affected side for blood pressure measurements, IVs, or injections.
   4. Turn only to back and unaffected side.
   5. Monitor client for bleeding, check under her.
   6. Begin range-of-motion exercises immediately on unaffected side.
   7. Start with simple movements on affected side: fingers and hands first, then wrist, elbow, and shoulder movements.
   8. Make abduction the last movement.
   9. Coordinate physical therapy if ordered.
   10. Teach client about any necessary life-style changes (special care of arm on affected side, monthly breast self-examination on remaining breast, use of prosthesis).
   11. Encourage/arrange visit from support group member.

C. Medical therapy
   1. Hormonal therapy: tamoxifen, anti-estrogen effect.
   2. Chemotherapy
   3. Radiation
   4. Chemotherapy and radiation used with lumpectomy

## Cancer of the Cervix

A. Detected by Pap smear, followed by tissue biopsy.
   1. Class I—normal pap smear
   2. Class II—atypical cells
   3. Class III—moderate dysplasia
   4. Class IV—severe dysplasia, cancer-in-situ
   5. Class V—Squamous cell carcinoma, invasive cancer

B. Preinvasive conditions may be treated by colposcopy, cryosurgery, laser surgery, cervical conization, or hysterectomy.

C. Invasive conditions are treated by radium therapy and radical hysterectomy.

## Cancer of the Uterus

A. May affect endometrium or fundus/corpus risk increased by unopposed estrogen.

B. Cardinal symptom: abnormal uterine bleeding, either pre- or postmenopause

C. Diagnosis: by endometrial biopsy or fractional curettage; cells washed from uterus under pressure may also be used for diagnosis

D. Usual intervention: total hysterectomy and bilateral salpingo-oophorectomy

E. Radium therapy and chemotherapy may also be used.

## Cancer of the Ovary

A. Etiology unknown.

B. Few early symptoms; palpation of ovarian mass is usual first finding.

C. Treatment of choice is surgical removal with total hysterectomy and bilateral salpingo-oophorectomy.

D. Chemotherapy may be used as adjuvant therapy.

## Cancer of the Vulva

A. Begins as small, pruritic lesions

B. Diagnosed by biopsy

C. Treatment is either local excision or radical vulvectomy (removal of entire vulva plus superficial and femoral nodes).

## Hysterectomy

A. General information
   1. Total hysterectomy: removal of uterine body and cervix only
   2. Subtotal hysterectomy: removal of uterine body leaving cervix in place (seldom performed)
   3. Total abdominal hysterectomy with bilateral salpingo-oophorectomy (TAH-BSO): removal of uterine body, cervix, both ovaries, and both fallopian tubes
   4. Radical hysterectomy: removal of uterine body, cervix, connective tissue, part of vagina, and pelvic lymph nodes

B. Nursing interventions
   1. Institute routine pre- and post-op care.
   2. Assess for hemorrhage, infection, or other postsurgical complications (e.g., paralytic ileus, thrombophlebitis, pneumonia).
   3. Support woman and family through procedure, encourage expression of feelings and reactions to procedure.
   4. Explain implications of hysterectomy.
      a. No further menses.
      b. If ovaries also removed, will have menopause and may need estrogen replacement therapy.
      c. Woman will be sterile after surgery; form signed by client stating awareness of not being able to become pregnant after hysterectomy.
   5. Allow woman (and partner) to verbalize concerns about sexuality postsurgery.
   6. Provide discharge teaching.

## Menopause

The time in a woman's life when menstruation ceases. Fertility usually ceases, and symptoms associated with changing hormone levels may occur. Reactions to menopause may be influenced by culture, age at menopause, reproductive and menstrual history, and complications.

## Assessment Findings

A. Symptoms related to hormone changes
 1. Vasomotor instability (hot flashes and night sweats)
 2. Emotional disturbances (mood swings, irritability, depression), fatigue, and headache
B. Physical changes include
 1. Atrophy of genitalia
 2. Dyspareunia
 3. Urinary changes (frequency/stress incontinence)
 4. Constipation
 5. Possibly uterine prolapse

## Interventions

A. Estrogen replacement therapy (ERT); many controversial issues
 1. Used to control symptoms, especially vasomotor instability and vaginal atrophy, and to prevent osteoporosis
 2. Women with family histories of breast or uterine cancer, hypertension, thrombophlebitis, or cardiac dysfunction are not good candidates for ERT.
 3. Women may need information about contraception, as ovulation and ability to conceive may continue for up to 12 months after menses cease.
 4. Sold under many pharmaceutical trade names; may be taken orally, or applied transdermally (patch).
 5. Women who still have a uterus must take progesterone to decrease risk of endometrial cancer. New studies have shown long-term use carries serious risk.
B. Alternatives to ERT include:
 1. Vitamin E: from dietary sources and supplements
 2. Herbs: varied relief with combinations of roots and herbs, such as licorice and dandelion
 3. Other medications: Bellergal (phenobarbital, ergotamine tartrate, and belladonna)
 4. Kegel exercises for genital atrophy: alternating constriction and relaxation of pubococcygeal muscles (muscles controlling the flow of urine) done at least three times/day
 5. Vaginal lubricants for genital atrophy: water-soluble lubricants can diminish dyspareunia
 6. Maintenance of good hydration: at least 8 glasses of water/day
 7. Good perineal hygiene

## Complications of Menopause
### Osteoporosis

A. Increased porosity of the bone, with increased incidence of spontaneous fractures.

B. Other symptoms in the postmenopausal woman include loss of height, back pain, and dowager's hump.
C. Diagnosis by X-ray is not possible until more than 50% of bone mass has already been lost.
D. Decreased bone porosity is inextricably linked with lowered levels of estrogen in the postmenopausal woman. Estrogen plays a part in the absorption of calcium and the stimulation of osteoclasts (new-bone-forming cells).
E. Treatment includes
 1. ERT unless contraindicated
 2. Supplemental calcium to slow the osteoporotic process (1 g taken daily at HS)
 3. Increased fluid intake (2–3 liters/day will help avoid formation of calculi)
 4. High-calcium/high-phosphorus diet with avoidance of excess protein
 5. Some exercise on a regular basis
F. Prevention includes:
 1. Not smoking
 2. Regular weight-bearing exercise
 3. Good nutrition, including sources of calcium and vitamin D
 4. Minimal use or exclusion of alcohol
 5. Regular physical examination

### Cystocele/Rectocele

A. Herniations of the anterior and posterior (respectively) walls of the vagina.
B. Usually the sequelae of childbirth injuries.
C. Herniation allows the bulging of the bladder and the rectum into the vagina.
D. Treatment is surgical repair of these conditions: anterior and posterior *colporrhaphy.*

### Prolapse of the Uterus

A. Usually the result of childbirth injuries or relaxation of the cardinal ligaments.
B. Allows the uterus to sag backward and downward into the vagina, or outside the body completely.
C. Vaginal hysterectomy is the preferred surgical intervention.
D. If condition does not warrant surgery, the insertion of a *pessary* (supportive device) will help to support and stabilize the uterus.

 **Sample Questions**

120. In collecting data for a health history of an infertility client, which of the following findings is most important?
 1. She is 5 ft 8 in tall and weighs 105 lb.
 2. She has never used any form of contraception.

3. She has been married for 3 years.

4. She has no brothers or sisters.

121. What teaching should be included to a woman who has just been fitted with her first diaphragm?
    1. Specific amount of spermicide to be used with diaphragm.
    2. Insertion at least 8 hours before intercourse.
    3. Specific cleaning techniques.
    4. Storage in the refrigerator.

122. A postmenopausal woman takes calcium supplements on a daily basis. What instruction should be given the woman to reduce the danger of renal calculi?
    1. Chewing her calcium tablets rather than swallowing them whole.
    2. Swallowing her calcium tablets with cranberry juice.
    3. Eliminating other sources of calcium from her diet.
    4. Drinking 2–3 quarts of water daily.

123. A postmenopausal woman is having a routine physical exam. Which of the following assessments would yield critical information as to her postmenopausal status?
    1. Asking about weight loss of more than 5 lb in the last year.
    2. Asking about her nightly sleep patterns.
    3. Asking about her cultural background.
    4. Asking about her last pregnancy.

124. A woman is admitted to the hospital for a panhysterectomy. Which nursing strategy should be included in the nursing care plan to meet her body-image perception changes?
    1. Allowing her time to work out her feelings on her own.
    2. Discouraging fears about weight gain.
    3. Helping her verbalize her concerns about her femininity.
    4. Insisting that she look at the scar.

125. Following a panhysterectomy, the woman is placed on estrogen replacement therapy. What is the primary purpose of estrogen replacement therapy following surgical menopause?
    1. Arthritis.
    2. Pregnancy.
    3. Breast cancer.
    4. Vasomotor instability.

126. A woman has advanced cancer of the breast. She is admitted to the medical unit for nutritional evaluation. She weighs 101 lb and is 5 ft 8 in tall. She is started on leucovorin (Wellcovorin). Which of the following would not be included in the assessment of her nutritional health?
    1. A diet history.
    2. Anthropometric measurements.
    3. Food preferences.
    4. Serum protein studies.

127. What is the nurse's primary role in relation to sexually transmitted disease?
    1. Case reporting.
    2. Sexual counseling.
    3. Diagnosis and treatment.
    4. Recognizing symptoms and teaching clients.

128. A female teen visits the local health clinic because her boyfriend was recently diagnosed as having gonorrhea. She asks the nurse about possible consequences if she went without treatment. What would be an appropriate answer?
    1. Disseminated systemic infections.
    2. Minor problems such as skin rashes.
    3. The need for delivery by cesarean section.
    4. Sterility, birth defects, and miscarriage.

129. Several adolescent girls are discussing sexual activity with the nurse at the STD clinic. Which comment indicates to the nurse that the client has not understood the teaching regarding safe sexual practices?
    1. "We use KY jelly on condoms."
    2. "I douche after intercourse."
    3. "I shower with my boyfriend."
    4. "We use condoms and birth control pills."

130. When discussing safe sex, which information about the use of condoms would be most helpful?
    1. Lambskin condoms do not interfere with sensation.
    2. Latex condoms help prevent the transmission of germs.
    3. Condoms are often inconvenient and unnecessary.
    4. Condoms prevent STDs but they are a poor choice for birth control.

131. A couple have come to your clinic because they have not been able to achieve a pregnancy after trying for 2 years without using any form of birth control. Which of the following tests could

determine that the woman is ovulating regularly?

1. Hysterosalpingogram.
2. Serial basal body temperature graph.
3. Postcoital test.
4. Semen analysis.

132. A woman is preparing to take Clomid to induce ovulation so she can have an in vitro fertilization. She asks if she should expect any side effects from the drug. Your *best* answer should include which of the following?

1. Weight gain with increased appetite and constipation.
2. Tingling of the hands and feet.
3. Alopecia (hair loss).
4. Stuffy nose and cold-like symptoms.

133. A couple have been using a diaphragm for contraception. Which of the following statements indicates they are using it correctly?

1. "We use K-Y jelly around the rim to help with insertion."
2. "I wash the diaphragm each time and hold it up to the light to look for any holes."
3. "I take the diaphragm out about 1 hour after intercourse because it feels funny."
4. "I douche right away after intercourse."

134. A 25-year-old wishes to take oral contraceptives. When taking her history, which of the following questions would determine whether she is an appropriate candidate for this form of birth control?

1. "Do you currently smoke cigarettes and, if so, how many?"
2. "Have you had any recent weight gain or loss?"
3. "Do you douche regularly after intercourse?"
4. "Is there any family history of kidney or gallbladder disease?"

135. A woman who is 18 weeks' pregnant is scheduled for a saline injection to terminate her pregnancy. She asks the nurse what she should expect. What would be the nurse's *best* answer?

1. "Contractions will begin immediately after the instillation of saline and will be mild."
2. "An amniocentesis will be performed with amniotic fluid removal and saline replacement."
3. "A tube will be inserted through the cervix and warm saline will be administered by continuous drip."
4. "The baby will be born alive but will die a short time later."

136. A woman comes to the office complaining of the following symptoms: fatigue, weight gain, pelvic pain related to menstruation, heartburn, and constipation. Which of the above symptoms might indicate a diagnosis of endometriosis?

1. Weight gain and fatigue.
2. Heartburn.
3. Constipation.
4. Pelvic pain related to menstruation.

137. A woman has been diagnosed with *Candida albicans*. Which of the following types of vaginal discharge would you expect to find?

1. Thin, greenish yellow with a foul odor.
2. Either a yellowish discharge or none at all.
3. Thick and white, like cottage cheese.
4. Thin, grayish white with a fishy odor.

138. A woman has just been diagnosed with genital herpes for the first time. You can expect which of the following treatments to be part of her plan of care?

1. Vaginal soaks with saline to keep the area moist.
2. Acyclovir 200 mg 5 times daily for 7–10 days.
3. Ceftriaxone 125 mg IM times 1 dose.
4. Topical application of podophyllin to the lesions.

139. A woman is 10 weeks' pregnant and tested positive for syphilis but has no symptoms. She asks you why she needs to be treated since she feels fine? Your *best* response to her would include which of the following?

1. "Syphilis can be transmitted to the baby and may cause it to die before birth if you are not treated."
2. "If you do not receive treatment before the baby is born, your baby could become blind."
3. "If syphilis is untreated, the baby may be mentally retarded at birth."
4. "Syphilis may cause your baby to have a heart problem when it is born."

140. A woman has been diagnosed with fibrocystic breast disease. Which of the following should be included in the teaching plan for her?

1. Limiting breast self-examinations to every 3 months because it may be painful.
2. Wearing a bra as little as possible because pressure on the breast may be painful.
3. Limiting caffeine and salt intake.
4. Using heat to the tender areas of the breast.

141. The local YWCA is having a series of seminars on health-related topics. You are invited to discuss breast self-examination (BSE) with the group. Which of the following would be appropriate to teach regarding when BSE should be performed by women of reproductive age?

1. At the end of each menstrual cycle.

2. At the beginning of each menstrual cycle.

3. About 7–10 days after the beginning of each menstrual cycle.

4. About 7–10 days before the end of the menstrual cycle.

142. You have been discussing breast self-examination (BSE) with a woman. Which of the following statements would *best* indicate she is doing BSE correctly?

1. "I begin to examine my breasts by placing the palm of my right hand on the nipple of the left breast."

2. "I don't like to press very hard because my breasts are very tender."

3. "I use the tips of the middle three fingers of each hand to feel each breast."

4. "I feel for lumps in my breasts standing in front of a mirror."

143. A woman had a simple mastectomy this morning. Which of the following should be included in your plan for her care?

1. Complete bed rest for the first 24 hours.

2. NPO with IV fluids for the first 48 hours.

3. Positioning on the operative side for the first 24 hours.

4. Keep patient-controlled anesthesia (PCA) controller within easy reach for the first 48 hours.

144. The nurse is teaching a woman who had a simple mastectomy. Which of the following would be appropriate to tell her?

1. She should wait to be fitted for a permanent prosthesis until the wound is completely healed.

2. Because she had a simple mastectomy, she will probably not feel the need to attend Reach for Recovery meetings.

3. She will have very little pain and the incision will heal very quickly.

4. She should refrain from seeking male companionship because she will be seen as less than a woman.

145. A group of women have gathered at the local library for a series of seminars about women's

health issues. In discussing cancer of the cervix, which of the following would be accurate?

1. This cancer is very rapid growing, so early detection is difficult to achieve.

2. A cervical biopsy is the screening test of choice for early detection of cervical cancer.

3. All women have an equal chance to develop cervical cancer because there are no high risk factors.

4. An annual Pap smear may detect cervical dysplasia, a frequent precursor of cervical cancer.

146. The nurse is talking to a woman who has been diagnosed with cancer of the ovary. She asks you what she could have done so that the cancer would have been found earlier. The best response should include which of the following?

1. She should have had more frequent, twice a year, Pap smears.

2. A yearly complete blood count (CBC) could have provided valuable clues to detect ovarian cancer.

3. Detection of ovarian cancer is easier if a yearly proctoscopy is done.

4. There is little more she could have done for earlier detection.

147. The nurse is caring for a woman who has had a vaginal hysterectomy and has an indwelling Foley catheter. After removal of the catheter, she is unable to void and has little sensation of bladder fullness. She is also constipated and is experiencing some perineal pain. Using a 2-part nursing diagnosis statement, which of the following would be appropriately paired with a diagnosis of altered urinary elimination?

1. Infection as evidenced by inability to void with frequency and urgency.

2. Retention as evidenced by inability to void and urinary distention.

3. Gastrointestinal functioning as evidenced by inability to void and constipation.

4. Dysuria as evidenced by inability to void and loss of bladder sensation.

148. A 42-year-old had a simple vaginal hysterectomy without oophorectomy due to uterine fibroids. You have completed your discharge teaching and she is preparing to go home. Which of the following statements indicates she understands the physical changes she will experience?

1. "I hope my husband will still love me since we can't have sexual intercourse anymore."
2. "I was hoping to stop having periods, but I guess that will need to wait a few more years."
3. "It will be so nice to not need to use birth control anymore."
4. "I just don't think I will ever feel feminine again since I can no longer experience orgasm."

149. The nurse has been discussing menopause with a 50-year-old woman who is experiencing some bodily changes indicative of the perimenopausal period. Which of the following statements indicates the client understands what is happening to her body?
    1. "Even though I am only having periods every few months, I should continue to use birth control until at least 6 months after my periods have stopped."
    2. "I am very upset to think that I will continue to have these hot flashes for the rest of my life."
    3. "Now that I am an old woman, I guess I'll be sick most of the time, so I should plan to move to a retirement home."
    4. "I may continue to bleed on and off throughout the next 25 years."

150. A 55-year-old woman who has ceased having menses has a family history of osteoporosis and increasing cholesterol levels over the past several years. Hormone replacement therapy (HRT) has been prescribed with estrogen and progesterone. She asks you why she should take the pills since she feels quite well. The nurse's answer would be:
    1. HRT is thought to help protect women from heart disease and osteoporosis.
    2. HRT will help to reestablish the menstrual cycle, thus providing natural protection against heart disease and osteoporosis.
    3. Even though she feels well now, she will soon begin having major health problems and HRT will protect her against those problems.
    4. She will be protected from breast cancer by HRT.

## Answers and Rationales

120. **1.** Because of the complex interaction between the hypothalamus, the ovary, and the amount of body fat, women who are underweight or who engage in strenuous physical activity over prolonged periods of time may experience changes in their menstrual cycle and their fertility.

121. **3.** The client must be instructed to clean the diaphragm with mild, plain soap, and warm water; dust it lightly with cornstarch; and store it in a cool, dry place. She should also be instructed to check it regularly for perforations or defects.

122. **4.** The ingestion of sufficient amounts of water by a woman taking calcium supplements is important to prevent renal calculi.

123. **2.** Postmenopausal women who are experiencing vasomotor instability may have night sweats and interrupted sleep.

124. **3.** Loss of the organs of reproduction are often equated with a loss of femininity. The client should be encouraged to explore her feelings and to adapt to body changes.

125. **4.** Low-dose estrogen therapy is used to relieve the vasomotor symptoms of menopausal women.

126. **3.** Food preferences are considered when planning a program to meet the client's nutritional requirement after the nutritional assessment has been completed.

127. **4.** Early recognition of sexually transmitted diseases (STDs) reduces the risk of serious sequelae. The primary role of the nurse is to recognize symptoms of STDs in order to teach clients how to comply with treatment and how to prevent reinfection.

128. **4.** Lack of treatment or inadequate treatment of gonorrhea can result in serious sequelae such as sterility, birth defects, and miscarriage. These are the most common complications and the ones most important to discuss.

129. **2.** Douching does not protect against infection and damages the natural protective barriers.

130. **2.** Condoms can prevent the transmission of many STDs. This information is very important to give.

131. **2.** Serial basal body temperature graphs are a baseline for determining when ovulation has taken place during a menstrual cycle. If ovulation has occurred, the temperature will be higher the second half of the cycle and lower the first half.

**132. 1.** Weight gain associated with increased appetite and constipation are fairly common side effects of Clomid.

**133. 2.** The diaphragm should be washed and dried and inspected for holes before being put away.

**134. 1.** Cigarette smoking significantly increases a woman's risk for circulatory complications and may contraindicate oral contraceptive use.

**135. 2.** The procedure begins with an amniocentesis where amniotic fluid is withdrawn and replaced with saline solution.

**136. 4.** Pelvic pain related to menstruation is the most common symptom of endometriosis. The pain usually ends following cessation of menses.

**137. 3.** Thick, white cottage cheese-like discharge is consistent with *Candida albicans*.

**138. 2.** This is the correct drug and dosage for an initial infection of genital herpes.

**139. 1.** Syphilis is associated with stillbirth, premature birth, and neonatal death.

**140. 3.** Most women benefit from caffeine and salt restriction because this reduces fluid retention and increases comfort.

**141. 3.** The breasts are softer, less tender, and swelling is reduced about a week after the beginning of the menstrual cycle.

**142. 3.** The ends of the three middle fingers are the most sensitive and should be used for BSE.

**143. 4.** Adequate pain relief is important and the use of PCA allows the client to control her own pain relief.

**144. 1.** The incisional site may change with time and healing, so a permanent prosthesis should be purchased only after complete healing has occurred.

**145. 4.** Cervical dysplasia is frequently a forerunner of cervical cancer and is readily detected by Pap smear; thus follow-up Pap smears allow for early detection and treatment of cervical cancer.

**146. 4.** Detection of ovarian cancer is very difficult because it gives only vague, subtle symptoms and there are no diagnostic screening tests.

**147. 2.** Retention of urine is common following vaginal hysterectomy due to stretching of musculature and proximity of the surgery to the bladder and its enervation.

**148. 3.** After the loss of the uterus, pregnancy is unachievable and birth control is not needed even if the ovaries remain.

**149. 1.** Even though ovulation is erratic and many periods are anovulatory, birth control should be continued for at least 6 months after the last menses.

**150. 1.** HRT appears to help protect many women from heart disease and osteoporosis if used with exercise and calcium supplements.

## REFERENCES AND SUGGESTED READINGS

Boyle, J. S., & Andrews, M. M. (2007). *Transcultural concepts in nursing care* (5th ed.). Philadelphia: Lippincott-Raven.

Littleton, L., & Engebretson, J. (2005). *Maternity nursing care* (1st ed.). Clifton Park, NY: Delmar Cengage Learning.

Lowdermilk, D., & Perry, S. (2007). *Maternity and women's health care* (9th ed.). St. Louis, MO: Mosby.

Munoz, C., & Luckmann, J. (2004). *Transcultural communication in nursing* (2nd ed.). Clifton Park, NY: Delmar Cengage Learning.

Olds, S., London, M., Ladewig, P., & Davidson, M. (2004). *Maternal-newborn nursing and women's health care* (7th ed.). Upper Saddle River, NJ: Prentice Hall.

Pillitteri, A. (2006). *Maternal and child health nursing* (5th ed.). Philadelphia: Lippincott.

White, L. (2004). *Foundations of maternal & pediatric nursing* (2nd ed.). Clifton Park, NY: Delmar Cengage Learning.

Wong, D., Perry, S., & Hockenberry, M. (2006). *Maternal child nursing care* (3rd ed.). St. Louis, MO Mosby.

# PSYCHIATRIC–MENTAL HEALTH NURSING

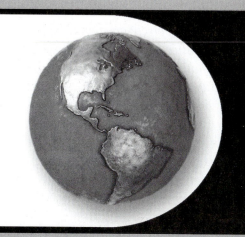

An important aspect of professional nursing is the use of therapeutic intervention for clients who are experiencing emotional distress. A client does not have to have a psychiatric diagnosis to be in emotional distress, and often clients and their families may respond to illness or injury with anxiety and fear that can be manifested in a variety of behaviors. The principles of psychiatric-mental health nursing and therapeutic interventions can be applied to any client, family, or group in need.

To plan appropriate interventions, nurses need to have an understanding and knowledge of personality development and other theories to analyze behaviors of the client or others. Theories, principles, the nursing process, and treatment modalities are the science of psychiatric-mental health nursing.

The manner the nurse selects to use the science of mental health nursing is based in part on that nurse's personal attributes. Personal experiences, the ability to implement principles and theories, and the willingness to use therapeutic communication constitute the art of psychiatric-mental health nursing. This creative aspect of each nurse is the therapeutic use of self involved in planning and implementing effective nursing interventions for dealing with clients who are experiencing emotional distress.

Implementing the art of psychiatric-mental health nursing is an important way to convey to clients the caring aspect of nursing. Perceiving clients' concerns and responding therapeutically will encourage clients to share more information with the nurse. Awareness of the client's attitudes, values, and fears will enable the nurse to individualize client care. Physical, psychologic, social, and spiritual needs should be the concern of a nurse who wants to provide holistic care. Nurses can determine specific client needs by assessing verbal and nonverbal behaviors. Application of the nursing process to meet client needs will ensure comprehensive nursing care.

The following principles of psychiatric-mental health nursing help form the basis of the therapeutic use of self:

- Be aware of your own feelings and responses
- Maintain objectivity while being aware of your own needs
- Use empathy (recognizing/identifying somewhat with client's emotions to understand behavior), not sympathy (close identification/duplication of client's emotions)
- Focus on the needs of the client, not on your own needs; be consistent and trustworthy
- Accept clients as they are; be nonjudgmental
- Recognize that emotions influence behaviors
- Observe a client's behaviors to analyze needs/problems
- Accept client's needs to use defenses/behaviors to deal with emotional distress
- Accept client's negative emotions
- Avoid verbal reprimands, physical force, giving advice, or imposing your own values on clients
- Avoid intimate relationships while maintaining a caring attitude
- Assess clients in the context of their social/cultural group
- Recognize that client communication patterns (verbal and nonverbal) vary with different cultural groups
- Teach/explain on client's level of capability
- Treat clients with respect, caring, and compassion

Asking yourself, "What is this client's need at this time?" can assist you in determining the best response to questions.

## THEORETICAL BASIS

### Medical-Biologic Model

**A.** Emotional distress is viewed as illness.
**B.** Symptoms can be classified to determine a psychiatric diagnosis.
**C.** DSM-IV-TR*
   **1.** Description of disorders
   **2.** Criteria (behaviors) that must be met for diagnosis to be made
   **3.** Axis: the dimensions and factors included when assessing a client with a mental disorder
      **a.** I and II: clinical syndromes (e.g., bipolar, antisocial personality, mental retardation)
      **b.** III: physical disorders and symptoms (e.g., cystic fibrosis, hypertension)
      **c.** IV: psychosocial and environmental problems: acute and long-term severity of stressors
      **d.** V: functioning of client, rating of symptoms and their effect on activities of daily living (ADLs) or violence to self/others
**D.** Diagnosed psychiatric illnesses are within the realm of medical practice and have a particular course, prognosis, and treatment regimen.
**E.** Treatment can include psychotropic drugs, electroconvulsive therapy (ECT), hospitalization, and psychotherapy.
**F.** There is no proven cause, but theory is that biochemical/genetic factors play a part in the development of mental illness. Theories with schizophrenia and affective disorders include:
   **1.** Genetic: increased risk when close relative (e.g., parent, sibling) has disorder
   **2.** Possible link to neurotransmitter activity

### Psychodynamic/Psychoanalytic Model (Freud)

**A.** Instincts (drives) produce energy.
**B.** There are genetically determined drives for sex and aggression.
**C.** Human behavior is determined by past experiences and responses.
**D.** All behavior has meaning and can be understood.
**E.** Emotionally painful experiences/anxiety motivate behavior.
**F.** Client can change behavior and responses when made aware of the reasons for them.

*American Psychiatric Association. (2000). *Diagnostic and Statistical Manual of Mental Disorders* (4th ed.), Text Revision.

**G.** Freud's theory of personality
   **1.** Id: present at birth; instinctual drive for pleasure and immediate gratification, unconscious. Libido is the sexual and/or aggressive energy (drive). Operates on pleasure principle to reduce tension or discomfort (pain). Uses primary process thinking by imagining objects to satisfy needs (hallucinating).
   **2.** Ego: develops as sense of self that is distinct from world of reality; conscious, preconscious, and unconscious. Operates on reality principle which determines whether the perception has a basis in reality or is imagined. Uses secondary process thinking by judging reality and solving problems.
      **a.** Functions of the ego
         **1)** Control and regulate instinctual drives
         **2)** Mediate between id drives and demands of reality; id drives versus superego restrictions
         **3)** Reality testing: evaluate and judge external world
         **4)** Store up experiences in "memory"
         **5)** Direct motor activity and actions
         **6)** Solve problems
         **7)** Use defense mechanisms to protect self
      **b.** Levels of awareness
         **1)** Preconscious: knowledge not readily available to conscious awareness but can be brought to awareness with effort (e.g., recalling name of a character in a book)
         **2)** Unconscious: knowledge that cannot be brought into conscious awareness without interventions such as psychoanalysis, hypnotism, or drugs
         **3)** Conscious: aware of own thoughts and perceptions of reality
   **3.** Superego: develops as person unconsciously incorporates standards and restrictions from parents to guide behaviors, thoughts, and feelings. Conscious awareness of acceptable/unacceptable thoughts, feelings, and actions is "conscience."
**H.** Freud's psychosexual developmental stages
   **1.** Oral
      **a.** 0–18 months
      **b.** Pleasure and gratification through mouth
      **c.** Behaviors: dependency, eating, crying, biting

d. Distinguishes between self and mother
e. Develops body image, aggressive drives
2. Anal
   a. 18 months–3 years
   b. Pleasure through elimination or retention of feces
   c. Behaviors: control of holding on or letting go
   d. Develops concept of power, punishment, ambivalence, concern with cleanliness or being dirty
3. Phallic/Oedipal
   a. 3–6 years
   b. Pleasure through genitals
   c. Behaviors: touching of genitals, erotic attachment to parent of opposite sex
   d. Develops fear of punishment by parent of same sex, guilt, sexual identity
4. Latency
   a. 6–12 years
   b. Energy used to gain new skills in social relationships and knowledge
   c. Behaviors: sense of industry and mastery
   d. Learns control over aggressive, destructive impulses
   e. Acquires friends
5. Genital
   a. 12–20 years
   b. Sexual pleasure through genitals
   c. Behaviors: becomes independent of parents, responsible for self
   d. Develops sexual identity, ability to love and work

# Psychosocial Model (Erikson)

A. Emphasis on psychosocial rather than psychosexual development
B. Developmental stages have goals (tasks)
C. Challenge in each stage is to resolve conflict (e.g., trust versus mistrust)
D. Resolution of conflict prepares individual for next developmental stage
E. Personality develops according to biologic, psychologic, and social influences
F. Erikson's psychosocial development tasks
   1. Trust versus mistrust
      a. 0–18 months
      b. Learn to trust others and self versus withdrawal, estrangement
   2. Autonomy versus shame and doubt
      a. 18 months–3 years
      b. Learn self-control and the degree to which one has control over the environment versus compulsive compliance or defiance
   3. Initiative versus guilt
      a. 3–5 years
      b. Learn to influence environment, evaluate own behavior versus fear of doing wrong, lack of self-confidence, overrestricting actions
   4. Industry versus inferiority
      a. 6–12 years
      b. Creative; develop sense of competency versus sense of inadequacy
   5. Identity versus role diffusion
      a. 12–20 years
      b. Develop sense of self; preparation, planning for adult roles versus doubts relating to sexual identity, occupation/career
   6. Intimacy versus isolation
      a. 18–25 years
      b. Develop intimate relationship with another; commitment to career versus avoidance of choices in relationships, work, or lifestyle
   7. Generativity versus stagnation
      a. 21–45 years
      b. Productive; use of energies to guide next generation versus lack of interests, concern with own needs
   8. Integrity versus despair
      a. 45 years to end of life
      b. Relationships extended, belief that own life has been worthwhile versus lack of meaning of one's life, fear of death

# Interpersonal Model (Sullivan)

A. Behavior motivated by need to avoid anxiety and satisfy needs
B. Sullivan's developmental tasks
   1. Infancy
      a. 0–18 months
      b. Others will satisfy needs
   2. Childhood
      a. 18 months–6 years
      b. Learn to delay need gratification
   3. Juvenile
      a. 6–9 years
      b. Learn to relate to peers
   4. Preadolescence
      a. 9–12 years
      b. Learn to relate to friends of same sex
   5. Early adolescence
      a. 12–14 years
      b. Learn independence and how to relate to opposite sex
   6. Late adolescence
      a. 14–21 years
      b. Develop intimate relationship with person of opposite sex

# Therapeutic Nurse-Client Relationship (Peplau)

A. Based on Sullivan's interpersonal model
B. Therapeutic relationship is between nurse (helper) and client (recipient of care). The goal is to work

together to assist client to grow and to resolve problems.
C. Differs from social relationship in which both parties form alliance for mutual benefit.
D. Therapeutic use of self
1. Focus is on client needs but nurse is also aware of own needs.
2. Self-awareness enables nurse to avoid having own needs influence perception of client.
3. Determine what client/family needs are at the time.
E. Three phases of nurse-client relationship
1. Orientation
   a. Nurse explains relationship to client, defines both nurse's and client's roles.
   b. Nurse determines what client expects from the relationship and what can be done for the client.
   c. Nurse contracts with client about when and where future meetings will take place.
   d. Nurse assesses client and develops a plan of care based on appropriate nursing diagnoses.
   e. Limits/termination of relationship are introduced (e.g., "We will be meeting for 30 minutes every morning while you are in the hospital.").
2. Working phase
   a. Client's problems and needs are identified and explored as nurse and client develop mutual acceptance.
   b. Client's dysfunctional symptoms, feelings, or interpersonal relationships are identified.
   c. Therapeutic techniques are employed to reduce anxiety and to promote positive change and independence.
   d. Goals are evaluated as therapeutic work proceeds, and changed as determined by client's progress.
3. Termination
   a. Relationship and growth in nurse and client are summarized.
   b. Client may become anxious and react with increased dependence, hostility, or withdrawal.
   c. These reactions are discussed with client.
   d. Feelings of nurse and client concerning termination should be discussed in context of finiteness of relationship.
F. Transference and countertransference
1. Transference: occurs when client transfers conflicts/feelings from past to the nurse. For example: Client becomes overly dependent, clinging to nurse who represents (unconsciously to client) the nurturing desires from own mother.
2. Countertransference: occurs when nurse responds to client emotionally, as if in a personal, not professional/therapeutic,

relationship. Countertransference is a normal occurrence, but must be recognized so that supervision or consultation can keep it from undermining the nurse-client relationship. For example: Nurse is sarcastic and judgmental to client who has history of drug abuse. Client represents (unconsciously to nurse) the nurse's brother who has abused drugs.
3. Interventions
   a. Reflect on reasons for behaviors of client or nurse.
   b. Establish therapeutic goals for this relationship.
   c. If unable to control these occurrences, transfer client to another nurse.

# Human Motivation/Need Model (Maslow)

A. Hierarchy of needs in order of importance
1. Physiologic: oxygen, food, water, sleep, sex
2. Safety: security, protection, freedom from anxiety
3. Love and belonging: freedom from loneliness/alienation
4. Esteem and recognition: freedom from sense of worthlessness, inferiority, and helplessness
5. Self-actualization: aesthetic needs, self-fulfillment, creativity, spirituality
B. Primary needs (oxygen, fluids) need to be met prior to dealing with higher-level needs (esteem, recognition).
C. Focus on provision of positive aspects such as feeling safe, having someone care, affiliation

# Behavioral Model (Pavlov, Skinner)

A. Behavior is learned and retained by positive reinforcement (e.g., more studying produces higher grades).
B. Motivation for behavior is not considered.
C. Behaviors that are not adequate can be replaced by more adaptive behaviors.

# Community Mental Health Model

A. Emotional distress stems from personal and social factors
1. Family problems (e.g., divorce, single parenthood)
2. Social factors (e.g., unemployment, lack of support groups, changing mores)
B. Health care a right
C. Decreased need for hospitalization, increased community care
D. Collaboration of social and health care services
E. Comprehensive services
1. Emergency care
2. Inpatient/outpatient services

3. Substance-abuse treatment
4. Transitional living arrangements (temporary residence instead of inpatient care)
5. Consultation and education to increase knowledge of mental health
F. Prevention
   1. Primary prevention
      a. Minimize development of serious emotional distress: promote mental health, identify persons at risk.
      b. Anticipate problems such as developmental crises (e.g., birth of first child, midlife crisis, death of spouse).
   2. Secondary prevention: early case finding and treatment (drug therapy, outpatient, short-term hospitalization).
   3. Tertiary prevention: restore client to optimal functioning; facilitate return of client to home and community by use of social agencies.

# NURSING PROCESS

A. Applies to all clients, not only to those with psychiatric diagnosis; incorporates holism.
B. Utilized in a unique manner for psychosocial assessment.
C. Sets goals (with client, whenever possible) that can be measured in behavioral terms (e.g., client will dress self and eat breakfast before 9 A.M.).
D. Uses principles of therapeutic communication for interventions.
E. Evaluates whether, how well goals were met.

## Physical Assessment

A. Subjective reporting of health history
B. Objective data (general status and appearance)
   1. Age: client's appearance in relation to chronologic age
   2. Attire: appropriateness of clothing to age/situation
   3. Hygiene: cleanliness and grooming, or lack thereof
   4. Physical health: weight, physical distress
   5. Psychomotor: posture, movement, activity level
   6. Sleep and rest
C. Neurologic assessment/level of consciousness

## Mental Status Assessment

### Emotional Status Assessment

Observation of mood (prolonged emotion) and affect (physical manifestations of mood). That is, sad mood may be evidenced by crying or downcast appearance;

joyful mood may be expressed by smiling or happy affect.
A. Appropriateness
B. Description: flat, sad, smiling, serious
C. Stability
D. Specific feelings and moods

## Cognitive Assessment

Evaluation of thought, sensorium, intelligence
A. Intellectual performance
   1. Orientation to person, place, and time
   2. Attention and concentration
   3. Knowledge/educational level
   4. Memory: short and long term
   5. Judgment
   6. Insight into illness
   7. Ability to use abstraction
B. Speech
   1. Amount, volume, clarity
   2. Characteristics: pressured, slow or fast, dull or lively
   3. Specific aberrations, i.e., echolalia (imitating and repeating another's words or phrases) or neologisms (making up of own words that have special meaning to client).
C. Thoughts
   1. Content and clarity
   2. Characteristics: spontaneity, speed, loose associations, blocked, flight of ideas, repetitions

## Social/Cultural Considerations

A. Age: assess for developmental tasks and developmental crises, age-related problems.
   1. 0–18 months: development of trust and sense of self, dependency
   2. 18 months–3 years: development of autonomy and beginning self-reliance, toilet training
   3. 3–6 years: development of sexual identity, relationships with peers, adjustment to school
   4. 6–12 years: mastery of skills, beginning self-esteem, identification with others outside family, social relationships
   5. 12–18 years: sense of self solidifies, separation and individuation often follow some disorganization and rebellion, substance abuse
   6. 18–25 years: identification with peer group, setting of personal and career goals to master future
   7. 25–38 years: take place in adult world, commitments made relating to career, marriage, parenthood
   8. 38–65 years: review of past accomplishments; may set new and reasonable goals; midlife crises when present achievements have not met goals set in earlier stages of development

9. 65/70 to death: loss of friends/spouse, retirement, loss of some social/physical functions
B. Family/community relationships
   1. Role of client in family
   2. Family harmony, family support for or dependency on client
   3. Client's perception of family
   4. Availability of community support groups to client (include government social agencies; religious, ethnic, and volunteer agencies)
C. Socioeconomic group/education
   1. Factors that relate to how client is approached and how client perceives own present state
   2. Determination of level of teaching and need for social services
D. Cultural/spiritual background
   1. Assess behaviors in context of client's culture.
   2. Avoid stereotyping persons as having attributes of their culture/subculture.
   3. Note client's religious/philosophic beliefs.

# ANALYSIS

Select nursing diagnoses based on collected data. Decide which is most important. Specific nursing diagnoses will be given when discussing particular disorders, but those nursing diagnoses generally appropriate to the client with psychiatric-mental health disorders include:
A. Anxiety
B. Chronic sorrow
C. Decisional conflict
D. Defensive coping
E. Deficient knowledge
F. Disturbed body image
G. Disturbed sleep pattern
H. Disturbed through processes
I. Dysfunctional family processes
J. Fatigue
K. Fear
L. Hopelessness
M. Impaired adjustment
N. Impaired social interaction
O. Impaired verbal communication
P. Ineffective coping
Q. Ineffective denial
R. Ineffective role performance
S. Ineffective therapeutic regimen management
T. Low self-esteem
U. Noncompliance
V. Powerlessness
W. Rape-trauma syndrome
X. Risk for injury
Y. Risk for violence
Z. Risk-prone health behavior
AA. Self-mutilation
BB. Social isolation
CC. Spiritual distress
DD. Stress overload

# PLANNING AND IMPLEMENTATION

## Goals

A. Client will:
   1. Participate in treatment program.
   2. Be oriented to time, place, and person and exhibit reality-based behavior.
   3. Recognize reasons for behavior and develop alternative coping mechanisms.
   4. Maintain or improve self-care activities.
   5. Be protected from harmful behaviors.
B. There will be mutual agreement of nurse and client whenever possible.
C. Short-term goals are set for immediate problems; they should be feasible and within client's capabilities.
D. Long-term goals are related to discharge planning and prevention of recurrence or exacerbation of symptoms.

## Interventions

The nurse will use therapeutic intervention and the nurse-client relationship to help the client achieve the goals of therapy. Interventions must be geared to the level of the client's capability and must relate to the specific problems identified for the individual client, family, or group.

### *Therapeutic Communication*

A. Facilitative: use the following approaches to intervene therapeutically
   1. Silence: client able to think about self/problems; does not feel pressure or obligation to speak.
   2. Offering self: offer to provide comfort to client by presence (*Nurse:* "I'll sit with you." "I'll walk with you.").
   3. Accepting: indicate nonjudgmental acceptance of client and his perceptions by nodding and following what client says.
   4. Giving recognition: indicate to client your awareness of him and his behaviors (*Nurse:* "Good morning, John. You have combed your hair this morning.").
   5. Making observations: verbalize what you perceive (*Nurse:* "I notice that you can't seem to sit still.").
   6. Encouraging description: ask client to verbalize his perception (*Nurse:* "Tell me when you need to get up and walk around." "What is happening to you now?").
   7. Using broad openings: encourage client to introduce topic of conversation (*Nurse:* "Where shall we begin today?" "What are you thinking about?").

8. Offering general leads: encourage client to continue discussing topic (*Nurse:* "And then?" "Tell me more about that.").

9. Reflecting: direct client's questions/statements back to encourage expression of ideas and feelings (*Client:* "Do you think I should call my father?" *Nurse:* "What do you want to do?").

10. Restating: repeat what client has said (*Client:* "I don't want to take the medicine." *Nurse:* "You don't want to take this medication?").

11. Focusing: encourage client to stay on topic/point (*Nurse:* "You were talking about . . .").

12. Exploring: encourage client to express feelings or ideas in more depth (*Nurse:* "Tell me more about . . ." "How did you respond to . . . ?").

13. Clarification: encourage client to make idea or feeling more explicit, understandable (*Nurse:* "I don't understand what you mean. Could you explain it to me?").

14. Presenting reality: report events/situations as they really are (*Client:* "I don't get to talk to my doctor." *Nurse:* "I saw your doctor talking to you this morning.").

15. Translating into feelings: encourage client to verbalize feelings expressed in another way (*Client:* "I will never get better." *Nurse:* "You sound rather hopeless and helpless.").

16. Suggesting collaboration: offer to work with client toward goal (*Client:* "I fail at everything I try." *Nurse:* "Maybe we can figure out something together so that you can accomplish something you want to do.").

B. Ineffective communication styles: the following nontherapeutic approaches tend to block therapeutic communication and are sometimes used by nurses to avoid becoming involved with client's emotional distress; often a protective action on part of nurse.

1. Reassuring: telling client there is no need to worry or be anxious (*Client:* "I'm nervous about this test." *Nurse:* "Everything will be all right.").

2. Advising: telling client what you believe should be done (*Client:* "I am going to . . ." *Nurse:* "Why don't you do . . . instead?" or "I think you should do . . .").

3. Requesting explanation: asking client to provide reasons for his feelings/behavior. The use of "why" questions should be avoided (*Nurse:* "Why do you feel, think, or act this way?").

4. Stereotypical response: replying to client with meaningless clichés (*Client:* "I hate being in the hospital." *Nurse:* "There's good and bad about everything.").

5. Belittling feelings: minimizing or making light of client's distress or discomfort (*Client:* "I'm so depressed about . . ." *Nurse:* "Everyone feels sad at times.").

6. Defending: protecting person or institutions (*Client:* "Ms. Jones is a rotten nurse." *Nurse:* "Ms. Jones is one of our best nurses.").

7. Approving: giving approval to client's behavior or opinion (*Client:* "I'm going to change my attitude." *Nurse:* "That's good.").

8. Disapproving: telling client certain behavior or opinions do not meet your approval (*Client:* "I am going to sign myself out of here." *Nurse:* "I'd rather you wouldn't do that.").

9. Agreeing: letting client know that you think and feel alike; nurse verbalizes agreement.

10. Disagreeing: letting client know that you do not agree; telling client that you do not believe he is right.

11. Probing: questioning client about a topic he has indicated he does not want to discuss.

12. Denial: refusing to recognize client's perception (*Client:* "I am a hopeless case." *Nurse:* "You are not hopeless. There is always hope.").

13. Changing topic: letting client know you do not want to discuss a problem by introducing a new topic (*Client:* "I am a hopeless case." *Nurse:* "It's time to fill out your menu.").

## *Therapeutic Groups*

Table 7-1 lists types of therapeutic groups.

A. Groups of clients meet with one or more therapists. They work together to alleviate client problems in:
   1. Interpersonal relations/communication
   2. Coping with particular stressors (e.g., ostomy groups)
   3. Self-understanding

B. Purposes
   1. Increase self-awareness
   2. Improve interpersonal relationships
   3. Make changes in behavior
   4. Deal with particular stressors
   5. Enhance teaching/learning

**Table 7-1** Types of Therapeutic Groups

| Type | Goal(s) | Example |
|---|---|---|
| Task | Accomplish outcome | Select field trip |
| Teaching/ learning | Gain knowledge/ skills | Identify side effects of medications |
| Social/support | Give and receive support | Postmastectomy clients |
| Psychotherapy | Insight/behavioral change | Resolve loss |
| Activity | Increase social interaction/ self–esteem | Grooming, manicures |

**C.** Structure of groups
  1. Leader(s) chosen
  2. Selection of members
  3. Size: 5 to 10 members
  4. Physical arrangements
  5. Time/place of meetings
  6. Open: accept members anytime
  7. Closed: do not add new members
**D.** Group dynamics
  1. System of interactions
  2. Collective activity
  3. Process: all activities/interactions
  4. Content: topics discussed
**E.** Stages of group development
  1. Beginning stage
     a. Anxiety in new situation
     b. Information given
     c. Group norms established
  2. Middle stage
     a. Group cohesiveness
     b. Members confronting each other
     c. Reliance on group member leading to self-reliance
     d. Sense of trust established
  3. Termination stage
     a. Individual member may leave abruptly
     b. Group decides work is done
     c. Ambivalence felt about termination
     d. Ideally, group members have met goals
**F.** Role of the nurse
  1. Explain purpose and rules of group
  2. Introduce group members
  3. Promote group cohesiveness
  4. Focus on problems of group and group process
  5. Encourage participation
  6. Role model
  7. Facilitate communication
  8. Set limits

## Family Therapy

**A.** Client is whole family, although a family member may be "identified client."
**B.** Purposes
  1. Improve relationships among family members
  2. Promote family function
  3. Resolve family problem(s)
**C.** Process
  1. Problem(s) are identified by each family member.
  2. Members discuss their involvement in problem(s).
  3. Members discuss how problem(s) affect them.
  4. Members explore ways each of them can help resolve problem(s).
**D.** Role of the nurse
  1. Assess interactions among family members
  2. Make observations to family members
  3. Encourage expression of feelings by family members to one another
  4. Assist family in resolving problems

## Milieu Therapy

**A.** Total environment (milieu) has an effect on individual's behavior, including:
  1. Physical environment (i.e., cleanliness, noise, colors, fresh air, light)
  2. Relationships of staff to staff, staff to clients, and client to clients
  3. Atmosphere of safety, caring, mutual respect (e.g., client-run community meeting, community-set standards for behaviors)
**B.** Purposes
  1. Improve client's behavior
  2. Involve client in decision making of unit
  3. Increase client's sense of autonomy
  4. Increase communication among clients and between clients and staff
  5. Set structure of unit and behavioral limits
  6. Form a sense of community
**C.** Role of the nurse
  1. Involve clients in decision making
  2. Promote involvement of all staff
  3. Promote development of social skills of individual clients (e.g., nurse serves as role model)
  4. Encourage sense of community in staff and clients

## Crisis Intervention

**A.** Client cannot resolve problem with usual problem-solving skills. Problem is so serious that functioning (homeostasis) is threatened. Crisis can be developmental (e.g., birth of first child), a sudden death (e.g., car accident), a result of interpersonal violence (e.g., arson), terrorist attacks and war (e.g., September 11, 2001), or situational (e.g., home destroyed by fire). Adapting to and coping with the crisis can be considered within the normal range up to 1 year.
**B.** Purposes
  1. Support client during time of crisis
  2. Resolve crisis
  3. Restore client at least to precrisis level of functioning or assist client to integrate the crisis and reinvest in life
  4. Allow client to attain higher level of functioning through acquiring greater skill in problem solving
**C.** Process
  1. Crisis event occurs: client unable to solve problem.
  2. Increase in level of client's anxiety.
  3. Client may use trial and error approach.
  4. If problem unresolved, anxiety escalates and client seeks help.
**D.** Role of the nurse
  1. Assess client's perception of problem: realistic/distorted

2. Determine situational supports (e.g., family, neighbors, agencies)
3. Explore previous coping behaviors of client
4. Offer support and education in resolving crisis
5. Enlist help of situational supports
6. Help client develop new, more effective coping behaviors
7. Convey hope to client that crisis can be resolved
8. Work with client as he resolves crisis
9. Encourage the client to attend a debriefing session (if one is available and appropriate for the crisis)

## Behavior Modification

A. Based on theory that all behavior is learned as a result of positive reinforcement. Behaviors can be changed by substituting new behaviors.
B. Purpose: change unacceptable or maladaptive behaviors
C. Process
  1. Determine the unacceptable behavior.
  2. Identify more adaptive behavior to replace the unacceptable behavior.
  3. Apply learning principles.
    a. Respond to unacceptable behavior by negative reinforcement (punishment) or by withholding positive reinforcement (ignore behavior).
    b. Determine what client views as reward.
  4. When desired behavior occurs, present positive reinforcement (reward).
  5. Consistently reward desired behavior.
  6. Consistently respond to unacceptable behavior with negative reinforcement/ignoring behavior.
D. Types
  1. Counterconditioning: specific stimulus evokes a maladaptive response that is replaced with a more adaptive response.
  2. Systematic desensitization
    a. Expose to small amount of stimulus while ensuring relaxation (client cannot be anxious and relaxed at same time).
    b. Continue relaxing client while increasing amount of stimulus.
    c. Fear response to stimulus is eventually extinguished.
  3. Token economy: Tokens (rewards such as candy) are used to reinforce desired behaviors.

## Psychotropic Medications

A variety of agents is used to control disordered thinking, anxiety, and mood disorders. Effects, side effects, and nursing implications are summarized with each disorder.

# EVALUATION

A. How well have goals been met? If not met, why not?
  1. Review prior steps of nursing process.
    a. Do you need more assessment data?
    b. Were nursing diagnoses prioritized?
    c. Were goals feasible and measurable?
    d. Were interventions appropriate?
  2. Revise goals as necessary.
B. Client
  1. Enrolled/participates in appropriate treatment program.
  2. Expresses concerns/needs and develops a therapeutic relationship with nurse.
  3. Identifies causes for behavior; learns and uses alternative coping mechanisms.
  4. Demonstrates ability to care for self at optimum level and to identify areas where assistance is needed.
  5. Does not engage in harmful behaviors; shows increased ability to control destructive impulses.
C. Client's behavior demonstrates optimal orientation to reality (e.g., can state name, place); interacts appropriately with others.

# BEHAVIORS RELATED TO EMOTIONAL DISTRESS

## Anxiety

A. General information
  1. One of the most important concepts in psychiatric-mental health nursing.
  2. Anxiety is present in almost every instance where clients are experiencing emotional distress/have a diagnosed psychiatric illness.
  3. Experienced as a sense of emotional or physical distress as the individual responds to an unknown threat or thwarting of unmet needs.
  4. The ego protects itself from the effects of anxiety by the use of defense mechanisms (see Table 7-2).
  5. Physiologic responses are related to autonomic nervous system response and to level of anxiety.
    a. Subjective: client experiences feelings of tension, need to act, uneasiness, distress, and apprehension or fear.
    b. Objective: client exhibits restlessness, inability to concentrate, tension, dilated pupils, changes in vital signs (usually increased by sympathetic nervous system response, may be decreased by parasympathetic reactions).

## Table 7-2 Defense Mechanisms

| Type | Characteristics | Examples |
|------|----------------|----------|
| Denial | Refusal to acknowledge a part of reality | A client on strict bed rest is walking down the hall; shows refusal to acknowledge need to stay in bed because of illness. A client states admission to the mental hospital is for reasons other than mental illness. |
| Repression | Threatening thoughts are pushed into the unconscious, anxiety and other symptoms are observed; client unable to have conscious awareness of conflicts or events that are source of anxiety | "I don't know why I have to wash my hands all the time, I just have to." |
| Suppression | Consciously putting a threatening/distressing thought out of one's awareness. | A nurse must study for the NCLEX, but she has had a heated argument with her boyfriend. She decides not to think about the problem until she finishes studying, then she will attempt to resolve it. |
| Rationalization | Developing an acceptable, justifiable (to self) reason for behavior | A friend tells you that he has been in an automobile accident because the car skidded on wet leaves in the road; you go to the scene of the accident, but there are no leaves; friend admits to you and to self that he was probably driving too fast. |
| Reaction-formation | Engaging in behavior that is opposite of true desires | A man has an unconscious desire to view pornographic films; he circulates a petition to close the theater where such films are shown. |
| Sublimation | Anxiety channeled into socially acceptable behavior | A student is upset because she received a failing grade on a test; she knows that she will feel better if she goes jogging and runs a few miles. |
| Compensation | Making up for a deficit by success in another area | A young man who cannot make any varsity teams becomes the chess champion in his school. |
| Projection | Placing own undesirable trait onto another; blaming others for own difficulty | A student who would like to cheat on an exam states that other students are trying to cheat; a paranoid client claims that the FBI had him committed to the mental hospital. |
| Displacement | Directing feelings about one object/person toward a less-threatening object/person | The head nurse reprimands you; you do not argue even though you do not agree with her reprimand; when you return home that evening you are hostile toward your roommate. |
| Identification | Taking onto oneself the traits of others that one admires | You greatly admire the clinical specialist in your hospital; unconsciously you begin to use the approaches she uses with clients. |
| Introjection | Symbolic incorporation of another into one's own personality | John becomes depressed when his father dies; John's feelings are directed to the mental image he has of his father. |
| Conversion | Anxiety converted into a physical symptom that is motor or sensory in nature | A young woman unconsciously desires to strike her mother; she develops sudden paralysis of her arms. |
| Symbolization | Representing an idea or object by a substitute object or sign | A man who was spurned by a librarian develops a dislike of books and reading. |
| Dissociation | Separation or splitting off of one aspect of mental process from conscious awareness | A student who prides herself on being prompt does not recall the times that she arrived late for class. |

*(continues)*

**Table 7-2** Defense Mechanisms *(continued)*

| Type | Characteristics | Examples |
|------|-----------------|----------|
| Undoing | Behavior that is opposite of earlier unacceptable behavior or thought | Joan tells an ethnic joke to a coworker, Sally; Sally, a member of that ethnic group, is offended; the following week Joan offers to work the weekend for Sally. |
| Regression | Behavior that reflects an earlier level of development; adults hospitalized with serious illnesses sometimes will engage in regressive behaviors | When a new baby is brought home, 5-year-old Billy begins to wet his pants although he had not done this for the past 2½ years. |
| Isolation | Separating emotional aspects of content from cognitive aspects of thought | A client discusses his terminal diagnosis in clinical terms. He does not express any emotion. |
| Splitting | Viewing self, others, or situations as all good or all bad | A client tells you that you are the best nurse. Later tells you that you are incompetent and she will report you. |

6. Anxiety can be viewed positively (motivates us to change and grow) or negatively (interferes with problem-solving ability and affects functioning).
   a. Trait anxiety: individual's normal level of anxiety. Some people are usually rather intense while others are more relaxed; may be related to genetic predisposition/early experiences (repressed conflicts).
   b. State anxiety: change in person's anxiety level in response to stressors (environmental or any internal threat to the ego).
7. Levels of anxiety
   a. Mild: increased awareness; ability to solve problems, learn; increase in perceptual field; minimal muscle tension
   b. Moderate: optimal level for learning, perceptual field narrows to pay attention to particular details, increased tension to solve problems or meet challenges
   c. Severe: sympathetic nervous system (flight/fight response); increase in blood pressure, pulse, and respirations; narrowed perceptual field, fixed vision, dilated pupils, can perceive scattered details or only one detail; difficulty in problem solving
   d. Panic: decrease in vital signs (release of sympathetic response), distorted perceptual field, inability to solve problems, disorganized behavior, feelings of helplessness/terror
B. Nursing interventions
   1. Determine the level of client's anxiety by assessing verbal and nonverbal behaviors and physiologic symptoms.
   2. Determine cause(s) of anxiety with client, if possible.
   3. Encourage client to move from affective (feeling) mode to cognitive (thinking) behavior (e.g., ask client, "What are you thinking?"). Stay with client. Reduce anxiety by remaining calm yourself; use silence, or speak slowly and softly.
   4. Help client recognize own anxious behavior.
   5. Provide outlets (e.g., talking, psychomotor activity, crying, tasks).
   6. Provide support and encourage client to find ways to cope with anxiety.
   7. In panic state nurse must make decisions.
      a. Do not leave client alone.
      b. Encourage ventilation of thoughts and feelings.
      c. Use firm voice and give short, explicit directions (e.g., "Sit in this chair. I will sit here next to you.").
      d. Engage client in motor activity to reduce tension (e.g., "We can take a brisk walk around the day room. Let's go.").

## Defense Mechanisms

Usually unconscious processes used by ego to defend itself from anxiety and threats (see Table 7-2).

## Disorders of Perception

Occur with increased anxiety, disordered thinking/impaired reality testing
A. Illusions
   1. General information: stimulus in the environment is misperceived (e.g., car backfiring is perceived as a gunshot; a bathrobe in an open closet is perceived as a person in the closet); may be visual, auditory, tactile, gustatory, olfactory.

2. Nursing intervention: show/explain stimulus to client to promote reality testing.
B. Delusions
1. General information: fixed, false set of beliefs that are real to client.
   a. Grandiose: false belief that client has power, wealth, or status or is famous person
   b. Persecutory: false belief that client is the object of another's harassment or harmful intent
   c. Somatic: false belief that client has some physical/physiologic defect
2. Nursing interventions
   a. Avoid arguing: client cannot be convinced, even with evidence, that the belief is false.
   b. Determine client's need (grandiose delusion may indicate low self-esteem; provide opportunities to succeed at task that will enhance self-concept).
   c. Reduce anxiety to encourage decreased need to use delusions.
   d. Accept client's need for delusion, present (but do not insist that client accept) reality.
   e. After therapeutic relationship has been established, you can express doubt about delusions to client.
   f. Direct client's attention to nondelusional, nonthreatening topics (e.g., current events, client's hobbies or interests).
C. Ideas of reference
1. General information: belief that events or behaviors of others relate to self (e.g., telephone rings in nurse's station, client believes "they" are calling for him; two nurses are talking and laughing, client believes nurses are talking/laughing at him).
2. Nursing interventions are the same as for Delusions.
D. Hallucinations
1. General information: sensory perceptions that have no stimulus in environment; most common hallucinations are auditory and visual (e.g., hearing voices; seeing persons, animals, objects).
2. Nursing interventions
   a. Encourage client to describe hallucination.
   b. Accept that this is a real experience for client.
   c. Present reality.
   d. Example: nurse sees client in listening attitude or responding to auditory hallucinations. *Nurse:* "You seem to be listening/talking." *Client:* "The voices are telling me to hurt myself." *Nurse:* "I don't hear the voices. Tell me what the voices are saying to you."

## Withdrawal

A. General information: withdrawal from social interaction by not talking, walking away, turning away, sleeping, or feigning sleep
B. Nursing interventions
1. Use silence.
2. Offer self.
3. Discuss nonthreatening topics that will not provoke increased anxiety.
4. Be consistent; keep promises, promote trust.

# Hostility and Aggression

A. General information
1. Hostile behavior: responding to nurse with anger, insults, threats.
2. Assaultive behavior: attempting to physically harm others.
3. Usually nurse is not real object of client's anger, but is convenient target for angry feelings/verbalizations.
B. Nursing interventions
1. Hostility
   a. Recognize own response of anger or defensiveness.
   b. Determine source of client's anger (e.g., intoxicated, psychotic, recent argument with parent).
   c. Accept angry feelings.
   d. Attempt to have client verbalize feelings and channel into acceptable behaviors.
   e. Assess the need for prn medications based on the possible source of the hostility.
2. Physical aggression/assaultive behaviors (client may act on increased anxiety by throwing objects or attempt to physically harm others)
   a. Assess for increased anxiety.
   b. Maintain distance, at least arm's length.
   c. Attempt to have client verbalize feelings.
   d. Talk client down.
   e. Obtain help if client becomes assaultive.

# Self-Mutilation

A. General information: behaviors cause physical injury but are not motivated by the desire to die.
B. Nursing interventions
1. Assess for suicide risk.
2. Offer support.
3. Protect client from carrying out self-mutilation actions.
4. Remove objects that can be used for self-harm.
5. Observe for changes in behaviors and attitudes.

# Suicide

A. General information
  1. Ideation: verbalization of wish to die (overt or disguised)
  2. Gestures: engaging in nonlethal behaviors (e.g., superficial scratches, ingestion of medication in amounts that are not likely to cause serious injury/death)
  3. Actions: engaging in behaviors or planning to engage in behaviors that have potential to cause death
  4. May or may not be associated with a psychiatric disorder
  5. Groups at risk (see Table 7-3)
B. Assessment findings
  1. Verbal cues
    a. Overt: "I'm going to kill myself."
    b. Disguised: "I have the answer to my problems."
  2. Behavioral cues
    a. Giving away prized possessions
    b. Getting financial affairs in order, making a will
    c. Suicidal ideation/gestures
    d. Indications of hopelessness, depression
    e. Behavioral and attitudinal changes (e.g., neat person becomes sloppy, depressed person suddenly becomes alert/positive, increased use of drugs and/or alcohol, alcohol withdrawal).
  3. For lethality assessment, see Table 7-4.
C. Nursing interventions
  1. Contract with client to report suicide ideation with intent and/or suicide attempt.
  2. Assess suicide risk.
    a. Ask client if he thinks about, intends to harm himself.

**Table 7-3** Groups at Increased Risk for Suicide

- Adolescents/young adults (ages 15–24)
- Elderly
- Terminally ill
- Persons who have experienced loss/stress
- Survivors of persons who have committed suicide
- Individuals with bipolar disorders
- Depressed persons (when depression begins to lift)
- Substance abusers
- Persons who have attempted suicide previously
- Schizophrenics
- More women attempt suicide; more men complete suicide

**Table 7-4** Lethality Assessment

- Plans for suicide: when? where? how?
- Means available: what will be used? Is it available to client?
- Lethality of means (e.g., tranquilizers are less lethal when used alone than when combined with alcohol; guns are more lethal than plan to cut wrists)
  - Most lethal: gunshot, hanging, jumping from high places, carbon monoxide, potent poisons (e.g., cyanide)
  - Less lethal: nonprescription drugs, wrist cutting, tranquilizers without CNS depressants
  - Males tend to use more lethal means
- Possibility of "rescue"
- Support systems available or sense of isolation
- Availability of alcohol or drugs
- Severe/panic level of anxiety
- Hostility
- Disorganized thinking
- Preoccupation with thought of suicide plan
- Prior suicide attempts

    b. Ask client if he has formulation of plan; if details are worked out, when? where? how?
    c. Check availability of method (e.g., gun, pills).
  3. Keep client under constant observation.
  4. Remove any objects that can be used in suicide attempt (e.g., shoe laces, sharp objects).
  5. Therapeutic intervention
    a. Support aspects of wish to live; clients often ambivalent: wish to live and wish to die.
    b. Use one-to-one nurse/client relationship (let client know you care for him).
    c. Allow client to express feelings of hopelessness, helplessness, worthlessness.
    d. Provide hope.
    e. Provide diversionary activities.
    f. Utilize support groups (e.g., family, clergy).
    g. Notify psychiatrist or responsible practitioner for the medical management of the client to evaluate medications and precaution level.
  6. Following a suicide
    a. Encourage survivors to discuss client's death, their feelings and fears.
    b. Provide anticipatory guidance to family who may experience problems at holidays, anniversaries.
    c. Hold staff meetings to ventilate feelings and provide a debriefing to process the event.

## Sample Questions

1. The nurse is talking with a mother to assess her child. A positive response to which question would indicate the child is in the anal stage of psychosexual development as described by Freud?
   1. "Does he put everything in his mouth?"
   2. "Does he say 'No!' to everything you say?"
   3. "Does he like to dress up and pretend to be his father?"
   4. "Does he seem jealous when you show affection to his father?"

2. The nurse is assessing a 70-year-old woman. Which statement by the client indicates that she has achieved integrity according to Erickson's stages of personality development?
   1. "My life has been wasted."
   2. "My children no longer visit me. I am just waiting to die."
   3. "I was a good nurse when I was younger, but now I am nothing."
   4. "I have a good life and I still enjoy it, but I feel ready to go when it is time."

3. Which cognitive skill would the nurse expect a 6-year-old child to be in the process of developing?
   1. Understanding of basic rules.
   2. Ability to understand abstract concepts.
   3. Recognition of object permanence.
   4. Imitation of others' actions.

4. The nurse is meeting a new client on the unit. Which action, by the nurse, is most effective in initiating the nurse-client relationship?
   1. Introduce self and explain the purpose and the plan for the relationship.
   2. Describe the nurse's family and ask the client to describe his family.
   3. Wait until the client indicates a readiness to establish a relationship.
   4. Ask the client why he was brought to the hospital.

5. An adult has just been brought to the psychiatric unit and is pacing up and down the hall. The nurse is to admit him to the hospital. To establish a nurse-client relationship, which approach should the nurse try first?
   1. Assign someone to watch him until he is calmer.

2. Ask him to sit down and orient him to the nurse's name and the need for information.
3. Check his vital signs, ask him about allergies, and call the physician for sedation.
4. Explain the importance of accurate assessment data to him.

6. A woman has been referred for help in managing her children. The woman arrives late for appointments and focuses on her busy schedule, the difficulty in parking, and other reasons for being late. How would the nurse best interpret this behavior?
   1. Transference.
   2. Counter-transference.
   3. Identification.
   4. Rationalization.

7. A woman has remained at the side of the nurse all day. When the nurse talked with other clients during dinner, the client tried to regain the nurse's attention and then began to shout, "You're just like my mother! You pay attention to everyone but me!" What is the best interpretation of this behavior?
   1. She is exhibiting sublimation.
   2. She has been spoiled by her family.
   3. The nurse has failed to meet her needs.
   4. She is demonstrating transference.

8. A nurse is part of a community task force on teenage suicide. The task force is considering all of the following steps in an effort to reduce teen suicide. Which action represents primary prevention?
   1. Encourage emergency room staff to request psychiatric consultation for adolescents who overdose.
   2. Educate teachers, counselors, and school nurses in recognition and early intervention with suicidal teens.
   3. Provide community programs, such as Scouts, which increase self-esteem for children and adolescents.
   4. Increase the number of inpatient adolescent psychiatric beds available in the community.

9. Two nurses are discussing plans for their client group. What should be in the plan to promote group cohesiveness?
   1. Let the group know which clients are behaving in ways approved by the nurses.
   2. Help the group identify group goals that are consistent with the individual members' goals.

3. Make most decisions about the group in advance and make each group member aware of the nurses' decisions.

4. Seat the most talkative members nearest the nurses where they can be more clearly heard by the group.

10. The nurse is the leader of a client group. The members of the group test each other and the group's rules, as well as compete for the nurse's attention. This behavior is typical of which phase of the nurse-client relationship?

1. Orientation.
2. Working.
3. Feedback.
4. Termination.

11. A family was referred to family therapy after their teenage son experienced behavioral problems in school. Which statement by the father indicates that he understands the purpose of family therapy?

1. "Our son will realize the consequences of his actions and try harder to behave."
2. "It will help us learn to communicate and problem solve better as a group."
3. "I expect the therapist to tell my wife how to discipline our son."
4. "The therapist will tell us how to make our son behave better in school."

12. A client walks in to the mental health outpatient center and states, "I've had it. I can't go on any longer. You've got to help me." The nurse asks the client to be seated in a private interview room. Which action should the nurse take next?

1. Reassure the client that someone will help him soon.
2. Assess the client's insurance coverage.
3. Find out more about what is happening to the client.
4. Call the client's family to come and provide support.

13. The nurse is caring for a client with anorexia nervosa who is to be placed on behavior modification. Which is appropriate to include in the nursing care plan?

1. Remind the client frequently to eat all the food served on the tray.
2. Increase phone calls allowed the client by one per day for each pound gained.
3. Include the family with the client in therapy sessions 2 times per week.
4. Reduce the client's TV time for any weight loss.

14. An adult is pacing about the unit and wringing his hands. He is breathing rapidly and complains of palpitations and nausea and he has difficulty focusing on what the nurse is saying. He says he is having a heart attack but refuses to rest. How would the nurse interpret his level of anxiety?

1. Mild.
2. Moderate.
3. Severe.
4. Panic.

15. Each time a client is scheduled for a therapy session she develops a headache and nausea. How would the nurse interpret this behavior?

1. Conversion.
2. Reaction formation.
3. Projection.
4. Suppression.

16. A man is admitted to the intensive care unit with chest pain, an abnormal ECG, and elevated enzymes. When the significance of this is explained to him, he says, "I can't be having a heart attack. No way. You must be mistaken." The nurse suspects the client is using which defense mechanism?

1. Sublimation.
2. Regression.
3. Dissociation.
4. Denial.

17. An adult is admitted for panic attacks. He frequently experiences shortness of breath, palpitations, nausea, diaphoresis, and terror. What should the nurse include in the care plan when he is having a panic attack?

1. Calm reassurance, deep breathing, and medication as ordered.
2. Teach him problem solving in relation to his anxiety.
3. Explain the physiologic responses of anxiety.
4. Explore alternate methods for dealing with the cause of his anxiety.

18. A client on an inpatient psychiatric unit refuses to eat and states that the staff is poisoning her food. Which action should the nurse include in the client's care plan?

1. Explain to the client that the staff can be trusted.
2. Show the client that others eat the food without harm.
3. Offer the client factory-sealed foods and beverages.
4. Institute behavior modification with privileges dependent on intake.

**19.** A woman is being treated on the inpatient unit for depression. She tells the nurse, "I don't see how I can go on. I've been thinking of ways to kill myself. I can see several ways to do it." What is the best initial action for the nurse to perform?

1. Notify her family about her statements.
2. Explain to the client the consequences of suicide on her family.
3. See that someone is with the client at all times.
4. Help the client identify alternate means of coping.

**20.** An adult has been admitted to the inpatient unit with a diagnosis of depression. He states that he continues to think of suicide. Which is most essential for the nurse to include in his nursing care plan?

1. Encourage the client to participate in all unit activities.
2. Ask the client if he has a knife.
3. Allow the client time alone to relax and think.
4. Have someone stay with the client 24 hours a day.

 ## Answers and Rationales

**1. 2.** Negativism is common to the toddler in the anal stage of development (age 1 to 3) who is learning to assert his independence and mastery.

**2. 4.** Integrity includes acceptance of changes; a sense of continuity of past, present, and future; and acceptance of death.

**3. 1.** Preoperational-preconceptual children (5 to 7 years old) are learning to integrate concepts based on relationships and can comprehend the basic rules.

**4. 1.** The client needs orientation to the nurse and the situation. An open, honest approach in sharing these initial data will set the tone for the relationship.

**5. 2.** Many clients are anxious at the time of admission and are often reassured by a calm, competent professional approach, which should always be tried first. If the client is unable to respond to this, then other measures, such as medication, may be necessary.

**6. 4.** Rationalization is characterized by providing the client acceptable reasons (to her) why she is having some difficulty.

**7. 4.** Transference is the unconscious transfer of qualities originally associated with another relationship to the nurse. These are often qualities associated with a parent or sibling and may provoke responses from the client that are not appropriate to the situation.

**8. 3.** Primary prevention involves making changes in the community that promote health and prevent disease.

**9. 2.** Goals that are best met by a group and that are consistent with the goals of the individual members foster cohesive groups.

**10. 1.** During the orientation phase, group members demonstrate these behaviors as they try to identify and develop trust with the group.

**11. 2.** Family therapy is aimed at improving communication and problem solving within the family group. The focus is on the family as a group, not on correcting the behavior of any one.

**12. 3.** The nurse must assess the client and his situation before the appropriate action can be determined.

**13. 2.** In behavior modification, rewards are tied to specific goals.

**14. 4.** Terror, physiologic changes, and inability to focus on the real world are characteristic of the most extreme form of anxiety, panic.

**15. 1.** Conversion changes anxious feelings into somatic symptoms.

**16. 4.** Denial helps the person escape unpleasant or intolerable reality by refusing to perceive the facts. It can serve as a normal protection in the early stages of crisis, but if the denial persists it will prevent the client from coping.

**17. 1.** Before any other interventions can be used, the client in panic must reduce his anxiety to a manageable level. The other interventions might be used when the client is less anxious.

**18. 3.** The client may be able to eat food if she knows the staff has not handled it.

**19. 3.** Maintaining client safety is the first priority. When a client is actively suicidal, one to one observation is necessary.

**20. 4.** The client who is actively suicidal needs constant observation to prevent him from carrying out his plan. Any objects that could be used in a suicide attempt would be automatically removed at admission.

# Psychiatric Disorders (DSM-IV-TR)

## DISORDERS OF INFANCY, CHILDHOOD, AND ADOLESCENCE

### Overview

A. A specific group of disorders beginning in infancy, childhood, or adolescence.
B. Clients in these age groups may also evidence other disorders such as depression or schizophrenia.
C. Intellectual, behavioral, and/or emotional dysfunction of the young client also has an effect on the family, which may require nursing intervention.

### Assessment

#### Newborn/Infants

A. Maturation
B. Developmental level
C. Sensorimotor capabilities
D. Bonding
E. Response to cuddling

#### Children/Adolescents

A. Motor skills
B. Communication abilities
C. Vocational/academic skills
D. Social and behavioral problems
E. Behavioral changes
F. Growth and development: physical/emotional
G. Self-concept
H. Knowledge of disorder

#### Parent/Family

A. Response to infant/child/adolescent with disorder
B. Guilt, sense of loss
C. Sibling jealousy/resentment
D. Knowledge of disorder
E. Expectations
F. Plans for future (home care/institutionalization)

### Analysis

Nursing diagnoses for a child/family with a psychiatric-mental health disorder may include:
A. Client
    1. Anxiety
    2. Deficient knowledge
    3. Deficient self-care

4. Disturbed sensory-perceptual
5. Fear
6. Ineffective coping
7. Low self-esteem
8. Risk for injury
9. Risk for violence
10. Sexual dysfunction
11. Total incontinence
B. Parents/family
    1. Anticipatory grieving
    2. Anxiety
    3. Deficient knowledge
    4. Disabled family coping
    5. Dysfunctional family process
    6. Impaired parenting
    7. Interrupted family processes
    8. Parental role conflict
    9. Risk for care-giver role strain

### Planning and Implementation

#### Goals

A. Client will:
    1. Communicate thoughts and feelings about self-concept.
    2. Perform tasks at optimal level of capability.
    3. Develop trusting relationship with caregivers.
B. Parents/family will:
    1. Communicate feelings and responses to child and to disorder.
    2. Demonstrate knowledge of disorder.
    3. Formulate plans for child's care.

#### Interventions

A. Client
    1. Establish a therapeutic relationship by accepting client and client's limitations.
    2. Promote communication by use of therapeutic techniques, play therapy.
    3. Encourage independence in task performance with guidance and support.
B. Parents/family
    1. Promote communication by accepting family responses.
    2. Provide information about disorder.
    3. Contact appropriate person/agency for consultation with family about care and assistance with the child.

### Evaluation

A. Client
    1. Demonstrates trust in caregivers.

2. Relates feelings about self verbally or symbolically.
3. Performs activities of daily living (ADLs) and tasks at optimal level.

**B.** Parents/Family
1. Relate positive/negative responses to child.
2. Demonstrate understanding of disorder and child's potential.
3. With consultant, formulate a plan for child's care.

## Specific Disorders

### Mental Retardation

*Note: This is coded on Axis II.*

**A.** General information
1. Significant subaverage intelligence (IQ of 70 or below) resulting in maladaptive behaviors with onset before age of 18 years
2. Etiology
   a. Heredity 5%
   b. Early alterations in embryonic development 30%
   c. Perinatal problems 10%
   d. Acquired in infancy/early childhood 5%
   e. Environmental/other mental disorders 15–20%
   f. Unknown etiology 30–40%
3. Degrees of retardation
   a. Mild mental retardation (IQ 50–70)
      1) 85% of cases
      2) Educable to 6th grade level
      3) Able to become self-supporting
   b. Moderate mental retardation (IQ 35–49)
      1) 10% of cases
      2) Educable to 2nd grade level
      3) Able to perform skills but will need supervision at work
   c. Severe mental retardation (IQ 20–34)
      1) 3–4% of cases
      2) May learn to talk/communicate
      3) Able to perform simple tasks and elementary hygiene
   d. Profound mental retardation (IQ below 20)
      1) 1–2% of cases
      2) Some speech/communication possible

**B.** Assessment findings
1. Intellectual impairment (determine degree)
2. Sensorimotor impairment
3. Communication, social, behavioral impairment
4. Lack of self-esteem and poor self-image
5. Sense of loss, guilt, nonacceptance or unrealistic expectations on part of parents/family

**C.** Nursing interventions
1. Promote optimal functioning in ADL and feelings of accomplishment, self-worth.

2. Provide opportunities for client/family to communicate thoughts, feelings.
3. Provide positive reinforcement for every success.
4. Accept client's limitations and set goals accordingly.
5. Provide support and information about disorder to family.
6. Accept family's response to client.

### Other Disorders of Childhood/Adolescence

**A.** General information
1. Separation anxiety: excessive anxiety and worry about being separated from person(s)/places to which child has become attached (e.g., refusal to leave mother/home to attend school)
2. Reactive/attachment disorder: reluctance to enter social relationships with others, creating an interference with social growth
3. Overanxious disorders: pervasive, unrealistic worry or concern about competency; somatic complaints without physical basis

**B.** Assessment findings: excessive anxiety related to separation, social interaction, and achievements

**C.** Nursing intervention: provide information regarding available mental health services for child and family.

### Disorders with Physical Manifestations

**A.** General information
1. Important to rule out any physiologic cause
2. Often related to stress or conflict in the family
3. May affect child's family/social interactions and development

**B.** Assessment findings
1. Enuresis: urinary incontinence (bedwetting) after age 5 not caused by physical disorder
2. Encopresis: fecal incontinence after age 4 not caused by physical disorder
3. Tics: involuntary, repetitive movements
4. Stuttering: repetition of sounds, words or frequent hesitations in speaking

**C.** Nursing interventions
1. Provide information about the disorders and emphasize that they are treatable.
2. Determine whether family therapy may be indicated, as well as individual therapy for child.
3. Offer support and help child/family overcome feelings of shame or guilt.
4. For enuresis and encopresis, utilize toilet training techniques.
5. Encourage discussion of client/family response to symptoms.

# PERVASIVE DEVELOPMENTAL DISORDERS

## Autistic Disorder

A. General information
   1. Usually develops prior to 3 years of age
   2. Categorized with a group of disorders known as autism spectrum disorders (ASD)
   3. 1 in 150 individuals is diagnosed with disorder; more common than pediatric cancer, diabetes, and AIDS combined
   4. Occurs in all racial, ethnic, and social groups; affects males to females 4:1
   5. Symptoms range from very mild to quite severe
   6. Fastest-growing serious developmental disability in the United States
   7. No known medical detection or cure
   8. Special education is necessary.
B. Assessment findings
   1. Infant not responsive to cuddling; may even show an aversion to being touched
   2. No eye contact or facial responsiveness
   3. Impaired or no verbal communication
   4. Echolalia (repetition of words/phrases spoken by others)
   5. Inability to tolerate change
   6. Ritualistic or repetive behavior
   7. Fascination with movement, spinning objects
   8. Labile moods
   9. Unresponsive or overresponsive to stimuli
   10. Symptoms may appear from 6 months to 2 years of age
   11. High risk for developing seizure disorders
   12. Medications that have been used to assist in treatment of behavior are haloperidol, clomipramine, and SSRIs.
C. Nursing interventions
   1. Provide parents/family with support and information about the disorder, opportunities for therapy and education for the child.
   2. Assist child with ADLs.
   3. Promote reality testing.
   4. Encourage child to develop a relationship with another person.
   5. Maintain regular schedule for activities.
   6. Provide constant routine for child (place for eating, sitting, sleeping).
   7. Controversial issues: Maintain a gluten-free or casein-free diet; multiple vaccines given at 18 months.
   8. Protect child from self-injury.
   9. Provide safe environment.
   10. Institute seizure precautions if necessary.
   11. Refer parents to support groups and websites.

## Eating Disorders

A. General information
   1. Gross disturbances in eating behaviors
   2. Pica: persistent eating of nonfood substances such as, paint, sand, ice, paper
   3. Bulimia nervosa: binge eating; the ingestion of large amounts of food in short time, often followed by self-induced vomiting. May be accompanied by affective disorders and fear of being unable to stop this behavior. Manifested by fluctuations in weight caused by binges of eating and fasting. Antidepressant medications can be used in the treatment of bulimia.
   4. Anorexia nervosa: refusal to eat or aberration in eating patterns, resulting in severe emaciation that can be life threatening. Characterized by a fear of becoming fat, and a body-image disturbance in which clients claim to feel fat even when extremely thin. This disorder is most common (95%) in adolescent and young adult females. There is a mortality rate of 7–18%. Antidepressant medications can be used in the treatment of anorexia.
B. Assessment findings (anorexia nervosa)
   1. Weight loss of 15% or more of normal body weight for age and height
   2. Electrolyte imbalance
   3. Depression
   4. Preoccupation with being thin; inability to recognize degree of own emaciation (distorted body image)
   5. Social withdrawal and poor family and individual coping skills
   6. History of high activity and achievement in academics, athletics
   7. Amenorrhea
C. Nursing interventions
   1. Monitor vital signs.
   2. Measure I&O.
   3. Weigh client 3 times per week at the same time (check to be sure client has not hidden heavy objects or water loaded before being weighed, weigh in hospital gown).
   4. Do not comment on weight loss or gain.
   5. Set limits on time allotted for eating.
   6. Record amount eaten.
   7. Stay with client during meals, focusing on client, not on food.
   8. Accompany client to bathroom for at least ½ hour after eating to prevent self-induced vomiting.
   9. Individual/family therapy may be necessary.
   10. Encourage client to express feelings.
   11. Help client to set realistic goal for self and to reduce need for being perfect.
   12. Encourage client to discuss own body image; present reality; do not argue with client.
   13. Teach relaxation techniques.
   14. Help client identify interests and positive aspects of self.

# DELIRIUM, DEMENTIA, AND OTHER COGNITIVE DISORDERS

## Overview

A. A group of disorders with a known or presumed etiology.
B. Frequently manifest as dementia or delirium.
C. May be substance induced (drugs or alcohol) or caused by a disease process; etiology may be unknown.
D. It is important for the nurse to assess behaviors rather than focus on medical diagnoses.
E. Behaviors related to impaired brain functioning may be temporary or permanent, with increasing degeneration and eventual loss of brain function.
F. Not exclusive to old age, may complicate illnesses in any age group.

## Types

A. Delirium/rapid development
   1. Manifested by reduced awareness of environment, disorders of perception, thought, speech, and attention deficits.
   2. Usually of brief duration.
   3. May occur postoperatively or following head injury, intoxication from drugs/alcohol, acute disease, or injury.
B. Dementia/gradual development
   1. Loss of intellectual abilities resulting in impaired social and occupational functioning.
   2. May be temporary, or progressive loss may occur.
   3. Found predominantly in elderly.
   4. Personality changes are usually an exaggeration of former character traits (e.g., suspicious, nontrusting person becomes paranoid); but alteration can also occur (e.g., formerly neat and orderly person pays no attention to hygiene, becomes sloppy and dirty).
   5. Memory impairment; short-term memory loss may be most obvious.
   6. Organic etiology may be known; conditions include intoxication, infections, tumors, circulatory disorders (cerebral atherosclerosis), trauma, Huntington's chorea, Korsakoff's syndrome, Creutzfeld-Jakob disease, neurosyphilis.
   7. Specific etiology may not be known (e.g., Alzheimer's disease, Pick's disease).
   8. Frequently these clients cannot perform basic ADLs.

## Assessment

A. Mental status assessment, especially orientation to time and place, memory, and judgment
B. Nutritional status
C. Ability to perform ADLs, self-care
D. Presence of confabulation (making up information to fill in memory gaps)
E. Behavioral/social changes
F. Disorders of perception
G. Impaired motor skills, coordination
H. Change in sleep patterns
I. Elimination: constipation/incontinence
J. Family response to client's condition

## Analysis

Nursing diagnoses for clients with these disorders may include:
A. Anxiety
B. Impaired verbal communication
C. Ineffective individual/family coping
D. Altered family processes
E. Risk for fluid volume deficit
F. Risk for injury
G. Imbalanced nutrition: less than body requirements
H. Self-care deficits
I. Low self-esteem
J. Disturbed sleep pattern
K. Disturbed thought processes
L. Risk for violence

## Planning/Implementation

### Goals

A. Client will:
   1. Be protected from injury.
   2. Retain optimal cognitive function and self-care abilities.
   3. Have fear/anxiety minimized.
   4. Maintain adequate nutrition/hydration.
B. Family will communicate feelings about client.

### Interventions

A. Institute safety measures: side rails, appropriate lighting in room, bed should be at lowest setting, frequent checks. Restraints should only be used as a last resort and for protection of client as ordered by physician and based on state and federal regulations.
B. Maintain reality orientation
   1. Client may not be capable of reality testing.
   2. Continue to address client by name.
   3. Maintain awareness of client's limitations in this area.
   4. Do not tell client to "remember"; severe memory loss may make client incapable of memory.
C. Assist/support with self-care needs; arrange for necessary assistive devices, help with feeding; encourage fluids.

D. Avoid "insight" therapy and discussion of impaired mental functioning as this may increase anxiety.
E. Provide spouse/family with information about client's capabilities.
F. Provide support for spouse/family; encourage continued interaction with client.
G. Administer ordered medications (based on etiology), assess response, and provide education to the client and family. Medications might include short-acting benzodiazepines, antidepressants, cholinesterase inhibitors, or low-dose antipsychotics.
H. Provide information on support organizations or groups.

## Evaluation

A. Client
1. Remains free from injuries.
2. Retains cognitive functions and self-care ability as far as possible; interacts with others appropriately.
3. Maintains appropriate weight.
B. Family
1. Expresses sense of loss or frustration related to client's condition.
2. Continues contact with client.
3. Participates in support or group organizations.

# SUBSTANCE USE DISORDERS

## Overview

A. The use of chemical agents (alcohol and drugs) to change behavior and mood
B. Abuse: continued use despite problems (social, occupational, psychologic) that are caused by substance or continued use in hazardous situations (e.g., operating machinery, driving)
C. Dependence
1. Need for larger amounts (tolerance)
2. Unsuccessful attempts to decrease/discontinue use
3. Inability to function as usual in work, social activities
4. Withdrawal symptoms (psychologic/physical distress when substance is reduced/discontinued)
D. Addiction: compulsive use of a substance; physiologic and psychologic dependence

# PSYCHOACTIVE SUBSTANCE-INDUCED ORGANIC MENTAL DISORDERS

The use of substances that result in intoxication or withdrawal syndromes, delirium, hallucinations, delusions, mood disorders.

## Assessment

A. Determine substances used, amount and last time taken, and if combined with other drugs
B. Pupillary changes, changes in vital signs or level of consciousness
C. Presence of dehydration
D. Presence of nutritional and vitamin deficiencies
E. Suicide potential: ideation, gestures
F. Level of anxiety
G. Use of denial/projection
H. Symptoms of overdose (will be drug-specific; see Table 7-5)
I. Drug-use patterns: what, when, why substances are used

## Analysis

Nursing diagnoses for clients with a psychoactive substance abuse disorder may include:
A. Anxiety
B. Ineffective coping
C. Fear
D. Risk for fluid volume deficit
E. Risk for injury
F. Imbalanced nutrition: less than body requirements
G. Self-care deficit
H. Low self-esteem
I. Disturbed sensory-perceptual
J. Sleep deprivation
K. Disturbed thought processes
L. Risk for violence
M. Ineffective denial

## Planning and Intervention

### Goals

Client will:
A. Be protected from injury.
B. Receive adequate hydration and nutrition.
C. Terminate use of substance being abused without withdrawal symptoms; emergency care will be provided if symptoms cannot be avoided.

**Table 7-5** Commonly Abused Drugs

| Drug | Effect | Dependence | Assessment Findings | Overdose | Nursing Interventions for Overdose |
|---|---|---|---|---|---|
| *Barbiturates*<br>Antianxiety drugs, hypnotics | Reduction in anxiety, escape from stress | Psychologic at first, then physiologic; withdrawal similar to alcohol withdrawal, to point of delirium; cross-tolerance to other depressants | Irritability, weight loss, changes in mood or motor coordination | Slurred speech, lethargy, respiratory depression, coma; use combined with alcohol can be lethal | Keep person awake and moving to prevent coma; maintain airway. |
| *Opioids/Narcotics*<br>Heroin, morphine, meperidine, methadone | Euphoria, dysphoria, and/or apathy | Psychologic dependence rapidly leading to physical; signs of withdrawal: cramps, nausea, vomiting, diarrhea; sleep disturbance, chills and shaking | Pinpoint pupils, mental clouding, lethargy, impaired memory and judgment, evidence of needle tracks, inflamed nasal mucosa if drug is snorted | Depressed consciousness and respirations, dilated pupils with anoxia or polydrug use | Provide emergency support of vital functions. In withdrawal, administer methadone or Narcan as ordered. |
| *Stimulant*<br>Cocaine/crack | Increased self-esteem, energy, sexual desire, euphoria; decreased anxiety | Dopamine deficiency results in psychologic dependency to produce feelings of well-being | Increased vital signs, headache, chest pain, depression and/or paranoia, inflamed nasal passages if snorted | Delirium, tremors, high fever (106+) convulsions, cardiac/ respiratory arrest | Emergency support of vital functions, reduce CNS stimulation. |
| *Amphetamines*<br>Amphetamine, dextroamphetamine, methamphetamine | Depressed appetite; increased activity, awareness, sense of well-being | Long-term use or high doses may produce delirium, paranoid-like delusions, withdrawal, depression, fatigue, sleep disturbances | Same as cocaine, plus suicidal ideation | Same as cocaine | Same as cocaine, plus suicide precautions. Observe for increased anxiety to panic, which may potentiate assaultive behavior. |
| Phencyclidine (PCP) | Euphoria, psychomotor agitation, emotional lability | Not reported | Vomiting, hallucinations, paranoid ideation, agitation | Violent behavior, suicide, respiratory arrest, delirium, coma, increased blood pressure and pulse | Monitor vital signs. Observe for suicidal or assaultive behavior. Provide nonthreatening environment, reality orientation, support. |
| *Hallucinogens*<br>LSD, mescaline | Disordered perceptions, depersonalization | Not reported | "Bad trip," high anxiety to panic; hallucinations may occur long after drug has been metabolized; flashbacks may produce long-lasting psychotic diorders | Reduced LOC | Same as PCP, plus talk client down. |

*(continues)*

**Table 7-5** Commonly Abused Drugs *(continued)*

| Drug | Effect | Dependence | Assessment Findings | Overdose | Nursing Interventions for Overdose |
|---|---|---|---|---|---|
| *Cannabis*<br>Marijuana, hashish, THC | Euphoria, intense perceptions, relaxation, lethargy | Not reported | Increased pulse rate and appetite; impaired judgment and coordination | Panic reaction, nausea, vomiting, depression and disorders of perception | In panic, talk down.<br>In severe depression, institute suicide precautions. |
| *Benzodiazepines*<br>Anti-anxiety drugs, muscle relaxants: clonazepam, diazepam, and others | Reduction in anxiety; anticonvulsant, reduces muscle spasms, reduces insomnia | Physical: dependence is low with oral dosing<br>Psychologic: withdrawal syndrome may resemble an anxiety disorder<br>Must differentiate withdrawal syndrome from anxiety disorders | Calm effect unless drug withdrawn abruptly<br>Mild withdrawal including confusion, anterograde amnesia (impaired recall of events after dosing), anxiety, diaphoresis, tremors<br>Effect may resemble alcohol intoxication | Mild sedation to stupor dependent on dose<br>CNS depression, sedation to stupor, dose dependent<br>Oral unlikely to cause significant respiratory depression without concomitant agents such as alcohol<br>Intravenous may cause severe respiratory depression and death | Support vital body functions.<br>Provide nonthreatening environment.<br>Administer Narcan as ordered. Must be closely monitored. |

**D.** Have decreased feelings of anxiety.

**E.** Receive information and consider help for substance-abuse disorder (e.g., AA or NA).

## Interventions

**A.** Assess drug use pattern: identity, recent use, and frequency of use of prescription and nonprescription drugs, other substances (e.g., alcohol, nicotine).

**B.** Support client during acute phase of detoxification or withdrawal.

1. Stay with client; reassure that current manifestations are temporary.
2. Monitor vital signs, level of consciousness.
3. Institute suicide precautions (if appropriate).
4. Administer medications (to prevent withdrawal) as ordered.
5. If client is experiencing panic, talk down, possibly with assistance of family/friends.
6. If client is hallucinating, reinforce reality, speak in a calm voice.
7. Confront client's use of denial.
8. Monitor your own responses of sympathy/anger.
9. Be aware of transference/countertransference.
10. Maintain course of action in plan of care; client must follow plan.

11. Involve staff in negotiating care plan revisions.

**C.** Rehabilitation/longer-term care
1. Provide nonthreatening environment.
2. Set limits on unacceptable behavior.
3. Provide adequate diet and fluids.
4. Provide information relating to substance abuse and rehabilitation programs.

## Evaluation

**A.** Client experiences no injury.

**B.** Vital signs are stable.

**C.** Withdrawal proceeded without symptoms; client remains drug/alcohol free.

**D.** Client can discuss substance-abuse problem and requests or agrees to consider rehabilitation/therapy for problem.

## Specific Disorders

### Alcohol Abuse/Dependence

**A.** General information
1. Alcohol is a legal substance and there are millions of social drinkers.

2. Alcohol is classified as a central nervous system depressant.
3. Alcohol abuse/dependence is a major problem in this country with over 18 million adults identified as alcohol abusers (see Table 7-6)
4. Only approximately 5% of alcohol abusers are the "skid row" type.
5. Incidence is increasing in women and adolescents.
6. Considered a disease that can be arrested but not cured.
7. Important to assess history of alcohol consumption for clients admitted to hospital for non–alcohol-related disorders, because they may go into withdrawal.
8. Socioeconomic as well as a physiologic problem, resulting in increased health care costs and loss of productivity if ability to maintain a job is impaired.
9. Alcohol used with other substances (barbiturates, antianxiety drugs) may have lethal consequences.
10. Long-term use may result in loss of health (gastritis, pancreatitis, cirrhosis, hepatitis, malnutrition, cardiac and neural disorders) and life (suicide, automobile accidents).
11. Directly related problems include withdrawal, delirium tremens, and alcohol-related dementia
    a. Withdrawal
       1) Alcohol consumption reduced/discontinued following continuous consumption for many days or longer
       2) Withdrawal is progressive and has four stages:
          I: At least 8 hours after last drink; symptoms include mild tremors, tachycardia, increased blood pressure, diaphoresis, nervousness
          II: Gross tremors, hyperactivity, profound confusion, loss of appetite, insomnia, weakness, disorientation, illusions, auditory and visual hallucinations
          III: 12–48 hours after last drink: symptoms include (in addition to those found in I and II) severe hallucinations, grand mal seizures
          IV: 3–5 days after last drink (24–72 hours if untreated): delirium tremens, confusion, agitation, severe psychomotor activity, hallucinations, insomnia, tachycardia
       3) Withdrawal may last less than a week or may evolve into alcohol withdrawal delirium (delirium tremens).
       4) 10–15% mortality rate from hypoglycemia/electrolyte imbalances.
    b. Delirium tremens (DTs)
       1) History of alcohol abuse usually for more than 5 years.
       2) May be preceded by seizures.
       3) Symptoms occur 2–3 days after alcohol reduced/discontinued.
       4) Signs include tachycardia, increased blood pressure, agitation, delusions, hallucinations.
    c. Alcohol hallucinosis: hallucinations only
    d. Alcohol-related dementia: caused by poor nutrition
       1) Korsakoff's psychosis is sometimes preceded by Wernicke's encephalopathy. Confusion and ataxia are predominant symptoms.
       2) Thiamine deficiency results in Korsakoff's dementia/psychosis; symptoms include chronic disorientation, confabulation. It is irreversible.
       3) Large doses of thiamine may prevent the development of Korsakoff's psychosis.
B. Medical management
   1. Vitamin and nutrition therapy
   2. Antianxiety drugs (Librium or Ativan)
   3. Disulfiram (Antabuse)
      a. Produces unpleasant reaction (thirst, sweating, palpitations, vomiting, dyspnea, respiratory and cardiac failure) when taken with alcohol.
      b. 500 mg/day for 1–2 weeks; usual maintenance dose is 250 mg/day.
      c. Duration of action is ½ to several hours; no alcohol should be taken at least 12 hours before taking drug.
      d. Increases effects of antianxiety drugs and oral anticoagulants.

**Table 7-6** Phases of Alcohol Addiction

| Phase | Features |
|---|---|
| Prealcoholic | Drink almost every day to reduce tension |
| | Increase in amount of alcohol ingested |
| Addiction | Blackouts |
| | Secret drinking |
| | Large amounts ingested |
| Dependence | Physical craving for alcohol |
| | Makes up reasons for drinking |
| | Reduced nutrition |
| | Aggressive behavior |
| | Pressure from family and/or employer to reduce/stop drinking |
| Chronic | Long periods of intoxication |
| | Impaired thinking |
| | Less alcohol produces sedation tremors |

e. Side effects include headache, dry mouth, somnolence, flushing.
f. Nursing responsibilities
1) Teach client the nature of severe reaction and importance of avoiding all alcohol (including cough medicine, foods prepared with alcohol, etc.).
2) Teach client to carry an identification card in case of accidental alcohol ingestion.
3) Monitor effects of antianxiety drugs if being taken at the same time.
4) Monitor for bleeding if taking oral anticoagulants.
4. High doses of chlordiazepoxide (Librium) to control withdrawal in acute detoxification.
C. Assessment findings
1. Dependent personality; often using denial as a defense mechanism
2. Tendency to minimize and underreport amount of alcohol consumed
3. Intoxication: blood alcohol level 0.15 (150 mg alcohol/100 mL blood). Legal level 0.08–0.10.
4. Signs of impaired judgment, motor skills, and slurred speech
5. Behavior may be boisterous, euphoric, aggressive, or may be depressed, withdrawn
6. Signs of withdrawal, DTs, or alcohol-related dementias
D. Nursing interventions
1. Stay with client.
2. Monitor vital signs and blood sugar levels.
3. Observe for tremors, seizures, increased agitation, anxiety, disorders of perception.
4. Administer medications as ordered; observe effects/side effects of tranquilizers carefully.
5. If disorders of perception occur, explain that these are part of the withdrawal process.
6. Provide fluids, adequate nutrition, and quiet environment.
7. When client is stable, provide information about rehabilitation programs (Alcoholics Anonymous); at this stage client may be willing to consider a program to stop drinking.
8. Provide information about Alanon (for spouse and adult family members), Alateen (for children), and ACOA (for adult children of alcoholics).

## Psychoactive Drug Use

A. General information
1. Drugs abused may be prescription or "street" drugs
2. Types of drugs frequently abused
a. Barbiturates, antianxiety drugs, hypnotics
b. Opioids (narcotics): heroin, morphine, meperidine, methadone, hydromorphone
c. Amphetamines (speed): amphetamine, dextroamphetamine, methamphetamine, some appetite suppressants
d. Cocaine, hydrochloride cocaine (crack)
e. Phencyclidine (PCP)
f. Hallucinogens: LSD, mescaline, DMT
g. Cannabis: marijuana, hashish, THC
B. Assessment findings and nursing interventions for overdoses vary with particular drug; see Table 7-5
C. Polydrug abusers
1. Common pattern of drug use.
2. Synergistic effect: drugs interact so that effect is greater than if each drug is taken separately.
3. Additive effect: two or more drugs with same action are taken together (e.g., barbiturates with alcohol will result in heavy sedation).

## Impaired Nurses

A. General information
1. Most nursing licenses are suspended or revoked for substance abuse while on duty.
2. Substances include alcohol and/or prescription drugs stolen from unit drug stocks.
3. Stealing drugs may result in criminal prosecution.
4. Work-related stress and easy access to drugs are factors relating to nurses' substance abuse.
5. Substance use results in impaired judgment and psychomotor abilities, resulting in unsafe nursing practice.
B. Assessment of impairment
1. Alcohol odor on breath
2. Frequent lateness/absences
3. Shortages in narcotics
4. Clients do not experience pain relief after "receiving" pain reduction medication from nurse
5. Nurse makes frequent trips to bathroom/locker room
6. Changes in locomotion, psychomotor skills, pupil size, and mood/affect
C. Nurses' responsibilities related to impaired nurse colleague
1. Client safety is first priority.
2. ANA code of ethics (and most state laws) require nurse to safeguard clients.
3. Interventions for suspected substance abuse by coworker
a. Obtain information about legal issues, treatment options, and institutional policies.
b. Document observations related to behaviors and narcotic charting.
c. If possible, have other coworkers verify your information.
d. Arrange meeting with peer(s), nurse, supervisor, nurse advocate (where possible) and confront nurse with documentation.
e. Let nurse know you care and will help.
f. Help nurse work through denial.
g. Provide plan to offer recovery program (e.g., include "recovering" nurse buddy).
h. Offer hope, support (moral and financial) to aid nurse in treatment.

i. Explain institutional policies regarding future employment.
j. If nurse continues to deny substance abuse, consider following steps:
  1) Advocate should protect nurse's rights.
  2) Suspension/dismissal from job.
  3) Report to licensing board.
  4) If theft of drug from unit has occurred, report to law enforcement agency.

# SCHIZOPHRENIA AND OTHER PSYCHOTIC DISORDERS

## Overview

A. Characterized by disordered thinking, delusions, hallucinations, depersonalization (feeling of being strange, not oneself), impaired reality testing (psychosis), and impaired interpersonal relationships.
B. Regression to the earliest stages of development is often noted (e.g., incontinence, mutism).
C. Onset is usually in adolescence/early adulthood (15 to 35 years of age).
D. Client may be seriously impaired and unable to perform ADLs.
E. Etiology is not known; theories include:
  1. Genetic: 1% of population.
  2. Biochemical: neurotransmitter dysfunction i.e., dopamine, serotonin.
  3. Interaction of predisposing risk and environmental stress.
F. Prior to onset (premorbid) client may have been suspicious, eccentric, or withdrawn.

## Classifications

A. Disorganized: incoherent; delusions are not organized; social withdrawal; affect blunted, silly, or inappropriate
B. Catatonic: psychomotor disturbances
  1. Stupor: mute, little reaction or movement
  2. Excitement: purposeless, excited motor activity
  3. Posturing: voluntary, inappropriate, bizarre postures
C. Paranoid: delusions and hallucinations of persecution/grandeur
D. Undifferentiated: disorganized behaviors, delusions, and hallucinations

## Assessment

A. Assess—"Four As"
  1. Affect: flat, blunted
  2. Associative looseness: verbalizations are disorganized
  3. Ambivalence: cannot choose between conflicting emotions
  4. Autistic thinking: thoughts on self, extreme withdrawal, unable to relate to outside world

B. Any changes in thoughts, speech, affect
C. Ability to perform self-care activities, nutritional deficits
D. Suicide potential
E. Aggression
F. Regression
G. Impaired communication

## Analysis

Nursing diagnoses for clients with schizophrenic disorders may include:
A. Anxiety
B. Disturbed sensory-perceptual
C. Disturbed sleep pattern
D. Disturbed thought process
E. Imbalanced nutrition; less than body requirements
F. Impaired verbal communication
G. Ineffective coping
H. Low self-esteem
I. Powerlessness
J. Risk for injury
K. Risk for violence
L. Self-care deficit
M. Social isolation

## Planning and Implementation

### Goals

Client will:
A. Develop a trusting/therapeutic relationship with nurse.
B. Be oriented, able to test reality.
C. Be protected from injury.
D. Be able to recognize impending loss of control.
E. Adhere to medication regimen.
F. Participate in activities.
G. Increase ability to care for self.

### Interventions

A. Offer self in development of therapeutic relationship.
B. Use silence.
C. Set time for interaction with client.
D. Encourage reality orientation but understand that delusions/hallucinations are real to client.
E. Assist with feeding/dressing as necessary.
F. Check on client frequently, remove potentially harmful objects.
G. Contract with client to tell you when anxiety is becoming so high that loss of control is possible.
H. Administer antipsychotic medications as ordered (see Table 7-7 for side effects and dosages); observe for effects.
  1. Reduction of hallucinations, delusions, agitation
  2. Postural hypotension
    a. Obtain baseline blood pressure and monitor sitting/standing.

## Table 7-7 Antipsychotic Medications

| Drug Classification | Dosages | | | Significant Side Effects |
|---|---|---|---|---|
| | Acute Symptoms | Maintenance/Day | Range/Day | |
| Chlorpromazine (Thorazine) | 25–100 mg IM q1–4h prn | 200–600 mg PO | 25–2000 mg PO | Sedation<br>Anticholinergic effects: dry mouth, blurred vision, constipation, urinary retention, postural hypotension |
| Fluphenazine HCl (Prolixin) | 1.25 mg IM, max 10 mg IM, divided doses | 1–5 mg PO | 1–30 mg PO | Extrapyramidal effects |
| Fluphenazine decanoate/enanthate (Prolixin) | – | 25 mg IM q2wk | 25–100 mg IM | Extrapyramidal |
| Trifluoperazine (Stelazine) | 1–2 mg IM q4h; 2–4 mg PO, max 10 mg qd | 2–4 mg PO | 2–80 mg PO | Extrapyramidal |
| Haloperidol (Haldol) | 2–10 mg IM in divided doses | 2–8 mg PO | 1–100 mg PO | Extrapyramidal |
| Thiothixene (Navane) | 8–16 mg IM in divided doses | 6–10 mg PO | 6–60 mg PO | Extrapyramidal |
| Loxapine (Loxitane) | – | 60–100 mg PO | 30–250 mg PO | Extrapyramidal |
| Olanzapine (Zyprexa) | 10–20 mg PO | 5–20 mg PO | 2.5–20 mg PO | Sedation, weight gain, increased glucose and lipid levels |
| Quetepine (Seroquel) | 400–800 mg PO | 200–600 mg PO | 25–800 mg PO | Sedation, may accelerate cataract formation |
| Ziprasidone (Geodon) | 40–80 mg PO BID with food or 10-20 mg IM BID | 20–80 mg PO BID | 20–80 mg PO BID 10–40 mg IM | Nausea, anxiety, insomnia (transient); QTC prolongation |
| Aripiprazole (Abilify) | 10–30 mg PO | 10–30 mg PO | 10–30 mg PO | Nausea, insomnia |
| Clozapine (Clozaril) | – | 300–450 mg PO | 75–700 mg PO | Agranulocytosis; sedation |
| Risperidone (Risperdal) | 2–6 mg PO | 2–6 mg PO | 0.25–8 mg PO | Increased prolactin levels, EPS at higher doses, sedation |

b. Client must lie prone for 1 hour following injection.
c. Teach client to sit up or stand up slowly.
d. Elevate client's legs while seated.
e. Withhold drug if systolic pressure drops more than 20–30 mm Hg from previous reading.

3. Photosensitivity
   a. Advise use of sun screen.
   b. Avoid exposure to sunlight.
4. Agranulocytosis
   a. Instruct client to report sore throat or fever.
   b. Institute reverse isolation if necessary.
5. Elimination
   a. Measure I&O.
   b. Check bladder distension.
   c. Keep bowel record.
6. Sedation
   a. Avoid use of heavy machinery.
   b. Do not drive.
7. Extrapyramidal symptoms (EPS)
   a. Dystonic reactions
      1) Sudden contractions of face, tongue, throat, extraocular muscles
      2) Administer antiparkinson agents prn (e.g., benztropine [Cogentin] 1–8 mg PO, IM, IV; diphenhydramine [Bendadryl] 10–50 mg PO, IM, IV; trihexyphenidyl [Artane] 3–15 mg PO only).
      3) Remain with client; this is a frightening experience and usually occurs when medication is started.

b. Parkinson syndrome
1) Occurs within 1–3 weeks
2) Tremors, rigid posture, masklike facial appearance
3) Administer antiparkinson agents prn.
c. Akathisia
1) Motor restlessness
2) Need to keep moving
3) Administer antiparkinson agents.
4) Do not mistake this for agitation; do not increase antipsychotic medication.
5) Reduce medications to see whether symptoms decrease.
6) Determine if movement is under voluntary control.
d. Tardive dyskinesia
1) Involuntary movements of tongue, face, extremities
2) May occur after prolonged use of antipsychotics
e. Neuroleptic malignant syndrome
1) Occurs days/weeks after initiation of treatment in 1% of clients
2) Elevated vital signs, rigidity, and confusion followed by incontinence, mutism, opisthotonos, retrocollis, renal failure, coma, and death
3) Discontinue medication, notify physician, monitor vital signs, electrolyte balance, I&O
f. Elderly clients should receive doses reduced by one-half to one-third of recommended level
I. Encourage participation in milieu, group, art, and occupational therapies when client able to tolerate them.

## Evaluation

Client
A. Stays with nurse prescribed period of time.
B. Is oriented to reality, can state name, place, and date.
C. Can feed/dress self with specified amount of assistance.
D. Has not attempted/will not attempt to injure self or others.
E. Adheres to medication regimen with minimal side effects.
F. Participates in activities.

# MOOD DISORDERS

## Overview

A. Characterized by disturbance in mood (affect) that is either depression or elation (mania); occur in a variety of patterns, alone or together (see Figure 7-1). Disturbance is beyond normal range of mood experienced by most people.

B. Bipolar disorder: components of both depression and elation (formerly called manic-depression)
C. Cyclothymic disorder: milder symptoms of both mania and depression, often separated by long periods of normal mood
D. Dysthymic disorder: long-standing symptoms of depression alternating with short periods of normal mood; client usually able to maintain roles in job, school, etc.
E. Etiology is unknown; theories include:
1. Genetic: approximately 7% of general population; risk is 20% if a close relative has depression
2. Biochemical: dysregulation in norepinephrine and serotonin
3. Psychoanalytic: anger turned inward (i.e., anger toward significant other is turned into anger toward self)

## Assessment

A. Mood: dysphoric; blue/sad or elated/aggressive
B. Presence of psychomotor agitation, retardation, or hyperactivity
C. Disorders of cognition: narrowed perception and interests, impaired concentration, grandiose delusions, flight of ideas in elation stage
D. Sexual functioning changes
E. Appropriateness of appearance/dress
F. Appetite
G. Potential for suicide

## Analysis

Nursing diagnoses for clients with affective disorders may include:
A. Constipation
B. Impaired verbal communication
C. Ineffective coping
D. Risk for injury
E. Imbalanced nutrition: less than body requirements
F. Self-care deficit
G. Disturbed self-esteem
H. Disturbed sleep pattern
I. Disturbed thought processes

## Planning and Implementation

### Goals

Client will:
A. Be protected from injury.
B. Receive adequate rest and sleep.
C. Maintain adequate intake of fluids and nutrients, regular elimination.
D. Develop trusting/therapeutic relationship with nurse.
E. Be oriented to reality.
F. Participate in planned activities.

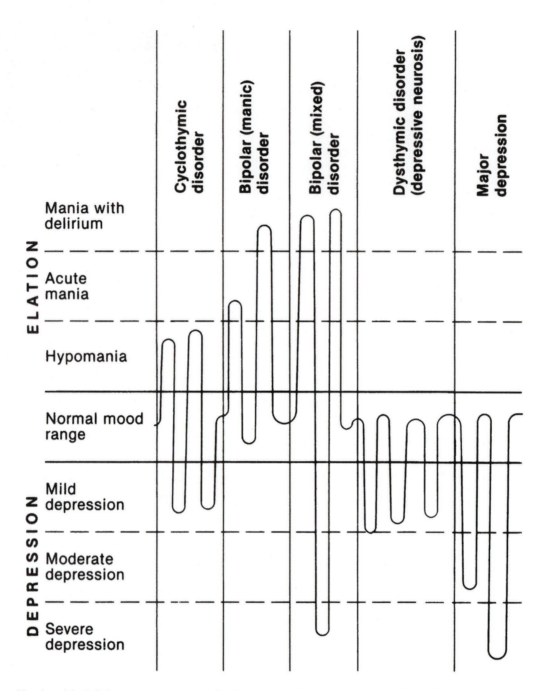

Mania with delirium: persecutory delusions, grandiose delusions, hallucinations
Acute mania: flight of ideas, impulsive behavior, bizarre dress and behavior, distractibility
Hypomania: decreased sleep, inflated self-esteem, increased activity, irritability
Mild depression: sadness, irritability, sleep disorders, social withdrawal, crying and tearful, low energy
Moderate depression: recurring thoughts of suicide, hopelessness, helplessness
Severe depression: delusions, hallucinations, psychomotor retardation and stupor, agitation (in depression with melancholia)

**Figure 7-1** Patterns of mood disturbances in affective disorders

## Interventions

A. Assess for suicide potential.
B. Encourage verbalization of feelings of hopelessness and helplessness.
C. Provide quiet environment for rest and sleep.
D. Provide small, attractive meals; encourage intake of fluids.
E. Maintain bowel record.
F. Use silence and broad openings, focus on client's verbal/nonverbal behaviors.
G. Present reality but accept client's need for delusions.
H. Accept client's negative responses, hostility.
I. Provide activities and tasks to raise client's self-esteem.
J. Assist with self-care as needed.
K. If client is agitated
   1. Work with client on a one-to-one basis.
   2. Walk with client; provide some diversional activity.
   3. Reduce environmental stimuli (e.g., quiet room, dim lights).

## Evaluation

Client
A. Has gained or maintained weight.
B. Reports any suicidal ideation.
C. Sleeps a specified number of hours.
D. Can meet own needs for ADLs.
E. Has realistic appraisal of self.

## Specific Disorders

### Bipolar Disorder (Manic Episode)

A. General information
   1. Onset usually before age 30
   2. Characterized by hyperactivity and euphoria that may become sarcasm or hostility
B. Assessment findings
   1. Hyperactivity to the point of physical exhaustion
   2. Flamboyant dress/makeup
   3. Sexual acting out
   4. Impulsive behaviors
   5. Flight of ideas: inability to finish one thought before jumping to another
   6. Loud, domineering, manipulative behavior
   7. Distractibility
   8. Dehydration, nutritional deficits
   9. Delusions of grandeur
   10. Possible short-term depression (risk of suicide)
   11. Hostility, aggression
C. Medical management
   1. Lithium carbonate (Eskalith, Lithobid, Lithotabs)
      a. Initial dosage levels: 600 mg TID, to maintain a blood serum level of 1.0–1.5 mEq/liter; blood serum levels should be checked 12 hours after last dose, twice a week.
      b. Maintenance dosage levels: 300 mg TID/QID, to maintain a blood serum level of 0.4–1.0 mEq/liter; checked monthly.
      c. Toxicity when blood levels higher than 2.0 mEq/liter: tremors, nausea and vomiting, thirst, polyuria, coma, seizures, cardiac arrest
   2. Antipsychotics may also be given for hyperactivity, agitation, psychotic behavior. Chlorpromazine (Thorazine) and haloperidol (Haldol) are most commonly used (see Table 7-7).
D. Nursing interventions
   1. Determine what client is attempting to tell you; use active listening.
   2. Assist client in focusing on a topic.
   3. Offer finger foods, high-nutrition foods, and fluids.
   4. Provide quiet environment, decrease stimuli.
   5. Stay with client, use silence.
   6. Remove harmful objects.
   7. Be accepting of hostile statements.
   8. Do not argue with client.
   9. Use distraction to divert client from behaviors that are harmful to self or others.
   10. Administer medications as ordered and observe for effects/side effects.
      a. Teach clients early signs of toxicity.
      b. Maintain fluid and salt intake.
      c. Avoid diuretics.
      d. Monitor lithium blood levels.
   11. Assist in dressing, bathing.
   12. Set limits on disruptive behaviors.

### Major Depression

A. General information
   1. Characterized by loss of ambition, lack of interest in activities and sex, low self-esteem, and feelings of boredom and sadness.
   2. Etiology may be physiologic or response to an actual or perceived loss.
   3. These clients are at high risk for suicide, especially when depressed mood begins to lift and/or energy level increases.
B. Medical management (see Table 7-8)
   1. Tricyclic antidepressants: amitriptyline HCl, etc.
   2. Monoamine oxidase inhibitors (MAOIs): isocarboxazid (Marplan), etc.
   3. Atypical antidepressants: fluoxetin (Prozac), sertraline (Zoloft), etc.
   4. Electroconvulsive therapy (ECT)
C. Assessment findings
   1. Feelings of helplessness, hopelessness, worthlessness
   2. Reduction in normal activities or agitation
   3. Slowing of body functions/elimination
   4. Loss of appetite
   5. Inappropriate guilt
   6. Self-deprecation, low self-esteem

**Table 7-8** Antidepressant Medications

| Drug | Initiating | Dosage Maintenance | Side Effects |
|---|---|---|---|
| *SSRIs* | | | |
| Fluoxetine (Prozac, Prozac Weekly) | 20 mg PO | 20–40 mg/day or 90 mg once per week (once stable) | Sexual dysfunction; nausea, diarrhea, headache, anxiety (transient) |
| Sertraline (Zoloft) | 50 mg PO | 50–200 mg/day | As above |
| Paroxetine (Paxil, Paxil CR) | 20 mg PO 25 mg PO | 20–40 mg/day 25–50 mg/day | As above |
| Citalopram (Celexa) | 20 mg PO | 20–80 mg/day | Sexual dysfunction; nausea, headache, nervousness (transient) |
| Escitalopram (Lexapro) | 10 mg PO | 10–20 mg/day | As above |
| Fluvoxamine (Luvox) | 50 mg PO HS | 50–300 mg HS | Tiredness, sexual dysfunction; headache, nausea, nervousness (transient) (used in treatment of OCD) |
| *Atypical Antidepressants* | | | |
| Bupropion (Wellbutrin SR) | 100 mg PO | 150 mg BID | Anxiety, insomnia; can lower seizure threshold in overdose |
| Mirtazapine (Remeron) | 15 mg PO HS | 30–45 mg HS | Sedation at 15 mg (less at higher doses); increased appetite |
| Nefazodone (Serzone) | 50 mg PO HS | 50–600 mg HS | Sedation, dry mouth, postural hypotension; liver toxicity |
| Venlafaxine (Effexor XR) | 37.5 mg PO | 75–375 mg | Sexual dysfunction; headache, nausea, nervousness; can increase BP at doses > 300 mg/day |
| Trazodone (Desyrel) | 150 mg PO in divided doses | 150–400 mg PO in divided doses | Sedation, anxiety, hypotension, priapism (commonly used as sleep aid) |
| *Tricyclics* | | | |
| Amitriptyline (Elavil, Endep) | 75–100 mg PO | 50–150 mg PO at bedtime; 80–100 mg IM in divided doses | Constipation, blurred vision, drowsiness, orthostatic hypotension, urinary retention, dry mouth, increased appetite, sexual dysfunction |
| Doxepine (Apo-Doxepin, Novo-Doxepin) | 25 mg PO TID (or up to 150 mg can be given at bedtime) | 75–150 mg/day | Sedation, confusion, constipation, decreased libido |
| Clomipramine (Anafranil) | 75–250 mg PO in divided doses at HS | 50–150 mg PO at HS | As above |
| Desipramine (Norpramin) | 50 mg HS | 100–150 mg HS | As above |
| Nortriptyline | 50 mg HS | 50–125 mg HS | As above |
| *Monoamine Oxidase Inhibitors (MAOIs)* | | | |
| Isocarboxazid (Marplan) | 30 mg PO in divided doses | 10–30 mg PO | As for tricyclics, plus angina, hypoglycemia, hypertensive crisis precipitated by ingestion of foods with tyramine or concurrent use of tricyclics |
| Phenalizine (Nardil) | 60 mg PO in divided doses | 30–60 mg PO | As above |

7

7. Inability to concentrate, disordered thinking
8. Poor hygiene
9. Slumped posture
10. Crying, ruminating (relates same incident over and over)
11. Dependency
12. Depressed children: possible separation anxiety
13. Elderly clients: possible symptoms of dementia
14. Somatic and persecutory delusions and hallucinations

D. Nursing interventions
1. Monitor I&O.
2. Weigh client regularly.
3. Maintain a schedule of regular appointments.
4. Remove potentially harmful articles.
5. Contract with client to report suicidal ideation, impulses, plans; check on client frequently.
6. Assist with dressing, hygiene, and feeding.
7. Encourage discussion of negative/positive aspects of self.
8. Encourage change to more positive topics if self-deprecating thoughts persist.
9. Administer antidepressant medications (see Table 7-8) as ordered.
   a. Tricyclic antidepressants (TCAs)
      1) Effectiveness increased by antihistamines, alcohol, benzodiazepines
      2) Effectiveness decreased by barbiturates, nicotine, vitamin C
   b. Monoamine oxidase inhibitors (MAOIs)
      1) Effectiveness increased with antipsychotic drugs, alcohol, meperidine
      2) Avoid foods containing tyramine (e.g., beer, red wine, aged cheese, avocados, caffeine, chocolate, sour cream, yogurt); these foods or MAOIs taken with TCAs may result in hypertensive crisis.
   c. Be sure client swallows medication. If side effects disappear suddenly, cheeking/hoarding may have occurred. These medications can be used to attempt suicide.
   d. Antidepressant medications do not take effect for 2–3 weeks. Encourage client to continue medication even if not feeling better. Be aware of suicide potential during this time.
   e. Warn client not to take any drugs without consulting physician.
10. Assist with electroconvulsive therapy as ordered.
   a. Give normal pre-op preparation, including informed consent (see Perioperative Nursing).
   b. Remove all hairpins, dentures.
   c. Ensure client is wearing loose clothing.
   d. Check vital signs after the procedure.
   e. Reorient and assure that any memory loss is temporary.
   f. Assist to room or to care of responsible party if outpatient.

### Dysthymic Disorder

A. General information: chronic mood disturbance of at least 2 years' duration for adults, 1 year for children
B. Assessment findings
   1. Normal moods for a period of weeks, followed by depression
   2. Insomnia/hypersomnia
   3. Social withdrawal
   4. Loss of interest in activities
   5. Recurrent thoughts of suicide and death
C. Nursing interventions: same as for major depression.

## NEUROTIC DISORDERS

In DSM-IV-TR, the disorders formerly categorized as neurotic disorders are included in Anxiety, Somatoform, and Dissociative Disorders. Reality testing is intact.

## ANXIETY DISORDERS

### Overview

A. Common element is anxiety, manifested in a variety of behaviors (see also Behaviors Related to Emotional Distress).
B. Therapy relates to reduction of anxiety; when anxiety is reduced, the symptoms will be alleviated.
C. Types include generalized anxiety disorder, panic disorder, phobic disorders, and obsessive-compulsive disorders.

### Assessment

A. Level of anxiety: may be to point of panic
B. Vital signs: may be elevated
C. Reality testing: should be intact; can recognize that thoughts are irrational but cannot control them
D. Physical symptoms: no organic basis
E. Memory: possible memory loss or loss of identity
F. Pattern of symptoms: chronic with a pattern of waxing and waning or sudden onset

### Analysis

Nursing diagnoses for the client with an anxiety disorder may include:
A. Anxiety
B. Deprivation of sleep

C. Disturbed thought processes
D. Fear
E. Ineffective coping
F. Ineffective tissue perfusion
G. Powerlessness

# Planning and Implementation

## Goals

Client will:
A. Develop a trusting/therapeutic relationship with nurse.
B. Recognize causes of anxiety and develop alternative coping mechanisms.
C. Reduce/alleviate symptoms of anxiety.

## Interventions

A. Encourage discussion of anxiety and relationship to symptoms.
B. Provide calm, accepting atmosphere.
C. Administer antianxiety medications (for short-term use only) as ordered and monitor effects/side effects.
   1. Diazepam (Valium): 5–20 mg PO daily; 2–10 mg IM or IV daily
   2. Chlordiazepoxide (Librium): 20–100 mg PO daily; 50–100 mg IM or IV daily
   3. Alprazolam (Xanax) 0.75–4 mg PO daily
   4. Oxazepam (Serax) 30–120 mg PO daily
   5. Triazolam (Halcion) 0.25–0.5 mg, PO HS
   6. Side effects
      a. Client may become addicted.
      b. Additive effect with alcohol.
      c. Dizziness may occur when treatment initiated.
      d. Lower doses for elderly client.
      e. Do not stop abruptly; taper doses.
D. Teach client about self-medication regimen and side effects.

# Evaluation

Client
A. Can discuss causes of anxiety with nurse.
B. Demonstrates constructive coping mechanisms and ability to reduce anxiety.
C. Demonstrates knowledge of effects and hazards of antianxiety medications.

# Specific Disorders

## Phobic Disorders

A. General information
   1. Irrational fears resulting in avoidance of objects or situations.
   2. Repressed conflicts are projected to outside world and eventually are displaced onto an object or situation.
   3. Client can recognize that fear of these objects/situations is irrational, but cannot control emotional response when confronting or thinking about confronting the particular object/situation.
B. Assessment findings
   1. Agoraphobia: most serious phobia; fear of being alone or in public places; may reach point where client panics at thought of being in public places and cannot leave home.
   2. Social phobias: fear of being in situations where one may be scrutinized and embarrassed by others.
   3. Specific phobias: irrational fear of specific objects/situations (e.g., snakes, insects, heights, closed places).
C. Nursing interventions
   1. Know that behavior modification and systematic desensitization most commonly used; client cannot be "reasoned" out of behavior.
   2. Do not force contact with feared object/situation; may result in panic.
   3. Administer benzodiazepines (alprazolam or clonazepam), SSRIs, venlafaxine, or buspirone as ordered.
   4. Instruct in and encourage use of relaxation techniques.

## Generalized Anxiety Disorder

A. General information
   1. Persistent anxiety for at least 1 month
   2. Cannot be controlled by client or displaced, remains free-floating and diffuse
B. Assessment findings
   1. Motor tensions: trembling, muscle aches, jumpiness
   2. Autonomic hyperactivity: sweating, palpitations, dizziness, upset stomach, increased pulse and respirations
   3. Affect: worried and fearful of what might happen
   4. Hyperalert: insomnia, irritability
C. Nursing interventions
   1. Stay with client.
   2. Encourage discussion of anxiety and its source.
   3. Provide calm, relaxing atmosphere.
   4. Administer antianxiety drugs, as ordered.
   5. Observe for effects and side effects.
   6. Monitor vital signs.
   7. Assess for level of anxiety.

## Panic Disorder (with/without Agoraphobia)

A. General information: acute, panic-like attack lasting from a few minutes to an hour.
B. Assessment findings
   1. Sudden onset of intense fear/terror
   2. Symptoms: include dyspnea, palpitations, chest pain, sensation of smothering or choking, faintness, fear of dying, dizziness

3. When severe, symptoms mimic acute cardiac disease that must be ruled out.
4. Client may be seen in ER.
C. Nursing interventions: same as for generalized anxiety disorder.

## Obsessive-Compulsive Disorder (OCD)

A. General information
   1. Obsession
      a. Recurrent thoughts that client cannot control; often violent, fearful, or doubting in nature (e.g., fear of contamination).
      b. Client cannot keep thoughts from intruding into consciousness; eventually resort to defense of undoing (performing ritual behavior).
   2. Compulsion
      a. Action (ritual behavior) that serves to reduce tension from obsessive thought.
      b. Client may not desire to perform behavior but is unable to stop, as this is the only relief from distress.
      c. May interfere with social/occupational functioning.
B. Nursing interventions
   1. Allow compulsive behavior, but set reasonable limits.
   2. Permit client to complete behavior once started; aggression may result if behavior is not allowed or completed.
   3. Engage client in alternative behaviors (client will not be able to do this alone).
   4. Provide opportunities to perform tasks that meet need for perfectionism (e.g., stacking and folding linens).
   5. As compulsive behavior decreases, help client to verbalize feelings, concerns.
   6. Help client to make choices, participate in decisions regarding own schedule.
   7. Administer clomipramine (Anafranil) as ordered. Gradual decrease in symptoms may take 2–3 months. Often used with behavior modification therapy (see Table 7-8).

## Post-Traumatic Stress Disorder (PTSD)

A. General information
   1. Disturbed/disintegrated response to significant trauma
   2. Symptoms can occur following crisis event such as war, earthquake, flood, airplane crash, rape, or assault
   3. Reexperiencing of traumatic event in recollections, nightmares
B. Assessment findings
   1. Psychic numbing: not as responsive to persons and events as to the traumatic experience
   2. Sleep disturbances (e.g., nightmares)
   3. Avoidance of environment/activities likely to arouse recall of trauma

4. Symptoms of depression
5. Possible violent outbursts
6. Memory impairment
7. Panic attacks
8. Substance abuse
C. Nursing interventions
   1. Arrange for individual or group psychotherapy with others who experienced same trauma (e.g., Iraq or Vietnam war veterans).
   2. Provide crisis counseling, family therapy as needed.
   3. Provide referrals.

# SOMATOFORM DISORDERS

## Overview

A. Anxiety is manifested in somatic (physical) symptoms.
B. There is organic pathology but no organic etiology.
C. Symptoms are real and not under voluntary control of the client.
D. Defense used is somatization or conversion: anxiety is transformed to a physical symptom.

## Specific Disorders

### Somatization Disorder

A. General information
   1. Multiple, recurrent somatic complaints (fatigue, backache, nausea, menstrual cramps) over many years
   2. No organic etiology for these complaints
B. Assessment findings
   1. Complaints chronic but fluctuating
   2. History of seeking medical attention for many years
   3. Symptoms of anxiety and depression
   4. Somatic complaints may involve any organ system
C. Nursing interventions
   1. Be aware of own response (irritation/impatience) to client.
   2. Rule out organic basis for current complaints.
   3. Focus on anxiety reduction, not physical symptoms.
   4. Minimize secondary gain.

### Conversion Disorder

A. General information
   1. Sudden onset of impairment or loss of motor or sensory function.
   2. No physiologic cause.
   3. Defenses used are repression and conversion; anxiety is converted to a physical symptom.
   4. Temporal relationship between distressing event and development of symptom

(e.g., unconscious desire to hit another may produce paralysis of arm).
5. Primary gain: client is not conscious of conflict. Anxiety is converted to a symptom that removes client from anxiety-producing situation.
6. Secondary gain: gain support and attention that was not previously provided. Tends to encourage client to maintain symptoms.

B. Assessment findings
1. Sudden paralysis, blindness, deafness, etc.
2. "La belle indifférence": inappropriately calm when describing symptoms
3. Symptoms not under voluntary control
4. Usually short term; symptoms will abate as anxiety diminishes

C. Nursing interventions
1. Focus on anxiety reduction, not physical symptom.
2. Use matter-of-fact acceptance of symptom.
3. Encourage client to discuss conflict.
4. Do not provide secondary gain by being too attentive.
5. Provide diversionary activities.
6. Encourage expression of feelings.

## *Pain Disorder*

A. General information: complaint of severe and prolonged pain
B. Assessment findings
1. Pain impairs social/occupational function
2. Pain often severe
3. Sleep may be interrupted by experience of pain
C. Nursing interventions
1. Pain management
2. Encourage participation in activities.

## *Hypochondriasis*

A. General information
1. Unrealistic belief of having serious illnesses.
2. Belief persists despite medical reassurance.
3. Defenses used are regression and somatization.
B. Assessment findings
1. Preoccupation with bodily functions, which are misinterpreted.
2. History of seeing many doctors, many diagnostic tests.
3. Dependent behavior: desires/demands great deal of attention.
C. Nursing interventions
1. Rule out presence of actual disease.
2. Focus on anxiety, not physical symptom.
3. Set limits on amount of time spent with client.
4. Reduce anxiety by providing diversionary activities.

5. Avoid negative response to client's demands by discussing in staff conferences.
6. Provide client with correct information.

# DISSOCIATIVE DISORDERS

## Overview

A. Sudden change in client's consciousness, identity, or memory.
B. Loss of memory, knowledge of identity, or how individual came to be in a particular place.
C. Defenses are repression and dissociation.

## Specific Disorders

### *Dissociative Amnesia*

A. General information: inability to recall information about self with no organic reason
B. Assessment findings
1. No history of head injury
2. Retrograde amnesia, may extend far into past
C. Nursing interventions
1. Rule out organic causes.
2. Reassure client that personal identity will be made known to client.
3. Provide safe environment.
4. Establish nurse-client relationship to reduce anxiety.

### *Dissociative Fugue*

A. General information
1. Client travels to strange, often distant place; unaware of how he traveled there, and unable to recall past.
2. May follow severe psychologic stress.
B. Assessment findings
1. Memory loss
2. May have assumed new identity
3. No recall of fugue state when normal functions return
C. Nursing interventions: same as for psychogenic amnesia.

# PERSONALITY DISORDERS

*Note: This is coded on Axis II.*

## Overview

A. Patterns of thinking about self and environment become maladaptive and cause impairment in social or occupational functioning or subjective distress.
B. Usually develop by adolescence.
C. Most common is borderline personality disorder.

## Specific Disorders

### Borderline Personality Disorder

A. General information: clients are impulsive and unpredictable, have difficulty interacting; characterized by behavior problems
B. Assessment findings
   1. Unstable, intense interpersonal relationships
   2. Impulsive, unpredictable, manipulative behavior; prone to self-harm
   3. Marked mood shifts from anger to dysphoric
   4. Uncertainty about self-image, gender identity, values
   5. Chronic intolerance of being alone, feelings of boredom
   6. Splitting: distinct separation of love and hate; views others as *all* good or *all* bad.
   7. Use of projection and regression
C. Nursing interventions
   1. Protect from self-mutilation, suicidal gestures.
   2. Establish therapeutic relationship, be aware of own responses to manipulative behaviors.
   3. Maintain objectivity.
   4. Use a calm approach.
   5. Set limits.
   6. Apply plan of care consistently.
   7. Interact with clients when they demonstrate appropriate behavior.
   8. Teach relaxation techniques.

### Antisocial Personality Disorder

A. General information
   1. Chronic history of antisocial behaviors (e.g., fighting, stealing, aggressive behaviors, substance abuse, criminal behaviors).
   2. These behaviors usually begin before the age of 15 and continue into adult life.
   3. May be hospitalized for injuries.
B. Assessment findings
   1. Manipulative behavior, may try to obtain special privileges, play one staff member against another
   2. Lack of shame or guilt for behaviors
   3. Insincerity and lying
   4. Impulsive behavior and poor judgment
C. Nursing interventions
   1. Provide model for mature, appropriate behavior.
   2. Observe strict limit-setting by all staff.
   3. Monitor own responses to client.
   4. Demonstrate concern, interest in client.
   5. Reinforce positive behaviors (socialization, conforming to limits).
   6. Avoid power struggles.

## Sample Questions

21. A 6-year-old has been diagnosed with enuresis after tests revealed no organic cause of bed wetting. The child's mother is upset and blames the problem on his father. "It's all his father's fault!" What is your initial response?
    1. "Why do you say that?"
    2. "It's usually nobody's fault."
    3. "You seem really upset by this."
    4. "Why are you blaming his father?"

22. An adolescent is admitted with anorexia nervosa. You have been assigned to sit with her while she eats her dinner. The client says to you, "My primary nurse trusts me. I don't see why you don't." What is your best response?
    1. "I do trust you, but I was assigned to be with you."
    2. "I'd like to share this time with you."
    3. "OK. When I return, I'll check to see how much you have eaten."
    4. "Who is your primary nurse?"

23. A teenager is hospitalized for the treatment of anorexia nervosa. She is 64 inches tall and weighs 100 pounds. What is the primary objective in the treatment of the hospitalized anorexic client?
    1. Decrease the client's anxiety.
    2. Increase insight into the disorder.
    3. Help the mother to relinquish control.
    4. Get the client to eat and gain weight.

24. A female adolescent is hospitalized for treatment of anorexia nervosa. While admitting the client, the nurse discovers a bottle of pills. She states they are antacids and she takes them because her stomach hurts. What would be the nurse's best initial response?
    1. "Tell me more about your stomach pain."
    2. "These do not look like antacids. I need to get an order for you to have them."
    3. "Tell me more about your drug use."
    4. "Some girls take pills to help them lose weight."

25. The nurse assesses an adolescent who has dropping grades, low motivation, somatic complaints, and dental caries. What disorder would the nurse suspect?
    1. Anxiety.
    2. Depression.

3. Acute mania.

4. Dissociative fugue.

26. An elderly client was recently admitted to a nursing home because of confusion, disorientation, and negativistic behavior. Her family states that she is in good health. The woman asks you, "Where am I?" What would be the best response from the nurse?

1. "Don't worry. You're safe here."

2. "Where do you think you are?"

3. "What did your family tell you?"

4. "You're at the community nursing home."

27. Which of the following would be an appropriate strategy in reorienting a confused client to where her room is?

1. Place pictures of her family on the bedside stand.

2. Put her name in large letters on her wristband.

3. Remind the client where her room is.

4. Let the other residents know where the client's room is.

28. An elderly client was recently admitted to a nursing home because of confusion, disorientation, and negativistic behavior. Which activity would you engage the client in at the nursing home?

1. Reminiscence groups.

2. Sing-alongs.

3. Discussion groups.

4. Exercise class.

29. A 78-year-old was recently admitted to a nursing home because of confusion, disorientation, and negativistic behavior. She has had difficulty sleeping since admission. Which of the following would be the best intervention?

1. Provide her with a glass of warm milk.

2. Ask the physician for a mild sedative.

3. Do not allow her to take naps during the day.

4. Ask her family what they prefer.

30. A middle aged client is on the verge of losing his job because of a drinking problem. He voluntarily enters an alcohol detoxification program. Along with the amount and type, what information is most important that he needs to inform the staff?

1. Time substances were taken over the past 24 hours.

2. Frequency of substances taken over the past week.

3. Frequency of substances taken over the past 2 weeks.

4. Frequency of substances taken over the past month.

31. What is a characteristic common to most substance abusers that is difficult for them to achieve?

1. Coping with stress and anxiety.

2. Interacting socially.

3. Performing in work-related settings.

4. Setting goals.

32. A client is developing impending alcohol withdrawal delirium. Besides tremors, what other signs and symptoms would be present?

1. Bradycardia and hypertension.

2. Bradycardia and hypotension.

3. Tachycardia and hypertension.

4. Tachycardia and hypotension.

33. What is the most widely accepted treatment modality for substance abuse?

1. Individual therapy with a psychodynamically oriented therapist.

2. Individual therapy with a systems-oriented therapist.

3. Group therapy with others with personality disorders.

4. Group therapy with other substance abusers.

34. A client was voluntarily admitted to the inpatient unit with a diagnosis of paranoid schizophrenia. As the nurse approaches the client, he says, "If you come any closer, I'll die." Which disorder of perception does this client exhibit?

1. Hallucination.

2. Delusion.

3. Illusion.

4. Idea of reference.

35. The nurse is approaching an adult client who is admitted with a diagnosis of paranoid schizophrenia. As the nurse approaches the client, he says, "If you come any closer, I'll die." What is the best response for the nurse to make to this behavior?

1. "How can I hurt you?"

2. "I am your nurse today."

3. "Tell me more about this."

4. "You're not going to die."

36. A young man admitted with a diagnosis of paranoid schizophrenia is pacing the halls and is agitated. The nurse hears him saying, "I have

to get away from those doctors! They are trying to commit me to the state hospital!" The nurse's continued assessment should include:

1. Clarifying information with the doctor.
2. Observing the client for rising anxiety.
3. Reviewing history of involuntary commitment.
4. Checking dosage of prescribed medication.

37. After 2 days in the hospital, the nurse assesses a client diagnosed with schizophrenia as exhibiting flat affect with little interest in other clients. What describes this characteristic of the schizophrenic process?

1. Paranoia.
2. Ambivalence.
3. Cyclothymic.
4. Undifferentiated.

38. What would be an appropriate activity for the nurse to recommend for a client who is extremely agitated?

1. Competitive sports.
2. Bingo.
3. Trivial Pursuit.
4. Daily walks.

39. A client who is diagnosed with a bipolar disorder is admitted to the hospital in the manic phase. What is the initial plan of care?

a. Put the client in seclusion.
b. Put the client on one to one for safety.
c. Provide a quiet environment for the client.
d. Stabilize the client on medication.

40. A 34-year-old is hospitalized with bipolar disorder. At 2 A.M. the nurse finds him phoning friends all across the country to discuss his new plan for eradicating world hunger. His excited explanations are keeping the entire unit awake, but he won't quiet down. Which drug is most likely to be prescribed for this client?

1. A tricyclic antidepressant.
2. An MAO-inhibitor antidepressant.
3. Lithium carbonate (Eskalith).
4. An antianxiety drug.

41. Which supportive therapy for a client who is exhibiting manic behavior would be inappropriate to use as treatment?

1. Psychoanalysis.
2. Cognitive therapy.
3. Interpersonal therapy.
4. Problem-solving therapy.

42. A 38-year-old was admitted to the psychiatric service after a failed suicide attempt by drug overdose. The client sought help when her husband informed her of his decision to leave her and the children after 19 years of marriage. Her suicide attempt was made after she and her husband had had a fierce argument about property settlement. Upon initial contact with the nurse, the client looked exhausted, affect was sad, movements and responses were slowed, and self-care impairments were evident. She is convinced that a blemish on her face is a melanoma that is invading her brain and eating away at the tissue. What type of disorder is being shown?

1. Bipolar disorder.
2. Depression with melancholia.
3. Dysthymic disorder.
4. Major depression.

43. An adult is admitted to the psychiatric service after a failed suicide attempt by drug overdose. She presents with a sad affect and moves and responds slowly. Which nursing diagnosis is of greatest priority at the time of her admission?

1. Imbalanced in nutrition: less than body requirements.
2. Ineffective coping.
3. Risk for violence: self-directed.
4. Bathing/hygiene self-care deficit.

44. An adult is admitted following a suicide attempt. She took sleeping pills. She has been receiving therapy for depression since her husband left her after 23 years of marriage. Upon admission she looks very tired, has a sad affect, and moves slowly. What intervention would be a priority in helping to stabilize the client?

1. Allow her to catch up on lost sleep for the first 3 days of her hospitalization.
2. Have her fully involved in all therapeutic activities.
3. Encourage her husband to visit for brief periods of time.
4. Schedule balanced periods of rest and therapeutic activity.

45. When a client is experiencing severe anxiety, what would be the priority nursing intervention?

1. Give the client medication immediately.
2. Offer the client psychotherapy to calm her down.
3. Isolate the client in a quiet environment.
4. Put the client in seclusion temporarily.

**46.** A client is admitted to the hospital because her family is unable to manage her constant handwashing rituals. Her family reports she washes her hands at least 30 times each day. The nurse noticed the client's hands are reddened, scaly, and cracked. What is the main nursing goal?

1. Decrease the number of hand washings a day.
2. Provide a milder soap.
3. Provide good skin care.
4. Eliminate the handwashing rituals.

**47.** An adult is admitted to the psychiatric hospital for handwashing rituals. The day after admission she is scheduled for lab tests. How will the nurse ensure that the client is there on time?

1. Remind the client several times of her appointment.
2. Limit the number of hand washings.
3. Tell her it is her responsibility to be there on time.
4. Provide ample time for her to complete her rituals.

**48.** An adult who is hospitalized with an obsessive-compulsive disorder washes her hands many times a day. Which of the following is an appropriate treatment for this client?

1. An unstructured schedule of activities.
2. A structured schedule of activities.
3. Intense counseling.
4. Negative reinforcement every time she performs the ritual.

**49.** A woman is admitted to the psychiatric hospital. She was found walking on a highway. She is unkempt and appears thin and dirty. What is the most thorough way to conduct a nursing assessment of her nutritional status?

1. Observe her at mealtime.
2. Request a medical consult.
3. Explore her recent dietary intake.
4. Compare current weight with her usual weight.

**50.** A client is admitted to the psychiatric unit. She was found wandering on a major four-lane highway and cannot recall her activities from the past 3 days. During the assessment, the nurse observes that her face and hands are very red and excoriated, her hair is matted and dirty, her clothing is dirty, and she is quite thin. When the client asked to be excused, she went directly to her room, and washed her hands and face. Within a very short while, it became apparent to

the nurse that the hand and face washing was quite repetitive and ritualistic. However, she refused to bathe or wash her clothing. Which nursing diagnosis describes the most prominent difficulty that the client is experiencing?

1. Impaired skin integrity.
2. Disturbed thought processes.
3. Ineffective coping.
4. Social isolation.

**51.** An adult is admitted because of ritualistic behavior. She is also constipated and dehydrated. Which nursing intervention would the client be most likely to comply with?

1. Drinking Ensure between meals.
2. Drinking extra fluids with meals.
3. Drinking 8 oz water every hour between meals.
4. Drinking adequate amounts of fluid during the day.

**52.** An adult is admitted because of excessive hand and face washing rituals. What would be the most effective way for the nurse to intervene with her hand and face washing?

1. Allow her a certain amount of time each shift to engage in this behavior.
2. Interrupt the activity briefly and frequently.
3. Lock the door to her room and restrict access to the bathroom.
4. Tell her to stop each time she is observed doing it.

**53.** A client was admitted for ritualistic behavior involving frequent hand and face washing. Upon admission, the client was also dehydrated and underweight. When will the nurse know to initiate discharge planning for this client?

1. The client's normal body weight is regained.
2. The client will express a desire to leave the hospital.
3. The client is able to start talking about her guilt and anxiety.
4. The client limits her hand and face washing to a few times a day.

**54.** A young adult was admitted on a voluntary basis to psychiatric services. During the last 3 years, he has been under psychiatric care and has a long history of petty crimes. Once on the unit, the client is difficult to manage because he is arrogant and manipulative. When a scheduled group therapy session is announced, he refuses to go. He uses other clients to his own ends and often pioneers causes that are disruptive to the milieu. What diagnostic title best describes his behavior?

1. Antisocial personality disorder.
2. Borderline personality disorder.
3. Somatization disorder.
4. Bipolar disorder.

55. An adult is admitted to a psychiatric unit with a diagnosis of antisocial personality disorder. In planning care for the client, which of the following would be least likely to occur?

1. Staff and client agree when setting treatment goals.
2. Staff and client are in a constant struggle for control of the milieu.
3. Allow client to set limits.
4. Staff and client use the same defense mechanisms when interacting.

56. A client is admitted with an antisocial personality disorder. Which key intervention would be contraindicated with this client?

1. Assisting him to identify and clarify his feelings.
2. Changing staff assigned to a client at his request.
3. Making expectations about his behavior clear as well as consequences for same.
4. Setting firm limits with clear consequences.

57. A client has been hospitalized with an antisocial personality disorder on a voluntary basis as an alternative to serving a jail sentence. Following discharge, what will be the most likely result of the client?

1. Be committed to another facility for a longer length of stay.
2. Be committed to a virtuous and socially acceptable lifestyle.
3. Continue to use sublimation.
4. Revert to pre-hospitalization behaviors.

58. A 28-year-old is admitted to the psychiatric unit under an involuntary petition after a perceived suicide attempt. Initially, she presented as very tearful and highly anxious. As the staff became more familiar with her, it became apparent that she had had many episodes of self-mutilation and would do so "so I can feel something." While she could appear quite intact most of the time, when stressed she would respond very impulsively, express anger, report hearing voices of a depreciative nature, and require a high level of observation. This client's symptoms can best be described as

fitting which of the following diagnostic categories?

1. Antisocial personality disorder.
2. Borderline personality disorder.
3. Generalized anxiety disorder.
4. Post-traumatic stress disorder.

59. A client is admitted to the psychiatric unit with a diagnosis of borderline personality disorder. Which of the following components would be needless to obtain for the history/data base?

1. Ego-strength assessment.
2. Social history.
3. Cognitive aspect of mental status exam.
4. Past psychiatric treatment history.

60. An adult was admitted to the psychiatric unit after cutting herself on the forearm. She has numerous scars which are from prior self-mutilation. Should the client attempt self-mutilation while in the hospital, which implementation should the nurse execute?

1. Focus on the how, when, and where of the injury.
2. Care for the injury and explore the client's activities and feelings immediately before the episode.
3. Care for the injury and leave the client alone for awhile to let her settle down.
4. Care for the injury and seclude, and possibly restrain, the client to prevent further injury.

61. A female client was admitted with a borderline personality disorder following an episode of self-mutilation. Her husband recently left her and she reports that she has injured herself in the past so she could feel something. Which of the following would be excluded during the discharge planning?

1. Cognition.
2. Identity.
3. Dealing with anger.
4. Separation/individuation.

62. While collecting data about a 7-year-old boy, the school nurse learned that he has minimal verbal skills and expresses his needs by acting out behaviors. The communication capabilities of this boy indicate which of the following levels of mental retardation?

1. Mild
2. Moderate.
3. Severe.
4. Profound.

63. What nursing care would be included for a 4-year-old boy with severe autistic disorder?
   1. Psychotropic medications.
   2. Social skills training.
   3. Play therapy.
   4. Group therapy.

64. The nurse makes the following assessment of a 14-year-old gymnast: underweight, hair loss, yellowish skin, facial lanugo, and peripheral edema. These findings are suggestive of which of the following disorders?
   1. Anorexia nervosa.
   2. Bulimia nervosa.
   3. Acquired immunodeficiency.
   4. Ulcerative colitis.

65. An adolescent gymnast presents in the eating disorders clinic severely emaciated, with sallow skin color, 20% body weight loss, amenorrhea for the past 12 months, and facial lanugo. Based on these findings, which one of the following nursing diagnoses would be most appropriate for the nurse to make?
   1. Impaired nutrition: less than body requirements.
   2. Impaired tissue integrity.
   3. Ineffective individual coping.
   4. Deficient knowledge, nutritional.

66. Which observation of the client with anorexia indicates the client is improving?
   1. The client eats meals in the dining room.
   2. The client gains 1 pound per week.
   3. The client attends group therapy sessions.
   4. The client has a more realistic self-concept.

67. A client with severe Alzheimer's disease has violent outbursts, wanders, and is incontinent. He can no longer identify familiar people or objects. In developing the nursing care plan, the nurse would give highest priority to which nursing diagnosis?
   1. High risk for injury.
   2. Impaired verbal communication.
   3. Self-care deficits.
   4. Altered pattern of urinary elimination: incontinence.

68. A client with Alzheimer's disease has a self-care deficit related to his cognitive impairment. Because the client has difficulty dressing himself, what would be the best action for the nurse to take?
   1. Have the client wear hospital gowns.
   2. Explain to the client why he should dress himself.

3. Give the client step-by-step instructions for dressing himself.
   4. Allow enough time for the client to dress himself.

69. Which question made by the family of a client with Alzheimer's disease indicates to the nurse an understanding of the prognosis?
   1. "Does another hospital have a better treatment?"
   2. "Will a change in diet help his memory?"
   3. "Won't his new medicine cure him?"
   4. "What supports are available for the future?"

70. A 75-year-old man was brought to the emergency room confused, incoherent, and agitated after painting his lawn furniture earlier in the day. He has no current history of illness. Which one of the following interpretations would be appropriate for the nurse to make about his condition?
   1. Depression related to aging.
   2. Dementia related to organic illness.
   3. Delirium related to toxin exposure.
   4. Distress related to unaccomplished tasks.

71. A student with a history of barbiturate addiction is brought to the infirmary with suspected overdose. Which of the following assessments is the nurse likely to make?
   1. Watery eyes, slow and shallow breathing, clammy skin.
   2. Dilated pupils, shallow respirations, weak and rapid pulse.
   3. Constricted pupils, respirations depressed, nausea.
   4. Responsive pupils, increased respirations, increased pulse and blood pressure.

72. A teenage girl is admitted to a detoxification unit with a history of cocaine abuse. Her pupils are dilated and she complains of nausea and feeling cold. She states that she is not addicted, but uses cocaine occasionally with friends. Which one of the following nursing diagnoses is appropriate for the nurse to make?
   1. Impaired verbal communication related to substance use as evidenced by giving untrue information.
   2. Altered growth and development related to substance use as evidenced by age of client.
   3. Perceptual alteration related to substance use as evidenced by distortion of reality.
   4. Ineffective denial related to substance use as evidenced in refusal to admit problem.

73. The nurse is caring for a client in early alcohol withdrawal. What would most likely be included in the nursing care plan?
   1. Using physical restraints.
   2. Providing environmental stimulation.
   3. Taking pulse and blood pressure.
   4. Administering antipsychotic medications.

74. A client in a detox program is being manipulative by trying to split staff. The client tells the nurse that he is the "best" staff member on the unit. What would be the best response from the nurse?
   1. Thank the client for the compliment.
   2. Identify the client's manipulative behavior.
   3. Ignore the client's comment.
   4. Ask the client why he feels that way.

75. In developing a teaching plan for adolescents on the topic of cocaine abuse, the nurse would highlight which of the following?
   1. Cocaine is a naturally occurring depressant.
   2. Cocaine's physical effects differ according to the method of ingestion.
   3. The body's peak reaction occurs 30 minutes after it is taken.
   4. Smoking cocaine is particularly dangerous to the cardiovascular system.

76. A 14-year-old male client is admitted to the emergency room after ingesting a high dose of PCP and subsequently injuring himself in a fall. What would be an effective action for the nurse to take?
   1. Attempt to talk the client down.
   2. Withhold fluids.
   3. Place the client in a quiet, dimly lit room.
   4. Administer a prn phenothiazine.

77. The nurse on a medical unit smells alcohol and notices that the relief nurse's words are slurred and she is giggling inappropriately. What is the best initial action for the nurse to take?
   1. Double assign the nurse's clients.
   2. Ask the relief nurse if she has been drinking.
   3. Report the nurse to the licensing board.
   4. Refer the nurse to an employee assistance program.

78. A nurse's coworker is argumentative and resistant to change. Her appearance has become sloppy over the last 6 months; she is frequently late for work and often calls in sick. When she is at work, she complains about everything. Which of the following is the most likely cause of these problems?
   1. The nurse is dissatisfied with her job.
   2. The nurse is having problems at home.
   3. The nurse may be abusing drugs or alcohol.
   4. The nurse realizes she is in the wrong profession.

79. A nurse is evaluating an adult client from the substance abuse unit. Which statement by the client reveals that the client may be ready for discharge?
   1. "I'll take my Antabuse when I need it."
   2. "I can't wait to hang out with my old buddies."
   3. "I'll drink in moderation and only on the weekend."
   4. "Attending daily AA meetings will help me not drink again."

80. Which of the following assessment findings would the nurse observe in a client with schizophrenia?
   1. Associative looseness, affect disturbance, ambivalence, autistic thinking.
   2. Euphoria, distractibility, dramatic mannerisms, energetic.
   3. Argumentative, anhedonia, poor judgment, manipulative.
   4. Psychomotor retardation, intense sadness, loss of energy, suicidal.

81. A client with a diagnosis of paranoid schizophrenia reports to the nurse that he hears a voice that says, "Don't take those poisoned pills from that nurse!" Which one of the following nursing diagnoses would it be appropriate for the nurse to make regarding this statement?
   1. Disturbed sensory perceptual: auditory, related to anxiety as evidenced by auditory hallucination.
   2. Disturbed thought processes related to anxiety as evidenced by delusions of persecution.
   3. Defensive coping related to impaired reality testing as evidenced by paranoid ideation.
   4. Impaired verbal communication related to disturbances in form of thinking as evidenced by use of symbolic references.

82. An adult is admitted with a diagnosis of catatonic schizophrenia, excited phase. She shouts and paces continuously and seems to be

responding to internal stimuli. What would be a short-term goal for the nurse to formulate?

1. The client will groom self daily.
2. The client will maintain adequate nutrition.
3. The client will sleep 8 hours per night.
4. The client will attend unit social activities.

83. A client with schizophrenia stops talking mid sentence and tilts her head to one side. The nurse suspects that the client is experiencing auditory hallucinations. What is an appropriate response from the nurse?

1. Ask the client what she is experiencing.
2. Change the topic of conversation.
3. Explain that hallucinations are not real.
4. Deny that she hears anything.

84. In teaching a client for whom clozapine (Clozaril) has been prescribed, the nurse would include which of the following?

1. The drug will be given every 4 weeks by intramuscular injection.
2. The drug will probably cause weight reduction.
3. There is a high incidence of extrapyramidal side effects.
4. Blood work may be required weekly.

85. An adult is to go on a 3-day pass and has his maintenance supply of chlorpromazine (Thorazine). Which statement indicates to the nurse that he understands instructions regarding his medication?

1. "I'll take my pills when I hear those voices."
2. "I'll drink beer but no wine while I'm away."
3. "I'll cover up when I go to the beach."
4. "I'll stop taking it if my mouth stays dry."

86. Which of the following behaviors indicates to the nurse that the client's antipsychotic medication is having a desired effect?

1. The client states that her "voices" are not as threatening.
2. The client reports having inner feelings of restlessness.
3. The client sleeps all day.
4. The client reports muscular stiffening in her face and arms.

87. A client taking trifluoperazine (Stelazine) exhibits severe extrapyramidal symptoms, a temperature of 40.5°C (105°F), and diaphoresis. The nurse suspects neuroleptic malignant syndrome. What is the nurse's best action?

1. Administer an antiparkinsonism medication.
2. Stop the neuroleptic medication.
3. Withhold fluids.
4. Administer an antianxiety medication.

88. A client with paranoid schizophrenia has a delusion of persecution. He tells the nurse, "The CIA is out to get me. They're spying on me." What is the nurse's best initial response?

1. "I don't want to hurt you."
2. "How would they spy on you here?"
3. "Tell me how they're trying to get you."
4. "I know the CIA wouldn't want to hurt you."

89. Which of the following statements indicates to the nurse that a client with obsessive-compulsive disorder has developed insight into her problem?

1. "I realize that the dangers are more in my mind."
2. "I don't hear the voices anymore."
3. "I check on my family 12 times every day."
4. "I slept 8 hours last night."

90. An adult is brought to the emergency room after he attempted to walk across the roof of a building in an attempt to "fly like a jet plane." In addition to impulsiveness, which of the following behaviors would the nurse assess in a client diagnosed as bipolar, manic type?

1. Hallucinations and delusions.
2. Euphoria and increased motor activity.
3. Paranoia and ideas of reference.
4. Splitting and manipulation.

91. During the focused assessment of a client with major depression, the nurse may ask which of the following questions?

1. "You seem to have a lot of energy; when did you last have 6 or more hours of sleep?"
2. "You seem to be angry with your family now; when was it that you last got along?"
3. "Have you had any thoughts of harming yourself?"
4. "You seem to be listening to something. Could you tell me about it?"

92. Which of the following nursing diagnoses would be most appropriate for a client who is diagnosed as bipolar I disorder, single manic episode and is intrusive, argumentative, and severely critical of peers?

1. Impaired social interaction related to narcissistic behavior as evidenced by inability to sustain relationships.

2. Risk for injury related to extreme hyperactivity as evidenced by increased agitation and lack of control over behavior.

3. Social isolation related to feelings of inadequacy in social interaction as evidence by problematic interaction with others.

4. Defensive coping related to social learning patterns as evidenced by difficulty interacting with others.

93. An adult is in an acute manic phase of bipolar disorder. He talks and paces incessantly, frequently shouting and threatening other clients. The nurse expects the client's care plan to include which of the following?

1. Monitor blood lithium levels.

2. Monitor client during phototherapy.

3. Monitor client after electroconvulsive therapy.

4. Teach client to avoid foods with tyramine.

94. The nurse is preparing to administer lithium (Eskalith) to a client with bipolar disorder. The client complains of nausea and muscle weakness, and his speech is slurred. His lithium level is 1.6 mEq/liter. What would be the nurse's best action?

1. Chart the client's symptoms after giving the lithium.

2. Explain that these are common side effects.

3. Withhold the client's lithium.

4. Administer a prn antiparkinsonism drug.

95. Which of the following behaviors indicates to the nurse that the client understands teaching related to lithium treatment?

1. Taking lithium 1 hour after meals.

2. Stopping taking her lithium when her mania subsides.

3. Going on a low-salt diet to counter weight gain.

4. Withholding her lithium if episodes of diarrhea, vomiting, and diaphoresis occur.

96. An adult is recovering from a severe depression. Which of the following behaviors alerts the nurse to a risk for suicide?

1. The client sleeps most of the day.

2. The client has a plan to kill herself.

3. The client loses 5 pounds.

4. The client does not attend unit activities.

97. A man has been severely depressed for 2 weeks. He had mentioned "ending it all" prior to admission. Which of the following questions should the nurse ask during the prescreen assessment?

1. "How long have you thought about harming yourself?"

2. "What is it that makes you think about harming yourself?"

3. "How has your concentration been?"

4. "What specifically have you thought about doing to harm yourself?"

98. A 19-year-old recently broke off her 1-year engagement. Her mother states, "She does nothing but cry and sit and stare into space. I can't get her to eat or anything!" She feels she can't go on without her boyfriend. The nurse should make which priority nursing diagnosis?

1. Impaired nutrition: less than body requirements.

2. Dysfunctional grieving.

3. Risk for self-directed violence.

4. Social isolation.

99. A client is admitted for treatment of a major depression. She is withdrawn, appears disheveled, and states, "No one could ever love me." What would the nurse expect to be ordered for this client?

1. Antiparkinsonism medication.

2. Suicide precautions.

3. A low-salt diet.

4. Phototherapy.

100. A man's wife complains that her husband's depression isn't any better after 1 week on amitriptyline (Elavil). What is the nurse's best response?

1. Tell her she will contact the physician.

2. Question the wife about what response she expects.

3. Explain that it may take 1 to 3 weeks to see any improvement.

4. Suggest that the client change antidepressants.

101. Which of the following behaviors indicates to the nurse that a client's major depression is improving?

1. Displaying a blunted affect

2. Losing an additional 2 pounds

3. Stating one "good" thing about himself

4. Sleeping about 16 hours per day

102. An adult is hospitalized for treatment of obsessive-compulsive disorder (OCD). The nurse recognizes which of the following as an

indication that the client's sertraline (Zoloft) is having the desired effect?

1. The client experiences nervousness and drowsiness.
2. The client's delusions are less entrenched.
3. The client engages in fewer rituals.
4. The client sleeps 4 hours per night.

103. A client with major depression is scheduled for electroconvulsive therapy (ECT) tomorrow. The nurse would plan for which of the following activities?

1. Force fluids 6 to 8 hours before treatment.
2. Administer succinylcholine (Inestine, Anectine) during pretreatment care.
3. Encourage the client's spouse to accompany him.
4. Reorient the client frequently during posttreatment care.

104. A severely depressed client received ECT this morning. Which of the findings listed below would the nurse *least* expect to assess posttreatment?

1. Headache.
2. Memory loss.
3. Paralytic ileus.
4. Disorientation.

105. A client for whom Nardil was prescribed for depression is brought to the ER with severe occipital headaches after eating pepperoni pizza for lunch. Which of the following interpretations is it important for the nurse to make regarding these findings?

1. Allergic reaction related to ingestion of processed food.
2. Hypertensive crisis related to drug and food reaction.
3. Panic anxiety related to unresolved issues.
4. Conversion disorder related to uncontrolled anxiety.

106. The nurse explains the major difference between neurotic and psychotic disorders. What is a major difference in clients with psychotic disorders?

1. The clients are aware that their behaviors are maladaptive.
2. The clients are aware they are experiencing distress.
3. The clients experience no loss of contact with reality.
4. The clients exhibit a flight from reality.

107. A client is prescribed buspirone hydrochloride (BuSpar). Which statement alerts the nurse that additional medication teaching is required?

1. "I'll take my drugs as soon as I feel anxious."
2. "I won't drink any alcohol."
3. "I'll report any troubles with my heart or seeing."
4. "I'll have my blood checked every month."

108. In teaching a client about her new antianxiety medication, alprazolam (Xanax), the nurse should include which of the following?

1. Caution the client to avoid foods with tyramine.
2. Caution the client not to drink alcoholic beverages.
3. Instruct the client to take the Xanax 1 hour after meals.
4. Instruct the client to double up a dose if she forgets to take her medication.

109. A client experiencing thanataphobia is afraid to leave her aging, ailing husband alone for any reason. She has not left her husband alone since her mother and sister died 4 years ago. Which of the following statements would be appropriate for the nurse to make during the initial assessment of this client?

1. "Are you afraid that your husband might die while you are away from him?"
2. "There must be someone you are able to trust to stay with your husband."
3. "Don't you have children who are willing to stay with your husband when you need to be away?"
4. "It must be very confining to have constantly attended to your husband for so long."

110. A newly admitted client is fearful of elevators. She needs to take one in 10 minutes to attend therapy on the 10th floor. Which of the following actions would be best for the nurse to take?

1. Explain to her that she needs to attend therapy.
2. Have another client go with her.
3. Accompany her to the 10th floor.
4. Explore with her why she is afraid of elevators.

111. A man, with a family of five, was recently laid off and now has financial concerns. He is experiencing muscle tension, breathlessness, and sleep disturbances. Which one of the following nursing diagnoses would be

appropriate for the nurse to make regarding his condition?

1. Post-trauma response related to loss of economic support as evidenced by job loss.
2. Parental role conflict related to perceived inability to meet his family's economic and physical needs as evidenced by job loss.
3. Ineffective individual coping related to recent unemployment as evidenced by physical manifestations.
4. Powerlessness related to inability to deal with anxiety as evidenced by physical manifestations.

112. A woman appears to be having a panic attack during group therapy. She is agitated, pacing rapidly, and not responding to verbal stimuli. What would be the nurse's initial intervention?

1. Remove her from the group.
2. Encourage her to express her feelings.
3. Facilitate her recognizing her anxiety.
4. Ignore her.

113. The nurse is assessing a client who presents with OCD. In addition to gathering information about the client's anxiety and rituals, the nurse should assess for which of the following?

1. Handwringing and foot-tapping behaviors.
2. Use of abusive substances and gambling.
3. Tics, stuttering, or other unusual speech patterns.
4. Diaphoresis and rapid breathing.

114. Which of the following statements by a client with delusions indicates to the nurse that the client is improving?

1. "I don't feel those crawling bugs anymore."
2. "I won't talk about my crazy thoughts at work."
3. "I feel less jumpy inside."
4. "I must check my room for bugs."

115. During the assessment phase of the nurse-client interaction, which of the following statements made by the client is suggestive of post-traumatic stress disorder?

1. "My dad had trouble swallowing before he died and I always feel as if I have a lump in my throat."
2. "After I contracted meningitis on vacation last summer, I can't control this horrible thought that all people who work in park restaurants are dirty."
3. "I continue to have the same dream over and over again."

4. "I had another horrible nightmare last night and went through the same trauma and anxiety all over again."

116. A client with OCD has an elaborate handwashing and touching ritual that interferes with her activities of daily living. She misses meals and therapy sessions. What effective strategy could the nurse initiate to limit her ritual?

1. Teach thought stopping techniques.
2. Prevent the ritualistic behavior.
3. Use adjunctive therapies for distraction.
4. Facilitate insight regarding the need for the ritual.

117. A client with an OCD has checking rituals and thoughts that her family will be harmed. Which of the following indicates to the nurse that the client is improving?

1. Obsessing about her family's health.
2. Adhering to the unit schedule.
3. Losing 2 pounds in 1 week.
4. Awakening 8 times during the night.

118. A 4-year-old girl, who is a victim of a bomb blast that demolished the building which housed her daycare, constantly builds block houses and blows them up. She also has nightmares frequently. Which one of the following diagnoses is appropriate for the nurse to make regarding this child?

1. Post-trauma response related to terrorist attack as evidenced by destructive behaviors and sleep disturbances.
2. Explosive disorder related to dysfunctional personality as evidenced by destructive behaviors.
3. Sleep disturbance related to emotional trauma as evidenced by nightmares.
4. Ineffective individual coping related to internal stressors as evidenced by destructive behaviors and nightmares.

119. The nurse recognizes that the client with post-traumatic stress disorder (PTSD) is improving when which of the following occurs?

1. States he feels "numb" most of the time.
2. Drinks alcohol to cope with his feelings.
3. Talks about a benefit of the traumatic experience.
4. Attends weekly group therapy.

120. A young woman is found wandering on campus after a fraternity party. She is disheveled and does not know who she is. She has no recollection of

the evening. At the student health service she is diagnosed with dissociative amnesia subsequent to a rape. What is the most appropriate nursing diagnosis for the nurse to formulate?

1. Ineffective individual coping.
2. Personal identity disturbance.
3. Anxiety related to alteration in memory.
4. Risk for violence, self-directed.

121. The nurse finds, during the initial assessment of the star player on the basketball team, that he is not concerned about the sudden paralysis of his "shooting arm." What is this behavior known as?

1. Secondary gain
2. La belle indifférence
3. Malingering
4. Hypochondriasis

122. A man's family brought him into the hospital because of his many somatic complaints. He has been seen by many medical specialists in the past without discovery of organic pathology. The nurse assesses that the client is probably experiencing which of the following problems?

1. Conversion disorder
2. Body dysmorphic disorder
3. Malingering
4. Hypochondriasis

123. An adult is hospitalized for treatment of a conversion disorder. She complained of paralysis of her right side after her husband threatened to leave her and their children. She seems unconcerned about her paralysis. What would be an appropriate long-term goal for the nurse to formulate for the client?

1. Cope effectively with stress without using conversion
2. Identify stressors
3. Express feelings about the conflict
4. Develop an increased sense of relatedness to others

124. An adult has hypochondriasis—believing he is dying of stomach cancer despite repeated and extensive diagnostic testing that has all been negative. He has become reclusive and is preoccupied with his physical complaints. The nurse would include which of the following in the nursing care plan as a client outcome?

1. Focus on the signs and symptoms of stomach cancer
2. Attend a support group for persons with cancer
3. Complete a contract to attend social and diversional activities daily

4. Receive secondary gain from his physical symptoms

125. A man is brought into the police station after he ran toward a boy who resembled his son. At the police station he was unable to recall any personal information. The prescreening nurse inferred that the man has which one of the following dissociative disorders?

1. Amnesia
2. Fugue
3. Personality disorder
4. Stress disorder

126. Which of the behaviors listed below would assist the nurse in establishing the diagnosis of borderline personality disorder?

1. Impulsivity
2. Hallucinations
3. Self-mutilation
4. Narcissism

127. A woman is admitted to the unit with a diagnosis of borderline personality disorder. She has angry outbursts and is impulsive and manipulative. She has lacerations on her arm from self-mutilation. Which of the following would be a priority nursing diagnosis?

1. Ineffective individual coping.
2. Disturbed body image.
3. Disturbed personal identity.
4. Risk for violence to self.

128. A client with borderline personality disorder tells the nurse she hates her doctor because he denied her a pass because she returned "high" from her last pass. What would be the nurse's best action?

1. Ask the client why she is feeling so angry.
2. Suggest that the client bring it up in community meeting.
3. Offer to contact the doctor and discuss the situation.
4. Set limits and point out that the denial is a consequence of her inappropriate behavior.

129. The nurse would formulate which of the following outcome criteria for a client with borderline personality disorder?

1. Displays anger frequently.
2. Acts out neediness.
3. Experiences troubling thoughts without self-mutilation.
4. Idolizes assigned nurse.

130. A client with antisocial personality disorder is charming, seductive, and highly manipulative. He has a history of multiple jobs and marriages, which have all failed, and problems with the law. Which of the following is an appropriate short-term goal for the nurse to formulate in relation to a nursing diagnosis of ineffective individual coping?

1. The client will avoid situations that provoke aggressive acts.
2. The client will adhere to unit rules.
3. The client will assume a leadership role in unit governance.
4. The client will acknowledge manipulative behaviors pointed out by staff.

131. Which of the following indicates to the nurse that a client with antisocial personality disorder is improving?

1. Complimenting the nurse for on outstanding job on the unit.
2. Testing the limits on personal behavior.
3. Acknowledging some manipulative behavior.
4. Sleeping 8 hours per night.

## Answers and Rationales

21. 3. Upon hearing her son's diagnosis, the mother is experiencing emotional turmoil and projecting blame. Acknowledging her feelings would build further trust and encourage her to discuss her thoughts and feelings.

22. 2. The nurse can offer himself to the client to establish trust. The nurse will stay with the client while eating.

23. 4. Because the anorexic client is experiencing starvation, her well-being is dependent on establishing an adequate nutritional state. Eating and gaining weight are the primary goals of hospitalization.

24. 1. While there might be some concern that the client is abusing drugs and possibly using them to induce further weight loss, the primary concern is that the client is experiencing abdominal pain. This may be a clue to an impending medical crisis needing further assessment.

25. 2. Dropping grades, low motivation, somatic complaints, and poor mouth hygiene are signs and symptoms of depression.

26. 4. Responding factually helps to orient the client.

27. 3. The nurse should be someone the client can turn to for guidance.

28. 4. Providing the client with structured activities will allow her to release tension. Exercises also help older people with balance and mobility and reduce falls.

29. 4. Including the family in the plan of care ensures a more effective plan.

30. 1. Although a complete substance abuse history is necessary eventually, on admission the most important information is the type and amount of substances taken by the client in the past 24 hours.

31. 1. While a substance abuser has difficulty in all areas listed, problems handling stress and anxiety underlie all the others.

32. 3. Delirium tremens is characterized by increased blood pressure, pulse, and respirations, and an increase in psychomotor activity.

33. 4. Group therapy with other substance abusers is the most highly prescribed therapy. It is the model for Alcoholics Anonymous, the most effective treatment group.

34. 2. A delusion is a fixed false belief.

35. 2. The nurse needs to present reality to the client and not encourage the delusion.

36. 2. Assessing increasing signs of anxiety and agitation gives clues to the client's ability to maintain control and suggests further nursing interventions to protect the client and others.

37. 2. There are four characteristics of schizophrenia that help in an assessment. One of the key indicators is the overwhelming attitude of ambivalence toward the environment and any emotional involvement with others. The other three indicators are affect, associative looseness, and autistic thinking.

38. 4. Daily walks provide time for the nurse to develop trust. Walking allows expenditure of energy without increasing paranoia.

39. 3. This client does not need additional stimuli from the environment.

40. 3. A drug frequently used to treat manic clients is lithium carbonate (Eskalith).

41. 1. Psychoanalysis is an in-depth, insight-oriented psychotherapy, not appropriate in treatment of bipolar disorders.

42. 4. The client shows many signs of classic depression as evidenced by psychomotor retardation, impairment of self-care, inability to sleep, a suicide attempt, and somatic delusion.

43. 3. The priority at this time is maintenance of client safety. This client is at particular risk for self-directed violence because of her recent failed suicide attempt and her obsession with what she perceives to be her impending death.

44. 4. Even though the client is probably exhausted, the most therapeutic plan would allow for both rest and activity.

45. 3. The client who is experiencing severe panic needs a quiet environment with supportive care to decrease anxiety enough to cope.

46. 1. Obsessive-compulsive behavior represents displacement of anxiety. A concrete measurable goal is to decrease the number of handwashings.

47. 4. Providing ample time for the client to complete her handwashing rituals will lessen her anxiety.

48. 2. Planning a structured schedule of activities provides the client with ways other than handwashing to reduce anxiety.

49. 4. Current weight as it relates to usual weight is the best determinant of nutritional status and weight change when the client is unable to be specific about recent activities and eating habits.

50. 3. Ineffective individual coping encompasses all of the other nursing diagnoses. This area will be the primary focus of nursing interventions, and positive changes in the client's ability to cope will be the criteria for discharge readiness.

51. 3. Building the intake of a specified amount of liquid into a daily schedule of activities is very consistent with the obsessive-compulsive client's need to control as many aspects of her life as possible.

52. 1. Allowing the client a certain amount of time to engage in the activity alleviates some of the client's anxiety.

53. 4. The major issue is control of behavior and thoughts. When the client is able to control her compulsive behavior, i.e., limit her hand and face washing to a few times a day, she will then be able to resume normal activities of daily living.

54. 1. A long history of petty crimes, a high level of manipulative behavior, use of other clients to his own end, and fostering behavior that is disruptive to the milieu are all signs of the diagnosis of antisocial personality disorder.

55. 1. The staff and client will most likely disagree when setting treatment goals.

56. 2. The client will compare and attempt to "split" staff, so it is very important to keep staff assignments as consistent as possible.

57. 4. People who have this type of personality disorder typically seek psychiatric care as a lesser of two evils. In this case in-hospital care is preferable to jail. The chances of this client making any great change in his lifestyle as a result of short-term hospitalization are slim. The client will likely be committed to another facility when he is again arrested for deviant behavior.

58. 2. The clustering of self-mutilation, impulsivity, transient psychosis, intense anger, and feeling empty is most typically found in borderline personality disorder.

59. 3. The mental status exam is conducted when the nurse suspects a client is disoriented. The client with a borderline personality disorder has, for the most part, intact reality testing.

60. 2. A matter-of-fact approach to the injury with emphasis on the events leading to the episode of mutilation is the most therapeutic approach.

61. 1. Impairments involving cognition are most commonly found in psychoses.

62. 3. Individuals with severe mental retardation possess minimal verbal skills. They often communicate wants and needs by acting out behaviors.

63. 3. Play therapy would be most effective given his developmental level and autism. In autistic disorder, communication with others is severely impaired. Through one-to-one play therapy, the therapist may establish rapport through nonverbal play.

64. 1. Anorexia nervosa, usually occurring in individuals ages 13–22 years, is an eating disorder characterized by self-starvation, weight loss (25% below normal weight), disturbance in body image, and physiologic and metabolic changes.

65. 1. The assessment data and history of the client support the diagnosis of altered nutrition related to anorexia.

66. 2. Weight gain is the best indication that the client's anorexia is improving. A realistic expectation is for the client to gain 1 pound per week.

67. 1. Safety is of highest concern for this client. His wandering and memory loss pose hazards for accidents, falls, and injuries.

68. 3. The client may need step-by-step instructions so he can focus on small amounts of information. This allows him to perform at his optimal level. Clients with dementia may not remember how to dress themselves.

69. 4. This response indicates that the family is expecting to need support during the process of the client's increasing cognitive impairment.

70. 3. Paint is a toxin that could cause delirium. Delirium is a state of mental confusion and excitement. The mind wanders, speech is incoherent, and the client is often in a state of continual, aimless physical activity. The onset is rapid (hours to days).

71. 2. The effects of overdose of barbiturates are shallow respirations, cold and clammy skin, dilated pupils, weak and rapid pulse, coma, and possible death.

72. 4. Denial is the minimizing or disavowing of symptoms or a situation to the detriment of health.

73. 3. Pulse and blood pressure should be checked hourly for the first 8–12 hours after admission. They are usually elevated during withdrawal and the pulse is a good indication of progress through withdrawal. Elevation may indicate impending alcohol withdrawal delirium.

74. 2. A priority in intervening in manipulative behavior is to identify it and then set limits by stating expected behaviors.

75. 4. A total cardiac collapse may occur. Smoking "crack" cocaine is the method that most often leads to myocardial infarction.

76. 3. Environmental stimuli need to be reduced for the client in PCP intoxication to reduce danger to self, paranoia, delusions, and hallucinations. These clients are sensitive to stimuli and quickly become combative and assaultive.

77. 2. There is usually a chain of command policy that begins with a direct discussion of the involved parties. If the relief nurse denies drinking, the nurse has a duty to intervene.

78. 3. Signs of possible substance abuse are social isolation; requesting to work nights; changes in appearance and mood; excessive tardiness, accidents, and absences; excuses for being unavailable when on duty; resistance to change; defensive when questioned about client complaints or drug discrepancies; failure to meet schedules and deadlines; and inaccurate and sloppy documentation. The situation requires further professional assessment. The nurse should follow agency policies and board of nursing guidelines to report his suspicions.

79. 4. Daily attendance at AA meetings is necessary for most discharged clients to remain sober and continue their rehabilitation.

80. 1. Eugen Bleuler's 4 As of schizophrenia are loosening of associations (L.O.A.), which are representative of thought disorders, disturbance in affect, ambivalence, and autistic thinking.

81. 1. Hallucinations are sensory experiences of perception without corresponding stimuli in the environment.

82. 2. It is important for the nurse to monitor dietary intake and weight so the person does not lose calories and fluids due to hyperactivity. "Finger foods" may need to be provided, e.g., sandwiches and fruit.

83. 1. The best initial action is to focus on the cues and elicit the client's description of her experience. It is important for the nurse to determine that she is hallucinating and the content. This is vital in relation to safety issues and command hallucinations.

84. 4. Weekly white blood cell counts may be required due to the side effects of possible life-threatening agranulocytosis.

85. 3. The client should avoid the sun or cover up and use sunscreen to protect himself from severe photosensitivity.

86. **1.** A desired effect of the antipsychotics is to reduce the disturbing quality of hallucinations and delusions.

87. **2.** The neuroleptic should be immediately discontinued. Medical treatment should be instituted because this is a potentially fatal syndrome.

88. **1.** The nurse should first clarify her intent and then empathize with the underlying feeling.

89. **1.** This statement indicates that the client has some insight into the underlying reason for her rituals.

90. **2.** The client diagnosed as bipolar, manic exhibits behaviors of elation, euphoria, and is full of energy, which may lead to exhaustion.

91. **3.** Clients with major depression are often suicidal. The first concern of assessment is the risk of suicide potential in the immediate future.

92. **2.** The client who invades the space of others, creates arguments, and attacks others is at risk for injury by those in the environment.

93. **1.** Lithium is the drug of choice for manic clients with an antimanic effectiveness of 78%. It reduces the intensity, duration, and frequency of manic and depressive episodes. Blood levels are monitored for therapeutic levels in the acute phase (1.0–1.5 mEq/liter) and during maintenance.

94. **3.** The client is exhibiting symptoms and signs of lithium toxicity. Another blood level should be drawn and the dose evaluated.

95. **4.** These are early signs of lithium toxicity. The drug should be withheld and a lithium blood level drawn and evaluated to determine an appropriate dosage.

96. **2.** Having a suicide plan is a risk factor. The lethality needs to be assessed. When a depression is "lifting," the client may have the energy and resources to carry out a plan. Behavioral, somatic, and emotional cues may be overt or covert.

97. **4.** This question assists in determining suicidal intent and lethality.

98. **3.** The depressed client often feels hopeless and helpless with self-directed anger. Suicidal ideations are often expressed and warrant immediate intervention.

99. **2.** Maintaining safety for the client is a priority because she may have suicidal ideation and/or a plan.

100. **3.** The client may need to take Elavil 1 to 3 weeks before any improvement or a therapeutic effect is noticed.

101. **3.** This behavior may indicate an increase in self-esteem that accompanies an improvement in depression. A depressed person often cannot problem solve or acknowledge any positive aspects of their lives.

102. **3.** Zoloft is a selective serotonin reuptake inhibitor (SSRI) that is effective in treating clients with obsessive-compulsive disorder. Using fewer rituals would indicate an improvement.

103. **4.** Common side effects of bilateral treatment include confusion, disorientation, and short-term memory loss. The nurse should provide frequent orientation statements that are brief, distinct, and simple.

104. **3.** ECT is treated as an operative procedure; however, paralytic ileus (intestinal obstruction, especially failure of peristalsis) frequently accompany peritonitis and usually result from disturbances in the bowel.

105. **2.** Severe occipital and/or temporal pounding headaches, manifestations of hypertensive crisis, occur when processed meats are eaten by individuals currently taking Nardil (MAOI).

106. **4.** In psychotic responses to anxiety, clients escape from reality into hallucination and/or delusional behavior.

107. **1.** BuSpar must be taken as a maintenance drug, not as a prn response to symptoms. Improvement may be noted in 7–10 days, but it may take 3 to 4 weeks to note therapeutic effects.

108. **2.** The depressant effects of alcohol and alprazolan will be potentiated and may cause harmful sedation.

109. **1.** Confronting fear diminishes the phobic response and the anticipatory anxiety that precedes it.

110. **3.** This is the best action because the nurse is conveying her support. Later, she would need to further assess the client's fear of elevators and respond accordingly.

111. **2.** Parental role conflict is the state in which a parent experiences role confusion and conflict in response to crisis. Loss of economic base constitutes a crisis state.

112. **1.** The nurse should remove the client from the group to provide a safe environment for her and others. The nurse should stay with the client and provide comfort and reality orientation.

113. **3.** There is comorbidity between Tourette's syndrome and obsessive-compulsive disorder.

114. **2.** Improvement in relation to delusional content includes a reduction in the disturbing quality of the delusions and the client's ability to control and/or not respond to them.

115. **4.** Symptoms of post-traumatic stress disorder range from emotional "numbness" to vivid nightmares in which the traumatic event is recalled.

116. **1.** Thought stopping techniques, flooding, and response prevention have proven effective in treating clients with OCD. Clients may shout or think "stop" or snap a rubber band on their wrist to dismiss the obsessive thought.

117. **2.** If the client adheres to the unit schedule, it is likely that her obsessions and compulsive rituals have lessened. They no longer preoccupy her to the point of interfering with activities.

118. **1.** Post-trauma response is the state of an individual experiencing a sustained painful response to an overwhelming traumatic event.

119. **3.** Cognitive treatment for PTSD includes redefining the event by considering benefits of the experience and finding meaning in the experience.

120. **2.** The client's behavior is indicative of personal identity disturbance related to a traumatic event, the rape. The client is unable to recall her identity, which is a factor in dissociative disorders. The person loses the ability to integrate consciousness, memory, identity, or motor behavior.

121. **2.** This lack of concern is identified as "la belle indifference" and is often a clue that the problem may be psychological rather than physical.

122. **4.** Hypochondriasis is excessive preoccupation with one's physical health, without organic pathology.

123. **1.** This is an appropriate long-term goal related to the client's ineffective coping (use of conversion symptom, paralysis) related to unresolved conflicts and anxiety.

124. **3.** This goal is related to the client's impaired social interaction in response to his preoccupation with illness.

125. **1.** In dissociative amnesia, an individual is unable to recall important personal information such as name, occupation, and relatives.

126. **3.** Self-mutilation is characteristic of borderline personality disorder.

127. **4.** A safe environment for the client is a priority. Her self-mutilation, poor impulse control, and temper are characteristic of persons with borderline personality disorder who have self-directed violence.

128. **4.** The client's acting out and demanding behavior indicates her need for ego boundaries and control, which the nurse provides.

129. **3.** Clients with borderline personality disorder frequently engage in impulsive suicidal or self-mutilating behaviors. The behavior described in choice 3 indicates less "acting-out" of feelings and less impulsiveness in response to more effective coping.

130. **4.** This is an appropriate short-term goal in relation to his use of manipulative behavior to meet his needs.

131. **3.** This would indicate that the client may be improving related to recognizing his manipulative behavior. This is a first step in reducing the need for manipulation and attaining more effective coping strategies.

# Psychologic Aspects of Physical Illness

## STRESS-RELATED DISORDERS

### Overview

A. Actual physiologic change in structure/function of organ or system
B. May be referred to as psychosomatic or psychophysiologic disorders
C. Theorized that client's response to stress is a factor in etiology of disease
D. Stress/anxiety not the sole cause but may be a causative factor in the development/exacerbation of physical symptoms
E. See Table 7-9 for types of disorders with a stress component.

### Assessment

A. Health history, family history
B. Physical symptoms
C. Social/cultural considerations
D. Coping behaviors

### Analysis

Nursing diagnoses for stress-related disorders may include any nursing diagnosis specific to the physiologic problem as well as:
A. Ineffective coping
B. Deficient knowledge
C. Health-seeking behaviors

### Planning and Implementation

#### Goals

Client will:
A. Receive appropriate treatment for any physical symptoms (e.g., maintenance of blood pressure within normal range).

**Table 7-9** Types of Stress-Related Disorders

| Systems | Examples |
| --- | --- |
| Respiratory | Asthma, common cold |
| Circulatory | Hypertension, migraine headaches |
| Digestive | Peptic ulcers, colitis |
| Skin | Hives, dermatitis |
| Musculoskeletal | Rheumatoid arthritis, chronic backache |
| Nervous | Fatigue |
| Endocrine | Dysmenorrhea, diabetes mellitus |

B. Recognize relationship of stress to physical symptom(s).
C. Acknowledge coping patterns that may affect recurrence of physical symptoms.
D. Recognize relationship of self-concept, self-esteem, role performance to disorder.
E. Develop alternative coping behaviors.

#### Interventions

A. Provide nursing care specific to physical symptoms.
B. Establish nurse-client relationship.
C. Encourage discussion of psychosocial problems.
D. Explain relationship of stress to physiologic symptoms.
E. Encourage client to devise alternative coping behaviors, changes in environment, attitude.
F. Role play new behaviors with client.

### Evaluation

A. Goals specific to client's physical symptoms have been met.
B. Client
  1. Is able to relate stress to physical symptoms.
  2. Develops alternative coping behaviors.
  3. Engages in role playing of new behaviors.

## VICTIMS OF ABUSE

### Overview

A. Abuse is physical or sexual assault, emotional abuse, or neglect.
B. Victims are helpless or powerless to prevent the assault on their bodies or personalities.
C. Sometimes victims blame themselves for the assault.
D. The abusers often blame the victims, have poor impulse control, and use their power (physical strength or weapon) to subject victims to their assaults.
E. Victims include children, spouse, elderly, or rape victims; each will be described separately.

### Child Abuse

#### Overview

A. Over one million cases reported each year
B. Suspected child abuse must be reported

**C.** Abusing adults (parents) often have been victims of abuse, substance abusers, have poor impulse control

**D.** Battered-child syndrome: multiple traumas inflicted by adult

**E.** Sexual abuse/incest: common types of child abuse

**F.** Health care workers often experience negative feelings toward abuser

**G.** See Child Abuse, Unit 5

### Assessment

**A.** Physical signs/behaviors of physical/sexual abuse (see Table 7-10)

**B.** Signs of neglect: hunger, poor hygiene/nutrition, fatigue

**C.** Signs of emotional abuse: habitual behaviors (thumb sucking, rocking, head banging), conduct/learning disorders

### Analysis

**A.** Situational low self-esteem

**B.** Fear

**C.** Pain

**D.** Altered parenting

**E.** Post-trauma response

**F.** Powerlessness

**G.** High risk for injury

### Planning and Implementation

**A.** Goals
  1. Client (child) will be safe until home assessment made by child welfare agency.
  2. Child will participate with nurse (therapist) for emotional support.
  3. Client (parent[s]) will be able to contact agencies to deal with own rage/helplessness.
  4. Parent(s) will participate in therapy (group or other required).

**B.** Interventions
  1. Provide nursing care specific to physical/emotional symptoms.

**Table 7-10** Symptoms of Child Abuse

| Physical Abuse | Sexual Abuse |
| --- | --- |
| Pattern of bruises/welts | Pain/itching of genitals |
| Burns (cigarette, scalds, rope) | Bruised/bleeding genitals |
| Unexplained fractures/ dislocations | Stains/blood on underwear |
| Withdrawn or aggressive behavior | Withdrawn or aggressive behavior |
| Unusual fear of parent/desire to please parent | Unusual sexual behaviors |

  2. Conduct interview in private with child and parent(s) separated.
  3. Inform parent(s) of requirement to report suspected abuse.
  4. Do not probe for information or try to prove abuse.
  5. Be supportive and nonjudgmental.
  6. Provide referrals for assistance and therapy.

**C.** Evaluation
  1. Physical symptoms have been treated.
  2. Child safety has been ensured.
  3. Parent(s) have agreed to seek help.

## Spouse Abuse

### Overview

**A.** Estimates of five million women assaulted by mate each year

**B.** Stages
  1. Tension builds: verbal abuse, minor physical assaults
     **a.** Abuser: often reduces tension with alcohol/drugs
     **b.** Abused: blames self
  2. Acute battering: brutal beating
     **a.** Abuser: does not recall incident
     **b.** Abused: depersonalizes, may seek separation/divorce
     **c.** Both parties in shock
  3. Honeymoon: make-up stage
     **a.** Abuser: apologizes and promises to control self
     **b.** Abused: feels loved/needed; forgives/believes abuser
  4. Cycle repeats with subsequent battering, usually more severe

### Assessment

**A.** Headache

**B.** Injury to face, head, body, genitals

**C.** Reports "accidents"

**D.** Symptoms of severe anxiety

**E.** Depression

**F.** Insomnia

**G.** X-rays reveal previously healed fractures/broken bones

### Analysis

**A.** Risk for injury

**B.** Anxiety

**C.** Pain

**D.** Disabled family coping

**E.** Ineffective coping

**F.** Spiritual distress

**G.** Fear

## Planning and Implementation

A. Goals
1. Client will admit self and/or children are victims of abuse
2. Client will describe plan(s) for own/children's safety
3. Client will name agencies that will assist in maintaining a safe environment

B. Interventions
1. Crisis stage
   a. Provide safe environment
   b. Treatment of physical injuries; document
   c. Encourage verbalization of actual home environment
   d. Provide referral to shelters
   e. Encourage decision making
2. Rebuilding stage: therapy (individual, family and/or group)

## Evaluation

Client will be protected from further injury.

# Elder Abuse

## Overview

A. Estimates one-half million to over one million cases per year.
B. Women, over age 70, with some physical/psychological disability are most frequent victims.
C. Neglect is most common, followed by physical abuse, financial exploitation, and sexual abuse/abandonment.
D. Victims do not always report abuse because of fear of more abuse/abandonment by caretaker(s).

## Assessment

A. Malnutrition
B. Poor hygiene, decubiti
C. Omission of medication/overmedication
D. Welts, bruises, fractures

## Analysis

A. Risk for injury
B. Fear
C. Anxiety
D. Imbalanced nutrition: less than body requirements
E. Powerlessness
F. Situational low self-esteem

## Planning and Implementation

A. Goals
1. Client will be free from injury.
2. Client will receive adequate nutrition, hydration, prescribed medication.

3. Client will notify nurse if further abuse takes place.
4. Caregiver will verbalize plans to meet own needs.
5. Caregiver will seek assistance to meet client's needs when necessary.

B. Interventions
1. Refer to state laws for reporting elder abuse and nurse's liability.
2. Obtain client's consent for treatment and/or transfer.
3. Document physical/emotional condition of client.
4. Refer client/caregiver to agencies for assistance.
5. Encourage client and caregiver to discuss problems.
6. Encourage communication between client and caregiver.

## Evaluation

A. Client will remain free of injury, effects of neglect.
B. Caregiver will utilize support systems for self.

# Rape

## Overview

A. Estimates of occurrence vary; only 10% reported
B. Most victims are female between ages of 15 and 24 years
C. Response to rape
1. Shock: panic to overly controlled
2. Outward adjustment: "manages" life but may make drastic changes (e.g., moves, leaves school/job)
3. Integration: acknowledges response (e.g., depression, fear, rage)

## Assessment

A. Physical injury
B. Emotional response: controlled/hysterical

## Analysis

A. Rape trauma syndrome
1. Compound reaction: immediate to 2 weeks (anger, fear, self-blame)
2. Long-term: nightmares, phobias, seeks support
B. Silent reaction: anxiety, changes in relationships with men, physical distress, phobias
C. Post-trauma response

## Planning and Implementation

A. Goals
1. Client will express response to assault
2. Client will verbalize plan to handle immediate needs

3. Client will seek assistance from rape counselor
4. Client will discuss need for follow-up counseling
5. Client will report (long-term) reduction of physical and emotional symptoms.

B. Interventions
1. Give emotional support in nonjudgmental manner.
2. Maintain confidentiality: client must give consent for reporting rape and for medical examination.
3. Listen to client, encourage expression of feelings.
4. Document physical findings. Put evidentiary garments in paper bag.
5. Provide referral to rape counselor and follow-up care.

## Evaluation

A. Client seeks support from family/agencies.
B. Client verbalizes emotional response to rape.
C. Long-term: client reports return to prerape lifestyle.

# CRITICAL ILLNESS

## Overview

A. Individuals in critical life-threatening situations have realistic fears of death or of permanent loss of function.
B. Clients and their families may respond to these crises with denial, anger, hostility, withdrawal, guilt, and/or panic.
C. Loss of control and a sense of powerlessness can be overwhelming and detrimental to chance of recovery.

## Assessment

A. Physiologic needs (first priority)
B. Anxiety level of client/family
C. Client/family fears
D. Coping behaviors of client/family
E. Social and cultural considerations

## Analysis

Nursing diagnoses for the psychologic component of critical illness may include:
A. Anxiety
B. Hopelessness
C. Ineffective coping
D. Deficient knowledge
E. Fear
F. Powerlessness

## Planning and Implementation
### Goals

A. Client will:
1. Receive treatment for physiologic problems.
2. Experience decrease in level of anxiety/fear.
3. Discuss anxiety/fears with nurse.
B. Family will:
1. Be informed of client's condition on regular basis.
2. Discuss anxiety/fears with nurse.
3. Provide appropriate support to client.

### Interventions

A. Provide nursing care specific to physiologic problems.
B. Stay with client.
C. Explain all procedures slowly, clearly, concisely.
D. Provide opportunities for client to discuss fears.
E. Provide opportunities for client to make decisions, have as much control as possible.
F. Encourage family to ask questions.
G. Recognize negative family responses as coping behaviors.
H. Encourage family members to support each other and client.

## Evaluation

A. Goals specific to client's physiologic status have been met.
B. Client
1. Demonstrates a decrease in anxious behaviors.
2. Is able to express fears verbally.
3. Has participated in decisions whenever possible.
C. Family members
1. Have discussed fears.
2. Demonstrate support for each other and for client.

# CHRONIC ILLNESS

## Overview

A. Chronic illnesses, such as diabetes mellitus, multiple sclerosis, or illnesses/injuries resulting in loss of function or loss of a body part necessitate adaptation to the inherent changes imposed.
B. Clients/families may respond to the losses associated with chronic illness with a variety of behaviors and defenses, including recurrent depression, anger and hostility, denial, or acceptance.

## Assessment and Analysis

Same as stress-related disorders as well as:

A. Ineffective coping
B. Risk for violence, self-directed
C. Spiritual distress

## Planning and Intervention

### Goals

A. Client will:
   1. Receive appropriate treatment for any physiologic symptoms.
   2. Be able/willing to discuss responses to illness.
   3. Recognize effect of illness on aspects of self-concept.
   4. Develop realistic plans for activities and role functions.
   5. Contract with nurse to report depression/suicidal ideation.
B. Family will:
   1. Be able to discuss responses to client illness.
   2. Develop plans to deal with alterations in client's behaviors and functions.

### Interventions

A. Provide nursing care specific to physiologic problems.
B. Develop nurse/client relationship through active listening, acceptance of positive and negative client responses.
C. Encourage client to plan activities within present capabilities.
D. Provide information about illness, suggestions for activities.
E. Contract with client to request support in times of depression and to report suicidal ideation.
F. Encourage family members to discuss their response to client's illness.
G. Be accepting and nonjudgmental of negative responses (e.g., anger, hopelessness).
H. Support family efforts to develop plans for their participation in client's care.

## Evaluation

A. Client
   1. Receives appropriate treatment for any physiologic problems.
   2. Recognizes/discusses positive and negative responses to illness.
   3. Understands effects of feelings about body image, self-esteem, role function.
   4. Agrees to report depression or suicidal thoughts.

B. Family
   1. Discusses positive and negative responses to client's illness.
   2. Plans/engages in appropriate activities with client.

## AIDS

### Overview

A. In the United States, many thousands of reported cases and deaths, estimates between 1 and 2 million infected.
B. Highest risk populations: homosexual/bisexual men, IV drug users and their sexual partners, hemophiliacs, newborns from infected mothers, and black females between the ages of 15 and 44 years.
C. Approximately 60% of persons with AIDS develop neurological symptoms.
D. Health care workers may have difficulty caring for these clients because of fear of contagion, knowledge deficit, bias against lifestyle, or burnout.
E. Families/partners will require support, education, and counseling.

### Assessment

A. Physical symptoms
   1. Fever
   2. Fatigue
   3. Weight loss
   4. Diarrhea
   5. Opportunistic infections
B. Neurological and emotional responses
   1. Depression
   2. Panic disorders
   3. Paranoid reaction
   4. HIV dementia complex
C. See AIDS (Unit 4) for other physical assessment findings.

### Analysis

A. Anxiety
B. Fear
C. Ineffective denial
D. Anticipatory grieving
E. Ineffective coping
F. Powerlessness
G. Risk for violence, self-directed
H. Social isolation

## Planning and Implementation

### Goals

A. Client will:
   1. Communicate responses (physical and psychologic) to disease process
   2. Maintain ADLs as long as possible
   3. Report suicidal ideation/impulses
B. Family/partners will:
   1. Seek support and education relating to care of HIV-positive client
   2. Communicate responses to client's illness to nurse/support group
C. Health care workers will:
   1. Discuss feelings of homophobia, addictophobia, and fear of infection
   2. Attend groups for education and support

### Interventions

A. Monitor cognitive and affective domain.
B. Encourage communication of fears and concerns.
C. Maintain nonjudgmental attitude.
D. Assist client/family through grieving process.
E. Provide opportunities for decision making to client and/or caregivers.

## Evaluation

A. Client participates in care decisions.
B. Client and caregivers discuss responses to illness.
C. Client expresses anger but does not harm self.

# DEATH AND DYING

## Overview

A. One of the most difficult issues in nursing practice
B. Often difficult for nurses to maintain objectivity because of identification and response to death based on own value system and personal experiences

## Assessment

A. Stage of dying (Kubler-Ross); see Table 7-11
B. Physical discomfort
C. Emotional reaction (withdrawal, anger, acceptance) and stage of dying

**Table 7-11** Stages of Dying

1. Denial and isolation
2. Anger
3. Bargaining
4. Depression
5. Acceptance

D. Desire to discuss impending death, value of own life
E. Level of consciousness
F. Family needs

## Analysis

Nursing diagnoses for the dying client may include:
A. Anxiety
B. Pain
C. Ineffective coping
D. Fear
E. Anticipatory grieving
F. Hopelessness
G. Impaired mobility
H. Powerlessness
I. Self-care deficit
J. Social isolation

## Planning and Implementation

### Goals

A. Client will:
   1. Be maintained in optimum comfort.
   2. Not be alone.
   3. Have opportunity to discuss what death means and to progress through stages of dying.
B. Family will have opportunity to be with client as much as they desire.

### Interventions

A. Recognize clients/families have own way of dealing with death and dying.
B. Support clients/families as they work through dying process.
C. Accept negative responses from clients/families.
D. Encourage clients/families to discuss feelings related to death and dying.
E. Support staff and seek support for self when dealing with dying client and grieving family.

## Evaluation

A. Client
   1. Takes opportunity to discuss feelings about impending death and eventually acknowledges inevitable outcome.
   2. Is comfortable and participates in self-care for as long as possible.
B. Family discusses feelings about loss of loved one.

# GRIEF AND MOURNING

## Overview

A. Response to loss (person, body part, role)
B. Biologic, psychologic, social implications
C. Family system effects

D. Mourning is process to resolve grief
1. Shock, disbelief are short term
2. Resentment, anger
3. Concentration on loss
   a. Possible auditory, visual hallucinations
   b. Possible guilt
   c. Possible fear of becoming mentally ill
4. Despair, depression
5. Detachment from loss
6. Renewed interest, investment in others/interests

## Assessment

A. Weight loss
B. Sleep disturbance
C. Thoughts centered on loss
D. Dependency, withdrawal, anger, guilt
E. Suicide potential

## Analysis

A. Ineffective coping
B. Hopelessness
C. Sleep pattern disturbance
D. Disturbed thought processes
E. Risk for violence, self-directed

## Planning and Implementation

### Goals

Client/family will:
A. Discuss responses to loss.
B. Resume normal sleeping/eating patterns.
C. Resume ADLs as they accept loss.

### Interventions

A. Encourage client/family to express feelings.
B. Accept negative feelings/defenses.
C. Employ empathic listening.
D. Explain mourning process and relate to client/family responses.
E. Refer client/family to support groups.

## Evaluation

Client/family
A. Express feelings.
B. Progress through mourning process.
C. Seek necessary support groups.

## Sample Questions

132. An 18-month-old has been admitted for second-degree burns surrounding the genital area. Her mother told the nurse that the child grabbed for the hot coffee cup and spilled it on herself. Legally, what is the nurse required to do?
    1. Testify in court on the injuries.
    2. Report suspected child abuse.
    3. Have the mother arrested.
    4. Refer the mother to counseling.

133. A toddler was admitted for second-degree burns surrounding the genital area. Her mother told the nurse that the child grabbed the hot coffee cup and spilled it on herself. The toddler's mother is 17 years old. In which of the areas would the nurse provide health teaching?
    1. Normal growth and development.
    2. Bonding techniques.
    3. How to childproof the apartment.
    4. Parenting skills.

134. A young woman was returning home from work late and was sexually assaulted. She was brought to the emergency room upset and crying. What is the nurse's main goal?
    1. Assist her in crisis.
    2. Notify the police of the alleged assault.
    3. Understand she will have a long recovery period.
    4. Provide support and comfort.

135. The nurse is caring for a young woman who was sexually assaulted. Which of the following is indicative of successful adjustment to the trauma?
    1. She moves to another city.
    2. She resumes her work and activities.
    3. She takes classes in the martial arts.
    4. She remains silent about the assault.

136. A young man has recently begun experiencing forgetfulness, disorientation, and occasional lapses in memory. The client was diagnosed with AIDS dementia. His family began sobbing on hearing the diagnosis. What would be an appropriate response from the nurse?
    1. "You must never give up hope."
    2. "He was in a high-risk group for AIDS."
    3. "I can understand your grief."
    4. "This must be very difficult for you."

137. The nurse is planning care for a young man who has AIDS dementia. What is the primary goal in his care?
    1. Enhance the quality of life.
    2. Teach him about AIDS.
    3. Discuss his future goals.
    4. Provide him with comfort and support.

**138.** What is one of the major fears experienced by people with AIDS?
1. Dying.
2. Debilitation.
3. Stigma.
4. Poverty.

**139.** A school nurse is assessing a second-grade child for symptoms of sexual abuse. Which of the following behavioral symptoms would support the possibility of sexual abuse?
1. Enuresis, impulsivity, decline in school performance.
2. Thumb sucking, isolating self from peers on playground, excessive fearfulness.
3. Hyperactivity, rocking, isolating self from peers on playground.
4. Stuttering, rocking, impulsivity.

**140.** A 21-year-old college student is seen in the ER following an incident of date rape. During the nursing assessment, the client describes the entire chain of events with a blank facial expression. She ends her comments by saying, "It's like it didn't happen to me at all." Which of the following statements most accurately explains that patient's reaction?
1. This client is using dissociation/isolation as a defense mechanism to cope with the attack.
2. This client is using denial as a defense mechanism to cope with the attack.
3. This client is in the shock phase of a crisis and is repressing feelings associated with the traumatic event.
4. This client is using reaction formation to manage the hostility she feels toward the attacker.

**141.** A 38-year-old mother of three children is seen in the medical clinic with complaints of chronic fatigue. The woman looks sad, makes only brief eye contact, and startles easily. The nurse acknowledges these observations and the woman says, "My husband has started to hold a gun to my head when I don't do exactly what he wants." Which of the following is the most appropriate response by the nurse?
1. "What is it you won't do that makes him do this?"
2. "Tell me what has influenced your decision to stay with your husband?"
3. "That is abusive behavior; there are resources which can help you."
4. "How often does this happen?"

**142.** Which of the following statements made by a victim of spouse abuse would indicate to the nurse that the woman was admitting that she was a victim of spousal abuse?
1. "It would be nice to be out of the situation, but I cannot afford to leave. I have no skills."
2. "My husband has never visited me when I've been in the hospital. He even said he will take me out more often."
3. "Last time it happened I tried to talk to his mother. She said he was never like this growing up."
4. "I have the shelter number and I've decided to work on my high school diploma while the kids are in school each day."

**143.** A 78-year-old male with a history of cancer of the prostate is admitted to the medical unit for the fourth time in 6 weeks. On admission, the client is confused and has a decubitis ulcer the size of a fifty cent piece on the sacral area. The client did not have this breakdown on discharge 10 days ago. The nurse also notes what appear to be friction burns on both wrists. Which of the following nursing diagnosis statements takes priority in the care of this patient?
1. Impaired skin integrity.
2. Disturbed thought processes.
3. Ineffective health maintenance.
4. Risk for injury.

**144.** A 27-year-old is admitted to the medical unit with severe abdominal pain, dehydration, and renal insufficiency associated with substance abuse. The patient's admitting chest X-ray shows diffuse interstitial infiltrates and the physician asks that the client give consent for HIV testing. The client consents and the test returns positive. After learning of the positive results, the client says to the nurse, "I never thought this would happen to me. I don't know if I can go through this." Which of the following nursing diagnosis statements is of highest priority for this patient?
1. Anticipatory grieving.
2. Risk for infection.
3. Risk for self-directed violence.
4. Thought process, altered.

**145.** The nurse is changing the dressing on a client who has had a modified radical mastectomy 2 days ago. The client refuses to look in the direction of the nurse or the operative site. The nurse notices a tear running down the client's cheek. Which of the following responses would most appropriately facilitate the client's grief resolution?

1. "You look very sad, it might help you feel better if you let yourself cry."

2. "Tell me what's the worst part about losing your breast."

3. "Everything is going to be all right; you can be fitted for a new bra and no one will notice."

4. "Are you crying because you are concerned about how your partner will respond?"

146. A 42-year-old male is admitted to the medical unit for insertion of an access site for hemodialysis. The client relates that his transplant graft failed, he has lost his job due to corporate downsizing, and his wife left him recently. He has now moved back into his parents' home. Which of the following nursing diagnosis statements takes priority in planning nursing care for this client?

1. Fluid volume deficit.

2. Ineffective denial.

3. Ineffective tissue perfusion; renal.

4. Powerlessness.

147. The condition of a client diagnosed with chronic obstructive pulmonary disease (COPD) and cor pulmonale is deteriorating. The client is very hypoxemic, obtunded, and easily fatigued by any activity. The nurse who has been working with this client throughout this hospitalization is repositioning the client. Which of the following remarks made by the client indicates that the client has come to terms with death?

1. "It is finally spring and that is my favorite time of year."

2. "Am I going to die?"

3. "I'm very tired, but content and ready to go."

4. "I'm feeling stronger by the moment today."

148. A family member whose mother is terminally ill asks to speak to the nurse. Which of the following statements made by this family member should indicate to the nurse that this family member understands the emotional response to death and dying?

1. "Mother seems very comfortable; so we're able to recall some of our good times spent together."

2. "My mother is irate because she says you all told her she had to have an advanced directive."

3. "My mother is talking about redoing her bedroom when she's discharged. Doesn't she know she's dying?"

4. "My mother is crying so much these days. Where's all this sadness coming from?"

## Answers and Rationales

132. 2. Legal statutes require health professionals to report suspected cases of child abuse. The burn pattern described is consistent with being placed in a tub of very hot water.

133. 4. Because the toddler's mother is only 17 years old, she needs information and role modeling on how to provide an emotionally and physically safe environment for her child. This response is more inclusive and includes the other responses.

134. 1. A sexual assault is a crisis situation that requires crisis intervention.

135. 2. The goal of adjustment is to have the woman return to her precrisis level of functioning.

136. 4. AIDS is an illness that generates intense emotional reactions and fears. Acknowledging these feelings allows the family to discuss them with the nurse in a nonthreatening environment.

137. 1. Because the client's illness has no cure and the progression is dependent on the body system affected, the primary goal is to ensure his personal dignity and make plans to fulfill personal goals.

138. 2. Research has found that many clients with AIDS are most fearful of the debilitating effects of the disease.

139. 2. Behavioral symptoms of children who are victims of sexual abuse include: regression (thumb sucking would be regressive behavior in a second-grade child who is probably around 7 years old), disturbed sleep patterns, clinging behaviors, lack of peer friendships, sexual acting out, running away or threats to do so, and suicide attempts.

140. 1. One of the defense mechanisms that a person can use to manage the anxiety associated with an attack/rape is dissociation/isolation in which the client strips an event of its emotional significance and affective content.

141. 3. This response identifies the husband's behavior as abusive and offers help for the wife if she is ready to consider other options. It does not cast judgment on her or question why she stays.

142. 4. This statement acknowledges that the victim has admitted the need for protection in case of emergency and is making plans to work on

establishing some degree of autonomy, which is a factor that keeps many women in abusive relationships.

143. **4.** The highest priority for this client based on the available data is the increased risk for injury because of confusion. The nurse's immediate concern must be the client's safety in the present environment.

144. **3.** Based on the patient's comment, the highest priority of care for this client immediately is the risk of suicide. He states he doesn't know if he can go through this. Suicide is a common reaction of persons who learn they are HIV-positive, which is associated with stigma and many losses. The client does not have a history of positive coping, which increases the risk of suicide.

145. **1.** This acknowledges the client's mood and gives her permission to cry. Crying puts the client in touch with the sadness/pain over the loss. Offering permission to cry facilitates expression of feelings related to the loss.

146. **4.** Powerlessness, or feelings of uncertainty about the future, may be present in this client due to the uncertainty about his future in several areas: job, another transplant, long-term hemodialysis, reconciliation in his marriage, whether he will have to be dependent on parents long term, and concern about their own possible declining health.

147. **3.** This response indicates that the client is exhausted and ready to let the natural processes take their course. The client is at peace.

148. **1.** This statement indicates that the family member and mother have been able to reminisce about good times together, acknowledging that

there may be few remaining times to share these memories. This sharing indicates both have accepted death of mother and its finality.

## REFERENCES AND SUGGESTED READINGS

American Psychiatric Association. (2000). *Diagnostic and statistical manual of mental disorders:* Text revision (4th ed.). Washington, DC: Author.

Antai-Otong, D. (2008). *Psychiatric nursing, biological and behavioral concepts* (2nd ed.). Clifton Park, NY: Delmar Cengage Learning.

Austism Speaks, Inc. (2008). Retrieved on Sept 7, 2008, from http://www.autismspeaks.org

Boyd, M. A. (2008). *Psychiatric nursing: Contemporary practice* (4th ed.). Philadelphia: Lippincott.

Centers for Disease Control and Prevention (2008). Autism Information Center. Retrieved on Sept. 7, 2008, from http://www.cdc.gov/ncbddd/autism.

Fortinash, K. M., & Holodey Worret, P. A. (2007). *Psychiatric mental health nursing* (4th ed.). St. Louis. MO: Elsevier Health Sciences.

Frisch, N. C., & Frisch, L. E. (2002). *Psychiatric mental health nursing* (3rd ed.). Clifton Park, NY: Delmar Cengage Learning.

Gorman, L., Sulton, D., & Raines, M. (2008). *Davis's manual of psychosocial nursing for general client care* (3rd ed.). Philadelphia: F. A. Davis.

Mullins, D. (2006). *501 human diseases.* Clifton Park, NY: Delmar Cengage Learning.

Sadock, B., & Sadock, V. (2007). *Kaplan and Sadock's synopsis of psychiatry: Behavioral sciences/clinical psychiatry* (10th ed.). Philadelphia: Lippincott, Williams & Wilkins.

Spratto, G. R., & Woods, A. L. (2009). *Delmar Nurse's Drug Handbook 2009.* Clifton Park, NY: Delmar Cengage Learning.

Townsend, M. C. (2008) *Nursing diagnosis in psychiatric nursing: care plans and psychotropic medications* (7th ed.). Philadelphia: F. A. Davis.

Varcarolis, E. M., Carson, V. B., & Shoemaker, N. C. (2006). *Foundations of psychiatric mental health nursing: A clinical approach* (5th ed.). Philadelphia: W. B. Saunders.

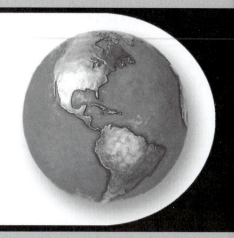

# APPENDIX

# SPECIAL DIETS

## APPENDIX OUTLINE

# Diabetic Diet and Exchange Lists

## DIABETIC DIET

### Description

A diabetic diet is prescribed for clients with diabetes mellitus. Purposes include: attain or maintain ideal body weight, ensure normal growth, and maintain plasma glucose levels as close to normal as possible. Food preparation includes:

- Distribution of kcal: protein 12–20%; carbohydrates 55–60%; fats (unsaturated) 20–25%.
- Daily distribution of kcal: equally divided among breakfast, lunch, supper, snacks.
- Foods high in fiber and complex carbohydrates.
- No simple sugars, jams, honey, syrup, frosting.

## EXCHANGE LISTS FOR MEAL PLANNING

### Food Exchange Lists*

| List | Measure | Carbohydrates (g) | Protein (g) | Fat (g) | Energy (kcal) |
|---|---|---|---|---|---|
| Milk, nonfat (see List 1) | 1 cup | 12 | 8 | trace | 80 |
| Milk, whole (see List 1) | 1 cup | 12 | 8 | 9 | 160 |
| Vegetables (see List 2) | ½ cup | 5 | 2 | | 25 |
| Fruits (see List 3) | Varies | 10 | | | 40 |
| Breads, cereals, and starchy vegetables (see List 4) | Varies | 15 | 2 | | 70 |
| Meat, low fat (see List 5) | 1 oz | | 7 | 2.5 | 50 |
| Meat, medium fat (see List 5) | 1 oz | | 7.5 | 5 | 75 |
| Meat, high fat (see List 5) | 1 oz | | 7 | 7.5 | 95 |
| Fat (see List 6) | Varies | | | 5 | 45 |

*Resource: Committees of the American Diabetes Association, Inc., and the American Dietetic Association: Exchange Lists for Meal Planning. Chicago: The American Dietetic Association and the American Diabetes Association, in cooperation with the National Institute of Arthritis, Metabolism and Digestive Diseases and the National Heart, Blood and Lung Institute, Public Health Service, U.S. Department of Health, Education and Welfare, 1976.

### List 1: Milk Exchanges

| | Amount to Use |
|---|---|
| **Nonfat, fortified** | |
| Use only this list for diets restricted in saturated fat. | |
| Skim or nonfat milk | 1 cup |
| Powdered (nonfat dry) | 1/3 cup |
| Canned, evaporated, skim | ½ cup |
| Buttermilk made from skim milk | 1 cup |
| Yogurt, made from skim milk, plain, unflavored | 1 cup |
| **Low fat, fortified** | |
| 1% fat, fortified (omit ½ fat exchange) | 1 cup |
| 2% fat, fortified (omit 1 fat exchange) | 1 cup |
| Yogurt made from 2% fortified, plain, unflavored (omit 1 fat exchange) | 1 cup |
| **Whole** | |
| Whole milk | 1 cup |
| Canned evaporated | ½ cup |
| Buttermilk made from whole milk | 1 cup |
| Yogurt made from whole milk, plain, unflavored | 1 cup |

## List 2: Vegetable Exchanges

One-half cup equals one exchange.

| | | |
|---|---|---|
| Asparagus* | Greens*† | Onions |
| Bean sprouts | Beet greens | Rhubarb |
| Beets | Chard | Rutabaga |
| Broccoli*† | Collards | Sauerkraut |
| Brussels sprouts | Dandelion greens | String beans, green or yellow |
| Cabbage* | Kale | Summer squash |
| Carrots† | Mustard greens | Tomatoes* |
| Celery | Spinach | Tomato juice |
| Cauliflower* | Turnip greens | Turnips |
| Cucumbers | Mushrooms | Vegetable juice cocktail |
| Eggplant | Okra | Zucchini |

*Good sources of ascorbic acid.
†Good sources of vitamin A.
These vegetables can be used as desired: chicory, Chinese cabbage, endive, escarole, lettuce, parsley, radishes, and watercress.
*See List 4, Bread Exchanges, for starchy vegetables.*

## List 3: Fruit Exchanges

| | Amount to Use | | Amount to Use |
|---|---|---|---|
| Apple | 1 small | Mango*† | ½ small |
| Apple juice | 1/3 cup | Cantaloupe* | ¼ small |
| Applesauce (unsweetened) | ½ cup | Honeydew* | 1/8 medium |
| Apricots, fresh† | 2 medium | Watermelon | 1 cup |
| Apricots, dried† | 4 halves | Nectarine | 1 medium |
| Bananas | ½ small | Orange* | 1 small |
| Blackberries | ½ cup | Orange juice* | ½ cup |
| Blueberries | ½ cup | Papaya*† | ¾ cup |
| Raspberries | ½ cup | Peach† | 1 medium |
| Strawberries | ½ cup | Pear | 1 small |
| Cherries | 10 large | Persimmon | 1 medium |
| Cider | 1/3 cup | Pineapple | ½ cup |
| Dates | 2 | Pineapple juice | 1/3 cup |
| Figs, fresh | 1 | Plums | 2 medium |
| Figs, dried | 1 | Prunes | 2 medium |
| Grapefruit* | ½ | Prune juice | ¼ cup |
| Grapefruit juice | ½ cup | Raisins | 2 tbsp |
| Grapes | 12 | Tangerine* | 1 large |
| Grape juice | ¼ cup | | |

*Good sources of ascorbic acid.
†Good sources of vitamin A.
Tanberries may be used as desired if no sugar is added.

## List 4: Bread, Cereal, and Starchy Vegetable Exchanges

| | Amount to Use | | Amount to Use |
|---|---|---|---|
| **Bread** | | English muffin, small | ½ |
| White (including French and Italian) | 1 slice | Frankfurter roll | ½ |
| Whole wheat | 1 slice | Hamburger bun | ½ |
| Rye or pumpernickel | 1 slice | Plain roll (bread) | 1 |
| Raisin | 1 slice | Dry bread crumbs | 3 tbsp |
| Bagel, small | ½ | Tortillas, 6 inch | 1 |

*(Continues)*

## List 4: Bread, Cereal, and Starchy Vegetable Exchanges (*Continued*)

| | **Amount to Use** | | **Amount to Use** |
|---|---|---|---|
| **Cereal** | | **Starchy Vegetables** | |
| Bran flakes | ½ cup | Corn | ⅓ cup |
| Other ready-to-eat unsweetened cereal | ¾ cup | Corn on cob | 1 small |
| Puffed cereal, unfrosted | 1 cup | Lima beans | ½ cup |
| Cereal, cooked | ½ cup | Parsnips | ⅔ cup |
| Grits, cooked | ½ cup | Peas (green, fresh, canned, or frozen) | ½ cup |
| Rice or barley, cooked | ½ cup | Potato, white | 1 small |
| Pastas, cooked | ½ cup | Potato, mashed | ½ cup |
| Popcorn, popped | 3 cups | Pumpkin | ¾ cup |
| Cornmeal, dry | 2 tbsp | Winter squash, acorn or butternut | ½ cup |
| Flour | 2½ tbsp | Yam or sweet potato | ¼ cup |
| Wheat germ | ½ cup | | |
| | | **Prepared Foods** | |
| **Crackers** | | Biscuit, 2 inch diam. (omit 1 fat exchange) | 1 |
| Arrowroot | 3 | Corn bread, 2 × 2 × 1 inch (omit 1 fat exchange) | 1 |
| Graham, 2½ inch | 2 | | |
| Matzoh, 4 × 6 inch | ½ | Corn muffin, 2 inch diam. (omit 1 fat exchange) | 1 |
| Oyster | 20 | | |
| Pretzels, 3⅛ inch × ⅛ inch | 15 | Crackers, round, butter type (omit 1 fat exchange) | 5 |
| Rye wafers, 2 × 3½ inch | 3 | | |
| Saltines | 6 | Muffin, plain, small (omit 1 fat exchange) | 1 |
| Soda, 2½ inch square | 4 | Pancake, 5 × ½ inch (omit 1 fat exchange) | 1 |
| **Dried Beans, Peas, and Lentils** | | Potatoes, french fried, 2 inch to 3½ inch (omit 1 fat exchange) | 15 |
| Dried beans, peas, and lentils cooked | ½ cup | | |
| Baked beans, no pork | ¼ cup | Waffle, 5 × ½ inch (omit 1 fat exchange) | 1 |

## List 5: Meat and Protein-Rich Exchanges

| | **Amount to Use** |
|---|---|

### *Lean Meat, Protein-Rich Exchanges*

Use only this list for diets low in saturated fat and cholesterol.

**Beef**

| | |
|---|---|
| Baby beef (very lean), chipped beef, chuck, flank steak, tenderloin, plate ribs, plate skirt steak, round (bottom, top), all cuts rump, spare ribs, tripe | 1 oz |

**Lamb**

| | |
|---|---|
| Leg, rib, sirloin, loin (roast and chops), shank, shoulder | 1 oz |

**Pork**

| | |
|---|---|
| Leg (whole rump, center shank), smoked ham (center slices) | 1oz |

**Veal**

| | |
|---|---|
| Leg, loin, rib, shank, shoulder, cutlets | 1 oz |

**Poultry without skin**

| | |
|---|---|
| Chicken, turkey, Cornish hen, guinea hen, pheasant | 1 oz |

**Fish, any fresh or frozen**

| | |
|---|---|
| Canned crab, lobster, mackerel, salmon, tuna | ¼ cup |
| Clams, oysters, scallops, shrimp | 5 or 1 oz |
| Sardines, drained | 3 |
| Cheeses containing less than 5% butterfat | 1 oz |
| Cottage cheese: dry or 2% butterfat | ¼ cup |
| Dried peas and beans (omit 1 bread exchange) | ½ cup |

|  | **Amount to Use** |
|---|---|
| *Medium-Fat Meal, Protein-Rich Exchanges* | |

### *Medium-Fat Meal, Protein-Rich Exchanges*

**Beef**

| Ground, 15% fat; comed beef, canned; rib eye, round, ground (commercial) | 1 oz |
|---|---|

**Pork**

| Loin, all cuts tenderloin, shoulder arm (picnic); shoulder blade, Boston butt, Canadian bacon; boiled ham | 1 oz |
|---|---|
| Liver, heart, kidney, and sweetbreads (high in cholesterol) | 1 oz |
| Cottage cheese, creamed | ¼ cup |

**Cheese**

| Mozzarella, ricotta, farmer's, Neufchâtel | 1 oz |
|---|---|
| Parmesan | 3 tbsp |
| Eggs (high in cholesterol) | 1 |
| Peanut butter (omit 2 fat exchanges) | 2 tbsp |

### *High-Fat Meal, Protein-Rich Exchanges*

| Beef brisket; corned beef brisket; ground beef (over 20% fat); hamburger (commercial); chuck, ground (commercial); rib roast, club and rib steak | 1 oz |
|---|---|
| Lamb, breast | 1 oz |
| Pork, spare ribs, loin (back ribs); pork, ground; country style ham, deviled ham | 1 oz |
| Veal, breast | 1 oz |
| Poultry: capon, duck (domestic), goose | 1 oz |
| Cheese: cheddar type | 1 oz |
| Cold cuts, 4½ × 1/8 inch | 1 slice |
| Frankfurter | small |

---

## List 6: Fat Exchanges

|  | **Amount to Use** |
|---|---|
| For a diet low in saturated fat and higher in polyunsaturated fat select only from this list. | |
| Margarine: soft, tub, or stick (made with corn, cottonseed, safflower, soy, or sunflower oil) | 1 tbsp |
| Avocado, 4 inch diam. | 1/8 |
| Nuts | |
|    Almonds* | 10 whole |
|    Peanuts* | |
|    Spanish | 20 whole |
|    Virginia | 10 whole |
|    Pecans* | 2 large, whole |
|    Walnuts | 6 small |
|    Other nuts* | 6 small |
| Oil, corn, cottonseed, safflower, soy, sunflower | 1 tsp |
| Oil, olive or peanut* | 1 tsp |
| Olives* | 5 small |
| Salad dressings, if made with corn, cottonseed, safflower or soy oil | |
|    French dressing | 1 tbsp |
|    Italian dressing | 1 tbsp |
|    Mayonnaise | 1 tsp |
|    Salad dressing, mayonnaise type | 2 tsp |

*(Continues)*

| | Amount to Use |
|---|---|
| The following fats should not be used on a diet low in saturated fat. | |
| Margarine, regular stick | 1 tsp |
| Butter | 1 tsp |
| Bacon fat | 1 tsp |
| Bacon crisp | 1 strip |
| Cream, light | 2 tbsp |
| Cream, sour | 2 tbsp |
| Cream, heavy | 1 tbsp |
| Cream cheese | 1 tbsp |
| Lard | 1 tsp |
| Salad dressings (permitted on restricted diets if made with allowed oils) | |
| French dressing | 1 tbsp |
| Italian dressing | 1 tbsp |
| Mayonnaise | 1 tsp |
| Salad dressing, mayonnaise type | 2 tsp |
| Salt pork | ¾ inch cube |

*Fat content is primarily monounsaturated.

# Renal Diet

## Description

A renal diet consists of controlling the intake of fluids, potassium, phosphorus, and sodium (salts). A typical renal diet could be written as "80-3-3," which means 80 grams of protein, 3 grams of sodium, and 3 grams of potassium a day.

## Food Preparation

Foods should be selected that are restrictive in sodium and potassium levels. Fluid intake will also need to be limited.

### Diet Guidelines

| Type of food | Allow | Avoid |
|---|---|---|
| Milk | Cool Whip, mocha mix, rice milk | Eggnog |
| Eggs | Egg substitute | |
| Cheese | All | More than one 4-oz serving |
| Meat, fish, poultry | Beef, chicken, fish, fresh pork, lamb, tuna, turkey | Bacon, bologna, canned meat, ham, sausage, hot dogs, lunchmeat |
| Vegetables, potatoes | | ½ cup baked, boiled, fried |
| Other vegetables | Beans, cabbage, cauliflower, celery, eggplant, leek, lettuce, mushrooms, onion, peppers, radishes, turnips | Artichoke, beet, dried beans, pumpkin, spinach, sweet potato, tomato, winter squash |
| Cereals | Dry, low salt; Cream of Rice, hominy grits, Malt-o-Meal, puffed rice, puffed wheat, wheat farina | |
| Bread | Bagels, hamburger, hot dog buns; hard or dinner rolls | Dark, whole, unrefined grains; croutons |
| Crackers | Unsalted | Salted crackers |
| Other cereal | Couscous, macaroni, noodles, rice, spaghetti | Chow mein noodles |
| Fats | Butter, canola oil, cream cheese, margarine, mayonnaise, Miracle Whip, nondairy creamers, olive oil, salad dressings, sour cream | |

(*Continues*)

| Type of food | Allow | Avoid |
|---|---|---|
| Fruits | Berries, cranberries, figs, fruit cocktail, grapes, lemons, limes, mandarin oranges, peaches, pears, plums, rhubarb | Avocado, bananas, dried fruits, kiwis, mangoes, melons, nectarines, oranges, tangeloes, papayas, raisins |
| Desserts | Animal crackers, cookies, hard candy, Fig Newtons | Banana pudding |
| Beverages | Coffee, fruit punch, grape juice, lemon/lime soda, tea | Orange juice, prune juice, unsalted tomato juice, dark-colored sodas |
| Sauces | | Bottled sauces |
| Soup | | Canned soups |
| Condiments | | |
| Sweets | Hard candy | Chocolate |

# Bariatric Diet

The bariatric diet is used for clients who have had bariatric surgery for obesity. Depending on the type of bariatric surgical procedure, some foods are restricted while others are limited. Weight loss is considerably faster with gastric banding and gastroplasty. To avoid nutritional problems, additional vitamin and mineral supplements may be needed.

## Food Preparation

Food intake is started in liquid form and progresses to a regular diet but with limited proportions.

Postoperative 1–2 days—Ice chips, water, sugar-free noncarbonated beverage (up to 4 oz per hour)

Postoperative 5–12 days—Additions to above; sugar-free popsicles, diet Jell-O, decaffeinated coffee/tea, chicken/beef broth. Client can avoid clumping syndrome by restricting high carbohydrate foods and drinking liquids between meals instead of with meals.

Diet Guidelines

| Type of food | Allow | Avoid |
|---|---|---|
| Milk | Nonfat, 1% milk, plain soy milk | High fat milk, yogurt |
| Eggs | Egg Beaters | Those prepared with fats other than vegetable oils |
| Cheese | Low-fat cheese | Whole milk cheese |
| Meat, fish, poultry | Turkey, chicken, fresh fish, low fat deli meat, water-packed tuna; reduced fat ham | Fatty meat or fish |
| Vegetables | Fresh vegetables; all (baked, boiled) Potatoes | Fried, French fries |
| Other vegetables | Vegetable broth | Fried vegetables |
| Cereals | Cream of Rice, Cream of Wheat, whole grain cereal, regular or unflavored oatmeal | Sugary cereals |
| Breads | Whole wheat or oat bran | White |
| Other cereal products | Pasta noodles, rice | |
| Fats | Spray olive oil, nonfat mayonnaise, light margarine, reduced-calorie salad dressing | Palm oil, full-fat condiments |
| Fruits | All fresh fruits | Canned in syrup fruit |
| Dessert | Sugar-free pudding, custard | Highly concentrated sweets (cakes, cookies, doughnuts) |
| Beverages | Unsweetened, pulp-free juice, coffee (no sugar), unsweetened tea, Crystal Light, bottled water, herbal tea | Sweetened juice, tea |

# High-Fiber Diet

## Description

The diet is essentially a normal diet with increased amounts of cellulose, hemicellulose, lignin, and pectin. It increases the volume and weight of the stool; increases gastrointestinal motility; and decreases intraluminal colonic pressure in clients suffering from increased pressure, including clients with constipation, hemorrhoids, and long-term management of diverticulosis.

## General Characteristics

Consume a regular diet with increased fiber content.

1. Include raw fruits and vegetables instead of canned or cooked ones.
2. Substitute whole-grain bread and cereals for refined grains.
3. Include dried fruits and nuts in meals. (Nuts may be eliminated in clients with diverticulosis.)
4. Prepare soups with high-fiber vegetables.
5. Eat a fresh vegetable or fruit salad daily.
6. Add 1–2 tablespoons of bran to other foods daily.
7. Initiate the high-fiber diet gradually to prevent gas and loose stools.

## Possible Complications

1. Osmotic diarrhea.
2. Decreased serum levels of minerals, such as iron, calcium, magnesium, etc.

# 1500-Kilocalorie Diet

## Description

1500-kcal diet will permit a steady weight loss of body fat without loss of body tissue and other essential body components. The diet meets the Recommended Dietary Allowances for the adult for protein, minerals, and vitamins.

## Food Preparation

Foods should be prepared without added sugar and flour, using only that amount of fat allowed in the diet. Meats may be broiled, braised, stewed, or roasted. All visible fat should be trimmed. The measure or weight of food refers to the food in its cooked form.

## Diet Guidelines

Food Exchange Lists

| | Daily Allowance |
|---|---|
| **List 1: Milk: 1 serving = 8 ounces**<br>Skim milk (1% fat)<br>Buttermilk (1% fat)<br>Yogurt made from<br>skim milk | 2 cups |

**Daily Allowance**

## List 2: Vegetables: 1 serving = ½ cup
3 servings

| | | |
|---|---|---|
| Asparagus | Cauliflower | Onions |
| Been sprouts | Celery | Sauerkraut |
| Beets | Eggplant | String beans |
| Broccoli | Greens | Summer squash |
| Brussels sprouts | Green peppers | Tomatoes |
| Cabbage | Mushrooms | Tomato/vegetable juice |
| Carrots | Okra | Turnips |
| | | Zucchini |

## List 3: Fruits (fresh or unsweetened)
5 servings

| | | |
|---|---|---|
| Small apple | 2 dates | Medium peach |
| 1/3 cup apple juice | ½ grapefruit | ½ cup pineapple |
| 2 apricots | ½ cup grapefruit juice | 1/3 cup pineapple juice |
| ½ small banana | 2 tbsp raisins | 2 plums |
| ½ cup berries | 12 grapes | 2 prunes |
| ¾ cup strawberries | 1/8 honeydew melon | ¼ cup prune juice |
| ¼ cantaloupe | Small orange | 1 cup watermelon |
| 10 cherries | ½ cup orange juice | Medium tangerine |

## List 4: Bread, Cereal, Starchy Vegetables
6 servings

| | | |
|---|---|---|
| 1 slice bread | ½ cup rice, grits | ½ matzoh |
| ½ bagel | ½ cup peas, beans | 25 small pretzels (3 1/8 long, 1/8 inch diam) |
| ½ English muffin | ¼ cup baked beans | 3 cups popcorn |
| ½ hamburger roll | ¼ cup sweet potato | ½ cup pastas |
| ¾ cup dry cereal | 2 graham crackers | 1 small potato |
| ½ cup cooked cereal | 6 saltine crackers | 1/3 cup corn |

## List 5: Meat and Poultry Foods Lean
3 oz total or ¾ cup

1 oz beef: leg, round, chipped, rump, loin
1 oz lamb; leg, rib, loin, sirloin
1 oz veal: leg, loin, rib, cutlets
1 oz pork: leg, rump, center slice
1 oz poultry: without skin (no duck or goose)
¼ cup tuna, salmon, crab, shrimp, lobster
¼ cup dry cottage cheese

## Medium Fat
3 oz total or ¾ cup

1 oz ground beef (15% fat)
1 oz pork shoulder, boiled ham, Canadian bacon
1 oz liver
1 egg
1 oz mozzarella, ricotta, farmer's cheese
¼ cup cottage cheese

## List 6: Fats
5 servings

| | | |
|---|---|---|
| 1 tsp butter | 10 peanuts | 1 tsp bacon fat |
| 1 tsp margarine | ¾ inch cube salt pork | 5 small olives |
| 1 tsp oil | 1 tbsp cream cheese | 1 tsp mayonnaise |
| 1 tbsp French dressing | 2 tbsp cream | 1 tsp lard |
| 1 tbsp Italian dressing | 1 slice crisp bacon | |

## Foods Allowed

| | | |
|---|---|---|
| Cucumbers | Dill pickles | Chinese cabbage |
| Endive | Escarole | Lettuce |
| Parsley | Radishes | Bouillon |
| Unflavored gelatin | Coffee | Tea |
| Spice | | |

# 1000-Milligram Sodium-Restricted Diet

## Description

The aim of this diet is to promote the loss of excess sodium and water from the extracellular fluid compartments of the body. It is used primarily for clients with ascites/edema associated with advanced liver or renal disease, clients in congestive heart failure, as a treatment for essential hypertension, and with clients receiving adrenocorticosteroids.

## Food Preparation

All food should be prepared without the addition of salt, regular baking powder, and baking soda. No salt should be used at the table.

## General Principles

Select foods that have not been processed or preserved with large amounts of salt. Include all fruits and fruit juices, fresh, canned, frozen, dried. Use only unsalted snack foods.

### Diet Guidelines

| Type of food | Allow | Avoid |
| --- | --- | --- |
| Milk | Whole or skim milk Limit: 9 cups/day | Milk shakes, malted milk, commercial chocolate, or buttermilk |
| Eggs | Any form prepared without the addition of salt. Limit: 4/week | |
| Cheese | Dry cottage cheese and low-sodium American cheese | All types except those allowed |
| Meat, fish, poultry | Meat or poultry without added salt or sodium products. Fresh or canned fish without added salt. Unsalted peanut butter. | Lunchmeat, sausage, hot dogs, shellfish, organ meats, bacon, ham, corned beef, dried beef, canned meat, anchovies, salted canned fish, dried cod |
| Soups and sauces | All made with allowed milk and vegetables | Broth, bouillon, gravy, canned soup, consomme, and cream sauce |
| Vegetables, potatoes | Fresh, frozen or canned white and sweet potatoes without added salt | Potato chips |
| Other vegetables | Unsalted asparagus, green beans, wax beans, corn, fresh or canned lima beans, eggplant, endive, escarole, lettuce, mushrooms, fresh or canned peas, squash, tomatoes. Also, if tolerated: broccoli, Brussels, sprouts, cabbage, cauliflower, turnips, onions, parsnips, radishes, rutabagas, and cucumbers<br>Following vegetables should be limited to one serving per day: beets, carrots, celery, spinach, or turnips | Beet greens, kale, frozen lima beans, olives, frozen peas, pickles, sauerkraut, Swiss chard, mustard greens, dandelion greens |
| Cereals | Puffed rice, puffed wheat, shredded wheat, and regular cooked whole-grain or enriched cereals | All other ready-to-eat cereals. Quick Cream of Wheat, quick-cooling farina, hominy |
| Bread | Regular white, whole wheat, or rye. Limit: 3 slices/day. If additional bread is desired, use low-sodium bread. | All others |
| Crackers | Unsalted crackers | All others |
| Other cereal | Macaroni, spaghetti products, noodles, rice | |
| Fats | Unsalted butter, margarine, oil | Salted butter or margarine, salad dressings, salt pork, bacon fat |

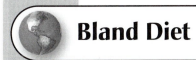

# Bland Diet

## Description

This diet excludes foods that may be chemically or mechanically stimulating or irritating to the gastrointestinal tract. Small, frequent meals may be indicated. Prescribed for clients with ulcers and postoperatively after some types of surgery.

## Food Preparation

Meats may be baked, broiled, stewed, or roasted, but not fried. Fruits and vegetables should be cooked or canned. Avoid meat extracts, pepper, and chili powder.

### Diet Guidelines

| Type of food | Allow | Avoid |
|---|---|---|
| Milk | Milk, buttermilk, cocoa, milk beverages | None |
| Eggs | Soft cooked, hard cooked, poached, steam scrambled | Fried, deviled |
| Cheese | Cottage cheese, cream, mild cheddar in sauces or in combination dishes | Strongly flavored cheese |
| Meat, fish, poultry | Tender beef, lamb, pork, liver, poultry, veal, fish, crisp bacon | Smoked, salted, or fatty meat or fish |
| Vegetables, potatoes | Baked (without skin), boiled, creamed, escalloped, or mashed white potatoes | Sweet potatoes, fried potatoes |
| Other Vegetables | Cooked asparagus tips, beets, carrots, peas, chopped spinach, winter squash, green beans, mushrooms, waxed beans, strained corn pudding | All others |
| Cereals | Cream of Rice, Cream of Wheat, farina, cornmeal, hominy grits, strained oatmeal, corn flakes, puffed rice, Rice Krispies, Special K | Bran, whole-grain cereals |
| Breads | White, Italian, French, rye bread without seeds, melba toast | Whole-grain breads |
| Crackers | Soda crackers, saltines | Graham crackers, crackers with seeds |
| Other cereal products | Macaroni, noodles, rice, spaghetti | |
| Fats | Butter, margarine, cream, salad oil | All others |
| Fruits | Avocado, ripe bananas, canned peaches, pears, Royal Anne cherries, peeled apricots, applesauce, baked apple (no skin), all strained fruit juices | Raw fruits except avocado and bananas; berries, figs, pineapple |
| Desserts | Plain sugar cookies, vanilla wafers, lady fingers, angel food cake, sponge cake, plain sherbet, plain ice cream, custard, Jell-O, Junket, Bavarian cream, simple puddings, fruit whips | Any containing fruits, nuts, or spices; pastries, pies, doughnuts |
| Beverages | Decaffeinated beverages | Caffeine-containing soft drinks, coffee, tea; alcohol |

# Low-Residue Diet

## Description

The low-residue diet is low in fiber, soft in texture, and easily digested. It decreases the weight and look of the stool.

## Food Preparation

Fruits and vegetables should be well cooked and pureed. Meats may be baked, broiled, stewed, or roasted. The meats that must be ground may be made from cooked meats that have had the gristle and excess fat removed, or ground meats may be purchased and made into patties or meatloaf. The food may be mildly seasoned.

### Diet Guidelines

| Type of food | Allow | Avoid |
|---|---|---|
| Milk | 1 pint | Any additional |
| Eggs | Hard cooked, soft cooked, steam scrambled, poached | All others |
| Cheese | Cottage, cream, mild American | All others |
| Meat, fish, poultry | Ground lean beef, lamb, veal, liver, sliced white meat of chicken or turkey, fish, crisp bacon, smooth peanut butter | Luncheon meats, sausages; smoked, highly seasoned or highly salted meats and fish |
| Vegetables, potatoes | White potato, strained sweet potato | Potato chips or fried potatoes |
| Other vegetables | Cooked and pureed: beets, peas, lima beans, squash, string beans, spinach, asparagus, pumpkin, whole asparagus tips and carrots cooked tender, mushrooms tomato juice | All others |
| Cereals | Cream of Rice, Cream of Wheat, farina, cornmeal, strained oatmeal, corn flakes, puffed rice, Rice Krispies, Special K | Whole-grain cereals |
| Breads | White bread, melba toast, zwieback | All others |
| Crackers | Soda crackers, saltines | All others |
| Other cereal products | Macaroni, noodles, refined rice, spaghetti | Whole-grain rice |
| Fats | Butter, margarine, cream, mayonnaise, salad oil, shortening | All others |
| Fruits | All canned or strained fruit juices, cooked or canned applesauce, Royal Anne cherries, peeled apricots, peaches, pears, bananas, peeled baked apple | All others |
| Desserts | Simple puddings, ice cream, sherbet, plain cakes and cookies, flavored gelatin, custards | All others. Allowed desserts with nuts, seeds, or coconut |
| Beverages | Coffee, tea, Postum, Sanka, carbonated beverages, fruit juices, milk in allowed amount | All others |

# 20-Gram Fat-Restricted Diet

## Description

The 20-gram fat-restricted diet is designed for clients with an acute intolerance for fat and for clients with high serum cholesterol levels. Lean meat is the only source of fat. For a 40-gram fat-restricted diet, add any combination of 4 teaspoons of the following: butter, margarine, shortening oil, mayonnaise.

| Type of food | Allow | Avoid |
|---|---|---|
| Yogurt, milk | Skim milk, skim milk yogurt, skim milk buttermilk | Whole milk, buttermilk, yogurt |
| Eggs | Egg whites only | Whole eggs and egg yolks |
| Cheese | Dry cottage cheese, skim milk cheese | Whole milk cheese |
| Meat, fish, poultry | Two 2-oz servings of lean beef, veal, pork, lamb, poultry, liver, or fish | Corned beef, sausages, goose, duck, fish canned in oil such as sardines, tuna fish, and salmon; fried meats, fish, and poultry |
| Vegetables, Potatoes | Sweet or white | Those prepared with fat |
| Other vegetables | All prepared without fat, oil, or cream | Frozen vegetables in butter or cream sauces, au gratin; potato chips; casseroles |
| Cereals | Cooked and ready-to-eat cereals | None |
| Bread | White, whole wheat, and rye bread; hard, water rolls, simple yeast buns | All others |
| Crackers | Saltine and graham | All others |
| Other cereal products | Macaroni, noodles, rice, and spaghetti | |
| Fats | None | All |
| Fruits | Any fruit or juice | Olives, avocados |
| Desserts | Fruit ices and sherbets, gelatin desserts, puddings prepared with skim milk, fruit whips made with egg whites, angel food cake | Pies, cakes, pastries, chocolate, rich desserts, ice cream, any containing nuts, whole milk, cream, or butter |
| Beverages | Coffee, tea, carbonated beverages | All beverages made with whole milk |
| Sauces | Tomato sauce and white sauce made with skim milk, gravy made with fat-free broth or drippings | Gravies with fat, cheese sauces, meat sauces, rich dessert sauces |
| Soups | Fat-free broth soups and creamed soups made with skim milk | Soups made with whole milk, cream, or additional fat |
| Condiments and miscellaneous | In moderation: salt, pepper, spices, herbs, flavoring extracts | Chocolate, nuts |
| Sweets | Sugar, jelly, honey, jams, syrups, molasses, plain hard candy | Candy with chocolate and nuts |

# Fat-Controlled Diet

## Description

The fat-controlled diet limits foods containing cholesterol and saturated fatty acids and increases foods high in polyunsaturated fatty acids. (Cholesterol intake should be limited to 300 mg daily if diet is followed.)

## Food Preparation

Only lean meats, fish, and poultry are used. The allowed vegetable oils may be used in preparing meats, fish, or poultry; used in salad dressings; or in baked products. A portion of the total fat is allowed in the form of margarine each day. Margarine labels should be read carefully to ensure that the one selected contains liquid polyunsaturated oils, preferably corn, soy, or safflower.

| Type of food | Allow | Avoid |
|---|---|---|
| Milk | Yogurt made from skim milk, skim milk, skim buttermilk | Whole milk and cream; creamed buttermilk |
| Eggs | Three whole eggs per week; egg whites as desired | Those prepared with fats other than vegetable oils |
| Cheese | Dry cottage cheese, skim milk cheese | All others, whole milk cheese |
| Meat, fish, poultry | Lean beef, veal, lamb, and pork limited to 9 oz/week; fish, poultry without skin | Fat meats such as bacon, duck, goose, sausages, luncheon meats, frankfurters, and spareribs; glandular and organ meats, caviar, and shrimp |
| Vegetables, Potatoes | Sweet or white | Those prepared with fats other than a special margarine or vegetable oil |
| Other vegetables | All | None |
| Cereals | All | None |
| Bread | White or whole grain, hot breads made with vegetable oil | Breads made with other shortenings and egg yolk |
| Crackers | Soda and graham | All others |
| Other cereal | Macaroni, rice, and spaghetti | Noodles made with egg |
| Fats | Margarine (polyunsaturated), corn oil, safflower oil, soybean oil; salad dressings made with these oils | Butter, mayonnaise, cream, lard, hydrogenated vegetable shortening, olive oil, coconut oil |
| Fruits | All | None |
| Desserts | Fruit ices, gelatin, fruits, angel food cake, puddings prepared with skim milk, fruit whips made with egg whites, and baked products made with allowed oils | Ice cream; sherbet; baked products made with egg yolk, shortening (other than vegetable oil) or cream; other desserts prepared with same |
| Beverages | Coffee, tea made with skim milk, carbonated beverages | Beverages made with whole milk or cream |
| Sauces | Tomato sauce and sauces made with skim milk | Gravies, meat sauces, and rich dessert sauces |
| Soups | Homemade fat-free soups made with allowed ingredients | Soups made with cream and whole milk |
| Condiments | All desired | No restrictions |
| Sweets | All except chocolate | Chocolate |

# COMPREHENSIVE
# PRACTICE TESTS

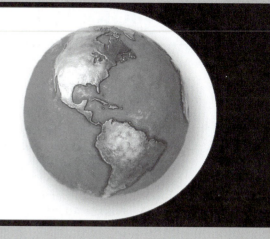

This section contains eleven 100-question tests similar in structure and content to those you will find on the NCLEX-RN® examination.

At the end of each test are the correct answers and a comprehensive rationale for the correct answers. Also included are identifiers for the phases of the nursing process, the categories of client needs, the cognitive level, and the subject area for each question.

Following the directions for test taking described in Unit 1, allow 100 minutes for each practice test. The following codes are used in the answers and rationales to categorize the test items.

| | | | | | |
|---|---|---|---|---|---|
| **NP** | = **PHASES OF THE NURSING PROCESS** | **He/3** | = Health Promotion and Maintenance | **CL** | = **COGNITIVE LEVEL** |
| **As** | = Assessment | | = Growth and Development Through the Life Span | **K** | = Knowledge |
| **An** | = Analysis | | = Prevention and Early Detection of Disease | **Co** | = Comprehension |
| **Pl** | = Planning | | | **Ap** | = Application |
| **Im** | = Implementation | **Ps/4** | = Psychosocial Integrity | **An** | = Analysis |
| **Ev** | = Evaluation | | = Coping and Adaptation | | |
| | | | = Psychosocial Adaptation | **SA** | = **SUBJECT AREAS** |
| **CN** | = **CLIENT NEED** | **Ph** | = Physiological Integrity | **1** | = Medical-Surgical |
| **Sa** | = Safe Effective Care Environment | **Ph/5** | = Basic Care and Comfort | **2** | = Psychiatric and Mental Health |
| **Sa/1** | = Management of Care | **Ph/6** | = Pharmacological and Parenteral Therapies | **3** | = Maternity and Women's Health |
| **Sa/2** | = Safety and Infection Control | **Ph/7** | = Reduction of Risk Potential | **4** | = Pediatric |
| | | **Ph/8** | = Physiological Adaptation | **5** | = Pharmacologic |

The above categories are discussed in more detail in Unit 1. The following sample answer should help you understand how to interpret these codes. The correct answer is given, followed by the comprehensive rationale. The codes are listed beside each question.

| ANSWER | RATIONALE | NP | CN | CL | SA |
|---|---|---|---|---|---|
| #1. 4. | Hemorrhagic reactions are a result of banked blood that is low in platelets and coagulation factors. The other choices describe allergic and hemolytic reactions, plus circulatory overload. | An | Ph/6 | Co | 1 |

The elements are as follows:

#1 is the question or item number in the test; 4 is the correct answer.

A comprehensive rationale explains the correct answer, and may include information on the incorrect answers.

The phase of the nursing process is analysis.

The category of client need is physiologic integrity; pharmacological and parenteral therapies.

The cognitive level is comprehensive.

The subject area is medical-surgical.

1. An adult who has a fractured right hip with 5 lb of Buck's traction needs to be transferred to another bed. What instructions should the nurse tell the team?

   1. Slowly lift the traction to release the weight, support the right leg, and lift the client to the new bed.
   2. Slowly lift the 5 lb weight from the traction set up, and apply 10 lb of manual traction during the move.
   3. It is not safe to move the client with Buck's traction. Support her position changes with pillows until traction is no longer needed.
   4. Decrease the weight of traction over a 2-hour period; then discontinue the traction and move the client into the new bed.

2. When assigning the proper precautions for a client with HIV, which of the following transmission-based precautions would be the most appropriate?

   1. Contact
   2. Airborne
   3. Universal
   4. Reverse

3. A two-year-old begins to scream, kick, and wave his arms angrily when the nurse lowers his side rails to take his temperature and other vital signs. The child and nurse are alone in the room. What is the best action for the nurse to take?

   1. Leave the child alone until his mother comes to visit and can be there to help hold him on her lap for the procedures.
   2. Immediately call another nurse to come and help hold the child still for the procedures.
   3. Hold the child and talk calmly while showing him something of interest and explain what is going to be done.
   4. Tell the child he will be left alone for 2 minutes without his toys and he must quiet down during that time.

4. The nurse is providing discharge instructions to an adult client who has had a cataract extraction with a lens implant performed on an outpatient basis. Which statement by the client indicates a need for further instruction?

   1. "I need to sleep with this metal eye shield at night, but I can wear my glasses during the day."
   2. "I should avoid coughing, sneezing, and vomiting."
   3. "It's okay to bend over to pick something up from the floor as long as I put the eye shield on."
   4. "I should call the doctor for any bad pain in my eyes that the pain medicine doesn't help, or if I start seeing double or light flashes."

5. A client is diagnosed with hypertension and prescribed hydrochlorothiazide (HCTZ). What teaching instruction by the nurse should be included?

   1. "Take this medication in the evening to prevent falls due to hypotension."
   2. "Make sure to eat a banana or salad everyday."
   3. "Notify your health care provider if your urine output increases."
   4. "Be aware that your heart rate may be slower."

6. A woman who has cystitis is receiving Pyridium 200 mg PO TID. Which assessment best indicates to the nurse that the medication is effective?

   1. The client's urine is reddish-orange in color.
   2. There is a decrease in pain and burning on urination.
   3. There is a decrease in the client's temperature.
   4. The client's white blood cell count has returned to normal.

7. An adult client is now ready for discharge following a bilateral adrenalectomy for treatment of Cushing's syndrome. Which statement the client makes indicates to the nurse that further discharge teaching is needed?

   1. "I will begin to look more normal soon."
   2. "I should not lift heavy objects for 6 weeks."
   3. "I will gradually discontinue the hormone pills in a few months when I feel better."
   4. "I will not go grocery shopping or run the vacuum cleaner until the doctor says I can."

8. An adult woman is recovering from a mastectomy for breast cancer and is frequently tearful when left alone. The nurse's approach should be based on which of these understandings?

   1. Clients need a supportive person to help them grieve for the loss of a body part.
   2. The client's family should take the leadership in providing the support she needs.
   3. The nurse should explain to the client that breast tissue is not needed by the body.
   4. The client should focus on the cure of her cancer rather than the loss of the breast.

9. An adult has been hospitalized for 1 week for severe depression and suicidal thinking. Last night, he was tearful with his wife present, but this morning he is relaxed and says, "Now I have it all figured out. I know exactly what I'm going to do." What does the nurse deduct from this statement?

   1. A sudden lifting of depression may indicate that the client has formed a suicide plan.
   2. Support from his wife may have convinced the man that life is worth living.
   3. Antidepressant drugs may require several weeks before an effect is felt.
   4. An absence of sadness and the ability to plan may indicate improvement in depression.

10. An adult client has visible jaundice and tests positive for asterixis. Palpation reveals hepatomegaly. The client's labs show an increase in AST, ALT, and LDH. Based on these findings, which nursing diagnosis should the nurse plan to address first?

   1. Activity intolerance related to weakness secondary to liver failure.
   2. Risk for injury related to reduced prothrombin synthesis and reduced vitamin K absorption.
   3. Ineffective health maintenance related to insufficient knowledge of etiology of condition and treatment.
   4. Fluid volume excess related to retention.

11. The nurse is evaluating a new mother feeding her newborn. Which observation indicates the mother understands proper feeding methods for her newborn?

   1. Holding the bottle so the nipple is always filled with formula.
   2. Allowing her 7-pound baby to sleep after taking 1½ ounces from the bottle.
   3. Burping the baby every 10 minutes during the feeding.
   4. Warming the formula bottle in the microwave for 15 seconds and giving it directly to the baby.

12. The nurse is assessing a woman admitted for a possible ectopic pregnancy. The nurse should ask the client about the presence of which of the following?

   1. Profuse, bright-red vaginal bleeding.
   2. Right or left colicky abdominal pain.
   3. Nausea and vomiting.
   4. Dyspareunia.

13. A 19-year-old woman is admitted with a diagnosis of anorexia nervosa. Which of the following should the nurse include in the care plan?

   1. Allow her as much time as she needs for each meal.
   2. Explain the importance of an adequate diet.
   3. Observe her during and one hour after each meal.
   4. Use a random pattern for surprise weights.

14. A 28-year-old client with schizophrenia is sitting alone in his room. He alternates quiet, listening behaviors with agitated talking. The nurse enters his room and observes this behavior. What should the nurse say first?

   1. "You need to come out to the day area with the group now."
   2. "Why are you hearing voices again?"
   3. "You appear to be listening to something."
   4. "I know you hear something but there is no one here."

15. A client has just returned to the surgical unit following a femoral arteriogram. Which assessment data would require immediate intervention by the nurse?

   1. The client is keeping the affected extremity straight.
   2. The client's right pedal pulse is 3+.
   3. The client is complaining of numbness in the right foot.
   4. The pressure dressing to the right femoral area is intact.

16. A 28-year-old client with schizophrenia has been taking a phenothiazine drug, chlorpromazine (Thorazine) 50 mg PO QID for 4 days. Which observation by the nurse indicates a desired effect of the drug?

   1. The client reports fewer episodes of hallucinations.
   2. Sleeping 10 hours at night plus a 2-hour afternoon nap.

3. The client reports feelings of stiffness in his neck and face.

4. The client is increasingly responsive to his delusional system.

17. The nurse is to give medication to an infant. What is the best way to assess the identity of the infant?

    1. Ask the mother what the child's name is.
    2. Look at the sign above the bed that states the client's name.
    3. Compare the bed number with the bed number of the MAR.
    4. Compare the ankle band with the name on the MAR.

18. An adult client sustained a fractured tibia 3 hours ago and had a long cast applied. The client is now complaining of increasing pain and the nurse suspects compartment syndrome. What initial action will the nurse take?

    1. Prepare for emergency fasciotomy.
    2. Raise the casted leg to the level of the heart and notify the physician.
    3. Administer the ordered pain medication.
    4. Instruct client to wiggle his foot and toes more frequently.

19. The nurse is caring for a client who is scheduled for an magnetic resonance imaging (MRI) study. Which statement made by the client warrants further assessment by the nurse?

    1. "I am allergic to iodine and seafood."
    2. "I had a total hip replacement 5 years ago."
    3. "I've been taking a blood thinner and bleed easily."
    4. "My doctor told me never to take laxatives."

20. An adult is admitted to the psychiatric unit with a diagnosis of obsessive-compulsive disorder. His hands are red and rough and he tells the nurse that he washes them many times a day. What would be an appropriate short-term goal for him?

    1. He would explain why his hand washing is inappropriate.
    2. He is prevented from accessing the sink in his room.
    3. He records the number of times he washes his hands each day.
    4. He verbalizes the anxiety underlying each episode of handwashing.

21. The nurse is caring for a client who has been placed in cloth wrist restraints. What should the nurse do to ensure the client's safety?

    1. Remove the restraints every 2 hours and inspect the wrists.
    2. Wrap each wrist with gauze dressing beneath the restraints.
    3. Keep the head of the bed flat at all times.
    4. Tie the restraints using a square knot.

22. An adult client is scheduled for gallbladder X-rays in the morning for suspected cholelithiasis. What question will be important for the nurse to ask the client in preparation for the X-ray?

    1. Have you ever had trouble with uncontrolled bleeding?
    2. Do you have any known allergies?
    3. Have you received teaching on the low-fat diet?
    4. Do you understand the procedure for local anesthesia?

23. A client is scheduled for a glycosylated hemoglobin assay (Hgb A1c). What explanation will the nurse provide to the client regarding the purpose for this test?

    1. It is used to diagnose thyroid levels.
    2. It reveals heart inflammation.
    3. It measures liver enzymes.
    4. It reflects blood glucose level over a 2–3 month period.

24. An adult client's telemetry monitor has been showing normal sinus rhythm with occasional PVCs. When there is a sudden change on the monitor screen to a ventricular fibrillation pattern, what should be the most appropriate action by the nurse?

    1. Administer a precordial thump.
    2. Obtain the defibrillator.
    3. Begin cardiopulmonary resuscitation.
    4. Check the client's ECG electrodes.

25. An adult client presents with the sudden onset of the appearance of "floating black spots" in her right eye. The client sees a black shadow in her peripheral vision. There is no pain but the client is very frightened. What should the nurse expect to do in the care of this client?

    1. Place patches on both eyes and plan for strict bed rest.
    2. Patch the right eye and let the client resume activity after 24 hours.

3. Plan for emergency surgery as the client is in danger of losing her eyesight.

4. Administer a cholinergic eye drop (Pilocarpine) to decrease intraocular pressure.

26. The nurse is caring for a woman in labor. When she is 8 cm dilated she tells her support person she wants "to go home for a few hours of sleep." The woman's statement reveals the woman's desire for what action?

1. Have others tell her what she needs.

2. Have a soothing back rub.

3. Be rid of this difficult situation.

4. Be left alone.

27. A 22-year-old woman comes into the obstetrics clinic requesting oral contraceptives. Which item in the nursing history would indicate that she is not a good candidate for this method of contraception?

1. She has a history of heavy menstrual periods.

2. She has diabetes mellitus.

3. The client reports a broken leg when she was 10 years old.

4. The client had a baby 6 months ago.

28. The nurse is caring for a client who has just had a craniotomy. The client has an intracranial pressure monitor in place and is becoming more lethargic. The intracranial pressure is high. How should the nurse position the client?

1. Elevate the head of the bed 90°. Position the client upright with pillow support under the head.

2. Place the client flat in bed with the legs elevated 15° on pillows.

3. Position the client on the left side with pillow support to the back.

4. Elevate the head of the bed 30°.

29. An adult will be administering daily insulin to her 84-year-old blind grandfather. The insulin dose is 15 units NPH, 5 units regular every morning at 0745. Which statement best indicates that the granddaughter needs further instruction in insulin administration prior to her grandfather's discharge from the hospital?

1. "The regular insulin acts quickly. NPH insulin is milky colored and lasts longer, usually the whole day."

2. "I need to keep track of where I give his insulin so that I don't use the same site over and over."

3. "If I can't get to Granddaddy's house until lunch time, I can give him a little more insulin in case his sugar went up in the morning."

4. "It's very important to keep insulin shots on schedule and for him to eat at regular times."

30. An elderly woman received digoxin 0.25 mg for treatment of her congestive heart failure. Which of the following physiological responses indicates that the digoxin is having the desired effect?

1. Increased heart rate.

2. Decreased cardiac output.

3. Increased urine output.

4. Decreased myocardial contraction force.

31. An adult is admitted to the hospital with anorexia, weight loss, and ascites. Serum SGOT (AST), SGPT (ALT), LDH, and total bilirubin are significantly elevated. Based on the lab results, what would the nurse expect to find while performing an admission assessment?

1. Pallor.

2. Dry mucous membranes.

3. Jaundice.

4. Peripheral edema.

32. The nurse is preparing a client for an IVP tomorrow. The client tells the nurse that she gets a rash and becomes short of breath after eating lobster. Given this information, what should the nurse plan for the client?

1. A dietitian should visit the client while in the hospital.

2. The client is not a candidate for IVP.

3. The client is at risk for an allergic reaction.

4. An antihistamine will be required before the IVP.

33. An elderly client requiring abdominal wound packing TID complains about his wound care to the nurse making morning rounds. He states that "everyone does it differently and at any time they feel like it." He is angry at being awakened at night for this procedure. What is the nurse's best response?

1. "The wound care is being done as ordered by your doctor."

2. "I understand you're upset at losing sleep. You can have medication to help you get back to sleep."

3. "Tell me what's really bothering you."

4. "After rounds I'll be back and we can plan your wound care."

34. The nurse is planning care for a client with cervical radiation implants. Which nursing intervention will be included in the plan of care?
    1. Implement strict isolation protocol.
    2. Provide a lead apron for the client.
    3. Use only disposable supplies and equipment in the client's room.
    4. Limit visitors to 30 minutes per day.

35. The nurse reviews a client's laboratory data and notes the following hematology values: hematocrit (hct) 43%; hemoglobin (Hgb) 15 g/dL; RBCs 5 million; WBCs 7500; platelet count 30,000. What nursing care is indicated in relation to these lab values?
    1. Plan a diet high in iron.
    2. Plan for frequent rest periods throughout the day.
    3. Avoid invasive procedures and injections.
    4. Implement protective isolation precautions.

36. The nurse is planning care for a client who is having a gastroscopy performed. What will be included in the plan of care for the immediate postgastroscopy period?
    1. Maintain nasogastric tube to intermittent suction.
    2. Assess gag reflex prior to administration of fluids.
    3. Assess frequently for pain and medicate according to orders.
    4. Measure abdominal girth every 4 hours.

37. An elderly client has suffered a cerebrovascular accident (CVA) and as a result has left homonymous hemianopia. Based on this fact, what measure will the nurse include in this client's plan of care?
    1. Supporting the client's left arm and hand with pillows.
    2. Applying a patch to the client's left eye.
    3. Encouraging the client to use his right hand for activities of daily living.
    4. Placing the client's meal on the right side of the overbed table.

38. A toddler is admitted with a history of vomiting and diarrhea for 2 days, accompanied by abdominal pain. The admitting diagnosis is gastroenteritis. What type of room assignment should the nurse make?
    1. A room near the nurses' station so that he can be checked frequently and heard if he vomits.
    2. A single room with a sink near the doorway for isolation use.
    3. A double room with another toddler who also has vomiting and diarrhea.
    4. A bed in the pediatric intensive care unit, in case dehydration develops.

39. The nurse is caring for a client who is to have a lumbar puncture (LP). How should the client be positioned during the procedure?
    1. Prone with head turned to the left.
    2. Side-lying in a fetal position.
    3. Sitting at the edge of the bed.
    4. Trendelenburg position.

40. The physician has ordered a Schilling test for a client with possible pernicious anemia. What implementation will be required by the nurse?
    1. Administer a mild laxative.
    2. Initiate a 24-hour urine collection.
    3. Administer an intramuscular dose of iron.
    4. Insert an intravenous catheter.

41. The nurse has given discharge instructions on how to care for a newly applied cast to an adult client. Which statement indicates the client understands the instructions?
    1. "I should pack the casted leg in ice for 24 hours to help it dry."
    2. "I can use my hair dryer to help the cast dry faster."
    3. "A good way to relieve the itching under the cast is to gently scratch under the cast with a soft knitting needle."
    4. "Putting the casted leg up on fabric-covered pillows is the best way to dry the cast."

42. The nurse is caring for a client who has just had a bone marrow biopsy. What is essential for the nurse to do at this time?
    1. Apply firm pressure over the puncture site.
    2. Maintain the client on bed rest for 24 hours.
    3. Apply an occlusive dressing to the puncture site.
    4. Refrigerate the biopsy specimen.

43. An adult client is one day post subtotal thyroidectomy. What intervention is most important for the nurse to include in the care plan?
    1. Carry out range-of-motion exercises to the neck and shoulders every shift.
    2. Maintain bed rest with client in supine position at all times.
    3. Ask client questions every hour or two to assess for hoarseness.
    4. Provide tracheostomy care every shift and suction prn to maintain a patent airway.

44. An adult client is 4 hours post-op abdominal hysterectomy. She has an IV at 125 mL per hour, an indwelling catheter that has drained 100 mL since surgery, and her pain is "3" out of "10." Which would be the priority nursing diagnosis?

 1. Alteration in comfort, pain.

 2. Alterations in patterns of elimination.

 3. Disturbance in self-concept, body image.

 4. Fluid volume deficit, actual or risk for.

45. An adult client has meperidine HCl (Demerol) 50 mg–100 mg IM every 3–4 hours ordered. He received Demerol 50 mg IM 3 hours ago but he's still complaining of pain at "8 out of 10." The client is asking for pain medication even before it is due and refuses to get out of bed "because of the pain." He was heard telling jokes to the cleaning personnel. What is the best action for the nurse to take?

 1. Give the client 50 mg of Demerol IM now.

 2. Wait 1 hour and give the client 75 mg of Demerol IM.

 3. Give the client 100 mg of Demerol IM now and repeat 100 mg Demerol IM in 3 hours if the pain is still greater than "5 out of 10."

 4. Do not medicate the client now. Laughing and joking behavior indicate the pain is not as severe as the client claims.

46. An elderly male with undiagnosed respiratory symptoms is to receive a diagnostic test for histoplasmosis. How will the nurse administer the histoplasmin skin test?

 1. Apply a patch to the skin on the forearm.

 2. Make a shallow scratch on the skin surface.

 3. Use a 25-gauge needle placed parallel to the skin.

 4. Use a 19-gauge needle and Z track injection.

47. A 35-year-old woman is admitted for treatment of depression. Which of these symptoms would the nurse be least likely to find in the initial assessment?

 1. Inability to make decisions.

 2. Feelings of hopelessness.

 3. Family history of depression.

 4. Increased interest in sex.

48. An adult male, who appears about 40 years old, is admitted to the psychiatric unit for alcohol detoxification. He is tremulous and irritable, and complains of nervousness and nausea. Which information is most important for the admitting nurse to obtain?

 1. The amount of alcohol and other drugs usually taken and the type and amount taken in the last few days.

 2. The events prompting the client to seek treatment.

 3. The factors that trigger the client's drinking episodes.

 4. Any work, legal, or family problems that relate to his use of alcohol.

49. A woman who is 9 months pregnant is attending a luncheon and fashion show. Suddenly, her membranes rupture and contractions come so rapidly that she yells, "The baby is coming." What is the most appropriate action for the nurse to take?

 1. Ask for boiled water, towels, string, and scissors.

 2. Ask someone to call her doctor.

 3. Take her via cab to the nearest hospital.

 4. Have her lie on her left side in a less-crowded area and be prepared to help with the delivery.

50. While attending a basketball game, a woman who is 9 months pregnant suddenly goes into labor and delivers her baby within 5 minutes. What is the most appropriate course of action for the nurse to take?

 1. Tie the cord with a shoelace and cut the cord with a penknife.

 2. Have the mother's friend hold the baby until an ambulance arrives.

 3. Place the naked baby on the mother's bare chest, cover both, and encourage breastfeeding.

 4. Ask people to clear the area so more air can circulate around the mother and baby.

51. A young man with newly diagnosed acquired immune deficiency syndrome (AIDS) is being discharged from the hospital. The nurse knows that teaching regarding prevention of AIDS transmission has been effective when the client expresses what thought?

 1. He verbalizes the role of sexual activity in spread of the disorder.

 2. He states he will make arrangements to drop his college classes.

 3. He acknowledges the need to avoid all contact sports.

 4. He says he will avoid close contact with his 3-year-old niece.

52. A client in the intensive care unit is on a volume-cycled mechanical ventilator. The high-pressure alarm (PAP) begins to sound repeatedly. The client is sleeping quietly. What is the most appropriate initial response by the nurse?
    1. Call the respiratory therapist to check the ventilator.
    2. Turn the client to stimulate coughing.
    3. Obtain arterial blood for blood gas analysis.
    4. Check the ventilator tubing.

53. A woman is 4 cm dilated and wants to walk about the labor and delivery nursing unit. Which of the following criteria will help the nurse determine whether she should walk?
    1. Whether her membranes are intact.
    2. Her contraction frequency.
    3. The fetal position.
    4. The fetal station.

54. Which statement by the client to her partner demonstrates understanding of the diaphragm as a contraceptive device?
    1. "It is good for 5 years."
    2. It has to be used with a condom."
    3. "It must be left in place for at least 6 hours after intercourse."
    4. "It has to be removed between each sexual intercourse encounter."

55. The nurse is caring for a woman four hours following a cesarean birth. Because there are surgical effects that hinder the woman's resumption of eating, the nurse should include which of the following in the plan of care?
    1. Ambulation at this time.
    2. Applying an abdominal binder.
    3. Administering a Dulcolax suppository.
    4. Listening for bowel sounds.

56. An adult client is admitted to the nursing care unit with intestinal obstruction and has a Miller-Abbott tube in place. How should the nurse assess for proper placement and function of the tube?
    1. Inject air and auscultate over the stomach.
    2. Aspirate the tube for stomach contents.
    3. Check the distance markings on the tube.
    4. Assess for signs of respiratory compromise.

57. An adult client who has rheumatoid arthritis reports that the pain and stiffness are greatest upon arising early in the morning. What advice should the nurse give to help the client decrease the pain?

1. Keep the salicylate medication at the bedside and take before getting out of bed.
2. Take a hot tub bath or shower upon rising.
3. Ask the physician to order splints to be worn at night to maintain anatomical position.
4. Increase activity to work out the stiffness.

58. An adult client has a central line placed for IV fluids. When the nurse enters the room the IV bottle is empty, the IV line is full of air, and the client is dyspneic. What is the best initial nursing action?
    1. Notify the physician and administer oxygen via nasal cannula immediately.
    2. Hang another IV bag as soon as possible, then remove the air from the IV line.
    3. Clamp the tubing and place the client on the left side with head down.
    4. Begin CPR and call the code team.

59. The nurse is caring for a client who has just returned to the nursing unit following a left above-the-knee amputation. How should the client be positioned?
    1. Place the stump on a pillow to decrease edema.
    2. Place the stump flat on the bed to prevent contractures.
    3. Place the client in a prone position to prevent contractures.
    4. Place the client in reverse Trendelenburg position to promote arterial flow.

60. The nurse is planning care for a child with diabetes. Which concept is essential to include when developing the care plan?
    1. Most of the family and child education about diabetes and its management takes place in the first 3 or 4 days after the initial diagnosis is made.
    2. The morning short-acting insulin dosage is usually determined by the previous day's late morning and noon blood glucose levels.
    3. The majority of the total daily dose of insulin is given in the evenings to cover the day's intake of food.
    4. Snacks for children with diabetes should be given during an exercise episode, rather than before it.

61. An adult has had diabetes mellitus for many years. When the nurse enters the room to administer the morning dose of regular and NPH insulin, the client complains of dizziness, diaphoresis, and nausea. The nurse does a blood glucose, which is 30. What is the next nursing action?

1. Give the usual dose of regular insulin and get the client's breakfast tray.
2. Hold the NPH insulin but give the regular insulin.
3. Hold the regular and NPH insulin and call the physician.
4. Give the client a glass of orange juice, hold all insulin, and call the physician.

62. An adult had a thyroidectomy this morning. The nurse assesses a positive Chovstek's sign and a positive Trousseau's sign. The nurse understands that the most common cause of these symptoms is which of the following?
    1. Inadvertent removal of the parathyroid glands during the thyroidectomy surgery.
    2. Overuse of radioactive iodine given preoperatively to clients undergoing thyroidectomy.
    3. A history of insufficient intake of iodine.
    4. Overstimulation of parathormone during the thyroid surgery.

63. The nurse is to begin bladder training with a young woman who has a T-2 spinal cord injury. What should the nurse plan to do?
    1. Teach her to change the indwelling catheter drainage bag to a leg bag at night.
    2. Plan a consistent intermittent catheterization schedule with her and teach her self-catheterization technique as she is able.
    3. Plan to place her on the bedside commode to void every 2 hours until consistent urination is achieved.
    4. Clamp the indwelling catheter for longer periods of time each day until a bladder capacity of 1500 mL is achieved.

64. An adult client has a comminuted fracture of the ulnar bone. He asks the nurse what type of fracture this is. The nurse's response is based on which of these understandings?
    1. The ulnar bone has been crushed and broken in several places.
    2. The two ends of the fractured ulnar bone are pulled apart and separated from each other.
    3. The ulnar bone has been broken in two and one end of the bone broke through the skin.
    4. Only one side of the ulnar bone is broken.

65. The nurse is caring for several clients with fractures. Which client is most at risk for fat embolus?
    1. A 4-year-old with a wrist fracture.
    2. A 20-year-old with a femur fracture.

3. A 35-year-old with an ulnar fracture.
4. A 75-year-old with rib fractures.

66. A man with a 10-year history of asthma presents with respiratory distress with labored breathing, use of accessory muscles, and audible inspiratory and expiratory wheezes. Which of the following would indicate his condition is worsening?
    1. Audible expiratory wheezes with lessening inspiratory wheezes.
    2. Increasing expectoration of thick, tenacious sputum with decreasing wheezing lung sounds.
    3. Absence of audible inspiratory and expiratory wheezes with increasing somnolence.
    4. Decreasing respiratory rate with decreased use of accessory muscles.

67. The nurse has instructed an adult in crutch-walking technique. Which statement best indicates that the client understands the proper way to bear weight on crutches while ambulating?
    1. "I should bear my weight on my hands while walking."
    2. "It's OK to lean on my crutches, bearing the weight under my arms, as long as I don't walk like that."
    3. "I should bear weight on my underarms while I walk."
    4. "I should avoid bearing weight on the crutch that is on my injured side as much as possible."

68. An adult has undergone a total hip replacement and is now ready for discharge. Which of his statements indicates good understanding of what activities are allowed?
    1. "I can't wait to see my daughter. She lives 8 hours away and until now my hip hurt too much to travel such a long distance."
    2. "I will really have to be careful not to cross my legs. That's the way I used to sit all the time."
    3. "It will be great to be able to put on my socks and shoes by myself."
    4. "As soon as I get home, I won't have to use this walker."

69. The nurse is giving discharge instructions to an adult client who is to be discharged taking hydantoin (Dilantin). Which of the following is correct and must be included in the discharge teaching?
    1. If there are problems with taking Dilantin orally, the drug is easily given intramuscularly.

2. Alcohol interferes with the absorption of Dilantin. Do not drink alcohol while taking Dilantin.

3. Dilantin builds up in the body and achieves blood levels that prevent seizures. Skipping a day or two will not affect the Dilantin blood levels.

4. Slurred speech and confusion are side effects of Dilantin and are normal while taking Dilantin.

70. An adult client underwent an exploratory laparotomy 24 hours ago. The nurse assesses her abdominal incision and observes a bulging area at the lower part of the midline abdominal incision. This finding most likely indicates which of the following?
    1. Normal postoperative incisional edema.
    2. A hematoma beneath the skin.
    3. Abdominal distention.
    4. Impending wound infection with purulent drainage.

71. An adult client is to receive a unit of whole blood. The client's vital signs before starting the transfusion are BP 120/70, P 80, and T 98.4°F. Five minutes after the transfusion was started the vital signs are: BP 100/70, P 100, and T 99.4°F. What should the nurse do initially?
    1. Slow down the rate of the transfusion, reassess the client in 15 minutes.
    2. Stop the transfusion, keep vein open with normal saline.
    3. Slow down the infusion, notify the physician immediately.
    4. Administer acetaminophen (Tylenol), continue to monitor closely throughout the transfusion.

72. A woman is in the outpatient clinic to have a pelvic sonogram for a suspected ovarian mass. What will the nurse ask the client to do in preparation for the sonogram?
    1. Sign a permit.
    2. Drink several glasses of water.
    3. Take a mild sedative.
    4. Completely empty her bladder.

73. The community health nurse is making an initial home visit for an elderly client to assess the client's ability to provide self-care in the home. Which one of the following areas of concern should be assessed for determining the client's ability to remain at home?
    1. Elimination.
    2. Cognitive abilities.

3. Exercise.
4. Metabolism.

74. Where would the nurse place the stethoscope to assess the client's apical pulse before administering a dose of digitalis?
    1. Left fifth intercostal space, midclavicular line.
    2. Right second intercostal space, midclavicular line.
    3. Site of carotid pulsation.
    4. Left third intercostal space, sternal border.

75. The nurse is assessing a person with long-standing chronic obstructive pulmonary disease (COPD). Which findings would the nurse expect to find?
    1. Low-grade fever.
    2. Weak, thready pulse.
    3. Increased chest diameter.
    4. Crepitus.

76. The nurse is assessing a female client who says she has gained a lot of weight recently, feels cold all the time and is always tired. In addition she reports her hair is falling out. Given the signs and symptoms, which of the following disorders is the woman most likely to have?
    1. Addison's disease.
    2. Cushing's syndrome.
    3. Myxedema.
    4. Graves' disease.

77. The nurse is caring for a client who underwent a total hip replacement yesterday. Which of the following assessments is inappropriate at this time?
    1. Presence of Homan's sign.
    2. Ability to flex and adduct affected hip.
    3. Temperature.
    4. Complaints of pain.

78. A client is admitted with the diagnosis of gout. What is the client most likely to relate when the history is taken?
    1. A slow gradual onset of pain, redness, swelling, and warmth of the affected joint.
    2. Waking up at night with severe pain in the foot.
    3. Pain and muscle spasms that occurred in the morning hours.
    4. A sudden onset of discomfort, redness, and swelling of the affected joint, occurring mostly during waking hours.

79. The nurse is caring for a person during a seizure. What is the priority assessment at this time?
   1. Presence of an aura.
   2. Length of the seizure.
   3. What precipitated the seizure.
   4. Type and progression of seizure activity.

80. The school nurse initiates a screening program for pediculosis capitis. What else might the nurse also find when searching for nits clinging to the hair shafts?
   1. Bites, pustules, and excoriated areas on the scalp from scratching.
   2. Pruritic, scaling, erythematous papules, plaques, and patches with well-defined borders.
   3. Beefy-red erythematous areas with a few surrounding papules and pustules.
   4. An inflammation of the hair follicles with pus-filled nodules.

81. An 8-year-old girl suffered a partial thickness scald burn over most of her anterior thigh and lower leg. What admission assessment would give the nurse the most data about the probability of shock occurring?
   1. Edema, weeping blisters, high serum potassium, low serum sodium.
   2. Tachycardia, hyperventilation, and a pale appearance.
   3. Variations in hyperthermia and hypothermia, and decreased gastric motility.
   4. Anemia from red blood cell loss through damaged capillaries.

82. The nurse is caring for a client on a hypothermia blanket. The nurse turns the client every 2 hours for which of the following reasons?
   1. The client will accept the treatment more readily if allowed to change positions.
   2. Turning frequently helps to prevent shivering.
   3. Frequent turning helps the client's autoregulatory mechanism to reestablish itself.
   4. Hypothermia causes vasoconstriction, which may result in skin damage.

83. The nurse is assessing a 26-year-old man whose diagnosis is schizophrenia. Which statement the client makes indicates he is experiencing hallucinations?
   1. "I don't get along very well with my mother."
   2. "I hear my mother talking to me when I'm alone."
   3. "That picture on the wall looks like my mother."
   4. "I think my mother plans to get rid of me."

84. A woman who is 32 years old and 35 weeks pregnant has had rupture of membranes for 8 hours and is 4 cm dilated. Because she is a candidate for infection, the nurse should include which of the following in the care plan?
   1. Universal precautions.
   2. Oxytocin administration.
   3. Frequent temperature monitoring.
   4. More frequent vaginal examinations.

85. A man is hospitalized with probable bacterial pneumonia. The physician has ordered a sputum specimen for culture and sensitivity. What should the nurse do to obtain a good specimen?
   1. Teach the client deep breathing and coughing techniques.
   2. Use nasotracheal suction.
   3. Obtain the specimen after starting antibiotics.
   4. Keep client NPO until sputum specimen obtained.

86. The nurse is caring for a mother and her newborn son. Which statement the mother makes indicates understanding of newborn care?
   1. "The face and neck are washed first, then the eyes, going from the outer corners inward."
   2. "As soon as the cord looks dried, my baby can sit in a tub bath instead of being sponged."
   3. "After applying alcohol to the cord once a day with the bath, the diaper is applied over the umbilicus to keep it dry."
   4. "The yellow-white covering over the end of the penis is part of the healing process and should not be removed, but washed gently with water."

87. The pregnant client with diabetes on insulin needs to be evaluated for correct medication dosage. What is the most effective method to assist the nurse in determining the client's need for insulin management?
   1. Home serum glucose testing.
   2. Weight gain.
   3. Daily dietary diary.
   4. Home urine glucose monitoring.

88. An adult is admitted for further evaluation of a very high white blood cell count, which may indicate leukemia. A bone marrow aspiration

and biopsy are scheduled. What is the purpose of this test?

1. Determine whether Reed-Sternberg cells are present in the marrow.
2. Identify the number and type of white blood cells in all stages of development.
3. Determine whether Epstein-Barr virus is present in the marrow.
4. Identify metastatic changes in the bone structure that are characteristic of leukemia.

89. A 4-year-old boy with acute epiglottitis is admitted to the emergency room. He has a fever of 102°F, is agitated, drools, and insists upon sitting up and leaning forward with the chin thrusting outward. The nurse expects which of the following?

1. Intravenous fluids and an antibiotic will be started before anything else is done.
2. The child will cry and resist lying supine when he needs to be examined and X-rayed.
3. The child will be intubated in the emergency room or operating room and then transferred to the pediatric intensive care unit.
4. A croup tent with an oxygen source available will be ordered on the regular pediatric unit.

90. A few days ago a child had red, swollen, itchy, poison ivy lesions that are now becoming fluid-filled vesicles. Which statement from the child demonstrates that she understands how to keep from getting poison ivy again?

1. "If I'm careful not to touch the leaves of the plant, I can play with the berries and pretend I'm baking."
2. "My shoes, clothes, and dolls all have to be washed to get the poison ivy off them so I won't get sores from touching them."
3. "Our dog doesn't get poison ivy when she lies in the plants, so I can hug her all I want."
4. "When I come inside from playing house, I have to scrub myself with soap and hot water."

91. An elderly client is in for her annual health checkup. Which of the following findings during the physical assessment is of greatest concern to the nurse?

1. Altered pupillary constriction and dilation.
2. Sluggish bowel sounds.
3. Kyphosis.
4. Hyperactive deep-tendon reflexes.

92. When working with groups of older clients in a day care setting, the nurse can promote socialization best by implementing which of the following interventions?

1. Grouping clients together by age and gender to encourage the development of friendships based on a common characteristic.
2. Assign a different nurse to group activities each day to familiarize client with staff.
3. Avoid discussion of client's life outside the day care setting to encourage participation in current activities.
4. Get to know the clients and accompany them to group events such as singing, crafts, communal meals, etc.

93. An elderly client who has diabetes mellitus and severe cataracts has been given instructions for administering insulin. Which of the following client behaviors signals to the nurse that he has a need for assistance with administration of his insulin?

1. He uses a magnifier to read the insulin syringe.
2. He states he will pinch the skin at the site and inject the insulin at a 90° angle.
3. He mixes NPH and regular insulins by drawing up the NPH first.
4. He rotates sites only after using all available areas within each site.

94. The nurse is teaching a client with an L-3 spinal cord injury regarding a bladder training regimen. Which of the following instructions should be included in the bladder training process?

1. Drink 1200–1500 mL of liquid a day.
2. Drink adequate fluids until 10:00 P.M. at night.
3. Tighten the abdominal muscles to void.
4. Pour cool water on the perineum.

95. A female was diagnosed with breast cancer 12 weeks ago. She was admitted to the hospital 4 days ago and is undergoing chemotherapeutic treatment of her cancer. Since her admission, she has communicated very little with the staff, stays in her room, eats almost none of the food provided, and is occasionally seen punching her pillow. While caring for her today, the nurse also finds out that she has not been sleeping and feels as though she is "somehow being punished for not doing regular breast-self exams." Based on the noted observations, which of the following nursing diagnoses should the nurse select as most appropriate for this client?

1. Anticipatory grieving.
2. Fear.

3. Ineffective individual coping.

4. Anxiety.

96. The nurse is reviewing the breast self-exam with a client who is being discharged after a spontaneous vaginal delivery. She is breastfeeding. The nurse should determine that the client understands which of the following?

1. Breast self-exam should not be done during lactation.

2. Breast should be examined between the 4th and 7th day after menstrual bleeding begins or at least once a month.

3. Breast self-exam should be done with the woman lying flat on her back.

4. The breasts must be checked in a circular method and assessed for any lumps or bumps.

97. An adult has been placed on coumadin therapy after prosthetic valve replacement. Which statement by the client demonstrates correct understanding of the teaching about coumadin therapy?

1. "If I miss a dose, I will double the next dose."

2. "I should eat plenty of green and leafy vegetables."

3. "If my arthritis flares up again, I'll take only two aspirins every 6 hours."

4. "I will use a soft toothbrush and stop flossing my teeth."

98. A 17-year-old female has been admitted with a diagnosis of anorexia nervosa. What is the most appropriate short-term nursing goal?

1. Client will admit that she has a fear of weight gain.

2. Client will adhere to a nutritionally balanced diet appropriate for her age.

3. Client will identify her problems and develop new coping methods to deal with them.

4. Client will accept herself as having self-worth.

99. The client has right hemiplegia as a result of a cerebrovascular accident. What finding indicates that the caregivers understand the importance of positioning a client with hemiplegia?

1. The right shoulder is adducted and internally rotated.

2. The right hip is externally rotated with knee flexion.

3. The right foot shows plantar flexion.

4. The right fingers are extended with the thumb abducted.

100. An adult is to have a pulse oximeter applied to assess arterial oxygen saturation level. What action will be included in the correct application?

1. Placement over the apical area of the chest.

2. Covering the probe with an opaque material.

3. Insertion of an arterial catheter.

4. Insertion of a venous catheter.

# Answers and Rationales for Practice Test 1

| ANSWER | | RATIONALE | NP | CN | CL | SA |
|---|---|---|---|---|---|---|
| #1. | 1. | Five to eight lb of traction is applied temporarily to provide immobilization prior to surgery. No additional treatment is required, such as manual traction or pillows. Once the transfer is complete, the weight should be maintained until no longer needed. | Im | Ph/7 | Ap | 1 |
| #2. | 3. | Universal precautions are utilized as the HIV virus is transmitted by body fluids, not by contact or airborne means. Reverse isolation would be used if a client was immunocompromised, in which case the client had AIDS and was more susceptible to infection. | Pl | Sa/2 | Ap | 1 |
| #3. | 3. | A 2-year-old may respond to distraction to regain some sense of control so he can listen to the explanation of what the nurse wants him to do. A comforting voice may help calm the child even if he cannot listen while screaming. Vital signs are essential to evaluate | Im | He/3 | Ap | 2 |

| ANSWER | RATIONALE | NP | CN | CL | SA |
|---|---|---|---|---|---|

ongoing treatment and must be performed whether or not the parent is present; another nurse in the room may foster more anger in the child; a time-out should only be used if discipline is required.

**#4. 3.** Bending over should be avoided as it increases intraocular pressure. The client should wear the eye shield at night to protect the eye from accidental injury during sleep; coughing, sneezing would increase intraocular pressure; and pain, double vision, or light flashes may indicate glaucoma or retinal detachment, in which case medical attention should be sought.  
Ev · Ph/7 · An · 1

**#5. 2.** HCTZ is a thiazide diuretic which acts on the distal tubules to block $Na^+$ reabsorption and increase potassium and water excretion; therefore, potassium-rich foods should be encouraged. The client should be aware that the medication should be taken in the morning to prevent interrupted sleep due to increased urine excretion. Tachycardia is a possible side effect.  
Im · Ph/6 · Ap · 5

**#6. 2.** Pyridium acts locally on the urinary tract mucosa to produce an analgesic effect. A side effect is the urine will turn reddish-orange, yet does not indicate a therapeutic effect, such as a decrease in pain. Pyridium does not have microbial properties, so the temperature or WBC will not be affected by it.  
Ev · Ph/6 · An · 5

**#7. 3.** Clients undergoing a bilateral adrenalectomy require lifelong glucocorticoid and mineralocorticoid replacement, not for just a few months. The client will gradually lose the Cushing's syndrome features as the hormones are adjusted. After abdominal surgery clients should abstain from lifting heavy objects or strenuous activity until given approval by the physician.  
Ev · Ph/7 · An · 1

**#8. 1.** The nurse must support the client through the steps and importance of grief by encouraging discussion of the loss, its meaning to the client, the reactions of others, and the ways of compensating. Families also may need support first before providing support to the client; and the loss of breast tissue may represent a loss of femininity and self-esteem.  
An · Ps/4 · Co · 3

**#9. 1.** Reassessment for suicide risk is essential when depression suddenly improves, as the client may appear to feel better once the decision to commit suicide has been made. Even if the wife's visit, medications, or ability to plan may have decreased the depression, it is still vital to reassess.  
An · Ps/4 · An · 2

**#10. 4.** The client's assessment findings point to cirrhosis of the liver. Fluid retention is the most immediate concern due to fluid/electrolyte fluctuations and overload. It would be expected that the client have fatigue and possible bleeding, so in following with Maslow's Hierarchy of Needs, the physiological problem would be addressed first.  
Pl · Sa/1 · An · 1

**#11. 1.** Holding the bottle so the nipple is always filled with formula prevents the baby from sucking air, which can cause gastric distention and intestinal gas pains. Based on the infant's weight, it should be 50 calories per pound, which would calculate to 2–3 oz per feeding. Burping could be performed halfway through the feeding and at the end; the temperature should be checked first before feeding.  
Ev · He/3 · An · 3

| ANSWER | RATIONALE | NP | CN | CL | SA |
|--------|-----------|-----|-----|-----|-----|

**#12. 2.** In ectopic pregnancy, the abdominal pain is usually on one side, is vague, cramping, or colicky from tubal distention, and lasts from one day to a week or longer. Other reports may be dark red blood as the uterine deciduas is sloughed off, nausea and vomiting after a rupture. Dyspareunia is not a complaint. — As — He/3 — An — 3

**#13. 3.** Left alone at mealtime, clients with anorexia nervosa may hide or discard food, or induce vomiting after a meal. Maladaptive behaviors may be reinforced if meal times do not have a time limit, or include discussing food. Weights of clients should always be done at the same time, wearing a hospital gown and voiding prior to weighing. — Pl — Ps/4 — Ap — 2

**#14. 3.** This response shares the nurse's observation and allows for validation by the client. Group participation may not be appropriate at this time; avoid using "why" questions which imply blame; validate whether the client is hallucinating and its content before confrontation with reality. — Im — Ps/4 — Ap — 2

**#15. 3.** Any neurovascular assessment data that are abnormal require intervention by the nurse; numbness may indicate decreased blood supply to the right foot. The affected leg should be kept straight for at least 6–8 hours (may vary) to prevent any arterial bleeding from the insertion site at the right femoral artery; +3 is a normal finding; and a normal finding would be an intact pressure dressing at the site. — As — Ph/7 — Ap — 1

**#16. 1.** Phenothiazine drugs, like chlorpromazine, are antipsychotic drugs and the desired action is to reduce the symptoms of psychosis, such as hallucinations. Drowsiness is a common side effect in early treatment and should diminish over time; a dystonic reaction with stiffness in the neck and face is also a side effect and can be treated with an antiparkinson drug; increased delusions indicate the psychosis may be worsening. — Ev — Ph/6 — Ap — 2

**#17. 4.** Two parameters are required to assure right client and medication. If a name band is missing, a new one should be put on as soon as possible. Mistakes may have occurred if the nurse only identifies the bed number or room. Always administer the 5 rights of medication for each client. — As — Sa/2 — Ap — 3

**#18. 2.** To decrease the pressure within the compartment, the affected extremity is raised to the level of the heart, and if this does not relieve pressure, a fasciotomy may be necessary. An accurate assessment should be performed before pain medication is given; foot exercises will not relieve the pressure from compartment syndrome. — Pl — Ph/8 — An — 1

**#19. 2.** Implanted medical devices (pacemaker, screws, pins, etc.) may render the client unsuitable for the MRI procedures. No contract media is utilized so allergies are not a concern; the MRI is a non-invasive procedure so bleeding is not a risk; and a bowel prep is not required. — As — Ph/7 — An — 1

**#20. 3.** The client participation in obtaining baseline data is the first step to decreasing that behavior. Clients with compulsive behavior cannot stop without increasing anxiety; physical prevention of the behavior may initiate a panic attack or other extreme behavior; verbalization is a long-term goal. — Pl — Ps/4 — Ap — 2

| ANSWER | | RATIONALE | NP | CN | CL | SA |
|---|---|---|---|---|---|---|
| #21. | 1. | Wrists must be inspected for breakdown/trauma. Wrist restraints are sufficiently padded; position of the head of the bed has no relation to use of restraints; even though a square knot is used, it does not ensure client safety. | As | Sa/2 | Ap | 1 |
| #22. | 2. | Iodine contract medium is used for gallbladder X-rays. The client must be assessed for a history of iodine allergy. This procedure is non-invasive; diet is recommended but not related to X-ray preparation; local anesthesia is not used. | As | Ph/7 | Ap | 1 |
| #23. | 4. | The Hgb A1c assay provides information about long-term control of DM. The assay reflects glucose level within erythrocytes, providing an average level over 2–3 months preceding the test. It is not related to thyroid, heart or liver findings. | An | Ph/7 | An | 1 |
| #24. | 4. | Sudden changes in ECG patterns may be a result of loose electrodes (artifact) rather than a lethal dysrhythmia. The client should be assessed upon any abnormal monitor activity. A precordial thump, defibrillation and cardiopulmonary resuscitation all could cause injury and would not be utilized unless the client has a true lethal dysrhythmia. | An | Ph/8 | An | 1 |
| #25. | 1. | The client is displaying signs of a detached retina, which requires patching of both eyes to minimize eye movement and bed rest with a flat or slightly raised head of bed to prevent separation of retina and choroid layers. Emergency surgery is not the initial plan, but scleral buckling or laser reattachment are treatment options; Pilocarpine is used for glaucoma. | Pl | Ph/8 | An | 1 |
| #26. | 3. | The pain may be unbearable and she wishes to get away from it. Her desires include to be in control, yet turn inward and shut out external stimuli; a back rub would be more appropriate in early labor. | An | He/3 | An | 3 |
| #27. | 2. | Diabetes is a contraindication for taking oral contraceptive, as DM is linked with cardiovascular disease. The contraceptives would decrease menstrual flow; the broken leg is too far in the past and the baby is old enough that contraceptives won't be a concern. | As | Ph/6 | An | 3 |
| #28. | 4. | Elevation to 30° to promote optimum venous outflow causing reduction in intracranial pressure and prevention of aspiration. Pillows should be avoided because they may cause head flexing, which decreases venous outflow. Avoid elevation above 30° or leg elevation which will increase blood to the brain. Side-lying does not affect intracranial pressure, but the choice does not specify elevation of head, as supine would be avoided. | Im | Ph/8 | Ap | 1 |
| #29. | 3. | It is important not to change insulin dosage without consulting the physician. This statement indicates that the client needs further instruction before her grandfather leaves the hospital. All other statements are correct statements. | Ev | Ph/6 | An | 1 |
| #30. | 3. | Urine output increases due to the increased cardiac output and myocardial contraction force, increasing perfusion of the kidney. The other choices are opposite from the true action of digoxin. | Ev | Ph/6 | An | 1 |

| ANSWER | RATIONALE | NP | CN | CL | SA |
|--------|-----------|-----|-----|-----|-----|

#31. 3. Elevated liver enzymes and total bilirubin, along with the symptoms, anorexia, weight loss, and ascites, all suggest liver disease. Jaundice occurs with liver disease because of the inability of diseased liver cells to clear bilirubin from the blood. Bile is deposited in the skin and sclera, producing the yellow discoloration. Pallor, dry mucous membranes, and peripheral edema are associated with anemia, dehydration, and congestive heart failure, respectively.
— An Ph/7 An 1

#32. 3. People who are allergic to shellfish (iodine) are at risk for allergic reactions to the contract material (iodine) used for an IVP. A dietitian is not needed, and the test can be performed using a less allergic contract material. The physician will be the one to order an antihistamine, which may be combined with steroids.
— An Ph/7 An 1

#33. 4. The nurse arranges to plan wound care with the client, thereby allowing him to participate in his own care and addressing the source of his anger. The other responses discount the client's feelings, only address part of the problem, and show a misunderstanding of the client's complaints.
— An Sa/1 Ap 1

#34. 4. Limited time in the client's room reduces exposure to radiation for nursing staff and visitors. Strict isolation is not needed; time and distance limits are needed. The lead apron could be worn for staff or visitors and disposable supplies and equipment are not necessary. Bed linens are handled according to radiation protocol.
— Pl Sa/2 Ap 1

#35. 3. The platelet count is low. Normal platelet count is 150,000–450,000. A low platelet count places the client at risk for bleeding. Trauma, injections, and invasive procedures should be avoided. All other values are within normal limits.
— Pl Ph/7 Ap 1

#36. 2. Because a local anesthetic is used to numb the pharyngeal area for gastroscopy, the nurse must be certain the client is able to swallow before giving food or fluids. It may take 2–4 hours for the gag reflex and swallowing ability to return. An NG tube or pain will not be present after the procedure, and measuring abdominal girth is not indicated following procedure.
— Pl Ph/7 Ap 1

#37. 4. This disorder involves blindness on the left half of the visual field of both eyes. Therefore, the client can only see objects placed within the right visual field. The other choices are related to hemiplegia or double vision.
— Pl Ph/7 Ap 1

#38. 2. The child should be placed on enteric isolation until the lab reports no contagious organisms in the stool. If the stool is infected, isolation is continued after the antibiotics are completed until 3 consecutive daily stool specimens are negative. Priority placement of room is dependent on prevention of communicability, not exposing other children, and dehydration can be managed on a regular floor.
— Pl Sa/2 Ap 4

#39. 2. The fetal position increases space between lumbar vertebrae, facilitating easier entry of the needle into the subarachnoid space. Sitting is a possible position but not for obtaining cerebrospinal fluid and may cause a headache. The prone and Trendelenburg are acceptable positions for this procedure.
— Im Ph/7 Co 1

| ANSWER | RATIONALE | NP | CN | CL | SA |
|---|---|---|---|---|---|
| #40. 2. | A Shilling test measures the percent of vitamin B12 excreted in a 24-hour urine sample following an intramuscular "loading" of vitamin B12 and a radioactive oral dose of vitamin B12. Laxatives could interfere with the B12 absorption, iron treats iron-deficiency anemia, and an intravenous catheter is not required. | Im | Ph/7 | Co | 1 |
| #41. 4. | Cloth-covered pillows or blankets are breathable materials that allow the cast to air dry. No plastic should be used. Ice should only be used in 20-minute intervals; the listed heat sources will cause uneven drying of the cast, and no objects should be inserted into a cast. | Pl | Ph/7 | Ap | 1 |
| #42. 1. | Bleeding may occur from the puncture site. Firm pressure is required for several minutes to prevent this. The client can resume normal activity after the sedation has worn off, no occlusive dressing is needed, and the specimen is sent immediately to the lab. | Im | Ph/7 | Ap | 1 |
| #43. 3. | Damage to the recurrent laryngeal nerve is a major complication of thyroid surgery. Hoarseness immediately following surgery is often related to intubation during surgery. However, report persistent or worsening hoarseness immediately to the physician because it may be the first sign of nerve injury. Semi-fowler's position is preferred with pillow support. A tracheostomy set should be available, but only used in emergency situations. | Pl | Ph/7 | Ap | 1 |
| #44. 4. | All abdominal surgery clients have a potential for third-spacing of fluids, causing a fluid volume deficiency. Post-op urine output should be maintained to at least 30 mL/hr. 100 mL indicates a beginning deficit. Remembering Maslow's Hierarchy of Needs, physiological needs are addressed first. | Pl | Ph/8 | Ap | 3 |
| #45. 3. | Pain is what the person says it is and occurs when the person says it does. The client's report of "8 out of 10" validates the nurse administering 100 mg of Demerol. The other responses do not meet the client's need for pain relief and clients use various mechanisms to deal with their pain, which may be laughter, exercise, or being quiet. | Pl | Ph/6 | Ap | 1 |
| #46. 3. | Using a 25-gauge needle inserted between the skin layers angling the needle parallel to the skin of the forearm. A patch, the scratch method, or the Z-track IM injection are not suitable methods for this test. | Im | Ph/7 | Co | 1 |
| #47. 4. | Interest in sex is markedly decreased in depression, not increased. The other symptoms are commonly found in clients with depression. | As | Ps/4 | Co | 2 |
| #48. 1. | Knowledge of the types and amounts of alcohol and other drugs consumed are necessary to plan the program of detoxification and anticipate physical complications. The other choices may be helpful to determine the reason for the episodes; however the staff will need to be on the alert for delirium tremors. As treatment progress, the additional information will be important in the later stages of the client's treatment. | As | Ps/4 | An | 2 |

| ANSWER | RATIONALE | NP | CN | CL | SA |
|--------|-----------|-----|-----|-----|-----|

#49. 4. Lying on the left side provides the best perfusion to the uterus and the infant while waiting for delivery. The nurse should have the mother in as clean and uncrowded a place as possible. It would be advisable to call her doctor after placing her in the left-side position, to keep her where she is rather than risk having the baby in transit to the hospital, and the umbilical cord would not be cut if hospital care is likely within 1 hour.  
Im   He/3   Ap   3

#50. 3. Skin-to-skin contact is recommended so that the mother's warm body will warm the infant. Covering both will help keep them warm. Breastfeeding will help contract the mother's uterus and reduce bleeding. The umbilical cord would not be cut if hospital care is likely within 1 hour.  
Im   He/3   Ap   3

#51. 1. The AIDS virus is spread through direct contact with body fluids such as blood, and through sexual intercourse. All the other activities are casual contact, which do not spread AIDS. Contact sports may post a risk if there is potential for direct contact with blood.  
Ev   Sa/2   An   1

#52. 4. Unless the client is coughing, has decrease airway compliance, or has an airway obstruction, a high pressure alarm usually indicates water collection in or kinking of ventilator tubing. The RN should check the tubing first.  
Ev   Ph/7   An   1

#53. 4. If the fetal station is engaged, that is, at 0 station or +1 or more, cord prolapse will be prevented whether her membranes are ruptured or not. The most important criteria is the fetal station. Presentation refers to the anatomical part of the fetus closest to the birth canal.  
As   He/3   Co   3

#54. 3. For effective action, the diaphragm must be left in place for 6–8 hours after intercourse. The diaphragm should have regular inspections, is more effective when used with other contraceptives, and should be removed at least once in a 24-hour period.  
Ev   He/3   An   3

#55. 4. Bowel sounds indicate a beginning return of peristalsis. Ice chips could be offered until either gas or bowel sounds are present.  
Pl   Ph/7   Ap   3

#56. 3. The Miller-Abbott intestinal tube is weighted with mercury to decompress the small intestine. As the tube moves through the intestine, progress can be assessed by comparing distance marking on the tube. The Salem-sump or feeding tube placement is assessed by either injecting air and auscultating or aspiration for stomach contents.  
Ev   Ph/7   Co   1

#57. 2. A hot tub bath/shower helps to shorten the period of stiffness. Salicylate should be avoided on an empty stomach, splints would decrease joint mobility, and activity may need to be decreased if pain is present.  
Im   Ph/5   Ap   1

#58. 3. Air embolism occurs frequently with central lines with sudden onset of dyspnea, hypotension, chest pain, and cyanosis. The best initial nursing action is to clamp the IV line, and turn the client on to the left side to trap the air on the right side of the heart, so it does not enter the pulmonary artery. Then call the physician and administer oxygen. The client does not warrant CPR at this time, another IV bag of fluids would be hung, but only after the tubing is unhooked from the client and re-primed.  
Im   Ph/8   Ap   1

| ANSWER | RATIONALE | NP | CN | CL | SA |
|---|---|---|---|---|---|
| #59. 1. | Elevating the stump will decrease edema. However, elevation on a pillow is indicated only for the first day, because prolonged hip flexion can lead to contracture. Following that, the foot of the bed should be elevated on shock blocks. Reverse Trendelenburg is contraindicated as it promotes venous congestion. | Im | Ph/7 | Co | 1 |
| #60. 2. | The morning short action insulin dosage is usually determined by the previous day's late morning and noon blood glucose levels. To depend on today's BG levels to determine dose of regular insulin, would put the child into a situation of constant overtreatment or undertreatment. Education is an ongoing activity, insulin is given before intake of food, and snacks would be given before exercise. | Pl | Ph/6 | Ap | 4 |
| #61. 4. | The symptoms indicate hypoglycemia. Ten grams of rapidly absorbing carbohydrate is the treatment for hypoglycemia. This should be repeated in 5 minutes if the client does not feel better. The physician should be notified for new orders if glucose and insulin parameters have not already been determined. Regular insulin should be held, as it will lower the blood glucose. | Pl | Ph/6 | Ap | 1 |
| #62. 1. | The symptoms suggest hypocalcemia. The four pea-sized parathyroid glands, which regulate calcium and phosphorus balance, are embedded in the thyroid. Inadvertent removal during a thyroidectomy is a common cause of post-operative hypocalcemia. Radioactive iodine is used to shrink the thyroid and causes hypothyroidism, insufficient intake of iodine may cause a goiter, and over stimulation of parathormone causes hyperthyroidism. | An | Ph/8 | Ap | 1 |
| #63. 2. | Early intermittent catherization is essential in bladder training. A high thoracic spinal cord injury may have some arm, shoulder, and hand movement that would enable client to learn self-catherization techniques. An indwelling catheter should be removed as soon as possible; the client will be able to void on her own; a clamp would be contradicted as an areflexic neurogenic bladder would accommodate the urine. | Pl | Ph/7 | Ap | 1 |
| #64. 1. | Comminuted fracture usually results from a crush injury and results in fractured and crushed bones. Bones pulled apart are displaced, compound fracture is through the skin, and greenstick involves only one side of the bone. | An | Ph/8 | Co | 1 |
| #65. 2. | Fat embolism occurs most often in the client with long bone lower extremity fractures or multiple fractures, regardless of age. | An | Ph/7 | Co | 1 |
| #66. 3. | Absence of audible wheezes can be a sign of improvement. However, when coupled with somnolence, a sign of hypercapnia, absence of wheezing is a sign of worsening bronchospasm. This is a respiratory emergency period. All of the other choices demonstrate improvements in respiratory function. | An | Ph/8 | An | 1 |

| ANSWER | RATIONALE | NP | CN | CL | SA |
|--------|-----------|-----|-----|-----|-----|

#67. 1. Client should be taught to support his weight on the crutch handpieces. Weight should be avoided on the axilla and should be placed on crutch side. — Ev — Ph/5 — Ap — 1

#68. 2. The client should not cross his legs or abduct or assume any position that requires acute flexion of more than 90 degrees. Traveling long distances should be avoided as the person remains in hip flexion for an extended time; and a walker will be used until sufficient muscle tone has developed. — Ev — Ph/7 — An — 1

#69. 2. Alcohol interferes with Dilantin and causes it to remain at subtherapeutic level causing the client to be prone to seizure activity. Dilantin is not given IM, it needs to be given on a consistent basis, and side effects include ataxia, nystagmus, hypotension, rash, gingival hyperplasia, and ventricular fibrillation. — Im — Ph/6 — Co — 1

#70. 2. A hematoma beneath the skin may cause the skin to bulge, but this does not mean the client has abdominal distention. This may require evacuation of the hematoma so that healing may take place. No evidence is given that an infection is present. — Ev — Ph/7 — An — 1

#71. 2. The symptoms suggest acute hemolytic transfusion reaction. The priority nursing action is to stop the infusion immediately, remove the existing tubing and blood, flush the IV site, and administer normal saline. The physician should be notified and blood tubing and remaining blood should be sent back to the lab. — Im — Ph/6 — An — 1

#72. 2. The bladder should be full for a pelvic sonogram to serve as a reference point and sonic window to the pelvic organs. The procedure is noninvasive (no permit needed) and a sedative is not required. — Ev — Ph/7 — Ap — 3

#73. 2. Alzheimer's disease is the most common cognitive impairment affecting older adults. As the disease progresses, it requires ongoing assessment to determine the client's ability to maintain himself in the home environment. All other needs will depend on his cognitive abilities. — As — He/3 — Ap — 1

#74. 1. This is the appropriate place for the stethoscope, as the others are used for aortic heart sounds and Erb's point (murmurs). — As — He/3 — Co — 1

#75. 3. The anterior-posterior diameter increases over time as compensation for chronic hypoxemia, and is known as a "barrel chest." Fever is associated with pneumonia; shock is associated with a weak pulse; and crepitus is associated with a pneumothorax. — As — Ph/7 — An — 1

#76. 3. Myxedema is a condition of the thyroid gland in which there is thyroid hypofunction. Addison's is hypofunction of the adrenal cortex (low blood sugar, hypotension, bronze-colored skin); Cushing's syndrome is the hyperfunction of the adrenal cortex (high blood sugar, hypertension, buffalo hump, moon face, hirsutism); Graves disease is hyperfunction of the thyroid gland (weight loss, tremor, tachycardia, tachypnea, heat intolerance). — As — Ph/7 — Co — 1

| ANSWER | RATIONALE | NP | CN | CL | SA |
|--------|-----------|-----|-----|-----|-----|

**#77. 2.** The client should not flex and adduct affected joint for 24 hours after surgery. Usually an abductor pillow maintains the hip in slight abduction to prevent dislocation. Nursing actions would include assessing for a deep vein thrombosis by checking for a positive Homan's sign, taking vital signs that could signal an infection, and administering pain medication as needed. (Note: Although a positive Homan's sign is still used in clinical practice, it is not used as the single diagnostic indicator for a deep vein thrombosis. Further tests include venography and ultrasonography.) — As Ph/7 Co 1

**#78. 2.** An acute attack of gout may be caused by trauma, alcohol ingestion, dieting, surgical stress or medications. It often occurs at night, which awakens the patient due to pain in the affected area. Osteoarthritis is associated with pain & muscles spasms upon rising in the morning hours. — As Ph/7 An 1

**#79. 4.** The priority nursing action should be to observe the type and progression of the seizure activity. It is also important to ensure the client is safe and does not injure himself during the seizure. The client can be asked about the presence of an aura when he is conscious. — As Ph/8 An 1

**#80. 1.** The scalp itches from the crawling and saliva of the adult louse. The child's fingernails scratch the skin, leaving red marks. The others describe ringworm, candidiasis, and folliculitis, respectively. — As Ph/7 Co 4

**#81. 1.** Shifts in fluid and electrolytes are caused by the loss of fluid and proteins through damaged tissues and blood vessels. Loss of protein causes the interstitial area to fill with fluid, decreasing the intravascular volume. Broken cells release potassium into the circulation. Sodium is retained when aldosterone is released into the bloodstream in response to stress. From the bloodstream, it goes into the interstitial spaces through broken capillaries, thus lowering serum levels and drawing more fluid from the circulating volume. Shock is a major complication during the first 1–2 days. #2 is related to pain; #3 is incorrect as tissue cannot maintain temperature balance; and #4 occurs 4–7 days after injury. — As Ph/8 An 4

**#82. 4.** Turning frequently reduces skin damage, as it does not prevent shivering or help autoregulatory systems. — An Ph/7 An 1

**#83. 2.** A hallucination is a sensory experience with no stimuli, as in hearing voices when alone. — As Ps/4 An 2

**#84. 3.** Temperature elevation will indicate beginning infection. This is the most important measure to help assess the client for infections, because the lost mucous plug and the ruptured membranes increase the potential for ascending bacteria from the reproductive tract. This will infect the fetus, membranes, and uterine cavity. — Pl He/3 Ap 3

**#85. 1.** Deep breathing and coughing are essential for obtaining mucus from the bronchi. The optimal collection time is early in the morning, after the client has brushed his teeth. The specimen should be obtained before antibiotics are given. NPO status is not necessary. — Im Ph/7 Ap 1

| ANSWER | RATIONALE | NP | CN | CL | SA |
|---|---|---|---|---|---|
| #86. 4. | This statement is correct, as soap may cause irritation if used. Eyes are washed first; the cord must have fallen off and the area healed completely before immersing in water; avoid placing diaper in contact with an unhealed umbilicus to prevent contamination by fecal organisms. | Ev | He/3 | An | 3 |
| #87. 1. | This is the best method as it is the only one that indicates metabolism of food and the body's response to intake. | Pl | Ph/7 | An | 3 |
| #88. 2. | Leukemia is diagnosed by identifying abnormal white blood cells and their precursors in the bone marrow and noting how many of these cells are present. Reed-Sternberg cells are found in Hodgkin's lymphoma and Epstein-Barr virus has not been shown to have a direct relation with leukemia. Metastasis is not found by a bone marrow test. | An | Ph/7 | Co | 1 |
| #89. 3. | Epiglottitis is always a medical emergency. Intubation is best facilitated in the operating room where all equipment is readily available, and where the epiglottis can be visualized with a laryngoscope. Laryngospasm is prevented by starting an IV after the intubation, keeping the child on the mother's lap, and antibiotics with the procedure. | An | Ph/8 | An | 4 |
| #90. 2. | Shoes, toys, and clothes can all transfer the oil (urushiol) to the skin, where it sets up an immediate reaction. Items that have touched any part of the plant should be washed in hot water and detergent. All parts of the plant are poisonous, including dried or burning leaves. The fur on animals can contain the plant oils. The first contact (within 15 minutes) should be with cool water, as soap will wash off the natural protective oils in skin. | An | He/3 | Ap | 4 |
| #91. 4. | Clonus is a phenomenon where reflexes are very hyperactive and suggests the presence of central nervous system disease. The client required further evaluation. The other findings are a normal process of aging. | An | He/3 | An | 1 |
| #92. 4. | Socialization is fostered when nurses and other caregivers take time to talk with the clients and show a genuine concern for their well-being, for their present and past life stories. There is no need to separate by age or gender and continuity of care has proven to enhance client outcomes. | Pl | He/3 | Ap | 1 |
| #93. 3. | The correct preparation of insulin should be the regular (clear) insulin is drawn up first, then the NPH (cloudy). This action is performed to keep the short-acting regular insulin free from potential "contamination" by the intermediate-acting NPH. Remember "clear to cloudy." The client would be correct in all the other actions. | An | Ph/6 | An | 1 |
| #94. 3. | Clients with injuries to the lumbosacral area usually have a lower motor neuron (flaccid) bladder. The emptying of the bladder may be achieved by performing a Valsalva maneuver or tightening the abdominal muscles. Fluid intake should be 2000–2500 mL during the day and decrease fluids after 6 P.M. Pouring water on the perineum may help clients with upper motor neuron injuries. | Im | Ph/7 | Ap | 1 |

| ANSWER | RATIONALE | NP | CN | CL | SA |
|--------|-----------|-----|-----|-----|-----|
| #95. 1. | Anticipatory grieving is the state in which an individual experiences multiple feelings in response to an expected significant loss. A client's behaviors may include emotional, physical, spiritual, social, and intellectual responses, in which the nurse recognizes the client is experiencing real grief related to the perception of potential loss. | An | Ps/4 | An | 3 |
| #96. 2. | This is the appropriate time when hormones have the least effect on the breasts, making them easier to examine. When not menstruating, breasts should be examined once a month, even when lactating. Proper positioning during a self-breast exam should be both lying and standing, using one of the 3 methods: circular, vertical strip, or wedge. | Ev | He/3 | Ap | 3 |
| #97. 4. | Clients should be cautious about any injuries while on anticoagulants, which may precipitate bleeding. Anticoagulants should not be increased without physician and/or lab indication. The foods mentioned contain vitamin K, which is the antidote for coumadin and should not be eaten in large amounts. Salicylate drugs, such as aspirin, produce inhibition of platelet aggregation and could cause further bleeding. | Ev | Ph/6 | Ap | 1 |
| #98. 1. | To aid in promoting positive expectations regarding body image, fears must be discussed openly before management can be approached. The other choices involve long-term goals in all or part of the selection. | Pl | Ps/4 | Ap | 2 |
| #99. 4. | Spasms in the flexors and adducts in a hemiplegic can result in flexion and adduction contractures. Proper positioning of joints in an extended, abducted position prevents contractures. The hand tends to form a fist around the thumb unless properly positioned in a semi-extended position. A pillow under the axilla, a trochanter roll by the hip, and a posterior split are additional positional supports. | Ev | Ph/7 | Ap | 1 |
| #100. 2. | The pulse oximeter is a painless, noninvasive procedure, in which the probe is attached over a pulsating vascular bed, such as the finger or earlobe. Covering the probe with an opaque material helps to prevent inaccurate readings from bright external lighting. | Im | Ph/7 | Ap | 1 |

# Practice Test 2

1. The nurse is administering medication in an extended care facility. The client answers to Mr. Smith and Mr. Brown. What is the best way for the nurse to correctly identify the client before administering the medications?
   1. Check with the picture identification on file.
   2. Check the arm band.
   3. Check the name on the bed.
   4. Check the name on the room door.

2. An adult is scheduled to undergo an exploratory laparotomy in 1 hour. The nurse has just received the order to administer his preoperative medication. What assessment is essential for the nurse before administering the medication?
   1. The client's ability to cough and deep breathe.
   2. Any drug hypersensitivity or allergy.
   3. The client's understanding of the surgical procedure.
   4. Whether the client's family is present and supportive.

3. The nurse is assessing a male client who has been admitted for treatment of alcoholism. Which question by the nurse is least appropriate?
   1. "How much do you drink?"
   2. "What other drugs do you use?"
   3. "How is your general health?"
   4. "Why do you drink so much?"

4. The nurse is planning care for a client who has a phobic disorder manifested by a fear of elevators. Which goal would need to be accomplished first?
   1. Demonstrates the relaxation response when asked.
   2. Verbalizes the underlying cause of the disorder.
   3. Rides the elevator in the company of the nurse.
   4. Role plays the use of an elevator.

5. Which statement would be least expected when the nurse assesses a client with post-traumatic stress disorder (PTSD)?
   1. "Sometimes my heart pounds and I can't get my breath."
   2. "I have nightmares about my time in the war."
   3. "I can't concentrate at work but I do fine at home."
   4. "My wife worries that I am drinking more now."

6. An adult client comes to the nurses' station complaining of shortness of breath, choking, dizziness, and nausea. He says, "I think I'm going crazy or dying or something. I don't know what happened. Help me, help me." When the nurse tries to ask about what happened, the client can only say, "Help me, help me." What level of anxiety is the client displaying?
   1. Mild.
   2. Moderate.
   3. Severe.
   4. Panic.

7. A woman completes a session with her psychotherapist and becomes increasingly anxious. The nurse talks with her and the physician orders Xanax (alprazolam) 0.25 mg PO. Which action by the nurse is appropriate for evaluating the effectiveness of this drug?
   1. Ask her whether she remembers not to drive or use alcohol.
   2. Assess her anxiety level 1 hour after giving the drug.
   3. Encourage her to use a relaxation tape along with the medication.
   4. Ask her if the medication caused her to be nauseated.

8. The nurse is assessing a client who was raped a month ago. The client cannot describe any feelings related to her rape. She focuses on the need for better law enforcement and rape prevention programs. The client is using which defense?
   1. Denial.
   2. Conversion.
   3. Introjection.
   4. Isolation.

9. A client confides to the nurse that he is being pursued by the Federal Bureau of Investigation because he has access to information that will prevent future wars. This behavior most likely represents which of the following?
   1. Ideas of reference.
   2. Delusions.

3. Hallucinations.

4. Dissociation.

10. A middle-age woman is admitted in the manic phase of bipolar disorder. She has eaten very little food from her meal trays and has lost 2 pounds in the 3 days since admission. Which approach by the nurse is most likely to meet her nutritional needs?

    1. Provide frequent snack foods that are high in nutrition.

    2. Limit her intake of between-meal snacks.

    3. Allow her to eat in the cafeteria and choose her own foods.

    4. Set up a system in which greater intake is rewarded by privileges.

11. An adult male was admitted to the psychiatric unit 3 days ago with a diagnosis of schizophrenia. Today the nurse finds him facing the window, and he seems to be talking and listening. After validating that the client is hallucinating, which is the best action by the nurse?

    1. Allow him to continue his conversation without interruption.

    2. Offer him a choice of IM or PO for his PRN medication.

    3. Tell him that his behavior is inappropriate and should stop.

    4. Involve him in some concrete game or other activity.

12. The nurse is evaluating a woman who has been treated for major depression for 3 weeks. Which is the best indication that her depression is improving?

    1. She takes her medication as prescribed.

    2. She says, "I think I can set more realistic goals now."

    3. Her husband demonstrates more understanding of his wife's condition.

    4. She ventilates about how sad and hopeless she feels.

13. The nurse enters the room of a depressed client to find the client poorly responsive and an empty pill bottle and water pitcher on the night stand. What is the best initial action by the nurse?

    1. Determine if the client is on suicide precautions.

    2. Check the client's level of consciousness and vital signs.

3. Ask the client what precipitated his overdose.

4. Find out how many pills were in the bottle.

14. During her first trimester, a woman experiences many physiological changes that lead her to think she is pregnant. Which of the following changes will the nurse most likely tell her are normal for an 8-week pregnancy?

    1. Dysuria.

    2. Colostrum secretion.

    3. Nosebleeds.

    4. Dependent edema.

15. The nurse is assessing a healthy neonate upon admission to the newborn nursery. Which characteristic would the admitting nurse record as normal?

    1. Hypertonia.

    2. Irregular respiratory rate of 50 breaths/minute.

    3. Head circumference measuring 31cm.

    4. High-pitched or shrill cry.

16. Following her baby's birth, the woman's uterine fundus is soft, midline, 2 cm above the umbilicus, and she has saturated two pads within 30 minutes. Which immediate need by the client should be addressed?

    1. Be cleaned and have another pad change.

    2. Empty her bladder.

    3. Have an increase in her intravenous fluids of Ringer's lactate.

    4. Have her fundus massaged.

17. The nurse is caring for a child with hemophilia who is actively bleeding. Which nursing action is most important in the prevention of the crippling effects of bleeding?

    1. Active range of motion.

    2. Avoidance of all dental care.

    3. Encourage genetic counseling.

    4. Elevate and immobilize the affected extremity.

18. The nurse is planning care for an infant with Hirschsprung's disease who is admitted to the hospital prior to surgery. Which would not be included in the nursing care plan?

    1. Measure abdomen every 4 hours.

    2. Administer tap water enemas until clear results.

    3. Begin colostomy care teaching with the parents.

    4. Complete daily intake and output.

19. The nurse is developing a care plan for a woman with cystitis. Which is most appropriate to include in the care plan?
    1. Testing urine for protein with a dipstick.
    2. Promoting elimination of excess fluid by maintaining NPO.
    3. Encouraging voiding every 2 to 3 hours.
    4. Telling her to take a tub bath to sooth the urethra.

20. A man underwent an exploratory laparotomy yesterday. He is on strict intake and output. Calculate his intake and output for an 8-hour period.

    | Intake | Output |
    |---|---|
    | IV—D$_5$LR at 125 mL/hr | Foley urine output 850 mL |
    | PO–1 ounce ice chips | NG tube–200 mL |
    | NG irrigant–NS 15 mL q 2 hr | |

    Intake _____    Output _____

21. An adult is receiving Coumadin (warfarin) 5 mg PO QD for treatment of a resolving deep vein thrombosis. When asked, the client states his gums have been bleeding when he brushes his teeth. Which nursing action is most appropriate?
    1. Administer the daily dose of Coumadin, then notify the physician so tomorrow's dose can be adjusted.
    2. Administer the daily dose of Coumadin. These are the expected side effects of Coumadin.
    3. Hold the Coumadin and notify the physician of the assessment findings.
    4. Hold the Coumadin until the next daily dose is due.

22. A client has had Parkinson's disease for several years. He exhibits all of the typical signs and symptoms of advanced Parkinson's. He is being discharged to his home with his 70-year-old wife as his primary caregiver. Which statement best indicates that his wife understands his symptoms and needs?
    1. "Since my husband is on Levodopa, I need to watch him closely for things like facial grimacing and involuntary movements of his trunk, legs, and arms."
    2. "It is very important for my husband to rest in bed or his chair most of the day."
    3. "My husband may have bad diarrhea due to his Parkinson's."
    4. "My husband may be embarrassed by his difficulties with eating so we should not go out like we used to do."

23. A client with a head injury is moaning and complaining of head pain. The family requests that some pain medication be given. The nurse explains that most pain medications are usually not given to clients with head injuries. The family says, "Aspirin won't hurt him." What is the best rationale for withholding the aspirin from a client with a head injury?
    1. Gastrointestinal distress.
    2. Tinnitus, making neuro assessments more difficult.
    3. Increased likelihood of intracranial bleeding.
    4. Constriction of the pupils, making pupil assessment more difficult.

24. A client has a closed head injury. Vital signs are T 103°F rectally; pulse 100; respirations 24; BP 110/84. Hourly urine output is 200 mL/hr. What is the best understanding of the cause of these findings?
    1. Damage to the hypothalamus resulting in decreased hormone production.
    2. Movement of fluid from the tissue into the intravascular space, resulting from sepsis.
    3. An increase in antidiuretic hormone (ADH) as a result of injury to the hypothalamus.
    4. Fluid shifts from the tissue into the intravascular space due to administration of normal saline used during fluid resuscitation.

25. An adult client has been on bed rest for several months. Which statement best describes the relationship between complications of prolonged bed rest and nursing interventions to prevent these complications?
    1. Turning and positioning will help decrease the potential for calcium loss from bones.
    2. Adequate fluid intake is vital to decrease the risk of brittle bones.
    3. Leg exercises are important to decrease the loss of calcium from the bones and the risk of pathological fractures.
    4. Encouraging milk intake will help decrease the loss of calcium from the bones.

26. An adult client had an exploratory laparotomy 3 days ago. The nurse assesses the client's incision and observes the following: edges of incision well approximated; a small amount of edema noted the entire length of incision; moderate amount of serosanguineous drainage. What do these findings indicate?
    1. That the wound is likely to develop an infection.
    2. An abnormal amount of wound drainage.

3. A healthy postoperative wound.

4. That the wound is infected.

27. An order is written to start an IV on a 75-year-old client who is getting ready to go to the operating room for a total hip replacement. What gauge of catheter would best meet the needs of this client?

    1. 18
    2. 20
    3. 21 butterfly
    4. 25

28. An adult client is taking prednisone. Which statement by the client best indicates understanding of the possible side effects of prednisone therapy?

    1. "I really need to limit how much potassium I take in since hyperkalemia is a side effect of this medicine."
    2. "I must take this medicine exactly as my doctor ordered it. I shouldn't skip doses or double up on them if I should forget."
    3. "This medicine will protect me from getting any colds or infections."
    4. "Since I'm taking prednisone, my incision will heal much faster."

29. The nurse is inserting an indwelling urinary catheter. Which action is essential to decrease the risk of complications associated with catheter insertion?

    1. Cleanse the female client using betadine-soaked 4 × 4s, cleaning from the rectal area to the clitoris.
    2. Utilize a catheter that is slightly larger than the external urinary meatus.
    3. Utilize clean technique.
    4. Test the retention balloon prior to insertion.

30. A client who is receiving tamoxifen (Tamofen) 20 mg PO BID asks the nurse the reason for this medication and what side effects are possible. What is the nurse's best response?

    1. "Tamoxifen is a vasodilator-antihypertensive. It will lower your blood pressure. The main side effects include dizziness, headache, nasal congestion, and nausea."
    2. "Tamoxifen will help you manage your nausea and vomiting associated with chemotherapy. It may cause you to be a little sleepy and constipated, and to have dry eyes."

3. "Tamoxifen is used to treat your breast cancer. It will help stop the tumor from growing. You may have some nausea, vomiting, and hot flashes from this drug."

4. "Tamoxifen is an antiulcer medication. Constipation is the major side effect."

31. An adult has terminal cancer. She is receiving morphine sulfate by PCA. She is grimacing and moaning occasionally. She sleeps for short intervals. Her respiratory rate is 20, heart rate 100, and BP 140/90. Which is the most accurate assessment of this client's pain?

    1. As long as the client is sleeping for short periods, the pain is manageable.
    2. The client may be hurting some, but her respirations should not be depressed any further.
    3. The client may need additional pain medication or an increase in dosage.
    4. As long as the client does not voice complaints of pain, the nurse can assume she is comfortable.

32. A child fell off her bicycle and was seen in the emergency room for a mild concussion. The X-rays and physical exam were normal and the child was discharged. Which statement indicates the parents have a need for further instruction?

    1. "I should let her sleep as much as possible since she needs the rest."
    2. "I should report any vomiting episodes."
    3. "She should be seen in 1 or 2 days for a follow-up exam."
    4. "I can give her Tylenol (acetaminophen) as needed for pain."

33. An adult is seen in the outpatient medical clinic for an upper respiratory infection. The physician prescribes erythromycin 500 mg PO q 8 h. Which statement indicates the client understands the possible side effects of erythromycin?

    1. "I may have to increase my theophylline dose while I'm taking this medication."
    2. "Erythromycin is supposed to cause constipation, so I should take it with a glass of fruit juice."
    3. "Taking antibiotics may cause me to get a yeast infection."
    4. "This drug may cause me to feel light-headed when I stand up."

34. An infant is being treated for talipes equinovarus. Which statement by the child's mother indicates the best understanding of the casting process?

1. "My child will have successive casts until the desired results are achieved."
2. "Wearing a cast is very painful, so I'll need to medicate her every 4 hours."
3. "Once the cast is on, it will remain on until the deformity is corrected."
4. "My child will be immobilized and confined to an infant seat."

35. The nurse is caring for an adult client with cirrhosis. What is the best explanation for the development of edema?

1. Shunting of the blood from the portal vessels into vessels with lower pressure.
2. Inadequate formation, use, and storage of vitamins A, C, and K.
3. Decreased concentration of plasma albumin.
4. Decreased production of aldosterone, causing sodium and water retention.

36. A man is admitted to the nursing care unit with a diagnosis of cirrhosis. He has a long history of alcohol dependence. During the late evening following his admission, he becomes increasingly disoriented and agitated. Which of the following would the client be least likely to experience?

1. Diaphoresis and tremors.
2. Increased blood pressure and heart rate.
3. Illusions.
4. Delusions of grandeur.

37. The nurse is caring for an adult client who is scheduled for an intravenous pyelogram (IVP). Which nursing intervention is most essential?

1. Encourage large amounts of fluids prior to the test.
2. Assess for any indications of allergies.
3. Administer a laxative.
4. Restrict fluids only in clients with marginal renal reserve or uncontrolled diabetes.

38. A child has chickenpox. Her mother calls a nurse friend to find out when the child can return to school. What is the best response for the nurse to make?

1. All the lesions must be completely gone before contact with others is resumed.
2. Within 2 to 3 weeks, the itching should be under control and good hand washing established so that contact with others can be started.

3. Your child can return 6 days after the first lesions appear, because the crusts will be formed.
4. Your child must first learn to cough with her mouth covered, put tissues in the trash, and wash her hands after touching her nose and mouth.

39. A 1-year-old child has a staph skin infection. Her brother has also developed the same infection. Which behavior by the children is most likely to have caused the transmission of the organism?

1. Bathing together.
2. Coughing on each other.
3. Sharing pacifiers.
4. Eating off the same plate.

40. The nurse is caring for a client who has a nasogastric tube attached to low wall suction. Which of the following is the nurse likely to note when assessing the client?

1. Client vomits.
2. Client has a distended abdomen.
3. There is no nasogastric output in the last 2 hours.
4. Large amounts of nasogastric output.

41. An adult was placed in four-point restraints 3 hours ago after he attempted to hit a nurse. Which observation by the nurse is the best indication that the client's restraints could be discontinued?

1. The client has had one hand and one leg free for the past hour and has made no aggressive moves.
2. The client apologizes to the nurse and explains that he doesn't want to hurt anyone.
3. The nurse has explained the importance of not striking out in anger and the client verbalized understanding.
4. The medication administered to the client has been effective and he is now sleeping.

42. The nurse is planning care for a client who has just had a renal biopsy. Which would the nurse expect?

1. The client's urine will be red.
2. The client will experience severe excruciating pain in the flank that radiates to the groin.
3. The client will be encouraged to drink at least 3000 mL of fluid per day.
4. The client will ambulate 4 hours after the procedure.

43. The nurse is planning care for an adult client who has just undergone a liver biopsy. Which nursing action is of highest priority?
    1. Making sure the client can void right away.
    2. Measuring and recording the client's blood pressure, pulse, and respiratory rate every 10 to 20 minutes.
    3. Positioning the client on his left side with a pillow placed under his costal margin.
    4. Ambulating the client to the chair, placing a pillow against his abdomen.

44. An elderly client was admitted with a diagnosis of left-sided heart failure. Furosemide (Lasix) 80 mg IVP was given. Which indication shows that the medication is not having the desired effect?
    1. Oliguria.
    2. Hypotension.
    3. Absence of rales.
    4. Polydipsia.

45. Zantac is ordered for an adult client. The nurse mistakenly administered Xanax. What is the most appropriate action for the nurse to take?
    1. Notify the physician, document in nurse's notes of error occurrence.
    2. Notify the supervisor, complete medication error report, and document in nurse's notes of error occurrence.
    3. Notify the charge nurse, assess client hourly, and document if adverse effects occur.
    4. Notify the physician, complete incident report, document notification of physician, and any assessments made.

46. A client who has ascites is admitted to the hospital and will be undergoing a paracentesis. What should be included in the nursing care plan?
    1. Monitor client closely for evidence of vascular collapse.
    2. Place client in Trendelenburg position for the procedure.
    3. Encourage client to drink plenty of fluids to distend the bladder prior to the procedure.
    4. Have client remain on bed rest for 24 hours following the procedure.

47. A client had an exploratory laparotomy 2 days ago and now has a new order for a soft diet. The nurse's assessment includes absence of bowel sounds in any quadrant. What is the best nursing action?
    1. Follow the physician's order and feed the client.
    2. Cancel the physician's order and make the client NPO.

3. Order clear liquids for the client.
4. Withhold food from the client at this time. The physician may be notified of the absence of bowel sounds.

48. An adult is receiving $O_2$ at 3 liters per nasal cannula. His roommate lights a cigarette and tosses the match, catching the curtain on fire. What is the priority action for the nurse?
    1. Turn off the oxygen.
    2. Sound the fire alarm.
    3. Try to extinguish the flames.
    4. Remove the clients from the room.

49. An 84-year-old male client has been bedridden for 2 weeks. Which of the following complaints by the client indicates to the nurse that he is developing a complication of immobility?
    1. Stiffness of the right ankle joint.
    2. Soreness of the gums.
    3. Short-term memory loss.
    4. Decreased appetite.

50. A woman has been diagnosed with cervical cancer and will be undergoing internal radiation in addition to surgery. The nurse is planning her nursing care. Check all that are appropriate in maintaining a safe environment.
    ___ Minimizing staff contact with the client.
    ___ Utilizing required shielding.
    ___ Encouraging staff to stay at the foot of the bed or at the entrance to the room.
    ___ Wearing isolation gowns when entering the room.

51. The lab results of a 68-year-old male reveal an elevated titer of *Helicobacter pylori*. Which of the following statements, if made by the nurse, indicates an understanding of this data?
    1. "Treatment will include Pepto-Bismol and antibiotics."
    2. "No treatment is necessary at this time."
    3. "This result indicates a gastric cancer caused by the organism."
    4. "Surgical treatment is indicated."

52. Which of the following nursing interventions indicate an understanding on the part of the nurse concerning proper care of pressure ulcers?
    1. Rub reddened skin to increase circulation.
    2. Use a heat lamp 4 times a day to dry the wound surface.

3. Cleanse a noninfected pressure ulcer with isotonic saline.

4. Cleanse a noninfected pressure ulcer with povodone-iodine.

53. A female client, scheduled for a mammogram, is called the day before regarding pre-procedure instructions. Which statement by the client best indicates adequate understanding of the preparation?
   1. "I know that I can't use deodorant, so I will use powder instead that morning."
   2. "I should eat a low-fat diet today and drink extra water."
   3. "I should not use deodorant, powders, or creams under my arms."
   4. "The technician will be able to tell me immediately if my mammogram is okay."

54. A client has been placed in blood and body fluid isolation. Which statement by the nursing assistant indicates the best understanding of the correct protocol for blood and body fluid isolation?
   1. Masks should be worn with all client contact.
   2. Gloves should be worn for contact with nonintact skin, mucous membranes, or soiled items.
   3. Isolation gowns are not needed.
   4. A private room is always indicated.

55. Autonomic dysreflexia may be manifested by flushed skin above the level of the lesion, pallor below; severe hypertension; tachycardia; and piloerection. How would these symptoms best be explained?
   1. Parasympathetic nervous system stimulation with release of epinephrine.
   2. Sympathetic nervous system hyperactivity with release of norepinephrine.
   3. Disruption in the communication between upper motor neurons and lower motor neurons.
   4. Muscles served by a lower motor neuron no longer receive stimuli and are unable to contract.

56. An adult client is to participate in a double-blind research study of a new medication. Which statement by the client indicates that the client does not understand the study risks?
   1. "I can drop out of the study at any time."
   2. "I must sign an informed consent form to be in the study."
   3. "They will tell me exactly what medication I am getting."
   4. "My confidentiality will be protected in the study."

57. A woman underwent a D&C under general anesthesia and was placed in lithotomy position during surgery. Because she was placed in lithotomy position, what assessment is essential in the immediate postoperative period?
   1. Check anxiety level.
   2. Check for foot drop.
   3. Check for sensation in lower extremities.
   4. Check for equal, bilateral radial pulses.

58. An adult will have to change the dressing on her injured right leg twice a day. The dressing will be a sterile dressing, using 4 × 4s, normal saline irrigant, and abdominal pads. Which statement best indicates that the client understands the importance of maintaining asepsis?
   1. "If I drop the 4 × 4s on the floor, I can use them as long as they are not soiled."
   2. "If I drop the 4 × 4s on the floor, I can use them if I rinse them with sterile normal saline."
   3. "If I question the sterility of any dressing material, I should not use it."
   4. "I should put on my sterile gloves, then open the bottle of saline to soak the 4 × 4s."

59. A teen has his arm in suspension traction. Which nursing assessment is highest priority?
   1. Skin integrity.
   2. Neurovascular status of the affected extremity.
   3. Level of discomfort.
   4. Knowledge about his injury.

60. A 74-year-old client has been admitted with a 3-day history of severe diarrhea. The nurse is assessing for fluid volume deficit. Which findings are seen in the client with a fluid volume deficit?
   1. Pedal edema.
   2. Orthostatic hypotension and tachycardia.
   3. Increased urine output.
   4. Elastic skin turgor.

61. The nurse is assessing a client who is developing slow progressive hydrocephalus. Which is the nurse least likely to find in the assessment?
   1. Client reports a headache.
   2. Client reports blurred vision.
   3. Rapid thready pulse.
   4. Decreased level of consciousness.

62. While assessing the client with a history of allergic asthma, the nurse questions the client about what precipitates an attack. Which is the client's response least likely to include?
   1. Climate changes.
   2. Exposure to animal dander.
   3. Exposure to high pollen and mold counts.
   4. Seasonal changes.

63. A young child is admitted with acute epiglottitis. Which is of highest priority as the nurse plans care?
   1. Assessing the airway frequently.
   2. Turning, coughing, and deep breathing.
   3. Administering cough medicine as ordered.
   4. Encouraging the child to eat.

64. A young child with bronchial asthma is admitted for the second time in 1 month. Cystic fibrosis is suspected. Which physiological assessment is most likely to be seen in the child with cystic fibrosis?
   1. Expectoration of large amounts of thin, frothy mucus with coughing, and bubbling rhonchi for lung sounds.
   2. High serum sodium chloride levels and low sodium chloride levels in the sweat.
   3. Large, loose, foul-smelling stools with normal frequency or a chronic diarrhea of unformed stools.
   4. Obesity from malabsorption of fats and polycythemia from poor oxygenation of tissues.

65. A physician has prescribed tetracycline 500 mg PO q 6 h. While completing the nursing history for allergies, the nurse notes that the client is also taking oral contraceptives. What is the most appropriate initial nursing intervention?
   1. Administer the dose of tetracycline.
   2. Notify the physician that the client is taking oral contraceptives.
   3. Tell the client she should stop taking oral contraceptives because they are inactivated by tetracycline.
   4. Tell the client to use another form of birth control for at least 2 months.

66. A client with an acute exacerbation of rheumatoid arthritis is admitted to the hospital for treatment. Which drug, used to treat clients with rheumatoid arthritis, has both an anti-inflammatory and immunosuppressive effect?
   1. Gold sodium thiomalate (Myochrysine)
   2. Azathioprine (Imuran)
   3. Prednisone (Deltasone)
   4. Naproxen (Naprosyn)

67. Which finding would alert the nurse to potential problems in a newly delivered term infant of a mother whose blood type is O negative?
   1. Pallor.
   2. Negative direct Coombs.
   3. Infant's blood type is O negative.
   4. Resting heart rate of 155.

68. A 10-year-old is admitted to the hospital with sickle cell crisis. Which client goal is most appropriate for this child?
   1. The client will participate in daily aerobic exercises.
   2. The client will take an antibiotic until the temperature is WNL.
   3. The client will increase fluid intake.
   4. The client will utilize cold compresses to control pain.

69. The nurse is caring for a client who has had a total gastrectomy. The client complains of weakness, palpitations, cramping pains, and diarrhea. He is also experiencing reactive hypoglycemia. What is the best explanation for these signs and symptoms?
   1. Rapid distention of the jejunal loop anastomosed to the stomach.
   2. Lack of fluid intake at mealtime.
   3. There is only a small opening from the gastric remnant to the jejunum.
   4. The hypotonic intestinal contents draw extracellular fluid from the circulating blood volume into the jejunum to dilute the high concentration of electrolytes and sugars.

70. An adult presents with severe rectal bleeding, 16 diarrheal stools a day, severe abdominal pain, tenesmus, and dehydration. Because of these symptoms the nurse should be alert for complications associated with which of these diseases?
   1. Crohn's disease.
   2. Ulcerative colitis.
   3. Diverticulitis.
   4. Peritonitis.

71. An adult underwent a below-the-knee amputation 4 days ago. He is complaining of burning, crushing pain in his amputated foot. What is the best action for the nurse to take in relation to administering his ordered pain medication?
   1. Explain to the client that he really is not having pain and encourage him to wait until later for his pain medication.

2. Acknowledge the client's pain and administer the pain medication.

3. Acknowledge the client's pain but tell him he really shouldn't use pain medication for his pain.

4. Explain to the client that he really is not having pain and administer his pain medication.

72. A client with antisocial personality uses manipulation to gain access to a vending room close to the hospital entrance, where he attempts to leave the hospital grounds. Which is the best nursing intervention for manipulative behavior?

1. Place client in restraints for attempting to escape.

2. Help client identify patterns of manipulative behaviors and the consequences as determined by the team plan.

3. Deal with each incident of client manipulation on individualized basis, dependent on the situation and nurse involved.

4. Restrict the client from all activities to reflect on social behavior.

73. An adult has undergone surgery for a detached retina. What is essential to include in the postoperative care plan?

1. Up ad lib with assistance.

2. Notify physician of severe pain or nausea/vomiting.

3. Bed rest in supine position.

4. Maintain a low carbohydrate diet.

74. A child is admitted to the rehabilitation center for gait training and use of adaptive devices. He has cerebral palsy and a history of falls related to spasticity. Which of the following nursing goals has highest priority?

1. Prevent deformity.

2. Prevent physical injury.

3. Establish locomotion.

4. Ensure a balanced diet.

75. A 2-year-old is admitted to the hospital with meningitis. What is the highest priority?

1. Inform the parents of the child's condition.

2. Maintain a quiet environment.

3. Monitor for changes in intracranial pressure.

4. Maintain bed rest.

76. Which of the following statements, if made by a 43-year-old female, would indicate to the nurse in a cancer health screening clinic that further follow-up is needed?

1. "My diet is low in fat and high in residue."

2. "My mother and uncle died of colon cancer."

3. "I have a yearly rectal exam."

4. "I was born and raised in a rural area."

77. A 2½-year-old child is hospitalized for severe otitis media. He was toilet trained prior to being hospitalized but is having "accidents" now that he is in the hospital. What is the best explanation for this change in behavior?

1. It is unrealistic for a child at age 2½ to be toilet trained.

2. The nurse did not show the child where the bathroom is located.

3. A child of this age needs a parent available to assist with toileting.

4. It is normal for a child to experience regressive behavior due to the stress of hospitalization.

78. The nurse has been instructing the parents of a toddler about nutrition. Which of the following statements best indicates the parents' understanding of an appropriate diet for a toddler?

1. "It's unusual for a toddler to be a picky eater."

2. "A multivitamin each day will meet my child's nutritional needs."

3. "A toddler needs servings from each food group daily."

4. "Toddlers should still be eating prepared junior foods."

79. The nurse is caring for a woman who is having labor induced with an oxytocin (Pitocin) drip. Which assessment of the client indicates there is a problem?

1. The fetal heart rate is 160 beats per minute.

2. The woman has three contractions in 5 minutes.

3. Contraction duration is 60 seconds.

4. Early fetal heart rate decelerations are occurring.

80. A client is in labor and taking three cleansing breaths followed by four slow, deep breaths with each contraction. She is experiencing much discomfort with her contractions. What action is most appropriate for the nurse to take?
   1. Demonstrate to the woman a different breathing pattern during contractions.
   2. Ask the physician for an order for pain medication.
   3. Have the man take a break and instruct the woman in another breathing pattern.
   4. Leave the couple alone as they have their routine established.

81. The nurse is teaching childbirth education classes. What topic should be included during the second trimester?
   1. Overview of conception.
   2. Medication usage and breastfeeding.
   3. Infant care.
   4. Strategies to relieve the discomforts of pregnancy.

82. A woman 30 weeks pregnant is admitted to the hospital with a diagnosis of placenta previa. She and the fetus are stable. To help achieve the goal of avoiding premature delivery, what intervention will be initiated?
   1. Receive a blood transfusion.
   2. Be placed on bed rest.
   3. Receive betamethasone.
   4. Avoid sexual intercourse upon discharge.

83. A 37-week-gestation neonate has just been born to a woman with insulin-dependent diabetes mellitus and is admitted to the term nursery. Which of the following is most essential when planning immediate care for the infant?
   1. Glucose monitoring.
   2. Daily weights.
   3. Supplemental formula feedings.
   4. An apnea monitor.

84. The nurse is caring for a woman in labor who suddenly complains of dizziness, becomes pale, and has a 30-point drop in her blood pressure with an increase in pulse rate. What is the most appropriate initial nursing action?
   1. Turn her to her left side.
   2. Have her breathe into a paper bag.
   3. Notify her physician.
   4. Increase her intravenous fluids.

85. A client on the labor and delivery unit has spontaneous rupture of membranes at 2 cm dilation. The nurse notes that the fetal heart rate has dropped to 80 and suspects a prolapsed cord. What is the most appropriate immediate nursing action?
   1. Call for an emergency cesarean section.
   2. Place the woman in knee-chest position.
   3. Place the expelled cord back into the vagina.
   4. Open up the main intravenous line.

86. A woman is 25% over her ideal weight of 140 pounds. She would like to lose weight before becoming pregnant. The woman is 2 months into her weight loss program. Which indicates she is following proper weight management principles?
   1. Carefully selects only carbohydrate and fat choices for meals.
   2. Has lost a total of 4 pounds.
   3. Is now 5% over her ideal weight.
   4. Goes to beginning aerobics 3 times a week.

87. The nurse is caring for a client admitted with herpes zoster, or shingles. What should the nurse expect to find during the initial assessment?
   1. Rhinorrhea, small red lesions, including some with vesicles that are widespread over the face and body.
   2. A painful vesicular eruption following a nerve pathway.
   3. Blisters on the lips and in the corners of the mouth.
   4. Painful fluid-filled vesicles in the genital area.

88. The mother of a 4-month-old who received his second DTP immunization yesterday calls the office nurse to report he has a temperature of 104°F and a hard red area as big as a quarter on his thigh. What is the best interpretation of these data about the child?
   1. Reacting normally to the immunization.
   2. May be allergic to the vaccine.
   3. Is developing symptoms of the disease.
   4. Has developed a secondary infection.

89. The nurse is administering insulin to an adult client. Which is the correct method of administering insulin?
   1. Administer via intramuscular injection holding the needle at a 90° angle.
   2. Inject via Z track intramuscular injection.
   3. Use a ½ inch 27-gauge needle at a 90° angle into subcutaneous tissue.
   4. Inject at a 10° angle into the intradermal area.

90. The nurse is caring for a client from an Asian culture. The client refuses to look at the nurse and does not maintain eye contact. What is the best interpretation of this behavior?
    1. The client is angry at the nurse.
    2. The nurse is not effective in communicating with the client.
    3. The client does not understand English.
    4. The client is treating the nurse with respect.

91. A male client tells the office nurse that his wife does not let him change his colostomy bag himself. Which response by the nurse indicates an understanding of the situation?
    1. "Your wife's need to help you is a reality you should accept."
    2. "Do you think your wife might benefit from counseling?"
    3. "You feel you need privacy when changing your colostomy?"
    4. "Have you discussed the situation with your doctor?"

92. Which of the following nursing interventions would the nurse perform prior to administering a tube feeding?
    1. Check for placement by aspirating for gastric contents with a syringe and test pH with Testape.
    2. Advance the tube 3–5 inches prior to the feeding.
    3. Instruct the client to swallow.
    4. Instill 30 mL of sterile water into the tube.

93. The nurse is caring for an adult who is 1-day post-op following an abdominal cholecystectomy. Which finding by the nurse indicates the patient-controlled analgesia (PCA) is controlling her pain?
    1. The client's vital signs have returned to preoperative status.
    2. The client is observed laughing and talking with her family.
    3. The client rates her pain as 8 on a 0–10 pain scale.
    4. The client states that she is comfortable.

94. An adult male is admitted to a medical floor with a diagnosis of "sepsis, dehydration." Which finding by the nurse indicates that he is now rehydrated within normal limits?
    1. His urine output is 40 mL per hour.
    2. His skin "tents" when it is pinched.

3. The specific gravity of his urine is 1.001.
4. His apical pulse is 120 and his blood pressure is 70/40.

95. Which statement by a postoperative client suggests that he is ready to learn how to care for his new ileostomy?
    1. "I think I'll be able to wear one of those pouches my doctor told me about without any problems. What do you think, Nurse?"
    2. "I want to know all about my ileostomy, right after you give me my pain medication."
    3. "I suppose I have to learn how to take care of this thing eventually, but it sure is disgusting."
    4. "My wife's always been the one to do the nursing in our house. She'll come in and learn how to take care of it and I'll watch."

96. An adult who is 1-day post abdominal cholecystectomy complains to the nurse that she is having abdominal pain. The nurse goes in to assess her pain utilizing a visual analog scale. Which action by the nurse would be initially most important?
    1. Have the client describe the type and location of pain.
    2. Check the chart for the pain medication order.
    3. Assess the client's abdomen.
    4. Ask the client to locate the pain on a linear scale.

97. An elderly widow is being discharged after treatment for chronic renal disease. Dietary teaching is being done to her daughter, with whom she lives. The physician has ordered a high-carbohydrate, low-protein, low-sodium diet. Which of the following choices best reflects the information the nurse should provide for the client's family?
    1. Avoid canned and processed foods, do not use salt replacements, substitute herbs and spices for salt in cooking, and when seasoning foods, call a dietitian for help.
    2. Use potassium salts in place of table salt when cooking and seasoning foods, read the labels on packaged foods to determine sodium content, and avoid snack foods.
    3. Limit milk and dairy products, cook separate meals that are low in sodium, and encourage increased fluid intake.
    4. Avoid eating in a restaurant, soak vegetables well before cooking to remove sodium, omit all canned foods, and remove salt shakers from table.

**98.** An adult client is being treated in the burn unit for partial- and full-thickness burns of the left foot, ankle, and leg. Skin autografts are taken from the right thigh and a skin graft is performed. The nurse planning care for the client on return from the operating room includes which of the following nursing interventions?

1. Change dressing on graft sites every shift.
2. Cover donor site with fine mesh gauze and expose to air.
3. Lubricate donor site with skin cream every shift.
4. Hydrotherapy to graft sites daily.

**99.** The client is being admitted with acute adrenal insufficiency (Addisonian crisis). Which assessment finding would be consistent with this diagnosis?

1. Pulse 70.
2. Respirations 12.

3. Blood pressure 80/50.
4. Complaints of constipation.

**100.** A client who weighs 380 pounds has had a Roux-en-Y gastric bypass surgery. When the client's sister asks questions about the procedure and the postoperative care, which will be a correct statement?

1. The stomach was removed.
2. Several pounds of extra skin were removed.
3. The client will be allowed 60 cc of fluid 6 times a day.
4. It will help reduce the client's ability to absorb nutrients and calories.

# Answers and Rationales for Practice Test 2

| ANSWER | RATIONALE | NP | CN | CL | SA |
|---|---|---|---|---|---|
| #1. 1. | Having a current picture ID for each resident allows the nurse to positively identify the client. This helps to decrease errors in a population that may not always be able to respond appropriately. The client may have taken off or put on another client's armband; the client may be on another client's bed or in another's room. The visual picture will be the most accurate verification. | As | Sa/1 | Ap | 1 |
| #2. 2. | Drug hypersensitivity and allergic reactions should be documented on every perioperative client before administration. Deep breathing exercises should have been taught at an earlier period as well as the surgeon's discussion of the procedure with the client. By this time, the family would have already seen the client and be in the waiting area. It is not the priority at this time if the family is supportive. | As | Ph/7 | Co | 1 |
| #3. 4. | Questions that begin with "Why" should be avoided, as it appears blaming. | As | Ps/4 | An | 1 |
| #4. 1. | The ability to use relaxation is basic to the treatment of phobia. Choices 3 and 4 are long-term goals. The client may not know the cause of the phobia. | Pl | Ps/4 | Ap | 2 |
| #5. 3. | Work and family life are usually both affected by PTSD. The other choices are symptoms of PTSD. | As | Ps/4 | An | 2 |
| #6. 4. | The client has typical symptoms of a panic attack, in which he cannot focus on the nurse's questions or current events. | An | Ps/4 | An | 2 |

| ANSWER | RATIONALE | NP | CN | CL | SA |
|--------|-----------|-----|-----|-----|-----|

Anxiety is categorized into four levels of mild, moderate, severe, and panic: mild—learning can occur; moderate—focus only immediate concerns; severe—perceptual field reduced; panic—unable to follow directions or communicate.

**#7. 2.** Because Xanax is an anti-anxiety medication, assessment is an appropriate action, and the only choice that evaluates the effectiveness. — Ev — Ps/6 — Ap — 2

**#8. 4.** Isolation is separating unacceptable feelings from one's thoughts. Denial is refusing to believe a stressful event has occurred; conversion is changing unacceptable feelings into physical symptoms; and introjection is taking in feelings/attitudes of another. — An — Ps/4 — An — 2

**#9. 2.** Delusions are fixed false beliefs. They occur when the client's unacceptable feelings are projected and rationalized. Ideas of reference occur when events are directly related to him; hallucinations are sensory perceptions without stimuli; and dissociation involves a change in consciousness, such as amnesia. — An — Ps/4 — An — 2

**#10. 1.** The nutritional problem in mania is the client's decreased attention span and difficulty sitting still long enough to eat. Snack foods that are easy to eat and have good nutritional value may prevent malnutrition until the client is in better control. The cafeteria may impose too much stimulation and her attention span does not allow goal-oriented rewards. — Pl — Ps/4 — Ap — 2

**#11. 4.** Involvement in reality may decrease the client's preoccupation with his hallucinations. Medication is offered only if a threat of danger to himself or others is apparent; a judgmental approach may increase the client's hallucinations and agitation. — Im — Ps/4 — Ap — 2

**#12. 2.** Clients with depression often have unrealistic expectations for themselves and cannot set goals that are possible to reach. Severely depressed clients may be unable to visualize any future and thus are unable to set any goals. The other choices do not show a true improvement in the condition. — Ev — Ps/4 — An — 2

**#13. 2.** Assessing the client's LOC will help determine the next actions. Whether the client is on precautions is irrelevant at this time; questions to the client will be asked later when a stable condition is obtained; determining the amount of medication is helpful, however assessment and treatment is performed first. — Im — Ph/8 — Ap — 2

**#14. 3.** Epistaxis (nosebleed) occurs in the first trimester. It is related to capillary dilation. Dysuria is an abnormal condition with urinary track infection; colostrum occurs at 16 weeks gestation; and dependent edema may occur in the third trimester. — As — He/3 — An — 3

**#15. 2.** The normal respiratory rate is between 30 and 60, characterized by shallow, irregular breaths, often interrupted by short periods of apnea lasting 5 to 15 seconds. Hypertonia or a high-pitched/shrill cry may indicate neurologic impairment or drug withdrawal and normal head circumference is 33–35 cm. — As — He/3 — An — 3

| ANSWER | RATIONALE | NP | CN | CL | SA |
|---|---|---|---|---|---|
| #16. 4. | Massaging the fundus is most important because her uterus is soft and higher than normal. Fundal massage causes uterine contraction leading to vasoconstriction, which will lead to decreased bleeding. Cleaning and pad change along with replacing IVF are important, but not before an action to decrease bleeding. Information given does not indicate the bladder is full. | An | He/3 | An | 3 |
| #17. 4. | Repeated hemarthrosis may result in flexion contractures and joint fixations. During bleeding episodes, the affected joint must be elevated and immobilized to prevent the crippling effects of bleeding. Active range of motion is contraindicated during a bleeding episode. Dental care and genetic counseling are both appropriate, but neither is a priority action during a bleeding episode. | Pl | Ph/7 | Ap | 4 |
| #18. 2. | Tap water enemas are contraindicated in children, as the hypotonic solution can cause rapid fluid shift and fluid overload. The other choices are appropriate interventions. | Pl | Ph/5 | Ap | 4 |
| #19. 3. | This prevents overdistention of the bladder and a compromised blood supply to the bladder wall. Protein is not in the urine in a client with cystitis; fluids should be increased to promote flushing out the bacteria; tub baths should be avoided due to the chance of bacteria in the water entering the urethra. | Pl | Ph/7 | Ap | 3 |
| #20. | Intake = 1090 mL; Output = 1050 mL. 125 mL/hr (125 × 8 hr) is 1000 mL. One ounce of ice chips is 30 mL; NG irrigant 15 mL q 2 (15 mL × 4) is 60 mL for a total of 1090 mL. Output is 850 mL urine and 200 mL of nasogastric drainage for a total of 1050 mL. | Im | Ph/6 | Ap | 1 |
| #21. 3. | The physician should be notified prior to administration because bleeding gums are an adverse side effect of Coumadin and may indicate overdose. The dose should be held until blood tests are performed. | Im | Ph/6 | Ap | 1 |
| #22. 1. | Dyskinesias (abnormal involuntary movements) are fairly common side effects of Levodopa. This may be due to the effect of the body's disappearance of dopamine. The dose of Levodopa may need adjusting. An exercise program is important; constipation is common due to inactivity or inadequate fluid intake; and drooling is common with Parkinson's. | Ev | Ph/6 | Ap | 1 |
| #23. 3. | Aspirin (ASA) is an anticoagulant and increased the client's potential for further bleeding. Large doses may cause GI bleeding or tinnitus. ASA does not cause constriction of the pupils. | An | Ph/6 | An | 1 |
| #24. 1. | Injury to the hypothalamus usually leads to decreased secretion of antidiuretic hormone (ADH), which is manifested by large amounts of very dilute urine output. The hypothalamus also controls temperature. Injury causes a very high temperature. | An | Ph/8 | An | 1 |
| #25. 3. | The ideal exercises will have some resistance of weight bearing as tolerated. Turning and positioning is essential for skin | An | Ph/7 | An | 1 |

| ANSWER | | RATIONALE | NP | CN | CL | SA |
|---|---|---|---|---|---|---|
| | | protection: fluids help mobilize pulmonary secretions; milk intake will not decrease loss of calcium. | | | | |
| #26. | 3. | The findings are typical of healing, common health incision. No evidence is present to indicate an infected wound. | Ev | Ph/7 | An | 1 |
| #27. | 1. | Clients going to the operating room ideally should have an 18 gauge catheter. This is large enough to handle blood products safely and to allow rapid administration of large amounts of fluid if indicated during the perioperative period. A 20 gauge would be a second choice, and the others are too small. | Im | Ph/6 | Ap | 1 |
| #28. | 2. | Prednisone should be taken exactly as ordered. It is very important not to skip doses. Stopping the medication suddenly may result in adrenal insufficiency manifested by anorexia, nausea, fatigue, weakness, hypotension, dyspnea, and hypoglycemia. If these appear, the physician should be notified immediately as this can be life threatening. Prednisone can cause hypokalemia, immunosuppression, and slow wound healing. | Ev | Ph/6 | An | 5 |
| #29. | 4. | The balloon should be checked for inflation and leaks prior to insertion, preventing repeated catherizations if the balloon fails. Sterile technique is used after cleansing from front to back, using a catheter slightly smaller than the meatus. | Im | Ph/7 | Ap | 1 |
| #30. | 3. | It is given following a mastectomy to prevent recurrence. Side effects include nausea, vomiting, hypercalcemia, and hot flashes. The medication suppresses tumor growth, and is not for use in hypertension, nausea, or ulcers. | Ev | Ph/6 | Ap | 5 |
| #31. | 3. | The client's actions of grimacing and moaning, along with the elevated vital signs may indicate that she has not had adequate pain relief. It would be advisable to assess whether she is using the PCA machine correctly, or if cultural issues are prohibiting the client from voicing complaints. Depending on the findings, the physician may need to be notified for a change in dosage. | Ev | Ph/6 | An | 1 |
| #32. | 1. | A child with a concussion should be aroused every 2 hours and evaluated for responsiveness. All the other actions are appropriate. | Ev | Ph/7 | Ap | 4 |
| #33. | 3. | Erythromycin may lead to superimposed infection including yeast infection. Other side effects include increased theophylline blood levels so the dose may need to be decreased; as diarrhea may also occur, extra water instead of juices should be encouraged to prevent a yeast infection; light-headedness is associated with antihypertensives. | Ev | Ph/6 | Ap | 5 |
| #34. | 1. | Cast changes will be repeated throughout the course of treatment, usually every 1–2 week period. Although casts may feel heavy, continuous pain would need to be reported to the physician. Age appropriate activity should be encouraged. | Ev | Ph/7 | An | 4 |
| #35. | 3. | The late symptoms of cirrhosis can be attributed to chronic failure of liver function. The concentration of plasma albumin is reduced, leading to the formation of edema. Fibrotic changes in the liver will cause the development of collateral vessels, which can form varices/ hemorrhoids; the vitamins noted are involved in the clotting factor; and overproduction of aldosterone causes sodium and water retention. | An | Ph/8 | An | 1 |

| ANSWER | RATIONALE | NP | CN | CL | SA |
|--------|-----------|----|----|----|----|
| #36. 4. | Delusions of grandeur are symptomatic of manic clients, not clients withdrawing from alcohol. The symptoms and history of alcohol abuse suggest this client is in alcohol withdrawal. | As | Ps/4 | Co | 1 |
| #37. 2. | The client should be assessed for allergic reactions to iodine, i.e., shellfish allergy or previous allergic reaction to contrast material. Liquids may be restricted up to 10 hours prior to the test to concentrate the urine; laxatives may have been administered the night before, but is not essential; fluids are generally not restricted in clients with renal or diabetic conditons to prevent dehydration. | As | Ph/7 | Ap | 1 |
| #38. 3. | Varicella zoster is found in the respiratory secretions of infected person and also in the skin lesions that are not scabbed over. Scabs are not infectious, which are usually crusted over by 6 days. | Im | He/3 | Co | 4 |
| #39. 1. | Direct contact is the mode of transmission for staphylococcus. | An | Sa/2 | An | 4 |
| #40. 4. | The purpose of the NG tube is to remove stomach contents, therefore the first three choices would be assessed as reasons that output is not occurring. If large amounts are present, then the tube is performing adequately. | As | Ph/7 | Ap | 1 |
| #41. 1. | The controlled behavior demonstrates an ability to remain in control. Apologizing, verbalizing, and sleeping do not demonstrate the capability to maintain behavior control. | An | Sa/2 | Ap | 1 |
| #42. 3. | Increasing fluid intake will decrease hematuria, unless the client has renal insufficiency. Gross hematuria should not be expected. Pain may be from a clot in the ureter; bed rest is recommended for 24 hours following the procedure. | Pl | Ph/7 | Ap | 1 |
| #43. 2. | Vital signs are the priority action, due to the possibility of hepatic bleeding. The client will be placed on his right side with a pillow under the costal margin and kept on bed rest for several hours to decrease the risk of bleeding. | Pl | Ph/7 | Ap | 1 |
| #44. 1. | Lasix is a loop diuretic that should increase urinary output. Oliguria is decreased urinary output. All the other symptoms would be expected during the diuresis. | Ev | Ph/6 | Ap | 1 |
| #45. 4. | This would be the proper protocol. The incident report will not be included in the client's medical record. It would be advisable to also inform the client of the error and to perform appropriate monitoring, i.e., vital signs, labs. | Im | Sa/1 | Ap | 5 |
| #46. 1. | Removing large amounts of fluid may cause vascular collapse, therefore vitals sign are essential. The position for the procedure is usually an upright position: the client voids before the procedure to minimize puncturing the bladder; bed rest is not necessary. | Pl | Ph/7 | Ap | 1 |
| #47. 4. | It would be advisable to withhold food as peristalsis is not present; food would set the patient up for nausea and a probable nasogastric tube if administered before the return of bowel motility. | Im | Ph/5 | Ap | 1 |
| #48. 1. | If the client is not in immediate danger, turn off the oxygen, then follow the RACE protocol: Rescue, Alarm, Contain, Extinguish. | Im | Sa/2 | Ap | 1 |

| ANSWER | | RATIONALE | NP | CN | CL | SA |
|--------|--|-----------|----|----|----|----|

**#49. 1.** Stiffness of a joint is the only choice that may indicate the beginning of a contracture and/or early muscle atrophy. — As, Ph/5, Co, 1

**#50.** All are appropriate except for wearing an isolation gown, which does not offer protection from radiation. — Pl, Ph/7, Ap, 3

**#51. 1.** *H. pylori* is the bacteria believed to cause most chronic gastritis or peptic ulcers. The use of these medications suppresses and eradicates the bacteria, which can be predisposing to cancer. — An, Ph/7, Co, 1

**#52. 3.** Cleansing should include an isotonic solution to prevent disruption of healing. Evidence-based practice has shown not to rub reddened areas; heat lamps are no longer used. — Im, Ph/5, Ap, 1

**#53. 3.** Aluminum chlorhydrate (found in many deodorants, powders, creams) may mimic calcium clusters, so the client is instructed not to wear these. Diet is not affected; results are received from the physician. — Ev, Ph/7, Ap, 3

**#54. 2.** Gloves would be protection from blood and body fluids, as the other choices would not be the correct protocol. — Ev, Sa/2, An, 1

**#55. 2.** This condition is usually seen above the 6th thoracic vertebra in spinal cord injuries. This results from uninhibited sympathetic discharge with release norepinephrine. Choice 3 is related to a client experiencing shock. — An, Ph/7, An, 1

**#56. 3.** A double-blind research study of a new medication generally will have a placebo and test drug. The client will not know which drug is being administered. — Ev, Sa/1, An, 1

**#57. 4.** Positioning changes can cause hypotension, so evaluation of cardiovascular stability is performed first, followed by the pulse circulation checks. Sensation would be assessed later when the client is more alert; footdrop occurs when pressure is placed on the peroneal nerve, which is unlikely in the lithotomy position. — As, Ph/7, An, 3

**#58. 3.** If there is any doubt about the sterility of an instrument or dressing, it should not be used. The sterile field will be within visual and physical proximity of the person performing the action. — Ev, Sa/2, An, 1

**#59. 2.** It is essential to first assess to the neurovascular status (color, temperature, capillary refill, edema, pulses, sensations, movement) frequently and to compare to unaffected extremity. — As, Ph/7, Ap, 4

**#60. 2.** These are seen in a volume depleted person. The other choices are apparent in a client with either proper hydration or fluid overload. — As, Ph/8, An, 1

**#61. 3.** A rapid thready pulse is a sign of shock, not hydrocephalus, which causes increased intracranial pressure. — As, Ph/8, An, 1

**#62. 1.** Exacerbation triggered by climate changes (cold air, air pollution) is most often associated with non-allergic allergy. The other choices can trigger an attack. — As, Ph/7, An, 1

**#63. 1.** Airway occlusion frequently occurs with epiglottis. No liquid medications or food should be administered at this time, because of the swelling of the infected tissue in the throat which may block the airway and cut off breathing. Turning, coughing and deep breathing are not a priority at this time as for a client with a lung condition, such as pneumonia. — Pl, Ph/7, Ap, 4

| ANSWER | RATIONALE | NP | CN | CL | SA |
|--------|-----------|-----|-----|-----|-----|

#64. 3. The obstruction of the pancreatic duct with thick mucus prevents digestive enzymes from entering the duodenum, thus preventing digestion of food. Undigested food (mainly fats and proteins) are excreted in the stool, increasing the bulk to twice the normal amount. Expectoration is very difficult because the excess mucus produced is tenacious and viscous. Elevated sweat chloride above 60 mmol/L is consistent with the diagnosis of cystic fibrosis.  
**As  Ph/7  An  4**

#65. 2. Tetracycline decreases the effectiveness of oral contraceptives. Document on nurse's notes or in chart that physician was notified. The client would not be instructed by the nurse to stop contraceptive use or use another method unless by physician order.  
**Im  Ph/6  An  5**

#66. 3. Prednisone is the only drug presented that has both properties. Gold and Imuran have only an immunosuppressive effect; naproxen has only an anti-inflammatory effect.  
**An  Ph/6  K  5**

#67. 1. When maternal sensitization occurs, maternal antibodies destroy the fetus's red blood cells, leading to anemia and pallor. Negative direct Coombs indicates no development of maternal antibodies; O negative would not present an incompatibility; HR of 155 is a normal finding.  
**An  Ph/7  An  3**

#68. 3. Adequate hydration prevents sickling and delays the stasis thrombosis-ischemic cycle. Exercise should be avoided because it causes cellular metabolism; antibiotics are given only for 7–10 days; and cold enhances vasoconstriction.  
**Pl  Ph/7  Ap  4**

#69. 1. The sign and symptoms suggest dumping syndrome. The exact cause is unknown, but rapid emptying in the small intestine is associated with the symptoms. It is prevented by taking in small meals at frequent intervals. Ingestion of fluids usually increases signs and symptoms; there is a large opening from the gastric remnant to the jejunum; intestinal contents are hypertonic.  
**An  Ph/7  An  1**

#70. 2. The signs and symptoms described are associated with ulcerative colitis. Less frequent diarrhea, crampy pain, and abdominal pains are associated with the other diseases, respectively.  
**An  Ph/8  An  1**

#71. 2. Phantom-limb pain is a commonly occurring complication of amputation. The nurse should recognize that the pain is real to the client and administer pain medication as ordered. The other choices are not therapeutic to the client.  
**Im  Ph/6  Ap  1**

#72. 2. Help the client to develop a relationship between his behavior and the consequences. Do address the client with a consistent team plan to minimize manipulation and to help the client understand and live within set limits. The client needs continued opportunities to interact with staff and peers.  
**Im  Ps/4  Ap  1**

#73. 2. The physician should be notified of any severe pain that does not respond to therapy, severe nausea, vomiting, swelling, cloudy vision, a halo around lights, or purulent or excessive mucoid drainage. Activity may be restricted to bed rest with bathroom privileges and may include face down or on the client's side if a gas tamponade is used (so that gas bubble will float into the best position). Diet is not a factor in the postcare instructions.  
**Pl  Ph/7  Ap  1**

| ANSWER | RATIONALE | NP | CN | CL | SA |
|--------|-----------|----|----|----|----|
| #74. 2. | All are important, but the history of falls and spasticity would initiate this as a priority nursing goal. | Pl | Ph/7 | Ap | 1 |
| #75. 3. | All are important: however, changes in intracranial pressure can be life-threatening. | Pl | Ph/7 | An | 4 |
| #76. 2. | A family history of colon cancer is a known risk factor. Susceptibility to some forms of colon cancer is inherited. The other choices are not risk factors. | As | He/3 | An | 3 |
| #77. 4. | Regressive behavior is frequently seen in children who are under stress. This age is appropriate for toilet-training and the child could be assisted by anyone. | An | He/3 | Ap | 4 |
| #78. 3. | Toddlers present a challenge to parents because they are picky eaters, so food choices would include a variety of food servings from all food groups. | Ev | He/3 | An | 4 |
| #79. 2. | If the woman has more than three contractions in 5 minutes, the oxytocin should be discontinued. Normal fetal heart rate is 120–160 beats/min; normal contraction is 40–90 seconds; early decelerations indicate fetal head compression but not distress. | Ev | Ph/6 | Ap | 3 |
| #80. 1. | Appropriate demonstration does not belittle the man or diminish his wife's confidence in him. This allows the man to maintain continued control in the situation. | Im | He/3 | Ap | 3 |
| #81. 4. | Many discomforts arise during the second trimester and information regarding relief will make pregnancy much more comfortable. The other topics would be discussed at other periods of pregnancy. | Pl | He/3 | Ap | 3 |
| #82. 2. | Restricted activity is the most important measure to minimize stress on the cervix and reduce chances of premature labor. The other choices do not prevent premature delivery. | Pl | He/3 | Ap | 3 |
| #83. 1. | Because the infant is no longer exposed to the mother's high circulating glucose levels and its own pancreas is still secreting insulin in response to the glucose, the infant is subject to hypoglycemia. | Pl | He/3 | Ap | 3 |
| #84. 1. | The signs and symptoms described are those of vena caval syndrome. It is most important to remove the gravid uterus from the interior vena cava and the aorta. Turning the woman to the left side will accomplish this. | Im | He/3 | Ap | 3 |
| #85. 2. | Knee-chest position removes pressure from the cord, which is caught between the presenting part and woman's pelvis. A cesarean will most likely be performed, but the first action will be to remove the pressure. | Im | Ph/8 | Ap | 3 |
| #86. 4. | Traditional weight loss programs combine dieting, exercise, psychosocial support, and behavior modification. Protein should be included in the diet; a 4 lb weight loss is inadequate for 2 months; or has occurred too quickly, respectively. | Ev | He/3 | An | 3 |
| #87. 2. | Herpes zoster (shingles) is an acute infectious disease caused by the Varicella zoster virus, accompanied by painful vesicular eruptions. The others choices are associated with true chicken pox, Herpes simplex I, and Herpes simplex II. | As | Ph/8 | An | 1 |

| ANSWER | RATIONALE | NP | CN | CL | SA |
|---|---|---|---|---|---|
| #88. 2. | The description is of an adverse reaction to the immunization, showing an allergic response. | An | He/3 | An | 4 |
| #89. 3. | Insulin is administered via a short needle at a 90° angle into the SQ tissue. In a person with adipose tissue, it can be administered at a 60° angle, but always in SQ tissue. Z-track is used only in IM injections. | Im | Ph/6 | Ap | 1 |
| #90. 4. | In many Asian cultures, a person does not look directly at a person who is in a position of authority or who is greatly respected. No evidence of anger or non-English speaking actions are indicated. | An | Ps/4 | An | 1 |
| #91. 3. | This type of communication technique, making an observation, enables the nurse to acknowledge that something exists or has changed in some way. This acknowledgement made by the nurse should open communication with the client. The nurse should avoid making assumptions and jumping to conclusion without involving the client. | An | Ps/4 | Ap | 1 |
| #92. 1. | Placement is always checked first before any administration of liquids, by either aspiration of gastric contents or auscultating over stomach area with injected air. Because the tube was initially placed in the stomach, no advancement is required and swallowing was performed during insertion of tube and does not assess placement. | As | Ph/7 | Ap | 1 |
| #93. 4. | The only true evidence that a client's pain is controlled is that the client says it is. | Ev | Ph/7 | An | 1 |
| #94. 1. | A normal urinary output is indicative of adequate hydration and renal perfusion. Urine output for adults should approximate 0.5 mL/kg/hr or 30 mL/hr. The other symptoms are associated with either overhydration or hypovolemic shock. | Ev | Ph/8 | An | 1 |
| #95. 1. | By soliciting the nurse's opinion, the client is indicating he is ready to learn. Pain inhibits the learning process; the Disturbed Body Image statement also inhibits learning; and lastly, the client is pushing care to someone else. | As | Ps/4 | An | 1 |
| #96. 4. | A visual analog pain scale is a line indicating the intensity of pain with visual anchors at either end, one end indicating the worse possible pain and the other end indicating no pain. The other actions will be performed also, but the questions pertains to using a visual analog scale. | As | Ph/7 | Ap | 1 |
| #97. 1. | Salt is used as a preservative in most canned and processed foods. Salt-substitutes may contain high potassium, which would be contraindicated. Limit milk and dairy products as they are high in protein; eating out in restaurants is possible as long as care in selections is utilized. | Pl | Ph/5 | Ap | 1 |
| #98. 2. | The donor site may be treated in a variety of ways, but the most common method is to cover the wound with a fine mesh gauze or impregnated gauze that is open to the air or exposed to a heat lamp to allow the wound to dry. Dressings are usually changed every 48–72 hours; the healed wound (not donor site) is lubricated to prevent drying and itching. Hydrotherapy is used in cleaning wounds, removing eschar and necrotic tissue, but autografts would be dislodged by the currents. | Pl | Ph/7 | Ap | 1 |

| ANSWER | RATIONALE | NP | CN | CL | SA |
|--------|-----------|----|----|----|----|
| #99. 3. | As Addisonian crisis develops, this condition is characterized by signs of cyanosis, shock, apprehension, rapid and weak pulse, rapid respiration, and low blood pressure with additional complaints of nausea and diarrhea. | As | Ph/8 | Co | 1 |
| #100. 4. | This procedure is recommended for long-term weight loss and is a combined and mal absorptive procedure. A small pouch will only allow approximately 30 mL of fluid to be ingested at a time. The jejunum is divided and anastomosed to the new pouch. After the client has lost 100+ pounds, the client may elect to have a panniculectomy, which will remove excess fat and skin. | As | Ph/8 | Ap | 1 |

1. A woman is admitted for a suspected duodenal ulcer. The nurse is interviewing her for an admission history. Which description of her pain would be most characteristic of a duodenal ulcer?
   1. Aching in the epigastric area that wakens her from sleep.
   2. Right upper quadrant pain that increases after meals.
   3. Sharp pain in the epigastric area that radiates to the right shoulder.
   4. A sensation of painful pressure in the midsternal area.

2. The nurse is playing with a 2-year-old child with tetralogy of Fallot, who suddenly squats on the floor. What is the best initial nursing action?
   1. Return the child to bed immediately.
   2. Allow the child to remain in that position.
   3. Place the child in a chair.
   4. Call the physician immediately.

3. The nurse is caring for a client with cirrhosis of the liver who has developed esophageal varices. The nurse understands that the best explanation for development of esophageal varices is which of the following?
   1. Chronic low serum protein levels result in inadequate tissue repair, allowing the esophageal wall to weaken.
   2. The enlarged liver presses on the diaphragm, which in turn presses on the esophageal wall, causing collapse of blood vessels into the esophageal lumen.
   3. Increased portal pressure causes some of the blood that normally circulates through the liver to be shunted to the esophageal vessels, increasing their pressure and causing varicosities.
   4. The enlarged liver displaces the esophagus toward the left, tearing the muscle layer of the esophageal blood vessels, which allows small aneurysms to form along the lower esophageal vessels.

4. An adult with esophageal varices begins to experience severe gastrointestinal bleeding. To meet the client's fluid needs, what priority should be included in the plan of care?
   1. Accommodating his frequent need for the bedpan.
   2. Maintaining the gastric pH.
   3. Monitoring vital signs on an hourly basis.
   4. Rapid blood and fluid administration.

5. An adult has just had a broken left ankle casted in the emergency department. He will be going home to a second floor apartment. What teaching instructions will be given on how to walk upstairs with crutches?
   1. Resting his weight on his right foot while he lifts the crutches and his left foot to the next step, then resting his weight on the crutches while he brings his right foot up onto the same step.
   2. Resting his weight on the crutches while he lifts his right foot to the next step, then moving the crutches and his left foot to the same step.
   3. Holding both crutches with his left arm and using the crutches to bear part of his weight while he lifts his right foot to the next step, then moving his crutches and his left foot to the same step.
   4. Sitting on the steps and using his right leg and left arm to lift his weight and place his buttocks on the next step, while pulling the crutches with his right hand.

6. A child has cerebral palsy and is hospitalized for corrective surgery for muscle contractures. What is the most important immediate postoperative goal?
   1. Ambulate using adaptive devices.
   2. Demonstrate optimal oxygenation.
   3. Verbalize pain control.
   4. Complete daily self-care needs.

7. A 5-year-old child with a terminal illness is talking to the nurse. Which of the following best reflects a 5-year-old's understanding of death?
   1. "I'll see Grandma in heaven."
   2. "Will it hurt when I die?"
   3. "Can Mommy go with me?"
   4. "It isn't fair. Why me? I'm too young to die."

8. The nurse is teaching the parents of a child who is being treated in clinic for otitis media. Which of the following statements is essential to include in the teaching?

   1. "Do not take acetaminophen as this is contraindicated."
   2. "Take the medication until the pain and fever are gone."
   3. "Do not apply heat to the ear."
   4. "Take all of the medication as ordered."

9. The nurse is planning care for a child who must remain in a croup tent continuously. Which goal is of highest priority?

   1. The tent will remain closed, except for feedings and hygiene.
   2. The child will maintain normal body temperature and have dry linens.
   3. The tent will deliver mist and cooled air simultaneously while the child is inside.
   4. The child will find entertainment within the tent to encourage compliance.

10. A woman comes to the prenatal clinic because she thinks she might be pregnant. She tells the nurse that her menstrual periods are irregular but, since her last menses 7 weeks ago, she's noticed some physiologic changes in her body. Which finding should the nurse expect when assessing the woman for a probable sign of pregnancy?

    1. Morning sickness.
    2. Urinary frequency.
    3. A positive pregnancy test.
    4. Auscultation of fetal heart sounds.

11. A woman in the prenatal clinic tells the nurse that the first day of her last normal menstrual period was June 15th. The nurse uses Nägele's rule to calculate the due date as being about _____.

12. A woman who is 6 months pregnant is seen in antepartal clinic. She states she is having trouble with constipation. To minimize this condition, what instruction would the nurse provide?

    1. Increase her fluid intake to 3 liters/day.
    2. Request a prescription for a laxative from her physician.
    3. Stop taking iron supplements.
    4. Take 2 tablespoons of mineral oil daily.

13. A nurse works 12 hour shifts in a hospital setting. What intervention would be beneficial for the nurse's health?

    1. Drink at least 1 liter of fluid per day.
    2. Elevate legs at least twice during the shift.

    3. Pull objects rather than push them.
    4. Wear supportive stockings when working.

14. The nurse is caring for a woman in labor. The woman is irritable, complains of nausea and vomits, has heavier show, and the membranes have ruptured. What does this indicate?

    1. The woman is in transition stage of labor.
    2. The woman is having a complication and the doctor should be notified.
    3. Labor is slowing down and the woman may need oxytocin.
    4. The woman is emotionally distraught and needs assistance in dealing with labor.

15. The nurse is caring for a woman who had a vaginal delivery an hour ago without complications. She has a boggy fundus after voiding 500 mL. What would be the highest priority for the nurse to address?

    1. Massaging the fundus until it is firm.
    2. Assessing the lochia.
    3. Adding Pitocin to the intravenous solution being administered.
    4. Calling the health care provider.

16. A client who is having a saline abortion is being cared for on the labor floor. The client's vital signs are temperature 101°F, pulse 100, respirations 24, blood pressure 120/90. How does the nurse interpret this data?

    1. The blood pressure is elevated from receiving the saline injection.
    2. The vital signs are within normal limits for a client undergoing saline abortion.
    3. The client is at extreme risk for shock.
    4. The client may be developing an infection, such as chorioamnionitis.

17. A woman who is taking oral contraceptives tells her nurse neighbor that she is experiencing a vaginal discharge. What would be the most appropriate advice the nurse should give the woman?

    1. Purchase an over-the-counter remedy.
    2. Change undergarments.
    3. See the physician as soon as possible.
    4. Stop taking the oral contraceptives.

18. The nurse is assessing a woman for sexually transmitted diseases. Which symptom would be most apt to be present in a woman with a *Trichomonas vaginalis* vaginal infection?

    1. A profuse, white, bubbly discharge.
    2. White cheese-like patches in the vagina.

3. A perineal deformity.

4. An ulcer or lesion of the vulva or vagina.

19. The nurse is assessing a newborn 5 minutes after birth. He has full flexion of the extremities, is acrocyanotic, has a heart rate of 124, a full, lusty cry, and resists the suction catheter. The nurse should record the Apgar score as _____.

20. A client in the active phase of labor has just been given continuous epidural anesthesia. Which assessment finding indicates to the nurse that the client is experiencing a common side effect of this type of anesthesia?

1. Blood pressure of 50/30.

2. Uterine pain.

3. Fetal heart rate of 140.

4. Euphoria.

21. An adult has had a cerebrovascular accident (CVA) and has severe right-sided weakness. She has been taught to walk with a cane. The nurse is evaluating her use of the cane prior to discharge. Which of the following reflects correct use of the cane?

1. Holding the cane in her left hand, the client moves the cane forward first, then her right leg, and finally her left leg.

2. Holding the cane in her right hand, the client moves the cane forward first, then her left leg, and finally her right leg.

3. Holding the cane in her right hand, the client moves the cane and her right leg forward, then moves her left leg forward.

4. Holding the cane in her left hand, the client moves the cane and her left leg forward, then moves her right leg forward.

22. The nurse is caring for a client who has just had a splenectomy. When planning care in the immediate postoperative period the nurse should avoid using which position?

1. Left side-lying.

2. Right side-lying.

3. Semi-Fowler's.

4. Supine.

23. A 23-year-old is admitted to the hospital after having taken LSD. What should the nurse assess for?

1. Dilated pupils, flushing, and tremors.

2. Pupillary constriction, constipation, and sleepiness.

3. Tremors, muscular weakness, and mask-like face.

4. Vertical and horizontal nystagmus.

24. A group of eight psychiatric clients have been together in group therapy for 12 sessions. There has been an expression of warm feelings, self-disclosure, and an awareness of events in the here and now. The group finds it difficult to deal with two members who must now join the group. The nurse recognizes that group members are experiencing which phase of the group process?

1. Beginning phase.

2. Transition phase.

3. Middle phase.

4. Termination phase.

25. An adult has been informed that he needs surgery for rectal cancer. His response is, "There's nothing wrong with me. I just have hemorrhoids." The nurse knows this response to be which defense mechanism?

1. Projection.

2. Repression.

3. Denial.

4. Displacement.

26. A female client is hospitalized for depression. One evening after an argument with her husband, she discusses with the evening nurse her intent to cut her wrists. Her husband has threatened to divorce her and retain custody of the children. What is the most appropriate initial action for the nurse to take?

1. Attempt to convince the client of the need to address her husband's threats instead of using self-destructive behavior.

2. Place the client on suicide precautions, which restrict her leaving the nursing unit.

3. Place the client on suicide precautions, requiring close observation and one-to-one monitoring by nursing staff.

4. Recognize the suicidal remarks as less serious because the client is in a safe environment.

27. A teen is brought to the emergency room in a semiconscious state. The friend who accompanies him reports that he fell while playing ball. The nurse assesses the client and notes Kussmaul respirations, hypotension, tachycardia, decreased reflexes, and an acetone odor to his breath. Which question does the nurse appropriately ask the friend at this time?

1. "Does he have diabetes?"

2. "Does he have epilepsy?"

3. "Did he hit his head?"

4. "Did he use drugs?"

28. An adult client has been passing blood in his feces. What would be the best way for the nurse to assess whether the hematochezia is a symptom of gastric bleeding?
    1. Ask him how long he has been bleeding.
    2. Check his vital signs.
    3. Monitor his laboratory results.
    4. Obtain his complete past medical history.

29. A construction worker complains of low back pain that increases when he bends over, coughs, or lifts objects. A diagnosis of herniated disc is made. When asked about the cause of his pain, the nurse's response is based on the knowledge that pain associated with a herniated disc results from what?
    1. Compression of the spinal nerve root.
    2. Spasms of the paraspinal muscles.
    3. A friction rub created by degeneration of vertebrae.
    4. Edema and swelling of nerve endings.

30. The nurse is caring for a client who is being transfused for severe gastrointestinal bleeding. How can the nurse decrease the danger of hypothermia?
    1. Administering blood with normal saline.
    2. Administering blood products through a central line.
    3. Giving only packed cells.
    4. Warming blood to body temperature before administering.

31. A client complains of a sudden onset of pain in the ankle, which is swollen, red, and extremely sensitive to pressure. The client asks the nurse about gout. What explanation will the nurse provide about gout?
    1. A metabolic disorder that results in elevated serum uric acid levels.
    2. An infection of the synovial membrane by microorganisms, resulting in inflammation.
    3. A disease of cartilage resulting in destruction of the cartilage and the underlying bone, causing severe pain.
    4. Inflammation of the bursal sac accompanied by formation of large calcium deposits, which cause swelling and joint pain.

32. A client is admitted to the hospital with congestive heart failure. She has shortness of breath and a +3–4 peripheral edema. What nursing strategies should be included in the plan of care to reduce the client's edema?
    1. Establishing limits on activity.
    2. Fostering a relaxed environment.
    3. Identifying goals for self-care.
    4. Restricting IV fluids.

33. An elderly woman admitted with congestive heart failure and +3–4 peripheral edema complains that she is always tired. Which of the following would be the most appropriate suggestion by the nurse while the client is still on bed rest?
    1. Continue to exercise your legs.
    2. Try not to think about the fatigue.
    3. Eat larger meals.
    4. Sleep as much as possible.

34. An adult is admitted with early left-sided congestive failure. Which symptom should the nurse expect to find?
    1. Bradycardia.
    2. Rales.
    3. Liver engorgement.
    4. Jugular vein distention.

35. An adult is given digoxin (Lanoxin) 0.25 mg daily. What signs of digitalis toxicity would the nurse provide to the client?
    1. Auditory hallucinations and bradycardia.
    2. Dry mucous membranes and diarrhea.
    3. Heart block and brittle hair and nails.
    4. Visual disturbances and premature heartbeats.

36. Which serum potassium level reported for an adult requires no immediate nursing intervention?
    1. 3.2 mEq/liter.
    2. 4.0 mEq/liter.
    3. 5.7 mEq/liter.
    4. 6.0 mEq/liter.

37. The mother of a newborn learns that her infant son has lost 8 ounces since his birth 2 days ago. The nurse explains that this weight loss is normal. What explanation will the nurse provide for the weight loss result?
    1. Feeding infants every 4 hours instead of every 3 hours.
    2. Loss of fluid from the cord stump.
    3. Limited food intake since birth.
    4. Regurgitation of feedings.

38. A 16-year-old Type 1 diabetic takes his morning dose of insulin and leaves for school. At 10 A.M. he feels faint and is brought to the nurse's office. He has tachycardia and diaphoresis and is unresponsive. What would be the appropriate intervention by the nurse at this time?
    1. 5 units regular insulin SC.
    2. 8 ounces of orange juice.
    3. Glucagon SC.
    4. Glucose 50% IV push.

39. A client is given discharge instructions following a thoracotomy. Which of the following would be included in the teaching?
    1. Cough when necessary.
    2. Keep arm of affected side in sling.
    3. Remove dressing from groin area after 24 hours.
    4. Explain the use of a Passy-muir valve.

40. The nurse in a well-baby clinic is assessing a 12-month-old child. He is 30 inches tall and weighs 30 lb. How does the nurse interpret this data?
    1. Normal height, increased weight.
    2. Normal height, decreased weight.
    3. Small for age, normal weight.
    4. Tall for age, but weight appropriate for height.

41. The nurse has been discussing promotion of growth and development with a family whose 15-month-old son has a cyanotic heart defect. Which statement by the father indicates a need for further teaching?
    1. "I need to feed him slowly and allow frequent rest periods."
    2. "I need to play quiet games and activities with my son."
    3. "I need to provide highly nutritious foods."
    4. "I need to limit my son's interactions with other children."

42. A child with hemophilia cut his hand while working on a craft project in the hospital play room. What will be the nurse's initial action?
    1. Apply pressure to the bleeding area for at least 10 to 15 minutes.
    2. Apply an ice pack.
    3. Cover the wound with a sterile dressing.
    4. Notify the physician immediately.

43. The nurse is caring for a woman in the fourth stage of labor. What should the woman be monitored for?
    1. Uterine contractions.
    2. Cervical dilation.

3. Birth of the baby and delivery of the placenta.
4. Readjustment to the nonpregnant state.

44. A female woman is diagnosed with somatization disorder. She experiences palpitations, nausea, abdominal pain, and headaches. Physical exam and diagnostic tests do not reveal pathology. The client comes to the nurse stating she has palpitations. Which plan of care by the nurse best reduces secondary gain?
    1. After investigation of her palpitations, do not continue to take her vital signs with each complaint of the problem.
    2. Inform her that the palpitations are not real and she must learn to relax.
    3. Convey an intense interest in her palpitations by encouraging her to talk about her symptoms.
    4. Reassure her that she will be assisted in meeting her dependency needs.

45. The nurse is assessing a client with borderline personality disorder. What behavior will the nurse assess for?
    1. Aggression.
    2. Depression.
    3. Sleep disturbances.
    4. Splitting.

46. An elderly woman is addicted to pain killers prescribed for her arthritis. She denies it is a problem because it was prescribed by her physician. What is the best interpretation of the client's view of her addiction?
    1. The client is using rationalization to support her denial.
    2. The client really does not have a problem; it is the physician who does.
    3. The client is transferring blame by denying she has a problem.
    4. The client is an uneducated woman so she couldn't understand her problem.

47. An adult is prepared for discharge following a bilateral adrenalectomy. Which statement by the client demonstrates understanding of the discharge teaching?
    1. "The surgery cured my disease, now I won't have to take any medications."
    2. "I should wear a Medic Alert bracelet or necklace at all times."
    3. "I will need to take replacement doses of steroids daily for 1 to 2 months."
    4. "I will probably develop a round face and gain weight now that I will take cortisol daily."

48. Sandra, an RN, reports to work looking unkempt. Nancy, another RN, approaches when she notices her using uncoordinated movements. Sandra's breath reeks of peppermints and Nancy suspects Sandra may be intoxicated. What is the best initial nursing action for Nancy to take?
    1. Call the supervisor and report Sandra.
    2. Confront Sandra with the concerns and relieve her of her nursing duties immediately.
    3. Ignore the situation.
    4. Give Sandra a lecture about substance abuse and do nothing else.

49. An adult is experiencing a panic attack. The nurse intervenes by escorting him to his room, using short sentences, and conveying a calm demeanor. Which action by the client indicates the nursing interventions are effective?
    1. Releases his anxiety by punching his fist on a bedside table.
    2. States he wants to be alone to deal with his feelings.
    3. Expresses verbally his demands to the nurse.
    4. Makes connections between events and his anxious response.

50. A young adult is readmitted to the rehabilitation unit after a T4 spinal cord injury that occurred 6 months ago. He is about to begin an intensive rehabilitation program. Which of the following statements made by this client best indicates that he understands the extent of his injury?
    1. "I want to use an electric wheelchair."
    2. "My goal is to be independent in transfers."
    3. "Soon I'll be walking."
    4. "There is little I can do, but I will try."

51. The nurse is caring for an adult with a T4 spinal cord transection. Which activity by the client indicates adequate learning regarding urinary tract care?
    1. Avoiding the Valsalva maneuver when the bladder is full.
    2. Cleaning the urinary meatus every 2 hours.
    3. Checking the bladder distention frequently.
    4. Limiting fluids to 100 mL per 24 hours.

52. To evaluate the effectiveness of bowel training for an adult with a T6 spinal cord injury, what should the nurse expect him to be able to do?
    1. Avoid laxatives and stool softeners.
    2. Experience no incontinence.
    3. Move his bowels daily.
    4. Resume previous bowel habits.

53. The nurse is caring for a client with severe back strain. The nurse administers diazepam (Valium) 10 mg QID. Which observation is most indicative of the need to reassess this order?
    1. Drowsiness.
    2. Hyperesthesia of the arms.
    3. Loss of appetite.
    4. Severe muscle spasms.

54. An adult has been receiving physical therapy following a cerebrovascular accident. His left leg is weak and he is instructed in the use of a cane. What documentation by the nurse shows the client's ability to use the cane correctly?
    1. Holds the cane in his left hand.
    2. Leans his body toward the cane when walking.
    3. Advances the left leg and cane simultaneously.
    4. Advances the right leg and cane simultaneously.

55. The nurse is caring for a client who is hypertensive. To facilitate the client's ability to lower his blood pressure to a normal range, the nurse should teach him to avoid which of the following foods?
    1. Cooked cereal.
    2. Broccoli.
    3. Catsup.
    4. Sugar.

56. An adult client has hypertension. The nurse takes his blood pressure in lying and standing positions. What condition is this test used for?
    1. Central nervous system depression.
    2. Malignant hypertension.
    3. Orthostatic hypotension.
    4. Vascular insufficiency.

57. The nurse is formulating a teaching plan for an adult client with severe emphysema. What are the recommended activities the nurse should instruct the client to select?
    1. Avoid movement.
    2. Build strength.
    3. Conserve energy.
    4. Test his limits of tolerance.

58. What is an appropriate expected outcome for a client with chronic obstructive lung disease (COPD)?
    1. Deemphasizes expirations.
    2. Increases his respiratory rate.

3. Reduces the use of his diaphragm.

4. Utilizes abdominal breathing.

59. An adult is hospitalized for treatment of deep electrical burns. Burn wound sepsis develops and mafenide acetate 10% (Sulfamylon) is ordered BID. What physiological response will the nurse inform the client to expect from the topical application?

1. Severe burning pain for a few minutes following application.

2. Possible severe metabolic alkalosis with continued use.

3. Black discoloration of everything that comes in contact with this drug.

4. Chilling due to evaporation of solution from the moistened dressings.

60. A client is admitted to the burn unit with partial and full thickness burns of both legs, which occurred when a charcoal grill tipped over on her. Blister formation and a large amount of fluid exudate is noted. Urine output is 30 mL/hr, BP 90/60, and pulse 110. What is the primary nursing diagnosis during the initial 48–72 hours following the burn?

1. Body image disturbance related to disfiguring burns of both legs.

2. High risk for infection related to skin breakdown.

3. Potential for ineffective airway clearance related to smoke inhalation.

4. Fluid volume deficit related to increased capillary permeability.

61. While assessing the client with burns on the back and trunk, the nurse notes areas that are not painful, grayish-white in color, and leathery in appearance. What type of burns will the nurse document?

1. Superficial burns.

2. Superficial partial thickness burns.

3. Deep partial thickness burns.

4. Full thickness burns.

62. A middle-aged woman has no memory of her past. She assumed the name Blanche as she created a new identity during her hospital stay. Why does the nurse feel it is important for her to do this?

1. It decreased the client's anxiety level.

2. All people need a name and a history.

3. The hospital needs to have a name for its records for payment purposes.

4. It increased the client's self-esteem by developing a possible self.

63. A high school student with a history of sexual abuse was admitted to the psychiatric unit experiencing depersonalization. What is an appropriate short-term goal for the nurse?

1. Help the client develop coping skills.

2. Orient the client to the staff and unit.

3. Place the client on q 15 minute checks.

4. Teach the client about her medications.

64. A delusional client is admitted to the hospital. What is the most appropriate action for the nurse to take?

1. Attempt to disprove the client's delusion.

2. Focus on the reality aspects of the client's communication.

3. Place the client on room restriction to decrease stimuli.

4. Agree with the delusion until psychotropic medications take effect, then focus on reality.

65. The nurse evaluates a delusional client for improvement. Which of the following statements indicates a positive outcome for a delusional client?

1. Client states he hears voices, but only when alone.

2. Client states people are observing him but are not talking about him.

3. Client expresses less fear in using the public phone on the hospital unit.

4. Client states he can now use the unit shower room because he realizes the shoe left by another client is not a rat.

66. A child who is 2 years and 6 months old has had one bout of nephrosis (nephrotic syndrome). His mother suspected a recurrence when she observed swelling around his eyes. The nurse helps to confirm this condition by recognizing what additional symptom?

1. Blood pressure of 140/90.

2. Marked proteinuria.

3. Cola-colored urine.

4. A history of positive streptococcal infection.

67. The nurse is evaluating a child who is being treated for nephrosis. Which observations indicate successful treatment of nephrosis?

1. Diuresis and weight loss.

2. Improved appetite and weight gain.

3. Increase in the sedimentation rate and urine specific gravity.

4. Return of temperature to normal and indications that the child is more comfortable.

**68.** The mother of a 2-year-old tells the nurse that her son has temper tantrums, demanding cookies in the supermarket, and asks how she can best handle these temper tantrums. What suggestion should the nurse give to the mother?

1. Buy one box of cookies for each shopping trip.
2. Leave him home while she goes shopping.
3. Remain calm and ignore his behavior.
4. Discipline the child immediately when he demands cookies.

**69.** A young woman is in her fifth month of pregnancy. She has been taking 20 units of NPH insulin for diabetes mellitus daily for 6 years. Which of the following statements indicates that the woman understands the teaching regarding her insulin needs during her pregnancy?

1. "Are you sure all this insulin won't hurt my baby?"
2. "I'll probably need my daily insulin dose raised."
3. "I will continue to take my regular dose of insulin."
4. "These finger sticks make my hand sore. Can I do them less frequently?"

**70.** A woman who delivered a healthy baby 18 hours ago has just been given Rho (D) immune globulin. Which finding indicates the need for administration of this medication?

1. The mother is Rho (D) negative with Rho (D) antibodies.
2. The infant is Rho (D) positive.
3. There is a positive indirect Coombs test of cord blood.
4. The mother is Rho (D) positive.

**71.** What would the nurse expect when evaluating the effectiveness of IV Pitocin for a client with secondary dystocia (uterine inertia)?

1. A precipitate delivery.
2. Cervical effacement without delivery.
3. Infrequent contractions lasting longer than 90 seconds.
4. Progressive cervical dilation with contractions lasting less than 90 seconds.

**72.** A client with type 2 diabetes delivered a 3700-gram live girl via cesarean delivery for a breech position 15 minutes ago. She wishes to breastfeed as soon as possible. The nurse caring for the infant makes the following assessments of vital signs: T 98.8°F, P 148, respirations 22,

color pink with tremors and irritability. What is the best nursing intervention at this time?

1. Feed the infant 5% dextrose water via gavage.
2. Take the infant to the mother to feed immediately.
3. Check the infant's blood sugar.
4. Ask a coworker to call the pediatrician immediately.

**73.** When caring for a client with a casted extremity, frequent assessments of neurologic and circulatory status of the affected extremity are required. Which of the following assessment findings should be recognized by the nurse as abnormal?

1. Client reports the extremity feels "like it's asleep."
2. Capillary refill time is less than 5 seconds.
3. The area distal to the cast is warm to touch.
4. Client reports dull aching in the casted extremity.

**74.** An adult is receiving peritoneal dialysis. His acid-base balance and electrolytes are now within normal limits. Which of the following best explains the mechanism of action for peritoneal dialysis?

1. Hypotonic fluid is instilled into the peritoneal cavity and waste products passively diffuse into it.
2. Sodium and bicarbonate from the dialysate in the peritoneal cavity are exchanged for excess potassium and hydrogen ions from the blood.
3. Increased intra-abdominal pressure caused by the dialysate solution in the abdomen creates a filtration pressure similar to that in the kidney, causing wastes and electrolytes to move out of the blood.
4. Glucose added to the dialysate solution increases the osmotic pressure of the dialysate, causing fluid to move from the blood into the dialysate along with wastes and electrolytes.

**75.** An adult with chronic renal failure is receiving peritoneal dialysis. His acid-base balance and electrolyte levels are now within normal limits. His hemoglobin is 9.2 and his hematocrit is 30. What is the most likely cause for his anemia?

1. Hemodilution secondary to fluid retention.
2. Eating insufficient protein due to taste changes that occur with dialysis.

3. Failure of his kidneys to produce the hormone necessary to stimulate bone marrow to produce red blood cells.

4. Hemolysis of red blood cells as they move past the membrane containing the dialysis solution.

76. An adult is scheduled for an intravenous pyelogram (IVP). What action should the nurse do before sending her to the test?
1. Ask if she is allergic to barium.
2. Ask if she is allergic to shellfish.
3. Give her a full glass of water.
4. Instruct her not to urinate until after the test.

77. A child is recovering from chickenpox. At what point will he be allowed to return to school?
1. After he has been on antibiotics for 48 hours.
2. After his temperature is normal and the itching has subsided.
3. When all lesions are crusted and scabbed.
4. When his skin is clear of all lesions.

78. A woman calls her neighbor, who is a nurse, to say that her 5-year-old has had a stomach virus with vomiting for 24 hours. The doctor recommended the child eat nothing for 4 to 6 hours. There has been no vomiting during that time and now she wants to know what is best to give him. What does the nurse recommend?
1. Broth and water.
2. Flat ginger ale and tea.
3. Jell-O and a soft boiled egg.
4. Skim milk and dry toast.

79. The nurse is assessing a child who is admitted with pyloric stenosis. Which of the following findings is most likely to be reported/observed?
1. The child has greenish-yellow mucus-like emesis that has a strong odor.
2. The vomiting began gradually and then increased until there is no retention of feedings.
3. The infant is content between feedings and shows hesitancy to feed.
4. There is a palpable lump in the epigastrum directly under the xyphoid process.

80. A family is planning a camping trip. The mother calls the clinic to obtain information regarding Lyme disease. Which information is appropriate for the nurse to give? Select all that apply.
___ Wear long pants and long-sleeved shirts when hiking.
___ Use a tick repellent.
___ Inspect hair and skin several times a day for ticks.
___ Look for bites that have a fine petechial rash.

81. An adult is scheduled for a liver biopsy. What should the nurse include when planning the postprocedure care?
1. Administering narcotic analgesics every 3 to 4 hours for the first 24 hours.
2. Positioning her on her right side for at least the first 2 hours.
3. Monitoring for pain referred to the left arm.
4. Changing the dressing over the puncture site frequently, until bile leakage has stopped.

82. The nurse is evaluating whether nonprofessional staff understand how to prevent transmission of HIV. Which of the following behaviors indicates correct application of universal precautions?
1. A lab technician rests his hand on the desk to steady it while recapping the needle after drawing blood.
2. An aide wears gloves to feed a helpless client.
3. An assistant puts on a mask and protective eye wear before assisting the nurse to suction a tracheostomy.
4. A pregnant worker refuses to care for a client known to have AIDS.

83. An adult is ready for discharge following creation of a sigmoid colostomy. Which of the following statements by the client should be evaluated by the nurse as an indication that he has understood his discharge instructions correctly?
1. "I will irrigate the colostomy with tap water every day."
2. "I can eat anything as long as I chew thoroughly."
3. "I will change the pouch every day."
4. "I should not drink more than six glasses of fluid a day."

84. The nurse is caring for a premature 33-week baby girl who is 5 days old and weighs 2000 grams. Which should be included in the nursing care plan?
1. Teach her parents how to do gavage feedings, because the baby has no sucking reflex.
2. Allow the mother to breastfeed when she visits.
3. Inform the parents that the infant will need to stay in an isolette until she is discharged.
4. Instruct the parents on how to take rectal temperatures.

85. The mother of an infant who has had a cleft lip repair has been taught the postoperative care needed. What does the nurse hope to see when evaluating this mother's understanding of this care?

1. Positioning the child on his abdomen to facilitate drainage of oral secretions.
2. Comforting the child as soon as he starts to fuss, to prevent his crying.
3. Using a regular bottle nipple to feed the infant in a semi-reclining position.
4. Cleaning the suture line with warm water and a washcloth once a day.

86. The school nurse is assessing a child who has fallen in the gymnasium. The child exhibits all of the following. Which finding indicates to the nurse that the child most likely has a fracture in addition to soft tissue injury?

1. Localized swelling.
2. Abnormal motion.
3. Ecchymosis.
4. Pain.

87. The nurse is planning care for a 3-year-old child who has just returned to the unit following a cardiac catheterization. The nurse should include which of the following on the care plan?

1. Monitor for response to general anesthetic.
2. Bed rest for 24 hours.
3. NPO for 12 hours.
4. Observe for severe pain and medicate as needed.

88. The school nurse is assisting a school teacher to understand the classroom capabilities of a child with athetoid cerebral palsy. What action will the child most likely demonstrate?

1. Exaggerated hyperactive reflexes.
2. Normal intelligence levels.
3. Slow, worm-like, writhing movements.
4. Unsteady gait and clumsy, uncoordinated upper extremity function.

89. A woman with severe pregnancy-induced hypertension was delivered 2 hours ago. Which nursing action should be included in the plan of care for her postpartum hospital stay?

1. Continuing to monitor blood pressure, respirations, and reflexes.
2. Encouraging frequent family visitors.
3. Keeping her NPO.
4. Maintaining an IV access to the circulatory system.

90. An adult has received one unit of packed red blood cells after sustaining severe trauma to his legs with profuse bleeding. What action will the nurse perform to evaluate the transfusion's effectiveness?

1. Take his blood pressure.
2. Auscultate lung sounds.
3. Check hemoglobin and hematocrit results.
4. Take his temperature.

91. A client who underwent a right total hip replacement arrived on the nursing unit from the post anesthesia care unit at 2 P.M. What should be the initial assessment by the 3 to 11 nurse during initial rounds at change of shift?

1. The dressing.
2. Urine output.
3. Circulation to the leg.
4. Breath sounds.

92. An adult who had gastric surgery is passing large amounts of blood via nasogastric suction. Which finding, if assessed by the nurse, is an early sign of shock?

1. Distended neck veins.
2. Rapid shallow breathing.
3. Bradycardia.
4. Constricted pupils.

93. The nurse is administering tracheostomy care to an adult. Which of the following should be included in the procedure?

1. Soaking the outer cannula with saline solution.
2. Performing the procedure utilizing medical asepsis.
3. Soaking the inner cannula in half-strength hydrogen peroxide solution.
4. Cutting a sterile gauze pad to place between the neck and the tracheostomy tube.

94. Which of the following teachings should the nurse include when establishing a bowel training regimen for a client with chronic constipation?

1. Avoid laxatives.
2. Decrease exercise.
3. Increase the fiber content of your diet.
4. Increase fluid intake 4500 to 5000 mL.

95. Medicare will pay for a limited number of home care visits for clients with hypertension. What must the nurse assess on an elderly hypertensive client on a regular basis?

1. Ability to ambulate.
2. Dehydration.

3. Effectiveness of medication.
4. Awareness of advanced directives.

96. The clinic nurse is teaching the client about breast cancer. Which one of the following risk factors for breast cancer should be assessed regularly by the nurse?
   1. Dietary habits.
   2. Socioeconomic status.
   3. Early menarche.
   4. Being over 30 years of age.

97. The home health nurse is visiting a 90-year-old man who lives with his 88-year-old wife. He is legally blind and suffered a broken hip 5 years ago. He ambulates with difficulty with the aid of a walker. What is the highest priority nursing diagnosis?
   1. Self-care deficit, toileting.
   2. Knowledge deficit regarding blindness.
   3. High risk for injury.
   4. Impaired adjustment.

98. A client with Guillain-Barré syndrome has been on a ventilator for 3 weeks and can communicate only with eye blinks because of quadriplegia. The intensive care nursing staff sometimes have no time for this tedious communication process. The client's family comes infrequently because they run a family-owned restaurant that does not close until visiting hours are over. How should the nurse respond to the family's request for exemption from visiting hours?

1. Arrange for a volunteer to stay with the client during the day to provide for socialization needs and to facilitate communication with staff.
2. Explain to the family that consistency in enforcing rules is important to prevent complaints from the families of other clients.
3. Suggest that the family visit in shifts during the normal visiting hours, because the client needs to sleep at night.
4. Make an exception to visiting regulations because of the long-term nature of the client's recovery and the need for family support.

99. An adult client has congestive heart failure and is receiving spironolactone (Aldactone). Which of the following is least appropriate for the nurse to teach the client about his medication?
   1. Use calcium-based salt substitutes.
   2. Swelling and tenderness of the breasts may occur with long-term therapy.
   3. Take the medicine in the morning if possible.
   4. Include high-potassium foods in the diet to decrease the possibility of hypokalemia.

100. A young child is admitted to the hospital with Tay-Sachs disease. What order can the nurse anticipate that this child will be placed on?
   1. Seizure precautions.
   2. A cooling blanket.
   3. Strict intake and output.
   4. Protective isolation.

# Answers and Rationales for Practice Test 3

| ANSWER | | RATIONALE | NP | CN | CL | SA |
|---|---|---|---|---|---|---|
| #1. | 1. | Pain from a duodenal ulcer is often aching or burning in character, and occurs when the stomach is empty. It is likely to occur in the mid-upper abdomen, whereas pain in the epigastric/shoulder area is characteristic of gallbladder disease and pain in the midsternal area with cardiac problems. | As | Ph/7 | An | 1 |
| #2. | 2. | The squatting position serves to decrease venous return by occluding the femoral vein through hip flexion, to lessen the workload on the right side of the heart, and to increase arterial oxygen saturation. Returning the child to bed or placing in a chair would not lessen the heart's workload as the squatting does. The physician would already be aware of this condition. | Im | Ph/7 | Ap | 4 |

| ANSWER | RATIONALE | NP | CN | CL | SA |
|--------|-----------|-----|-----|-----|-----|
| #3. 3. | The fibrosed liver obstructs flow through portal vessels, which normally receive all blood circulating from the gastrointestinal tract. The increased pressure in portal vessels shunts some of the blood into the lower pressure veins around the lower esophagus. Because these veins are not designed to handle the high-pressure portal blood flow, they develop varicosities, which often rupture and bleed. | An | Ph/8 | An | 1 |
| #4. 4. | Administration of blood and fluid is vital in maintaining blood volume in a client with severe gastrointestinal bleeding. Vital signs would need to be monitored more frequently than hourly. A client with severe bleeding would have decreased urine output, so the bedpan would not be used frequently as with diuretics and the gastric pH is not related to the client's fluid needs. | Pl | Ph/8 | An | 1 |
| #5. 2. | When going up steps the client must always provide for either the crutches or the unaffected leg to be bearing his weight at all times. Moving the unaffected leg up first allows the strong leg muscle of the unaffected leg to do the lifting to raise him to the next step. The other choices involve positions that would place the arms trying to lift the body, cause the client to lean and be off balance or sitting down which would be difficult to raise back up; all placing the client at risk for falling. | Im | Ph/5 | Ap | 1 |
| #6. 2. | Oxygenation is the most important immediate goal. Remember the ABCs of client care. The other choices are appropriate goals, but not as important as oxygenation. | Pl | Ph/7 | Ap | 1 |
| #7. 3. | Children ages 3 to 5 often think of death as sleep or a departure. To them, death is reversible. Children ages 5 to 9 view death as irreversible and permanent; children ages 7 to 10 view death as inevitable and final. Teenagers view life in the present and can become angry at the injustice of death. | An | He/3 | An | 4 |
| #8. 4. | To prevent reinfection, the entire prescribed antibiotic needs to be taken, with a course of treatment lasting 7 to 10 days. Acetaminophen is the drug of choice instead of aspirin; heat helps to decrease pain. | Im | Ph/6 | Ap | 4 |
| #9. 3. | The delivery of room air and oxygen will keep carbon dioxide levels decreasing, preventing hypoxia. The humidity will prevent the drying of the mucous membranes and subsequent edema. The tent can be opened or even remain open with the understanding that the treatment will not be as effective. | Pl | Ph/7 | Ap | 4 |
| #10. 3. | The nurse would be looking for *objective* signs which would be a positive urine test. Morning sickness would be a subjective sign; urinary frequency could also be a sign of a urinary tract infection; and fetal heart tones would not be auscultated this early. | As | He/3 | An | 3 |

| ANSWER | RATIONALE | NP | CN | CL | SA |
|---|---|---|---|---|---|
| #11. | March 22. Nägele's rule for calculating the estimated date of confinement (EDC) or birth is to add 7 days to the first day of the last menstrual period, subtract 3 months, and add 1 year. | As | He/3 | Ap | 3 |
| #12. 1. | In pregnancy, constipation results from decreased gastric motility and increased water reabsorption in the colon caused by increased levels of progesterone. Prenatal vitamins have iron in them, which also contributes to constipation. The best instruction is to increase fluid intake and to avoid laxatives as they may cause cramping. | Pl | He/3 | Ap | 3 |
| #13. 4. | Supportive stockings will help circulate blood flow back to the heart because the nurse will be standing for most of the shift. They will also help prevent varicose veins. It would be beneficial to drink more than 1 liter for the entire shift; elevation could be done at home, but not usually done on a working shift; proper body mechanics would entail pushing objects, not pulling them. | Pl | Ph/7 | An | 1 |
| #14. 1. | These signs and symptoms describe the transition phase of labor. | An | He/3 | Co | 3 |
| #15. 1. | Gentle massage of the uterine fundus is indicated. The bladder, lochia, fundal firmness and placement should be assessed. If uterine atony is not resolved, the physician or midwife should be called for further evaluation. | Im | He/3 | Ap | 3 |
| #16. 4. | There is risk of infection from saline abortion because saline is injected into the amniotic sac. The woman also may labor at length with ruptured membranes. The elevated temperature and blood pressure are associated with infection. | An | Ph/7 | An | 3 |
| #17. 3. | Vaginal discharge can be from Chlamydia infection and can be seen in conjunction with other infections such as gonorrhea or trichomonas. Cultures and blood studies are needed and contacting a physician is necessary. | Im | Ph/6 | Ap | 3 |
| #18. 1. | The discharge would also be foul-smelling, Choice 2 is associated with monilia infection; warts or ulcers are usually seen in herpes simplex virus types I and II and in syphilis. | As | Ph/7 | Co | 3 |
| #19. | Nine (9). The baby gets 2 points for full flexion of the extremities, 1 point for being acrocyanotic, 2 points for heart rate, 2 points for respirations (full, lusty cry), and 2 points for resisting the suction catheter. | As | He/3 | Ap | 3 |
| #20. 1. | The most common side effect of epidural anesthesia is a sudden drop in material blood pressure, which can compromise fetal blood flow. | Ev | Ph/6 | An | 3 |
| #21. 1. | When a person with weakness on one side uses a cane, there should always be two points of contact with the floor. When the client moves the cane forward, she has both feet on the floor. As she moves the weak leg, the cane and the strong leg provide support. Finally, the cane, which is even with the weak leg, provides stability while she moves the strong leg. | Ev | Ph/5 | An | 1 |

| ANSWER | RATIONALE | NP | CN | CL | SA |
|--------|-----------|-----|-----|-----|-----|
| #22. 4. | Supine position would provide less room for lung expansion and cause increased pressure of abdominal organs. The most beneficial position would be semi-Fowler's to allow for lung expansion. | Pl | Ph/7 | Co | 1 |
| #23. 1. | These are characteristics seen with someone taking hallucinogens. The other choices are characteristic of opioid use, Parkinson's, and PCP, respectively. | As | Ps/4 | An | 2 |
| #24. 3. | The cohesiveness is apparent in the group. Joining or leaving the group results in strong emotions due to disruption of the sharing group. In the beginning phase, members are getting to know each other, transition is not a phase in group process; termination phase may bring various emotions, but not what is described. | An | Ps/4 | An | 2 |
| #25. 3. | Denial is the blocking out of thoughts or feelings perceived as painful. Projection is blaming others; repression is a forgotten memory; and displacement is the expression of emotion on to another person or object. | As | Ps/4 | Co | 1 |
| #26. 3. | Suicide attempts are more common on evenings, night shift or weekends when the unit structure is lessened. The client feels threatened from her husband's actions and is expressing "tunnel vision" in regards to her situation. The safety of the client is the first concern and all suicidal remarks and gestures must be taken seriously. Therapeutic sessions will be held at a later time. | Im | Ps/4 | Ap | 2 |
| #27. 1. | All the findings suggest diabetic ketoacidosis. However, a negative answer does not rule out diabetes. The other choices would include a seizure noted; or manifestations of increased intracranial pressure (slow, labored respirations, bradycardia, pupillary dysfunction, changes in motor function); a drug overdose would present with shallow respiration, constricted pupils, and circulatory collapse. | An | Ph/8 | An | 4 |
| #28. 4. | Hematochezia (blood in the stool) may come from a source in either the upper or lower GI tract. The client's past medial history will aid in determining the location of the bleeding, as the others will not suggest a location. | As | He/3 | An | 1 |
| #29. 1. | In herniation of the disc, the nucleus of the disc protrudes into the annulus, which causes pain in the nerve distribution. Paraspinal muscles are next to the spine and spasms will cause the muscles to tighten up, causing a painful, burning sensation; the third choice is related to arthritis of the spine in which pain comes and goes; edema and swelling occur after a spinal cord injury. | An | Ph/8 | Co | 1 |
| #30. 4. | Hypothermia with cardiac arrhythmias may occur when infusing the large quantities needed in GI bleeding. Blood warming equipment should be used to prevent this problem. | Im | Ph/6 | Ap | 1 |
| #31. 1. | Gout, or gouty arthritis, is a systemic disease in which urate crystals are deposited in joints and other body tissues. | An | Ph/7 | Co | 1 |

| ANSWER | RATIONALE | NP | CN | CL | SA |
|---|---|---|---|---|---|
| | Elevated uric acid levels occur as a result of improper metabolism of purines, resulting in excessive production of uric acid, which the kidneys are unable to adequately eliminate. It is not an infection; osteoarthritis is a destruction of bone and cartilage; bursitis is an inflammation of the bursa and is usually the result of trauma or strain to the joint. | | | | |
| #32. 4. | Fluid restrictions should be implemented to reduce excess vascular volume. The other activities do not affect the edematous state. | Pl | Ph/7 | Ap | 1 |
| #33. 1. | Active and passive leg exercises are important with clients on bed rest as a method of preventing thrombophlebitis. It will be therapeutic to allow the client to verbalize her feelings about fatigue or other problems associated with the disease process. | As | Ph/7 | An | 1 |
| #34. 2. | Left-sided failure caused by ventricular dysfunction, results in increased pressure in the pulmonary veins, which leads to the development of rales. Choices 3 and 4 are associated with right-sided heart failure, and tachycardia would be present in both. | As | Ph/8 | An | 1 |
| #35. 4. | Digitalis toxicity would include nausea/vomiting, irregular pulse, diarrhea, and yellow vision. | Ev | Ph/6 | Ap | 5 |
| #36. 2. | Normal serum potassium levels are 3.5–5.3 mEq/L. Immediate interventions are required for all the other levels and the physician should be notified. The client also should be placed on cardiac monitoring. | An | Ph/7 | An | 1 |
| #37. 3. | Weight loss occurs through excessive extracellular fluid loss, meconium loss, and limited food intake. Infants take in small amounts of feedings and energy expenditure exceeds intake. | An | He/3 | An | 3 |
| #38. 3. | Glucagon is the drug of choice in the treatment of hypoglycemia due to excess insulin when the client cannot safely take glucose by mouth. Glucagon begins to raise the blood sugar within 5 minutes, whereby raising the level of consciousness to allow the client to eat carbohydrates. | Im | Ph/6 | Ap | 4 |
| #39. 1. | Coughing is necessary to move retained secretions. A sling is not necessary, whereas arm and shoulder exercises are to be performed to regain previous range of motion; the dressing will be on the thoracic area and not the groin (as in a cardiac catherization); a Passy-muir is an assistive device used after a tracheostomy for speaking purposes. | Im | Ph/8 | Ap | 4 |
| #40. 1. | Normal height is 29–32 inches; normal weight is between 19 and 27 pounds. | An | He/3 | An | 4 |
| #41. 4. | The parents should be encouraged to foster normal socialization of their child. Parents may need additional information regarding fears they may have. Resting periods while feeding and engaging in quiet activities will reduce energy expenditure; a good diet will foster growth and development. | Ev | He/3 | An | 4 |

| ANSWER | | RATIONALE | NP | CN | CL | SA |
|---|---|---|---|---|---|---|
| #42. | 1. | Applying pressure to allow for clot formation is the initial action. | Im | Ph/8 | Ap | 4 |
| #43. | 4. | The fourth stage of labor is the first hour or two after delivery and is a critical period for maternal systems to stabilize after giving birth. The other choices are in various other stages of labor. | Pl | He/3 | An | 3 |
| #44. | 1. | The plan is to reduce secondary gain, which is the avoidance of an unpleasant activity. Focusing on symptoms only promotes secondary gain. Somatic symptoms are perceived as real to the client and not under voluntary control. Goals would be to show an interest in the client rather than symptoms and to foster independence. | Pl | Ps/4 | Ap | 2 |
| #45. | 4. | Splitting is the primitive defense mechanism, seen in clients with borderline personality disorder, that presents as an inability to integrate both good and bad aspects of self and others into an integrated whole. This results in both an idealization and a devaluation of others and self. | As | Ps/4 | An | 2 |
| #46. | 1. | Denial is often used for maintaining self-esteem when control is lost. The physician should have been monitoring the situation closer to prevent its occurrence. | An | Ps/4 | An | 2 |
| #47. | 2. | The Medic Alert bracelet is essential to warn health care providers that his adrenals have been removed and that glucocorticoid and mineralocorticoid replacement is essential for life. Failure to supply replacement doses will precipitate severe hypotension, shock, coma, and vasomotor collapse. Careful adjustment of the replacement hormones can prevent the "moon face," weight gain, and edema that is associated with steroid use. | Ev | Ph/7 | An | 1 |
| #48. | 2. | Sandra needs to be relieved from her duties, as client safety is the primary concern. Notifying the supervisor will be the secondary measure, as the supervisor may not be available right away. Ignoring the situation is against the professional code of conduct for nurses and Sandra would not benefit from a lecture in her condition. | Im | Sa/1 | Ap | 1 |
| #49. | 4. | With reduced levels of anxiety, the client's perceptual field broadens, allowing the client to focus on the cause of anxiety and to connect the cause with his anxious response. He is able to learn from the experience. High levels of anxiety, as expressed in the other choices, prevent this from occurring. | Ev | Ps/4 | Ap | 2 |
| #50. | 2. | Clients with a T4 injury will have sufficient upper extremity strength to master the technique of independent transfer and not need an electric wheelchair. Given the level of the spinal injury, he will not be walking, but will still be able to do a great deal. | As | Ph/7 | An | 1 |
| #51. | 3. | Bladder distention may cause urinary tract infections, distention of the ureters and renal pelvis, and autonomic dysreflexia. Checking for bladder distention should be | Im | Ph/7 | Ap | 1 |

| ANSWER | RATIONALE | NP | CN | CL | SA |
|--------|-----------|----|----|----|----|
| | done every 3–4 hours and assessing whether intermittent self-catherization is required, especially if this is on a scheduled basis. The Valsalva maneuver can help to expel urine, but is dangerous for clients with cardiovascular disease. Cleaning is only necessary 2–3 times a day and fluid intake of 2500 mL/day is encouraged. | | | | |
| #52. 2. | The goal with this client is to prevent incontinence by having the client control defecation. The client should not need laxatives, nor expect a bowel movement every day. | Ev | Ph/7 | An | 1 |
| #53. 4. | The muscle spasm indicates that the Valium is not effective as a muscle relaxant. Choices 1 and 3 are possible side effects of Valium. Hyperesthesia (sensitivity to touch or painful stimuli) is not seen with Valium administration. | Ev | Ph/6 | An | 1 |
| #54. 3. | The cane should be held in the hand opposite the affected leg and should be advanced at the same time as the weak leg is advanced to maximize support. | Ev | Ph/5 | An | 1 |
| #55. 3. | Catsup, like all canned tomato products, is high in sodium and should be avoided. The cooked cereals are low in sodium; broccoli is high in vitamins A, K, calcium, and fiber and should be eaten regularly; sugar may be restricted if weight reduction is desired or diabetes is present. | Pl | Ph/5 | Ap | 1 |
| #56. 3. | A decrease in systolic blood pressure when the client moves from a lying to a standing position is evaluated and will result in the client reporting dizziness (also known as postural hypotension). A neurological exam would be performed for CNS depression; malignant HTN is characterized by elevated BP in both standing and lying positions; vascular insufficiency involves occlusion of vessels with atherosclerotic plaques. | Im | He/3 | Co | 1 |
| #57. 3. | The client must work hard to breathe, so the plan of care should structure a balance between rest and activity. | Pl | Ph/7 | Ap | 1 |
| #58. 4. | Abdominal breathing elevates the diaphragm, thereby improving breathing effectiveness in clients with COPD. | Ev | Ph/7 | An | 1 |
| #59. 1. | Because of the burning pain upon application, an analgesic may be required before ointment application. Sulfamylon is a strong carbonic anhydrase inhibitor that affects the renal tubular buffering system, resulting in metabolic acidosis. | Im | Ph/6 | Co | 1 |
| #60. 4. | Fluids are a primary intervention to replace lost fluids and prevent irreversible shock. The critical hours after the burn are characterized by a rapid shift of fluid from the vascular compartment into interstitial spaces. As the burns are located on the lower extremities, the client is not at risk for pulmonary inhalation problems. After the primary goals are met, then care of the wounds and infection begins, usually 48–72 hours once the client has stabilized. Dealing with the psychological aspects of disfiguring of a burn is a long-term goal. | An | Ph/8 | An | 1 |

| ANSWER | RATIONALE | NP | CN | CL | SA |
|--------|-----------|----|----|----|----|
| #61. 4. | The epidermis and dermis are destroyed in full thickness burns. Because the nerve endings are destroyed, there is an absence of pain. | An | Ph/8 | An | 1 |
| #62. 4. | By developing an identity the client is able to reckon with negative and positive feelings to establish self-esteem. This should provide motivation to cope. | An | Ps/4 | An | 2 |
| #63. 2. | The client experiencing depersonalization sees herself as changed or the situation as unreal. It is essential to orient the client to the unit to create a sense of reality and security in her environment. | Pl | Ps/4 | Ap | 2 |
| #64. 2. | Delusions are fixed false beliefs. The nurse focuses on reality aspects of communication in an effort to promote health rather than focus on delusions, which could become further entrenched. The nurse should not disprove or agree with the delusion. | Im | Ps/4 | Ap | 2 |
| #65. 2. | The intensity of the ideas of reference has diminished, showing improvement in the client's delusional thinking. The other choices reflect auditory hallucination, phobia, and illusions. | Ev | Ps/4 | An | 2 |
| #66. 2. | In nephritic syndrome, plasma proteins are excreted in the urine due to an abnormal permeability of the glomerular basement membrane of the kidney to protein molecules, particularly albumin. The cause of nephrosis is unknown, with the average age of onset at 2½ years, more commonly in boys than girls. Blood pressure and dark urine is not associated in nephritic syndrome. A history of strep infection is associated with glomerulonephritis. | As | Ph/8 | An | 4 |
| #67. 1. | The primary goal in the treatment of nephritic syndrome is to control edema. Diuretics are used to promote diuresis and subsequent weight loss. Corticosteroids are also given. A decrease will be seen in the sedimentation rate and urine specific gravity; temperature elevations are not common. | Ev | Ph/8 | An | 4 |
| #68. 3. | The best technique for handling temper tantrums includes being consistent, remaining calm, and ignoring the behavior. It is advisable to explain to the child how to act in the store before entering and to have one or more "trial runs" in educating the child how to behave in a public place. | Im | He/3 | Ap | 4 |
| #69. 2. | As a result of placenta maturation and placental production of lactogen, insulin requirements begin increasing in the 2nd trimester and may double or even quadruple by the end of pregnancy. Newer glucometers allow blood glucose to be taken from other areas beside the fingers only. | Ev | Ph/6 | An | 3 |
| #70. 2. | Rho (D) immune globulin is given to prevent maternal sensitization by promoting destruction of Rh positive red blood cells circulating in the mother's bloodstream. Two of the criteria for administration of the Rho (D) immune globulin are: Rho (D) negative mother without Rh antibodies (nonsensitized) and an Rho (D) positive infant. | An | Ph/6 | An | 3 |

| ANSWER | RATIONALE | NP | CN | CL | SA |
|---|---|---|---|---|---|
| #71. 4. | Intravenous Pitocin should produce progressive cervical dilation with contractions lasting no longer than 90 seconds. Longer contractions may be dangerous to the unborn baby. | Ev | Ph/6 | An | 5 |
| #72. 3. | The infant has signs of hypoglycemia: tremors, irritability, and a decreased respiratory rate. Checking the blood sugar is necessary to determine whether hypoglycemia is the problem before any other interventions are done. | Im | Ph/7 | Ap | 3 |
| #73. 1. | Paresthesias, such as numbness or tingling occur when compression of the tissues deprives the nerves of part of the circulation or when something presses directly on the nerve. The capillary refill is normally 5 seconds or less; dull aching would be expected. | Ev | Ph/7 | An | 1 |
| #74. 4. | This is the correct explanation of peritoneal dialysis (PD), in which it removes toxic substances from the body. PD can be dangerous and may cause death if not done with adequate supervision of body fluid and electrolyte balance. | An | Ph/8 | An | 1 |
| #75. 3. | In chronic renal failure the hormone, erthythropoietin, is not produced, which stimulates red blood cell production. The trade name is Epogen. Hemodilution can produce a drop in hematocrit, however sodium would also be lower, which it is not in this case. Renal clients need to monitor their protein intake. Hemolysis does not occur as RBCs do not move outside the client's own blood vessels. | An | Ph/8 | An | 1 |
| #76. 2. | Dye is injected intravenously, and it contains iodine. Allergy to shellfish often reflects iodine allergy and would place the client at high risk. If this is the case, the physician would need to be notified for further orders. | As | Ph/7 | Ap | 1 |
| #77. 3. | Once chickenpox lesions are crusted over, they are no longer infectious. Antibiotics are not ordered. | Ev | Sa/2 | Ap | 4 |
| #78. 2. | These are well tolerated and not irritating to the gastrointestinal tract after a stomach virus. Broth could be irritating and the other choices are harder to digest. | Pl | Ph/5 | Ap | 4 |
| #79. 2. | Although there is variability in the pattern and type of vomiting, it usually starts gradually, rather than suddenly and becomes more projectile (1 to 4 feet away) and more frequent with the tightening and further obstruction of the pyloric channel. It takes about 4 to 6 weeks for complete obstruction to occur. Greenish-color emesis is indicative of an obstruction below the stomach level; an infant will want to feed after a vomitus episode. | As | Ph/8 | An | 4 |
| #80. 1,2,4 | All are correct except a Lyme disease rash is characterized by a papule with a circular border, known as the "bull's eye rash." | Pl | He/3 | Ap | 4 |
| #81. 2. | The client will need to be positioned on her right side for the first 2 hours or longer, to put pressure on the liver. Pressure will decrease the bleeding from the very vascular liver and also reduce leakage of bile into the peritoneal cavity (which would not be present on the outside of the body). Pain, which | Pl | Ph/7 | Ap | 1 |

| ANSWER | RATIONALE | NP | CN | CL | SA |
|--------|-----------|----|----|----|----|

may be referred to the right shoulder, should not persist
up to 24 hours, nor be severe enough to require narcotics.
The pressure dressing on the site should be not disturbed,
and bile leakage would be an abnormal finding.

**#82. 3.** Universal precautions will be utilized with all clients, and always if there is a risk the transmission of blood and body fluids. The other choices are inappropriate for the situation given, unless blood/body fluids are going to be a transmission risk.  — Ev | Sa/2 | Ap | 1

**#83. 2.** There are no dietary restrictions with a colostomy, but high flatulence foods may be limited due to the odor produced. Irrigation should only be used as an enema would be used; the pouch should last 3 to 5 days to prevent skin excoriation; and fluid intake should be encouraged to prevent constipation.  — Ev | Ph/7 | Ap | 1

**#84. 2.** At 33 weeks, the infant's sucking reflex is developed and breastfeeding should be encouraged if this is the mother's wish. The move to a crib is appropriate, rectal temps are avoided due to the risk of perforation.  — Pl | He/3 | Ap | 3

**#85. 2.** Crying pulls the edges of the suture line and may widen the scar line. The baby should be prevented from crying as much as possible by keeping the infant's needs met and providing postoperative analgesia. Prone position is avoided as the infant can move the face back and forth on the bed, putting tension on the sutures and Logan bar. Drainage secretions are suctioned by a bulb syringe or placing the infant on his side. Special nipples are available to allow closure of the jaw without damaging the lip repair. Cleaning is performed as a sterile procedure with the use of cotton applications dipped in saline (as ordered).  — Ev | Ph/7 | Ap | 4

**#86. 2.** Following a fracture or break in a bone, the extremity cannot be used and tends to move unnaturally instead of remaining rigid as it normally would. Swelling, ecchymosis, and pain does not differentiate between a fracture or a soft tissue injury, as they are present in all.  — As | Ph/8 | An | 4

**#87. 2.** The prolonged bed rest is to prevent bleeding at catherization insertion site. Mild sedation, not general anesthesia, is used; fluids are encouraged to flush out the injected dye; pain would not be an expected syndrome.  — Pl | Ph/7 | Ap | 4

**#88. 3.** Athetoid cerebral palsy (CP) is characterized by involuntary, purposeless movements. Normal intelligence is common in this type of disorder; hyperactive reflexes and unsteady gait are seen with spastic CP.  — As | Ph/7 | Co | 4

**#89. 1.** Post delivery management of the mother includes close observation for BP elevation, CNS irritability (visitors are limited), and respiratory function. The client is at risk for seizure for 24 hours after delivery.  — Pl | He/3 | Co | 3

| ANSWER | RATIONALE | NP | CN | CL | SA |
|---|---|---|---|---|---|
| #90. 3. | Hemoglobin and hematocrit are expected to rise. All the other choices are interventions that are performed during the transfusion. | Ev | Ph/6 | An | 1 |
| #91. 4. | Respiratory function is always of prime importance in assessing a postoperative client. The other choices are essential also, after the respiratory assessment. Post-operative clients are at risk for pneumonia and pulmonary embolism. | As | Ph/7 | Ap | 1 |
| #92. 2. | Shock is a syndrome in which the peripheral blood flow is inadequate to return sufficient blood to the heart for normal function. The most outstanding symptoms are skin paleness, cyanosis, staring of the eyes, pulse weak and rapid, and rapid breathing rate is increased and shallow. | As | Ph/8 | Ap | 1 |
| #93. 3. | Using a sterile technique, the inner cannula is removed utilizing sterile gauze and is soaked in the hydrogen peroxide solution, cleaned with a small brush/pipe cleaner, then rinsed with normal saline and dried. Outer cannulas are not removed; gauze is not cut due to risk of filaments working their way into the stoma. | Im | Ph/7 | Ap | 1 |
| #94. 3. | Bowel training is to manipulate factors within the client's control (food, fluid, exercise, time for defecation) to produce the elimination of a soft formed stool at regular intervals. Chronic laxative use will create a dependency on them. | Im | Ph/5 | Ap | 1 |
| #95. 3. | In clients with cardiovascular disease, the effectiveness of medications, as well as side effects, should be monitored. This is the highest priority. The others are related to management of hypertension. | As | He/3 | Ap | 1 |
| #96. 1. | Dietary habits is the only risk factor that can be assessed. A high-fat diet put the woman at risk for breast cancer as well as other cancer, so a high-fiber, low-fat diet is recommended. | As | He/3 | Ap | 1 |
| #97. 3. | The fact that the client is legally blind and has difficulty ambulating place him at extreme risk for injury. | An | Sa/2 | Ap | 1 |
| #98. 4. | Guillain-Barré syndrome is characterized by the onset of ascending paralysis, which may include respiratory muscles. The client may be ventilator-dependent for weeks but may have full consciousness. The prognosis is good but dependent upon the level of supportive care during the acute stage. | Im | Sa/1 | Ap | 1 |
| #99. 4. | Aldactone is a potassium sparing diuretic so dietary potassium should be limited, not increased. Substitutes used should contain calcium versus potassium; breast swelling may occur with long-term therapy; morning administration prevents sleep deprivation due to voiding. | Pl | Ph/6 | An | 5 |
| #100. 1. | Tay-Sachs disease is a degenerative neurologic disorder, which is often characterized by seizures. The other choices are not indicated for this disease. | Pl | Ph/7 | An | 4 |

# Practice Test 4

1. Which statement by the client would suggest the client has hyperthyroidism?
   1. "I feel more nervous than usual."
   2. "I have had to wear a sweater all the time."
   3. "My appetite has really been decreased lately."
   4. "Should I be taking a laxative to prevent this constipation?"

2. An 8-year-old is admitted with rheumatic fever. Which clinical finding indicates to the nurse that the client needs to continue taking the salicylates he had received at home?
   1. Chorea.
   2. Polyarthritis.
   3. Subcutaneous nodules.
   4. Erythema marginatum.

3. The nurse is caring for a client with advanced cancer of the breast. She complains of hypoguesia. What recommendation should the nurse give?
   1. Eating dry crackers.
   2. Monitoring intake and output.
   3. Using spices to enhance food flavors.
   4. Weighing her before and after meals.

4. An adult is admitted to the hospital to undergo a stapedectomy for the treatment of otosclerosis. Which findings elicited during physical assessment are most indicative of otosclerosis?
   1. Bone conduction is greater than air conduction.
   2. Bone conduction is equal to air conduction.
   3. Air conduction is greater than bone conduction.
   4. Sound lateralizes to the unaffected ear.

5. The nurse is caring for a client who has had a stapedectomy. What will be appropriate postoperative communication by the nursing staff?
   1. Overarticulate.
   2. Shout in the affected ear.
   3. Speak at a moderate rate.
   4. Use long, easily understood phrases.

6. A 4-year-old has been blind since birth. She has been attending a nursery program for the visually impaired. When her lunch tray arrives, what action by the nurse will continue independence in her ADLs?
   1. Offer to feed her.
   2. Explain that foods on her tray are set up like a clock.
   3. Put food on her fork and hand her the fork.
   4. Tell her that two foods are in front of her, one at the top of the tray and one at the bottom.

7. A nurse identifies that an infant displays the abduction, extension, and adduction of arms to an embracing position when startled. How would this finding be explained to the parent?
   1. "This is a normal occurrence of the Babinski reflex."
   2. "Your child needs to see a neurologist."
   3. "This is called the Moro reflex and disappears around 3–4 months."
   4. "Placing your child on his abdomen will help reduce these twitches."

8. Discharge instructions are given to a woman who had been admitted with placenta previa. Which statement by the client to her husband best demonstrates she understands the teaching?
   1. "We can't have sex."
   2. "I have to return in a few days for a vaginal exam."
   3. "I will have to have a cesarean for this and other pregnancies."
   4. "I can go back to part-time work beginning tomorrow."

9. Which of these statements would be appropriate for a nurse to give to a client who is scheduled to have surgery in 15 minutes?
   1. "You need to remove your underwear now."
   2. "You may have sips of water for that dry mouth."
   3. "Let me show you how to use an incentive spirometer (IS)."
   4. "How long have you smoked?"

10. A young adult is involuntarily admitted to the psychiatric unit in a manic state. Upon arrival on the unit he is unable to sit, he is very difficult to understand because of his rapid rate of speech, and he refuses to eat or drink. What area of disturbance poses the greatest physical danger to this client?

1. Activity.
2. Perceptual.
3. Sensory.
4. Social.

11. A young man was arrested by the police for indecent exposure, loitering, and disturbing the peace. He was also reported stripping off his clothes at his mother's grave (who has been deceased for 12 years). Upon admittance to the psychiatric unit, he was speaking rapidly, refusing food or drink, and refusing to sit. Which nursing diagnosis would describe the behavior that is of greatest concern?

1. Anxiety.
2. Potential for violence.
3. Spiritual distress.
4. Alteration in nutrition: less than body requirements.

12. A young woman with a history of bipolar disorder is admitted to the psychiatric unit. She is talking excitedly and walking rapidly around the unit. What intervention would most likely be initiated during the initial period of hospitalization?

1. Encourage the client to participate in group and therapeutic activities.
2. Observe the client closely until she calms down.
3. Place the client in four-point restraints for protection of self and others.
4. Place the client in seclusion but maintain frequent one-to-one contact with her.

13. Which of the following is least likely to influence the potential for a client to comply with lithium therapy after discharge?

1. The impact of lithium on the client's energy level and lifestyle.
2. The need for consistent blood level monitoring.
3. The potential side effects of lithium.
4. What the client's friends think of his need to take medication.

14. A teen who is 20 weeks pregnant has attended a prenatal nutrition course at her high school. Which meal chosen by the female would warrant further instruction on proper protein intake?

1. Roast chicken sandwich and ice cream cone.
2. Roast beef sandwich and vanilla pudding.
3. Fruit salad with cottage cheese and frozen yogurt.
4. Bacon, lettuce, and tomato sandwich and an apple.

15. The nurse in the delivery room is caring for the newborn. Which action is the most important and most immediate action for the nurse to take?

1. Do the Apgar score.
2. Dry the baby completely.
3. Place identification bracelets on the infant and the mother.
4. Prevent infection by doing eye care.

16. The nurse caring for a mother who is breastfeeding her full-term 2-day-old baby boy instructed her on proper breast care this morning and wishes to evaluate her learning. Which of the following would demonstrate that the mother has an adequate knowledge base?

1. She states she should not be concerned if hard lumps develop in her breasts at home because engorgement may cause lumps.
2. She states she will continue to feed the infant as she has been, even if mild skin breakdown occurs on the nipple.
3. She assesses her nipples carefully before and after each feeding.
4. She states she does not have to worry about good hand washing because her baby is not premature.

17. The nurse is caring for a 30-weeks gestation baby girl who is currently receiving 15 mL of breast milk via oral gastric tube every 3 hours. As part of the routine assessment the nurse should assess which of the following?

1. Assess for heme in the stool at each bowel movement.
2. Assess abdominal girth once every 3 days.
3. Assess for residual once per shift.
4. Assess for tube placement once every 24 hours.

18. The nurse is caring for a 2-week-old baby who is showing clinical manifestations of heart murmur, widened pulse pressure, cardiomegaly, bounding pulses, and tachycardia. The assessment findings indicate that which of the following shunt systems from fetal circulation has failed to close?

1. Ductus venosus.
2. Ductus arteriosus.

3. Ligamentum arteriosum.

4. Foramen ovale.

19. The nurse is caring for a 48-hour full-term infant whose mother abused cocaine and heroin throughout pregnancy. The mother does not wish to go into rehabilitation at this time. The nursing care plan should include which of the following?

1. Feeding the infant whenever the infant cries or acts hungry.

2. Allowing extra time to assist the woman with breastfeeding and promote attachment.

3. Organizing all necessary care around feeding times.

4. Covering the baby loosely with a blanket to allow the body to cool down from the fever.

20. A mother brings her baby in for his 1-month checkup. The mother reports that she has difficulty spreading the baby's right leg when she is diapering him. The nurse suspects a dislocated hip. Further assessment for the possibility of a dislocated hip on the right side would include what observation?

1. Absence of Ortolani's sign.

2. Presence of Trendelenburg's sign.

3. An increase in skin folds on the unaffected side.

4. Shortening of the affected femur when supine with knees bent.

21. A client is receiving intravenous (IV) therapy for correction of a fluid volume deficit. Which observation by the nurse indicates infiltration of the IV has occurred?

1. Pallor at the infusion site.

2. Increased temperature at the infusion site.

3. Erythema around the infusion insertion device.

4. Seepage of blood around the infusion insertion device.

22. An adult woman is admitted to an isolation unit in the hospital after tuberculosis was detected during a pre-employment physical. Which method would be responsible for the contamination?

1. Hands.

2. Droplet nuclei.

3. Milk products.

4. Eating utensils.

23. An adult is receiving rifampin (Rifadin). Teaching by the nurse should include alerting the client to which of the following common side effects?

1. Vertigo.

2. Skin rash.

3. Tingling in the feet.

4. Orange-tinged body fluids.

24. The nurse is caring for an elderly woman who has been admitted to the hospital. The woman is upset and confused and repeatedly tells the nurse she is worried about being constipated while in the hospital. Which question by the nurse would elicit information about the client's bowel status?

1. "Do you realize you are confused?"

2. "What laxative do you take at home?"

3. "When was your last bowel movement?"

4. "Why are you so worried about your bowels?"

25. An elderly client has had Buck's traction applied while awaiting surgery for repair of a fractured left hip. Which intervention must be included in the plan of care?

1. Turn from side to side every 2 hours.

2. Maintain high-Fowler's position.

3. Remove boot every shift.

4. Use footboard to position left foot.

26. The nurse is caring for a client who has just returned to the nursing unit from the recovery room (postanesthesia care unit) after surgery. What is the first action the nurse should perform?

1. Take vital signs.

2. Administer pain medication.

3. Connect drainage systems.

4. Check dressings.

27. An adult client received a kidney transplant 8 days ago. During this first period when an acute rejection of the kidney could occur, what is an essential assessment?

1. Increased output of very dilute urine.

2. Hypotension.

3. Anemia.

4. Fever.

28. What advice by the school nurse would ensure a safe health care environment for the child with impetigo?

1. "You need to see your doctor this week to get started on some antibiotics so the sores on your face will clear up."

2. "It's O.K. to share personal items, such as towels, with the rest of the family, because good handwashing will prevent the spread of impetigo."

3. "Be sure to drink 6 to 8 glasses of fluid each day and let me know right away if your urine turns dark like the color of cola."

4. "If the itching bothers you, put some rubbing alcohol on your face several times a day."

29. A male client is admitted to the emergency department with a medical diagnosis of closed-angle glaucoma. He is placed on miotic therapy and receives 75% glycerin (Glycol). In planning care for the client, which of the following should be a teaching priority during the acute phase of his illness?

    1. Eyedrop administration.
    2. Eye patch changes every hour.
    3. Measuring intake and output.
    4. Keeping bright lights on in the room.

30. Which nursing action represents unsafe nursing care for a client with closed-angle glaucoma?

    1. Administering morphine sulfate 8 mg IM prn for pain.
    2. Allowing him to ambulate to the bathroom with assistance.
    3. Occluding the puncta during the administration of eye drops.
    4. Wearing unsterile gloves when examining the eye.

31. A client who has glaucoma is receiving pilocarpine (Pilocar). Which of these statements would assure the nurse that the client understands the reason for treatment?

    1. "It will reduce my intraocular pressure."
    2. "It will improve my vision."
    3. "It will relieve the pain."
    4. "It will restore my peripheral vision."

32. An elderly man has closed-angle glaucoma. He tells the nurse that he has heard that glaucoma may be hereditary. When he expresses concern about his children, which is the most appropriate response for the nurse to make?

    1. "Are your children complaining of eye problems?"
    2. "There is no need for concern because glaucoma is not a hereditary disorder."
    3. "There may be a genetic factor with glaucoma and your children should be screened."
    4. "Your son should be evaluated because he is over 40."

33. A woman develops disseminated intravascular coagulation (DIC) following childbirth. Lab studies show she has elevated prothrombin time (PT), elevated activated partial thromboplastin time (APTT), and decreased platelet count and fibrinogen level. What would be the explanation for the occurrence of these changes?

    1. Formation of clots in small blood vessels throughout the body has used up her clotting factors.
    2. Damage to her liver during childbirth has resulted in impaired production of clotting factors.
    3. Exposure to fetal blood of a type different from hers has caused her to form antibodies, which are attacking her bone marrow.
    4. Internal bleeding has resulted in loss of the clotting factors from the intravascular space into the interstitial spaces.

34. A 4-year-old girl was in a car accident with her family. Upon arrival in the emergency room, she is noted to have lacerations on her head and arms, a temperature of 39°C, BP 158/102, pulse 60, and sluggish pupil reactions. She is crying and does not recognize her family. With what condition would the nurse suspect these manifestations to be associated?

    1. Elevated intracranial pressure.
    2. Reye's syndrome.
    3. Guillain-Barré syndrome.
    4. Anxiety attack related to being in a strange environment.

35. An adult male is admitted in alcohol withdrawal. The nurse plans his care to include all of the following. What is the most important goal to approach first?

    1. Client will be able to identify reality.
    2. Client will remain free from injury.
    3. Client will remain free of alcohol use.
    4. Client will maintain optimal nutrition intake.

36. A man is admitted with a diagnosis of antisocial personality. He has a long history of fights, incarcerations for stealing and forgery, lying, lack of remorse for his actions, inconsistent employment, and impersonal relationships with others. As a child, he was often truant, in trouble with school officials, and cruel to his family dog. Based on his background, which explanation is associated with antisocial personality?

    1. A low I.Q.
    2. Failure to develop a stabilized and socialized ego and superego during early childhood.
    3. Rebelliousness despite parental discipline and moral values in the home.
    4. Poverty and resulting need to meet basic needs independent of family.

37. A young adult suffered from depression and was withdrawn when admitted to the unit. She has responded well to treatment and, though still depressed, now attends unit group meetings. How can the nurse best determine whether the client's condition has improved?
   1. The client has been compliant with her medications.
   2. Ask another client if she has improved in her participating in the milieu.
   3. Observe whether she socializes appropriately with other clients outside of unit group meetings.
   4. Observe that the client attends unit group meetings.

38. A child is admitted with idiopathic thrombocytopenic purpura with a platelet count of 18,000/mm³. What will the nurse expect to be ordered for this child?
   1. Aspirin every 4 hours.
   2. Seizure precautions.
   3. Restricted activity level.
   4. Tracheostomy set at bedside.

39. A older client with arthritis is experiencing increased alterations in mobility. In planning her care, which of the following measures would be the best approach for the nurse to safeguard the client?
   1. Using a vest restraint at all times.
   2. Teaching crutch walking.
   3. Removing excess room furniture and clutter.
   4. Placing the bedside table away from the client.

40. An adult client states that it hurts too much to cough and deep breathe following abdominal surgery. Which of the following approaches would the nurse take first?
   1. Inform the client that coughing is not a matter of choice and must be done.
   2. Call the respiratory therapist in to talk with the client.
   3. Notify the surgeon that the client refuses to cough.
   4. Coordinate a pain medication and respiratory exercise schedule.

41. An adult client has been admitted to the psychiatric unit. She is convinced that a blemish on her face is a malignant melanoma. By the end of the third day of hospitalization, her fear of dying from the melanoma has reached psychotic proportions. What would be the most adaptive way she might try to deal with this situation?
   1. Attempt thought-control methods to decrease pervasiveness of thoughts.
   2. Request prn medication whenever such thoughts intrude.
   3. Share her concerns with another client whenever they arise.
   4. Withdraw to her room whenever such thoughts arise.

42. Several clients are participating in group therapy. Which is least likely to be a benefit of group therapy for clients?
   1. Focusing strictly on personal situations.
   2. An increase in the sense of belonging and worthiness.
   3. A decrease in isolation and an increase in reality testing.
   4. The opportunity to ventilate and problem solve.

43. The nurse is caring for a woman who is 35 weeks pregnant. She comes to the emergency department with painless vaginal bleeding. This is her third pregnancy and she states that this has never happened to her before. What would be avoided in caring for this client?
   1. Allowing her husband to stay with her.
   2. Keeping her at rest.
   3. Shaving the perineum.
   4. Performing a vaginal examination.

44. The nurse is caring for a woman with a placenta previa who has been hospitalized for several weeks. She is now at 38 weeks' gestation and her membranes have ruptured. The amniotic fluid has a greenish color and the woman has started to bleed again. What would be the nurse's first action?
   1. Administer oxygen.
   2. Place her in Trendelenburg's position.
   3. Call the physician and prepare for a cesarean birth.
   4. Move her to the delivery room immediately.

45. A child has been brought to the emergency room with an asthma attack. What signs and symptoms would the nurse expect to see?
   1. A prolonged inspiratory time and a short expiratory time.
   2. Frequent productive coughing of clear, frothy, thin mucus progressing to thick, tenacious mucus heard only on auscultation.

3. Hypoinflation of the alveoli with resulting poor gas exchange from increasingly shallow inspirations.

4. Swelling of the bronchial mucosa, with wheezes starting on expiration and spreading to continuous.

46. A 2-month-old baby who has a rash on his cheeks, trunk, and extremities that won't heal is brought in for a well checkup. Infantile eczema is diagnosed and the nurse provides educational teaching for this problem. Upon returning for the 3-month checkup, what reported activity indicates the mother has been properly caring for the baby's skin?

1. She bathes him twice a day to remove crusts.

2. She leaves his skin exposed to air whenever possible.

3. She gently pats lubricant into the skin.

4. She uses only natural fibers against his skin.

47. The parents of a 2-month-old infant who has an apnea monitor are visiting the pediatrician for a checkup. When asked how the monitoring is going at home, the parents indicate dissatisfaction with the process, saying it keeps everyone awake and on edge while the baby is okay. What can the nurse do to promote a safe, effective health care environment for this infant?

1. Order another monitor for them, because there are several brands to choose from.

2. Ask the parents to apply the monitor and turn it on, so the nurse can see what happens.

3. Stress the importance of continuation of monitoring during the first year for all high-risk infants.

4. Recommend that the infant's crib be placed beside the parents' bed so the baby can be heard if any distress occurs.

48. The nurse is caring for a woman who has had a lumbar laminectomy with a spinal fusion. Immediately after surgery, which of the following should the nurse expect the client to manifest?

1. Absence of lower extremity movement.

2. Response to pinprick sensation.

3. Severe muscle spasms.

4. Weak pedal pulses.

49. The nurse is caring for a client who has had a spinal fusion. The donor site for the graft begins to hemorrhage and then ooze blood. What is the most appropriate way to determine whether nursing interventions to stop bleeding have been effective?

1. Monitoring output.

2. Taking hourly vital signs.

3. Asking the client if she feels dizzy.

4. Outlining drainage on the dressing and noting the time.

50. A woman who has had a lumbar laminectomy and a spinal fusion is getting out of bed for the first time. What action by the client will indicate that the teaching plan is considered effective?

1. Bends only from the waist.

2. Moves rapidly.

3. Thinks through every movement.

4. Refuses to use a walker.

51. A 16-year-old client has acute infectious mononucleosis. Which statement by the client indicates to the nurse that he understands the necessary home care?

1. "I'm excited about going to the football game tonight."

2. "My friends are coming over here to help me with my school work."

3. "I plan to work out with the swim team tomorrow."

4. "I have to stay in bed all the time."

52. A 70-year-old woman with severe macular degeneration is admitted to the hospital the day before scheduled surgery. What would the nurse's preoperative goals include for her?

1. Independently ambulating around the unit.

2. Reading the routine preoperative education materials.

3. Maneuvering safely after orientation to the room.

4. Using a bedpan for elimination needs.

53. The nurse is caring for a client with a newly implanted pacemaker. When monitoring pacemaker functioning, which of the following should the nurse initially assess?

1. Electrocardiogram.

2. Pulse.

3. Blood pressure.

4. Incision site.

54. The nurse is assessing a child with conjunctivitis (pink eye). Which of the following findings would the nurse most likely observe?

1. Serous drainage from the eyes.

2. Crusting of the eyelids.

3. Severe eye pain.

4. Only one eye is affected.

55. An adult client is receiving cancer chemotherapy. Which action the client makes

indicates a need for further instruction to prevent stomatitis?

1. Brushing teeth with a soft bristle brush.
2. Lubricating lips with petroleum jelly.
3. Avoiding hard or spicy foods.
4. Rinsing with an alcohol-based mouthwash.

56. The nurse is conducting a mental status examination. What is used in the component of the examination that tests for the client's ability to think abstractly as well as reason?

1. Proverbs.
2. Item identification.
3. Presidents' names.
4. Serial sevens.

57. A young adult was seen by the psychiatric nurse and the client states he hears the voice of his former girlfriend calling to him to help her. In an attempt to find her, he breaks into various buildings and enters others' homes uninvited. He rarely sleeps and has lost a job; afraid he will miss a visit or call from her. He now lives with his parents who have threatened to evict him if he does not get help. Which of the following nursing diagnoses is least appropriate?

1. Altered thought processes.
2. Bathing hygiene self-care deficit.
3. Sensory/perceptual alterations.
4. Sleep pattern disturbance.

58. A young adult was seen in outpatient clinic. He states he hears the voice of a former girlfriend calling to him to help her. He does not sleep and has lost his job because he is afraid he will miss a visit or a phone call. What would the nurse plan to do using the community mental health model?

1. Encourage the client to admit himself to a community hospital psychiatric unit.
2. File a petition for involuntary commitment.
3. Maintain the client in treatment in a community-based setting.
4. Refer the client to a psychiatrist for medication as sole treatment.

59. The nurse is preparing to administer 2 units of packed red blood cells. Which action should be included at this time?

1. Prime the blood administration tubing with 3% saline solution.
2. Add prescribed antibiotics when blood is infusing to ensure proper distribution throughout the body.

3. Inform client that most reactions usually do not occur until the end of the administration.
4. Gather blood filter tubing and IV catheters with a 18 to 20 gauge needle.

60. An adult is admitted for bipolar illness, manic phase, after assaulting his landlord in an argument over the client staying up all night playing loud music. The client is hyperactive, intrusive, and has rapid, pressured speech. He has not slept in 3 days and appears thin and disheveled. Which of the following is the most essential nursing action at this time?

1. Providing a meal and beverage for him to eat in the dining room.
2. Providing linens and toiletries for the client to attend to his hygiene.
3. Consulting with the psychiatrist to order a hypnotic to promote sleep.
4. Providing for client safety by limiting his privileges.

61. The nurse is assessing a 2-year-old child with tetralogy of Fallot. Which of the following is most characteristic of a child with this condition?

1. Normal growth and development.
2. Hypotonia of upper extremities.
3. Epistaxis.
4. Assuming a squatting position.

62. A client has had a radical neck dissection. He is having difficulty breathing and secretions are visible in the laryngectomy tube. What should be the initial nursing intervention?

1. Obtain the vital signs.
2. Notify the physician.
3. Remove the secretions.
4. Start oxygen via a tracheostomy collar.

63. The nurse is caring for a client who has had a total laryngectomy. What is nursing management in the early postoperative period directed toward?

1. Alleviation of pain.
2. Decreasing the client's concern about appearance.
3. Improving the nutritional status of the client.
4. Observing the client for hemorrhage.

64. The nurse is caring for a toddler who has infantile eczema. What will be included in the nursing care plan?

1. Applying the emollient preparation to the skin before allowing the child to sit in the bathtub to protect the skin from water damage.

2. Removing the gloves, cotton stockings, or elbow protector devices when the child is sleeping.

3. Measures to protect the family from the child's lesions.

4. Teaching the parents that permanent remission will usually take place around age 2 or 3.

65. The nurse is assessing a newborn baby girl and finds the following: in a supine position with hips and knees flexed, the right knee is higher than the left; there are more gluteal and thigh folds on the left than the right. What is the best interpretation for this data?

1. The right hip is dislocated.

2. The left hip is dislocated.

3. Both hips are dislocated.

4. The baby has normal newborn joint laxity.

66. A client with schizophrenia is admitted to the hospital experiencing auditory hallucinations that others are after him and intend to harm him. What should the nursing plan of care include?

1. Seclusion until hallucinations lessen.

2. Placement in a reality-oriented therapy group.

3. Advising the client that antipsychotic drugs will cure him.

4. Presenting reality by stating that the nurse does not hear the voices.

67. An adult client underwent a cardiac catherization in which atherosclerotic plaque formations were seen on his coronary arteries. Blood work revealed cholesterol of 260 and HDL of 30. After dietary teaching, the client states "I can eat red meat as long as I don't see any fat on it." Which nursing diagnosis is most appropriate related to the client's statement?

1. Altered nutrition: risk for more than body requirements.

2. Altered nutrition: dysfunctional eating behaviors.

3. Knowledge deficit: lack of information.

4. Knowledge deficit: information misinterpretation.

68. One liter of fluid every 6 hours is ordered for an adult client. If the adminstration set delivers 10 gtts/mL, then the drip rate is _____.

69. The nurse is caring for a woman who is 1 day post radical mastectomy. What must be included in the care plan?

1. Elevate the arm on the operative side for 24 to 48 hours.

2. Maintain complete bed rest for 24 to 48 hours.

3. Do not allow the client to perform any self-care activities for 48 hours.

4. Maintain the client NPO for 24 hours.

70. A young woman comes to the gynecology clinic to be fitted for a diaphragm. Which nursing action would best prevent incorrect placement of a diaphragm when the client is inserting it for the first time?

1. Allowing her supervised practice time.

2. Providing a brochure.

3. Teaching her to lie on her back.

4. Teaching her sex partner to insert it.

71. The nurse in the gynecology clinic is assessing a young woman. The client states that she gets her menstrual period every 18 days. She states that her flow is very heavy and lasts 6 days. How does the nurse identify this pattern?

1. Dysmenorrhea.

2. Dyspareunia.

3. Menorrhagia.

4. Metrorrhagia.

72. A young woman is seen in the woman's clinic. She states that she has "many little blisters on my privates." After examining her labia and perineum, the nurse finds multiple vesicles, some ruptured and crusted over. There is no unusual vaginal discharge. What would the nurse suspect?

1. Chlamydia.

2. Gonorrhea.

3. Herpes.

4. Syphilis.

73. A young child is admitted to the hospital with a diagnosis of Reye's syndrome. Which of the following would the nurse expect to see in the child's history?

1. Temperature elevations of 103°F or higher in the past 8 hours.

2. Enlarged spleen.

3. Influenza 1 week ago.

4. Family history of Reye's syndrome.

74. An older man with a 10-year history of Parkinson's disease is admitted to the hospital because his condition is deteriorating. What is an obvious symptom of Parkinson's disease that could be present on admission?

1. Confusion.

2. Intention tremor.

3. Pallor.

4. Pill rolling.

75. Amantadine hydrochloride (Symmetrel) is prescribed for a client with Parkinson's disease. The client asks how the drug works. What response by the nurse indicates the correct action of the drug?
   1. The drug allows accumulation of dopamine.
   2. The drug corrects mineral deficiencies.
   3. The drug elevates the client's mood.
   4. The drug replaces enzymes.

76. The nurse is planning care for an elderly client who has severe Parkinson's disease. Which of the following is of highest priority?
   1. Positioning.
   2. Encouraging independence.
   3. Increasing activity.
   4. Preventing aspiration.

77. In planning care for a client with advanced Parkinson's disease, which activity is most likely to be effective in alleviating fatigue?
   1. Getting him to bed on time.
   2. Avoiding high-carbohydrate foods.
   3. Collaborating with him when scheduling activities.
   4. Providing for morning and afternoon naps while he is in the hospital.

78. What intervention should the nurse include when planning care for the client with multiple myeloma?
   1. Fluid restriction.
   2. Administration of potassium supplements.
   3. Assisting with mobility.
   4. Administration of aspirin to control bone pain.

79. The nurse is evaluating a client who has been in a long leg cast for 3 weeks. Which finding indicates the client is free of neurological or circulatory complications?
   1. The toes on the casted foot are cool to the touch.
   2. The nail beds have a blue tinge when pressed lightly.
   3. The client reports pain under the cast near the fracture site.
   4. The dorsalis pedis pulse is +3.

80. An unlicensed assistive personnel (UAP) is assisting children in play. Which action by the UAP would need further instruction by the RN?
   1. Works a puzzle with a child recovering with Reye's syndrome.
   2. Places an infant in side-lying position due to diaper rash.

   3. Provides ROM exercises with the child admitted with rheumatic fever.
   4. Positions the head of bed slightly elevated for a child diagnosed with bacterial meningitis.

81. An adult is admitted to the hospital with a femoral neck fracture of the left leg. A total hip replacement is performed. While planning care for 2 days following the surgery, the nurse includes which of the following nursing interventions?
   1. Ambulate in room with weight bearing on both legs for 5 minutes.
   2. Out of bed in the chair for 1 hour, elevating both legs on another chair.
   3. Turn from side to side q 2 h, support upper leg with pillows from thigh to heel.
   4. Turn from supine to right side q 2 h while maintaining the left leg in abduction.

82. An elderly client is admitted with the following problems: oliguria, extreme fatigue, dyspnea. Vital signs are as follows: T 100.2°F (oral), HR 62, R 28, BP 152/94. Assessment reveals 3+ bilateral pedal edema, crackles in bilateral lungs fields, blood glucose of 150, hypoactive bowel sounds, and a pressure ulcer on the left lateral ankle. Which nursing diagnosis would be assigned the highest priority?
   1. Activity intolerance.
   2. Ineffective breathing patterns.
   3. Constipation.
   4. Skin integrity impairment.

83. An adult client is hospitalized for treatment of diabetes insipidus. The nurse is performing the initial assessment. Which finding should the nurse expect?
   1. Daily urine output of 10 liters.
   2. Urine specific gravity of 1.050.
   3. Serum sodium levels of 120 mEq/liter.
   4. Daily fluid intake of 1–2 liters.

84. A 1-day-old infant is admitted to the intensive care nursery. She is suspected of having esophageal atresia. What assessment findings should the nurse expect to find?
   1. Bile-stained vomitus and a weak cry.
   2. Diarrhea and colicky abdominal pain.
   3. Excessive drooling and immediate regurgitation of feedings.
   4. Visible peristaltic waves and projectile vomiting.

85. The nurse is assessing a 6-month-old child. Which developmental skills are normal and should be expected?
   1. Speaks in short sentences.
   2. Sits alone.
   3. Can feed self with a spoon.
   4. Pulling up to a standing position.

86. The parents of a 1-year-old are discussing the safety needs of their daughter with the nurse. Which statement indicates a need for further education on safety practices?
   1. "We should fence in our yard soon."
   2. "One of us will always be with her while she is in the bathtub."
   3. "We don't need the stair gate anymore; she's so good at walking."
   4. "The safest position for her car seat is in the middle of the back seat."

87. The nurse is caring for a client with Raynaud's phenomenon. The nurse should instruct the client to avoid which of the following situations?
   1. Living in a warm climate.
   2. Active exercising.
   3. Exposure to cold temperatures.
   4. Alcohol consumption.

88. The nurse is caring for an elderly client who has been diagnosed as having sundowner's syndrome. The nurse asks the client and his family to list all of the medications, prescription and nonprescription, he is currently taking. What is the primary reason for this action?
   1. Multiple medications can lead to dementia.
   2. The medications can provide clues regarding his medical background.
   3. Ability to recall medications is a good assessment of the client's level of orientation.
   4. Medications taken by a client are part of every nursing assessment.

89. The nurse must report to another nurse about a client's problem and is using the SBAR technique for communication. Which of the following would be included in this particular type of communication?
   1. S – sensory capabilities
   2. B – background information
   3. A – ADLs
   4. R – respiratory status

90. An adult has continued slow bleeding from the graft after repair of an abdominal aortic aneurysm and is in the intensive care unit. The client insists on having a visit from a medicine man whom the family visits regularly. How should the nurse interpret this request?
   1. The principle of justice prohibits giving one client a privilege that other clients are not permitted.
   2. Faith healers do not meet the standards for clergy exemption from visitation rules.
   3. Medicine men are not approved by the hospital as legitimate health care providers.
   4. Provision of holistic care requires that the client's belief system is honored.

91. The nurse is caring for a client who had a left knee replacement. The nurse is adjusting the passive motion device on his third post-op day. Which of the following indicates correct technique?
   1. Allow passive motion prn as desired.
   2. Monitor alignment at hinged joint of machine.
   3. Monitor pressure areas on shins.
   4. Allow client to choose speed and degree of extension.

92. An adult is admitted to the surgical floor with a diagnosis of a tumor, right lung. Upon return to the surgical unit following a right pneumonectomy, the nurse should place the client in which position?
   1. Left lateral decubitus.
   2. Right lateral decubitus.
   3. Semi-Fowler's.
   4. High-Fowler's.

93. An adult comes to the clinic because she has a productive cough. She smokes two packs of cigarettes a day and has a family history of lung cancer and emphysema. Using the principles of health promotion, the nurse would make what interpretation of the client's behavior?
   1. Using denial to deal with being at high risk for lung cancer.
   2. Not assuming self-responsibility for her health.
   3. Exhibiting a laissez-faire attitude toward smoking and her risk of cancer.
   4. Demonstrating passive suicidal tendencies.

94. The nurse is teaching an adult who has ulcerative colitis. In developing the teaching plan which of the following foods should the nurse plan to instruct the client to avoid?
   1. Roast chicken and cooked spinach.
   2. Broiled liver and white rice.

3. Cottage cheese and canned apricots.

4. Pork chop and brown rice.

95. A 46-year-old female with chronic constipation is assessed by the nurse for a bowel training regimen. Which factor indicates further information is needed by the nurse?

   1. The client's dietary habits include foods high in bulk.

   2. The client's fluid intake is between 2500–3000 mL per day.

   3. The client engages in moderate exercise each day.

   4. The client has bowel sounds in all four quadrants.

96. A 26-year-old obese female is assessed for a weight reduction diet by a clinic nurse. Which of the following statements by the client presents most concern to the nurse?

   1. "I understand the food pyramid."

   2. "My family is in support of my weight reduction."

   3. "I have gained and lost weight over the last 5 years."

   4. "I do not have diabetes."

97. A man suffered a traumatic amputation of his left arm in a factory accident about 7 months ago and has had severe chronic phantom pain for the last 6 months. Which statement, if made by his wife, who assists her husband with his daily care, indicates an understanding of this client's pain?

   1. "Phantom pain is not real pain; his body is just tricked into thinking he has pain."

   2. "Because he lost his arm so long ago, his pain must be caused by something besides his injury."

3. "I believe he is having pain and I want to help him deal with it."

4. "If he continues taking pain medication, he will become a drug addict even though he really has pain."

98. The nurse is assessing a client following hemodialysis. Which of the following findings indicates the treatment was effective?

   1. Hypertension.

   2. Hyperkalemia.

   3. Fluid volume decrease.

   4. Cardiac dysrhythmias.

99. The nurse is discontinuing an intravenous catheter. Which action should be included at this time?

   1. Apply a tourniquet proximal to the catheter insertion site.

   2. Flush the catheter with a heparin solution to ensure patency of the catheter before removal.

   3. Assess the insertion site for signs of infiltration or inflammation.

   4. Wear only sterile gloves to perform the procedure.

100. The client diagnosed with asthma has visible oral candidiasis. What question should the nurse ask this client?

   1. "Will you show me how you use your inhaler?"

   2. "When was your last dentist visit?"

   3. "Have you had respiratory infection lately?"

   4. "Do you floss your teeth daily?"

# Answers and Rationales for Practice Test 4

| ANSWER | RATIONALE | NP | CN | CL | SA |
|---|---|---|---|---|---|
| #1. 1. | Excess output of the thyroid hormones increase the metabolic rate causing an increased demand for food. Other symptoms are the presence of a goiter, fine tremor of the fingers, increased nervousness, weight loss, altered bowel activity, heat intolerance, excessive sweating and increased heart rate. | An | Ph/8 | An | 1 |

| ANSWER | RATIONALE | NP | CN | CL | SA |
|--------|-----------|----|----|----|----|
| #2. 2. | Polyarthritis is characterized by swollen painful, hot joints that respond to salicylate. Chorea is irregular movement; SC nodules and erythema marginatum (nonpruritic rash) are typical with rheumatic fever. | An | Ph/6 | An | 4 |
| #3. 3. | It is thought that hypoguesia (altered taste sensation) occurs when cancer cells release substances that resemble amino acids and stimulate the bitter taste buds. Food-enhancing seasoning can mask the taste alternations. This phenomenon is also reported in the aging population. | As | Ph/5 | Ap | 3 |
| #4. 1. | Otosclerosis is the formation of spongy bone in the capsule of the ear labyrinth. As it advances, it causes progressive fixation of the footplate of the stapes. With oval window obstruction by otosclerosis, hearing by air conduction is reduced. | As | Ph/8 | An | 1 |
| #5. 3. | Speaking at a moderate rate allows the client to observe the lips of the speaker and to hear normal voice tones, while using short phrases and speaking slowly. | Ev | Ph/7 | Ap | 1 |
| #6. 4. | Placing the food in a recognizable location fosters autonomy as well as independence. The 4-year-old is too young to understand the clock method. | Im | Ph/5 | Ap | 4 |
| #7. 3. | The nurse recognizes a normal occurrence in a 1–3 month old infant, known as the Moro reflex. No abnormality is occurring that warrants seeing a neurologist; a Babinski reflex involves the feet; and it is recommended that infants are not placed prone (unless otherwise indicated). | An | He/3 | An | 4 |
| #8. 1. | Sexual intercourse is avoided as it causes uterine contractions, contributing to further placental separation or dislodge the placenta. The client will not have vaginal examinations (as it can cause further separation of the placenta); cesarean will be evaluated at a later time; bed rest is recommended. | Ev | He/3 | An | 3 |
| #9. 1. | The usual requirement for dress to the operating room is a hospital gown, with all jewelry, dentures, and contact lenses removed. Liquids are contraindicated to prevent aspiration (unless ordered specifically by the physician or anesthesiologist); IS instructions should have given at a previous time as the client may be experiencing some anxiety at this time; although it is important to know the client's smoking habits, which will influence postoperative healing, this information would already be known when obtaining a client history. | Im | Ph/7 | An | 1 |
| #10. 1. | The client's high activity level poses the most danger because it can lead to absence of food, fluid, and rest with resultant dehydration, electrolyte imbalance, and physical collapse. | An | Ps/4 | An | 2 |
| #11. 2. | Many characteristics of a client who is manic (i.e., irritability, excitement, agitation, provocative behavior) contribute to the potential for violence. Maintaining the safety of the client and those around him is the greatest priority. | An | Ps/4 | An | 2 |
| #12. 4. | Manic clients cannot calm down without assistance. Decreasing the level of sensory stimulation is of paramount importance and provides the greatest therapeutic effect until proper medication | Im | Ps/4 | Ap | 2 |

| ANSWER | RATIONALE | NP | CN | CL | SA |
|--------|-----------|-----|-----|-----|-----|
| | levels (often lithium) are established. Restraints would further agitate the client. | | | | |
| #13. 4. | While the client's social network can influence the client in terms of compliance, the influence is typically secondary to that of the other factors listed. Side effects of lithium include fine tremor, drowsiness, diarrhea, polyuria, thirst, weight gain, and fatigue, which can be disturbing to the client. | Ev | Ph/6 | An | 5 |
| #14. 4. | This is the only choice that only has one source of protein, whereas the others have two sources. | Ev | Ph/5 | An | 4 |
| #15. 2. | Drying prevents heat loss and reducing of body temperature, the most important part of newborn care. The other interventions will be done following the drying or within 1 hour after birth. | Im | He/3 | Ap | 3 |
| #16. 3. | Careful assessment of the breasts before and after each feeding is extremely important for noting any early skin breakdown, which can get infected. A lump can signify a clogged duct; position changes may be needed if skin breakdown is occurring; handwashing is appropriate for all infants. | Ev | He/3 | An | 3 |
| #17. 1. | Heme in the stool can be an early warning sign of necrotizing enterocolitis. All the other activities should be assessed prior to each feeding. | As | Ph/7 | An | 4 |
| #18. 2. | The baby shows clinical manifestations of patent ductus arteriosus (PDA): failure of the fetal ductus arteriosus to completely close after birth. The ductus venous is a major blood channel that develops through the embryonic liver from the left umbilical vein to the inferior vena cava; after the ductus arteriosus closes, the remains are called the ligamentum arteriosus; the foramen ovale closes at birth, failure of closure is manifested by dyspnea. | An | Ph/7 | An | 3 |
| #19. 3. | Because infants born to addicted mothers are highly irritable, it is best to organize all care around the feedings and then try to disturb them as little as possible. The infants also have a strong sucking reflex, may have frequent vomiting, and are prone to temperature instability, so it is advisable to keep the infant wrapped snugly to maintain temperature. Breastfeeding would not be recommended as drugs will cross the breast milk. | Pl | He/3 | Ap | 3 |
| #20. 4. | Gravity will cause the head of the femur to drop toward the bed, causing the affected thigh to appear shorter. Ortolani's sign (a popping sensation when hip joint is internally and externally rotated) is normal; Trendelenburg's sign is seen with an abnormality of the pelvis associated with congenital hip dislocation; skinfolds would be increased in the affected thigh. | As | Ph/7 | An | 4 |
| #21. 1. | Infiltration is the infusion of fluid into tissue. The accumulation of fluid causes pressure, which reduces circulation to the area, resulting in pallor. Increased warmth or redness at the site would suggest phlebitis or infection. Blood seeping around the needle may be from anticoagulant overdose or the insertion site has been stretched and needs restarting at a new site. | Ev | Ph/6 | An | 1 |

| ANSWER | RATIONALE | NP | CN | CL | SA |
|--------|-----------|----|----|----|----|
| #22. 2. | The most frequent means of transmission of the tubercle bacillus is droplet nuclei. The bacillus is present in the air as a result of coughing, sneezing, laughing, singing, and expectorating of sputum by an infected person. | Pl | Sa/2 | Co | 1 |
| #23. 4. | A side effect of rifampin is orange-tinged tears, sweat, urine, and it may stain soft contact lenses. Tingling in the feet is a side effect of isoniazid (INH), which is sometimes taken in conjunction with rifampin. | Im | Ph/6 | Co | 5 |
| #24. 3. | Determining when the client had her last bowel movement provides baseline data as a first part of bowel history. Avoid questions that begin with "why" as it may appear threatening to the client. | As | Ph/5 | Ap | 1 |
| #25. 3. | The boot should be removed at least once a shift for skin care and to assess for skin breakdown and nerve damage. The left leg must be immobilized by one person and traction applied while the second person removes the boot, provides the skin care, and performs the assessment. Turning may cause bone fragments to move against each other resulting in damage to blood vessels and nerves. A trapeze would be placed for the client to lift herself, while also being encouraged to cough and deep breathe. | Pl | Ph/5 | Ap | 1 |
| #26. 1. | Monitoring vital signs is the most important aspect of assessing respiratory and cardiovascular status. All the other actions would follow assessment. | Im | Ph/7 | Ap | 1 |
| #27. 4. | Sign and symptoms of acute rejection include temperature of 100°F or greater, enlarged tender kidney, fluid retention, increased blood pressure, fatigue and lethargy. Anuria or oliguria, not polyuria, occurs with acute rejection. An increase in blood pressure would increase, not decrease, due to the fluid overload. Anemia is a symptom of chronic renal failure, not acute rejection. | As | Ph/7 | Co | 1 |
| #28. 3. | Several weeks after the lesions have healed, the child who had beta-hemolytic streptococci infection is at risk for acute glomerulonephritis. Puffiness around the eyes would also be seen. Medical referral is needed promptly. An antibiotic would be started after the infection is diagnosed; personal items do not need to be separate, as secretions harbor the organism; Neosporin could be a topical antibiotic applied several times a day. | Im | Ph/7 | An | 4 |
| #29. 3. | Because glycerin, a rapid-acting osmotic diuretic, is being used, the client's intake and output would be monitored. During the acute phase, eye patches may not be present and bright lights would be irritating. Eyedrop administration would be done at a later time. | Pl | Ph/6 | Ap | 1 |
| #30. 1. | Morphine is contraindicated for a client with glaucoma because it is constipating. Straining at stool raises intraocular pressure. Occluding the puncta prevents the eye medication from entering the systemic circulation. Unsterile gloves can be worn to prevent exposure of viruses to the examiner. | An | Ph/6 | Ap | 1 |
| #31. 1. | Pilocar is a cholinergic agent that reduces intraocular pressure by producing miosis (constriction of the pupil), thus increasing outflow of aqueous humor. It will not perform any of the other choices. | An | Ph/6 | Co | 5 |

| ANSWER | RATIONALE | NP | CN | CL | SA |
|---|---|---|---|---|---|
| #32. 3. | There is a strong hereditary factor in glaucoma. Therefore, family members of all ages should have intraocular pressures measured yearly. | Im | He/3 | Co | 1 |
| #33. 1. | The pathophysiology of DIC includes formation of multiple microscopic clots in very small vessels, which uses up the clotting factors, leaving the client vulnerable to bleeding at other sites. The abnormal lab values are the indication of the cause of the problem. | An | Ph/7 | An | 3 |
| #34. 1. | Head injury is one situation that may cause elevated intracranial pressure, as evidence by the manifestations listed. Reye's syndrome affects the central nervous system; Guillain-Barré presents with ascending paralysis; and the child's crying would be expected, but the presenting assessment would point to a different problem. | An | Ph/8 | An | 4 |
| #35. 2. | Safety is the highest priority. A client in withdrawal suffers from altered cognition and sensory disturbances, as well as tremors, which increase the potential for injury. | Pl | Ps/4 | Ap | 2 |
| #36. 2. | This is the psychodynamic view and usually begins prior to age 15. His antisocial personality stems from a failure to develop a stabilized and socialized ego and superego during early childhood. A low I.Q. is associated with mental retardation, however many antisocial persons have an above average intelligence. A child with the stated behaviors are the result of a lack of consistent or effective behavior, which also does not provide an atmosphere to instill society morals and values. Poverty is not a direct link to antisocial personality. | An | Ps/4 | An | 2 |
| #37. 4. | The client's attendance displays that she is a participant in her treatment and has made a step forward from her withdrawn behavior. | Ev | Ps/4 | An | 2 |
| #38. 3. | Prevention of injury, bruising, and bleeding is high priority when the platelet count is low. As normal is 150,000–500,000/mm$^3$, this child's count is extremely low. Aspirin is contraindicated in bleeding disorders; seizure precautions are associated with a central nervous system disorder, not thrombocytopenic; there is not a risk for airway obstruction. | Pl | Ph/7 | Ap | 1 |
| #39. 3. | Removing excess items from the room is the best way to safeguard the client. Crutch walking would be difficult due to the arthritis and the bedside table should be close to avoid overreaching and the chance of injury or falling. | Pl | Ph/5 | Ap | 1 |
| #40. 4. | Pain medication should be given when available, even on a PRN basis. If the pain is lessened the client will be more cooperative and achieve the goal of coughing and deep breathing. | Pl | Ph/7 | Ap | 1 |
| #41. 1. | Thought-control methods are applicable to this situation and are the least restrictive method of achieving symptom control which is designed to subvert an individual's control of her own thinking, behavior, emotions, or decisions. | Im | Ps/4 | An | 2 |
| #42. 1. | This action is handled in individual therapy, not group therapy. All the other choices are a beneficial goal of group therapy. | An | Ps/4 | An | 2 |

| ANSWER | RATIONALE | NP | CN | CL | SA |
|---|---|---|---|---|---|
| #43. 4. | Painless vaginal bleeding is symptomatic of placenta previa. Vaginal exams are contraindicated before 36 weeks unless done in the delivery room set up for emergency cesarean section if needed. Bed rest is essential and shaving is not necessary. | Im | He/3 | Ap | 3 |
| #44. 3. | Green amniotic fluid is indicative of fetal distress. This combined with bleeding from the placenta previa may require a cesarean section. Oxygen and movement to the delivery room may be performed, but notifying the physician would be a definite plan. | Pl | He/3 | Ap | 3 |
| #45. 4. | Asthma causes spasm of the smooth muscles in the bronchi and bronchioles, resulting in prolonged exhalation. Inspirations increase in rate in an effort to relieve hypoxia. The cough would begin as nonproductive, then progress to a profuse mucous; gas trapping is caused by allowing more air to enter the alveoli than can escape, which causes increased depth and rate of respirations. | As | Ph/8 | Co | 4 |
| #46. 3. | Lubricants applied to the skin after bathing seal in moisture and rehydrate, lubricate, and moisturize the skin. Wool is an example of a natural fiber, which would not be used. | Ev | Ph/7 | Ap | 4 |
| #47. 2. | The nurse should observe how the family applies and positions the monitor's leads. This will provide the nurse more data to rule out faulty technique. When monitors frequently alarm for breathing infants, it is usually due to loose leads or low batteries. | Ev | Ph/7 | Ap | 4 |
| #48. 2. | Sensation and movement should be present, along with normal pedal pulses. Spasms are indicative of nerve damage during surgery. | As | Ph/7 | An | 1 |
| #49. 4. | It will be important to outline the drainage so that a quantitative measure can be obtained. | Ev | Ph/7 | An | 1 |
| #50. 3. | Good body alignment and avoiding sudden movements will be to her advantage as she thinks through her moves. A walker may not be indicated, but does not indicate effective teaching. | Ev | Ph/5 | Ap | 1 |
| #51. 2. | Rest is a primary treatment; however adolescents have a great need for socialization with peers. Activities during the acute phase should be restricted. | Ev | Ph/7 | Ap | 4 |
| #52. 3. | This is a realistic goal to be oriented to the room and bathroom, as the others could either cause injury or not be able to be seen well enough to read. | Pl | Sa/2 | Ap | 1 |
| #53. 1. | The ECG reflects the heart rate, pacer spikes, and dysrhythmias. | As | Ph/7 | Ap | 1 |
| #54. 2. | This is associated with purulent drainage and is usually bilateral. Serous drainage is characteristic of a viral infection and pain is characteristic of a foreign body in the eye. | As | Ph/7 | Ap | 4 |
| #55. 4. | An alcohol-based mouthwash will break down the tissues. All the other choices are appropriate. | Ev | Ph/7 | Ap | 1 |
| #56. 1. | The use of proverbs test for the client's ability to abstract meaning as well as reason. Item identification tests knowledge of object in the environment; presidents' names test long-term memory; serial sevens tests calculation ability. | As | Ps/4 | Co | 2 |

| ANSWER | RATIONALE | NP | CN | CL | SA |
|---|---|---|---|---|---|
| #57. 2. | There is nothing in the case information to support the diagnosis of a self-care deficit. The client does exhibit all the other diagnoses. | An | Ps/4 | An | 2 |
| #58. 3. | As the client is unlikely to admit himself to a psychiatric unit, he would best be managed in a community setting with partial hospitalization and outpatient care, as he will need psychotherapy as well as medication. | Pl | Ps/4 | Ap | 2 |
| #59. 4. | The large bore needle prevents lysis of the red blood cells, and the special blood filter prevents emboli or contamination matter from flowing into the bloodstream. Blood tubing is always primed with normal saline (0.9%), and no medications are infused with the blood. Blood reactions mostly occur during the first 15 to 60 minutes of an infusion. | Pl | Ph/6 | Ap | 1 |
| #60. 4. | It is reasonable to expect that client may be assaultive with peers and staff. His mental illness produces a hyperactive state and poor judgment and impulse control. External controls such as limiting of unit privileges will assist in feelings of security and safety. His hyperactivity interferes with food and hygiene needs; he will receive an evaluation before medication is ordered. | Im | Ps/4 | Ap | 2 |
| #61. 4. | This position allows for relief of dyspnea, which improves the hemodynamics. Children with tetralogy have poor growth; hypotonia and epistaxis may be present, but these are not the most characteristic manifestations. | As | Ph/7 | Ap | 4 |
| #62. 3. | Secretions that are visible in the tube may be partially occluding the airway and should be removed by suctioning. After removing secretions, oxygen may be required, but if no relief is obtained, the physician would be called to report the condition and provide vital signs. | Im | Ph/7 | Ap | 1 |
| #63. 4. | Life-threatening disorders such as hemorrhage and breathing difficulties are a priority in the immediate period. The others are important, but remember the ABCs of nursing care. | Pl | Ph/7 | Ap | 1 |
| #64. 4. | Until the time of spontaneous remission, there will be many exacerbations and remissions. Sometimes these children develop asthma-type respiratory reactions or other allergies. Lotion is applied after the bath; protector devices are left on to prevent scratching; and eczema runs in families. | Pl | Ph/7 | Ap | 4 |
| #65. 2. | The shorter leg is on the affected side, because the femur head slips further upward into the acetabulum. This causes the extra skin folds in the thigh on the affected leg. | An | Ph/7 | An | 3 |
| #66. 4. | Reality is presented to decrease fear in the client which results from internal stimuli. Seclusion and group therapy will not be beneficial at this time; antipsychotic drugs do cure the problem. | Pl | Ps/4 | An | 2 |
| #67. 4. | The client is displaying denial or has misinterpreted the information given to him by the dietitian. He should abstain from red meat as it contains hidden fat that is not visible. | An | Ph/5 | An | 1 |

| ANSWER | RATIONALE | NP | CN | CL | SA |
|---|---|---|---|---|---|
| #68. | 28 gtts/min. Using the formula: amount of solution in mL ÷ time in minutes x the drop factor, the correct rate of low is 28 gtts/min.<br><br>6 hrs × 60 min. = 360 min.<br><br>$\dfrac{1000 \text{ mL}}{360} = 2.8 \times 10 = 28$ | Im | Ph/6 | Ap | 5 |
| #69. 1. | It is elevated and placed at a right angle to the chest. Early ambulation and post operation exercises are encouraged to promote functioning of all body systems and to prevent postoperative complications. Food and fluid are also encouraged. | Pl | Ph/7 | Ap | 3 |
| #70. 1. | Correct placement is accomplished best if the client is allowed time to practice insertion of the device under professional supervision. Lying on the back is not necessary and the client needs to take responsibility for proper insertion. | Im | He/3 | Ap | 3 |
| #71. 3. | This is abnormal menstrual flow. Dysmenorrhea is painful menstruation; dyspareunia is painful intercourse; and metrorrhagia is uterine bleeding other than that caused by menstruation. | As | Ph/7 | K | 3 |
| #72. 3. | This condition is descriptive of genital herpes, which is highly contagious and causes severe morbidity and recurrences. There is no cure, but acyclovir helps to reduce the number of occurrences. Chlamydia has a non-odorous white discharge; gonorrhea has yellowish-green discharge; and syphilis has a cancre present. | As | Ph/7 | Co | 3 |
| #73. 3. | Reye's syndrome follows a common viral illness such as influenza or varicella and an enlarged liver may accompany the condition. There is no genetic predisposition for Reye's syndrome. | As | Ph/7 | Co | 4 |
| #74. 4. | Rhythmic flexion and contraction of the muscles cause a characteristic tremor called a "pill rolling" tremor. A staring mask-like facial expression may be apparent due to muscle tension. Confusion and pallor are not characteristics of Parkinson's disease; tremors are unintentional at rest and tend to disappear with motion. | As | Ph/7 | Ap | 1 |
| #75. 1. | Because Parkinson's disease is characterized by a dopamine deficiency, the medication allows dopamine to accumulate in extracellular or synaptic sites. The disease is not related to mineral or enzyme deficiencies, or mood disorders. | An | Ph/6 | Ap | 5 |
| #76. 4. | Clients with advanced Parkinson's disease usually have difficulty swallowing and are in danger of choking. Families need much instruction on this slowly progressing disorder, as the swallowing disorder may require hospitalization. Preventing aspiration pneumonia must be a high priority. | Pl | Ph/7 | Ap | 1 |
| #77. 3. | Scheduling activities in collaboration with the client will allow him to proceed at his own pace and maximize his strength. All activities, including naps, should be planned with the client, as well as providing a high-carb diet to provide energy. | Pl | Ph/7 | Ap | 1 |
| #78. 3. | Mobility is important for the client with multiple myeloma. Weight bearing promotes movement of calcium back into | Pl | Ph/7 | Ap | 1 |

| ANSWER | RATIONALE | NP | CN | CL | SA |
|--------|-----------|----|----|----|----|

weakened bones, helping to maintain their strength. This will also reduce the risk of hypercalcemia, which is a common complication with multiple myeloma. Fluids are encouraged to prevent renal failure due to the high levels of uric acid released as plasma cells are destroyed; aspirin is avoided due to decreased platelet count from chemotherapy, which would predispose to bleeding.

**#79. 4.** The casted extremity should have palpable pulses of +2 to +3, feel warm to touch, the toes should be able to move freely, have pink nail beds, and a report of decreasing pain at fracture. Increasing pain would indicate a warning of complications, such as compartment syndrome.    Ev   Ph/7   Ap   1

**#80. 3.** Rheumatic fever is an inflammatory disease that may develop after an infection with streptococcus bacteria and develops as a type of arthritis. To relieve discomfort due to the arthritic pain, the child should not perform ROM exercises, should not be massaged or have splints applied, as these treatments will cause additional pain. The other actions are appropriate for the specified diagnosis.    Pl   Ph/5   An   4

**#81. 4.** The leg must be maintained in abduction and the hip is not to be flexed more than 45–60°. Recommended activities would include standing on nonoperative leg and weight bearing when permitted and turning to the right side. Activities to avoid would be sitting in a chair that requires more than a 60° bend at the hip or elevating the legs on a chair.    Pl   Ph/7   Ap   1

**#82. 2.** All nursing diagnoses are appropriate for the client; however the need for air is a priority, cited on Maslow's Hierarchy of Needs, as a physiological need. The need for air is a higher priority than activity, bowel movements or skin impairment.    An   Ph/7   An   1

**#83. 1.** Clinical manifestations in diabetes insipidus include marked polyuria, extreme dilution of the urine resulting in a specific gravity of 1.000–1.005, polydipsia, high serum osmolarity, and hypernatremia. This disorder is caused by a deficiency of vasopressin.    As   Ph/7   Co   1

**#84. 3.** The esophagus is closed at some point and there is a fistula to the trachea. Because of the blockage, excessive mucus builds up in the nasopharynx and the child has difficulty breathing and becomes cyanotic. After being suctioned, the baby becomes pink again. As food is not getting to the intestine, there would be no evidence of diarrhea or colicky abdominal pain.    As   Ph/7   Co   3

**#85. 2.** A 6-month-old is learning to sit alone. Language skills begin between ages 1 and 3; spoon use begins at 12–15 months; and pulls himself to a standing position at 8–12 months.    As   He/3   K   4

**#86. 3.** Most children at 12 months are not proficient walkers. They may know how to climb upstairs but not how to come down. Their sense of balance is not stable and they lack judgment.    Ev   Sa/2   Ap   4

**#87. 3.** Raynaud's phenomenon (excessive and prolonged painful vasoconstriction of the extremities, especially the hands) is precipitated by exposure to cold and aggravated by smoking. The other activities do not cause an attack.    Im   Ph/7   Ap   1

| ANSWER | | RATIONALE | NP | CN | CL | SA |
|---|---|---|---|---|---|---|
| #88. | 1. | Polypharmacy (concurrent use of several drugs) increases the potential for adverse side effects, one being dementia. Sundowner's syndrome involves behaviors that are seen in the late afternoon or early evening when the sun sets, which include disorientation, emotional upset, or confusion. | An | Ph/6 | An | 1 |
| #89. | 2. | The SBAR technique for communication is a method that helps guide required information to be passed on to another. The acronym is as follows:<br><br>S – Situation – identify the client's name and problem<br><br>B – Background – state pertinent background information<br><br>A – Assessment – state concern<br><br>R – Recommendation – state what you want | Im | Sa/1 | Ap | 1 |
| #90. | 4. | The client's spiritual needs must be met within the framework of his personal belief systems, even if those beliefs differ from those of the nursing staff. | An | Sa/1 | An | 1 |
| #91. | 2. | It is imperative that correct alignment at the knee joint is regarded while in the continuous passive motion (CPM) machine. The client will complain of increased pain if alignment is not maintained, so frequent checking is necessary. The CPM time and degrees are ordered by the physician. No pressure is exerted on the shins. | Im | Ph/7 | Ap | 1 |
| #92. | 3. | Semi-Fowler's position would promote respiratory function. High-Fowler's would probably cause too much fatigue for the client; decubitus is a lying down position. | Im | Ph/7 | Ap | 1 |
| #93. | 2. | There are four principles of health promotion: self-responsibility, nutrition, stress management, and exercise. Self-responsibility includes avoiding high-risk behaviors, such as smoking, abusing alcohol, overeating or driving while intoxicated. | An | He/3 | An | 1 |
| #94. | 4. | A low-fiber diet is recommended, which will be limited in high roughage content (which stimulates peristalsis and makes symptoms of ulcerative colitis worse). Foods to avoid would include whole grains, nuts, raw fruits and vegetables, caffeine, alcohol, tough meats, pork, and highly spiced meats. | Pl | Ph/5 | Co | 1 |
| #95. | 4. | Even though the client has positive bowel sounds in all four quadrants, this does not provide information about bowel habits of the client. This information would help the nurse determine the normal patterns of the client at present. | An | Ph/5 | Co | 1 |
| #96. | 3. | To design an effective care plan for an obese client, the nurse should be aware of past weight problems, along with eating behaviors, exercise habits, medical diagnoses, family support, and reasons for desiring weight loss. | An | Ph/5 | Ap | 1 |
| #97. | 3. | Nurses and caregivers must realize that pain is whatever the client says it is, when it is. Phantom pain can last for many years. Addiction is the seeking of drugs for a psychic, not physical, action. | Ev | Ph/7 | Ap | 1 |
| #98. | 3. | One of the cardiovascular manifestations of chronic renal failure and uremia is fluid volume excess. Blood pressure | Ev | Ph/7 | An | 1 |

| ANSWER | RATIONALE | NP | CN | CL | SA |
|--------|-----------|----|----|----|----|
| | and potassium would decrease following hemodialysis, due to the fluid reduction. | | | | |
| #99. 3. | Extravasation of intravenous fluid may cause tissue ischemia or necrosis. A catheter is inserted using a tourniquet, heparin is used when flushing a PICC or central line, and this is not a sterile procedure. | Im | Ph/6 | Ap | 1 |
| #100. 1. | This condition appears as a cheesy white plaque on the tongue and is also called thrush. The client may not be using the metered dose inhaler (MDI) without a spacer. After using the spacer with the medication, the mouth should be rinsed to further prevent thrush. The other choices would not be the cause for thrush. | As | Ph/6 | An | 1 |

# Practice Test 5

1. An adult client is admitted to the hospital with a diagnosis of tuberculosis. Which room assignment is most appropriate for a client with active tuberculosis?
   1. A semiprivate room.
   2. A room with laminar flow.
   3. A reverse isolation unit.
   4. A negative pressure room.

2. A sputum specimen is ordered for a client. What is an important factor to consider when obtaining a sputum specimen for culture?
   1. A copious amount must be collected.
   2. Sputum collected must not be diluted.
   3. It should be coughed up from deep in the lungs.
   4. The specimen must be refrigerated immediately.

3. An adult client with tuberculosis asks the nurse if she needs to follow any special diet. Which suggestion would be most appropriate for the nurse to give?
   1. Eat a high-carbohydrate diet.
   2. Eat a low-calorie, low-protein diet.
   3. Eat frequent small, high-calorie meals.
   4. Consume only high-carbohydrate liquids.

4. An adult has been in the burn unit 3 days following second- and third-degree burns of both legs. The nurse plans to assess the client for indications of the complication that is the major cause of death in this period and includes which of the following?
   1. Monitor arterial blood gases (ABGs) daily.
   2. Monitor intake and output every shift.
   3. Monitor results of wound cultures daily.
   4. Monitor daily caloric intake.

5. An adult is admitted to the surgical ICU following a left adrenalectomy. An IV containing hydrocortisone is running. The nurse planning care for him knows it is essential to include which of the following nursing interventions at this time?
   1. Monitor blood glucose levels every shift to detect development of hypo- or hyperglycemia.

2. Keep flat on back with minimal movement to reduce risk of hemorrhage following surgery.
3. Administer hydrocortisone until vital signs stabilize, then discontinue the IV.
4. Teach him how to care for his wound because he is at high risk for developing postoperative infection.

6. When a 10-year-old went to see the school nurse about a circle of ringworm on his scalp, he was asked some questions for a data base. Which of his environmental factors most likely contributed to the child's acquisition of ringworm?
   1. He rides a public bus to and from school each day and likes to sit behind the driver so they can talk about baseball.
   2. He has a pet kitten that stays outside during the day but comes inside to sleep with him at night.
   3. He loaned his baseball hat to a friend last week but hasn't gotten it back yet.
   4. He forgets to wash his hair sometimes, and his mother has to remind him.

7. When planning immediate postoperative care for the adolescent with a Harrington rod insertion, what would be the priority nursing focus?
   1. Assessment of paralytic ileus.
   2. Cast care and repair of rough edges.
   3. Neurological assessments.
   4. Vital signs and urinary output.

8. When a child vomits a bright-red liquid several hours after a tonsillectomy, the nurse needs to determine whether the child is bleeding from the operative site. Which nursing action would be most informative?
   1. Visualizing the posterior throat with use of a tongue depressor and flashlight.
   2. Asking if the child had received red Koolaid for oral intake during the last hour.
   3. Taking vital signs, including the blood pressure, and checking oral mucous membranes for color changes.
   4. Examine the blood to see if the membrane from the operative site is present.

9. The nurse has been teaching the family of a child with croup about emergency care. Which statement made by the parent indicates that teaching was effective?
   1. "If he wakes up coughing a barky cough, I'll try sitting in a steamy bathroom with him. If he isn't better in an hour, I'll bring him to the hospital for an aerosol of epinephrine."
   2. "If the X-ray shows no swelling of the epiglottis, we can probably go back home and use the humidifier there."
   3. "Symptoms of breathing hard, inward movement of the ribs and neck with breathing, and a continuous loud breathing noise, are usual signs of spasmodic croup and can be treated at home."
   4. "If he has an episode of loud, labored breathing and retractions, becomes frightened, sweaty, and thrashes around, then falls asleep, the croup attack is over."

10. The nurse is assisting a child with congestive heart failure (CHF). Which of the following would the child be least likely to manifest?
    1. Weakness and fatigue.
    2. Dyspnea.
    3. Tachycardia.
    4. Oliguria.

11. A woman is scheduled for radiation therapy following a mastectomy. What symptoms can the nurse expect the client to report?
    1. Increased energy after treatment.
    2. Increased appetite after treatment.
    3. Skins changes at radiation site.
    4. Diarrhea.

12. The nurse is assessing an elderly client who wears glasses and a hearing aid and is in generally good health. What is a common theme in the physical assessment and evaluation of the elderly client?
    1. The elderly are living a shorter period of time.
    2. Reserve capacity is diminished.
    3. Changes are usually related to disease.
    4. Clients with good health habits experience few age-related changes.

13. The nurse is performing a cardiovascular assessment on an elderly client. What findings would be expected?
    1. A bounding radial pulse.
    2. An early systolic murmur.

3. First-degree heart block.
4. Frequent bursts of tachycardia.

14. When caring for an elderly client it is important to keep in mind the changes in color vision that may occur. What colors are apt to be most difficult for the elderly to distinguish?
    1. Red and blue.
    2. Blue and gold.
    3. Red and green.
    4. Blue and green.

15. Which statement by the client who has Type 2 diabetes mellitus requires additional teaching on foot care?
    1. "I should use a mirror to examine all surfaces of my feet for cuts, cracks, or redness."
    2. "I should wear shoes that fit well and allow room for my toes to wiggle."
    3. "I should use a bath thermometer to ensure that my bath water is between 85° and 90° before I step into the tub."
    4. "I should remove corns and calluses by using the special medicated pads available at the drugstore."

16. An elderly client is diagnosed as having sick sinus syndrome and is being prepared for the insertion of a demand pacemaker. What explanation will be provided to the client on how the pacemaker works?
    1. It senses changes in blood pressure.
    2. It stimulates the SA node at 60 beats per minute.
    3. It beats when there is decreased coronary blood flow.
    4. It senses the heart rate and starts a beat as needed.

17. Which information would be most accurate when describing pacemakers to a client who is to receive a pacemaker?
    1. Batteries are no longer necessary.
    2. Today's pacemakers are smaller than earlier models.
    3. The generator will be implanted in the upper arm.
    4. Modern pacemakers can be inserted in the client's room.

18. Which information should the nurse include in the discharge teaching plan of a client who had a pacemaker implanted?
    1. Remember to take all medications as directed.

2. Avoid sudden changes in temperature.

3. Keep the pacemaker insertion site covered.

4. Follow a low-cholesterol diet carefully.

19. The nurse is teaching a client about symptoms of pacemaker failure. Which symptoms would be excluded in the teaching?

    1. Nausea.

    2. Syncope.

    3. Dizziness.

    4. Palpitations.

20. The client has a 2-year history of back pain and sciatica. Which of the following is he least likely to report having been included during conservative therapy for his back problem?

    1. Analgesics.

    2. Enzymes.

    3. Muscle relaxants.

    4. Anti-inflammatory agents.

21. What is a correct statement about an objective approach for eliciting the severity of pain from a client?

    1. Asking the client to describe the pain on a 0–10 scale, record the information, and base future assessments on it.

    2. Asking the client to compare the current pain experience to that of previous experiences.

    3. The pain experience is a subjective one and not amenable to a standardized assessment approach.

    4. The best approach is to medicate the client sufficiently to control the pain.

22. What assessment finding would be expected in a client with polycythemia?

    1. Pallor.

    2. Tachycardia.

    3. Leg pain with exercise.

    4. Shortness of breath.

23. Which of the following actions should the nurse take in assisting an above-the-knee amputee who is 2 weeks post-op and experiencing phantom pain?

    1. Provide and encourage client activities.

    2. Keep the client on bed rest.

    3. Tell the client the pain will disappear in one week.

    4. Instruct the client to ignore the pain.

24. A mother brings her 6-month-old daughter to the well-baby clinic for her regular checkup. Which

diseases would the nurse explain that routine childhood immunizations protect against?

    1. Poliomyelitis, *Haemophilus influenzae* type B, and mononucleosis.

    2. Measles, mumps, rubella, and herpes simplex.

    3. Diphtheria, tetanus, and Calmette-Guérin bacillus.

    4. Poliomyelitis, *Haemophilus influenzae* type B, and pertussis.

25. The mother of a child in well-baby clinic asks the nurse which immunizations contain live virus. What is the nurse's best response?

    1. MMR and varicella.

    2. Hib and PPV.

    3. DTaP and IPV.

    4. DTaP and Hib.

26. A 6-month-old child is seen in well-baby clinic. The child has had the routine immunizations up to this point. At this visit, which immunizations should the nurse expect to administer?

    1. IPV.

    2. MMR.

    3. DTaP.

    4. Smallpox.

27. What nursing intervention should be included prior to electroconvulsive therapy (ECT)?

    1. Providing an opportunity for the client to ask questions and express concerns about ECT.

    2. Telling the client that it is not helpful to concentrate on the therapy.

    3. Reassuring the client that ECT is no worse than having a venipuncture.

    4. Telling the client she will recover completely as a result of ECT.

28. The nurse is discussing electroconvulsive therapy (ECT) with a client who asks how long it will be before she feels better. How soon will the nurse state the beneficial effects of ECT occur?

    1. 1 week.

    2. 3 weeks.

    3. 4 weeks.

    4. 6 weeks.

29. Nursing assessment before electroconvulsive therapy (ECT) is aimed at establishing parameters that reflect the client's mental and physical status. Which assessment is excluded in the assessment before ECT therapy?

    1. Activity level.

    2. Bowel habits.

3. Pain tolerance.

4. Sleep habit.

30. What side effects would the nurse expect to be present following electroconvulsive therapy (ECT)?

1. Cardiac arrhythmias, elevated SED rate, and fractures of the spine.

2. An increase in norepinephrine at synapses of the brain, an increase in MAO platelet levels, and euphoria.

3. Slowing of electrical impulses in the brain, temporary amnesia, and confusion.

4. Mild organic changes in the neurons of the brain, dementia, and mild aphasia.

31. The nurse is planning care for a client who has had a bowel resection. It is important for the nurse to assess the client for which complication after this type of surgery?

1. Atelectasis.

2. Parotitis.

3. Temporary ileus.

4. Transient ischemia.

32. The nurse is to irrigate a nasogastric tube every 2 hours. Which solution should the nurse select to irrigate the tube?

1. Normal saline.

2. Tap water.

3. Ringer's lactate.

4. Half-strength peroxide.

33. To prevent postoperative pulmonary complications, which of the following will be most effective in helping a client who has had abdominal surgery to breathe deeply?

1. Oxygen via nasal prongs.

2. Incentive spirometry.

3. Periodic ambulation.

4. Verbal encouragement.

34. An adult has received albumin to treat ascites secondary to cirrhosis. What action will the nurse perform to evaluate if the albumin has been effective?

1. Assess whether pedal edema has decreased.

2. Observe whether the client is less short of breath.

3. Measure the client's abdominal girth.

4. Check lab study results for an increase in serum albumin.

35. An adult who has had an abdominal perineal resection asks the nurse when he can expect his bowel function to return. Which answer by the nurse would be most appropriate?

1. Upon returning to the floor from the post recovery unit.

2. After voiding once.

3. In approximately 6 hours.

4. In 2 to 3 days.

36. An elderly female client is dying from heart failure. The client's daughter only cries when alone with the nurse, not in front of her mother. Which statement made by the daughter indicates to the nurse that the daughter is adjusting to the dying process her mother is experiencing?

1. "I'm so depressed. I try to do my best but I find myself crying a lot of the time."

2. "My mother isn't dying. She has so many relatives to live for."

3. "I really don't know what I would do if mother died."

4. "We don't talk about death. It's a morbid topic."

37. The nurse is caring for an adult client who had an abdominal resection. On the fourth postoperative day, the client's wound dehisces. What is the appropriate nursing intervention at this occurrence?

1. Cover the wound with sterile, moist saline dressings.

2. Approximate the wound edges with tape.

3. Irrigate the wound with sterile saline.

4. Hold the abdominal contents in place with a sterile, gloved hand.

38. An adult client has been experiencing double vision and frequent headaches. Which diagnostic procedure most likely would be used to confirm the presence of a brain tumor?

1. A CT scan.

2. A myelogram.

3. Skull X-rays.

4. A lumbar puncture.

39. The nurse is caring for an adult admitted with a diagnosis of a brain tumor. Shortly after her admission, the client suffers a seizure. What will the nurse's initial intervention be directed toward?

1. Controlling the seizure.

2. Protecting the client.

3. Restraining the client.

4. Reducing circulation to the brain.

40. Following a craniotomy, the client asks the nurse why a bone flap is necessary. What explanation does the nurse give for the purpose for removing the bone flap?
    1. Allow for the insertion of an ICP bolt.
    2. Accommodate postoperative brain swelling.
    3. Allow free flow of fluid into the Jackson-Pratt (JP) drain.
    4. Permit reoperation if necessary as access will be easier.

41. The nurse is caring for a client who had a craniotomy performed this morning. What is the importance of positioning the client's head?
    1. Maintain a patent airway.
    2. Facilitate venous drainage.
    3. Provide for client comfort.
    4. Prevent hemorrhage from the suture line.

42. Following craniotomy, which of the following measures is contraindicated for postoperative pulmonary toilet?
    1. Coughing.
    2. Deep breathing.
    3. Turning.
    4. Suctioning.

43. Following a craniotomy, what is the rationale for giving glucocorticoid dexamethasone (Decadron)?
    1. It creates a feeling of euphoria, which is beneficial in the early postoperative period.
    2. It promotes excretion of water, which aids in reducing ICP.
    3. It enhances venous return and thus reduces ICP.
    4. It reduces cerebral edema, thus reducing ICP.

44. An adult client is diagnosed as having psychogenic amnesia. The nurse would find which of the following symptoms during the assessment?
    1. Client states he feels detached from his body.
    2. Client states he can recall some things but not everything.
    3. Client states he can't move his arm since he saw a man killed.
    4. Client states he's told he does things that he can't remember.

45. A newly admitted client with a conversion disorder says he cannot move his legs. What is the best nursing response?
    1. "The physical tests and examinations state no physiological reason for your paralysis."
    2. "Let me help you out of bed to the wheelchair. I will show you where the dining room is. Dinner is served at 5:30 P.M. I'll be telling you more about the typical routine later."
    3. "I'll plan to have your meals served to you in bed. Because of your physical problem you will receive special privileges."
    4. "You are here to get an understanding of how your physical symptoms related to the conflicts in your personal life. Maybe you should reflect on this awhile and I'll be back in one hour to discuss it with you."

46. Which of the following assessments made by the nurse would be essential in understanding behavior of a client with a conversion disorder?
    1. Physical symptoms are not under voluntary control.
    2. Physical symptoms are under voluntary control but without intent to reduce secondary gain.
    3. Physical symptoms are experienced as a means to manipulate others to meet narcissistic needs.
    4. Physical symptoms are produced through purposeful means to reduce anxiety and maintain dependency.

47. After a young woman witnesses a traumatic vehicle accident, she suddenly reports changes in her vision and claims to be developing blindness. A conversion disorder is diagnosed, when no physical problems are present. Which of the following responses by family members indicate to the nurse that they understand their daughter's symptoms?
    1. "She's afraid to get involved as a witness of the event, so she claims to be blind."
    2. "She's trying to avoid her civic responsibilities, so she's manipulating the situation and being childish."
    3. "Seeing the accident was very traumatic for her."
    4. "Perhaps the physical examinations aren't true. Maybe glass splinters are in her eyes and are too small to be seen."

**48.** Which of the following would best indicate to the nurse that a depressed client is improving?

1. Reduced levels of anxiety.
2. Changes in vegetative signs.
3. Compliance with medications.
4. Requests to talk to the nurse.

**49.** In assessing a client for posttraumatic stress disorder (PTSD), which symptoms would the nurse perceive as key in the client's response to trauma?

1. Emotional numbing and detachment followed by irritability, anxiety, aggressiveness, and hyperalertness.
2. Depression and social withdrawal.
3. Intrusive, hyperactive behavior and use of alcohol to soothe symptoms.
4. Drug-seeking behavior and sexual promiscuity as a means to cope.

**50.** The nurse is talking with a young female client in the health clinic who is concerned she may have a sexually transmitted disease. What reason does the nurse provide for the delayed treatment of the majority of STDs?

1. The client is embarrassed.
2. Symptoms are thought to be caused by something else.
3. Symptoms are ignored.
4. The client never has symptoms.

**51.** A female client tells the nurse that her boyfriend has told her he has gonorrhea and they had their last sexual experience three days ago. How long should the nurse tell the client to expect symptoms from the initial infection?

1. 2 to 5 days.
2. 5 to 7 days.
3. 1 to 2 weeks.
4. 2 to 3 weeks.

**52.** What organism is linked with up to 90% of cervical malignancies and may be linked to other genital cancers?

1. *Neisseria gonorrhoeae*.
2. *Chlamydia trachomatis*.
3. Human papilloma virus.
4. Herpes simplex virus.

**53.** The nurse is teaching a client about the treatment for gonorrhea. What explanation does the nurse provide on why follow-up cultures are taken after treatment?

1. Evaluate for complications.
2. Check the lab's work.
3. Validate eradication of the infection.
4. Provide an opportunity for sexual counseling.

**54.** A client has newly diagnosed Type 1 diabetes and asks when she will have to test her urine for ketones. For what condition will the nurse state this action needs to be done?

1. She is overhydrated.
2. She begins to gain weight.
3. The glucometer reading is abnormal.
4. Her blood glucose level is more than 240 mg/dL for 6 hours.

**55.** The nurse is discussing ketones with a newly diagnosed client with Type 1 diabetes. In answering the client's question about how ketones will affect her, the nurse should base the answer on which concept?

1. The client with diabetes is no different from others in the capacity to handle ketones.
2. Ketones overpower the client's adaptive mechanisms.
3. Most clients with diabetes are allergic to the by-products of ketone metabolism.
4. It is impossible to predict the reaction to ketones.

**56.** Which special precaution must the nurse take when assisting a client with self-monitoring of blood glucose?

1. Give the client a machine for his use only.
2. Wear gloves when performing the test.
3. Rinse the lancet between uses.
4. Recalibrate the glucometer before each use.

**57.** An adult client's insulin dosage is 10 units of regular insulin and 15 units of NPH insulin in the morning. What will the nurse state as the first insulin peak?

1. As soon as food is ingested.
2. In 2 to 4 hours.
3. In 6 hours.
4. In 10 to 12 hours.

**58.** Dietary teaching for a client with Type 1 diabetes includes information on the glycemic impact of a meal. Which statement by the client indicates she has a good understanding of the teaching?

1. "Foods high in protein raise blood sugar rapidly."
2. "Simple sugars or carbohydrates cause a predictable rise in blood sugar."

3. "The protein, fat, and carbohydrate composition of a meal affect the blood glucose level."

4. "Dairy beverages contain lactose, which dramatically increases the need for insulin."

59. Teaching a client who is insulin-dependent will include guidelines for managing sick days. What is the recommended treatment for an insulin dependent diabetic if nausea is present?
    1. Take the prescribed insulin.
    2. Go to the emergency department.
    3. Administer regular insulin only.
    4. Take nothing by mouth if vomiting.

60. An adult with Type 1 diabetes tells the clinic nurse that she plans to accompany her husband on a business trip. When traveling, the client can use which food or beverage as a substitute for a delayed meal?
    1. Diet cola.
    2. Raisins.
    3. A candy bar.
    4. A glass of wine.

61. An adult with Type 1 diabetes tells the nurse that she would like to lose 15 pounds. What would be the best way for the client to lose weight?
    1. Increase her insulin dosage.
    2. Reduce calories and walk daily.
    3. Do an aerobic exercise program daily.
    4. Restrict all carbohydrates from diet.

62. The nurse is caring for a adult client who has been taking insulin for 8 months. Which diagnostic study is the most valuable in evaluating long-term management of a diabetic client?
    1. A 2-hour postprandial test.
    2. A 6-hour glucose tolerance test.
    3. A glycosylated hemoglobin test.
    4. The diary of glucometer test results.

63. An adult client known to have diabetes is brought to the emergency department with complaints of fever, vague abdominal pain, nausea, and vomiting for the past several days. For what sign of ketoacidosis would the nurse be particularly observant?
    1. Polyuria.
    2. Abnormal reflexes.
    3. Increased thirst.
    4. Mental deterioration.

64. The nurse is assessing an adult client admitted in ketoacidosis. What would be the expected condition of the client's skin?
    1. Clammy.
    2. Flushed.
    3. Diaphoretic.
    4. Silky.

65. The nurse is caring for an adult client who is admitted in diabetic ketoacidosis. The client was diagnosed 10 months ago. This is the first episode of ketoacidosis since the client was diagnosed. What focus should be discussed?
    1. An extremely poor prognosis.
    2. The client's noncompliance.
    3. Reinforcement of client teaching.
    4. The potential for a long, painful, chronic disorder.

66. The nurse is doing discharge teaching with an adult client who had diabetic ketoacidosis. What reminder should the client be given?
    1. The symptoms of ketoacidosis can vary; therefore, all changes in status should be monitored.
    2. Weight loss and fatigue are early symptoms of ketoacidosis.
    3. Headache is a serious diagnostic sign of ketoacidosis.
    4. In ketoacidosis mucous membranes will be pale.

67. In assessing adult clients for early signs of cancer, which of the following findings reported to the nurse would indicate a priority for follow-up?
    1. Bowel movements twice a day for the past 5 years.
    2. Monthly breast self-exam.
    3. Lingering cough 1 week after a cold.
    4. Mole that has become larger in the past 4 weeks.

68. The nurse is caring for the mother of a newborn. What action by the mother indicates to the nurse that more teaching is needed?
    1. Keeps the cord exposed to the air.
    2. Washes her hands before sponge bathing her baby.
    3. Washes the cord with water at each diaper change.
    4. Checks the cord daily for bleeding and drainage.

69. What is recommended to minimize discomfort and embarrassment when the nurse is assessing an adolescent girl?
    1. Make sure a parent is present.
    2. Provide a gown and private area.
    3. Examine two adolescents at the same time.
    4. Postpone the exam until the adolescent is older.

70. A 10-month-old child is brought to the clinic for the first time. During the assessment interview, the mother states that her baby is allergic to eggs. The child will need testing before receiving which immunization?
    1. DTaP.
    2. Smallpox vaccine.
    3. OPV.
    4. MMR.

71. Which of the following interventions would be appropriate to add to the plan of care for a client diagnosed with cancer, who is receiving radiation and chemotherapy?
    1. Provide air sprays to mask odors.
    2. Administer Demerol IM for complaints of pain.
    3. Encourage rinsing sore mouth with commercial mouthwashes.
    4. Avoid fresh fruit and vegetables.

72. What should the nurse do when an elderly client with sundowner syndrome becomes mildly disoriented?
    1. Ignore the disorientation.
    2. Prepare a normal saline IV.
    3. Turn off the lights in the room.
    4. Remind him where he is and why he is there.

73. A young male is admitted to the emergency department suffering from a gunshot wound. What assessment finding would be of most concern to the nurse?
    1. Nausea.
    2. Headache.
    3. BP 104/54.
    4. Tracheal deviation.

74. When assessing the client with the diagnosis of chronic obstructive pulmonary disease (COPD), which data would require the nurse to take immediate action?
    1. Large amounts of thick white sputum.
    2. Oxygen via nasal cannula set on 8 liters.

    3. Use of accessory muscles during inspiration.
    4. Presence of barrel chest and dyspnea.

75. Which statement by the client indicates the discharge teaching for the client diagnosed with pulmonary embolus is effective?
    1. "I am going to use a regular-bristle toothbrush."
    2. "I will avoid being around large crowds."
    3. "I will take enteric-coated aspirin if I have a headache."
    4. "I will drink extra fluids while on long trips."

76. What should the nurse include in the care plan for a client with sundowner syndrome regarding his room environment during his sleeping hours?
    1. Keep the room brightly lit.
    2. Use subdued lighting.
    3. Keep the room dark with a night light.
    4. Ask the client how he is most comfortable.

77. The nurse is caring for a client who is having a panic attack. Which symptom will the client be least likely to exhibit?
    1. Bradycardia.
    2. Sweating.
    3. Chest pain.
    4. Fear of going crazy.

78. The nurse is caring for a man who has angina. He complains of chest pain. For what reason is nitroglycerin given?
    1. Slows and strengthens the heart rate.
    2. Assists smooth muscles to contract.
    3. Increases venous return to the heart.
    4. Reduces both preload and afterload.

79. To combat the most common adverse effects of chemotherapy, what medication would the nurse administer?
    1. Antibiotic.
    2. Antiemetic.
    3. Anticoagulant.
    4. Anti-inflammatory.

80. Discharge teaching for an adult client with angina includes a complete review of nitroglycerin usage. After opening, what time frame does the nurse tell the client that the nitroglycerin may be used in?
    1. 1 week.
    2. 1 month.
    3. 4 months.
    4. 6 months.

81. What advice should the nurse give an adult client who takes a sublingual nitroglycerin tablet without relief of pain?
    1. Go to the emergency department.
    2. Take another tablet sublingually.
    3. Take two more tablets orally.
    4. Double the strength of the next dose.

82. Which statement indicates the need for further teaching for the client diagnosed with sleep apnea?
    1. "I'm trying to lose weight and stop smoking."
    2. The continuous airway pressure prevents the collapse of my airway."
    3. "Using the CPAP at night will help me stay awake during the day."
    4. "I'm glad they found out I have sleep apnea from all the X-rays they took of my mouth."

83. What would be an expected assessment finding in a client with iron-deficiency anemia?
    1. Bradycardia.
    2. Jaundice.
    3. Hunger.
    4. Fatigue.

84. The nurse has been teaching self-care to an adult client who is receiving external radiation therapy to the facial area. Which of the following client actions indicates a need for further teaching?
    1. Sitting next to his wife and holding hands.
    2. Applying lotion and powder to the radiated site.
    3. Gently cleaning mouth and teeth with a sponge.
    4. Resting between activities.

85. The nurse is caring for a 28-week-premature infant on a ventilator. Which action is essential for the nurse to take?
    1. Assess the oxygen saturation of the infant once per 8-hour shift using a pulse oximeter.
    2. Notify the physician if the oxygen saturation falls below 95% on the pulse oximeter, and plan to increase the oxygen settings.
    3. Notify the physician if the oxygen saturation is continually above 95%.
    4. Suction the infant every 2 hours around the clock.

86. To prevent complications for a client who has developed thrombocytopenia secondary to radiation therapy, what instruction will the nurse provide to the client?
    1. Brush the teeth with a hard bristle brush.
    2. Shave with an electric razor.
    3. Continue with sports activities.
    4. Continue with intramuscular pain medications.

87. A laboring client has just been told that she will be delivering her baby by cesarean birth because of a contracted pelvis. To ensure a positive outcome for the parents, what will be given the highest priority by the nurse?
    1. Keeping the woman clean and dry.
    2. Keeping the woman informed.
    3. Escorting the husband to the waiting room.
    4. Maintaining comfort.

88. Following circumcision of a 1-day-old infant, what is the most effective strategy for ensuring urinary elimination?
    1. Feeding the infant.
    2. Having nonconstrictive gauze over the penis.
    3. Keeping the infant on his side.
    4. Checking for first void postcircumcision.

89. An adult client is scheduled for gallbladder surgery in 4 weeks. During his preadmission office visit he states that he smokes two packs of cigarettes a day. What instructions will the nurse give to the client about this activity?
    1. Demonstrate how to use an incentive spirometer.
    2. Try to decrease smoking.
    3. Stop smoking now.
    4. Join a nonsmoker's group and reschedule surgery.

90. An adult had abdominal surgery 2 days ago. Which of the following statements would indicate to the nurse that normal bowel peristalsis is returning?
    1. "My belly seems bigger this afternoon."
    2. "I keep burping."
    3. "I passed some rectal gas today."
    4. "I feel like vomiting."

91. A client was admitted with a diagnosis of left-sided cerebrovascular accident (CVA) and placed on cardiac monitoring. There were indiscernible P waves and the QRS complex was normal but the ventricular rhythm was irregular with a rate of between 100 and 180 beats per minute. What is the supraventricular arrhythmia associated with CVA called?
    1. Wide complex junctional tachycardia.
    2. Sinus tachycardia.
    3. Second-degree AV block referred to as Wenckebach.
    4. Atrial fibrillation initiated by an ectopic focus outside the SA node.

92. An adult is admitted with a diagnosis of probable Graves' disease with thyrotoxic crisis. Which of the following assessments will provide the nurse with the best measure of the severity of the client's disease?
    1. Blood glucose.
    2. Heart rate.
    3. Urine output.
    4. Blood pressure.

93. An adult with diabetes mellitus has a glycosolated hemoglobin (hemoglobin A1c) reading of 10% and the blood glucose reading is 100 mg/dL. How should the nurse proceed?
    1. Ask the client for daily blood glucose monitoring records, and ask the client to describe self-care practices.
    2. Congratulate the client on the excellent level of diabetic control achieved and suggest that the client continue the present regimen.
    3. Observe the client for the signs and symptoms of diabetic ketoacidosis and refer the client to the physician immediately.
    4. Observe the client for signs and symptoms of hypoglycemia and provide orange juice immediately.

94. An elderly client with Type 2 diabetes mellitus lives alone. Admission assessment includes the following information: eats one meal a day (mostly carbohydrate foods); wears poor fitting shoes and often goes barefoot. Which nursing diagnosis would be appropriate if the client is receptive to a change in these behaviors?
    1. Impaired home maintenance management related to declining health.
    2. Activity intolerance related to pedal pain.
    3. Feeding self-care deficit related to poor food choices.
    4. Altered health maintenance related to inadequate health teaching.

95. An adult client with hemiplegia and right hemianopia expresses concern about how to operate the vacuum cleaner and washing machine at home. Which of the following nursing diagnoses is appropriate for this client?
    1. High risk for injury related to right-sided weakness.
    2. Impaired home maintenance management related to paralysis and visual impairment.
    3. Altered health management related to altered mobility and sensory perception.
    4. Hygiene and self-care deficit related to inability to operate appliances.

96. Which assessment is the most important to include in an older client with a family history of diabetes mellitus?
    1. Palpation of pedal pulses and auscultation for carotid bruit.
    2. Palpation of liver and observation of sclera.
    3. Palpation of spleen and pulse oximetry.
    4. Palpation of abdomen and auscultation of breath sounds.

97. The nurse is teaching a male client to examine his testicular area for abnormal masses. Which of the following would be included in the appropriate assessment of the scrotum?
    1. Observing that the right side is lower than the left.
    2. Including the inguinal and femoral areas for bulges.
    3. Requesting he inhale during the exam.
    4. Holding the penis down during the exam.

98. The nurse is discussing risk factors for osteoporosis with a middle-aged client. Which assessment finding indicates a risk factor for osteoporosis?
    1. The client has lactose intolerance and does not drink milk, but eats cheese and dark green vegetables.
    2. The client is 5 feet 2 inches tall and weighs 90 pounds.
    3. The client participates in aerobics classes twice weekly.
    4. The client has been taking estrogen since her ovaries were removed 2 years ago.

**99.** The nurse is performing a breast examination for a nonpregnant woman during her annual gynecological visit. The nurse will be concerned if which one of the following findings is present?

1. Nipple discharge.
2. Tail of Spence.
3. Soft axilla.
4. Consistent patterns of veins.

**100.** The nurse is assessing an adult client who has had a kidney transplant. Which of the following assessment findings would indicate to the nurse that the client might be developing acute rejection of the kidney?

1. Oliguria.
2. Temperature range of 37.2°C (98.6°F) – 37.7°C (99.8°F).
3. Blood pressure of 110/76.
4. Serum Creatine of 0.8 and BUN at 12.

# Answers and Rationales for Practice Test 5

| ANSWER | RATIONALE | NP | CN | CL | SA |
|---|---|---|---|---|---|
| #1. 4. | A negative pressure room is always a private room, in which the air is vented to the outside, ensuring that contaminated air cannot escape from the room into other parts of the facility. This type of room usually also has a separate side room in which to enter that has a sink and personal protective equipment (PPE) is housed. | Pl | Sa/2 | Ap | 1 |
| #2. 3. | The client should be instructed the day before how to cough and obtain the specimen, as the best time secretions are easily obtainable is early in the morning. The client may brush the teeth first, but not swallow. The specimen will be taken to the lab where it will be placed on an appropriate culture medium and incubated for at least 24 hours. | Im | Ph/7 | Ap | 1 |
| #3. 3. | The goal will be to maintain normal weight or allow for weight gain. Weight lost may have occurred during the disease process, so small, frequent meals would be tolerated best. | Pl | Ph/5 | Ap | 1 |
| #4. 3. | Infection, which begins in the burn wound and travels to the bloodstream, is the primary cause of death in persons who survive the first few days following extensive burns. Cultures are taken to monitor the colonization of the wound by organisms, alerting staff to early detection of infection and treatment with antibiotics. ABGs would indicate a need for intubation; fluid overload is monitored to prevent congestive heart failure; and a high-calorie, high-protein diet is ordered. | Pl | Ph/7 | Ap | 1 |
| #5. 1. | Hydrocortisone promotes gluconeogenesis and elevates blood glucose levels. Following adrenalectomy the normal supply of hydrocortisone is interrupted and must be replaced to maintain the blood glucose at normal levels. The medication will be changed when the client is able to take it by mouth and will be necessary for 6 months to 2 years until his remaining gland recovers. Wound care will be done at a more appropriate time. | Ev | Ph/6 | Ap | 1 |
| #6. 2. | It is common for children to acquire ringworm from their pets, especially if the pets are outside during the day and only spend the night in the house. The pet will also need to be assessed for ringworm lesions. The child is most likely leaning forward while talking with the bus driver (not placing head on headrest); the | An | He/3 | Ap | 4 |

child who has his hat should be checked for ringworm. Not washing the hair is not the cause for the current infection.

| | | | | | |
| --- | --- | --- | --- | --- | --- |
| #7. 3. | Any sign of paresthesia or paralysis needs to be reported promptly. Spinal nerve damage is a risk and may require emergency removal of the instrumentation. It is also imperative to monitor kidney perfusion which could result in acute renal failure, and would be a good second choice. A paralytic ileus is not an immediate complication, but if it occurs, treatment would be nasogastric intubation. Cast care is addressed 8 to 12 days postoperatively, when the child is removed from the immobilization of the Stryker frame bed. | Pl | Ph/7 | Ap | 4 |
| #8. 1. | Because the operative site can be visualized, the nurse should look for oozing of blood using good lighting and a tongue depressor. The surgical membrane does not pull apart until 4–10 days after surgery. | Im | Ph/7 | Ap | 4 |
| #9. 1. | Laryngotracheobronchitis (LTB) will fatigue the child unless the airway is opened more. In worsening signs of respiratory distress, epinephrine is given to cause vasoconstriction and a reduction of airway swelling. The child will require monitoring in a hospital setting for side effects and any rebound signs and symptoms. No swelling of the epiglottis is present with LTB; "breathing hard" describes stage II of the progression of symptoms of LTB, which necessitates being observed in a croup tent along with an oximeter to indicate oxygenation status. | Ev | Ph/7 | Ap | 4 |
| #10. 4. | Due to the administration of diuretics in CHF, oliguria is usually not seen. All the others are expected symptoms seen in CHF. | As | Ph/8 | Ap | 4 |
| #11. 3. | Skin changes would include thinning, altered pigmentation, ulceration, or necrosis. The client should be taught only to use creams/lotions approved by the radiation oncologist. Fatigue and anorexia are expected after treatment, and diarrhea would be expected if the intestinal area were being radiated. | Pl | Ph/8 | Ap | 3 |
| #12. 2. | Body organs experience a decrease in functional capacity as the individual ages; the cardiac and respiratory system are particularly vulnerable to decline. Changes are always related to disease and good health habits may help prevent disease. | As | He/3 | Ap | 1 |
| #13. 2. | Cardiac valves thicken and stiffen with age which can be a cause of the common systolic murmur heard in the elderly. The pulse may become weaker with age and tachycardia would not be constant, but have frequent bursts. | As | He/3 | An | 1 |
| #14. 4. | The elderly have poor blue-green discrimination because of the difference in wavelengths. This is due to the yellowing of the lens with age. | An | He/3 | K | 1 |
| #15. 4. | The client did not hear the importance of seeing a podiatrist for the treatment of problems of the foot. Special shoes may be necessary to prevent recurrence of these problems. | Ev | Ph/7 | Ap | 1 |
| #16. 4. | A pacemaker is an electrical device that provides repetitive electrical stimuli to the heart muscle for the control of heart rate. It is set at a rate determined individually for each client and is | Im | Ph/7 | Ap | 1 |

| ANSWER | RATIONALE | NP | CN | CL | SA |
|--------|-----------|-----|-----|-----|-----|
| | either inhibited by ventricular response or initiated by the atria. It is not able to sense coronary blood flow. | | | | |
| #17. 2. | The pulse generators are smaller in size, but still require a battery, usually a lithium cell that lasts 8–12 years. The generator is a smooth, lightweight case containing a tiny computer and a battery which is implanted under the collarbone in a pocket underneath the skin. The insertion is done by fluoroscopic control in a cardiovascular laboratory or operating room. | Im | Ph/7 | Ap | 1 |
| #18. 1. | Many clients will require cardiac medication following the insertion of a pacemaker. Avoidance of sudden changes in temperature and covering the site is not necessary. The diet will depend on the client's serum cholesterol level. | Im | Ph/7 | Ap | 1 |
| #19. 1. | Nausea is the only symptom listed that is usually not associated with pacemaker failure. | Ev | Ph/7 | An | 1 |
| #20. 2. | Conservative treatment would not include enzyme therapy. Chemonucleolysis is a surgical procedure that injects an enzyme in the nucleus pulposus of the intravertebral disc. | As | Ph/7 | An | 1 |
| #21. 1. | A numerical scale can be used to compare it with future assessments. As the goal of pain management is to use as little medication as possible to control pain, alternative methods should be used in conjunction with drug-induced analgesia. | Im | Ph/7 | Ap | 5 |
| #22. 4. | Polycythemia is an excess of red blood cells, in which blood viscosity is increased, making circulation through capillary beds sluggish. The decreased oxygenation of the tissues leads to shortness of breath, headache, flushing of the face, and paresthesias. Leg pain with exercise is associated with intermittent claudication. | As | Ph/7 | Ap | 1 |
| #23. 1. | Phantom pain may occur several months after amputation and the caregiver should acknowledge the pain as real, providing medication and client activities. | Im | Ph/7 | Ap | 1 |
| #24. 4. | Routine childhood immunizations are given to prevent poliomyelitis, diphtheria, pertussis, tetanus, *Haemophilus influenzae* type B, measles, mumps, and rubella. There are no vaccines for mono or herpes simplex; the Calmette-Guérin bacillus (BCG) is given in some countries to protect against tuberculosis. | Pl | He/3 | Ap | 4 |
| #25. 1. | The measles, mumps, and rubella vaccine (MMR) and varicella (chickenpox) contain live virus. | An | He/3 | Ap | 4 |
| #26. 3. | DTaP is given at 2, 4, 6, 18 months and between 4 and 6 years of age. IVP is given at 2, 4, and 18 months and between 4 and 6 years of age. MMR is given at 15 months and between 11 and 12 years of age. The smallpox vaccine is no longer given since the disease's eradication in the United States in 1972. | Im | He/3 | Ap | 4 |
| #27. 1. | The opportunity to ask questions helps to reduce anxiety and misinformation while enlisting the client and family's support and cooperation in the treatment. The treatment often results in significant reduction in depression but the results cannot be guaranteed. | Im | Ps/4 | Ap | 2 |

| ANSWER | RATIONALE | NP | CN | CL | SA |
|--------|-----------|----|----|----|----|
| #28. 1. | Treatments are administered at intervals of 48 hours, with beneficial effects usually evident after the first several treatments, which is within 1 week. | Ev | Ps/4 | Co | 1 |
| #29. 3. | Pain is not associated with ECT, but activity level, bowel habits, and sleep habits and/or depression provide insight into the client's physical and mental status. | As | Ps/4 | An | 2 |
| #30. 3. | Common side effects of ECT include slowing of electrical impulses in the brain and temporary confusion and amnesia. | As | Ph/7 | Co | 1 |
| #31. 3. | An ileus is a result of bowel manipulation during surgery. Bowel sounds need to be assessed as measures will need to be taken if they are not present within the first few days following surgery. Atelectasis is possible after any surgery, however an ileus is a complication that is associated with abdominal surgery. Parotitis is an inflammation of the parotid gland and a TIA is a episode of cerebrovascular insufficiency. | As | Ph/7 | An | 1 |
| #32. 1. | Normal saline will not cause a loss of sodium when it is removed by suction. Tap water would cause the cells to swell, and sodium would be lost when fluid is suctioned. Ringer's lactate (or Lactated Ringer's) is used intravenously to replace electrolytes; hydrogen peroxide is not indicated for internal use. | Pl | Ph/7 | Ap | 1 |
| #33. 2. | Incentive spirometry (IS) will help the client to breathe deeply by providing visual reinforcement to the breathing effort. Ambulation will be encouraged, but the IS can be performed on an hourly basis. | An | Ph/7 | Ap | 1 |
| #34. 3. | Because ascites is the accumulation of fluid in the abdominal cavity, measuring the girth before and after treatment will be the most effective way to determine success of treatment. | Ev | Ph/7 | An | 1 |
| #35. 3. | Peristalsis (bowel motility) usually occurs within 6 hours after surgery and food absorption is tolerated. All segments of the bowel may take up to 3 to 4 days to achieve full motility. The nurse should assess that bowel sounds and flatulence is present before liquids or food is given. | Ev | Ph/7 | An | 1 |
| #36. 1. | Depression is a response to impending loss, chronic illness, or death. The daughter recognizes this as a healthy response in adjusting to this life event. The other statements show the daughter is not adjusting. | Ev | Ps/4 | Ap | 2 |
| #37. 1. | This action prevents infection and drying of the wound until the physician arrives and decides on a plan of action. | Im | Ph/8 | Ap | 1 |
| #38. 1. | Computerized tomography (CT scan) is a highly accurate neurological diagnostic test that provides definitive information on presence, size, and location of brain tumors. A myelogram is associated with the spinal cord, skull x-rays would only view the bones, and a lumbar puncture would examine the cerebrospinal fluid. | An | Ph/7 | An | 1 |
| #39. 2. | Safety is the first priority of care during a seizure. Protect head/body from hitting other objects and turn client to the side if vomiting occurs. | Im | Ph/7 | Ap | 1 |

| ANSWER | RATIONALE | NP | CN | CL | SA |
|--------|-----------|-----|-----|-----|-----|
| #40. 2. | A bone flap allows for accommodation of postoperative brain tissue swelling. It can be removed, preserved in a freezer, and re-implanted several months later. The ICP bolt is inserted through the skull without removing a bone flap; a JP drain is inserted during surgery; removal only occurs should postoperative brain swelling is present. | An | Ph/8 | An | 1 |
| #41. 2. | Elevating the head of the bed 30–45° promotes venous return and improves cerebrospinal circulation, thus minimizing the most serious potential problem of increased intracranial pressure. This is the one case in which maintenance of a patent airway is secondary to facilitating venous drainage. | Im | Ph/7 | Ap | 1 |
| #42. 1. | Coughing or sneezing will elevate intra-abdominal or intrathoracic pressure, preventing venous return from the cranial vault, resulting in increased intracranial pressure. Suctioning would be performed through the nose for no longer than 10–15 second intervals. | Pl | Ph/7 | Co | 1 |
| #43. 4. | Decadron has an anti-inflammatory action that is effective in reducing cerebral edema, which reduces ICP. | An | Ph/6 | An | 5 |
| #44. 2. | Selective amnesia is recalling some things but not everything. Depersonalization is feeling detached; conversion reaction is associated with no organic reason for the inability to move the arm; multiple personality disorder may be the reason for not remembering what's been said. | As | Ps/4 | An | 2 |
| #45. 2. | Explanation of normal routine reduces anxiety and decreases secondary gain. It is too early in the relationship to uncover the conflict underlying the conversion. | Im | Ps/4 | Ap | 2 |
| #46. 1. | The disorder is a loss or alteration in physical functioning due to psychological causes, but the symptoms are not produced on a conscious level. Symptoms are involuntary. | As | Ps/4 | An | 2 |
| #47. 3. | This response shows an understanding of the traumatic event and the conflict she feels in terms of the consequences of being a witness to it. | Ev | Ps/4 | Ap | 2 |
| #48. 2. | Vegetative signs such as insomnia, anorexia, psychomotor retardation, constipation, diminished libido, and poor concentration are biological responses to depression. Improvement in these signs indicates a lifting of the depression. | Ev | Ps/4 | Co | 2 |
| #49. 1. | Psychic numbing and detachment are followed by somatic and cognitive symptoms. Depression and social withdrawal can occur in other disorders; alcohol is common in response to PTSD, but the described behavior is typical of manic depressive; and sexual activity is not a symptom of PTSD. | An | Ps/4 | Ap | 2 |
| #50. 4. | Chlamydia is the #1 STD and clients are asymptomatic. Many females with *Neisseria gonorrhea* and syphilis are asymptomatic also. | Ev | He/3 | An | 3 |
| #51. 1. | The usual incubation period between infection and onset of symptoms is 2–5 days. | An | Ph/7 | K | 3 |
| #52. 3. | Human papilloma virus (genital warts) has been strongly linked to cervical malignancies, as a shift from the Pap test to the HPV | An | He/3 | An | 3 |

| ANSWER | RATIONALE | NP | CN | CL | SA |
|--------|-----------|-----|-----|-----|-----|
| | test is being recommended to be the primary detection method for cervical cancer. | | | | |
| #53. 3. | A repeat culture is important to validate eradiation of disease, thus preventing spread of infection. | Ev | He/3 | An | 3 |
| #54. 2. | The urine should be tested for ketone bodies when there is a persistent increase in the blood sugar. Ketones in the urine signal that the body is breaking down fat stores for energy. | Ev | Ph/7 | An | 1 |
| #55. 2. | A lack of insulin stimulates ketoacidosis. The hyperglycemia of ketoacidosis produces large fluid losses (polyuria) and the client becomes thirsty (polydipsia). The body is unable to compensate for the renal losses and dehydration results. | An | Ph/7 | An | 1 |
| #56. 2. | Gloves, and any additional PPE, should be worn any time contact with blood or body fluids is anticipated. | Pl | Sa/2 | Ap | 1 |
| #57. 2. | Regular insulin is classified as rapid acting and will peak 2 to 4 hours after administration. The second peak will be 6 to 12 hours after the administration of NPH insulin. This is why a snack should be eaten mid-morning and also 3–4 hours after the evening meal. | Ev | Ph/6 | An | 1 |
| #58. 3. | The glycemic index is the result of research that revealed that factors other than chemical composition impact the blood glucose level. The protein and fat composition of a meal appears to delay gastric emptying, resulting in a slower rise in blood sugar. Protein foods raise blood sugar slowly, simple sugars cause a rapid rise, and lactose does not increase the need for insulin. | Ev | Ph/5 | Ap | 1 |
| #59. 1. | Sick-day procedure includes taking all prescribed insulin as usual to prevent diabetic ketoacidosis (DKA). The physician will need to be notified if vomiting is consistent and fluids cannot be tolerated. Sick-day rules consist of liquids or soft foods. | Pl | Ph/6 | Ap | 1 |
| #60. 2. | Nonperishable foods such as raisins are the most appropriate food to serve as a substitute for a delayed meal. One-quarter cup provides one fruit exchange, containing 10 grams of carbohydrate and 40 calories. The other choices would either elevate the blood sugar too quickly followed by a rebound fall or does not provide any sustained carbohydrates. | Pl | Ph/5 | Ap | 1 |
| #61. 2. | Clients who need to lose weight should have a reduced-calorie diet plan. Exercise must be carefully selected and used in combination with diet control. Increased insulin might cause hypoglycemia, and restricting carbs would not balance the diet plan. Fifty to sixty percent of calories must be derived from carbs and help maintain blood glucose levels. | Pl | Ph/5 | Ap | 1 |
| #62. 3. | This test is also referred to as the A1c, which shows a pattern of blood glucose levels over a 3-month period. The other methods are used for a more current glucose reading. | Ev | Ph/7 | An | 1 |
| #63. 4. | The buildup of ketone bodies causes a decline in tissue perfusion, resulting in hypoxia. Early detection of cerebral hypoxia is achieved by assessing orientation of person, place and time, along with simple questions and commands. Identifying the subtle changes in these | As | Ph/8 | An | 1 |

| ANSWER | RATIONALE | NP | CN | CL | SA |
|---|---|---|---|---|---|
| | areas can facilitate the early diagnosis and initiate treatment of ketoacidosis and prevent progression to coma. Slow reflexes are a late sign of ketoacidosis. Polyuria and polydipsia would be expected to be present. | | | | |
| #64. 2. | Ketoacidosis causes dehydration resulting in flushed, dry skin. Clammy and diaphoresis is seen in hypoglycemia. | As | Ph/8 | Co | 1 |
| #65. 3. | Because this is the first time in 10 months that the client has had any problems, reinforcement of client teaching is the priority to avoid future episodes. | Pl | Ph/7 | Ap | 1 |
| #66. 2. | Symptoms include fatigue, weight loss, polydipsia, polyuria, nausea, vomiting, flushed membranes, and change in the level of consciousness (LOC). Physical examination reveals dehydration and fruit odor of the breath, with a blood sugar greater than 250 mg/dL. | Im | Ph/7 | Ap | 1 |
| #67. 4. | The seven warning signals of cancer are: | As | He/3 | Ap | 1 |
| | C: Change in bladder/bowel habits | | | | |
| | A: A sore that does not heal | | | | |
| | U: Unusual bleeding or discharge | | | | |
| | T: Thickening or presence of lump | | | | |
| | I: Indigestion/difficulty swallowing | | | | |
| | O: Obvious changes to moles or warts | | | | |
| | N: Nagging cough or hoarseness that lingers | | | | |
| #68. 3. | Wetting the cord keeps it moist and predisposes it to infection. Air exposure helps to dry the cord. | Ev | He/3 | Ap | 3 |
| #69. 2. | Meeting with the adolescent alone, and providing gown and private area would be recommended to ensure privacy needs are met. | Im | He/3 | Ap | 4 |
| #70. 4. | The measles, mumps and rubella (MMR) vaccine is the only choice that contains eggs. Any child who is allergic to eggs should receive a skin test before receiving the vaccine. If the child tests positive, the vaccine would be given in very small doses at 20-minute intervals with adrenaline available should anaphylaxis occur. | An | He/3 | Ap | 4 |
| #71. 4. | If the client's WBC is < 1000/mm3, fresh fruits and vegetables may harbor bacteria and increase the risk of infection. Refrain from sprays which may stimulate nausea/vomiting; avoid IM infections to prevent intramuscular bleeding; alcohol content in mouthwashes will potentiate breakdown. | Pl | Ph/7 | An | 1 |
| #72. 4. | When the client's cognitive level declines, the nurse should provide clear and simple explanations and cues to minimize confusion and disorientation. Turning the lights off may produce more confusion during this time of day when the occurrence is most frequent (late afternoon or early evening). | Im | Ps/4 | Ap | 1 |

| ANSWER | RATIONALE | NP | CN | CL | SA |
|--------|-----------|-----|-----|-----|-----|
| #73. 4. | The wound in the chest wall may cause air to be trapped and not be expelled during expiration, thereby causing the lung to collapse and the heart, vessels, and trachea to shift toward the unaffected side of the chest. This would compromise respirations and circulatory function. | As | Ph/7 | An | 1 |
| #74. 2. | A client with COPD is usually treated with low-flow oxygen delivery of 2 L/min to avoid depressing the respiratory drive in some clients. Nasal cannula is used for oxygen flow up to 6 liters, and then a different type mask would be used. The other choices are expected to be present in a client with COPD. | As | Ph/6 | An | 1 |
| #75. 4. | Extra fluids will help avoid hemoconcentration if there is a fluid deficit while traveling or in warm weather. The client may be taking warfarin (Coumadin) for several weeks following the incident and should not take aspirin, or any NSAIDs, while on the ordered anticoagulant. A soft-bristle toothbrush will prevent gum injury/bleeding. | Ev | Ph/7 | An | 1 |
| #76. 3. | The lighting in the room should be adjusted for normal circadian rhythm. Darkening the room will signify bedtime and a night light is a safety measure to prevent falls. | Pl | Sa/2 | Ap | 1 |
| #77. 1. | A panic attack stimulates the sympathetic nervous system, resulting in increased heart rate, chest pain, anxiety, and choking. | An | Ps/4 | An | 2 |
| #78. 4. | Nitrates can cause venous pooling, resulting in reduced blood return to the heart. This reduces preload. The systemic arterial bed is also relaxed, causing a fall in blood pressure. The result is decreased afterload. Digitalis therapy slows and strengthens the heart. | An | Ph/6 | Ap | 1 |
| #79. 2. | Antiemetics are used for nausea and vomiting, which are common side effects of chemotherapy, and may persist from 24 to 48 hours. Antibiotics are used for infection, anticoagulants are used in blood coagulation, and anti-inflammatory medications are used for inflammatory problems. | Pl | Ph/6 | Ap | 1 |
| #80. 4. | Nitroglycerin may be used up to 6 months after the vial is opened, but should be kept in a cool, dark place. | Im | Ph/6 | Ap | 1 |
| #81. 2. | Up to three sublingual nitroglycerin tablets should be taken at 5-minute intervals before the client seeks further medical intervention for the relief of pain. | Ev | Ph/6 | Ap | 5 |
| #82. 4. | Diagnosis of sleep apnea is based on clinical features plus polysomnographic findings from a sleep study. Using the CPAP at night while sleeping will prevent the nocturnal hypoxemia; this may result in cardiac problems. | Ev | He/3 | An | 1 |
| #83. 4. | Fatigue is often the only symptom of the condition in its early stages. Inadequate iron stores result in inadequate production of red blood cells. This decreases the amount of oxygen carried to all tissues. When anemia is severe enough to affect heart rate, the change will be seen in tachycardia, as the heart is trying to compensate to increase the amount of oxygen to reach tissues. Jaundice may be seen in sickle cell anemia, hemolytic anemia or hepatic diseases. | As | Ph/7 | Ap | 1 |

| ANSWER | RATIONALE | NP | CN | CL | SA |
|---|---|---|---|---|---|
| #84. 2. | Lotions and powders are not applied as they may cause skin irritation. Clients receiving external radiation are not radioactive; oral hygiene is done to prevent irritation; fatigue is a common side effect. | Ev | Ph/7 | Ap | 1 |
| #85. 3. | If the infant continually has high pulse oxygenation readings and other vital signs are stable, the infant may be ready to be weaned to lower oxygen settings. Hyperoxemia increases the potential for retrolental fibroplasia. The oxygen saturation is monitored on an hourly basis; check connections first if pulse ox drops; suctioning would be on a prn basis. | Im | Ph/7 | Ap | 4 |
| #86. 2. | All precautions to prevent bleeding must be taken: using electric razors, soft bristle toothbrush, stopping sports activities, and discontinuing IM injections (due to decreased platelets from radiation). | Im | Ph/7 | Ap | 1 |
| #87. 2. | A couple may be prepared for cesarean delivery at the last minute. The nurse should make the birth experience a positive one by making collaboration between client and staff a priority. Maintaining comfort is important, but given the new planned action, anxiety will be reduced with providing information. | Im | He/3 | Ap | 3 |
| #88. 1. | The infant has had feeding restrictions prior to the circumcision so feeding him afterwards will satisfy his nutritional needs and provide him with fluid to help him void. The gauze is to prevent irritation/friction from covers on the penis; side-lying position has no influence on the urethra to expel urine; the first void is an evaluate measure and does not lead to voiding as feeding would. | Pl | Ph/7 | Ap | 3 |
| #89. 3. | All clients should be encouraged to stop smoking 4–6 weeks before surgery, with explanation to the client that the cessation will decrease the chances of respiratory complications during and after surgery. | Pl | Ph/7 | Ap | 1 |
| #90. 3. | Passage of flatus is usually a sign of positive peristaltic activity. It is after this finding that the client may start eating. | Ev | Ph/7 | Ap | 1 |
| #91. 4. | Atrial fibrillation is the most rapid of atrial dysrhythmias. The atria beat chaotically at rates of 350 to 600 beats per minute. Cardiac output is reduced due to loss of atrial kick. Mural thrombi tend to form, resulting in pulmonary or cerebral thrombosis. Atrial fibrillation is characterized by no definite P wave and an irregular ventricular rhythm. | An | Ph/8 | An | 1 |
| #92. 2. | The metabolic rate and body temperature are elevated in Graves' disease (hyperthyroidism). The client's heart rate increases to provide additional oxygen required to meet metabolic demands. Thyrotoxic crisis (thyroid storm) is a state of extreme hyperthyroidism characterized by a heart rate over 130 beats per minute. Because it can be fatal if untreated, it must be recognized immediately. | As | Ph/7 | Co | 1 |
| #93. 1. | Glycosylated hemoglobin is formed each time blood glucose levels are elevated and remains attached to the red blood cell for up to 120 days. Although the reading is normal this day, the Hgb A1c reflects the average levels of diabetic control over the past | An | Ph/7 | Ap | 1 |

| ANSWER | RATIONALE | NP | CN | CL | SA |
|--------|-----------|----|----|----|----|

three months. Asking the client for more information about daily self-care will reveal the cause of the poor control. The Hgb A1c values should range between 4 and 6%. The normal reading at the present rules out ketoacidosis or hypoglycemia.

#94. 4. This would be the appropriate diagnosis as the client expresses a desire to learn better health management techniques. Poor nutrition and unsafe foot care habits place a client with diabetes at risk for complication of diabetes, such as infection, vascular disease, hyperglycemic hyperosmolar nonketotic coma, nephropathy, neuropathy, and retinopathy.  
An　Ph/7　Ap　1

#95. 2. Hemiplegia is one-sided paralysis. Hemianopia (or hemianopsia) is the loss of one-half of the visual field in each eye. The diagnosis would be appropriate when a client expresses concern about the ability to maintain the home properly.  
An　Ph/7　Ap　1

#96. 1. The vascular complications of diabetes may be so mild that detection of the disease is delayed. Pedal pulses may be absent in the presence of peripheral vascular disease of the lower limbs. The presence of a carotid bruit may indicate partial occlusion of the carotid artery related to arteriosclerosis. Other organs typically affected in diabetes include the eye, kidney, and nerves.  
As　He/3　Ap　1

#97. 2. In teaching the client to examine the scrotal area, it is important to also inspect the inguinal and femoral areas for bulges that indicate herniation. The left testicle is usually lower than the right; inhaling would make palpation more difficult; the penis is held up during the exam.  
Im　He/3　Ap　1

#98. 2. Women who are short and slender are at increased risk and should be encouraged to increase their source of calcium, perform weight-bearing exercises, and take estrogen if prescribed.  
An　He/3　Ap　1

#99. 1. A woman who is not pregnant or lactating who has nipple discharge should be further evaluated. The Tail of Spence is the tissue of the mammary gland that extends into the axillary region and becomes enlarged premenstrually and during lactation. The other choices are normal findings.  
As　He/3　Ap　3

#100. 1. Acute rejection of a kidney transplant can be differentiated from chronic rejection. Oliguria or anuria are signs of acute rejection. The other choices are values within normal limits.  
As　Ph/7　An　1

1. The nurse is caring for a middle-age client whose blood pressure over the past 2 months has ranged between 140/88 and 148/94. When explaining the condition to the client, which limit would be viewed as normal systolic pressure?
   1. 110 mm Hg.
   2. 120 mm Hg.
   3. 135 mm Hg.
   4. 145 mm Hg.

2. An adult client is diagnosed with mildly elevated blood pressure. According to the Joint Committee which of the following studies would be excluded in evaluating this client?
   1. An ECG.
   2. A urinalysis.
   3. Serum calcium levels.
   4. White blood cell count.

3. An adult client's blood pressure (BP) has ranged between 142/90 to 148/96. She is 55 lb overweight for her height and age. What lifestyle change should the nurse suggest for this client?
   1. Lose weight as rapidly as possible.
   2. Plan a gradual exercise program.
   3. Begin vigorous exercise immediately.
   4. Avoid exercise until your blood pressure is within the normal range.

4. A client diagnosed with primary hypertension asks the nurse what is the cause. What is the nurse's best response?
   1. Atherosclerosis.
   2. Renal disease.
   3. Diabetic vessel changes.
   4. The cause is unknown.

5. The nurse is discussing dietary teaching with an overweight woman who has mild hypertension. What should the nurse advise the woman to do?
   1. Eat fewer vegetables.
   2. Reduce calcium intake.
   3. Read contents labels on processed foods.
   4. Add a water softening system for drinking water.

6. A patient with a chest tube needs to leave the floor for another procedure. When the person comes to transport the patient he asks the nurse to clamp off the suction so the patient can leave the room, what would be the nurse's response?
   1. "Ok, but have him back as soon as possible to be put back on suctioning."
   2. "We will have to call the doctor and get an order before we can do that."
   3. "It should be clamped already to maintain lung pressure."
   4. "No, I cannot clamp the suction tube; let me get a portable suction that you can take with you."

7. A adult who has mild hypertension asks if blood pressure medicine is needed. When is pharmacologic therapy usually added to the therapeutic regime?
   1. When symptoms appear.
   2. Any time a client is noncompliant with diet therapy.
   3. When the history indicates the client is at risk for cardiovascular disease.
   4. When the difference between systolic and diastolic blood pressure is greater than 60 mm Hg.

8. The nurse is teaching a client who has mild hypertension. What is the major goal of treatment in a teaching plan for an adult with hypertension?
   1. Control of the disease.
   2. A healthier lifestyle.
   3. Avoidance of renal complications.
   4. Restoration of her prior state of health.

9. The gynecologist has referred a young couple to the infertility clinic. They have been married for 5 years, are in their late 20s, and have been trying to conceive a child for over a year. What is a primary tool in the initial assessment of this infertile couple?
   1. A complete history and physical.
   2. A psychological examination.
   3. An explanation of all surgical options.
   4. Hormonal assessment of ovulatory function.

10. What is the purpose of a semen analysis for a couple in an infertility clinic?
    1. Chromosomal disorders.
    2. Hormone levels.
    3. Sperm motility.
    4. Temperature.

11. The nurse in an infertility clinic is discussing tests that will be done to evaluate an infertile couple. What does the nurse provide in the teaching plan that is a simple method of determining ovulatory function?
    1. Laparoscopy.
    2. Cervical mucous testing.
    3. Postcoital sampling.
    4. Testing urine LH levels.

12. When the cuff pressure from an endotracheal tube is too high, above 20 mm Hg, which of the following would be excluded in possible complications?
    1. Risk of aspiration.
    2. Tracheal bleeding.
    3. Pressure necrosis on the trachea.
    4. Ischemia of the tracheal lining.

13. A woman who is being evaluated and treated for infertility is instructed to graph her ovulatory function by taking her basal body temperature upon awakening each morning. What other information should be documented at this time?
    1. All food consumed.
    2. Her daily weight.
    3. The temperature of the room.
    4. The presence of a sore throat.

14. An infant who is fitted with a Pavlik harness is given home care instructions. Which of the following would be excluded from the instructions?
    1. Turn her every 3 to 4 hours.
    2. Keep her off the affected side.
    3. Watch for signs of skin breakdown.
    4. Give her sponge baths, not tub baths.

15. After a newborn has spent 6 weeks in the Pavlik harness, an open reduction is planned. Awaiting surgery, the newborn is in Bryant's traction to bring the femoral head fully into position. What position of traction will demonstrate that the mother understands the placement?
    1. The hips will be flexed at a 45° angle.
    2. The buttocks will be flat.
    3. The buttocks will be slightly elevated off the bed.
    4. The knees will be bent.

16. An infant who has congenital hip dysplasia not responding to a Pavlik harness is placed in Bryant's traction prior to surgery. The baby's mother asks the nurse if she can take the baby out of traction for feeding. What is the nurse's best response?
    1. "Yes, but only for feedings."
    2. "Yes, this is intermittent traction."
    3. "No, parenteral feedings will be given."
    4. "No, continuous traction is necessary to bring the femoral head fully into position."

17. The nurse is caring for an infant who has had a hip spica cast applied. What should the nurse do to keep the cast free of urine and stool?
    1. Use a Bradford frame.
    2. Use a Denis Browne splint.
    3. Catheterize the baby prn.
    4. Insert an indwelling catheter.

18. The nurse is caring for an infant who is in a hip spica cast. Which action is least appropriate for the nurse to take to prevent skin irritation at the edges of the baby's cast?
    1. Give meticulous skin care.
    2. Petal the edges with moleskin.
    3. Use baby powder around the edges.
    4. Tuck plastic wrap under the edges.

19. Adult clients with acute pancreatitis often have $H_2$ blockers or antacids ordered. What is the primary purpose of giving these drugs to a client with pancreatitis?
    1. Coat the stomach to protect it from the effects of bile reflux.
    2. Reduce gastric pH to inactivate digestive enzymes.
    3. Counteract excessive gastric acid secretion stimulated by release of gastrin from the damaged pancreas.
    4. Raise gastric pH to decrease stimulation of excessive release of pancreatic enzymes.

20. In caring for an adult client with varicose veins, which of the following measures is most essential for the nurse to include in the plan of care?
    1. Discussing cosmetic techniques to improve appearance.
    2. Discouraging stair climbing or walking.
    3. Teaching activities to promote circulation.
    4. Encouraging activities that cause venous stasis.

21. After swallowing a dime, a 22-month-old toddler is brought to the emergency room by her frightened mother. What assessment would alert the nurse to the possibility of esophageal blockage?

1. Dim breath sounds in upper right lobe.
2. Choking, gagging, wheezing, and coughing.
3. Increased salivation, painful swallowing.
4. Inability to speak, cyanosis, and collapse.

22. Which of the following manifestations indicates to the nurse that an infant needs further fluid therapy for dehydration?
    1. Fontanel level with skull and sutures.
    2. Liquid, loose stools.
    3. Specific gravity of 1.010.
    4. Urinary output 1–2 mL/kg/hour.

23. The nurse is caring for an adult client with chronic venous insufficiency. He now has deep, draining, foul-smelling ulcers on his legs. The nurse can anticipate that the client is likely to be given which of the following vitamins?
    1. Vitamin A.
    2. B complex vitamins.
    3. Vitamin C.
    4. Vitamin D.

24. The treatment of an adult client with chronic venous insufficiency and severe leg ulcers includes the application of a gelatin bandage around the stasis ulcers. What is the correct term for this bandage?
    1. A Jobst stocking.
    2. An Unna's paste boot.
    3. A specialized Ace bandage.
    4. A plaster of Paris bandage.

25. A client with chronic venous insufficiency is given discharge instructions. What activity will he be told to avoid?
    1. Walking.
    2. Sexual intercourse.
    3. Elevating the legs.
    4. Standing for long periods.

26. The nurse is discussing the prevention of osteoporosis with a group of adult clients. The nurse explains factors required to keep bones strong. What information is excluded from the nurse's discussion?
    1. An adequate calcium intake.
    2. Maintenance of a low weight.
    3. Sufficient estrogen levels.
    4. Weight-bearing exercise.

27. A client whose mother has developed osteoporosis asks the nurse if there was anything that would have indicated her mother had osteoporosis. What is the nurse's best response?
    1. "Did she experience cramps after exercising?"
    2. "Were her nails and hair brittle?"
    3. "Is she shorter now than she was in the past?"
    4. "Had she been eating less and still gaining weight?"

28. When teaching about osteoporosis, the nurse stresses the importance of prevention. What vitamin would the nurse emphasize that the client's diet should include?
    1. Vitamin A.
    2. Vitamin D.
    3. Vitamin E.
    4. Vitamin K.

29. The nurse is teaching a client about osteoporosis. The client reports all of the following. Which should the nurse recommend the client stop doing to help reduce the risk of osteoporosis?
    1. Smoking.
    2. Overeating.
    3. Biting her nails.
    4. Skipping breakfast.

30. The nurse has been teaching a client about factors to reduce the risk of development of osteoporosis. Adding which food to her diet indicates that the client understands the role of nutrition in preventing osteoporosis?
    1. Oatmeal.
    2. Peaches.
    3. Canned salmon.
    4. Poached flounder.

31. An elderly man was admitted for surgery for benign prostatic hypertrophy. Preoperatively he was alert, oriented, cooperative, and knowledgeable about his surgery. Several hours after surgery, the evening nurse found him acutely confused, agitated, and trying to climb over the protective side rails on his bed. What will be the most appropriate nursing intervention that will calm an agitated client?
    1. Limit visits by staff.
    2. Encourage family phone calls.
    3. Position in a bright, busy area.
    4. Speak soothingly and provide quiet music.

32. A young woman is admitted to the eating disorders clinic for treatment of bulimia. What is the primary issue for the bulimia client?
    1. Delusions.
    2. Depersonalization.
    3. Fear and suspicion of others.
    4. Poor impulse control.

33. The nurse is assessing a client with bulimia. Which characteristic is least likely to be evident in the history?
    1. Repeated crash dieting.
    2. Repeated weight fluctuations.
    3. Rigorous exercise regimens.
    4. Self-induced vomiting.

34. In planning care for a client with bulimia, the nurse expects that the client may be given which pharmacologic agent?
    1. An anticonvulsant.
    2. An antidepressant.
    3. A major tranquilizer.
    4. A minor tranquilizer.

35. The nurse is caring for a client admitted with severe diarrhea. Why should the nurse observe this client for hyponatremia?
    1. Sodium is concentrated in gastrointestinal fluid.
    2. Water lost in diarrhea causes sodium to follow it.
    3. Diarrhea triggers renal mechanisms to waste sodium.
    4. Hyponatremia occurs as a result of treatment for diarrhea.

36. A client with Type 1 diabetes mellitus is diagnosed with peripheral arterial disease. How would the nurse expect the client to describe his discomfort?
    1. Incapacitating.
    2. Throbbing.
    3. Mild.
    4. Aching weakness in the lower extremities.

37. An older adult with a long history of Type 1 diabetes mellitus is being evaluated for peripheral arterial disease. The nurse assesses his feet after elevating them for 30 seconds and notes the color is pale. How would the nurse correctly interpret the color?
    1. Normal.
    2. Dependent rubor.
    3. Pregangrenous.
    4. Cadaveric pallor.

38. The nurse is examining the feet of an older man suspected of having peripheral arterial disease (PAD). Which finding indicates an inadequate nutritional supply to the feet?
    1. Coarse body hair.
    2. Muscle hypertrophy.
    3. Thick, ridged nails.
    4. Rough, reddened skin.

39. When you read a client's chart and see that a syngeneic bone marrow transplant is scheduled in the morning, who would you automatically know the donor is?
    1. The client.
    2. The client's identical twin.
    3. A family member.
    4. A friend of the client.

40. The nurse understands that a client with a long history of diabetes is at increased risk for developing peripheral arterial disease due to what occurrence?
    1. Hypoglycemic episodes.
    2. Capillary rupture.
    3. Early atherosclerotic changes.
    4. Fluctuating levels of insulin.

41. A client has peripheral arterial disease and long-term diabetes mellitus. If the client develops diabetic neuropathy, why is the risk of complications of peripheral arterial diseases increased because of diabetic neuropathy?
    1. It dilates peripheral vessels.
    2. It decreases sensation.
    3. It increases cardiac output.
    4. It alters renal function.

42. The nurse is caring for a client with long-standing diabetes. Which finding is most consistent with damage to the autonomic nervous system?
    1. Flushed, warm extremities.
    2. Dry, cracked skin.
    3. Absent pulses.
    4. Burning sensation on the soles of the feet.

43. The nurse is teaching a client with diabetes mellitus and peripheral arterial disease how to care for his feet. Which instruction should the nurse include?
    1. Avoid deodorant soaps.
    2. Examine your feet weekly.
    3. Use only hot water.
    4. Soak your feet daily.

44. The nurse is caring for a client who is scheduled for surgery tomorrow. It is expected that he will have patient-controlled analgesia (PCA) following surgery. Which statement by the nurse provides the primary reason for using the PCA?
    1. "It is very cost effective."
    2. "It requires less pain medication."
    3. "It allows for families to assist in pain management."
    4. "It allows clients to control their own pain."

45. The nurse knows that which criteria is most important in determining whether a client is a good candidate for PCA?
    1. He is alert.
    2. He is not overweight.
    3. His pain will be constant.
    4. His surgical procedure will be relatively short.

46. What information will the nurse provide that explains why the possible side effect of respiratory depression is reduced using a PCA?
    1. It eliminates peaks in serum drug levels.
    2. It uses drugs without respiratory side effects.
    3. It requires very little medication for pain relief.
    4. There are intervals when the client receives no medication.

47. The nurse is caring for a client who is at risk for developing deep venous thrombosis. Which nursing care measure is not appropriate?
    1. Careful leg massages.
    2. Elastic stockings.
    3. Elevating the legs.
    4. Leg exercises.

48. The nurse is caring for a client who has a deep venous thrombosis. Which nursing care measure would be excluded in the care?
    1. Nursing measures to help the client avoid straining at stool.
    2. Telling the client to avoid sudden movements.
    3. Assisting the client to dangle on the side of the bed 3 times a day.
    4. Teaching the client to avoid bumping the legs against other objects.

49. A client with deep vein thrombosis is started on heparin therapy. Which of the following actions would be inappropriate during heparin administration?

1. Having vitamin K available if bleeding occurs.
2. Observing for hematomas at IV puncture sites.
3. Suggesting that the client use a soft bristled toothbrush.
4. Using an IV control device for drug administration.

50. Two days after admission with deep venous thrombosis (DVT), an adult client develops a cough with slight hemoptysis and complains of shortness of breath and sharp pain under the right shoulder blade. What will the ventilation/perfusion scan show if the client has a pulmonary embolism (PE) but no other pulmonary disease?
    1. Decreased ventilation; decreased perfusion.
    2. Decreased ventilation; normal perfusion.
    3. Normal ventilation; decreased perfusion.
    4. Normal ventilation; normal perfusion.

51. The nurse is caring for a small child. Child abuse is suspected. Who does the nurse know is most frequently the abuser of small children?
    1. Babysitter.
    2. Relative.
    3. Teacher.
    4. Casual acquaintance.

52. In evaluating risk factors for child abuse, which family would be at least risk for abusing?
    1. Moves frequently.
    2. Owns their own home.
    3. Has experienced divorce.
    4. Has problems with chronic illnesses.

53. The nurse is assessing a 4-year-old girl who has been brought to the emergency room with a high fever. Child abuse is suspected. Which test is least likely to indicate that the child has been sexually abused?
    1. A Pap smear.
    2. Urine culture.
    3. Throat culture.
    4. Vaginal culture.

54. What should the nurse do when interviewing a child suspected of being sexually abused?
    1. Ask leading questions.
    2. Have the parents present.
    3. Have a security guard present.
    4. Use the child's words to describe body parts.

55. An adult client has a diagnosis of severe hypovolemia. The medication administration record (MAR) states that the client should receive a hypertonic solution. How should the nurse respond to the order?
    1. Hold the solution until further clarification from the physician.
    2. Administer the solution as ordered.
    3. It doesn't matter if the solution is hypertonic or hypotonic, as long as the patient is getting the necessary fluids.
    4. The nurse should question the order because the client has too much fluid and should not be getting any more.

56. A 4-year-old girl is brought to the emergency room with a high fever. She is clinging to two dolls and has them engaging in explicit sexual behaviors. What will be the nurse's interpretation of this activity?
    1. The child is mimicking behavior seen on TV.
    2. She is acting out a personal experience.
    3. Such play is a healthy expression of sexual development.
    4. The child needs to be directed to more appropriate play.

57. When child abuse is suspected, what is the least appropriate nursing action to initiate?
    1. Take a wait-and-see position.
    2. Call a local social service agency for help.
    3. Prevent the child's return to a dangerous environment.
    4. Confront the parent with security present.

58. Which question is least useful in the assessment of a client with AIDS?
    1. Are you a drug user?
    2. Do you have many sex partners?
    3. What is your method of birth control?
    4. How old were you when you became sexually active?

59. When planning care for the client with *Pneumocystis carinii* pneumonia (PCP), what is the nurse aware of?
    1. It is usually fatal.
    2. The client has few symptoms.
    3. It is highly contagious.
    4. Treatment is more successful now than in the past.

60. What is the drug of choice for treatment of *Pneumocystis carinii* pneumonia?
    1. Amphotericin B (Fungazone).
    2. Ethambutol (Myambutol).
    3. Pentamidine (Pentam).
    4. Zidovudine (Retrovir).

61. The nurse is planning care for an adult client who has *Pneumocystis carinii* pneumonia and AIDS. If this client were to participate in IV drug use, why would he be at risk for infective endocarditis?
    1. HIV-associated arrhythmias.
    2. Increased workload on the heart.
    3. Resistance of bacteria to antibiotics.
    4. Introduction of bacteria into the bloodstream.

62. The nurse is planning care for an HIV-infected drug abuser. Which goal is unrealistic?
    1. Quitting the drug addiction.
    2. Cooperating with unit goals.
    3. Learning to clean drug equipment.
    4. Remaining for the full treatment course.

63. The nurse is assessing a client who has infective endocarditis secondary to AIDS. Which symptoms indicate that the client is experiencing endocarditis?
    1. A pronounced $S_1$ and $S_2$.
    2. Chronic low-grade fever.
    3. Tachycardia and hypertension.
    4. Shortness of breath and chest pain.

64. A 6-year-old is brought to the emergency department unconscious after having been hit by a car. Which of the following would be absent from a baseline neurologic exam?
    1. Motor function.
    2. Visual acuity.
    3. Vital signs.
    4. Level of consciousness.

65. A young adult has Type 1 diabetes mellitus. If she should plan to have a child, what will be of primary importance for her to consider?
    1. Perform a review of the dietary modifications that will be necessary.
    2. Seek early prenatal medical care.
    3. Look into adoption instead of conception.
    4. Knowing that pregnancy is a major health risk to the mother.

66. A young woman who has Type 1 diabetes mellitus is pregnant. She asks the nurse how

much weight she can gain during her pregnancy. What is the nurse's best response?

1. 10 to 15 pounds.
2. 25 to 30 pounds.
3. Less than 40 pounds.
4. The weight of the baby plus 3 pounds.

67. The nurse is teaching a pregnant woman who is also diabetic about her diet during pregnancy. What statement conveys to the nurse that the client understands her dietary needs?
    1. "I will eat a low-protein, low-salt diet."
    2. "I will continue my normal intake of simple carbohydrates."
    3. "I will increase my water consumption."
    4. "I will eat lots of fruits, vegetables, and grains."

68. The nurse is caring for a pregnant woman who is also diabetic. What statement conveys to the nurse that the client understands her blood sugar levels during pregnancy?
    1. "I will keep my blood sugar between 80 to 110 mg/dL."
    2. "My blood sugar should stay within 150 to 200 mg/dL."
    3. "My goal should be between 200 and 250 mg/dL."
    4. "I will not allow my blood sugar to go over 300 mg/dL."

69. The nurse is assessing a client with diabetes for signs and symptoms of hyperglycemia. Which symptom is least likely to be stated by a client with hyperglycemia?
    1. "I am very tired."
    2. "I am voiding more than normal."
    3. "I am very thirsty."
    4. "My bed needs to be remade, as I am sweating so much."

70. A pregnant woman asks the nurse if there are any special problems that she might encounter during labor and delivery because she has diabetes. Which condition will the nurse state that may develop during the birth process?
    1. Hypoglycemia.
    2. Hyperglycemia.
    3. Metabolic alkalosis.
    4. Hyperosmolar nonketotic coma.

71. Which would be of the most importance when inserting an indwelling urinary catheter?
    1. Putting the catheter bag on the lowest part of the bed.
    2. Maintaining aseptic technique.

3. Taping the catheter to the top of the client's leg.
4. Filling the balloon up with normal saline.

72. What would be a short-term goal (to be met in 1 week following admission) planned by a nurse for a delusional client?
    1. Reduce the frequency and intensity of the delusional thinking.
    2. Verbalize why he uses delusions to deal with life.
    3. Communicate in only reality-oriented terms.
    4. Recognize his delusions as nonreality-based statements.

73. The nurse and a severely depressed client mutually plan a short-term goal regarding self-esteem needs. Which of the following would be appropriate to meet in 1 week?
    1. The client will be able to describe one positive attribute about himself to the nurse.
    2. The client will be able to attend and fully participate in all groups and therapeutic activities.
    3. The client verbalizes to the nurse that he is now able to solve his problems.
    4. The client verbalizes to the nurse that he feels good enough to run the next community meeting.

74. An adult client states, "That TV newsman is talking about me." The nurse recognizes the statement as what type of thought process?
    1. Thought broadcasting.
    2. Delusion of reference.
    3. Thought insertion.
    4. Delusion of persecution.

75. Which statement would indicate further discharge teaching is required for a client who is prescribed warfarin (Coumadin)?
    1. "I am going to have to keep coming back to get my blood tested."
    2. "An electric razor would be better to shave with."
    3. "I will use less salt when cooking my food."
    4. "I will contact my doctor if I see blood in my bowel movements."

76. Which of the following behaviors indicates to the nurse that the client with agoraphobia is improving?
    1. Client is able to offer complaints to the boss regarding the workload.
    2. Client is able to travel five flights on an elevator.

3. Client is able to shop alone at a local mall without intense anxiety.

4. Client is able to resist washing hands after touching a dirty object.

77. A client has just completed the detoxification process and is due for discharge. His nurse must evaluate his comprehension of the long-term nature of his addiction. Which statement indicates the best understanding?

1. "I can have a social drink for special holidays without a problem."

2. "I must attend 90 AA meetings in 90 days."

3. "I know I must never drink alcohol again."

4. "Once I finish the 12 stages, I'm cured."

78. An adult has been taking tricyclic medication for a week with no improvement in mood. What is the nurse's best explanation for this situation?

1. The client has been ordered an antidepressant that is ineffective due to client insensitivity.

2. The client should consider electroconvulsive therapy for a more rapid change in mood.

3. The client needs to wait longer because drug onset takes 7 to 10 days.

4. The client requires a second opinion with regards to her medical diagnosis and treatment.

79. A client with a spinal cord injury develops the signs and symptoms of autonomic dysreflexia. What would be the nurse's initial action?

1. Administer an analgesic to relieve the headache.

2. Instruct the client on preventive measures.

3. Examine the rectum for a fecal mass.

4. Sit the client up to lower the blood pressure.

80. A client who is scheduled for a bowel resection tomorrow has just completed preoperative teaching by the nurse. Which of the following statements to the nurse indicates the client needs further instruction on postoperative care?

1. "I know I'll have pain after surgery, but I can call the nurses for medicine."

2. "They will be taking my pulse and blood pressure many times after the operation."

3. "The intravenous needle will come out in the recovery room."

4. "I'll show you how I can deep breathe and cough."

81. An 11-year-old girl is ready for hospital discharge after being newly diagnosed with Type 1 diabetes mellitus. Which statement by the child alerts the nurse to do further teaching before the child leaves?

1. "I never know when my sugar is low, because I don't feel any different, so I guess I'll really have to use my blood glucose monitor on schedule."

2. "On my constant carb diet I can have a dessert every day, as long as I eat it at the same time each day."

3. "I need to pinch up my skin for the injections because if the insulin gets into my muscle instead of fat it won't work right."

4. "I think I'll have Mom get me some of those glucose tablets to carry with me, because I won't be tempted to eat them for snacks, like I would with Life Savers."

82. An adult has acute cholecystitis secondary to cholelithiasis. Which factor in the history is most often associated with cholelithiasis?

1. Low-fat diet for many years.

2. A period of unusually strenuous exercise.

3. Use of oral hypoglycemic drugs.

4. Being a descendant of the Pima Indians.

83. An adult client was discharged following treatment for partial and full thickness burns of the upper body, and an elastic pressure garment was prescribed. When examining the wounds a year later, how will the nurse document that the wounds are healing without complications?

1. Red, raised, and hard.

2. Pink, flat, and soft.

3. Hard, raised, and shiny.

4. Open, pink, and draining.

84. A child with head lice is seen in the clinic and receives home care instructions. Which statement reflects understanding of the teaching?

1. "I'm really embarrassed about this situation, because our home isn't a dirty place."

2. "I guess we'll have to wash all the towels and sheets in the house, along with all your clothes!"

3. "I'll have to get seven bottles of this special shampoo and use one every day for a week on my child's hair. Then she can return to school."

4. "I'm supposed to leave this special shampoo on her for 10 minutes, rinse, and then comb out the nits with a fine-toothed comb."

85. Knowing that a test for phenylketonuria (PKU) is conducted on all babies in the United States, what instructions does the nurse provide to the mother?
    1. Keep the infant NPO before the test.
    2. Maintain the infant's feeding schedule.
    3. Request that it be done within 8 hours of delivery.
    4. Give the infant water before the test.

86. The nurse has just completed education with parents of a newborn recently diagnosed with phenylketonuria. Which statement the parents make indicates the best understanding of phenylketonuria?
    1. "The child only needs to be on a special diet until the age of 1 year."
    2. "The child must eat a diet low in phenylalanine."
    3. "There is medicine that the child can take to avoid being on any special diet."
    4. "The child must avoid all foods that contain phenylalanine."

87. The nurse has just completed teaching a woman regarding the use of the diaphragm and is assessing her understanding. Which statement demonstrates correct learning by the client?
    1. "I will use Vaseline to lubricate the rim of the diaphragm prior to insertion."
    2. "I should get refitted for the diaphragm if I gain or lose more than 5 pounds."
    3. "I should put spermicide only on the rim of the diaphragm before insertion."
    4. "I will leave the diaphragm in place at least 6 hours after intercourse."

88. An elderly client has reported to a local health department to receive a flu shot. The nurse should make which one of the following assessments prior to administering the flu vaccine?
    1. Mental status.
    2. Gastrointestinal system.
    3. Integumentary system.
    4. Egg allergies.

89. While teaching self-testicular examination, when does the nurse instruct as the best time to perform the exam?
    1. After a warm bath or shower.
    2. In the morning before getting out of bed.
    3. At bedtime.
    4. After exercise.

90. The nurse is administering CPR. Which is most important for the nurse to evaluate to determine whether the procedure is being done effectively?
    1. Feeling the carotid pulse during compressions.
    2. Observing the chest rise and fall during rescue breathing.
    3. Monitoring arterial blood gases.
    4. Monitoring the electrocardiogram rhythm.

91. The nurse is assessing an elderly client in a long-term care facility. Which is a normal finding?
    1. Deposits of melanin.
    2. Thickening of the epidermis.
    3. Increase in hair follicles.
    4. Increase in subcutaneous tissue.

92. An adult has had a left hip replacement. He is now 3 days post-op. Which parameter should the nurse monitor to determine if the client is meeting goals related to the nursing diagnosis of high risk for infection?
    1. Nutrition status.
    2. Hemoglobin and hematocrit.
    3. Vital signs every 4 hours.
    4. Amount and character of drainage from incision.

93. The nurse suspects a complication in a client who is receiving peritoneal dialysis. Which of the following observations would support this evaluation?
    1. Pain during the inflow of dialysate.
    2. Occasional diarrhea.
    3. Cloudy or opaque effluent.
    4. Clear or light yellow effluent.

94. The clinic nurse is administering tuberculin skin tests. When administering the purified protein derivative (PPD), which angle and location will the nurse select?
    1. 90° angle into the deltoid.
    2. 45° angle into the subcutaneous tissue of the arm.
    3. 60° angle into the hypodermal space of the gluteal.
    4. 10° angle into the forearm.

95. A client received a PPD 72 hours ago. Assessment finds an erythematosus circle of 10 mm in diameter and an induration of 1.5 mm. How will the nurse interpret these findings?
    1. Meaningless, as the test must be read at 24 and 48 hours. The test will need to be repeated.
    2. Possible exposure to tuberculosis because of the size of the erythema.

3. Positive for active tuberculosis because there is an induration and erythema.

4. There is no evidence of tuberculosis because the induration is small.

96. A tracheostomy was performed and mechanical ventilation instituted on an adult. What will the nurse include when performing tracheal suctioning?

1. Wearing clean gloves, goggles, and a mask.

2. Applying constant suction while inserting the catheter.

3. Hyperoxygenating the client with 100% oxygen only after the procedure is completed.

4. Applying intermittent suction and rotating the catheter as the suction catheter is drawn from the tracheostomy tube.

97. The physician has ordered total parenteral nutrition to be delivered through the central venous line. When changing the tubing to institute the TPN, the nurse should perform which of the following activities to prevent the occurrence of an air embolism?

1. Cleanse the central line insertion site with povidone-iodine ointment.

2. Wrap sterile Vaseline gauze around the hub of the open central venous line while priming the TPN line.

3. Clamp the central venous line while connecting the primed TPN administration set.

4. Place an alcohol wipe over the open end of the central venous catheter while preparing to insert the primed TPN tubing.

98. An adult was admitted to the coronary care unit (CCU) for complaints of substernal chest pain of one-hour duration unrelieved by nitrogylcerin.

Hardwire cardiac monitoring was instituted using lead sites for MCL[1]. What anatomical point will the nurse identify to properly place the electrodes?

1. McBurney's point.

2. Angle of Louis.

3. Suprasternal notch.

4. Costovertebral angle.

99. The nurse provides instructions on a low-fat, high-fiber diet. Which of the following food choices, if selected by the client, indicate an understanding of a low-fat, high-fiber diet?

1. Tuna salad sandwich on whole wheat bread.

2. Vegetable soup made with vegetable stock, carrots, celery, and legumes served with toasted oat bread.

3. Chef's salad with hard-boiled eggs and fat-free dressing.

4. Broiled chicken stuffed with chopped apples and walnuts.

100. An adult female asks the nurse why she should have a mammogram. What is the nurse's best response?

1. "Mammograms can diagnose breast cancer with nearly 100% accuracy."

2. "Every sexually active woman needs to have a mammogram, since there is a correlation between sexual intercourse and breast cancer."

3. "You are 38 years old. This is the appropriate time to have a baseline mammogram done."

4. "The dye, or contrast medium, used when you have a mammogram helps the radiologist see the difference between a tumor and a cyst."

# Answers and Rationales for Practice Test 6

| ANSWER | RATIONALE | NP | CN | CL | SA |
|---|---|---|---|---|---|
| #1. 2. | Current upper limit for normal systolic blood pressure is 120 mm Hg. | Im | He/3 | Co | 1 |
| #2. 4. | A white blood cell count is not necessary, as it is associated with an infection. The Joint National Committee recommends: an electrocardiogram; urinalysis; blood glucose; hematocrit; serum potassium, creatinine, calcium, lipid profile. | An | He/3 | An | 1 |

| ANSWER | RATIONALE | NP | CN | CL | SA |
|---|---|---|---|---|---|
| #3. 2. | Exercise would be the best choice, but one that will not be too vigorous for the cardiovascular system. Rapid weight loss would not be healthy. | Pl | He/3 | Ap | 1 |
| #4. 4. | Primary hypertension is a disorder in which the cause cannot be identified. The other conditions cause hypertension. | An | He/3 | Co | 1 |
| #5. 3. | Salt and fat in the diet should be limited. Processed foods usually have a high sodium and fat content. Vegetables and calcium are encouraged, as they are low in sodium and fat and help to reduce blood pressure. If a water softening system has added sodium, it should be avoided. | Im | He/3 | Ap | 1 |
| #6. 4. | Clamping can result in a tension pneumothorax. The chest tube should not be clamped unless ordered by the physician. | Im | Ph/7 | Ap | 1 |
| #7. 3. | First-line drugs used in the management of hypertension are added when the client is considered high risk for cardiovascular disease. | Ev | Ph/6 | An | 1 |
| #8. 1. | The goal is to control the disease with diet, exercise and possibly medication, and to avoid complications involving other organs. | Pl | He/3 | Ap | 1 |
| #9. 1. | After a thorough history is taken, and both partners have expressed concerns, possible surgical intervention will be discussed at a later time. | As | He/3 | Ap | 3 |
| #10. 3. | Motile sperm (20–120 million per mL) should compose at least 50% of the specimen sent for analysis. | Ev | He/3 | Ap | 3 |
| #11. 4. | Ovulation occurs 16–30 hours after the luteinizing hormone (LH) surge. Testing the urine on a daily basis throughout the cycle helps to pinpoint the time of ovulation. Cervical mucous testing gives an indication of when ovulation occurs but is not as accurate as testing urine for LH levels. | Pl | He/3 | Ap | 3 |
| #12. 1. | Risk for aspiration is a problem that occurs when the cuff is inflated below what is recommended. | An | Ph/7 | An | 1 |
| #13. 4. | A sore throat may be indicative of a cold or other infection, which will distort the interpretation of the graph. The other items do not affect the basal body temperature. | Ev | He/3 | An | 3 |
| #14. 2. | The infant in a Pavlik harness can be turned from back to abdomen but should not be positioned on either side. | Pl | Ph/7 | Ap | 4 |
| #15. 3. | The buttocks need to be raised slightly off the bed and the hips are flexed at a 90° angle. | Im | Ph/7 | Ap | 4 |
| #16. 4. | Continuous traction is needed to bring the femoral head into position. The child easily learns to play with toys tied to the crib and to eat in this position. | Im | Ph/5 | Ap | 4 |
| #17. 1. | The Bradford frame facilitates collection of urine and stool for an infant or child in a spica cast. The Denis Browne splint is a splint used for the correction of club foot. | Im | Ph/7 | Ap | 4 |

| ANSWER | RATIONALE | NP | CN | CL | SA |
|--------|-----------|----|----|----|----|
| #18. 3. | Baby powder coats the skin and causes skin irritation. It is also not advised in infants as it can cause respiratory irritation. | Im | Ph/7 | Ap | 4 |
| #19. 4. | In acute pancreatitis, the pancreas itself is exposed to the digestive action of pancreatic enzymes. During the acute phase it is desirable to remove the stimulation to release these enzymes and thus reduce autodigestion. NPO and H$_2$ blockers are also commonly ordered for this reason. | An | Ph/6 | An | 5 |
| #20. 3. | The client should be taught activities that include walking and climbing stairs, promote circulation and avoid activities that decrease circulation (or venous stasis). | Pl | Ph/7 | Ap | 1 |
| #21. 3. | A dime-size object usually can pass through the gastrointestinal tract and be eliminated in the stool within a week. However, if it occludes the esophagus, the child will not be able to swallow saliva effectively and will begin drooling. Swallowing causes pain from the tightening motion of esophageal tissues around the coin. A foreign object in the air passageway could be evident by choking, gagging, or the inability to speak. | As | Ph/8 | Ap | 4 |
| #22. 2. | Liquid, loose stools contribute to dehydration in infants and would warrant further liquid therapy. | Ev | Ph/8 | Ap | 4 |
| #23. 3. | Vitamin C, the healing vitamin, will aid wound healing through mechanisms that maintain capillary integrity. Vitamin A is for skeletal growth; the B complex vitamins aid in normal metabolism; and Vitamin D aids in absorption of calcium and phosphorus. | Pl | Ph/7 | An | 1 |
| #24. 2. | An Unna's paste boot is a gelatin-based bandage that is frequently used to treat stasis ulcers occurring in a client with venous insufficiency. A Jobst stocking is a custom-made support hose; an Ace bandage provides support to the extremity; and a plaster of Paris bandage dried into a cast is used to support a fractured bone. | An | Ph/7 | K | 1 |
| #25. 4. | Pain and venous congestion can be the result when standing for a long period of time which aggravates venous insufficiency. | Im | Ph/7 | Ap | 1 |
| #26. 2. | Low weight is not a requirement for bone strength. It is indicated for persons with osteoarthritis. Calcium intake should be started in childhood and continued through all ages. Weight-bearing exercise is vital to maintaining bone strength. | Pl | He/3 | An | 1 |
| #27. 3. | There is a loss of height in clients with osteoporosis. Leg cramps relate to arterial insufficiency; brittle hair and nails may indicate iron deficiency anemia; and weight gain may indicate hypothyroidism. | As | He/3 | An | 1 |
| #28. 2. | Vitamin D is a fat-soluble vitamin essential for the normal formation of bone and teeth and for the absorption of calcium and phosphorus from the gastrointestinal tract. It is present in saltwater fish, sardines, organ meats, fish liver oils, and egg yolk. However, requirements are usually met from vitamin D-fortified breads, milk, and dairy products and by exposure to sunlight. Vitamin A is for skeletal growth; Vitamin E is for reproduction and muscle development; and Vitamin K is involved in the clotting of blood. | Pl | He/3 | An | 1 |

| ANSWER | RATIONALE | NP | CN | CL | SA |
|---|---|---|---|---|---|
| #29. 1. | Smoking causes a decrease in bone density. | As | He/3 | Ap | 1 |
| #30. 3. | Canned salmon is a good source of calcium if the bones are not removed. The other food choices are not high in calcium, but contain grains (oatmeal), vitamin A and vitamin C (peaches), and protein (flounder). | Ev | He/3 | An | 1 |
| #31. 4. | The environment is an important factor in the prevention of injuries. Talking softly and providing quiet music have a calming effect on the agitated client. | Pl | Sa/2 | An | 1 |
| #32. 4. | The bulimic client's awareness of the inappropriateness of the eating pattern coupled with the client's inability to control eating activity indicates lack of impulse control. The other choices describe paranoia or schizophrenia. | An | Ps/4 | An | 2 |
| #33. 3. | This activity is seen in anorexia nervosa. The others are commonly associated with bulimia. | As | Ps/4 | An | 2 |
| #34. 2. | Antidepressants have been found to be the most promising pharmacologic treatment of bulimia. The others listed are for seizure, psychotic, and anxiety disorders, respectively. | Pl | Ph/6 | Ap | 2 |
| #35. 1. | Gastrointestinal fluid has a high concentration of sodium, as water follows sodium. Treatment for diarrhea helps restore electrolyte balance. | As | Ph/8 | Ap | 1 |
| #36. 4. | Intermittent claudication is pain occurring when walking that subsides with rest. Resulting from inadequate blood supply, it may be due to arterial spasm, atherosclerosis, arteriosclerosis obliterans, or an occlusion of an artery to the extremity. "Aching weakness" is a common description. | As | Ph/7 | An | 1 |
| #37. 4. | When the extremities of a client with peripheral arterial disease are elevated for 30 seconds, a cadaverous pallor (skin color is pale gray) often results. Dependent rubor is when the leg is held in a dependent position and becomes reddened in color. Pregangrenous would present as cyanotic, cold skin, and absent pulses. | An | Ph/7 | An | 1 |
| #38. 3. | Due to a lack of nutrients to the area, the nails are often thick and hardened. A client with peripheral arterial disease (PAD) would reveal thin, shiny, hairless, and muscular atrophy in extremities. | An | Ph/7 | An | 1 |
| #39. 2. | Syngeneic means that the donor is the client's identical twin. Autologous means that the donor would be the client and allogeneic means the donor is either a family member or a matched donor. | As | Sa/1 | An | 1 |
| #40. 3. | The client with diabetes often experiences early atherosclerotic changes due to alterations in fat and carbohydrate metabolism. | An | Ph/7 | An | 1 |
| #41. 2. | Decreased sensation is the only choice that can lead to injury or the client may be unaware of injury. Healing is slow in persons with peripheral arterial disease. | An | Ph/7 | An | 1 |

| ANSWER | RATIONALE | NP | CN | CL | SA |
|--------|-----------|-----|-----|-----|-----|

**#42. 2.** The blood vessels of the skin constrict in response to impulses from the autonomic nervous system. The result can be dry, cracked skin when vascular constriction is of a long-standing nature. The damage to the feet would be indicative of diabetic neuropathy related to the central nervous system.  
As — Ph/7 — An — 1

**#43. 1.** To prevent drying and cracking, only mild soaps should be used on the feet. Feet should be examined every day, using a mirror if needed; avoid hot water, especially if decreased sensation is present; soaking too frequently may cause the skin to become too soft, and meticulous care to dry the feet, especially between the toes.  
Pl — Ph/7 — Ap — 1

**#44. 4.** Current research shows that pain medication is more effective when it is given before the client's pain gets too intense. The client can stay on top of pressing the button to receive some medication before the pain escalates. Instructions are given that only the client is the one to push the button for medication.  
Pl — Ph/6 — Ap — 5

**#45. 1.** The use of a PCA is best in a client who is alert enough to activate the system. Short periods of sleep may occur, but when the client awakes, he should be reminded to perform deep breathing exercises.  
Pl — Ph/6 — An — 1

**#46. 1.** A PCA is set up to only give small doses, thus eliminating peaks in the serum drug levels. The client still needs monitoring regarding respiratory depression, as the dose may be too high or family members may be pushing the PCA button when the client is asleep. Deep breathing between pushing the button should be encouraged.  
An — Ph/6 — An — 5

**#47. 1.** Leg massages are contraindicated for deep venous thrombosis or those at risk because of the danger of dislodging part of the clot and causing it to become an embolus. The other choices would be ordered for this client.  
Pl — He/3 — Ap — 1

**#48. 3.** A client with a DVT should be on bed rest. Dangling would promote movement of the clot and formation of additional clots by putting pressure on the leg veins. The client would be instructed to avoid straining (which causes the Valsalva maneuver and could dislodge the clot), or sudden movements.  
Im — Ph/7 — Ap — 1

**#49. 1.** The antidote for heparin is protamine sulfate. Vitamin K is the antidote for Coumadin. Bleeding tendencies would be monitored and heparin should always be administered via an IV pump.  
Im — Ph/6 — Ap — 5

**#50. 3.** Pulmonary embolism causes a decrease in perfusion due to obstruction of the vascular system from the clot. Ventilation will be normal.  
An — Ph/7 — An — 1

**#51. 2.** In 90% of child physical abuse cases, the abuser is a relative whom the child trusts.  
An — Ps/4 — An — 4

| ANSWER | RATIONALE | NP | CN | CL | SA |
|---|---|---|---|---|---|
| #52. 2. | The family who owns their own home provides some stability and is less likely to be at risk for abusing their children. Risk factors in child abuse include isolation, unemployment, poverty, marital problems, or chronic illness. | As | Ps/4 | An | 4 |
| #53. 1. | A Pap smear does not detect sexual abuse, but detects changes in cells that may indicate cancer and precancer changes. | As | Ps/4 | An | 4 |
| #54. 4. | Using words the child uses to describe body parts ensure that the child understands what is being said. The child should be asked to describe things in her own words, and in a private interview so the child will feel free to express her feelings. | Im | Ps/4 | Ap | 4 |
| #55. 1. | Hypovolemia means that the client is lacking water or is dehydrated so an isotonic solution should be administered to expand the extracellular fluid. The client's lab values should be given to the physician so a correct solution could be ordered. | Pl | Ph/6 | An | 1 |
| #56. 2. | Demonstrating explicit sexual activity is not within the normal 4-year-old's realm of understanding. These are acts that could only have been known through actual experience, not seen on TV. Observation of this action will help the nurse to be able to explore feelings with the child. | An | Ps/4 | An | 4 |
| #57. 1. | The primary goal is to prevent further abuse and to ensure the child's safety. Taking a wait-and-see stance can prove deleterious to the child. If the situation indicates, the nurse may confront the parents in a nonjudgmental manner with a security guard present. | Im | Ps/4 | An | 4 |
| #58. 4. | The age at which sexual activity began is not relevant as an identifier for a risk factor for AIDS. Drug use and multiple sex partners are risk factors. | As | Sa/2 | Ap | 1 |
| #59. 4. | Great progress has been made in the treatment of PCP, and research is continuing. It is not highly contagious in a person with an intact immune system. | Pl | Ph/7 | An | 1 |
| #60. 3. | Pentam is used in the treatment of PCP. The other choices are used as an antifungal, antitubercular, and antiviral, respectively. | Pl | Ph/6 | An | 5 |
| #61. 4. | The direct introduction of bacteria into the bloodstream increases the risk of the IV drug user developing infective endocarditis. | An | Ph/7 | An | 1 |
| #62. 1. | Counseling may be insufficient to obtain desired behaviors when the negative consequences seem distinct. Objectives must take into consideration the lifestyle of the individual and where changes can be made with the client's cooperation. Therefore, quitting the drug addiction can be unrealistic or inappropriate for clients seeking only care for their medical problems. | Pl | Ps/4 | An | 1 |
| #63. 4. | Signs of endocarditis include shortness of breath, chest pain, murmurs, high fever, and tachycardia (but not hypertension). | As | Ph/7 | An | 1 |
| #64. 2. | A neurological exam would include level of consciousness (LOC), motor function and vitals signs, but it is impossible to assess visual acuity in an unconscious client. | As | Ph/7 | An | 4 |

| ANSWER | RATIONALE | NP | CN | CL | SA |
|---|---|---|---|---|---|
| #65. 2. | Pregnancy makes metabolic control of diabetes more difficult. It is essential that prenatal care starts early so that potential complications can be controlled or minimized. In a pregnant woman with diabetes, the greater risk is to the fetus. | Pl | He/3 | An | 1 |
| #66. 2. | The woman of average size should gain between 25 and 30 pounds during pregnancy. | Pl | He/3 | Ap | 3 |
| #67. 4. | The recommended diet for diabetes is high fiber, low fat. The pregnant client with diabetes should follow a high-fiber, moderate-fat diet with adequate amount of protein. | Ev | Ph/5 | Ap | 3 |
| #68. 1. | The ideal goal is to maintain blood sugar as near to a normal level as possible, 80 to 110 mg/dL. | Ev | Ph/7 | Ap | 1 |
| #69. 4. | Sweating is a symptom of hypoglycemia. | An | Ph/7 | An | 1 |
| #70. 1. | The metabolic demands on the mother during labor and delivery are great and glucose may be insufficient to meet these demands. Blood sugars will be monitored every hour to detect hypoglycemia. | An | Ph/7 | An | 3 |
| #71. 2. | While all the components of inserting a catheter are important, maintaining aseptic technique is most important because it limits the chances for infection and extended hospital stays. | Pl | Sa/2 | Ap | 1 |
| #72. 1. | Within one week, there may be minimal to moderate changes in thought process, depending on the client's diagnosed mental illness. An appropriate goal is for the client to feel less threatened and less anxious, lessening the requirement for delusional thought. If the client is compliant with psychotropic medications, the client may respond positively by decreased frequency and intensity of delusions after 1 week of medications. The other choices are long-term goals. | Pl | Ps/4 | Ap | 2 |
| #73. 1. | Stating a positive attribute about himself is the only choice that would be possible to meet within 1 week. Additional symptoms of depression, pessimisms, or thoughts of failure will prohibit the client from accomplishing the other tasks listed. As self-esteem improves, the client's activity involvement should advance. | Pl | Ps/4 | Ap | 2 |
| #74. 2. | A delusion of reference is a fixed false belief that events or people are directly related to the individual person. The other choices are a disturbance in thought pattern or a belief that others are attempting to harm a person. | As | Ps/4 | An | 2 |
| #75. 3. | Limiting sodium is not necessary for a patient on Coumadin. Dietary recommendations for foods high in vitamin K would be given. | Im | Ps/4 | Ap | 5 |
| #76. 3. | Agoraphobia is the fear of open or public places. The other choices are social, simple, and compulsive phobia, respectively. | Ev | Ps/4 | Ap | 2 |
| #77. 3. | Stating and abstaining from alcohol for life will be essential to his long-term addiction and recovery. | Ev | Ps/4 | Ap | 2 |
| #78. 3. | Drug onset with tricyclic antidepressants begins between 7 and 10 days after initial treatment with full effects taking up to 1 month. | An | Ph/6 | Ap | 5 |

| ANSWER | RATIONALE | NP | CN | CL | SA |
|--------|-----------|-----|-----|-----|-----|
| #79. 4. | Autonomic dysreflexia is an emergency situation which may be triggered by distension of the bladder or colon. The priority action is to lower the blood pressure by placing the client in a sitting position and monitoring blood pressure and other vital signs until the episode is resolved. Then check bladder and/or rectum for distension as the possible triggering response. | Im | Ph/8 | Ap | 1 |
| #80. 3. | Intravenous fluids are necessary post-op to maintain fluid and electrolyte balance and as a route for medications. The intravenous infusion will be kept in place until fluids can be taken by mouth. | Ev | Ph/7 | Ap | 1 |
| #81. 2. | The principle of the constant carbohydrate diet is to keep the CHO intake consistent by time of day, each day. But the "dessert" may differ considerably in content from day to day. | Ev | Ph/7 | Ap | 4 |
| #82. 4. | Seventy-five percent of elderly Pima Indians have evidence of gallstones. Cholelithiasis is also more common in people of northern European descent. A high-fat or high-cholesterol diet, sedentary lifestyle are associated with gallbladder disease. | As | Ph/7 | Ap | 1 |
| #83. 2. | The continuous use of the elastic pressure garment is designed to reduce vascularity and cellularity of the scar tissue and promote the growth of soft, pale scar tissue that is free of collagen nodules. A red wound indicates the development of hypertrophic scars, a hard area would be characteristic of keloid formation, and an open area indicates failure to heal. | Ev | Ph/7 | Ap | 1 |
| #84. 4. | The shampoo loosens the nits and kills the adult lice. The fine-tooth comb pulls the nits from the hair shaft. People from all socioeconomic groups get head lice; only wash items that have had direct contact and place into the dryer on a hot cycle; one initial shampooing is sufficient with a possible additional one 7–10 days later. | Ev | He/3 | An | 4 |
| #85. 2. | The infant's feeding schedule should be maintained because phenylalanine is an essential amino acid that is converted into tyrosine by the enzyme phenylalanine hydroxylase. Therefore, protein in the diet is necessary to see if phenylalanine is converted. | Im | He/3 | An | 4 |
| #86. 2. | A diet low in phenylalanine is necessary for an indefinite period of time and possibly throughout life. If initiated within the first days of life, a low-phenylalanine diet ensures a normal development and life span. | Ev | He/3 | Ap | 3 |
| #87. 4. | It should be left in for at least 6 hours after the last intercourse to allow the spermicidal cream or jelly to work. Vaseline is avoided as it can cause breakdown of the latex; a weight loss/gain of ± 25 lb would necessitate a refitting; spermicide is applied on the rim and inside the dome. | Ev | He/3 | Ap | 3 |
| #88. 4. | Because of the albumin in the influenza vaccine, it should be not given to individuals who are allergic to eggs or egg products. The other choices are not essential to flu shot administration. | As | He/3 | Co | 1 |
| #89. 1. | The most appropriate time for examination is when the scrotum is relaxed, as after a warm bath/shower. | Im | He/3 | Ap | 1 |

| ANSWER | RATIONALE | NP | CN | CL | SA |
|---|---|---|---|---|---|
| #90. 2. | If the airway is open and breaths are being delivered correctly, then the chest is rising and falling. Oxygen being delivered to the lungs is the most important factor during CPR. | Ev | Ph/8 | Ap | 1 |
| #91. 1. | As the skin ages, there is an increase in melanin. These are commonly called "age spots." The other choices are opposite occurrences of what happens in aging. | As | He/3 | Co | 1 |
| #92. 3. | Monitoring vital signs would provide the first means of detecting an infection that is not otherwise visible or obvious. Hgb and Hct provide information on loss of blood/bleeding, not infection. | Ev | Ph/7 | Ap | 1 |
| #93. 3. | The major complication for peritoneal dialysis is peritonitis. Cloudy or opaque effluent (the flowing outward liquid) is an early sign, along with fever, rebound abdominal tenderness, malaise, nausea, and vomiting. | Ev | Ph/7 | Ap | 1 |
| #94. 4. | The PPD skin test should always be given intradermally. When injected properly, the PPD will form a wheal just beneath the skin surface. | Im | Ph/7 | Co | 5 |
| #95. 4. | Indurations less than 5 mm are not significant and erythema is always insignificant. Further assessment is required of indurations of 10 mm or more, which is highly suggestive of tuberculosis; indurations of 5–9 mm are inconclusive and should be repeated in another site. If the client is at high risk for tuberculosis, further testing should be initiated. | Im | Ph/7 | An | 1 |
| #96. 4. | The method described is the proper way for tracheal suctioning. The procedure is sterile; suction should not be applied while inserting the catheter; hyperoxygenation should be performed before and after suctioning. | Im | Ph/7 | Ap | 1 |
| #97. 3. | Clamping the central venous line will prevent air embolism and blood backup. The tubing is always primed before attachment to the existing line. Cleaning helps to prevent infection. | Im | Ph/7 | Ap | 1 |
| #98. 2. | The sternal notch or Angle of Louis identified the second rib and thereby assists in locating the fourth intercostal space. McBurney's point is associated with appendix location; suprasternal notch is located above the sternum; costovertebral refers to the joining of a rib and vertebral and assessing kidney pain. | Im | Ph/7 | Ap | 1 |
| #99. 2. | The choice of a low-fat soup (which would have been higher in fat if made with chicken or beef stock) and high-fiber bread are correct choices. Mayonnaise in tuna salad is high in fat; hard-boiled eggs are high in fat; walnuts are high in fat. | Ev | Ph/5 | An | 1 |
| #100. 3. | The schedule for mammogram testing recommend by the American Cancer Society is a baseline between the ages of 35 and 40; once every 1–2 years between 40 and 50; yearly after age 50. The test can detect tumors and lesions that are still too small to be palpated but should not be promised as 100% accurate; a strong family history of cancer would initiate a mammogram performed at a younger age, not sexual activity; no contrast media is used. | Im | He/3 | Co | 3 |

1. An adult client has been taking aluminum hydroxide (Amphojel) for hyperphosphatemia. What will the client need to be taught about this medication?
   1. To inform the physician if he has constipation.
   2. The tablets tend to be more effective than the liquid.
   3. To take large amounts of water to ensure passage of the medication to the stomach.
   4. To report signs of muscle weakness, anorexia, and malaise.

2. An adult client has chronic idiopathic hypoparathyroidism. Which is not appropriate to include in the nursing care plan?
   1. Low-calcium, high-phosphorus diet.
   2. Oral calcium (Os-Cal) for chronic hypocalcemia.
   3. Seizure precautions.
   4. Private room to reduce environmental stimuli.

3. An adult has hyperthyroidism and is scheduled for a thyroidectomy. The physician has ordered Lugol's solution for the client. What is the primary reason for giving Lugol's solution preoperatively?
   1. Decrease the risk of agranulocytosis postoperatively.
   2. Prevent tetany while the client is under general anesthesia.
   3. Reduce the size and vascularity of the thyroid and prevent hemorrhage.
   4. Potentiate the effect of the other preoperative medication so less medicine can be given while the client is under anesthesia.

4. The nurse is caring for a client who had a thyroidectomy this morning. The nurse must monitor for possible adverse effects. Which is least likely to occur in this client?
   1. Chvostek's sign.
   2. Laryngeal damage.
   3. Brudzinski's sign.
   4. Trousseau's sign.

5. The nurse is caring for an older adult widow whose husband died 6 months ago. Which action best indicates to the nurse that the client is making progress in resocialization?

   1. She does biweekly grocery shopping.
   2. She has stopped attending a widow support group.
   3. She babysits her two grandchildren whenever asked.
   4. She participates in a local senior citizen group.

6. An adult resident is in a long-term care facility with a medical diagnosis of organic brain syndrome. Her mental status assessment documents an untidy, suspicious, easily agitated woman who speaks in nonsense syllables. In caring for her, the nurse should anticipate which nursing actions to promote socialization?
   1. Limiting visitation by family and friends.
   2. Utilizing the pet-animal companion program.
   3. Discussing the need for a speech therapist.
   4. Touching the client only when necessary.

7. In completing an assessment of an elderly client who has been a victim of abuse, who does the nurse know is at the highest risk?
   1. A Caucasian female who is physically or cognitively impaired.
   2. A Caucasian male who has a physical disability.
   3. An African-American female whose physical or mental conditions cause dependency on family members.
   4. An African-American male whose cognitive impairment causes behavioral problems.

8. Which would best indicate to the nurse that a client is depressed?
   1. Feelings of worthlessness.
   2. Poor hygiene and grooming.
   3. Intense anxiety.
   4. Thought insertion.

9. The nurse in an outpatient mental health clinic has identified marital discord as a significant problem for one of the clients. A client with this type of problem would be most likely to be dealing with issues in which developmental phase?
   1. Trust vs. mistrust.
   2. Identity vs. role confusion.
   3. Intimacy vs. isolation.
   4. Generativity vs. stagnation.

10. Which of the following statements best indicates that the client understands the nurse's teaching about effective coping mechanisms?

    1. "Talking to you really helped me put things into perspective."
    2. "Talking to you really helped me solve my problems."
    3. "I don't have time at home to do the relaxation techniques."
    4. "The relaxation techniques helped me to go right to sleep."

11. An adult was admitted to the chemical dependency unit with a history of daily alcohol use for the past 15 years. Which of the following nursing diagnoses should the admitting nurse select to be the primary focus during the initial phase of his treatment?

    1. Sensory/perceptual alteration related to withdrawal seizures secondary to alcohol cessation.
    2. High risk for injury related to suicidal thoughts secondary to alcohol cessation.
    3. Ineffective denial related to inability to identify effect of alcohol on life secondary to alcohol use.
    4. High risk for injury related to withdrawal seizures secondary to alcohol cessation.

12. The labor and delivery unit called to give report on a woman who delivered a full-term live baby girl 2 hours ago via spontaneous vaginal delivery. She had a first-degree laceration, which was repaired. She plans to breastfeed. Both mother and infant will be coming to the mother baby unit. What should the nurse expect will be included in the care plan?

    1. Keep the client NPO for 24 hours.
    2. An order for ice packs to the breasts.
    3. An order for ice packs to the perineum prn for 4 hours.
    4. An indwelling catheter that will remain in place for 12 hours.

13. The nurse has been giving a mother who is at risk for having a baby with Rh incompatibility instruction about preventing isoimmune hemolytic disease in future neonates. Which statement indicates that she understands the need for Rho(D) immune globulin in the future?

    1. The mother asks when her baby will get the shot.
    2. The mother verbalizes a need for a shot after donating blood.
    3. The mother verbalizes a need for a shot after giving birth to an Rh-positive baby.
    4. The mother verbalizes a need for a shot after breastfeeding.

14. A client who is 25 weeks pregnant with no previous medical or obstetrical problems is admitted to the hospital in premature labor. The nurse can expect that orders for this client, in addition to bed rest, will include which of the following?

    1. A fetal monitor and a tocolytic.
    2. A fetal monitor and a tranquilizer.
    3. A maternal cardiac monitor and fluid therapy.
    4. A fetal monitor and a maternal cardiac monitor.

15. Upon admission, a client tells the nurse that she has "weak blood" but doesn't know the name of her disease. She has been taking vitamin $B_{12}$ injections for 5 years. The nurse explains that vitamin $B_{12}$ is the drug management for which type of anemia?

    1. Iron deficiency anemia.
    2. Aplastic anemia.
    3. Pernicious anemia.
    4. Hemolytic anemia.

16. A client has been admitted with possible pernicious anemia. Various diagnostic tests are ordered. What test will the nurse expect to give a definitive test?

    1. A positive Schilling test.
    2. A gastric analysis with decreased free HCl acid.
    3. A bone marrow biopsy showing abnormal erythrocyte and defective leukocyte maturation.
    4. An elevated LDH.

17. An adult male is hospitalized for urolithiasis. A stone he passed in his urine was sent to the laboratory this morning. The lab identifies the stone as an oxalate stone. Which modifications should the nurse teach him to make in his diet?

    1. Limit milk and dairy products.
    2. Limit intake of tea, chocolate, and spinach.
    3. Eat an acid ash diet to keep his urine acidic.
    4. Limit food high in purine.

18. The nurse is teaching an older teen how to perform a testicular self-exam. Which is an abnormal finding that indicates he should see his physician?

    1. His left testis hangs lower than his right testis.
    2. His testes feel smooth, rubbery, and oval shaped.

3. His left testis is larger than his right testis.

4. His testes are slightly tender when he examines them.

19. An adult is in acute renal failure and must undergo hemodialysis. Which medication must the nurse withhold prior to dialysis?
    1. NPH insulin.
    2. Pilocarpine.
    3. Dipyridamole (Persantine).
    4. Cholestyramine (Questran).

20. The nurse is monitoring an adult who is undergoing hemodialysis. The client suddenly becomes cyanotic and complains of dyspnea and chest pain. His blood pressure is 70/40 and his pulse is weak and rapid. The nurse calls the physician immediately because the signs and symptoms suggest which complication of dialysis?
    1. Disequilibrium syndrome.
    2. Air embolism.
    3. Internal bleeding.
    4. Hemorrhage at the shunt.

21. An adult who has urolithiasis is being treated conservatively in hopes that surgery will not be necessary. Which of these nursing measures should the nurse plan to do?
    1. Provide fluid intake of 3000 mL or more.
    2. Restrict citrus juices and milk products.
    3. Insert an indwelling catheter as ordered.
    4. Administer ordered narcotic analgesics whenever the client requests them.

22. Prior to discharge, the client with COPD will need to be taught self-care. The nurse should plan to include which instruction to the client?
    1. Increase the oxygen flow rate to 4 liter/min. when you plan to exercise.
    2. Stay indoors if possible when the weather is very cold.
    3. Limit fluid intake to 200 mL or less.
    4. When short of breath, sit in a recliner chair with the backrest at a semi-Fowler's position.

23. An adult has developed dumping syndrome following a subtotal gastrectomy. Which should the nurse include in the plan of care?
    1. Sit upright for at least 30 minutes after meals.
    2. Take sips of fluid between bites of solid food.
    3. Eat something every 2 to 3 hours.
    4. Reduce the amount of simple carbohydrate in the diet.

24. An adult client is scheduled for a variety of tests for diarrhea and other gastrointestinal complaints. The doctor has ordered an antacid prn for upset stomach. Which antacid is least likely to be ordered for this client because it may have a laxative effect?
    1. Aluminum hydroxide (Amphogel).
    2. Kaopectate.
    3. Magnesium hydroxide (MOM).
    4. Dihydroxy-aluminum sodium carbonate (Rolaids).

25. An adult client is admitted for bowel surgery. The nurse teaches the client what to expect in preparation for surgery. Which is least likely to be included in the nurse's explanation?
    1. Cleansing enemas will be given the night before surgery.
    2. Antibiotics are given 3 to 5 days preoperatively to decrease bacteria in the intestine.
    3. A nasogastric tube will be inserted on the morning of surgery.
    4. Laxatives will be given the morning of surgery to relax the bowel.

26. A client recovering from rectal surgery is ordered Colace. What action does Colace have on the bowels?
    1. Attracts and hold large amounts of fluids, thereby increasing the bulk of stools.
    2. Coats the feces with an oily film and prevent the colon from reabsorbing water from the feces.
    3. Softens stool to prevent straining during defecation.
    4. Stimulates peristalsis.

27. An adult client is diagnosed with a hiatal hernia. He has listed all of the following on his admission form. Which activity is most likely to be aggravating his condition?
    1. Experiencing added stress because he gave up smoking recently.
    2. Lying down and falling asleep on the couch after a big dinner each evening.
    3. Taking an antacid before and after each meal.
    4. Eating six small meals a day.

28. When planning care for the client during the immediate postoperative period after a total laryngectomy, which of these measures would be included in the plan of care?
    1. Provision of a nonverbal means of communication.
    2. Positioning the client on the side with the head of the bed flat.

3. Administering cough suppressants.

4. Suctioning the tracheostomy every 4 hours.

29. Which common side effect should the nurse anticipate for a client receiving chemotherapy?

    1. Nausea and vomiting.

    2. Cardiac arrhythmias.

    3. Paralytic ileus.

    4. Diuresis.

30. An adult suffered a detached retina of the right eye while playing racquetball. He presents in the emergency department with which symptom?

    1. Sharp pain OD.

    2. Redness OU.

    3. Increase in intraocular pressure OD.

    4. Blank areas in the field of vision.

31. An adult has undergone surgery to correct a detached retina. What does the postoperative care plan include?

    1. Turn, cough, and deep breathe every 2 hours.

    2. Position on the operative side to keep the retina next to the choroid.

    3. A patch over the operative eye to prevent further detachment.

    4. Administer pilocarpine eye drops for pupil constriction.

32. The nurse is admitting a client with probable Ménière's disease. Which symptom is the client most likely to exhibit?

    1. Vomiting.

    2. Tinnitis.

    3. Nystagmus.

    4. Blurred vision.

33. An adult has Ménière's disease. Which statement indicates that more teaching about the management of her disease is needed?

    1. "I was trying to stop smoking anyway, so I'm glad to have to now."

    2. "I have to remember to move slower even when I'm in a hurry on my job."

    3. "I'm going to miss using a lot of salt on my food."

    4. "I'll have to fit in the extra fluid I need to drink throughout the day so I don't feel bloated all at once."

34. A term newborn is admitted to the nursery with excessive drooling, coughing, and sneezing. How will the nurse assess for esophageal atresia?

    1. Check the mother's prenatal record for a history of oligohydramnios.

    2. Pass a catheter gently into the esophagus to detect resistance.

    3. Give 10 mL of glucose water to check for swallowing and color changes with feeding.

    4. Place the infant with the head in a downward position to drain mucus.

35. The nurse performs a cardiovascular assessment on an elderly client which reveals a blood pressure of 162/86. The finding is a likely result of what problem?

    1. Less muscle mass.

    2. Calcification of arteries.

    3. Dehydration.

    4. Impaired lung capacity.

36. A 2-year-old child with congestive heart failure has been receiving digoxin for one week. What occurrence will alert the nurse to an early sign of digitalis toxicity?

    1. Bradypnea.

    2. Failure to thrive.

    3. Tachycardia.

    4. Vomiting.

37. A 5-year-old child is being discharged to home after a bone marrow transplant. Which of the following statements to the nurse by the child's mother indicates understanding of home care for this child?

    1. "My child needs to wear a mask when contact with others is necessary."

    2. "My child can return to school tomorrow."

    3. "My child should stay in bed."

    4. "My child will need a nurse 24 hours a day."

38. The nurse working in the newborn nursery notices that a newborn has one foot that curves inward. What information does the nurse know about congenital clubfoot?

    1. It rarely occurs in boys and is usually a bilateral defect.

    2. It can be manipulated to various range-of-motion positions if muscle stretching exercises are performed first.

    3. It will not need to be actually diagnosed until the infant is ready to be dismissed from the hospital.

    4. It is most commonly of the equinovarus type with plantar flexion and inversion of the ankle and foot.

39. A nurse on the orthopedic ward takes report on four clients in traction. Of the four, which client's traction is intermittent and can be released?
    1. A 1½-year-old in Bryant's traction for hip dislocation.
    2. A 24-year-old in Russell traction for a fractured femur.
    3. A 40-year-old in Buck's extension traction for a fractured hip.
    4. A 32-year-old in cervical traction for cervical disc disease.

40. The nurse is caring for an obese male client who has had a herniorrhaphy for a strangulated hernia. Which is important postoperative care and teaching?
    1. Turn, cough, and deep breathe every 2 hours, making sure to splint the incision.
    2. Assess for a distended bladder.
    3. Place a heating pad on the scrotal area to reduce the swelling.
    4. Restrict physical activities for 2 weeks.

41. A mother has brought her daughter to the pediatrician's office for her 9-month checkup. The nurse assesses the baby and finds all of the following data. Which finding would cause the nurse to be concerned about developmental delay?
    1. The child plays with a toy for only a few minutes, then moves on to something else.
    2. The child cannot pull herself up to a standing position.
    3. She does not sit up without assistance.
    4. When something is taken away from her, she cries and protests.

42. A 6-year-old is in the hospital for surgery. He has preoperative medications ordered by injection. When the nurse brings it to him, he cries, "No, I won't be bad! Don't give me a shot!" What is the nurse's best response?
    1. "You have to have this shot, but if you are good, there won't be any more."
    2. "What have you done that makes you say you are bad?"
    3. "You need this shot to get ready for your operation. It has nothing to do with being good or bad."
    4. "I know you try to be good. I'll call the doctor and ask if you really have to have this shot."

43. A young child is admitted with rheumatic fever. His mother must go home and child does not want his father staying with him, stating "I want Mommy! I am going to marry Mommy!" His mother is embarrassed saying, "I don't know where he gets such ideas." What is the nurse's most appropriate response?
    1. "It's pretty normal behavior for a 4-year-old."
    2. "Are you and your husband having difficulties in your marriage?"
    3. "If you discipline him when he says that, he will stop and eventually forget about it."
    4. "Have you considered getting counseling for Sam? It is not normal to want to marry your mother."

44. A 2-month-old infant is admitted to the pediatric unit in congestive heart failure. He has a history of ventricular septal defect diagnosed at birth. He is placed on digoxin by mouth in liquid form. Before administering this medication, what is the nurse's most appropriate action?
    1. Placing the medication in a small amount of formula and having the infant suck.
    2. Taking the apical heart rate and withholding if the rate is below 70.
    3. Drawing the medication up in a syringe and verifying the correctness with a second nurse.
    4. Giving the medication when the mother is available to hold the infant and preventing him from spitting it out.

45. A 2-month-old infant is admitted with a history of projectile vomiting for the last 2 weeks. The infant has gone from a birth weight of 9 lb to a current weight of 8 lb. He looks emaciated, acts hungry, and is crying. Given this data, which nursing diagnosis is appropriate for this client?
    1. Alteration in growth and development related to poor food intake.
    2. Alteration in fluid and electrolyte balance due to vomiting and poor intake.
    3. Potential for altered family process related to situational crisis.
    4. Nutritional deficit.

46. For a school nurse in a junior high school, it is important to check young teenage girls for scoliosis. What is the best way for the nurse to assess for this problem?
    1. Have each girl walk in a straight line.
    2. Have each girl bend over and measure shoulder height.
    3. Run fingers down the spine to feel for abnormalities.
    4. Watch as each girl does physical education activities to see if any abnormality is evident.

47. A 5-year-old boy is admitted in acute respiratory distress. He is sitting upright, drooling, unable to swallow, with a look of panic on his face. The nurse plans to place which essential equipment at the bedside?

1. Croup tent.
2. Padded bedsides for seizure precautions.
3. Tracheotomy set.
4. Suction.

48. A patient is admitted with an ulcer due to venous insufficiency. What characteristics would the nurse expect to find on assessment?

1. Location on the toes or heels.
2. Circular in shape.
3. Black in color, dry, and gangrenous.
4. Moderate to severe edema.

49. An 18-year-old has been sexually active for 2 years and has come to the clinic for birth control pills. Her history reveals she is 15 pounds underweight, a nonsmoker, exercises 3–4 times per week, and has numerous sexual partners. Which of the following would be the least appropriate birth control device?

1. Oral contraceptives.
2. Condoms and foam.
3. Intrauterine device.
4. Diaphragm.

50. A woman has just been admitted to the postpartum after delivery of a baby girl. When the nurse brings in the baby to assist her in breastfeeding, the mother states she does not want to try yet and begins talking about how difficult her labor and delivery was. The nurse recognizes this is indicative of what type of behavior?

1. Risk for alteration in parenting related to the mother's lack of interest in her baby's needs.
2. Fatigue from labor and delivery.
3. Inability to accept the reality of parenthood.
4. Normal developmental phase of taking-in during the early puerperium.

51. While caring for a newborn baby boy, the nurse notices the foreskin on the penis cannot be retracted. The baby's mother asks if this means her baby must be circumcised immediately. What is the nurse's best response?

1. "It is normal for a newborn. You cannot retract the foreskin until he is older."
2. "Yes, the foreskin should retract or bacteria can grow and cause infection."

3. "It is a good indication he'll need to be circumcised, but there is no hurry."
4. "Discuss this with your pediatrician. Circumcision is controversial."

52. A client who is 24 hours post cesarean delivery has orders to advance diet as tolerated. She has been on full liquids and asks if she can have real food. Which question is most appropriate for the nurse to ask before changing her to a regular diet?

1. "Have you had a bowel movement yet?"
2. "Are you passing gas?"
3. "Do you notice rumblings in your belly?"
4. "Are you still hungry after eating your liquid tray?"

53. A client is admitted to labor and delivery for an induction of labor. She is receiving Pitocin and has progressed to 5 cm dilation. Her contractions have steadily become stronger and longer until the nurse notices a contraction lasting 2 minutes. What is the nurse's best initial action?

1. Assess the fetal heart rate and observe a little longer.
2. Turn the client on her left side and encourage transition breathing.
3. Give the client oxygen through a nasal cannula and decrease the rate of the infusion.
4. Stop the pitocin infusion.

54. A woman who is 30 weeks pregnant has been diagnosed with gestational diabetes. Her physician has ordered a 2000-calorie ADA diet, moderate exercise, and weekly appointments for prenatal care. She is very upset and wants to know everything about her condition and how she can have a healthy baby. Which of the following is an appropriate goal for the client at this time?

1. Discuss how pregnancy causes diabetes.
2. Demonstrate insulin injections.
3. Keep a food diary for 48 hours.
4. Identify risks to her fetus if she doesn't follow her diet rigidly.

55. A woman is admitted to the antepartal unit with pregnancy-induced hypertension. Assessment findings include: 34 weeks gestation, BP 160/100, +3 protein in urine, generalized edema, headache, "seeing spots" before her eyes. She states concern about her two preschool children who are with a neighbor. What would be the priority nursing diagnosis?

1. Alteration in fluid volume.
2. Powerlessness.

3. Ineffective family coping.

4. Alteration in tissue perfusion.

56. A woman has been in labor for 8 hours, pushing for 1½ hours without progress and is extremely tired and discouraged. The fetus remains at minus one station. The nurse suggests changing to a nontraditional position. Which assessment is most important to make before proceeding?

1. The condition of the fetal membranes.

2. The level of maternal fatigue.

3. Effacement and dilation.

4. Status of maternal bladder.

57. A newborn is admitted to the nursery 20 minutes after birth. His vital signs are stable. He is crying vigorously. The nurse begins the admission procedure. Which of the following is most appropriate?

1. Wear latex gloves during the admission.

2. Do the admission in an open crib with good light.

3. Wear mask and gown when approaching the infant.

4. Perform the admission procedures while the infant is asleep.

58. An infant has just been delivered with a myelomeningocele. The infant is immediately transferred to the nursery. The nurse should place the infant in what position?

1. Semi-sitting with support of an infant seat.

2. Side-lying with his head lower than the rest of his body to promote drainage.

3. Supine to place counterpressure on the defect.

4. Prone to reduce the risk of rupture and infection.

59. Shortly after administering Prolixin (fluphenazine) 10 mg PO to a client who has schizophrenia, the nurse notices that he is pacing, appears restless, is drooling, and complains that his tongue feels thick. Which of the following prn orders would the nurse administer to alleviate these symptoms?

1. Ativan (lorazepam) 2 mg IM.

2. Atropine 4 mg IM.

3. Cogentin (benztropine mesylate) 2 mg IM.

4. Thorazine (chlorpromazine hydrochloride) 50 mg IM.

60. The nurse is evaluating the effectiveness of antipsychotic medication 2 weeks after starting treatment in a client who has paranoid schizophrenia. If the medication is effective, what would the nurse expect to see?

1. Decreased hallucinations and decreased sleep.

2. Increased sleep and improved personal hygiene.

3. Decreased suspiciousness and increased appetite.

4. Decreased hallucinations and decreased suspiciousness.

61. A physically abused wife says to her nurse, "I'd be nothing without my husband." To increase the woman's self-esteem, which statement by the nurse would be most appropriate?

1. "I see you as a survivor in a difficult situation."

2. "It sounds like you don't think you are important."

3. "Let's not talk about that right now."

4. "I can see that you're upset."

62. The nurse is planning nursing interventions for parents who abuse their children. What will be important for the nurse to recall about abusive parents?

1. They plan ahead as to when and how to abuse their children.

2. They ask for help generally only after feeling overwhelmed with the problem.

3. They usually feel no guilt concerning the abuse.

4. They are always a product of abuse themselves.

63. The nurse is caring for a client with antisocial personality. What behavior exhibited by the client would indicate an improvement?

1. Attending therapeutic groups daily.

2. Compliance with antipsychotic medications.

3. Abiding by hospital rules and regulations.

4. Interacting with peers in the day room.

64. The nurse is caring for an adult client who is to undergo a cystoscopy in the morning. What should be included in the plan of care?

1. Explaining that this is a painless test.

2. Instructing the client to drink several glasses of water prior to the test.

3. Giving instructions to breathe rapidly and deeply throughout the procedure.

4. Telling the client to administer a small package enema in the evening before the test.

65. A young woman is to undergo a Tensilon test. The nurse is explaining the test to the client.

Which statement the client makes indicates the best understanding of the test?

1. "A positive test will be evident within 1 minute of the Tensilon injection."
2. "The test is of diagnostic value in only about 20% of persons with myasthenia gravis."
3. "If the test is positive I will feel an immediate decrease in muscle strength."
4. "My blood sugar will decrease to a normal level after the test."

66. The client asks why it is necessary to have a serum creatinine and BUN drawn before the CT scan. What is the nurse's best response?

1. "These tests will determine if you are allergic to iodine contrast media."
2. "The tests determine if the kidneys are functioning and can eliminate contrast media."
3. "The tests serve as baseline information to determine if the scan has caused damage."
4. "The blood tests give additional information about the presence of possible tumors."

67. The nurse is performing an ophthalmologic examination on an elderly client. The client states, "my peripheral vision is decreased." What is the nurse's best response during the exam?

1. "You should be grateful you are not blind."
2. "As one ages, peripheral vision decreases. This is normal."
3. "You should rest your eyes frequently."
4. "You may be able to improve your vision if you move slowly."

68. An adult is admitted with post cerebral vascular accident (CVA) with right-sided paralysis. What documentation will be correct if the client is having difficulty speaking due to the impairment of the facial muscles?

1. Semantic aphasia.
2. Receptive aphasia.
3. Dysarthria.
4. Dysphagia.

69. The nurse is assessing a client for local inflammation following an injury. What is one of the cardinal signs the nurse should observe?

1. Fever.
2. Confusion.
3. Impaired function.
4. Malaise.

70. The nurse is caring for a client who is scheduled for a ureterosigmoidostomy. Which information is inappropriate and will not be a part of the preoperative teaching plan?

1. Liquid diet for 24 hours prior to the surgery.
2. Assessment of the adequacy of the rectal sphincter.
3. Administration of neomycin sulfate for 3 days prior to surgery.
4. Application of full-length elastic stockings.

71. An adult client who has chronic obstructive lung disease needs frequent monitoring of arterial blood gases. What is an essential action that should be performed after the drawing of arterial blood gases?

1. Encourage the client to cough and deep breathe.
2. Apply pressure to the puncture site for 5 minutes.
3. Shake the vial of blood before transporting it to the lab.
4. Keep the client on bed rest for 2 hours.

72. A client with chronic obstruction pulmonary disease (COPD) is on oxygen by nasal cannula at 2 liters per minute. Which is most useful in assessing the success of the oxygen therapy?

1. Respiratory rate.
2. Color of mucous membranes.
3. Pulmonary function tests.
4. Arterial blood gases.

73. The nurse is interpreting the results of a blood gas analysis performed on an adult client. The values include pH of 7.35, pCO$_2$ of 60, HCO$_3$ of 35, and O$_2$ of 60. Which interpretation is most accurate?

1. The client is in metabolic acidosis.
2. The client is in compensated metabolic alkalosis.
3. The client is in respiratory alkalosis.
4. The client is in compensated respiratory acidosis.

74. An elderly woman is admitted with a fractured left hip after a fall in her home. During the nursing assessment, the nurse would expect to see which of the following?

1. The client cannot move her left leg but can wiggle her toes.
2. The left leg will have internal rotation and appear longer.

3. The client can voluntarily move the left leg without pain.

4. The left leg will have involuntary tremors.

75. The nurse is evaluating the care given to a client who has had a total hip replacement. Which position indicates the client has been positioned appropriately?

1. The affected leg is abducted and externally rotated.

2. The affected leg is adducted and externally rotated.

3. The affected leg is abducted and internally rotated.

4. The affected leg is adducted and internally rotated.

76. A male client is admitted with Guillain-Barré syndrome and complains of severe weakness, numbness in both hands, and is extremely anxious. What would be the priority nursing action?

1. Raise the head of the bed to high-Fowler's to prevent increased intracranial pressure.

2. Place respiratory support equipment at the bedside.

3. Reassure the client that in time the strength will return to his legs.

4. Place the client in reverse isolation to prevent spreading the virus.

77. The nurse is assessing an adult who has a cataract in his right eye. What symptom is the client likely to exhibit?

1. Acute eye pain.

2. Redness and itching in the right eye.

3. Gradual blurring of vision.

4. Severe headaches and dizziness.

78. An adult is scheduled for a magnetic resonance imaging (MRI) test because of a back injury. Which question is it essential for the nurse to ask the client before the procedure?

1. "Are you allergic to iodine or shellfish?"

2. "Are you afraid of heights?"

3. "Do you get dizzy easily?"

4. "Do you have any metal in your body?"

79. An adult was born and raised in another country and received the BCG vaccine as a child. Upon taking a tuberculin skin test, a positive result is seen. What information will the nurse base a response on?

1. The only cause for a positive skin test and negative chest X-ray is exposure to the tubercle bacillus without development of tuberculosis infection.

2. The skin test is only a screening test.

3. BCG vaccine is not effective against tuberculosis.

4. BCG vaccine stimulates formation of antibodies against tuberculosis.

80. An adult has had a low-sodium, low-fat diet prescribed for heart disease. The nurse is evaluating her understanding of the diet. Which statement she makes indicates a need for further instruction?

1. "Whenever I go out to eat at a restaurant, I get the salad bar and use vinegar for a dressing."

2. "When I eat chicken, I take the skin off and broil the chicken in the oven."

3. "I like to put catsup on my noodles."

4. "We use skim milk for drinking and cooking."

81. The nurse is administering eyedrops to an elderly client. Which action is least appropriate for the nurse to take?

1. Inform the client that the drops may cause blurred vision and difficulty focusing for a period of time.

2. Apply gentle pressure to the nasolacrimal canal for 1 to 2 minutes after instillation to prevent systemic absorption.

3. Encourage the client to lie down with eyes closed after instillation to prevent systemic absorption.

4. Gently pull the lower lid down and place the medicine in the center of the lid.

82. A woman is admitted for internal radiation for cancer of the cervix. The nurse knows the client understands the procedure when she makes which of the following remarks the night before the procedure?

1. She says to her husband, "Please bring me a hamburger and french fries tomorrow when you come. I hate hospital food."

2. "I told my daughter who is pregnant to either come to see me tonight or wait until I go home from the hospital."

3. "I understand it will be several weeks before all the radiation leaves my body."

4. "I brought several craft projects to do while the radium is inserted."

83. The nurse is teaching auxiliary staff on the unit about standard precautions. Which statement

made by one of the aides indicates the best understanding of the procedure?

1. "I should wear gloves when I give an enema to a client who can't hold it."
2. "If I see a blood spill I will get iodine immediately and wipe up the spill."
3. "When I see used needles in the treatment room or the client's room, I will recap them and put them in the Sharps box."
4. "I will wear a gown and mask whenever I go into the room of a person with AIDS."

84. The nurse is caring for a client who has patches on both eyes following eye surgery. When entering the room the nurse should do which of the following?

1. Announce presence and name clearly before entering the room.
2. Speak in a louder tone than usual.
3. Enter the room quietly and touch the client before speaking.
4. Refrain from saying things like "I see" to the client.

85. A client is admitted after being stabbed by a knife and a chest tube is inserted. Immediately following insertion of the chest tube, which observation by the nurse best indicates the drainage system is functioning adequately?

1. There is no bubbling in the water seal chamber.
2. The fluid level in the suction control chamber fluctuates with each respiration.
3. The collection chambers are filling with sanguinous drainage.
4. The client reports pain relief.

86. An adult is admitted to the medical unit with symptoms of angina. Nitroglycerin is administered. Which assessment indicates the client is responding positively to the administration of nitroglycerin?

1. The client's blood pressure drops.
2. The client reports he has developed a headache.
3. The client asks to be discharged because his pain is relieved.
4. The client reports he has developed nausea.

87. The nurse is caring for several clients. Which client may need an order for wrist restraints?

1. An elderly woman who is confused and pulls out her intravenous line.
2. An adult man who refuses to have an intravenous line started.

3. A 1-year-old child who keeps pulling up in the crib and tries to climb out.
4. An adult who is supposed to be on bed rest following surgery who tried to get up during the night.

88. The nurse is to administer an intramuscular injection to a 1-year-old child. Which site is most appropriate for the nurse to select?

1. Dorsal gluteal.
2. Ventral gluteal.
3. Ventral forearm.
4. Vastus lateralis.

89. An adult client is being treated for hypertension. A low-sodium, low-fat diet is prescribed. The nurse knows the client understands his diet when he selects which of the following menus?

1. Fried chicken, mashed potatoes, green beans, and milk.
2. Macaroni and cheese casserole, tossed salad with dressing, and hot chocolate.
3. Baked chicken, steamed broccoli and cauliflower, steamed rice, and hot tea.
4. Steak, baked potato, peas, and hot coffee.

90. An adult client is to have a pelvic sonogram today to diagnose possible ovarian cysts. When she arrives in the clinic area, which question is the most important for the nurse to ask?

1. "When was your last menstrual period?"
2. "What have you had to drink this morning?"
3. "When was your last bowel movement?"
4. "Did you use powder or deodorant today?"

91. The nurse is working with a nursing assistant (NA). Which action should be delegated to the NA?

1. Ask the NA to apply the ice bag while the nurse performs decubitus ulcer care.
2. Ask the NA to assess the bowel sounds before feeding the client.
3. Ask the NA to perform decubitus care while the nurse applies an ice bag.
4. Ask the NA to feed the first meal to a client after surgery.

92. A man on the phone states he is a government official who needs access to a client's medical file. He states his name and position in the

government. According to HIPPA, what should the nurse do next?

1. Give him the information, as all government officials are allowed access.
2. Ask for a number to reach the official and contact the charge nurse with the information.
3. Inform the official that only the medical staff are allowed access to the file.
4. Ask the client why the government official is needing information about their file.

93. A middle-aged client was admitted for treatment of secondary hypertension that has not responded to lifestyle modifications over the last 5 weeks. Using the stepped-care approach, the medications included in his treatment were furosemide (Lasix) and quinipril hydrochloride (Accupril). What type of information should the nurse include in the discharge teaching?

1. Cholesterol restriction, weight reduction.
2. Potassium restriction, limited activity.
3. Sodium restriction, increased activity.
4. Magnesium restriction, limited alcohol intake.

94. A client's renal disease has progressed and has decided with his physician to use continuous ambulatory peritoneal dialysis (CAPD) as his treatment option. Which of the following choices best reflects the information that the nurse should include in the CAPD teaching plan?

1. Low-sodium diet and Foley catheter care.
2. Low-protein/high-carbohydrate diet and care of the AV shunt site.
3. Complications and aseptic technique for the Tenckhoff catheter.
4. Assessing for the bruit and thrill daily.

95. A client has been admitted to the coronary care unit with the diagnosis of an anterior wall myocardial infarction. While on telemetry, his rhythm strip demonstrates frequent premature ventricular beats as well as occasional episodes of second-degree heart block episodes. Which alterative drug to suppress the ventricular ectopic beats is most likely to be prescribed?

1. Atenolol (Tenormin).
2. Calcium gluconate.
3. Verapamil (Calan).
4. Diltiazem (Cardizem).

96. A client is 2 days post-op surgery. He is now complaining of shortness of breath and had a positive Homan's sign yesterday. How will the nurse interpret the findings?

1. The client is showing normal signs of pain and anxiety after surgery.
2. The client may be in the early stages of congestive heart failure.
3. The client will need to perform active range-of-motion exercises for his legs.
4. The client may be experiencing a pulmonary embolus.

97. An unconscious client is receiving a transfusion of whole blood. Upon assessment, the nurse finds a weak pulse, fever, and hypotension. What would be the priority nursing action?

1. Notify the physician.
2. Stop the blood transfusion.
3. Recheck the vital signs.
4. Check the amount of urine output.

98. The nurse is caring for an adult who has had an acute myocardial infarction. The nurse finds him very restless with a heart rate of 110, respiratory rate of 28, and blood pressure 80/50. What is the most appropriate nursing action?

1. Prepare for administration of vasoconstrictive drugs.
2. Limit IV intake to 100 mL the first 2 hours.
3. Prepare for insertion of CVP or pulmonary artery catheter.
4. Prepare to apply MAST trousers/suit.

99. The nurse is visiting a client at home and is assessing him for risk of a fall. What is the most important factor to consider in this assessment?

1. Illumination of the environment.
2. Amount of regular exercise.
3. The resting pulse rate.
4. Status of salt intake.

100. An elderly client who lives at home is alert and oriented and being treated for polyarthritis, primary biliary cirrhosis, mild hypertension, and glaucoma. He is prescribed four different medications, some of which are prescribed once a day, some twice a day and one at different times of the day. He states, "I'm not used to taking all these medicines and sometimes I miss them all." Which of the following suggestions would be most beneficial to the client to promote his medication regimen?

1. Purchase a pill sorting box to arrange dosages.
2. Make arrangements for the public health nurse to visit daily.
3. Require family members to administer medications.
4. Explain the importance of these medicines and tell the client he needs to find a better way to remember.

# Answers and Rationales for Practice Test 7

| ANSWER | | RATIONALE | NP | CN | CL | SA |
|---|---|---|---|---|---|---|
| #1. | 4. | These are symptoms of hypophosphatemia that may occur with prolonged use of Amphojel. Constipation is an expected side effect; the liquid tends to be more effective; large amounts of liquid would dilute the medicine. | Pl | Ph/6 | Ap | 5 |
| #2. | 1. | Hypoparathyroidism results in decreased calcium and increased phosphorus levels. A high-calcium, low-phosphorus diet will be prescribed, as well as the other interventions listed. | Pl | Ph/7 | Ap | 1 |
| #3. | 3. | Lugol's solution (iodine solution) may be given 10 to 14 days before surgery to decrease vascularity of the thyroid and thus prevent excess bleeding. | An | Ph/6 | Ap | 1 |
| #4. | 3. | Brudzinski's sign is flexion at the hip and knee in response to forward flexion of the neck and may be present in a client with meningitis. Chvostek's sign and Trousseau's sign may occur due to the parathyroid glands being inadvertently removed and in response to hypocalcemia; the laryngeal nerve may be damaged during the surgery, in which sudden hoarseness develops. | As | Ph/7 | Co | 1 |
| #5. | 4. | The client's social network is expanded by attending a local senior citizen group, and socializing with others outside of the family. | Ev | Ps/4 | Ap | 2 |
| #6. | 2. | Pets can provide an opportunity for touching and can promote socialization and speech when it otherwise would not be performed by the client. Family and friends are encouraged to visit; speech therapy cannot correct the progression of organic brain syndrome. | Pl | Ps/4 | Ap | 2 |
| #7. | 1. | According to the National Elder Abuse Incident Study of 1998, the elderly Caucasian female who has physical and/or cognitive impairment is at greatest risk for elder abuse by a family member. | As | Ps/4 | Co | 2 |
| #8. | 1. | Depressive symptoms include exaggerated feelings of sadness, dejection, worthlessness, hopelessness, and emptiness. Poor grooming and hygiene are signs of mental decompensation in mental illness such as in dementia and schizophrenia. Intense anxiety alone is not a symptom and thought insertion is a symptom of schizophrenia. | As | Ps/4 | Co | 2 |
| #9. | 3. | This stage of Erickson's developmental stages targets intimate relationships. Trust vs. mistrust is in the infant stage; identity vs. role confusion is in the adolescent stage; generativity vs. stagnation is in the middle adult stage with concerns related to productivity and contributing to society. | An | Ps/4 | Ap | 2 |
| #10. | 1. | The client learned a method to use in dealing with problems/ stressors such as verbalization rather than looking to quick and sometimes superficial answers to problems. | Ev | Ps/4 | Ap | 2 |

| ANSWER | RATIONALE | NP | CN | CL | SA |
|--------|-----------|----|----|----|----|

#11. 4. Using Maslow's hierarchy of needs as well as basic concepts of alcohol detoxification, the nurse needs to initially assess and attend to the potential for physical problems associated with withdrawal. There is no data to support suicidal thoughts; ineffective denial would be a focus later in treatment after safe detoxification has been achieved. — An Ps/4 Ap 2

#12. 3. An ice pack helps to soothe the area by constricting vessels and reducing inflammation. NPO status would be appropriate following a cesarean section until bowel sounds are audible; ice packs to the breasts would suppress lactation and are not appropriate for a woman who plans to breastfeed; a catheter is usually in place for a woman undergoing a cesarean section until the first postpartum day so bed rest can be maintained. — Pl He/3 Ap 3

#13. 3. Rho(D) should be given within 72 hours of delivery to the mother when the mother is Rho(D) negative and the infant is Rho(D) positive. Rho(D) is indicated following the termination of a pregnancy, after amniocentesis, after abdominal trauma during pregnancy, and after receiving a transfusion of Rho(D) positive blood. — Ev Ph/6 Ap 3

#14. 1. Monitoring fetal heart rate assesses fetal well-being and fetal distress. A tocolytic is administered to relax the smooth muscles of the uterus and inhibit uterine contractility. A tranquilizer may depress the neonate's respiratory center. — Pl He/3 Ap 3

#15. 3. Persons with pernicious anemia are unable to absorb vitamin $B_{12}$ from the gastrointestinal tract, in which injections must be taken for life. Iron is taken for iron deficiency anemia; blood transfusion and corticosteroids help manage aplastic and hemolytic anemias. — An Ph/6 Ap 1

#16. 1. A Schilling test utilizes radioactive vitamin $B_{12}$ for gastrointestinal absorption of vitamin $B_{12}$. The other choices do not provide a definitive diagnosis. — An Ph/7 Co 1

#17. 2. With an oxalate stone, the client should limit excess intake of food high in oxalate and maintain an alkaline ash diet for alkaline urine. Foods high in purine are limited for persons with uric acid stones or gout. — Pl Ph/7 Ap 1

#18. 3. A warning sign of testicular cancer is a slight enlargement or change in the consistency of the testes. The other findings are considered normal. — Ev He/3 An 4

#19. 3. Persantine is a peripheral vasodilator and should be withheld, along with antihypertensives and sedatives, to prevent a hypotensive episode. The other medications listed are not contraindicated before dialysis. — Im Ph/6 Ap 1

#20. 2. Air embolism is a potentially fatal complication characterized by sudden hypotension, dyspnea, chest pain, cyanosis and weak, rapid pulse. Complications of disequilibrium include: headache, muscle twitching, backache, nausea, vomiting, seizures; internal bleeding and hemorrhage present as restlessness; pale, cold clammy skin; rapid, weak, thready pulse; increased respiration. — An Ph/8 Ap 1

| ANSWER | RATIONALE | NP | CN | CL | SA |
|--------|-----------|-----|-----|-----|-----|
| #21. 1. | The goal of conservative treatment is to pass the stone without need for invasive procedures. Fluids will be forced to help flush the stone through the urinary tract quickly and dilute the urine to reduce the risk of forming additional stones. If obstruction is present, conservative treatment would not be selected. Narcotic analgesics would be required for severe pain on an ordered schedule. | Pl | Ph/7 | Ap | 1 |
| #22. 2. | Very cold air, especially if it is dry, is likely to cause brochospasms, which make breathing even more difficult. Oxygen flow rate is typically kept at 2–3 liter/min because high oxygen levels can reduce the hypoxic drive to breathe. Fluid will help to liquefy the secretions and make them easier to clear from the airways. The position of choice is a forward-leaning position or high-Fowler's. | Pl | Ph/7 | Ap | 1 |
| #23. 4. | Large amounts of simple carbohydrates in the diet produce a high osmotic pressure within the intestine, which draws fluid into the intestine from surrounding cells, causing the early dumping syndrome. The hypoglycemic effect noted in late dumping syndrome develops from production of large amounts of insulin when the intestinal contents are high in simple carbs. Reducing dietary carbs, using complex carbs, increasing fat and protein delays gastric emptying time. The client should be encouraged to lie on the left side, withhold fluid during the meal and eat six small meals rather than three large ones to slow gastric emptying. | Pl | Ph/7 | Ap | 1 |
| #24. 3. | Antacids containing magnesium have diarrhea as a side effect. Choices 1 and 4 cause constipation; 2 is an antidiarrheal. | An | Ph/6 | Co | 5 |
| #25. 4. | Laxatives are given, if needed, the night before surgery to help cleanse the bowel. | Im | Ph/7 | Ap | 1 |
| #26. 3. | Colace is a stool softener and the laxative of choice for clients who should not strain during defecation. It causes water and fats to penetrate the stool, making it easier to move the feces along. A bulk-forming laxative would hold a large amount of water, such as Metamucil; mineral oil is a laxative that retards colonic absorption of water; Lactulose is a laxative that retards colonic absorption of water and increases colonic peristalsis. | An | Ph/6 | Ap | 1 |
| #27. 2. | A hiatal hernia is a structural defect of a weakened diaphragm and is aggravated by reclining and activities that cause an increase in intra-abdominal pressure. The client should be instructed to wait at least 2 hours after eating before lying down. | An | Ph/7 | Ap | 1 |
| #28. 1. | A total laryngectomy leaves the client unable to speak, so it will be important to plan ahead for an alternate method of communication. | Pl | Ph/7 | Ap | 1 |
| #29. 1. | Nausea and vomiting are the most common side effects of cancer chemotherapy, the other choices are not. | Pl | Ph/6 | Ap | 1 |
| #30. 4. | There is no pain, bilateral redness, or increase in intraocular pressure with a detached retina. Symptoms include gaps in vision, flashes of light floating particles before the eyes, a curtain over the field of vision, and blindness, if not treated. | As | Ph/8 | An | 1 |

| ANSWER | | RATIONALE | NP | CN | CL | SA |
|---|---|---|---|---|---|---|
| #31. | 2. | Positioning to keep the retina next to the choroid and the area of detachment dependent is important. This may be on the operative or the nonoperative side depending on the position of the detachment. The client is to avoid coughing, wear patches on both eyes, and eyedrops are given for dilation and to paralyze the eye muscles postoperatively. | Pl | Ph/7 | Ap | 1 |
| #32. | 2. | Ménière's disease is a chronic disease of the inner ear characterized by recurrent episodes of vertigo, tinnitus, and progressive unilateral nerve deafness. Nausea may result from the vertigo the client experiences. | As | Ph/7 | An | 1 |
| #33. | 4. | Client's with Ménière's disease are on a restricted fluid intake and may also be on diuretics. Other management includes smoking cessation, moving slowly, and a low-sodium diet. | Ev | Ph/7 | Ap | 1 |
| #34. | 2. | The catheter should be sufficiently stiff so as not to coil in the esophageal pouch and should never be forced when resistance is felt. Air can be instilled into the stomach or gastric contents aspirated to confirm a patent esophagus. Placing the infant with head downward is an intervention rather than an assessment. If the defect is the most common type (upper atresia with lower fistula into the trachea), air will collect in the stomach with crying, causing upward pressure on the diaphragm. Because air rises, the infant's head should be elevated to reduce gastric distension from air. Continuous suction of the pouch with a catheter in place keeps the mucus away from the upper trachea. | As | Ph/7 | Ap | 3 |
| #35. | 2. | Increased systolic pressure is a result of fibrosis of blood vessels and calcification and elongation of arteries, which frequently occur in aging. Dehydration is likely to cause hypotension. Less muscle mass or impaired lung capacity are both normal occurrences in aging but do not cause increased systolic pressure. | As | He/3 | An | 1 |
| #36. | 4. | The earliest sign of digitalis toxicity is vomiting, although one episode does not warrant discontinuing medication. Bradycardia is also associated with digitalis toxicity. | Ev | Ph/6 | Ap | 4 |
| #37. | 1. | It is of the utmost importance to protect the child from infections, by wearing a mask and avoiding crowded areas. The child's energy level can dictate his activity; and family can learn the specifics of care required. | Ev | Ph/7 | Ap | 4 |
| #38. | 4. | Talipes equines refers to plantar flexion, which lowers the toes below the level of the heel. Talipes varus refers to the inversion of the whole foot. Boys have a 2:1 higher incidence of clubfoot than girls. Manipulation and casting are usually begun immediately upon discovery of the defect, as the infant's bones are most flexible during the newborn period. | As | Ph/7 | An | 3 |
| #39. | 4. | Cervical traction for cervical disc disease is the only one listed that can be intermittent. | Im | Ph/7 | An | 1 |
| #40. | 2. | The two major complications of a herniorrhaphy are a distended bladder and scrotal swelling. It is important to assess for difficulty in urinating postoperatively. | Im | Ph/7 | Ap | 1 |

| ANSWER | RATIONALE | NP | CN | CL | SA |
|--------|-----------|-----|------|-----|-----|
| #41. 3. | All of the choices are normal for a 9-month-old except sitting up without support and would need further investigation. | An | He/3 | Ap | 4 |
| #42. 3. | The nurse is firm in carrying out the order and separating it from behavior. | Im | He/3 | Ap | 4 |
| #43. 1. | This is known as the oedipal stage, in which it is normal for the child to want to marry the parent of the opposite sex. The child will outgrow this and only needs to be reminded that he can't marry his parent. | Im | He/3 | Ap | 4 |
| #44. 3. | A syringe is used for accuracy. A second nurse should always verify potent drugs that require measurement. Placing medication in formula will alter the taste causing the infant to refuse it and it may be unknown whether all the medication is ingested. The apical pulse should not be below 100 to 110 for a young infant. The nurse is responsible for giving the medication and will demonstrate to the mother as part of discharge teaching. | Im | Ph/6 | Ap | 4 |
| #45. 2. | All the diagnoses are relevant at some point in the care of this child, but the fluid and electrolyte balance is the most immediate concern. | An | Ph/7 | Ap | 4 |
| #46. 2. | A quick assessment is to look for uneven shoulders. Ask the girl to bend over and look at bra strap marks to see if one side is deeper. Walking a straight line, palpating the spine, or watching physical activities are all unreliable assessments. | As | He/3 | An | 4 |
| #47. 3. | The biggest risk to this child is that his airway will close off. If this occurs, a tracheotomy will be necessary to save his life. Suctioning could be dangerous as it may irritate, increase swelling, and cause complete blockage of the airway. | Pl | Ph/7 | Ap | 4 |
| #48. 4. | This is the only correct answer that would be found related to venous ulcers. The other choices are descriptors of arterial insufficiency. | As | Ps/4 | An | 1 |
| #49. 3. | An intrauterine device is least appropriate. With a history of numerous partners, she is at increased risk of infection, a common problem with IUDs. There are no risk factors presented that would contraindicate the use of oral contraceptives; condoms, foams or the diaphragm are acceptable methods but do require motivation to use. | An | He/3 | Ap | 3 |
| #50. 4. | Reva Rubin identified the phases of adjustment following delivery as taking-in, taking-hold, and letting-go. Lack of interest in infant care and the need to talk about herself are perfectly normal in this initial phase of taking-in. | An | He/3 | An | 3 |
| #51. 1. | It is rare to be able to retract the foreskin of a newborn. This does not indicate a need for circumcision. | Im | He/3 | An | 3 |
| #52. 2. | Passing flatus would indicate normal peristaltic activity. It would be unlikely to have a bowel movement so soon; the nurse would assess the bowel sounds with a stethoscope, (not by asking the client to describe them); hunger alone is not a criterion for the beginning of eating solid foods. | As | Ph/5 | Ap | 3 |

| ANSWER | RATIONALE | NP | CN | CL | SA |
|---|---|---|---|---|---|
| #53. 4. | A contraction lasting longer than 90 seconds increases the risk of fetal distress and uterine rupture. Safe practice requires the nurse to immediately discontinue the Pitocin. | Im | Ph/6 | Ap | 3 |
| #54. 3. | Assessment is done first by seeing what her normal eating habits are. The diet can then be individualized to her needs and compliance will be better. Insulin is not needed at this time. | Pl | Ph/7 | An | 3 |
| #55. 4. | All choices are appropriate but the most important is the risk of seizures and the probability of already suffering intrauterine growth retardation. Her physical well-being and that of the fetus are in jeopardy. | An | Ph/8 | An | 3 |
| #56. 4. | Given the mother is pushing, the cervix is already completely effaced and dilated. A full bladder may hold the fetus back. Most likely the fetal membranes are ruptured. | As | He/3 | An | 3 |
| #57. 1. | Wearing gloves is part of standard precautions, especially since the newborn is coated with amniotic fluid. The admission is usually done under a warmer and is it not practical to wait until the newborn is sleeping, although it is better to obtain heart rate and respiratory rate while the infant is quiet. | Im | Sa/2 | Ap | 3 |
| #58. 4. | Prone is the best position for minimal pressure on the defect. Rupture presents a surgical emergency and all efforts are taken to avoid it. | Im | Ph/7 | An | 3 |
| #59. 3. | The symptoms described are side effects of antipsychotic medication and are not the symptoms of agitation often seen in a schizophrenic client. Cogentin is the only medication listed that will decrease the side effects of the antipsychotic medication. | Im | Ph/6 | An | 5 |
| #60. 4. | Because the DM-IV-TR criteria for paranoid schizophrenia focus on delusions and suspiciousness, a decrease in these symptoms would be the expected outcome from antipsychotic medication. | Ev | Ph/6 | An | 2 |
| #61. 1. | This response points out the client's strength in a realistic manner and is an attempt to improve self-concept. The other choices are examples of judging, rejecting, or not promoting self-esteem. | Im | Ps/4 | Ap | 2 |
| #62. 2. | Abusive behavior often occurs when parents lose control or feel overwhelmed. | Pl | Ps/4 | An | 2 |
| #63. 3. | The most important improvement would be the client's ability to live within the guidelines, rules, and regulations, as well as a decrease in testing limits. | Ev | Ps/4 | An | 2 |
| #64. 2. | A cystoscopy is the examination of the bladder with the lighted cystoscope. Water may be drunk the night before, as the client is likely to be NPO after midnight. Enemas are given if the bowels are examined. | Pl | Ph/7 | Ap | 1 |
| #65. 1. | A Tensilon test yields immediate result in evaluating myasthenia gravis. If positive, the client almost immediately has an increase in muscle strength by increasing the amount of acetylcholine available. | Ev | Ph/7 | An | 1 |
| #66. 2. | Serum creatinine and blood urea nitrogen (BUN) are tests of kidney function. Before giving contrast media, it is essential to be sure the kidneys can excrete the dyes. | An | Ph/7 | An | 1 |

| ANSWER | RATIONALE | NP | CN | CL | SA |
|--------|-----------|----|----|----|----|
| #67. 2. | As one ages, the eyes undergo changes including a decreased ability to focus on near objects, increased difficulty with color discrimination, and a lessened field of peripheral vision. | As | He/3 | Ap | 1 |
| #68. 3. | Dysarthria is the term used to describe difficulty speaking when muscle impairment is present. Semantic is the inability to understand the meaning of words; receptive aphasia is the inability to understand spoken or written words; and dysphagia is difficulty swallowing. | As | Ph/7 | Ap | 1 |
| #69. 3. | Swelling, heat redness, impaired function, and pain are cardinal signs of local inflammation. Fever and malaise are signs of systemic inflammation. Confusion could be a sign of a systemic infection, impaired oxygenation or brain dysfunction, not a local inflammation. | As | Ph/7 | An | 1 |
| #70. 1. | A liquid diet should be given for 5 days prior to surgery to ensure adequate cleansing of the bowel before surgery. | Pl | Ph/7 | Ap | 1 |
| #71. 2. | Arterial blood gases are usually done by the respiratory therapist, however, it is essential that pressure is applied to the puncture site for 5 minutes to ensure the client does not bleed from the arterial puncture. | Im | Ph/7 | Ap | 1 |
| #72. 4. | The ABGs provide the most specific information about the adequacy of the oxygen therapy. Other factors may influence the other choices. | Ev | Ph/7 | An | 1 |
| #73. 4. | A pH of 7.35 is on the acid side of normal. All the other values are abnormal so the client has compensated. The $CO_2$ is sharply elevated and will lower the pH. The $HCO_3$ is also elevated and is responsible for bringing the pH up to the normal range. An abnormal $O_2$ suggests that the problem is a respiratory one. | An | Ph/7 | An | 1 |
| #74. 1. | The client should be able to move the toes, but be unable to move and will complain of pain if the leg is moved. The injured extremity will appear shorter and be in external rotation. | As | Ph/8 | Ap | 1 |
| #75. 1. | To keep the hip in the socket, the affected leg should be kept abducted and externally rotated. An abduction pillow can be used to achieve the position. | Ev | Ph/7 | An | 1 |
| #76. 2. | Guillain-Barré is characterized by an ascending paralysis that usually paralyzes the respiratory muscle before descending. It is thought to be an autoimmune response following a viral infection. If the client receives good respiratory support, the paralysis will descend after a few days. | Im | Ph/7 | Ap | 1 |
| #77. 3. | Cloudy vision and gradual blurring are symptomatic of cataracts. The other choices are from a foreign body, acute glaucoma, infection, allergy, or migraine headaches. | As | Ph/8 | An | 1 |
| #78. 4. | Metal in the body, such as pacemakers, aneurysm clips, and hip prostheses can cause serious injury and/or cause artifacts in the images. Dye is not used, but the client will be placed in a cylindrical scanner so explain that some suffer a feeling of claustrophobia, and they will have to remain totally still. | As | Ph/7 | Ap | 1 |

| ANSWER | RATIONALE | NP | CN | CL | SA |
|--------|-----------|----|----|----|----|
| #79. 4. | BCG vaccine is given in many parts of the world to immunize against tuberculosis. It causes formation of antibodies and consequently a positive reaction to a tuberculin skin test. A positive skin test indicates the vaccine is working and producing antibodies. | An | **He/3** | An | 1 |
| #80. 3. | Catsup is high in sodium so other choices should be suggested. | Ev | Ph/5 | Ap | 1 |
| #81. 3. | Lying down is not required after eyedrops. The other choices are correct information. | Im | Ph/6 | Ap | 5 |
| #82. 2. | Pregnant visitors and children under 16 are not allowed in the room if internal radiation therapy is used. The client will be on a clear liquid or low residue diet; the client will no longer be contaminated with radioactivity once the source is removed (probably 36 to 72 hours after insertion); crafts may require sitting, but the client will need to lie flat with very little head elevation. | Ev | Sa/2 | An | 1 |
| #83. 1. | Fecal material is a body fluid and could transmit AIDS or hepatitis. Blood spills are cleaned with chlorine bleach; needles are never recapped; a gown and mask are unnecessary to wear in an AIDS client's room unless contact is to be made with body fluids. | Ev | Sa/2 | Ap | 1 |
| #84. 1. | Announcing one's name will prevent the client from being startled, especially before touching the client. A normal tone of voice and language is the most appropriate method. | Im | Sa/2 | Ap | 1 |
| #85. 3. | Filling of the collection chambers with sanguinous (bloody) drainage indicates the drainage system is functioning. There should be intermittent bubbling in the water seal chamber. Absence of bubbling shortly after the chest tube insertion indicates an obstruction in the tubing. Fluid level fluctuation with respiration may occur in the fluid in the water seal chamber. | Ev | Ph/7 | Ap | 1 |
| #86. 3. | The purpose of administering nitroglycerin is to improve blood flow to the myocardium and relieve chest pain. Side effects of nitroglycerin may cause a blood pressure drop and a headache. Nausea is an unwarranted symptom and may indicate the condition is getting worse. | Ev | Ph/6 | Ap | 1 |
| #87. 1. | Wrist restraints may be indicated for a confused client who is pulling out essential lines; however the least restraint possible should be used for the shortest period of time. | As | Sa/2 | Ap | 1 |
| #88. 4. | The vastus lateralis is the most appropriate site as the other sites are not used until the child has been walking and develops some muscle, and there is danger of hitting vessels and nerves. The forearm is for skin tests. | Im | Ph/6 | Ap | 5 |
| #89. 3. | All the foods are low in sodium and low in fat. Fried chicken and milk are high in fat, as is the cheese, salad dressing, hot chocolate, and steak. A baked potato is acceptable without butter, cheese, or sour cream. | Ev | Ph/5 | Ap | 1 |
| #90. 2. | Persons having a pelvic sonogram should drink several glasses of water before the procedure so the bladder is full. No bowel prep is required and the procedure is safe even if pregnant. | As | Ph/7 | Ap | 1 |

| ANSWER | RATIONALE | NP | CN | CL | SA |
|--------|-----------|----|----|----|----|

#91. 1. Delegation of routine care is given to nonprofessional staff. An Sa/1 Ap 1
All activities, except applying ice, require assessment, skills, or safety precautions that the registered nurse should perform.

#92. 2. The medical staff has access to the client's file only if they As Sa/1 Ap 1
are assigned to that particular client. This does not mean that government officials are not allowed access. Sometimes police/courts need access for legal reasons. The nurse should first alert the charge nurse, who will handle the situation or contact her superior for further decision making.

#93. 3. Discharge information should include reducing sodium in Pl Ph/7 Ap 1
the diet, losing weight, increasing exercise, avoiding tobacco use, and reducing stress, along with the actions and side effects of drug therapy. There is no need to limit activity, restrict potassium or magnesium.

#94. 3. In addition to review of the disease process, a brief review of Pl Ph/7 Ap 1
anatomy and physiology is needed and the importance of good handwashing with aseptic technique during the exchange procedure. Possible complications and appropriate responses are also essential parts of the teaching plan. The client will not have an indwelling Foley catheter, nor an AV shunt or fistula.

#95. 1. A cardioselective beta blocker is less likely to cause or worsen Ev Ph/6 Co 5
the heart block while still effectively suppressing the ventricular ectopic beats. Calcium gluconate is contraindicated in ventricular fibrillation; verapamil is contraindicated in AV block; diltiazem is contraindicated in second-degree heart block.

#96. 4. There is a risk of developing a pulmonary embolism as a result As Ph/7 An 1
of venous thrombosis in the lower extremity following surgery. The Homan's sign is pain in the calf when the foot is passively dorsiflexed, which may indicate a deep vein thrombosis. More diagnostic testing should follow. Shortness of breath may indicate the thrombosis has traveled and may be in the lungs. Emergency intervention should be initiated.

#97. 2. The symptoms are indicative of a transfusion reaction. When Im Ph/6 An 1
a reaction is suspected, the transfusion should be stopped immediately and the IV line kept open with normal saline. The physician should be notified and the blood and tubing will be sent back to the lab. Vital signs will continue to be recorded.

#98. 3. A CVP or pulmonary artery catheter monitor fluid levels in the Im Ph/8 An 1
blood, which will provide early detection of high or low levels and promote management of complication. Fluids may or may not be restricted and MAST (Medical Anti-Shock Trousers) trousers are indicated if severe abdominal blood is occurring to slow the progress of shock.

#99. 1. Nightlights would help the client see to prevent falls. Other As Sa/2 An 1
factors to assess include removing loose scatter rugs, cleaning up spills, and installing handrails/grab bars as appropriate. The other choices are not related to preventing falls.

#100. 1. Older adults make medication administration errors for many reasons, the most common of which is forgetfulness. Pill boxes come in an assortment of styles and are very useful in organizing dosages, and are used for any client who is taking several medications either daily or more than once each day. The client should be able to be responsible for his own medication because he is alert and oriented. Encouragement, teaching, and follow-up are important to promote adherence to medication regimens.

Pl    Ph/7    Ap    1

# Practice Test 8

1. The nurse is assessing an elderly client. Which finding is most apt to be seen in the elderly client with dementia?
   1. Good hygiene and grooming.
   2. Rapid mood swings.
   3. Agnosia.
   4. Phobias and unwanted thoughts and behaviors.

2. An adult is being treated for second- and third-degree burns over 25% of his body and is now ready for discharge. The nurse evaluates his understanding of discharge instructions relating to wound care and is satisfied that he is prepared for home care when he makes which statement?
   1. "I will need to take sponge baths at home to avoid exposing the wounds to unsterile bath water."
   2. "If any healed areas break open I should first cover them with a sterile dressing and then report it."
   3. "I must wear my Jobst elastic garment all day and can only remove it when I'm going to bed."
   4. "I can expect occasional periods of low-grade fever and can take Tylenol every 4 hours."

3. The nurse is developing a care plan for a 2-year-old girl with Hirschsprung's disease. Which would be contraindicated for the care plan interventions?
   1. Administer stool softeners.
   2. Give isotonic enemas.
   3. Have client follow a low-fiber diet.
   4. Place on fluid restriction.

4. A 2-year-old is admitted with flu and dehydration. The history assessment reveals high fevers, little food or fluid intake for several days, has slept almost constantly, and weight has dropped from 30 lb to 21 lb. The mother has given him baby aspirin, decongestants, and leftover amoxicillin from a past ear infection. What fact increases his risk for Reye's syndrome?
   1. The use of aspirin.
   2. His high fevers.
   3. The use of antibiotics previously prescribed.
   4. Severe dehydration as evidence by weight loss.

5. A young child is brought to the emergency room by her parents with a fractured arm, which they say she sustained when she fell down the stairs. Which of the following would the nurse expect to find in the assessment of the child if she has been abused?
   1. A child who is very trusting of her nurse since she has not been able to trust her parents.
   2. The child will be constantly asking for her parents to comfort her even if they abused her.
   3. A child who doesn't cry much and who responds very little to her environment.
   4. The child will be bouncing around, feeling safe and happy to be away from an abusive home.

6. A pregnant woman is diagnosed as being anemic. Her physician has told her to eat an iron-rich diet and to take iron supplements BID. What instruction should the nurse plan to give about taking iron?
   1. Iron should be taken only on an empty stomach at least 1 hour before meals.
   2. It is good to increase consumption of dairy products while taking iron.
   3. Citrus juice taken with iron will increase absorption.
   4. Iron supplements often cause diarrhea and should be discontinued if diarrhea develops.

7. During parenting classes, the nurse teaches parents the importance of immunizations and the schedule that will be implemented. Which of the following findings indicate the nurse's teaching has been effective?
   1. The parents are able to list three reasons to immunize and when to begin immunization.
   2. Taking the infant for his first immunization at 2 weeks of age.
   3. The parents state their intent to follow a printed immunization schedule.
   4. By 6 months of age, the infant has received the recommended immunizations.

8. A woman delivered her first baby 12 hours ago. She calls the nurse in tears stating that she has been unable to get the baby to nurse. "All she does is cry when I try to get her to nurse." The

nurse comes to assist her. What is the nurse's best initial action?

1. Explain the basics of breastfeeding to the client.
2. Assess her nipples and the measures she has tried.
3. Demonstrate proper positioning of mother and baby.
4. Find out if she really wants to breastfeed or would rather bottle-feed.

9. A postpartum client complains of sore nipples, a sore bottom, cramping, fatigue, and lack of ability to satisfy her newborn, who is crying. Based on these data, which of the following would be an appropriate nursing diagnosis?

1. Ineffective parenting.
2. Alteration in comfort.
3. Anxiety related to new role of parenting.
4. Knowledge deficit.

10. A client in labor has been taught to use breathing to help her cope with the discomfort of contractions. How would the nurse best evaluate the effectiveness of teaching?

1. Ask the client to demonstrate each of the techniques and state the appropriate time in labor to use it.
2. Observe the client's use of breathing with contractions.
3. Have the client list the two main respiratory techniques and the variations.
4. Identify the client's request for pain medications or refusal as evidence of good breathing.

11. The nurse is to give Coumadin (warfarin) 10 mg PO. The nurse is comparing the anticoagulants Coumadin and heparin. Which statement is correct regarding the therapies?

1. Heparin is measured in mg; Coumadin dosage is measured in units.
2. Both have few drug interactions.
3. Heparin therapy is monitored by APTT; Coumadin therapy is monitored by PT.
4. Heparin dissolves existing clots; Coumadin does not.

12. An adult is post-op abdominoperineal resection (AP resection) for colon and rectal cancer. Which statement indicates to the nurse that he requires further teaching concerning his recovery?

1. "I'm glad this colostomy is only temporary."
2. "I'll have to cut back on eating coleslaw, my favorite type of salad."

3. "The warm sitz baths relieve the discomfort I feel from the incision on my bottom."
4. "This T-binder helps support my abdominal incision."

13. An adult had a tuberculin skin test, which the nurse reads as positive. Which of the following is true about the tuberculin skin test?

1. The intradermal test does not differentiate active tuberculosis from dormant infections.
2. The induration is measured in cm.
3. A positive test has a diameter of 5 mm.
4. Results of a tuberculin skin test must be read within 24 hours.

14. A man fractured his femur yesterday. In writing his care plan, the nurse notes to observe for a fat embolism from the long-bone fracture. Which of the following is likely to be seen with a fat embolism?

1. Bradycardia.
2. Dyspnea.
3. Edema in lower extremities.
4. Altered level of consciousness.

15. An adult has chronic renal failure. She begins complaining to the nurse of increasing numbness of her right hand and leg cramps. Of the medications ordered, which is the appropriate medication for the nurse to administer to help alleviate these symptoms?

1. Lasix.
2. Amphojel.
3. Dilantin.
4. Magnesium sulfate.

16. An adult had a barium enema for complaints of chronic diarrhea, right lower quadrant pain, weight loss, and weakness. The enema revealed the characteristic string sign. Which inflammatory disorder would the nurse suspect?

1. Ulcerative colitis.
2. Crohn's disease.
3. Diverticulosis.
4. Gastritis.

17. A baby boy who is 8 hours old is in his mother's room. Which finding by the nurse indicates the newborn needs his environment altered to promote adjustment to extrauterine life?

1. The baby just regurgitated his formula.
2. Petechiae are present on his head.
3. His hands and feet have a blue-tinged color.
4. His axillary temperature is 36°C (96.8°F).

18. A 3-year-old child has been diagnosed with Wilms' tumor and is scheduled for surgery. The nurse performing the preoperative assessment must modify the usual procedure. Which procedure would be contraindicated for this child?
    1. Auscultation of the lungs.
    2. Assessment of parents' understanding of the child's condition.
    3. Measurement of vital signs.
    4. Palpation of abdomen.

19. An elderly client is being treated for chronic open-angle glaucoma. Which medication is contraindicated for her?
    1. Pilocarpine eyedrops.
    2. Diamox.
    3. Mannitol.
    4. Neo-Synephrine eyedrops.

20. The nurse is caring for an adult who has just returned to the nursing care unit following a radical neck dissection for squamous cell carcinoma of the mouth. Which nursing action would be inappropriate during the early postoperative period?
    1. Provide mouthwash and lemon and glycerin swabs at the bedside to maintain the client's comfort and oral hygiene.
    2. Place the client in a side-lying position initially, then in Fowler's position.
    3. Place oral fluids in the back of the throat with an asepto syringe.
    4. Monitor for facial drooping and circumoral numbness or tingling.

21. A client is suffering from rejection of a kidney transplant and is told that kidney dialysis is the next treatment of choice. The client states, "I'm not going on that machine. My kidneys will hold out until I find another kidney." The nurse recognizes what defense mechanism is being used?
    1. Rationalization.
    2. Intellectualization.
    3. Denial.
    4. Suppression.

22. A 10-month-old is totally unresponsive to his parents talking to him or being cuddled by them. What will the nurse most likely find upon assessment if the child's behavior is a product of infant autism?
    1. The child is responsive to other adults.
    2. Babble is less than usual.

23. He will not rock back and forth as he tries to crawl.
    4. Though he won't cuddle, his body is relaxed when picked up.

23. What would be an appropriate intervention for a young child who has atopic dermatitis?
    1. Avoid bathing until condition has subsided.
    2. Avoid all eggs and milk products.
    3. Keep socks on hands.
    4. Use lotions with a higher water content.

24. When a client who is experiencing a conversion disorder exhibits paralysis, the nurse should provide which therapeutic approach?
    1. Develop trust through a therapeutic one-to-one relationship in which acceptance of the disorder is conveyed.
    2. Confront the client gently about the fact that no physical basis exists for the conversion.
    3. Probe into the nature of the recent conflict-producing event and the resultant paralysis.
    4. Provide a treatment approach in which the paralysis receives negative reinforcement so the client will eventually give up the symptom.

25. What would be important for the nurse to provide for a newly admitted client with schizophrenia?
    1. An environment that makes minimal demands on the client.
    2. An environment that provides maximal stimulation for the client.
    3. A climate in which the client can reflect on her problems.
    4. A climate of social relatedness for the client.

26. A middle-aged client is admitted following an overdose of prescribed antidepressant medication. He tells the nurse he may be losing his job and he would "rather die" than be faced with unemployment. What is the most appropriate short-term goal for him?
    1. To look at the help-wanted ads in the local newspaper every day.
    2. To identify one new adaptive coping mechanism by the end of the week.
    3. To contract for safety while on the unit.
    4. To contact his supervisor at work to discuss job possibilities within the company by the time of his discharge.

27. What would be an appropriate short-term goal for a client with borderline personality disorder?
   1. Discuss feelings of self-destruction with the nurse rather than to act out impulses.
   2. State ability to use problem solving as a means to deal with life problems.
   3. Control impulses through use of prn medications.
   4. Identify the process of splitting before acting out the behaviors.

28. A client with a history of alcoholism is admitted for pneumonia. What will be the nurse's reason for investigating the amount of alcohol the client has consumed during the 24 to 48 hours before admission?
   1. To determine how far the disease has progressed.
   2. To determine the severity of withdrawal.
   3. To determine whether the client will experience delirium tremens.
   4. To recommend Alcoholics Anonymous.

29. The nurse is assessing a 17-year-old female who is admitted to the eating disorders unit with a history of weight fluctuation, abdominal pain, teeth erosion, receding gums, and bad breath. Which of the following assessments will be the least useful as the nurse develops the care plan?
   1. Information regarding recent mood changes.
   2. Family functioning using a genogram.
   3. Ability to socialize with peers.
   4. Whether she has a sexual relationship with a boyfriend.

30. The mother of a 6-day-old breastfed infant calls the nurse and asks how she can be sure her baby is getting enough milk since she cannot see how much milk there is. He is breastfeeding approximately every 3 hours. The nurse would tell the mother to evaluate the effectiveness of breastfeeding by what action?
   1. Weigh the baby before and after feedings.
   2. Offer the baby water after a feeding to determine if he is still hungry.
   3. Compare the amount of time the baby cries with his contented time.
   4. See if the baby has at least 6 wet diapers in 24 hours.

31. A client is administered furosemide (Lasix) 100 mg IV. What finding would signal a possible complication is occurring?

1. The presence of edema.
2. Complaints of pain in great toe.
3. Urine output increased.
4. Decreased blood pressure.

32. The nurse is interviewing the mother of a child who is scheduled for a tonsillectomy. Which question is most essential for the nurse to ask the mother?
   1. "Have you had your tonsils out?"
   2. "Does your child get colds easily?"
   3. "Does your child have any bleeding tendencies?"
   4. "Has your child ever had an operation?"

33. A client is showing sinus tachycardia on the telemetry monitor. Which medication would the nurse expect to give?
   1. Atropine.
   2. Lidocaine.
   3. Diltiazem.
   4. Epinephrine.

34. A 2-year-old is to be admitted to the pediatric unit. His diagnosis is febrile seizures. In preparing for his admission, which of the following is the most important nursing action?
   1. Order a stat admission CBC.
   2. Place a urine collection bag and specimen cup at the bedside.
   3. Place a cooling mattress on his bed.
   4. Pad the side rails of his bed.

35. The nurse is caring for a 2-year-old who is admitted for febrile seizures. Which of the following is the primary goal of nursing care following admission?
   1. Recognition of abnormal signs or behavior indicative of a neurological deficit.
   2. Early detection and recognition of elevated temperatures.
   3. Identification of the etiology of the child's febrile condition.
   4. Promotion of rest and comfort in an atmosphere of limited stimulation.

36. A 2-year-old child is admitted with febrile seizures. A Tylenol (acetaminophen) suppository was given as ordered. Which intervention should be included in the care plan?
   1. Remove extra blankets to decrease the metabolic rate.
   2. Ask the mom to report any seizure activity.

3. Retake the temperature in 30 minutes.

4. Prepare an ice collar for the child.

37. A new graduate is to administer 2 units of PRBC (packed red blood cells) for a client whose hemoglobin is 7.2. What action will warrant intervention by the observing nurse?

    1. The blood tubing has been primed with normal saline.

    2. The blood is piggybacked into the tubing with the client's maintenance fluids of D5 ½ NS.

    3. The client has signed a consent for the administration of blood products.

    4. The graduate only obtains 1 unit of blood from the blood bank.

38. When implementing any method to reduce a child's fever, chilling should be avoided. Which of the following best explains the reason for this principle?

    1. Chilling makes the child irritable and uncooperative.

    2. Chilling causes peripheral vasodilation.

    3. Chilling can lead to shivering.

    4. Chilling can lessen the child's ability to fight infection.

39. The nurse is caring for a client admitted with pneumococcal pneumonia in the left lower lobe. Percussion of the client's left lower lobe would most likely produce which of the following findings?

    1. Rales.

    2. Rhonchi.

    3. Hyperresonance.

    4. Dullness.

40. Percussion and vibration are ordered as part of chest physical therapy for a client who has pneumonia. How often does the nurse understand that percussion should be performed?

    1. Intermittently during postural drainage.

    2. At each bronchopulmonary segment immediately prior to postural drainage.

    3. At each bronchopulmonary segment immediately following postural drainage.

    4. Only during the expiratory phase of respirations.

41. A mother calls the emergency department, stating her daughter has just taken 8 to 10 children's aspirin. After verifying the child is awake, what question would the nurse ask before telling her the child needs to be brought to the emergency department?

    1. "Do you have syrup of ipecac in your house?"

    2. "How much does your child weigh?"

    3. "When was the child's last bowel movement?"

    4. "When did your child last eat?"

42. A child has taken approximately 10 children's aspirin. The physician places a nasogastric tube in the child and administers activated charcoal. The mother asks the nurse what the charcoal is used for. What is the nurse's best response?

    1. "It induces vomiting."

    2. "It will correct electrolyte imbalances."

    3. "It will absorb the aspirin in the stomach."

    4. "It will prevent bleeding tendencies."

43. A child who has swallowed several aspirin is admitted to the emergency room. Aquamephyton is ordered. For what reason does the nurse tell the mother that it is given?

    1. To promote metabolism of aspirin.

    2. To prevent bleeding.

    3. To decrease absorption of aspirin.

    4. To prevent hepatotoxicity.

44. The nurse is giving instructions to a client who has a prescription for penicillin V potassium (Pen Vee K) 500 mg tablets to be given 4 times a day. Which statement by the client indicates the best understanding of the instructions regarding taking this medication?

    1. "I will take the pill with a full glass of orange juice to make it work better."

    2. "I will call my doctor when I feel better so I can stop taking the medicine."

    3. "I should take the pill 1 or 2 hours before meals or 2 to 3 hours after meals."

    4. "I know I could get a rash, so I won't worry if I start to itch."

45. The nurse is caring for a client who had major abdominal surgery. At 3:00 P.M. the day following surgery, the client's temperature is 102.6°F. What should the nurse do first to determine the most likely cause of the temperature elevation?

    1. Auscultate the lungs.

    2. Obtain a urine sample for culture.

    3. Culture the wound.

    4. Ask the client about exposure to communicable diseases.

46. The charge nurse observes a new staff nurse who is changing a dressing on a surgical wound. After carefully washing her hands the nurse

dons sterile gloves to remove the old dressing. After removing the dirty dressing, the nurse removes the gloves and dons a new pair of sterile gloves in preparation for cleaning and redressing the wound. What would be the most appropriate action of the charge nurse?

1. Interrupt the procedure to inform the staff nurse that sterile gloves are not needed to remove the old dressing.
2. Congratulate the nurse on the use of good technique.
3. Discuss dressing change technique with the nurse at a later date.
4. Interrupt the procedure to inform the nurse of the need to wash her hands after removal of the dirty dressing and gloves.

47. An adult male is scheduled for exploratory surgery this morning. After he is premedicated for surgery the nurse reviews his chart and discovers that he has not signed a consent form. The nurse's action is based on which of the following understandings?

1. Because the client came to the hospital, consent is implied even if the consent for the surgery has not been signed.
2. All invasive procedures require a consent form.
3. The nurse should have him sign a consent form immediately.
4. The nurse should have the next of kin sign the necessary consent form.

48. The nurse has administered an intramuscular injection. Following the procedure which is the best technique to use for disposal of the needle and syringe?

1. Recap the needle and discard in the waste container in the client's room.
2. Recap the needle and dispose of the entire unit in a special container in the utility room.
3. Carefully break the needle before placing the needle in a needle box and the syringe in a plastic-lined container.
4. Do not recap the needle, and place syringe with needle attached in a puncture-resistant container.

49. The nurse is evaluating the infection control procedures on the unit. Which finding indicates a break in technique and the need for education of staff?

1. The nurse aide is not wearing gloves when feeding an elderly client.
2. A client with active tuberculosis is asked to wear a mask when he leaves his room to go to another department for testing.

3. A nurse with open, weeping lesions of the hands puts on gloves before giving direct client care.
4. The nurse puts on a mask, a gown, and gloves before entering the room of a client on strict isolation.

50. A young adult is admitted to the emergency room. He is comatose. Initial assessment shows a pulse of 90 and respirations of 32 and deep. His face is flushed and his skin is dry. He is wearing a medical alert bracelet identifying him as diabetic. What initial order for this client would the nurse expect?

1. Administration of glucagon.
2. Oxygen at 6 liters/minute.
3. Administration of sweetened orange juice.
4. Starting an IV of normal saline.

51. A young adult is admitted to the emergency room with a rapid pulse, rapid, deep respirations, flushed face, and dry skin. He is known to be diabetic. He responds to treatment and regains consciousness. Which statement he makes is most likely related to the onset of his current problem?

1. "I've been eating at a lot of restaurants since I moved into my own apartment."
2. "I like my new job at the manufacturing plant."
3. "I recently joined the health club and I work out 3 times a week."
4. "I have a new kitten that I like a lot."

52. A client with diabetes who was admitted in ketoacidosis receives 30 units of regular insulin at 0730. When is he most likely to experience a hypoglycemic reaction?

1. Midmorning.
2. At the midday meal.
3. Midafternoon.
4. At the evening meal.

53. The nurse is caring for a client with diabetes. One morning at 1000 he becomes very irritable to the nurse. What is the nurse's first priority to determine?

1. What is actually upsetting the client.
2. When he took his insulin and if he ate his breakfast.
3. How well he slept the previous night.
4. Which of the nurse's behaviors is upsetting the client.

54. The nurse is teaching a young adult who is diabetic about management of his disease.

Which statement indicates the greatest need for further instruction?

1. "I'm glad I'll be able to eat out sometimes."
2. "I will take a snack when I go to the health club to exercise."
3. "I'll be glad when I get off the shots and start the pills."
4. "It's hard for me to remember to read labels on cans and boxes."

55. A client had a cystectomy with ileal conduit for a diagnosis of bladder cancer. During the first 48 hours post-op which symptoms should be reported to the physician?
    1. Absence of urinary output over a period of 1 to 2 hours.
    2. Swelling of the abdominal stoma.
    3. Pain along the incision site.
    4. Absent bowel sounds.

56. The nurse is teaching an adult who had a cystectomy and ileal conduit. Which statement made by the client indicates a need for further instruction?
    1. "Now that I've had the surgery, I'll have to be careful that I don't get frequent urinary tract infections."
    2. "My stoma is 1½ inches in size now, but I understand it will get smaller. Therefore, I will need to measure it again in several weeks."
    3. "I'm glad that once I get home and am better regulated, I will only have to wear an appliance at night."
    4. "I certainly don't want the stoma to close up so I will gently dilate it with my finger once a week."

57. An adult client has an IV infusing. The current fluid order is for Ringer's lactate 1000 mL to run in over an 8-hour period. The drop factor is 12 gtt/mL. What is the drip rate?_____gtt/min.

58. An adult client is admitted with a diagnosis of urinary tract calculi. The physician's orders read: vital signs every shift, morphine 10 mg for pain, Probanthine (propantheline bromide) 15 mg PO with meals, OOB as tolerated, limit fluid intake to 1000 mL/24 hours, strain all urine. Which medical order should the nurse question?
    1. Morphine 10 mg.
    2. Limit fluid intake.
    3. OOB as tolerated.
    4. Strain all urine.

59. An adult client is scheduled for a magnetic resonance imaging test. Before scheduling the test it is most essential for the nurse to ask the client which question?
    1. Are you afraid of heights?
    2. Do you have any metal in your body?
    3. Are you allergic to shellfish?
    4. Are you pregnant?

60. A 24-hour urine specimen is ordered for an adult client. The nurse goes to the client at 8:00 A.M. to start the specimen collection. What does the nurse instruct the client to do?
    1. Empty her bladder and save the specimen. Collect all urine until 8:00 A.M. tomorrow.
    2. Empty her bladder and discard the specimen. Collect all urine for 24 hours including that voided at 8:00 A.M. tomorrow.
    3. Drink large amounts of fluid during the test. Collect all urine for the next 24 hours.
    4. Note the time when she next voids and collect urine for 24 hours from that time. Notify the nurse when the collection is completed.

61. An adult client had a stapedectomy and has just returned to the nursing care unit following an uneventful stay in the postanesthesia care unit. What is essential for the nurse to include in the care plan?
    1. Instruct the client to ask for help when wanting to get out of bed.
    2. Encourage the client to drink plenty of fluids during the day.
    3. Remind the client to remain in bed for 24 hours.
    4. Tell the client to speak only when it is essential for the next 24 hours.

62. The nurse is performing an admission assessment on a client admitted for outpatient surgery today. In addition to obtaining vital signs, what information is most essential for the nurse to obtain?
    1. Time and amount the client last voided.
    2. Characteristics of client's stools.
    3. When the client last had anything to eat or drink.
    4. The client's understanding of the surgical procedure to be performed.

63. The nurse is performing an admission assessment on a client admitted with a diagnosis

of pernicious anemia. Which assessment is the nurse most likely to find?

1. Pallor, gingivitis, and fever.
2. Jaundice, hepatomegaly, and fatigue.
3. Ruddy complexion, ecchymotic areas, and distended veins.
4. Glossy red tongue, paresthesias, and fatigue.

64. An infant was born 3 months ago to a mother who was diagnosed with syphilis late in her pregnancy. Which information would be most useful in determining if the baby has congenital syphilis?

1. Irritability.
2. Red rash around anus.
3. Rhinitis.
4. Positive serology.

65. The nurse is caring for an infant who has congenital syphilis. The baby is started on penicillin. Which statement is true about the baby's ability to transmit the disease now that treatment is started?

1. She will not be contagious after 48 hours of penicillin therapy.
2. After 10 days of antibiotic therapy she will not be contagious.
3. She will always be infected and be contagious.
4. Congenital syphilis is not contagious.

66. The nurse is caring for an infant who is being treated for congenital syphilis. The baby develops vesicular lesions on the soles of her feet and has a rash on her face. What is the most appropriate initial intervention for the nurse?

1. Call the physician immediately.
2. Apply Neosporin ointment to the rash.
3. Cover the infant's hands with mittens.
4. Give Benadryl (diphenhydramine) by mouth.

67. The nurse is caring for a child with eczema. To prevent infection, what will be important use with the bath?

1. Baby oil.
2. Tepid water.
3. Bubble bath.
4. Perfumed soap.

68. The nurse is caring for a 4-year-old child who has eczema. Which toy is most appropriate to give to this child while she is in the hospital?

1. Fuzzy teddy bear.
2. Tabletop toy piano.
3. Stuffed doll.
4. 1,000-piece jigsaw puzzle.

69. A female teenager is admitted in sickle cell crisis. She is anemic, has painful joints, abdominal pain, a leg ulcer, and hematuria. What should the nurse expect to include in the nursing care plan during the acute stage?

1. Promotion of hydration.
2. Application of cold to swollen and painful joints.
3. Administration of aspirin for pain.
4. Active exercises to involved joints.

70. An adult client is scheduled for a colonoscopy. Which statement by the client indicates he understands the prescribed preparation regimen?

1. "All I need to do is give myself a packaged enema the morning of the procedure."
2. "I will eat only jello and drink clear liquids for 2 days before the test."
3. "I will take the dye tablets with water the night before the test."
4. "All I have to do is not eat anything after midnight the night before the test."

71. The nurse is caring for a woman who had a vaginal hysterectomy 2 days ago. The indwelling catheter has been removed. The nurse has performed a catheterization for residual urine. Which urine amount indicates the client is without complications?

1. 30 mL.
2. 150 mL.
3. 300 mL.
4. 500 mL.

72. An 11-month-old infant is brought to the pediatric clinic. The nurse suspects that the child has iron-deficiency anemia. Because iron-deficiency anemia is suspected, which of the following is the most important information to obtain from the infant's parents?

1. Normal dietary intake.
2. Relevant sociocultural, economic, and educational background of the family.
3. Any evidence of blood in the stools.
4. A history of maternal anemia during pregnancy.

73. The nurse is assessing a 6-month-old infant. He has acquired all the expected developmental milestones. Which will he have acquired most recently?

1. Imitates sounds.
2. Balances head well in a sitting position.
3. Smiles at mirror image.
4. Is able to grasp objects voluntarily.

74. The nurse is assessing a 2-month-old infant. The mother says the baby has colic. Which of the following is the most appropriate initial step in managing colic?
    1. Obtain a detailed history of normal daily events surrounding the infant.
    2. Eliminate cow's milk from the infant's diet or from the diet of the lactating mother.
    3. Request that the physician prescribe antispasmodic and antiflatulent medication and instruct the mother on its use.
    4. Identify the mother's feelings regarding mothering and the infant.

75. The nurse is talking with the parents of a normal 2-month-old. Which of the following should be included in anticipatory guidance for the next month of life?
    1. Stranger anxiety will begin.
    2. The posterior fontanel will close.
    3. The first tooth will erupt.
    4. The child will begin to show awareness of strange situations.

76. The clinic nurse is performing anticipatory guidance with parents of a 2-month-old infant. Instruction aimed at the prevention of accidents would best be planned with which as a reference?
    1. Mouthing of objects is very prominent.
    2. Grasps and manipulates objects well.
    3. Dislikes being restrained.
    4. Crawling and Moro reflexes are present.

77. A young woman had surgery today. Her father, a physician but not her surgeon, enters the nursing station and asks for her chart. What is the best action for the nurse to take?
    1. Allow him to read the chart as requested.
    2. Do not allow him to read the chart.
    3. Ask the attending surgeon for permission for him to read the chart.
    4. Ask the client if she wants him to read the chart.

78. An adult client is being prepared for abdominal surgery. She refuses to remove her plain gold wedding band before going to surgery. What is the best action for the nurse to take?
    1. Firmly insist that it must be removed or surgery cannot be performed.
    2. Ask her husband to assist you in discussing this with his wife.
    3. Cover the wedding band with adhesive tape and tape it to her finger.
    4. Premedicate her and remove the wedding band after she falls asleep.

79. The client has had a central venous access device (Hickman catheter) inserted. Correct placement has been confirmed by X-ray. The nurse is to set up parenteral nutrition to be connected to the Hickman catheter. The nurse should place the client in which position for the procedure?
    1. Trendelenburg.
    2. Semi-Fowler's.
    3. Side lying.
    4. Supine.

80. An adult client has an order for a nasogastric tube. Before inserting the tube the nurse measures the amount of tube needed. How would the nurse determine the amount of tube needed?
    1. Measure from the forehead to the ear and from the ear to the umbilicus.
    2. Measure from the chin to the back of the throat and from the back of the throat to the umbilicus.
    3. Measure from the mouth to the xiphoid process and add 2 inches.
    4. Measure from the tip of the client's nose to his earlobe and from the earlobe to the xiphoid process.

81. An adult client is admitted with an asthma attack. Aminophylline IV is prescribed. How will the nurse know if the desired results are achieved in the client?
    1. Pulse rate increases.
    2. Breathing effort is less.
    3. Pain is relieved.
    4. Respiratory rate increases.

82. An adult client has just returned to the nursing care unit following a gastroscopy. Which notation is essential for the nurse to include on the nursing care plan?
    1. Throat lozenges PRN for sore throat.
    2. Supine position for 6 hours.
    3. NPO for 4 hours.
    4. Clear liquid diet for 24 hours.

83. An adult has myasthenia gravis and is admitted in myasthenic crisis. The nurse should include which of the following on the nursing care plan immediately after admission?
    1. Suction equipment at bedside.
    2. Active exercises QID.
    3. Give medicines following meals.
    4. Prepare client for the Tensilon test.

84. The nurse is evaluating a client who is receiving total parenteral nutrition (TPN) therapy. Which observation best indicates the client is having the desired therapeutic effects from TPN?

1. The client has regular bowel movements.
2. The client maintains blood sugars in the normal range.
3. The client is gaining weight.
4. The client has normal urine output.

85. A man fractured his right ankle, which was plaster casted in the emergency room. Before discharge from the emergency room the nurse gives him instructions for his care. Which statement by the man indicates a need for further instruction?

1. "I will keep my foot elevated when I go home."
2. "My wife's hair dryer should work well to dry the cast."
3. "I won't let anyone sign my cast for a couple of days."
4. "It is okay to wiggle my toes on my right foot."

86. A woman who is 40 weeks pregnant, is admitted to the labor suite. While the nurse is assessing her, her membranes rupture. The nurse immediately performs a vaginal exam. During the exam, the nurse feels a loop of cord protruding into the vagina. What is the best immediate action for the nurse to take?

1. Attempt to lift the fetal head off the cord.
2. Prepare for immediate vaginal delivery.
3. Call the physician.
4. Place the tocometer on the mother's abdomen.

87. An adult is in acute renal failure secondary to hemorrhagic shock. Which statement by his wife best indicates to the nurse that she understands her husband's condition?

1. "I understand my husband will need dialysis for the rest of his life."
2. "I need to watch our son for evidence of renal failure as he grows up."
3. "My husband will be on a special diet for a long time."
4. "My husband has a good chance to recover normal kidney function."

88. The nurse is planning care for an adult who has just had a liver biopsy. What would be the proper positioning for the client?

1. On the left side
2. On the right side

3. In semi-Fowler's
4. Prone

89. An adult is to have a pelvic sonogram tomorrow. The nurse knows the client understands preprocedure instruction when which statement is made?

1. "I won't eat for 12 hours before the procedure."
2. "I will take a laxative the night before the procedure."
3. "I will empty my bladder immediately before the test."
4. "I will drink several glasses of water just before I come."

90. An adult has had a total hip replacement and is to be discharged home. The client can ambulate with a walker. The nurse is evaluating the home care environment. Which finding alerts the nurse to a potential safety problem?

1. The bathroom has a shower but not a tub.
2. The bathroom door is narrow.
3. The kitchen is equipped with a microwave.
4. There are scatter rugs on the floor in the entrance hall and the living room.

91. A young adult is admitted for a broken arm, ruptured spleen, increased intracranial pressure, and damage to the spinal cord at the level of C-5 and C-6 from a motor vehicle accident. His Glasgow Coma scale score is 10 and he is aphasic at present. Which nursing diagnosis would be the highest priority?

1. Impaired verbal communication.
2. Self-care deficit.
3. High risk for infection.
4. Decreased intracranial adaptive capacity.

92. An adult client was experiencing vertigo and severe headaches and a blood pressure of 180/104. The medication orders include furosemide (Lasix) and quinipril hydrochloride (Accupril). What specific drug information should the nurse include in the discharge plan of this client?

1. Take the Lasix in the morning and the Accupril at bedtime.
2. Change positions slowly and increase dietary potassium.
3. Discontinue the Lasix once blood pressure is within normal range and increase fluid intake.
4. Increase sodium intake and monitor blood pressure monthly.

93. An adult was admitted to the respiratory floor with COPD. The nurse finds him extremely restless, incoherent, and showing signs of acute respiratory distress. He is using accessory muscles for breathing and is diaphoretic and cyanotic. What is the nurse's best initial action?
    1. Administer oxygen as ordered.
    2. Assess vital signs and neural vital signs.
    3. Administer medication which has been ordered for pain.
    4. Call respiratory therapy for a prescribed arterial blood gas (ABG) analysis.

94. The nurse is evaluating an adult with respiratory disease. Which finding, if observed, indicates compliance with breathing exercises?
    1. Decreased use of pursed lip breathing.
    2. Decreased coughing after exhalation when using resisted breathing exercises.
    3. Increased coughing after exhalation when using resisted breathing exercises.
    4. Inhaling through the mouth and exhaling through the nose.

95. The nurse is caring for a client who has an order for a cooling blanket. What does the nurse need to assess before starting the procedure?
    1. If the client is improperly exposed.
    2. The skin for areas of breakdown.
    3. The amount of shivering the client exhibits.
    4. The skin color for cyanosis.

96. The nurse is instructing a homebound client how to apply a warm compress to her wrist. Which comment by the client indicates to the nurse that she understands the safety aspects of the procedure?
    1. "I will take my temperature before and after applying the compress."
    2. "If the pain is not reduced by the compress I will call the nurse."
    3. "I will make sure the water temperature is not over 37.7°C (100°F)."
    4. "If the compress begins to get cool, I can warm it up by putting my arm under the hot water faucet."

97. An elderly client lives alone at home and has a history of hypertension and constipation, but takes no medications. Which of the following assessment statements by the nurse will help to devise a strategy to help the client?
    1. "When did you have your last bowel movement?"
    2. "Tell me what you had to eat yesterday."
    3. "Why do you not take any antihypertensives?"
    4. "Tell me how much you walk during the day."

98. The nurse is assessing an elderly woman. Which statement by the client indicates an abnormal finding and one that needs to be further evaluated?
    1. "I move a little slower these days."
    2. "I can't seem to remember what's going on now."
    3. "I enjoy reading, but have to use a magnifying glass."
    4. "My skin is thin and dry and there are little brown spots on my hands."

99. The nurse is instructing a client how to perform Kegel's exercises. Which is most appropriate for the nurse to include in the instructions?
    1. Squeeze your buttocks.
    2. Hold your urine as long as possible before voiding.
    3. Push down on your lower abdomen while holding your breath.
    4. Practice stopping your urine in midstream.

100. The school nurse is called to the playground where an 8-year-old child is lying on the ground with bright red blood spurting from a wound in his thigh. He says he was climbing on the swings when he caught his leg on something. What is the nurse's most appropriate action?
    1. Assess the child's level of consciousness.
    2. Apply an ice pack.
    3. Call the rescue squad.
    4. Apply firm pressure to the bleeding leg.

# Answers and Rationales for Practice Test 8

| ANSWER | RATIONALE | NP | CN | CL | SA |
|--------|-----------|----|----|----|----|
| #1. 3. | Agnosia, the inability to identify familiar objects, is a key finding in dementia. The client may not be able to recognize a key or pencil and know what they do. The other choices are associated with delirium and depression. | As | Ps/4 | Ap | 1 |
| #2. 2. | The client will be taught to report changes in wound healing such as blister formation, signs of infection (fever, redness, pain, warmth at area or foul-smelling drainage), and opening of a previously healed area. Showering is permitted which will cleanse and remove dead tissue; Jobst garments must be worn 23 hours a day to promote constant pressure on the new forming tissue. | Ev | Sa/2 | Ap | 1 |
| #3. 4. | Hirschsprung's disease is a motility disorder of the bowel in which peristalsis is absent and feces accumulates proximal to the defect, leading to bowel obstruction. Fluid restriction would not help her condition, as the other selections would be indicated. | Pl | Ph/7 | An | 4 |
| #4. 1. | Aspirin ingestion associated with flu or chickenpox increases the risk of Reye's syndrome. Reye's syndrome is thought to occur when a child who has a viral infection receives aspirin. | An | Ph/7 | An | 4 |
| #5. 3. | The abused child doesn't cry because that has probably resulted in more abuse for her. She has learned to turn inward and not expect good things from her environment. | As | Ps/4 | An | 4 |
| #6. 3. | Vitamin C taken with iron increases absorption. Iron does absorb more readily when taken on an empty stomach, but may need to be taken with meals to avoid gastrointestinal distress. A common side effect of iron is constipation and darker stools. | Pl | Ph/6 | An | 3 |
| #7. 4. | The best way to evaluate that teaching has been effective is to see the desired behavior. Verbalizing is a strong indicator but not as strong as the behavior being demonstrated. | Ev | He/3 | An | 4 |
| #8. 2. | The nurse will need to know what the client has tried and if her nipples are flat or inverted before planning the appropriate intervention. Assessment is always done first. | As | He/3 | Ap | 3 |
| #9. 2. | Specific data (sore nipples, sore bottom, crying) are the supporting evidence for selected diagnosis. There is either a lack of information for the other choices or pain/comfort would be a priority. | An | He/3 | An | 3 |
| #10. 2. | The best way to evaluate is to watch the client demonstrate the use of the breathing techniques. | Ev | He/3 | Ap | 3 |
| #11. 3. | The lab values, APTT (Activated Partial Thromboplastin Time) and PT (Prothrombin Time) monitor blood coagulation for heparin and Coumadin, respectively. Heparin is measured in units and administered by IV or SQ. Coumadin is measured in mg and available in IV, but predominately given in pill form. Neither of the two medications dissolves clots. | An | Ph/6 | An | 5 |

| ANSWER | RATIONALE | NP | CN | CL | SA |
|---|---|---|---|---|---|
| #12. 1. | The distal sigmoid colon, rectum, and anus are removed and a permanent colostomy is created. | Ev | Ph/7 | Ap | 1 |
| #13. 1. | The tuberculin skin test measures the presence of antibodies against tuberculosis. Both dormant and active infections will give a positive skin test. A positive test shows an induration of 10 mm or more, with results read in 48 to 72 hours following the administration. | An | He/3 | An | 1 |
| #14. 4. | A fat embolism occurs 12 to 48 hours after injury with typical symptoms of fever, rash, tachycardia, tachypnea, blood-tinged sputum, cyanosis, anxiety, restlessness, altered level of consciousness, convulsions, and coma. | Pl | Ph/7 | Ap | 1 |
| #15. 2. | Paresthesias, muscle cramps, abnormal reflexes, and seizures are symptoms of hyperphosphatemia. A phosphate binder such as Amphojel or Renegal must be given with each meal so that they can bind with the phosphorus in newly consumed food and prevent its absorption into the body and bloodstream. It is imperative to prevent high levels of phosphorus that can weaken the bones and can cause them to break easily. | An | Ph/6 | An | 5 |
| #16. 2. | A barium enema shows the characteristic "string sign" which is a narrowing of the lumen revealed on X-ray ending at the ileo-caecal junction. The client's other symptoms are also indicative of Crohn's disease. | An | Ph/7 | Co | 1 |
| #17. 4. | A temperature of 36°C (96.8°F) is below the normal range of 36.1°–37.2°C (97° to 99°F) and may indicate a cold environment. The skin color is normally pink but petechiae, which are hemorrhagic spots on the skin from increased intravascular pressure in capillaries, may result from pressure on the presenting part at delivery. Acrocyanosis is a normal condition caused by vasomotor instability and poor peripheral circulation found in the newborn. | Ev | He/3 | An | 3 |
| #18. 4. | Wilms' tumor is an encapsulated tumor and palpation may cause the tumor to rupture and scatter cancer cells in the abdomen, so palpation would be avoided. | As | Ph/7 | Ap | 4 |
| #19. 4. | Neo-Synephrine is a mydriatic and contraindicated with open-angle glaucoma. Medications are given to constrict the pupil and increase the outflow of aqueous humor. | Im | Ph/6 | Co | 1 |
| #20. 1. | This choice would be contraindicated, as they would be chemically irritating to the client's mouth. Mouth irrigation would consist of sterile water, diluted peroxide, normal saline, or sodium bicarbonate. The other choices would be appropriate. | Im | Ph/7 | Ap | 1 |
| #21. 3. | Denial is occurring because the news of a chronic course to this client's illness is too painful to address at this time. Rationalization is the attribution of plausible reasons for one's behavior to deal with disappointment; intellectualization involves a separation of emotion from the event; suppression is a conscious attempt to forget something until a later time. | As | Ps/4 | An | 1 |
| #22. 2. | Babble, an early form of communication, is less than usual in autistic children. Autistic children treat people as inanimate objects, may demonstrate a rocking behavior, and stiffen their bodies when trying to be held. | As | Ps/4 | An | 4 |

| ANSWER | RATIONALE | NP | CN | CL | SA |
|--------|-----------|-----|-----|-----|-----|
| #23. 3. | Atopic dermatitis is a chronic, relapsing inflammation of the dermis, also known as "eczema." Treatment focuses on control of symptoms to relieve itching and hydration of the skin, which socks would prevent the child scratching. It is recommended to bath the child each day with warm water and apply a water-in-oil or lipid-based moisturizer to seal in moisture. As the condition may run in families, the exact etiology is unclear. | Im | Ph/8 | Ap | 4 |
| #24. 1. | The nurse must first accept the client where he is. Conversion reactions are due to a conflict-producing situation and are involuntary in nature. Presence of paralysis assists the client in avoiding some unpleasant situation. This needs to be brought out in psychotherapy at the client's pace. Analysis of the relationship between anxiety and conversion symptoms helps the nurse choose the correct response. | An | Ps/4 | An | 2 |
| #25. 1. | A newly admitted client with schizophrenia needs decreased stimulation/demands due to sensory perceptual alternation and an inability to process information correctly. | Pl | Ps/4 | An | 2 |
| #26. 3. | Using Maslow's hierarchy of needs, the issue of physical safety is the only appropriate short-term goal. The nurse is concerned about a possible suicide attempt and should have the client contract to notify the nurse if he feels like harming himself. | Pl | Ps/4 | Ap | 2 |
| #27. 1. | Clients with borderline personality need to remain in a safe environment and learn to discuss self-destructive feelings rather than acting out self-destructive impulses. Choices 2 and 4 are long-term goals; prn meds will be given but attempts will be made to problem-solve. | Pl | Ps/4 | Ap | 2 |
| #28. 2. | The amount of alcohol consumed recently will help to determine how much medication the client will need to relieve withdrawal symptoms. Delirium tremens may appear from 24 to 72 hours from cessation of alcohol intake, but the nurse's reason will be for medication reasons to prevent withdrawal symptoms. | As | Ps/4 | An | 2 |
| #29. 4. | It is inappropriate to ask her about sexual relationships. The other information will be important to assess. | An | Ps/4 | An | 2 |
| #30. 4. | Mothers should be taught to count the number of diapers that are wet each day, which would indicate adequate hydration. | Ev | He/3 | Ap | 4 |
| #31. 2. | A high dose of Lasix may cause rapid diuresis and if the client has a history of gout, uric acid may be underexcreted causing the painful condition. Edema would most likely be found in a client receiving a high dose of Lasix to rid the body of excess fluids via urine and it would be expected that blood pressure would decrease as the body excretes excess fluid. | As | Ph/8 | An | 1 |
| #32. 3. | Bleeding tendencies are especially significant in a child who is to have a tonsillectomy, as the most common complication is hemorrhage. | As | Ph/7 | Ap | 4 |
| #33. 3. | Diltiazem, a calcium channel blocker, is given to control the tachycardia occurrence. It will inhibit the influx of calcium through the cell membrane, resulting in a depression of automaticity and conduction velocity in cardiac muscle. Atropine is given for | Im | Ph/8 | Ap | 1 |

| ANSWER | RATIONALE | NP | CN | CL | SA |
|--------|-----------|-----|-----|-----|-----|

bradycardia; lidocaine is given for ventricular tachycardia; and epinephrine is given for ventricular fibrillation.

**#34. 4.** Precautions should be initiated to prevent injury and promote safety. A cooling blanket must be ordered by the physician and is usually not used unless other methods for fever reduction are unsuccessful. — Pl | Sa/2 | Ap | 4

**#35. 2.** Febrile seizures occur in association with a fever and are a common transient neurologic disorder of childhood. The height and rapidity of temperature elevation are important factors in the onset. Seizures are more likely to occur during a rise in temperature rather than after it has been elevated for a prolonged period. — Pl | Ph/7 | Ap | 4

**#36. 3.** The first concern is to reduce the fever, so the effectiveness of the Tylenol suppository will need determination. Removing blankets does not decrease the metabolic rate; the temperature may decrease via convection. It is a nursing responsibility to observe and report seizure activity; ice collars are typically used for a child who has had a tonsillectomy. — Pl | Ph/8 | An | 4

**#37. 2.** Blood administration is infused only with normal saline. Dextrose solutions may lyse RBCs and decrease RBC survival. Blood transfusions require a consent from the client, along with side effects explained. One unit of blood is obtained as needed, as each unit is only allowed to be at room temperature for a maximum of 4 hours. The 2$^{nd}$ unit would be obtained after the 1$^{st}$ unit has infused. — Im | Sa/2 | An | 1

**#38. 3.** Shivering is a normal compensatory mechanism used by the body to warm itself by increasing the body heat. Therefore, allowing the child to become chilled and shiver defeats the purpose of fever reduction activities. Chilling causes vasoconstriction, not vasodilation and it does not lessen the child's ability to fight infection. — An | Ph/7 | An | 4

**#39. 4.** When pneumonia is localized in a single lobe, consolidation or infiltration of exudates into the alveoli can be expected. Percussion reveals dullness over the lobe where the consolidation has occurred. — As | Ph/7 | An | 1

**#40. 1.** The technique of postural drainage is more effective when used in conjunction with percussion and vibration. Percussion performed intermittently during postural drainage loosens tenacious secretions so that they will flow more freely. — Im | Ph/7 | Ap | 1

**#41. 2.** The child's weight can help the nurse determine how emergent the situation is. The toxicity will be affected by the child's weight, elevated toxicity for a smaller weight. The nurse may decide for the mother to call 911 versus driving the child to the emergency department. Syrup of ipecac is not sold over the counter and should only be given by healthcare providers, as the vomiting may cause aspiration. The last bowel movement or food is not the immediate concern. — Im | Ph/8 | Ap | 4

**#42. 3.** Charcoal is an absorbent and will absorb the aspirin in the stomach. It will not induce vomiting, does not effect electrolytes, or prevent bleeding. — An | Ph/6 | Ap | 4

**#43. 2.** Aquamephyton is vitamin K, which promotes clotting. — An | Ph/6 | An | 4

| ANSWER | RATIONALE | NP | CN | CL | SA |
|--------|-----------|-----|-----|-----|-----|
| #44. 3. | Food may interfere with absorption. The medication should be given with a full glass of water, as juice (acid) will inactivate the drug and the full course of medication should be taken. | Ev | Ph/6 | Ap | 5 |
| #45. 1. | The most likely cause of a low-grade temperature elevation 24 to 48 hours after surgery is pulmonary infection, and the presence of rales or rhonchi should be ausculted in the lungs. A urinary tract infection occurs typically 48 to 72 hours and wound infection 72 hours following surgery. | As | Ph/7 | An | 1 |
| #46. 4. | The staff nurse is doing two things incorrectly. Nonsterile gloves are adequate to remove the old dressings. However, the use of sterile gloves does not put the client in danger so discussion of this can wait until later. However, the nurse should wash her hands after removing the soiled dressing and before donning sterile gloves to clean and dress the wound. Not doing this compromises client safety and should be brought to the immediate attention of the nurse. | Im | Sa/2 | Ap | 1 |
| #47. 2. | All invasive procedures require informed consent. The surgery is prescheduled and described as exploratory and therefore is not an emergency. If the client is an adult and has not been declared incompetent the client must sign the form. When the client has been premedicated, he cannot give legal consent when under the influence of mind-altering drugs. | An | Sa/1 | Ap | 1 |
| #48. 4. | The proper procedure is to place the needle in the puncture-resistant container (Sharps box) immediately after use. Some syringes now have safety features that cover the needle before placing it in the Sharps box. | Im | Sa/2 | Ap | 1 |
| #49. 3. | Persons with exudative lesions or weeping dermatitis should not give direct client care or handle client-care equipment until the condition resolves. | Ev | Sa/2 | An | 1 |
| #50. 4. | Initial assessment of this client reveals classic signs of hyperglycemia and metabolic ketoacidosis. Normal saline does not contain glucose. The client needs to blow off carbon dioxide. | Pl | Ph/8 | An | 1 |
| #51. 1. | Hyperglycemia and ketoacidosis may be caused by a change in eating patterns. Restaurant food is apt to be high in carbohydrates and fats. Exercise is apt to cause hypoglycemia. | An | Ph/8 | Ap | 1 |
| #52. 1. | Regular insulin is short-acting insulin, peaking in 2 to 4 hours after administration. Hypoglycemia is most apt to occur at peak action of insulin. | Pl | Ph/6 | Ap | 1 |
| #53. 2. | Irritability is a classic sign of hypoglycemia. The time suggests it might be hypoglycemia due to insulin reaction. The nurse must assess when he took his insulin and if he ate his breakfast. | As | Ph/6 | Ap | 1 |
| #54. 3. | A young adult would have Type 1 diabetes mellitus. Insulin is not produced and will always need insulin replacement. Oral agents that stimulated the pancreas will not be an option for him, therefore, his statement indicates a lack of understanding. | Ev | Ph/7 | Ap | 1 |
| #55. 1. | Absence of urine indicates poor renal perfusion. Urine output below 30 mL/hr is unacceptable and considered shock. Swelling, pain and absent bowel sounds are normal during the first 48 hours. | As | Ph/7 | Ap | 1 |

| ANSWER | RATIONALE | NP | CN | CL | SA |
|---|---|---|---|---|---|
| #56. 3. | An ileal conduit drains urine continuously, so an appliance must be worn at all times. It is true that urinary tract infections are apt to be more frequent, that the stoma will shrink in time, and the stoma should be dilated every week to keep it patent. | Ev | Ph/7 | An | 1 |
| #57. | 25 gtt/min. To calculate the drip rate, first determine the number of mL per hour. 1000 mL/8 hours = 125 mL/hr. Next, divide 125 mL/hr by 60 min per hour and multiply by the drop factor of 12 gtt/mL. The correct answer is 25 gtt/min. | Im | Ph/6 | Ap | 5 |
| #58. 2. | The nurse should encourage fluids from 3000–5000 mL in 24 hours to help flush the stones out of the urinary system. | An | Ph/7 | An | 1 |
| #59. 2. | MRI testing is based on magnetic fields that are affected by and can affect metal in the body such as pacemakers, hip prostheses, skull plates, etc. It is essential to ask the question, and to also inform the client about the claustrophobic environment, in case a mild sedative might be needed. | As | Ph/7 | Co | 1 |
| #60. 2. | The bladder is emptied and the specimen discarded at the beginning of the 24-hour collection. Urine in the bladder was made prior to the start of the collection time. The bladder will be emptied at the end of the time because it was made during the 24-hour period. Placing signs in and on doors of the bathroom will alert the entire staff to collect the urine. | Im | Ph/7 | Ap | 1 |
| #61. 1. | A stapedectomy is removal of the stapes (the small bone in the ear next to the inner ear) and insertion of prosthesis. The client may experience dizziness with a change in position or ambulation. | Pl | Ph/7 | Ap | 1 |
| #62. 3. | It is essential the client has maintained NPO status for at least 6 to 8 hours prior to surgery to prevent the possibility of aspiration. | As | Ph/7 | Ap | 1 |
| #63. 4. | A glossy red tongue is characteristic of pernicious anemia. The client lacks the intrinsic factor, which is necessary for absorption of vitamin $B_{12}$. $B_{12}$ is necessary for the manufacture of red blood cells and for proper functioning of the nervous system. Paresthesias, changes in sensation, are frequently seen in pernicious anemia. Fatigue occurs because the oxygen-carrying capacity is diminished when red blood cell count is decreased. Jaundice and hepatomegaly are seen in hemolytic anemias such as sickle cell and a ruddy complexion is seen with polycythemia vera. | As | Ph/7 | Co | 1 |
| #64. 4. | Congenital syphilis is difficult to diagnose until the infant develops her own antibodies. A positive serology confirms the diagnosis of congenital syphilis. | As | Ph/7 | An | 4 |
| #65. 1. | Until the 48 hours of penicillin therapy is complete, the infant should be in isolation. | An | Sa/2 | Ap | 4 |
| #66. 3. | Covering the infant's hands will minimize trauma to her skin from scratching, then the physician can be notified. | Im | Sa/2 | Ap | 4 |
| #67. 2. | Tepid water is the best substance to use for this condition when bathing. The others would be too irritating. | Im | Ph/5 | Ap | 4 |

| ANSWER | | RATIONALE | NP | CN | CL | SA |
|---|---|---|---|---|---|---|
| #68. | 2. | It would be advisable to avoid fuzzy, stuffed toys that may be allergenic, and the selected toy is age-appropriate. | Im | He/3 | Ap | 4 |
| #69. | 1. | Hydration is very important, because dehydration causes sickle cell crisis. The client will usually have both IV and PO fluids. Heat is used to dilate vessels and promote circulation; ASA is contraindicated; painful joints would be rested during the acute phase. | Pl | Ph/7 | Ap | 4 |
| #70. | 2. | The client is given laxatives for 24 to 48 hours before the procedure and will only have clear liquids the night before. He will be NPO after midnight the night before the procedure. | Ev | Ph/7 | Ap | 1 |
| #71. | 1. | The urine volume obtained during a catherization for residual urine should be 50 mL or less. | Ev | Ph/7 | Ap | 3 |
| #72. | 1. | Iron-deficiency anemia occurs commonly in children 6 to 24 months of age. For the first 4 to 5 months of infancy, iron stores laid down for the baby during pregnancy are adequate. When fetal iron stores are depleted, supplemental dietary iron needs to be supplied to meet the infant's rapid growth needs. Iron deficiency may occur in the infant who drinks mostly milk, which contains no iron, and does not receive adequate dietary iron or supplemental iron. | As | Ph/5 | An | 4 |
| #73. | 1. | This is the only correct choice. Choice 2 is typical of a 4-month-old, choices 3 and 4 are typical of a 5-month-old. | As | He/3 | Ap | 4 |
| #74. | 1. | The initial step should be an investigation of identifying factors that contribute to the cause of colic. The nurse would obtain a detailed history on diet of the infant and lactating mother, frequency and time of attacks, and activity of the mother surrounding the time of attacks. Assess first, then treat. | As | Ph/7 | Ap | 4 |
| #75. | 4. | Showing awareness would be expected, as the other occurrences would occur at 6 to 8 months, 2 months, and 5 to 6 months, respectively. | Pl | He/3 | Ap | 4 |
| #76. | 4. | These reflexes can propel the infant forward unexpectedly, causing injury from falling. | Pl | He/3 | Ap | 4 |
| #77. | 2. | Because he is not the client's physician and does not have a medical need to see her chart, he should not be allowed to read the chart without written permission from the client, who is above the age of 18. | Im | Sa/1 | Ap | 1 |
| #78. | 3. | It is preferred that all jewelry be removed before surgery and either be sent home with family or placed in the hospital safe. However, if a client has a plain wedding band with no stones and wants to keep the ring on, or if it's too tight to remove, it can be covered with adhesive tape and taped to the fingers. Rings with stones should not be taped, as the stones may loosen and dislodge. If swelling will occur on the hand, the ring must be removed. | Im | Sa/2 | Ap | 1 |
| #79. | 1. | Placing the client in Trendelenburg's position reduces the likelihood of an air embolism occurring during the procedure. | Im | Ph/7 | Ap | 1 |
| #80. | 4. | The best way to determine the amount of tube needed to reach the pylorus is to measure from the tip of the client's nose to his earlobe and from the earlobe to the xiphoid process. | Im | Ph/7 | Ap | 1 |

| ANSWER | RATIONALE | NP | CN | CL | SA |
|---|---|---|---|---|---|
| #81. 2. | Aminophylline is a bronchodilator. When it is effective, the breathing effort is less. It is expected the pulse rate will increase but is not the desired effect. Pain is not the problem with asthma. | Ev | Ph/7 | An | 5 |
| #82. 3. | Because a local anesthetic is used during the procedure, the client must be NPO until the gag reflex returns, which is usually 2 to 4 hours. Semi-Fowler's position will facilitate drainage of saliva and prevent aspiration. | Pl | Ph/7 | Ap | 1 |
| #83. 1. | Myasthenia gravis (MG) causes extreme muscle weakness. A person in myasthenia crisis will likely need vigorous respiratory support including possibly a tracheotomy, positive pressure breathing, and vigorous suctioning. The Tensilon test is used in diagnosing MG. | Pl | Ph/8 | Ap | 1 |
| #84. 3. | Weight gain should occur if the client is getting adequate nutrition. Blood sugars are checked every 6 hours due to the TPN solution. | Ev | Ph/6 | Ap | 1 |
| #85. 2. | The cast should be allowed to air dry. Fiberglass casts may be dried with a hair dryer on the cool setting. | Ev | Ph/7 | Ap | 1 |
| #86. 1. | Keeping the fetal head from compressing the cord will allow circulation through the cord to the fetus to continue and save the baby's life. The baby will be delivered as soon as possible by cesarean section. | Im | He/3 | Ap | 3 |
| #87. 4. | The client will have good chance of complete recovery if well cared for during the acute renal failure episode. In the acute episode, the other choices would not be a problem, as they would if the client was in chronic renal failure or end-stage renal failure. | Ev | Ph/8 | Ap | 1 |
| #88. 2. | The client should be positioned on his right side with a pillow under the costal margin and to remain in that position for several hours, avoiding coughing or straining. This will reduce the likelihood of bleeding. | Pl | Ph/7 | Ap | 1 |
| #89. 4. | The client should have a full bladder, which will act as a landmark and reflect sound waves. It is not necessary to be NPO or take a laxative, as for a colonoscopy. | Ev | Ph/7 | Ap | 1 |
| #90. 4. | Scatter rugs can be a hazard for anyone, but especially for a person with a walker. They should be removed for the client's safety. | Ev | Sa/2 | Ap | 1 |
| #91. 4. | Prioritization is first aimed at meeting basic physiologic needs for survival before meeting high level needs (Maslow's). The client is at high risk for alterations in basic body functioning secondary to pressure on the brain tissue. Once the intracranial pressure has been stabilized, the priority list would be reviewed. | Pl | Ph/8 | An | 1 |
| #92. 2. | Lasix is a potent loop diuretic that can cause potassium depletion unless dietary supplements are given. Early morning administration is recommended so that sleep is not disturbed by nocturia. Both medications can cause lightheadedness and orthostatic hypotension because of vasodilation and decreased vascular volume. Sodium intake should be decreased as it will hold more water and blood pressure should be monitored daily then weekly. | Pl | Ph/6 | Co | 5 |

| ANSWER | RATIONALE | NP | CN | CL | SA |
|---|---|---|---|---|---|
| #93. 1. | The client's symptoms are indicative of hypoxemia. Oxygen administration should be started followed by vital signs. Pain is not the primary problem and ABGs may be indicated, but not before administration of oxygen. | Im | Ph/8 | Ap | 1 |
| #94. 3. | Resisted breathing is one kind of breathing exercise than can be taught to clients with respiratory disease. Noncompliance is common and is suspected when clients do not have typical results. A cough is expected after the exhalation phase of resisted breathing. Pursed lip breathing is encouraged to lengthen the exhalation. | Ev | Ph/7 | Co | 1 |
| #95. 2. | The cooling blanket will cause vasoconstriction, which decreases the peripheral blood supply. Skin care and assessment should be carried out every hour to prevent skin breakdown. The client should not be unduly exposed, but this is not essential. After the blanket's initiation, shivering may occur and the skin will be assessed for any white areas, which may suggest frostbite. | As | Ph/7 | Ap | 1 |
| #96. 3. | It is the temperature of the compress that is important, which should be below 37.7°C (100°F). | Ev | Ph/7 | Ap | 1 |
| #97. 2. | The nurse should assess the client for dietary habits. A diet that is high in fiber helps to prevent constipation. It is not unusual for the elderly and those living by themselves not to eat fresh fruits and vegetables. Her blood pressure can be controlled with lifestyle changes instead of medications, and even though mobility helps prevent constipation, this is not the first assessment. | As | Ph/5 | An | 1 |
| #98. 2. | Recent memory loss can be a sign of organic brain disease and needs further investigation. The other choices are normal aging occurrences. | An | He/3 | An | 1 |
| #99. 4. | Stopping the urine while voiding requires the use of the pubococcygeus (PG) muscle—the muscle Kegel's exercises are designed to strengthen. Stopping the urine while voiding helps to identify the PG muscle so the client can learn to contract and relax it. | Im | Ph/7 | Ap | 3 |
| #100. 4. | Bright red blood spurting from a wound signals arterial bleeding. Firm pressure is necessary to stop the bleeding. The nurse should delegate someone to call the emergency rescue squad. | Im | Ph/8 | Ap | 4 |

# Practice Test 9

1. A child is suspected of having infective endocarditis (IE). Which of these questions during a client's history would most likely reveal the cause of the condition?
   1. "How long have you had this prolonged fever?"
   2. "Have you been to the dentist lately?"
   3. "When did the conjunctival infection start?"
   4. "How long has your blood pressure been high?"

2. A pregnant woman is experiencing physiologic anemia of pregnancy. What foods could the nurse recommend for this condition?
   1. Cheese omelet.
   2. Milk and ice cream.
   3. Apricots and prunes.
   4. Cottage cheese and fruit.

3. The physician has ordered 10 mEq/L IV push over 2 minutes. The nurse checks the client's serum potassium level as 2.7 before administering. What would be the nurse's best action?
   1. Give the medication as the potassium is very low.
   2. Explain to the client that the medication will cause diuresis.
   3. Hold the medication and page the physician.
   4. Verify the correct amount has been drawn up in the syringe.

4. The client's arterial blood gases show a high pH and a low $CO_2$. Which of the following conditions is the client most likely experiencing?
   1. Airway obstruction
   2. Panic attack
   3. Renal failure
   4. Vomiting

5. The new graduate nurse in orientation admits a client with a diagnosis of tuberculosis. Which finding from the assessment would the precepting nurse question?
   1. Visible skin lesions.
   2. Client reports weight loss.
   3. Client reports night sweats.
   4. Temperature of 37.7°C (100°F).

6. The nursing assistant (NA) is making rounds and reports that a client has oxygen saturation at 84%, respirations of 20. What would be the nurse's best action?
   1. Ask the NA to place the client on oxygen.
   2. Order an ABG from the respiratory therapist.
   3. Notify the charge nurse.
   4. Check the client with another pulse oximeter.

7. The nurse has completed an admission assessment on the client with left-sided heart failure. Which of the following would be expected for this type client?
   1. Crackles in the lungs.
   2. Distended abdomen.
   3. Pitting edema in extremities.
   4. Polyuria.

8. The nurse has admitted a client complaining of calf tenderness. Which finding would the nurse expect to find?
   1. Skin is cool to touch at calf area.
   2. Absence of Homan's sign.
   3. Edema and redness at calf area.
   4. Decreased urine output.

9. The client is given instruction on how to manage problems associated with a hiatal hernia. Which intervention should the nurse provide?
   1. "Lie down for about 20 minutes after a meal."
   2. "You will need to take medication for the *H. pylori* bacteria."
   3. "Bleeding from the stools is common, so call if it increases."
   4. "You can elevate the head of your bed."

10. The client is ordered an occult blood test of the stool to determine whether there is gastrointestinal bleeding. Which statement by the client indicates that additional instruction is required?
    1. "I'm allergic to seafood."
    2. "I'm glad this is an inexpensive test."
    3. "I will call you when I have a bowel movement."
    4. "I have held my usual dose of aspirin this week."

11. The nurse is monitoring a client who complains of right lower quadrant pain, low-grade temperature and nausea/vomiting. What actions does the nurse anticipate will occur?
    1. The client will sign a consent for surgery.
    2. The nurse will provide instructions for a high-fiber diet.
    3. Give laxatives and enemas to clean out the bowel.
    4. A 10–14 day regimen of antibiotics and PPIs will be ordered.

12. The client has started eating following gastric surgery and complains of weakness, dizziness, palpitations, diaphoresis, and cramping pains. What additional information should the nurse obtain related to these complaints?
    1. When was the client's last bowel movement?
    2. Is the client having trouble voiding?
    3. What was the client's last blood sugar?
    4. What is the client's temperature?

13. A client takes his own diuretic medications after the nurse administered the scheduled dose. After notifying the physician of the occurrence, what would be the nurse's best action?
    1. Monitor the client's potassium and magnesium levels.
    2. Scold the client for taking his own pills.
    3. Call the family and tell them to sit with the client.
    4. Bring the client a banana.

14. A client is scheduled for surgery. Assessment information states the client is 50 pounds overweight and has a 20-year smoking history. What is a potential complication during or after his surgery?
    1. Dehydration
    2. Fluid and electrolyte imbalance
    3. Atelectasis
    4. Latex allergy

15. A client states pain and cramping when walking, but it goes away at rest. What underlying condition does the nurse suspect the client has that is causing this problem?
    1. Diabetes mellitus
    2. Ischemic rest pain
    3. Atherosclerosis
    4. Venous insufficiency

16. A mother reports her 1-year-old child is taking a 2-hour nap and sleeping 11 hours at night. What would be the nurse's best response?

    1. This a normal schedule for a healthy 1-year-old.
    2. Wake the child up at least once during that time frame to change the diaper.
    3. Wake the child up to feed it at least once.
    4. Provide more noise so the child will awake more easily.

17. The 3-year-old child is crying saying she doesn't want to take her medicine. What would be an appropriate method to accomplish this task?
    1. Pinch the nose while administering the medication.
    2. Measure the medicine in the spoon the child used for pudding.
    3. Place medicine in a syringe for the child to squirt into her mouth.
    4. Give the medication to the mother to give to the child.

18. Which statement by the mother of a 4-month-old infant would raise concern from the nurse?
    1. "My baby's mouth is wet and pink."
    2. "I can wipe the tears from my baby when he cries."
    3. "I only have to change a wet diaper every 9 hours."
    4. "My baby awakens easily when I pick him up."

19. A nurse is preparing to give a client Motrin. Which item should be checked first?
    1. The temperature of the client
    2. The identification bracelet
    3. The pulse
    4. Whether the client is pregnant

20. A nurse teaches a client with chronic obstructive pulmonary disease (COPD) to use pursed lip-breathing. What is the rationale for teaching this action?
    1. It will increase airway pressure.
    2. It will decrease airway pressure.
    3. It increases the $HCO_3$ level.
    4. It increases the pH level.

21. The client is given instructions for a 24-hour urine test starting at 0700 this morning. What instructions will the nurse give to the client?
    1. Void and keep the first 0700 specimen.
    2. Void and discard the first 0700 specimen.
    3. Add in the last specimen at 0800 tomorrow morning.
    4. Discard the last specimen at 0700 tomorrow morning.

22. Which factor is more likely to cause the formation of renal calculi?
    1. Hyperkalemia
    2. Ingestion of calcium channel blocker
    3. Changes in pH balance
    4. Hyponatremia

23. Which of the following statements alerts the nurse that the client is displaying the defense mechanism of repression?
    1. "I don't know why but I have to drive in the right lane."
    2. "I will go play tennis to get my mind off this test."
    3. "I yelled at my husband after my boss critiqued my work."
    4. "I hate reading because a librarian was mean to me."

24. A nurse is administering Mucomyst for a client recently admitted to the emergency department with acute poisoning. The nurse knows besides being used as a mucolytic, Mucomyst is also used for treating which overdose?
    1. Morphine
    2. Aspirin
    3. Tylenol
    4. Codeine

25. A 2-day post-op client is on a morphine PCA and has also been prescribed fentanyl PRN for breakthrough pain. What other PRN medication would the nurse expect to be prescribed?
    1. Phenergan
    2. Ambien
    3. Lidocaine
    4. Naloxone

26. In which setting would a maternal-neonatal nurse practice?
    1. Free-standing birthing center.
    2. Labor and delivery ward.
    3. Operating room.
    4. Long-term care.

27. The nurse is caring for a client at risk for atelectasis. Which nursing measure is most important in preventing atelectasis?
    1. Administer prescribed opioids and sedatives.
    2. Teach appropriate technique for incentive spirometry.
    3. Frequent changes in position especially from supine to upright.
    4. Give them a bath.

28. Which of the following statements by the client indicates that teaching the purpose of TED hose was successful?
    1. "These hose are to keep my legs warm."
    2. "These help blood circulation."
    3. "These keep my legs protected from skin tears."
    4. "I take these off before putting on the sequential compression device."

29. A client tells the nurse that she has not had a period in several months. Which question should the nurse ask first?
    1. "Are you sexually active?"
    2. "Where are your parents?"
    3. "Do you live at home?"
    4. "Do you have a boyfriend?"

30. A client with diabetes is discharged home and will have a home care assistant visit once a day. Which service is contraindicated for the assistant to perform?
    1. Provide assistance with meal planning.
    2. Monitor the client's diet and snack habits.
    3. Assist client in and out of the bathtub.
    4. Provide foot care by cutting toenails.

31. A client is to receive digoxin (Lanoxin) via IV. What finding would alert the nurse to hold the medication?
    1. Hx of renal failure.
    2. BP is 89/72.
    3. HR is 58 bpm.
    4. Temp is 37.0°C (98.6°F).

32. A client is admitted for a left below-the-knee amputation. Which of the following nursing diagnoses would be appropriate to list on the care plan?
    1. Risk for depression.
    2. Disturbed body image.
    3. Risk for constipation.
    4. Diminished nutritional status.

33. Which statement by the client with diabetes indicates successful teaching regarding diet and meal planning upon discharge?
    1. "I have to eat full meals and snacks as prescribed to control my blood sugar."
    2. "I need to increase my fats in my diet."
    3. "Now that I am on medication, I can eat whatever I want."
    4. "My protein intake should be at least 50% each day."

34. The nurse suspects that a client receiving care regularly in an outpatient clinic has been battered by her spouse. Which action should the nurse take to find out whether the client is involved in a violent relationship?
    1. Ask a close friend of the client if she is being abused or battered.
    2. Look for signs such as bruises, broken teeth, wearing long sleeves in hot weather, wearing sunglasses indoors.
    3. Ask the client if she has been battered.
    4. Report suspicions to the police and ask them to question the client's husband.

35. What will the nurse use to remove an insect from a client's ear?
    1. Tweezers
    2. Normal saline
    3. Water
    4. Mineral oil

36. Two clients with dementia are seated near the nurse's station for close observation. Phones ringing or other noises cause the clients to yell out, disturbing the work environment. What is the most likely cause of the problem?
    1. The clients have dementia, so their behavior is unpredictable.
    2. The clients do not like sitting next to each other.
    3. The clients know they will get attention when they yell.
    4. The clients are receiving too much stimulation at the busy nurse's station.

37. Water-soluble vitamins are not stored in the body. Which would be an appropriate food choice to replace this needed vitamin?
    1. Carrots
    2. Broccoli
    3. Eggs
    4. Fortified milk

38. The nurse provided teaching to a mother on instilling eardrops in a 2-year-old child's ear. Which action would indicate successful teaching?
    1. Pull the earlobe up and back.
    2. Pull the earlobe down and back.
    3. Lie the child on his side with the ear up.
    4. Place medicine on a Q-tip and rub in ear.

39. A client refuses to follow the physician's orders and leaves the hospital against medical advice. What risk is the client assuming?

40. 
    1. Non-payment by their insurance company.
    2. Assuming the risk for her health state.
    3. Acting irresponsibly.
    4. Violating the physician's orders.

40. The nurse identifies a prolapsed cord. In which position should the nurse most likely place the client?
    1. Lithotomy
    2. Genupectoral
    3. Left lateral
    4. Low-Fowler's

41. The nurse knows that human immunodeficiency virus (HIV) and hepatitis B (Hep B) are spread by similar modes of transmission. Which of the following statements is the most accurate?
    1. Hepatitis B gradually destroys the liver and immune system.
    2. HIV gradually destroys the liver and immune system.
    3. HIV is not as infectious as hepatitis B.
    4. Hep B always develops into AIDS, a fatal disease.

42. A client is admitted with a diagnosis of possible tuberculosis. Until the diagnosis is confirmed, the client is placed in an airborne precautions room. Which of the following signs and symptoms would the client most likely report?
    1. Nausea
    2. Vomiting
    3. Night sweats
    4. Nasal drainage

43. A neonate is being closely monitored for anemia and hyperbilirubinemia. What process is occurring?
    1. Rh isoimmunization
    2. Leukemia
    3. Jaundice
    4. RBC deficiency

44. The school nurse assesses an 8-year-old boy who has dropping grades, low motivation, somatic complaints, and increasing proneness to accidents. What condition does the nurse suspect?
    1. Anxiety
    2. Depression
    3. Physical illness
    4. Boredom

**45.** Which statement by the client would the nurse expect to hear from a client with hypothyroidism?

1. "I have gained a lot of weight recently."
2. "My hair is falling out more than normal."
3. "I get very hot sometimes."
4. "I have been having diarrhea."

**46.** While getting the morning medications together for a client, the nurse notes the client will be going to dialysis in 1 hour. What should the nurse do if the client is scheduled for an antihypertensive?

1. Give the scheduled medication because dialysis will cause blood pressure to rise.
2. Give the medication because it is scheduled on the medication administration record (MAR).
3. Hold the medication because the client is going to dialysis soon.
4. Hold the medication until the client is leaving for dialysis.

**47.** A client with a history of atherosclerosis and emphysema states he felt a tearing sensation in his stomach and it still hurts. What would be the nurse's best action?

1. Ask the NA to obtain a set of vitals.
2. Assess the abdomen by palpation and auscultation.
3. Administer a PRN pain medication.
4. Visually inspect abdomen, obtain vital signs, and auscultate.

**48.** What would be an expected outcome for a client diagnosed with renal calculi?

1. Client demonstrates oxygen saturation within normal limits.
2. Client maintains normal weight.
3. Client will attain optimal level of mobility.
4. Client denies pain.

**49.** A client is admitted 1 hour after having a bronchoscopy. What nursing intervention should be performed?

1. Have the client brush teeth.
2. Check for a gag reflex.
3. Give the client's dentures back.
4. Provide client with ice chips.

**50.** A client presents at 38 weeks showing signs and symptoms of placenta previa. In addition to regular admission procedures, what other action should the nurse initiate?

1. Insert a Foley catheter.
2. Place the client on NPO status.

3. Collect a sterile urine sample.
4. Perform a sterile vaginal exam.

**51.** What is the primary purpose for the instillation of erythromycin in a newborn's eyes?

1. Protect against bacteria encountered in the birthing process.
2. Protect against blindness caused by gonorrhea.
3. Protect against blindness caused by syphilis.
4. Establish antibodies for the first 6 months.

**52.** A client is indifferent and aloof to the staff and other clients, and he has a difficult time establishing eye contact. Which personality disorder would the nurse know is being displayed?

1. Passive-aggressive personality.
2. Compulsive personality.
3. Antisocial personality.
4. Schizoid personality.

**53.** The physician tells the client that a therapist will assist with biofeedback techniques to relieve pain. The client asks the nurse the purpose of biofeedback. What explanation will the nurse provide?

1. It is a form of distraction.
2. It applies the principles of therapeutic touch to relieve pain.
3. It involves using post-hypnotic suggestion for pain relief.
4. It instructs the client to control physiologic variables relating to pain.

**54.** In assisting a client to plan care, the nurse considers that, according to Maslow, the client's unmet needs will cause what occurrence?

1. Frustration
2. Motivation
3. Low self-esteem
4. Hopelessness

**55.** A client confides to the nurse that she was raped and fears contracting AIDS. She is also afraid to tell her husband. What is the nurse's best action in this situation?

1. Inform the client's husband and encourage him to get an HIV test.
2. Counsel the client to get an HIV test, address her concerns, and say nothing.
3. Inform the physician of the problem and ask him to order an HIV test.
4. Document the information in the medical record.

56. A client, who has been on long-term ventilation and has a tracheostomy, is being discharged home with a portable ventilator. What is the priority teaching at the time of discharge?
    1. Discuss ways to reduce anxiety during the transfer home.
    2. Provide instructions on skin care.
    3. Assess the family's financial situation and provide resources.
    4. Develop a daily activity calendar for the caregiver.

57. The nurse assesses a client who begins to take stock in life and look to the future. Which of Erikson's developmental stages is this client displaying?
    1. Industry vs. inferiority.
    2. Trust vs. mistrust.
    3. Integrity vs. despair.
    4. Generativity vs. stagnation.

58. A client is one day postoperative after abdominal surgery. What priority action should be emphasized?
    1. Give pain medication every 4 hours.
    2. Assure client is eating meals.
    3. Ambulate at least TID.
    4. Use incentive spirometer (IS) every 4 hours.

59. A client is admitted with diabetes mellitus (DM) Type 1. Which finding will the nurse most likely obtain during the initial assessment?
    1. Weight gain
    2. Weight loss
    3. A goiter in the neck area
    4. Bronzelike pigmentation of the skin

60. A client was given 5-mg Haldol IM about 45 minutes ago and is beginning to experience a stiff neck and facial distortions. What would be the nurse's best reaction?
    1. Realize that he is experiencing acathisia.
    2. Discontinue the medication.
    3. Explain to the client that tardive dyskinesia is a side effect of the mediation.
    4. Question if the client is pretending a fake reaction.

61. The nurse makes a decision to apply restraints to a client. On which of the following criteria should the nurse most often base the decision to use restraints?

1. The client is restless.
2. The confused, post-op patient is trying to get out of bed.
3. There is a court order.
4. The family has requested it.

62. What nursing concern would be the top priority of nursing care for a client who is terminally ill?
    1. Risk for aspiration.
    2. Social isolation.
    3. Impaired comfort.
    4. Imbalanced nutrition.

63. One of the nurse's coworkers comes to work with a strong smell of alcohol but does not seem to be impaired. What action should the nurse take in this situation?
    1. Say nothing because the coworker's actions seem appropriate.
    2. Advise the coworker that no report will be filed this time, but will be next time.
    3. Report the suspicion according to agency policy and board of nursing requirements.
    4. Monitor the coworker for safe and appropriate actions.

64. The nurse is caring for a client's injuries when the client admits that she has been abused. She tells the nurse that she fears for her life. What is the best action to take first?
    1. Advise the client that the abuse is not her fault and that she will be helped.
    2. Tell the client that the abuse will be reported to the proper authorities.
    3. Inform the client that the social workers will be contacted to help her.
    4. Give the client the telephone number of the local women's shelter.

65. A client delivered a healthy infant 2 hours ago. She had an epidural block during the delivery. The client calls and tells the nurse that she is having severe lower abdominal pain. She requests something strong to eliminate the pain. Which of the following is the best action to take?
    1. Take the vital signs then administer an analgesic immediately.
    2. Assess the reason for the pain, checking the fundus and bladder for distention.
    3. Ask the client if she has had a bowel movement recently.

4. Position the client on her side, give her a backrub and tell her to breathe slowly through her mouth to relax her abdominal muscles.

66. The facility strives to enhance their continuous quality improvement (CQI) program. Which of the following would be included in this process?
    1. Scientific, data-driven approaches to study work processes.
    2. The nurse strives to do the right things well.
    3. The staff nurse uses a problem-solving approach to quality care.
    4. Teamwork and leadership goals are implemented.

67. The American Nurses Association (ANA) now recognizes nursing informatics as a specialty. How will this specialty help further nursing?
    1. It integrates the medical as well as the nursing science.
    2. It utilizes nursing and computer science.
    3. It allows nurses to chart using flow sheets.
    4. It promotes the study of medical information.

68. A nurse is providing care to a client who has had a transient ischemic attack (TIA). Which intervention would be included in the care plan?
    1. Obtain consent for a carotid endarterectomy.
    2. Determine whether the client has hypertension.
    3. Provide the client with information on smoking cessation.
    4. Educate the client that this may be a precursor to a stroke.

69. When communicating with a potentially violent client, which of the following is most important?
    1. To control the client's behavior and prevent injury
    2. To avoid judging and making assumptions about the client
    3. To make decisions about the client's welfare
    4. To respect the client's rights and maintaining dignity

70. A child suffers burns over 36% of her body. What is a potential cause of death in the first 24 hours?
    1. Hemorrhage
    2. Respiratory distress
    3. Hypovolemic shock
    4. Cardiac distress

71. As the child begins to recover from burns involving the arms, what activity should be included in the nursing care plan to promote optimal rehabilitation?

1. Make a game of moving around, such as throwing a ball.
2. Allow the child to put puzzles together.
3. Allow the child to play with other children.
4. Keep the child restricted as much as possible.

72. The nursing assistant is interested in becoming a nurse and asks what is the difference between certification and licensure. What is the nurse's explanation?
    1. Certification means the person has obtained permission from a local government to perform particular nursing tasks.
    2. Certification is given by a professional nursing organization to be able to teach nursing students.
    3. Licensure means the person has met the minimal level of safe practice as deemed by the government.
    4. Licensure is given once a person has completed nursing school.

73. A client is told she must take folic acid during her pregnancy. She asks the nurse for more information about this. What would be the nurse's best response?
    1. Poultry and milk will help to potentiate the B complex vitamins.
    2. Seafood and fresh fruit are essential for placenta functioning.
    3. Orange juice and green vegetables will help to increase red blood cell (RBC) production.
    4. Beef and dairy will prevent hemorrhaging during delivery.

74. A client has sprained an ankle and has been told to use the "RICE" method? When the nurse is asked to explain this, what would be an appropriate response?
    1. R means to observe the redness or discoloration that appears.
    2. I means to place ice on the area.
    3. C means to provide "comfort" by taking some pain medication.
    4. E means to exercise the area as soon as possible.

75. A client is complaining of weight gain. During the assessment, the nurse notes pitting edema in the lower extremities and jugular vein distention. What condition does the nurse suspect is occurring?
    1. Atherosclerosis
    2. Left-sided heart failure

3. Right-sided heart failure

4. Venous insufficiency

76. A middle-aged client complains of anxiety and has increased blood pressure and heart rate. What question should the nurse ask that would be related to this condition?
   1. "Have you been constipated also?"
   2. "Do you feel cold most of the time?"
   3. "Has your skin seemed extra dry?"
   4. "Have you had any vision changes?"

77. After receiving the morning report, which client should the nurse assess first?
   1. The client with a weight gain of 2 lbs in 2 days.
   2. A client whose hemoglobin is 15 gm/dL and hematocrit is 45%.
   3. A client who states pain of "10" on a 1–10 scale.
   4. A client whose chest tube has 450 mL of blood in the last 4 hours.

78. A nurse reports that a pregnant client is showing severe abruptio placentae. What assessment finding would the nurse most likely expect?
   1. Abdominal discomfort
   2. Anemia
   3. Hypertension
   4. Rigid, board-like abdomen

79. A client had a chest X-ray, electrocardiogram (ECG), a peripheral vascular study, an arterial blood gas (ABG) analysis, and a ventilation-perfusion scan. Based on these tests, what condition would the nurse suspect the client is experiencing?
   1. A pulmonary embolus
   2. Tuberculosis
   3. Myocardial infarction
   4. These are routine pre-operative tests.

80. A client being treated for a bipolar disorder is taking lithium. What instruction will the nurse give the client about the necessity of maintaining an adequate diet?
   1. Maintain a constant level of salt intake.
   2. Limit your sugar intake.
   3. Eat extra fiber.
   4. Take a vitamin E supplement every day.

81. A client is newly diagnosed as having various allergies. What would be a suggestion by the nurse to help control the exposure in the home?

1. Install wall-to-wall carpeting.
2. Dust and vacuum each day.
3. Remove feather-containing pillows and comforters.
4. Use a humidifier or vaporizer.

82. A client is in a state of metabolic alkalosis. What compensatory mechanism does the nurse know will help to correct this acid-base problem?
   1. Hypoventilation
   2. Hyperventilation
   3. Increased urine excretion
   4. Retaining the bicarbonate $HCO_3$

83. A nurse is caring for the following: a 10-year-old client newly diagnosed with diabetes; a 6-year-old client in skeletal traction for a fractured femur; and a 1-month-old infant with respiratory syncytial virus (RSV) infection. Which of these clients should the nurse assign to the nursing assistant for care?
   1. The 10-year-old client with diabetes
   2. The 6-year-old client in skeletal traction
   3. The 1-month-old infant with RSV
   4. None of these children

84. A client with dementia becomes agitated at the same time each day. Which of the following approaches should the nurse try first?
   1. Avoid the client at times when he is known to be agitated.
   2. Attempt to determine the cause of the agitation and eliminate it.
   3. Use therapeutic touch to calm the client.
   4. Ask other staff to approach the client and evaluate his response to different faces.

85. A new mother is concerned that her newborn is losing weight. The nurse explains that initially a newborn will lose some birth weight, but will regain it in how many days?
   1. 3 days
   2. 7 days
   3. 10 days
   4. 1 month

86. A client is being discharged after having cataract surgery. What condition will the nurse provide to the client as to when to notify the physician?
   1. Blurred vision
   2. Eye pain
   3. Glare
   4. Itching

87. A client with a tracheostomy is admitted with pneumonia. The client is given a nursing diagnosis of ineffective airway clearance. Which intervention would be most appropriate?
   1. Ambulate every hour.
   2. Suction every hour.
   3. Suction as needed.
   4. Request an order for suctioning.

88. A client is in need of blood and has blood type AB. Which blood type(s) can the client receive?
   1. A only
   2. B only
   3. AB only
   4. A, B, AB, or O

89. The client has one intravenous line and has blood infusing. The physician orders an antibiotic to be hung "NOW." What would be the nurse's best action?
   1. Start another IV site.
   2. Wait for the blood to finish, then hang the antibiotic.
   3. Stop the blood, run the antibiotic, then finish the blood.
   4. Call the physician to alert him the client is receiving blood.

90. The client is having a glycosylated hemoglobin (Hgb A1c) procedure done. The client asks how the procedure works. What is the nurse's best response?
   1. The normal life span of a healthy blood cell is 120 days.
   2. The kidneys do not excrete all the sugar out.
   3. The fasting test measures how fast the blood coagulates.
   4. After drinking the liquid, the blood sugar will rise.

91. Bulimia can cause serious health problems because it upsets a critical electrolyte balance within the body. Which lab values would be indicative of this occurrence?
   1. Serum sodium 141
   2. Serum potassium 3.0
   3. Blood pressure 140/90
   4. Serum calcium 9.0

92. When a client is diagnosed with tuberculosis, which occurrence will place the staff most at risk?
   1. The patient sneezes during a bed bath.
   2. The patient walks through the hall with a mask.

3. The staff changes the client's linens.
   4. The staff does not wear a mask in the room.

93. The nurse is teaching a class on cancer prevention. Which food choices would be most commonly associated with colon cancer and should be avoided or limited?
   1. White rice, hamburger
   2. Apple, baked potato
   3. Grilled chicken, granola cereal
   4. Cheese omelet

94. The nurse instructs a mother about nutrition for her toddler. The mother tells the nurse that the toddler loves milk and drinks about a quart-and-a-half each day. Instruction by the nurse should include which of the following regarding milk?
   1. Milk is an excellent source of calcium and is good for the child.
   2. The milk consumption is normal for a child of this age.
   3. Excessive milk consumption increases the risk of anemia.
   4. Toddlers are active and need extra calories, so milk is a good choice.

95. The pregnant client asks the nurse about the function of amniotic fluid. What is the nurse's best response?
   1. It provides antibodies to the fetus.
   2. It gives nutrients to the fetus.
   3. It gives protection for the fetus.
   4. It provides a smoother passage during delivery.

96. The nurse is performing an initial assessment on a woman who is 2 months pregnant. Which question will the nurse ask to determine whether she is at risk for developing toxoplasmosis?
   1. "Do you have a cat?"
   2. "Do you eat a lot of salt?"
   3. "Are you depressed?"
   4. "What is your normal blood pressure?"

97. A nurse is caring for 4 clients. After receiving report, which client should be assessed first?
   1. A client who has a serum sodium of 144.
   2. A client who had a PICC line inserted yesterday.
   3. A client with a chest tube whose pulse oxygen shows 94%.
   4. A client with hypertension complaining of a headache.

**98.** Which of the following laboratory findings would you expect to see in the client with hypothyroidism due to Hashimoto's thyroiditis?

1. Elevated T3 and T4.
2. Elevated TSH.
3. Elevated ACTH.
4. Decreased blood cholesterol.

**99.** Which of the following interventions is appropriate for the client with left-sided hemiplegia and dysphagia?

1. Obtain a referral by speech therapist.
2. Allow the client to eat soft foods.

3. Provide a clear liquid diet until swallowing ability improves.
4. Instruct the client and family that tube feedings will be necessary.

**100.** The nurse is performing a shift assessment on a client who has been taking haloperidol (Haldol) 2 mg BID. The nurse must monitor for which of the following common adverse reactions in the client who is taking Haldol?

1. Blood pressure 190/96.
2. Pill-rolling tremors of hands.
3. Dry mucous membranes.
4. Blood sugar of 70.

# Answers and Rationales for Practice Test 9

| ANSWER | | RATIONALE | NP | CN | CL | SA |
|---|---|---|---|---|---|---|
| #1. | 2. | IE is caused by an initial bacteremia that can occur following an invasive procedure such as dental work, or HI/HR surgery. The most common organisms are group A streptococci and *Staphylococcus aureus*. A prolonged fever is a symptom, not a cause of the IE; conjunctival infection is a redness of the conjunctiva common in Kawasaki disease; hypertension puts children and adults at risk for cardiovascular disease, but not IE. | An | Ph/8 | An | 1 |
| #2. | 3. | Apricots and prunes are high in iron. Milk products decrease iron absorption, and foods rich in vitamin C increase absorption. | As | Ph/5 | Co | 3 |
| #3. | 3. | Potassium is never given as IV push. | Pl | Ph/6 | An | 5 |
| #4. | 2. | A common cause of respiratory alkalosis is a panic attack in which hyperventilation is occurring, and a loss of carbon dioxide has occurred. | As | Ph/8 | An | 1 |
| #5. | 1. | All are symptoms of tuberculosis except visible skin lesions. | As | Ph/8 | An | 1 |
| #6. | 4. | Assessment by the nurse should be done first, as equipment may be faulty. Nursing assistants are not licensed to put clients on oxygen. An ABG would require a physician's order. | Im | Ph/8 | An | 1 |
| #7. | 1. | In left-sided heart failure, the left ventricle loses its ability to effectively pump oxygenated blood into the systemic circulation. | As | Ph/8 | An | 1 |
| #8. | 3. | The symptoms are indicative of a deep vein thrombosis, which is an inflammation of the vessel wall with formation of a clot. Other symptoms include pain, tenderness, and a positive Homan's sign. | As | Ph/8 | Ap | 1 |

| ANSWER | RATIONALE | NP | CN | CL | SA |
|--------|-----------|-----|------|-----|-----|

**#9. 4.** A hiatal hernia occurs when the portion of the stomach has slid upward in the diaphragm. Elevating the bed will help with gravity to keep the hernia in a lower position. — Im — Ph/8 — An — 1

**#10. 1.** Occult blood test for the presence of blood in the stool as an indicator of gastrointestinal bleeding. A small feces specimen is placed on a sample area. ASA is held which may cause bleeding. — As — Ph/8 — An — 1

**#11. 1.** The client's complaints are indicative of appendicitis and unless rupture has occurred, the client will be prepared for surgery either that day or the next and a consent form will need to be signed. — Pl — Ph/8 — An — 1

**#12. 3.** These are symptoms of dumping syndrome, which occurs with the abrupt emptying of stomach contents into the intestine. The body reacts by releasing excessive insulin, which in turn causes hypoglycemia. The client is told that the discomfort will last for 20–60 minutes. Blood sugars will need to be monitored. — As — Ph/8 — An — 1

**#13. 1.** Monitoring is the priority action. Clients are encouraged to have family members take their medications home so double dosage won't occur. The nurse should also verify the client has not taken any meds before administration. — Im — Ph/8 — An — 1

**#14. 3.** The client's weight and smoking habit will hinder deep breathing and coughing technique after surgery. — Ev — Ph/8 — An — 1

**#15. 3.** This is descriptive of intermittent claudication due to arterial occlusive disease, usually caused by atherosclerosis. — As — Ph/8 — An — 1

**#16. 1.** This is a normal sleep pattern, as the other choices are not recommended. — Im — He/3 — Ap — 4

**#17. 3.** The child may enjoy using the syringe and take the medication. Pinching the nose may cause aspiration and should be avoided; using a dietary spoon will not be the exact dosage; the mother is not responsible for giving the medication. — Im — Ph/6 — Ap — 4

**#18. 3.** Fewer wet diapers signals dehydration and further assessment is warranted. An infant can become dehydrated much more quickly than an older child or adult. — An — Ph/5 — An — 4

**#19. 2.** The nurse should always check the right patient to the right medication, along with the other medication rights. — Pl — Ph/6 — Ap — 5

**#20. 1.** Pursed lip-breathing causes delayed dynamic compression and minimizes the effects of airway trapping. — An — Ph/8 — An — 1

**#21. 2.** The first specimen is discarded as it has been sitting in the bladder. The last specimen at 0700 the next morning will be added as it is part of the 24-hour test. — Im — Ph/7 — Ap — 1

**#22. 3.** Renal calculi are favorable in conditions with consistent alkalinity or acidity. — An — Ph/8 — Ap — 1

**#23. 1.** Repression is pushing threatening thoughts into the unconscious. The others are examples of sublimation, displacement, and dissociation, respectively. — An — Ps/4 — Ap — 2

**#24. 3.** Tylenol overdose is treated orally with Mucomyst. — Im — Ph/8 — Ap — 5

| ANSWER | RATIONALE | NP | CN | CL | SA |
|--------|-----------|-----|------|-----|-----|
| #25. 4. | Both morphine and fentanyl are opioid analgesics, which are CNS depressants and can cause respiratory depression. Naloxone (Narcan) is an opioid antagonist and can reverse respiratory depression. | An | Ph/6 | Ap | 5 |
| #26. 1. | Maternal-neonatal nurses can practice in many facilities including physicians' offices, hospitals, clinics, and private homes. | An | He/3 | Ap | 3 |
| #27. 3. | Frequent changes in position promote ventilation and prevent secretions from accumulating. Although 1 and 2 are both measures the nurse could take, they would not be the primary concern. | Im | Ph/8 | An | 1 |
| #28. 2. | TED hose increase venous return and decrease pooling. They can be used with sequential compression device (SCDs). | Ev | Ph/8 | An | 1 |
| #29. 1. | Finding out whether the patient is sexually active will help to determine whether pregnancy tests need to be done. If she is not sexually active, her condition of amenorrhea will require further investigation. | Ev | He/3 | An | 3 |
| #30. 4. | All diabetic foot care should be managed by a podiatrist, to prevent injury to the feet, which could produce serious complications. | Pl | He/3 | Ap | 1 |
| #31. 3. | Heart rate should be greater than 60 before digoxin is given. | Im | Ph/6 | Ap | 5 |
| #32. 2. | The client who loses a limb is at risk for disturbed body image due to changes in appearance and body function. | An | Ph/4 | Ap | 1 |
| #33. 1. | The client will need instruction on correct food choices and the ratios to include from each food group. Snacks may be needed when the blood sugar may tend to fall. Carbohydrates should make up 50% of the diet, protein 20%. | Ev | He/3 | Ap | 1 |
| #34. 2. | This is a difficult situation requiring further investigation. The client will usually not admit that she has been battered for fear of the consequences. The best approach is to monitor for these specified occurrences or actions. | As | Ps/4 | Co | 2 |
| #35. 4. | Mineral oil causes the least amount of trauma to the ear canal. Water could cause the insect to swell and make it more difficult to remove. | Im | Ph/8 | Ap | 1 |
| #36. 4. | Clients with dementia commonly react to noise and confusion in the environment. If they are overstimulated by other clients or by environmental noise and confusion, they often display agitated behavior, including yelling and striking out. | Ev | Ps/4 | An | 2 |
| #37. 2. | Vitamin C needs to be replenished every day because it is not a fat-soluble vitamin; therefore, the body does not store it. | As | Ph/5 | Ap | 1 |
| #38. 2. | Until age 3, pull the earlobe down and back because the child's canal is shorter. For older children and adults, pull the earlobe up and back. | Ev | He/3 | Ap | 4 |
| #39. 2. | The client has the right to refuse medical treatment. But if this is done, the client must accept responsibility for any illness and possible injury. It is true that the insurance company will not pay | As | Sa/1 | Co | 1 |

| ANSWER | RATIONALE | NP | CN | CL | SA |
|---|---|---|---|---|---|
| | for the hospital stay, but the priority concern is the client's health status. | | | | |
| #40. 2. | The client may be put in knee-chest, or Trendelenburg, position to relieve the pressure of the presenting part away from the cord. | Im | He/3 | Ap | 3 |
| #41. 3. | According to the Centers for Disease Control and Prevention, the hepatitis B virus is more infectious than the HIV virus, which causes acquired immunodeficiency syndrome (AIDS). | Im | He/3 | Ap | 1 |
| #42. 3. | Of the signs and symptoms listed, night sweats are commonly seen in clients with tuberculosis. Other common signs and symptoms are fatigue, fever, weight loss, cough, expectorating blood-tinged sputum, chest pain, and dyspnea. | As | Ph/8 | Co | 1 |
| #43. 1. | Anemia results from the hemolysis of the erythrocytes. Hyperbilirubinemia results in the liver's inability to excrete the excess bilirubin. | An | Ph/8 | Ap | 4 |
| #44. 2. | Dropping grades, low motivation, somatic complaints, and increasing proneness to accidents are signs and symptoms of depression in childhood. | As | Ps/4 | Co | 2 |
| #45. 2. | Alopecia and coarse hair are symptoms of hypothyroidism. | An | Ps/4 | Ap | 1 |
| #46. 3. | Antihypertensives should be held before dialysis to avoid hypotension due to the combined effect of the medication and dialysis. Medications can be given after dialysis as long as vital signs are appropriate. | Pl | Sa/2 | An | 1 |
| #47. 4. | The client may be experiencing an abdominal aortic aneurysm. Light palpation may reveal the pulsating area, but heavier palpation could cause rupture, leading to a possible fatal condition. | Im | Ph/8 | An | 1 |
| #48. 4. | The goal will be for the kidney stone to either pass or be removed, which eliminates the pain. | Ev | Ph/8 | An | 1 |
| #49. 2. | Because of the preoperative sedation and local anesthesia, the laryngeal reflex and swallowing can stay impaired for several hours. Before the client is given anything by mouth, the client needs to have an active gag reflex making that the priority assessment for the nurse. | Im | Ph/7 | Ap | 1 |
| #50. 2. | A client with placenta previa will probably be taken to surgery and needs to be NPO as soon as possible. | Im | He/3 | Ap | 3 |
| #51. 2. | Erythromycin kills gonorrhea organisms that cause blindness in infants. Erythromycin also protects the newborn from the *Chlamydia* organisms. | As | Ph/6 | Co | 4 |
| #52. 4. | The client with a schizoid personality likes to stay aloof and withdrawn with as little activity with others as possible and will never initiate interpersonal communication or relationships. | An | Ps/4 | An | 2 |
| #53. 4. | Biofeedback involves giving the client information about changes in body functions. Some clients may use this information to control previously involuntary functions. It is often used for pain management. | Im | Ph/5 | Ap | 1 |

| ANSWER | RATIONALE | NP | CN | CL | SA |
|---|---|---|---|---|---|
| #54. 2. | Maslow has identified that unmet needs are strong motivating factors in healthy personalities and that satisfied needs do not motivate behavior. | Pl | He/3 | Co | 1 |
| #55. 2. | Keeping promises to clients involves fidelity. This is the ethical foundation of the nurse-client relationship. Keeping the information confidential is in keeping with the nondisclosure laws for HIV and AIDS and keeps the nurse's promise to the client. In this case, the information is harmful directly to the client and indirectly to others. | Im | Sa/1 | An | 1 |
| #56. 2. | A client on a portable ventilator will be sitting or lying down most of the time. Meticulous skin care, including around the tracheostomy, is the priority concern to prevent infection that could further decrease the client's function level. It is also appropriate for the nurse to discuss anxiety reducing options and to create an activities calender to help assist the caregiver with necessary duties. It is not the nurse's responsibility to assess for financial concerns, but could provide resources or contact the social worker to speak with the family. | Pl | Sa/1 | Ap | 1 |
| #57. 3. | According to Erikson, when adults begin to reflect on their lives, they are in the integrity vs. despair stage. | As | He/3 | Co | 1 |
| #58. 3. | Postoperative clients are at risk for deep vein thrombosis (DVTs) and should ambulate as soon as possible, if not on the day of surgery. Pain medication is given as the client requests, and the IS should be used every 1–2 hours. Food should not be given until the client has positive bowel sounds and is passing flatus. | Im | Ph/7 | An | 1 |
| #59. 2. | In Type 1 DM, the cells are starving and the client experiences hunger with weight loss. | As | Ph/8 | An | 1 |
| #60. 2. | The symptoms are indicative of dystonia, which is often a sudden adverse reaction to psychotropic medications, especially when given in large doses intramuscularly. Dystonia can usually be resolved by discontinuing the drug and administering an anticholinergic or Benadryl. Acathisia is the inability to sit down because of severe anxiety. Tardive dyskinesia is displayed as slow, rhythmical movements as a result of certain psychotropic drugs. | Im | Ph/6 | An | 5 |
| #61. 2. | When a client's safety is jeopardized, the use of restraints is warranted. This particular client may fall and cause injury to the new operative site. | An | Sa/2 | An | 1 |
| #62. 3. | The most important intervention for the client who is terminally ill is comfort and palliative nursing care. | An | Ph/5 | An | 1 |
| #63. 3. | The ANA Code of Ethics states that nurses have an ethical obligation to do everything possible to prevent anyone from taking advantage of clients or working with clouded objectivity, thereby jeopardizing client safety. Most state boards of nursing require nurses to report other nurses who are on duty and who are under the influence of alcohol or other substances. | Im | Sa/1 | An | 1 |
| #64. 1. | Depending on the circumstances, any of the approaches listed may be appropriate during the care of this client. However, the best first action is to tell the client that the abuse is not her fault. Abused women often hear that they are responsible for | Im | Ps/4 | An | 2 |

| ANSWER | RATIONALE | NP | CN | CL | SA |
|--------|-----------|-----|-----|-----|-----|

the abuse. Telling the client that she will be helped shows her that she is not alone and demonstrates that the nurse is concerned for her safety.

**#65. 2.** Before administering an analgesic, the nurse should assess the client carefully. A distended bladder is a common cause of lower abdominal pain in postoperative clients and those who have had spinal anesthesia.  Im  Ph/8  An  3

**#66. 1.** CQI uses scientific approaches to study work processes. Plans are developed based on this information, leading to system improvement. CQI has also evolved into systems that encompass process improvement and performance improvement.  As  Sa/1  Ap  1

**#67. 2.** This specialty incorporates nursing, science, and information sciences to manage and communicate data and information for use in nursing practice, and is supported by the use of information technology.  An  Sa/1  Ap  1

**#68. 4.** A TIA is caused from a temporary loss of blood supply to a part of the brain and the deficits usually resolve within 24 hours. It is also referred to as "ministrokes" and are an indication that medical management is essential.  Pl  Ph/8  An  1

**#69. 4.** The underlying principle of all therapeutic communication is respect for the client's rights and dignity.  An  Ps/4  An  2

**#70. 3.** There is a greater potential for fluid loss in a child who has a large body surface in proportion to weight. The largest areas represented on a child's body are: face & scalp 9%, back 18%, arm 9%, front 18%, each upper arm 9%, each lower leg 9%.  An  Ph/8  Ap  4

**#71. 1.** To prevent contractures, the child must move around as much as possible. Making a game of it will increase the child's participation in the plan of care.  Pl  Ph/8  An  4

**#72. 3.** Once nursing students graduate from an accredited school of nursing, they must sit for the national examination and upon passing will be awarded their license to practice nursing.  As  Sa/1  An  1

**#73. 3.** Folic acid is required for the structure of both RBCs and WBCs. A rapid division of cells is required because the blood volume doubles during pregnancy. Green leafy vegetables and orange juice are the best sources. Other good sources are liver, legumes, and wheat germ.  Im  Ph/6  An  3

**#74. 2.** The correct acronym is R:Rest, I:Ice, C:Compression, E:Elevation.  Im  Ph/8  An  1

**#75. 3.** These are symptoms of right-sided heart failure, which could also include ascites, fatigue, and a third heart sound may be present.  An  Ph/8  An  1

**#76. 4.** The symptoms are indicative of hyperthyroidism. The first 3 choices are symptoms of hypothyroidism except that a client may experience vision changes, exophthalmos, and a staring gaze with hyperthyroidism.  As  Ph/8  An  1

**#77. 4.** This is equivalent to a pint of blood loss and could indicate the client is hemorrhaging. It would take precedence over the pain complaint, as the pain is not life-threatening.  Im  Ph/8  An  1

| ANSWER | | RATIONALE | NP | CN | CL | SA |
|--------|--|-----------|----|----|----|----|
| #78. | 4. | A client with abruptio placentae would normally show symptoms of shock, moderate vaginal bleeding, pain in the abdomen or back, and abdominal tightening, with or without contractions. | As | Ph/8 | Ap | 3 |
| #79. | 1. | These tests are part of the initial diagnostic workup to verify whether a pulmonary embolus is present. | An | Ph/7 | An | 1 |
| #80. | 1. | Lithium and salt are interrelated. The constant level of salt will prevent fluctuation in lithium activity. It is recommended that the client on lithium consume normal amounts of salt to maintain the proper balance of sodium, lithium, and potassium. | Im | Ph/6 | Ap | 5 |
| #81. | 3. | Bedding made out of synthetic material is less likely to harbor allergies than feathers. Humidifiers would increase mite breeding, if present. | Im | He/3 | An | 1 |
| #82. | 1. | Hypoventilation would help retain the carbon dioxide, but treatment should be aimed at the underlying problem. Breathing in and out of a paper bag is one method of retaining carbon dioxide. | An | Ph/8 | An | 1 |
| #83. | 2. | The 6-year-old in traction is the most stable of the three clients and requires less careful monitoring. The 10-year-old client with diabetes must be carefully monitored for blood glucose changes, and the 1-month-old infant with RSV requires close respiratory status assessment. | Im | Sa/1 | An | 4 |
| #84. | 2. | Stay out of the client's personal space and avoid touching him. Invading space and touching the client when he is clearly agitated increases the nurse's risk of injury. The best approach is to determine the cause of the agitation and eliminate it. | Im | Ph/8 | An | 1 |
| #85. | 3. | A healthy newborn should regain weight, lost through insensible water loss and increased metabolism, within 10 days. | As | Ph/8 | Co | 4 |
| #86. | 2. | Pain should not be present after cataract surgery, but the other symptoms are normally present. | Im | Ph/8 | Ap | 1 |
| #87. | 3. | Suctioning should only be done as needed as it could cause trauma. It does not require a physician's order. | Im | Ph/8 | Ap | 1 |
| #88. | 4. | An individual with type AB is called a universal recipient; one with type O is called a universal donor. | As | Sa/2 | Ap | 1 |
| #89. | 1. | Medications are never added to blood products. Blood transfusions should not be stopped unless there is an adverse blood reaction. | Im | Ph/6 | An | 1 |
| #90. | 1. | The glucose is attached to the red blood cells and is the best indicator of the average blood glucose level for a 3-month period. | Im | Ph/7 | An | 1 |
| #91. | 2. | Frequent vomiting creates a deficiency of potassium, resulting in hypokalemia. | As | Ph/8 | An | 1 |
| #92. | 4. | Tuberculosis is spread by droplet nuclei through talking, coughing, sneezing, laughing, or singing. The staff should *always* be wearing a mask when in the room. | As | Sa/2 | Ap | 1 |

| ANSWER | RATIONALE | NP | CN | CL | SA |
|--------|-----------|-----|-----|-----|-----|
| #93. 1. | This choice is a combination of low fiber and high fat which increases the chance of constipation and is a risk factor for colon cancer. A low-fat, high-fiber diet is recommended such as in choice 3. | Im | He/3 | Ap | 1 |
| #94. 3. | Toddlers should drink 2 to 3 cups of milk each day for an adequate calcium intake. Excessive milk consumption increases the risk of anemia because it limits the amount of other nutrients consumed. | Im | Ph/5 | An | 4 |
| #95. 3. | In addition to providing protection, the amniotic fluid and sac keep the fetus at an even temperature. | As | Ph/8 | Co | 3 |
| #96. 1. | Cats are intermediate hosts for toxoplasmosis. | Im | He/3 | Ap | 3 |
| #97. 4. | This client may have the potential problem of a stroke, if the blood pressure is too elevated. The other clients have stable conditions. | Im | Ph/8 | Ap | 1 |
| #98. 2. | Hypothyroidism is a condition; Hashimoto's thyroiditis is a disease. This condition is rare in the United States due to the iodine in our salt products. An elevated thyroid-stimulating hormone will be greater than 1, as the T3 results may be in the normal range. | As | Ph/8 | Ap | 1 |
| #99. 1. | Dysphagia is impairment in swallowing and places the client at risk for aspiration, dehydration, and malnutrition. The speech therapist will perform a bedside swallowing evaluation to determine whether a barium swallow study is needed. | Im | Sa/1 | An | 1 |
| #100. 2. | One of the most common adverse reactions of Haldol is involuntary movements of the extrapyramidal system. The signs are pill-rolling tremors of hands, drooling, unsteady gait, and muscle rigidity. | As | Ph/6 | Co | 5 |

# Practice Test 10

1. The client's serum potassium is 6.0 mEq/L. Which medication would the nurse be prepared to administer?
   1. 0.9% sodium chloride (NS) with 20 mEq/L of potassium
   2. 3% sodium chloride (NS)
   3. Calcitonin
   4. Kayexalate

2. The nurse suspects that a client with pneumonia is experiencing hypoxemia. Which of the following assessment findings would be detected?
   1. Inspiratory crackles
   2. Productive cough
   3. Temperature of 38.3°C (101°F)
   4. Nail beds are cyanotic

3. The client with congestive heart disease (CHF) has lab results that show the client is in metabolic alkalosis. What findings would the nurse expect to find on the ABG lab results?
   1. pH – 7.25    $CO_2$ – 50    $HCO_3$ – 23
   2. pH – 7.37    $CO_2$ – 40    $HCO_3$ – 25
   3. pH – 7.55    $CO_2$ – 25    $HCO_3$ – 24
   4. pH – 7.52    $CO_2$ – 42    $HCO_3$ – 32

4. What type of oxygen delivery system would the nurse bring if the client is ordered flow rate of 8 liters/min, $FiO_2$ 40%?
   1. Simple mask
   2. Venturi mask
   3. Partial rebreathing mask
   4. Nonrebreathing mask

5. The nurse educates a client on the American Cancer Society's warning signals of cancer. Which statement by the client would require further clarification?
   1. Nagging cough or hoarseness
   2. Change in bowel or bladder habits
   3. Repetitive viral infections
   4. A sore that does not heal

6. The client states his annual ankle-brachial index (ABI) was checked, with the result of 0.95. Based on this finding, what would be an appropriate intervention for the client?
   1. Instruct the client to elevate his legs often.
   2. Encourage routine walking.
   3. Educate the client on the benefits of stent placement.
   4. Instruct the client to wash the feet daily.

7. The nurse is teaching a class on venous insufficiency. Which of the following would be included in this teaching session?
   1. Avoid elastic or compression stockings during the day.
   2. Elevate the legs every two hours.
   3. Use a heating pad to increase warmth and circulation.
   4. Ulcers may first appear on the tips of toes.

8. The nurse is giving pre-procedure instructions to a client who will undergo a colonoscopy. Which statement, if made by the client, indicates further instruction is needed?
   1. "I will be positioned on my left side."
   2. "The barium may turn my stools a white color."
   3. "My wife will be driving me home."
   4. "I won't eat after midnight the night before."

9. A client is diagnosed with peptic (duodenal) ulcer. Which of the following would most likely relieve the pain?
   1. Suppress emesis
   2. Eating tolerable food
   3. Drinking a milk shake
   4. Take an NSAID

10. The client is given discharge instructions for a new ileostomy placement. Which statement by the client demonstrates successful teaching?
    1. "The stool from this ostomy will be formed."
    2. "The bag will need to be emptied and cleaned once a day."
    3. "Foods high in fiber may need to be restricted at times."
    4. "I'm glad I won't have to wear the bag all the time."

11. A nurse is planning the assignment for the day. Which of the following clients is most appropriate to assign to the nursing assistant?
    1. A client who had gastric surgery today.
    2. A client with Alzheimer's disease and a colostomy.

3. A client who is "NPO" for a hernia repair.

4. A client complaining of angina.

12. The client will be having a colonoscopy under conscious sedation (moderate sedation). What would be an expected occurrence related with this procedure?

   1. The client may have a headache afterward.
   2. An oral airway will be inserted.
   3. The client can respond to verbal and physical stimuli.
   4. The client will be able to push the button for pain medication.

13. The client is scheduled for a transthoracic echocardiogram and asked what the purpose of this test is and whether it is uncomfortable. What would be the nurse's best response?

   1. This is a test to determine exercise tolerance and requires walking on a treadmill until tired.
   2. This is a test to examine the heart valves and is painless.
   3. This is a test to determine whether coronary arteries are obstructed with plaque and it will require slight sedation.
   4. This is a test to look at the cardiac rhythm and rate of your heart, and will require sticky pads to be placed on your chest.

14. A client has been taking an anticholinergic for 3 months before arriving to the urgent care with complaints of decreased sweating, constipation, and dry mouth. What does the nurse suspect is occurring?

   1. These are within normal limits for this medication.
   2. The client is having an adverse reaction to the medication.
   3. The client is in hypovolemic shock.
   4. The client is not taking the medication as ordered.

15. Which structure prevents fetal heat loss?

   1. Placenta
   2. Cervix
   3. Lanugo
   4. Amniotic fluid

16. Which ACE inhibitor-associated reaction usually leads to therapy disruption?

   1. Hemorrhage
   2. Bradycardia
   3. Diarrhea
   4. Cough

17. A postoperative client has returned from surgery with a gastrostomy tube and intravenous line. The client keeps gesturing toward the tubes, and the nurse is concerned the client will pull them out. Which of the following approaches should the nurse take first?

   1. Apply wrist restraints.
   2. Try other methods of keeping the client's hands away from the tubing.
   3. Contact the physician or nursing supervisor for advice.
   4. Administer a sedative.

18. A client has a positive polysomnogram. What recommendations would the nurse expect the client to be given?

   1. Lose weight if obese.
   2. Driving should not be allowed.
   3. Wear the CPAP only during the day.
   4. Encourage client to sleep prone.

19. What type of immunity will a client have after recovering from bacterial meningitis?

   1. None
   2. Natural
   3. Active acquired
   4. Passive acquired

20. The client is given discharge instructions for a new colostomy. Which food choice would show the client understands the teaching?

   1. "I can continue to drink milk."
   2. "Coffee may give me heartburn now."
   3. "Cabbage may need to be limited."
   4. "Cheese will cause too much constipation."

21. A new mother who is 3½ days postpartum complains of foul-smelling lochia. Which of the following nursing interventions is indicated?

   1. Check the color of lochia.
   2. Tell her this is normal.
   3. Check bladder distention.
   4. Check temperature and fundus.

22. A client with an ileostomy was recently admitted for dehydration. Which statement reveals to the nurse the cause of this problem?

   1. "I drink at least a quart of fluid each day."
   2. "I drink a lot while I am jogging."
   3. "My stools are always loose."
   4. "I clean my bag several times a day."

23. Where would be the best place for the nurse to place a victim of cardiac arrest to facilitate CPR?
    1. In a chair
    2. On a mattress
    3. On the floor
    4. On a compression board

24. Which of the following is a major developmental task of middle adulthood?
    1. Making a living
    2. Developing intimacy
    3. Resolving the past
    4. Reexamining life goals

25. A client admits that she has been abused but insists on returning home. She tells the nurse that her husband will not hurt her again for a few weeks. Before discharging the client, what is the nurse's next step?
    1. Tell the client to call the hospital if help is needed.
    2. Discharge the client as requested.
    3. Discuss where the client can go if she needs to flee.
    4. Conduct a safety assessment.

26. A client has a chest tube for a pneumothorax. The client turns over and accidentally pulls the chest tube out from the sutured site. What would be the highest priority action for the nurse?
    1. Place the tube back into the hole in the chest, then notify the physician.
    2. Tape an occlusive dressing over it taped on three sides.
    3. Instruct the client to hold his hand over the area until the physician can reinsert it.
    4. Instruct the client to lie still in bed while the physician is notified.

27. Children experience different fears at each stage of development. What are they most likely to fear at age 12?
    1. Enuresis
    2. Nightmares
    3. Their own death
    4. A parent's death

28. A client has receptive aphasia. What intervention will the nurse include in the care plan?
    1. Offer paper and pencil to write on.
    2. Have the client repeat the names of objects on a picture board.

3. Ask the client to practice writing simple words and sentences.
4. Give only one direction or ask one question at a time.

29. Which nursing diagnosis is a priority with a client who has been diagnosed with epilepsy?
    1. Impaired mobility related to seizure activity
    2. High risk for injury related to seizure activity
    3. Impaired adjustment related to incontinence during seizure
    4. High risk for activity intolerance related to fatigue post-seizure

30. A 16-year-old female asks for birth control information from the school nurse and confides to the nurse that she is pregnant and her parents do not know. Which of the following responses is most appropriate?
    1. "I'm sorry, but because you are a minor I cannot give you any birth control information."
    2. "I know it is difficult, but it would be best if your parents know about the pregnancy; I encourage you to talk to them."
    3. "I cannot help you myself, but I can give you the number of Planned Parenthood."
    4. "It is too late for birth control for you, but come back and see me after you have had the baby."

31. A client is having a lumbar puncture (LP) performed. Which intervention would be a priority for the nurse?
    1. Place client in prone position with slight Trendlenburg.
    2. Inform the client that a consent is not needed.
    3. Instruct client to keep a full bladder before and during the procedure.
    4. Assist client to a lateral recumbent position with knees flexed.

32. A new graduate nurse is aware of the HIPAA privacy rules. Where would the nurse expect information about the client's name, diagnosis, condition, and room number be found?
    1. In the medication area
    2. In the nurse's station
    3. Where is it least accessible to the public view
    4. Where only those needing to know that information can access it

33. Which of the following statements would be appropriate to include in a nurse-to-nurse report?
    1. "The client's blood sugar was 75 at 1030."
    2. "The client had a CT last month."
    3. "She has had a good day today."
    4. "The urine output has been really low today."

34. In assessing an older adult client, the nurse realizes that an individual grows from influences. What would be an appropriate question/statement that would help determine what the person's philosophy of life is most likely based on?
    1. "Tell me what values your parents stressed with you."
    2. "Did you follow what your peers did?"
    3. "Do you feel you have had demands from society?"
    4. "Tell me about personal experiences in your life."

35. The nurse observes the interaction between a nursing assistant (NA) and a hearing-impaired client. What action would prompt the nurse to provide instruction to the NA?
    1. The NA faces the client when speaking.
    2. The NA encourages the client to interrupt for clarification.
    3. The NA turns down the lights.
    4. The NA speaks in a normal volume.

36. Which of the following assessments should the nurse perform first in the client who is experiencing autonomic dysreflexia?
    1. Palpate for bladder distention.
    2. Check for Chvostek's sign.
    3. Auscultate for bilateral breath sounds.
    4. Check the client's blood glucose level.

37. The nurse is teaching new mothers about problems that can occur in children with spina bifida. Which statement requires further clarification?
    1. "I will limit my child's caloric intake to manage weight."
    2. "I will maintain a latex-free environment at home and school."
    3. "I will enroll my child in gymnastics early on."
    4. "I will find out if there is a support group to help deal with my child's anger."

38. A client has experienced brain death. Which underlying condition of the client will prevent organ transplantation?

1. Anemia
2. Bipolar disease
3. Breast cancer
4. Uncontrolled seizures

39. A client who has had a stroke asks the nurse the rationale for taking aspirin. What would be the nurse's best response?
    1. "Aspirin decreases the likelihood of a clot in the brain circulation."
    2. "Aspirin prevents the brain from swelling after a stroke."
    3. "Aspirin is given to alleviate the muscle pain associated with therapy."
    4. "Aspirin causes more blood to flow to the brain."

40. The client comes to the emergency department complaining of abdominal pain and the pain has been assessed positive at McBurney's point. What condition does the nurse suspect the client has?
    1. Ectopic pregnancy
    2. Peritonitis
    3. Diverticulitis
    4. Appendicitis

41. A client diagnosed with metastasis to the bone is being discharged. What should be included in the teaching instructions?
    1. Morphine is available only by instant-relief and will help your pain quickly.
    2. When the diarrhea starts, an anti-diarrhea medication will be prescribed.
    3. An NSAID may be added to your medications instead of more morphine.
    4. The medication should only be taken when pain increases.

42. Which pregnant woman would the nurse expect is at highest risk for having a newborn who is below average birth weight?
    1. One who is a diabetic
    2. One who exercises daily
    3. One who is a grand multipara
    4. One who smokes a pack of cigarettes a day

43. The nurse is instructing the new graduate nurse on the roles of a rehabilitation nurse. Which statement by the new nurse will require correction?
    1. "The rehab nurse will be a client advocate."
    2. "The rehab nurse will coordinate the client's care."

3. "The rehab nurse will develop the treatment plans."
4. The rehab nurse will act as a liaison to other team members."

44. Which is a priority nursing diagnosis for the client with Guillian-Barré syndrome?
   1. Ineffective breathing pattern related to skeletal muscle weakness
   2. Risk for impaired skin integrity related to physical immobilization
   3. Self-care deficit related to skeletal muscle weakness
   4. Powerless related to health care environment and illness

45. A client is going into shock. Which clinical sign would alert the nurse that the client is showing signs of compensatory shock?
   1. Agitation
   2. Bradycardia
   3. Decreased respirations
   4. Hyperactive bowel sounds

46. In treating croup, what is the rationale for cold humidification rather than steam?
   1. Cold infiltrates the lungs more effectively.
   2. Steam could cause accumulations in the lungs.
   3. Steam could increase fever.
   4. Steam is an ineffective humidifier.

47. The client is being seen for an annual checkup and is negative for the known risk factors for coronary artery disease. Because the fasting homocysteine was elevated, what instruction will be given to the client?
   1. Restrict foods that contain Vitamin $B_{12}$.
   2. Eat more foods that contain folic acid.
   3. Purchase the OTC supplements that you need.
   4. Stop smoking.

48. Which of the following statements is true regarding back injuries in nursing?
   1. Education on lifting techniques reduces back injuries.
   2. Injuries to nurses can be prevented by careful screening of nurses before hiring.
   3. The use of back belts reduces risk to health care providers.
   4. Adopt standardized assessment protocols for client handling and movement.

49. In managing a client with phlebitis, what would be included in the care plan?

1. Use the largest catheter possible in the largest vein available.
2. If phlebitis occurs, discontinue the catheter and restart further up the arm.
3. Place a warm compress on the affected area.
4. Speed up the infusion to complete administration before phlebitis occurs.

50. The nurse is providing psychotherapy to a client who is having difficulty recognizing the problem. In order to promote client self-awareness, which quality must the nurse possess?
   1. Understanding
   2. Sympathy
   3. Values
   4. Self-awareness

51. A client is admitted with Parkinson's disease. Which of the following nursing diagnoses would have the highest priority?
   1. Activity intolerance
   2. Altered body image
   3. Risk for injury: falls
   4. Self-care deficit

52. A client with osteoarthritis has been taking over-the-counter (OTC) ibuprofen several times a day for pain relief for 2 months. What reported symptoms could indicate a complication from this medication?
   1. Fever and malaise
   2. Muscle pain and weakness
   3. Stomach pain and indigestion
   4. Hematuria and burning on urination

53. The nurse is caring for a client who has an implant for internal radiation therapy for endometrial cancer. Which should the nurse include in the client's care?
   1. Spend extra time with the client to prevent social isolation.
   2. Ambulate the client in the room several times each day.
   3. Combine nursing activities to allow reduced entry into the room.
   4. Remove soiled linens from the room as soon as possible.

54. A client tells the nurse that she plans to deliver her infant at home with a midwife in attendance. Which presents the greatest risk of infection?
   1. Presence of bloody show
   2. Seeping of stool during contractions

3. Premature rupture of membranes

4. Inability to change the sheets on the bed before delivery

55. The nurse has been asked to speak at a school program about safety for parents of 7- to 10-year-old children. Which is the greatest safety concern in children of this age group?

1. Ingestion of hazardous substances

2. Injuries to children who are passengers in automobile accidents

3. Abduction by strangers

4. Experimenting with electrical hazards

56. The client with terminal cancer tells the nurse, "When my time comes, just let me go." What would be the nurse's best response?

1. "I will document this request in your chart."

2. "I will notify your family about your wishes."

3. "Tell me what you want done or not done."

4. "It is my responsibility to provide life-saving efforts to you."

57. Which comment by the client indicates the need for further instruction regarding a scheduled cardiac catheterization?

1. "This is an invasive diagnostic procedure."

2. "The catheter will be inserted through a blood vessel."

3. "I will use a urinal during my bedrest afterwards."

4. "I won't need an IV and I will be discharged an hour after it's done."

58. Which of these clients should receive priority in the morning assessment?

1. A young adult rating moderate pain after a tonsillectomy.

2. Hypertensive client with blood pressure 160/80.

3. A client with Type 2 diabetes with blood sugar of 360.

4. A client who is 2 days post-op prostatectomy.

59. The desired therapeutic effect is to prevent infection in a catheterized client. What is the nurse's best action against infection?

1. Use aseptic technique during insertion of catheter.

2. Have the client perform hand-washing.

3. Have only one nurse present during the insertion.

4. Tape the catheter to the right leg instead of the left.

60. Which of these clients would be more prone to develop osteoporosis?

1. Premenopausal, obese woman

2. Premenopausal, thin woman

3. Postmenopausal, obese woman

4. Postmenopausal, thin woman

61. Which statement describes the presence of a pathological fracture?

1. "I was just walking and I went down."

2. "The car wreck caused the bone to break and pierce the skin."

3. "My ankle broke but I didn't feel any pain."

4. "I have had this infection for a long time."

62. A mother calls and states that her child has just developed a rash. The nurse learns that the child has just started taking penicillin in the last 24 hours. How would the nurse interpret this information?

1. A normal reaction

2. A sign of some other disease process

3. A sign of the penicillin taking effect

4. An allergic reaction to penicillin

63. Which laboratory findings would indicate the client is at risk for displaying a positive Trousseau's sign?

1. Serum sodium 135 mEq/L

2. Serum potassium 4.1 mEq/L

3. Serum calcium 8.0 mg/dL

4. Serum magnesemia 3.0 mEq/L

64. The new graduate is interviewing a client who is in the early stages of liver failure. Which question would be contraindicated during the assessment?

1. "Have you had a respiratory infection lately?"

2. "How much Tylenol or Dilantin do you take?"

3. "Do you drink alcohol?"

4. "Have you traveled to China or any foreign countries?"

65. Which agency issues Sentinel Event Alerts due to medical errors?

1. American Medical Association (AMA)

2. Food and Drug Administration (FDA)

3. Joint Commission (JCAHO)

4. Institute for Safe Medicine Practices (ISMP)

66. When a client is admitted in active labor, what should be the initial action the nurse performs?

1. Perform Leopold maneuvers.

2. Catheterize for urine specimen.

3. Take vital signs and check fetal heart tones (FHT).
4. Assess for ruptured membranes.

67. The nurse notes that the client's flow sheet reports a pressure ulcer as "partial-thickness skin loss." Which stage would the nurse be aware is present?
    1. Stage I
    2. Stage II
    3. Stage III
    4. Stage IV

68. A client with chronic schizophrenia is taking Clozaril and has a history of seizure disorder. What instructions should the nurse give to the client?
    1. Status epilepticus is a common adverse reaction.
    2. A special diet will be necessary.
    3. Blood work will be required regularly.
    4. Clozaril raises the seizure threshold.

69. The client with congestive heart failure has been given instructions about the diagnosis. Which of these statements made by the client would indicate that the client has correct understanding of the instructions?
    1. "I should not be awakened at night to urinate."
    2. "I will notify my doctor if I lose 5 pounds in a week."
    3. "I will weigh myself every evening before bed."
    4. "I will notify my doctor if 1 gain 2 pounds overnight."

70. A client is two days post-operative bariactric surgery. What diet will the nurse make sure the client receives?
    1. The client should still be NPO until day 3.
    2. Full liquids, 2–3 ounces every hour.
    3. Pureed food, six small meals per day.
    4. Mechanical soft food, 5–6 meals per day.

71. Which signs/symptoms would make the nurse suspect that the client is experiencing atelectasis?
    1. Hypoactive bowel sounds.
    2. The client is very sleepy.
    3. Dyspnea and/or tachycardia.
    4. Nausea and abdominal pain.

72. When obtaining a health history on a female client diagnosed with breast cancer, what risk factor might the nurse expect to hear from the client?

1. Pregnancy before age 20.
2. An aunt who had breast cancer.
3. Hormone replacement therapy (HRT).
4. Performs exercise 3–5 times per week.

73. An adolescent female confides in the nurse that once a month she has headache, fatigue, weight gain, irritability, and crying spells. Which of the following conditions is most likely to cause these cyclic problems?
    1. Menarche
    2. Premenstrual syndrome (PMS)
    3. Puberty
    4. Normal hormonal changes

74. A 14-month-old child is hospitalized for acute asthma. She does not cry or exhibit any other signs or symptoms of separation anxiety from her mother. What nursing evaluation is indicated?
    1. Ignore the behavior as it is normal.
    2. Become suspicious of the mother-child relationship.
    3. Assess her as a well-behaved, good child.
    4. Assume she is accustomed to being away from her mother.

75. From children age 4 through adolescence, a major stressor related to hospitalization is loss of control. What nursing intervention focuses on alleviating this problem?
    1. Allow the child as many choices as possible.
    2. Minimize stress related to the loss of control.
    3. De-emphasize the control issue by ignoring it.
    4. Ask the family to give the child more control.

76. A physician prescribes Inderal for a client that is extremely nervous when performing in front of a crowd. What instruction should the nurse provide?
    1. "Get up slowly when lying or sitting."
    2. "Take this medication with orange juice."
    3. "Take your heart rate before taking this drug."
    4. "Decrease your salt intake."

77. A middle-aged client states having had to buy reading glasses to see smaller print. Which response by the nurse would be most appropriate?
    1. "This is a normal aging process called myopia."
    2. "You need to have your eyes checked for glaucoma."

3. "This sounds like you might have macular degeneration."

4. "As long as you can see distance, the reading glasses will be fine."

78. The nurse is admitting a client with glaucoma. Which assessment data would the nurse expect?
    1. Low intraocular pressure
    2. A dark spot in the middle of the vision
    3. Multicolored halos around lights
    4. Steroid use

79. A client reports vomiting along with severe, constant right upper quadrant abdominal pain that is radiating to the right shoulder. The client states this has happened before, "just not this bad." What is the most appropriate question for the nurse to ask next?
    1. "When did you have your last bowel movement?"
    2. "Do you have a history of hepatitis C?"
    3. "What did you last eat?"
    4. "What color is your urine?"

80. The nurse needs to suction a client's airway via the endotracheal tube. Which action would be done first?
    1. Place the client in supine position.
    2. Hyperoxygenate the client with 100% oxygen for 30 seconds.
    3. Place thumb on suction control and gently insert into airway.
    4. Apply suction for 10–20 seconds.

81. A client with Alzheimer's disease is delusional. She tells the nurse that she is going home to make dinner for her children. The nurse knows that the client's children are grown and live out of town. Which of the following is the best approach to take with the client?
    1. Tell the client she cannot leave the health care facility.
    2. Ask the client what she likes to cook, and talk to her about cooking.
    3. Inform the client that the children are grown and live out of town.
    4. Distract the client by giving her a magazine to read.

82. The nurse is talking with a client who is scheduled for dialysis. Which information by the client warrants further investigation?
    1. "Dialysis will clean my blood."
    2. "It takes 4 hours, but it keeps me alive."

3. "I can drink as much as I want now."
4. "My fistula is in my left upper arm."

83. Which finding would concern the nurse the most regarding a pregnant woman in her third trimester?
    1. Client states she is voiding more than normal.
    2. Client is not performing her Kegal exercises.
    3. Client is experiencing breast tenderness.
    4. Fetal heart rate of 94.

84. The client's lab values are as follows: Na$^+$ 139, K$^+$ 3.5, Ca$^+$ 9.2. The client will be treated by a diet recommendation. Which of the following should be added to the meal tray?
    1. Cheeses
    2. Sardines
    3. Dried fruits
    4. Canned soup

85. The nurse and a certified nursing assistant (CNA) are caring for a group of clients on a medical unit. Which information provided by the assistant warrants immediate assessment by the nurse?
    1. The client diagnosed with cancer of the lung has a small amount of blood in the sputum collection cup.
    2. The client diagnosed with chronic emphysema is sitting on the side of the bed and leaning over the bedside table.
    3. The client with an asthma attack whose wheezing has stopped.
    4. The client who has clubbing of the fingers and a barrel chest.

86. Which of the following interventions would be appropriate to add to the plan of care for a client diagnosed with cancer, who is receiving radiation and chemotherapy?
    1. Provide air sprays to mask odors.
    2. Administer Demerol IM for complaints of pain.
    3. Encourage rinsing sore mouth with commercial mouthwashes.
    4. Avoid fresh fruit and vegetables.

87. A child is placed in a spica cast and has just returned to the room. In what position should the nurse place the child?
    1. Prone
    2. High-Fowler's
    3. Supine
    4. Side-lying

88. The client is diagnosed with urolithiasis. Which nursing diagnosis is appropriate for this client?
    1. Altered urinary elimination
    2. Disturbed body image
    3. Interrupted family processes
    4. Ineffective airway clearance

89. The nurse has been alerted that the client's serum albumin level is low. Which explanation would be appropriate for the nurse to give to a client who has been prescribed albumin?
    1. "Albumin is an indicator of your cardiac problem."
    2. "Albumin is an indicator for the beginning of retinopathy in diabetic clients."
    3. "This will be given fairly rapidly."
    4. I will take your vital signs when the mediation is finished."

90. A newly admitted client is placed on fall precautions. What measures should be taken to ensure client safety?
    1. Make sure the call light is within reach while the client is in the bathroom.
    2. Inform the family they will need to stay with the client at all times.
    3. Offer the client the bedpan in toileting.
    4. Provide nonslip footwear.

91. The new graduate nurse has attended an in-service on methicillin-resistant *Staphylococcus aureus* (MRSA). When explaining what was taught, which statement will need correction?
    1. "Community-associated MRSA tends to cause skin infections like boils and blisters."
    2. "Health care-associated MRSA starts out looking like a spider bite."
    3. "All of the staff need to wash their hands after glove removal."
    4. "Dialysis clients are at risk, as well as IV drug abusers."

92. The nurse caring for the newborn, delivered by cesarean section, will monitor the infant carefully for which possible problem?
    1. Crib death syndrome
    2. Neurological deficits
    3. Failure to thrive syndrome
    4. Respiratory distress syndrome

93. A client is diagnosed with cancer and has a good prognosis. The physician informs her that the tumor should respond to chemotherapy. The client refuses all medical care and states that she is putting her faith in a higher power. Which right is she exercising?
    1. Paternalism
    2. Veracity
    3. Self-determination
    4. Nonmaleficence

94. A client is scheduled for surgery at 8:00 a.m. tomorrow. She was given a sedative several hours ago, but she is unable to sleep. The physician has not ordered a repeat sedative. She will be NPO in another hour. Which of the following actions are most appropriate for helping the client sleep?
    1. Administer another sedative immediately, and instruct the client to drink a carton of milk after the medication.
    2. Inform the client that the nurse will check on her frequently during the night.
    3. Tell the client to take slow, deep breaths and to call if she needs anything.
    4. Straighten the bed and give the client a backrub and a warm decaffeinated beverage, such as milk.

95. A client is admitted with foul-smelling wound drainage. A drug-resistant pathogen is suspected so a culture is obtained. The nurse knows that the client should be in isolation until the results of the culture are returned. Which of the following types of isolation precautions are used for this client?
    1. Contact precautions
    2. Drainage and secretion precautions
    3. Airborne precautions
    4. Droplet precautions

96. A client has developed thrombophlebitis and is being treated with a continuous heparin drip. Which morning lab result will determine if the heparin drip should be adjusted?
    1. Clotting time
    2. Prothrombin time (PT)
    3. Partial thromboplastin time (PTT)
    4. Serum sodium

97. The client is diagnosed with Ménière's disease. When experiencing an attack, what is the client at risk for?
    1. Falling
    2. Dyspnea
    3. Hypertension
    4. Cardiac arrhythmias

**98.** The client is given teaching on atrial fibrillation. Which statement, if made by the client, would indicate additional teaching is required?
1. "This is a common condition."
2. "My heart rate will not be consistent all the time."
3. "They don't know the cause of why I have this condition."
4. "There are no major complications associated with this condition."

**99.** The client with cystitis is prescribed to take phenazopyridine (Pyridium). What instructions will the nurse provide with this treatment?
1. It is an antibiotic that will cure the infection.
2. Limit your fluid intake while taking this medication.

3. Your urine will become dark orange and stain your clothes.
4. It will make you very sleepy.

**100.** The nurse admits a client with fibromyalgia. Which nursing diagnosis would be appropriate to include in the care plan?
1. Impaired gas exchange
2. Fatigue
3. Decreased cardiac output
4. Overflow urinary incontinence

# Answers and Rationales for Practice Test 10

| ANSWER | RATIONALE | NP | CN | CL | SA |
|---|---|---|---|---|---|
| #1. 4. | Kayexalate allows the exchange of sodium for potassium ions in the gut. It can be given by PO or PR. Loose bowel movements following administration are indicative of successful treatment. Insulin IV could also be given. | Pl | Ph/6 | Ap | 5 |
| #2. 4. | If a decrease occurs in the arterial oxygen in the blood, it leads to the impaired gas exchange of hypoxemia. | As | Ph/8 | An | 1 |
| #3. 4. | Metabolic acidosis can result from diuretic therapy that promotes the excretion of potassium. The client may also show signs of volume depletion and hypokalemia. | Ev | Ph/8 | An | 1 |
| #4. 2. | The Venturi mask delivers oxygen in a specified fraction of inspired ($FiO_2$) at 24, 28, 35, 40, or 60. The others would have oxygen ordered in liters. | Pl | Ph/8 | Ap | 5 |
| #5. 3. | All are inclusive of the warning signals except viral infections. | Im | He/3 | Ap | 1 |
| #6. 4. | The ABI determines a ratio of the systolic blood pressure in the ankle to the systolic blood pressure in the arm. This finding is indicative of a significant narrowing in one or more blood vessels in the legs. | Im | Ph/8 | An | 1 |
| #7. 2. | Pain usually occurs when the legs are in dependent position, so elevation will allow the blood to flow from the lower extremities by gravity. Heating pads should be avoided as they may cause a burn and ulcers on the tips of toes are common in arterial insufficiency. | Im | Ph/8 | An | 1 |
| #8. 2. | The only incorrect instructions are related to the barium, which would be given if the client were having a barium enema with | Ev | Ph/8 | An | 1 |

| ANSWER | RATIONALE | NP | CN | CL | SA |
|---|---|---|---|---|---|
| | X-rays or a barium swallow. The colonoscopy will be done by a flexible tube that looks into the colon. | | | | |
| #9. 2. | A duodenal ulcer is described as pain in the mid-epigastrium, occurs 2–4 hours after meals and is relieved by food. Vomiting is more common with gastric ulcers; heavy milk products tend to aggravate the problem; NSAIDs may cause bleeding. | Pl | Ph/8 | Ap | 1 |
| #10. 3. | The fecal drainage from the ileostomy will be liquid and the client will need to adjust to particular fiber foods. Because liquid may seep out at any time, the bag will need to be worn all the time and cleaned several times a day. | Ev | Ph/8 | An | 1 |
| #11. 2. | The nursing assistant is capable of emptying and caring for a colostomy. A client who has had surgery will need assessment and monitoring from the nurse, a client who is NPO will need teaching and a consent signed pre-op, and angina will require assessment and pain management. | An | Sa/1 | An | 1 |
| #12. 3. | The client will be induced by pharmacologic agents. A headache may be present after spinal anesthesia; general anesthesia would require an oral airway; the client is not awake enough to push the pain button. | Ev | Ph/7 | Ap | 1 |
| #13. 2. | The other choices describe the treadmill, a cardiac catherization, and an electrocardiogram. | An | Ph/7 | Ap | 1 |
| #14. 2. | The client is experiencing dose-related adverse reactions to the anticholinergics, which will usually decrease as treatment continues. | Ev | Ph/8 | An | 5 |
| #15. 4. | Amniotic fluid preserves fetal temperature as well as prevents heat loss. | As | He/3 | Ap | 3 |
| #16. 4. | Cough disrupts the sleep pattern in approximately 15% of clients who use ACE inhibitors, and will need evaluation. | As | Ph/6 | Ap | 5 |
| #17. 2. | Before applying restraints, all other interventions should be tried first. Other disciplines should be consulted to see whether they have a solution to the problem. If a restraint is necessary, a physician's order must be obtained and documentation in the medical record must support the need for it. The least restrictive device that provides safety should be used for the least amount of time possible. The nurse must obtain a physician order for restraints or apply them only in an emergency, according to facility policy. | An | Sa/2 | Ap | 1 |
| #18. 1. | A positive polysomnogram diagnoses obstructive sleep apnea. The first conservative method of treatment is to lose weight, change sleeping positions, and wear a CPAP (continuous positive airway pressure) machine at night. | As | Ph/7 | Ap | 1 |
| #19. 3. | An active immunity is developed because the body produces antibodies against specific antigens that were introduced into the body with the meningitis. | As | He/3 | Ap | 4 |
| #20. 3. | Cabbage is a gas-producing food that may cause client problems with odor control and ballooning of the ostomy bag, sometimes breaking the seal. | Ev | He/3 | Ap | 1 |

| ANSWER | RATIONALE | NP | CN | CL | SA |
|--------|-----------|----|----|----|----|
| #21. 4. | Odorous lochia after the third day is indicative of infection; therefore, the client's temperature and fundus must be checked. | Im | He/3 | An | 3 |
| #22. 1. | Fluid intake is particularly important in clients with an ileostomy. Because the ileostomy drains from 1200–1500 mL of liquid each day, the client must increase fluid intake to offset the loss, thus preventing dehydration. The other choices are correct statements. | As | Ph/5 | Ap | 1 |
| #23. 4. | To achieve proper compressions, the victim should be placed on a solid, flat surface such as a compression board. | As | Ph/7 | Ap | 1 |
| #24. 4. | An important developmental task for the middle-aged adult is to examine life goals with some degree of satisfaction. | As | He/3 | Co | 1 |
| #25. 4. | Before discharging the client, conduct a safety assessment to ensure that discharge will be safe. However, before releasing the client, discuss where she can go if she needs to flee quickly. | Pl | Ps/4 | An | 2 |
| #26. 2. | This occlusive dressing should be placed over the site immediately. The one side not taped will allow air to escape and reduce the risk for a tension pneumothorax. The physician should be notified immediately after. | Im | Ph/8 | An | 1 |
| #27. 4. | At age 12 the child realizes the finality of death and fears a parent might die and leave. This fear may create feelings of anger toward the parents. | As | Ps/4 | K | 4 |
| #28. 4. | Receptive aphasia is when a client is unable to understand what is being said or what is written, being a comprehension problem. Clients will have difficulty expressing their needs. Gestures may be helpful. | Im | Ps/8 | Ap | 1 |
| #29. 2. | Epilepsy is a seizure disorder which can start with a loss of consciousness, placing the client at risk for a fall or airway obstruction. | An | Sa/1 | Ap | 1 |
| #30. 2. | The adolescent needs help concerning her current pregnancy more than birth control at this time. As a pregnant teen, she is an emancipated minor and can make independent decisions; however, having the help and support of her family is very important. | Im | He/3 | Ap | 3 |
| #31. 4. | This is the preferred position for access to the L4 and L5 space to obtain CSF for analysis. The client will have signed a consent and after a good intake of fluids, has emptied the bladder. | Im | Ph/7 | Ap | 1 |
| #32. 4. | The Health Insurance Portability and Accountability Act of 1996 calls for all healthcare providers to protect unauthorized uses and disclosures of personal medical information. Even dietary workers should only be given the diet order, not the client's condition. | An | Sa/1 | Ap | 1 |
| #33. 1. | A good verbal report should include basic information about the client, diet, intravenous fluids, recent surgery, and current client status. Information should not be outdated or speculative. Accurate data should be communicated. | As | Sa/1 | Ap | 1 |
| #34. 4. | Each individual is influenced by all the factors listed, but the reality created for oneself through personal experience is what shapes one's philosophy. | An | Ps/4 | An | 2 |

| ANSWER | RATIONALE | NP | CN | CL | SA |
|---|---|---|---|---|---|
| #35. 3. | Turning down the lights will inhibit the client if able to lip-read. All the other actions are acceptable. | Im | He/3 | Ap | 1 |
| #36. 4. | The most common noxious stimulus that triggers the autonomic response in a spinal cord injury client is a distended bowel which is stimulated by a massive discharge of sympathetic responses. | As | Sa/1 | An | 1 |
| #37. 3. | A child with spina bifida will have orthopedic problems that can sometimes lead to impaired mobility. The child will need a prescribed and supervised rehabilitation program. | Ev | He/3 | An | 4 |
| #38. 3. | The organ procurement organization (OPO) should be contacted when there is a suspicion of brain death or when family is considering withdrawing mechanical ventilation. The OPO will ask questions which will determine if the client is medically suitable. | An | Sa/1 | An | 1 |
| #39. 1. | Aspirin produces inhibition of platelet aggregation. | An | Ps/6 | An | 5 |
| #40. 4. | Appendicitis can be difficult to identify because clients seek medical help at varying stages of the condition. McBurney's point is located midway between the anterior superior iliac spine and the umbilicus in the right lower quadrant. | An | He/3 | An | 1 |
| #41. 3. | The addition of an adjuvant medication rather than giving more of the opioid is many times more helpful in controlling pain. Constipation is an adverse side effect of morphine, which is available in a variety of forms. As clients build up a tolerance to opioid side effects, such as nausea and respiratory depression, the medication should be given on a continuous basis instead of PRN. | An | Ph/6 | An | 5 |
| #42. 4. | Studies indicate that nicotine has a direct impact on the weight of the fetus. Infants born to smoking mothers are usually below average weight. | Im | He/3 | Co | 3 |
| #43. 3. | A physiatrist is a physician specializing in physical medicine and rehabilitation who will develop a plan for rehabilitation that includes physical therapy, occupational therapy, and speech therapy. | Im | Sa/1 | Ap | 1 |
| #44. 1. | Guillian-Barré syndrome is a peripheral nerve disorder which usually begins in the legs and ascends sometimes to the muscles of respiration. | An | Ph/8 | An | 1 |
| #45. 1. | The compensatory stage is a result of the sympathetic nervous system in which there is a decrease in pulmonary blood flow that leads to hypoxemia which contributes to restlessness and agitation; an increase in respirations and heart rate occurs to increase the cardiac output; there are hypoactive bowel sounds due to blood being shunted from the GI track to the heart and brain. | As | Ph/8 | An | 1 |
| #46. 3. | Steam could create a much warmer environment, increasing body temperature. | An | Ph/8 | Co | 4 |
| #47. 2. | Homocysteine is a naturally occurring amino acid found to be elevated in clients with vascular disease. An elevated homocysteine is seen in clients with deficiencies of folic acid or vitamin $B_{12}$. The recommendation will be to eat a balanced diet that includes foods with folic acid and $B_{12}$. The presenting | Im | Ph/5 | Co | 1 |

| ANSWER | RATIONALE | NP | CN | CL | SA |
|--------|-----------|-----|-----|-----|-----|
| | information already states the client is negative for risk factors, which would include smoking. | | | | |
| #48. 4. | This is the only true statement, as the others have proven that injuries still occur even with education and assistive devices. | As | Sa/2 | An | 1 |
| #49. 3. | The IV site would be discontinued, a warm compress applied, a new one started in the opposite arm, and if the rate must be slowed, a central line may need to be inserted. | Pl | Ph/6 | Ap | 1 |
| #50. 4. | A helping relationship is most effective when the nurse has come to terms with the client's issues and problems through the nurse's own process of self-awareness. | An | Ps/4 | Ap | 2 |
| #51. 3. | The client has a muscle rigidity that leads to a shuffling gait, which makes the client prone for falls. | An | Sa/1 | An | 1 |
| #52. 3. | NSAIDs, such as ibuprofen (Motrin), can cause an increased risk of serious GI adverse events such as bleeding, ulceration, and perforation of the stomach or intestines, which can be fatal. The complaints need to be further investigated. | Ev | Ph/6 | An | 5 |
| #53. 3. | Clients receiving this form of treatment can emit radiation while the implant is in place, so contact with the staff and family needs to be limited. The client will be on bedrest and all material in the room with be handled per protocol for radiation precautions. | Im | Sa/1 | An | 1 |
| #54. 3. | The membranes are a defense mechanism against infection. Premature rupture of membranes eliminates the protective mechanism, increasing the risk of infection. | An | He/3 | An | 3 |
| #55. 3. | School-age children are most commonly injured during play, sports activities, and as passengers in automobile accidents. Abductions by strangers are common in this age group. Of the choices listed, abduction by strangers is the greatest safety concern. | An | He/3 | An | 4 |
| #56. 3. | This is a form of therapeutic communication of exploring which will encourage the client to express feelings more in-depth. | Pl | Ps/4 | An | 2 |
| #57. 4. | The client will require an IV for the mild sedation medication that is given and bedrest can be from 1–6 hours depending on the physician's form of closure. The client will be monitored at the insertion site, which is usually the femoral artery and the affected leg will remain straight for the allotted time. | Ev | Ps/7 | An | 1 |
| #58. 3. | The blood sugar of 360 is the most critical occurrence as insulin would be required. | Pl | Ps/7 | An | 1 |
| #59. 1. | Aseptic technique is a must for catheter insertion to prevent a nosocomial infection. | Pl | Ps/7 | An | 1 |
| #60. 4. | Osteoporosis is more prevalent in the postmenopausal woman who has a decrease in estrogen production. Prevention is recommended through weightbearing activities, and the thinner woman would have less weightbearing than the obese woman. | As | Ps/8 | An | 1 |
| #61. 1. | A pathologic fracture occurs when a bone breaks in an area that is weakened by another disease process, such as osteoporosis. | An | Ps/7 | An | 1 |

| ANSWER | RATIONALE | NP | CN | CL | SA |
|---|---|---|---|---|---|
| #62. 4. | Usually the first sign of an allergic reaction to penicillin occurs in the first 72 hours of administration of the drug. The nurse should instruct the mother to take the child to the physician's office because complications could include laryngeal edema and anaphylactic shock. | Ev | Ph/6 | An | 4 |
| #63. 3. | Hypocalcemia causes increased muscle contraction and excitability which can be seen by a carpopedal spasm. | An | Ph/7 | An | 1 |
| #64. 1. | All of the other questions would be associated with liver failure. The first complaints are often nonspecific, such as malaise, loss of appetite, fatigue, and nausea. A client who has visited a foreign country may have been exposed to hepatitis B. | As | Ph/7 | An | 1 |
| #65. 3. | A Sentinel Event Alert identifies specific sentinel events, describes their common underlying causes, and suggests steps to prevent occurrences in the future. | As | Sa/2 | Co | 1 |
| #66. 3. | The initial action should be assessment of vital signs and FHT. | Im | He/3 | An | 3 |
| #67. 2. | Stage II involves the epidermis, dermis, or both. It presents as an abrasion, blister, or shallow crater. | Im | He/3 | Co | 1 |
| #68. 3. | Clients with schizophrenia respond to and function very well with Clozaril. However, adverse reactions include agranulocytosis, leukopenia, and other blood dyscrasias. Clozaril lowers the seizure threshold and clients with a history of seizure disorder are very likely to experience seizures once Clozaril reaches a therapeutic level. | Im | Ph/6 | An | 5 |
| #69. 4. | The client will most likely be discharged home with diuretics and vasodilators, which will help to circulate the needed blood throughout the body. If this action is blocked, blood either backs up in the peripheral or dependent areas (right-sided) or causes a fluid accumulation in the lungs (left-sided). The client should be instructed to weigh every morning after initial voiding. | Ev | Ph/8 | An | 1 |
| #70. 2. | Once bowel sounds have returned, the client will start out with clear liquids then advance to a regular diet, but with small portions. Liquids should be taken in between meals instead of with them, to prevent dumping syndrome. | Im | Ph/7 | An | 1 |
| #71. 3. | Atelectasis is a diminished volume or lack of air in part or the entire lung, which could be present from an obstruction inflammation or tumor. Airflow to the alveoli is blocked, impairing oxygenation. | As | Ph/8 | Ap | 1 |
| #72. 3. | HRT has become controversial in its use, but has been linked with breast cancer from some studies. Very few breast cancers are caused by inherited factors. Chances of breast cancer are also decreased with pregnancy before age 20 and exercising. | As | Ph/8 | Ap | 1 |
| #73. 2. | This situation requires further investigation. The nurse should advise the client to keep a journal for at least two menstrual cycles to determine a pattern. Signs of premenstrual syndrome are headache, backache, fatigue, irritability, weight gain, and crying spells. PMS is a complex condition that occurs in approximately 85% of American women, however, most | An | Ph/8 | An | 3 |

women have symptoms that are mild and do not require treatment. Three to eight percent of menstruating women may have a more serious form of PMS which requires medication treatment.

| #74. 2. | When a child this age does not exhibit the normal signs of anxiety separation, such as crying, then the nurse should become suspicious that there may be a potential problem, such as abuse. | Ev | He/3 | An | 4 |
|---|---|---|---|---|---|
| #75. 2. | Minimize stress by allowing the child to have reasonable control in situations when possible. | Im | He/3 | Ap | 4 |
| #76. 1. | Inderal is a beta-blocker that blocks the beta-adrenergic receptors in the sympathetic nervous system, causing a relaxation response. There may be a possibility of orthostatic hypotension. | Im | Ps/6 | An | 5 |
| #77. 2. | Presbyopia is what the client is experiencing as part of the natural part of aging. | Im | He/3 | Ap | 1 |
| #78. 3. | Glaucoma is an optic neuron disease that results from inadequate drainage of the aqueous humor from the eye. It is diagnosed by an elevated intraocular pressure reading above 21 and the client's report of pain or halos around lights. | As | Ps/8 | Ap | 1 |
| #79. 3. | The symptoms reported are indicative of cholecystitis (gallbladder obstruction) and it presents itself after eating a heavy meal. | As | Ps/8 | An | 1 |
| #80. 2. | The only correct statement is pertaining to hyperoxygenating the client, which is done before and after suctioning. The client is placed in semi-Fowler's position, the thumb is applied when the suction catheter is withdrawn from the client, for a maximum of 10 seconds. | Im | Sa/1 | Ap | 1 |
| #81. 2. | The client is probably looking for a state of mind, not a physical location. By talking to her about cooking, the nurse will restore the state of mind the client is seeking. | Im | Ps/4 | An | 2 |
| #82. 3. | Dialysis is the process of filtering toxins and extra fluid from the blood, usually 3 times a week (since the kidneys are not functioning); therefore, the individual should monitor the amount of fluid intake. | Ev | Ps/8 | An | 1 |
| #83. 4. | A fetal heart rate (FHR) of 94 should cause great concern, as the FHR baseline should range from 110 to 160. Increased voiding is normal; Kegal exercises help, but it is the client's choice not to do them; breast tenderness is normal. | An | Ph/7 | An | 3 |
| #84. 3. | $K^+$ (potassium) is the only abnormal value, and is just on the low side of normal. A diet increased in potassium foods, such as dried fruits and bananas should increase the value. | Im | He/3 | An | 1 |
| #85. 3. | A client with asthma normally has wheezing, but as the obstruction worsens, the wheezing may disappear and may signal an impending respiratory failure. | An | Ph/8 | An | 1 |
| #86. 4. | Fresh fruits and vegetables can harbor bacteria not removed by ordinary washing and the client's immunologic response is already altered due to treatment. | Im | He3 | An | 1 |

| ANSWER | RATIONALE | NP | CN | CL | SA |
|---|---|---|---|---|---|
| #87. 3. | The child should be supine, preferably on a firm mattress. Any other position would be awkward or unreasonable for the child. | Pl | Ph/8 | Ap | 4 |
| #88. 1. | Urolithiasis refers to stones in the urinary tract. If the stones block the flow of urine, obstruction causes a desire to void, yet little urine is passed. | An | Ph/8 | Ap | 1 |
| #89. 3. | Albumin is the major protein found in the blood. It is used to detect protein deficit in adults and to treat shock. It is a blood product that is usually infused quicker than other medications; however, vital signs are taken before, during, and after administration. | An | Ph/8 | Ap | 1 |
| #90. 4. | This is one of many steps to take to prevent or reduce client falls. A high-risk client should not be left alone in the bathroom or other treatment area; it is not the family's responsibility to prevent a fall; staff should assess the client every 1–2 hours to assess positioning, pain, and toileting. | Im | Sa/2 | Ap | 1 |
| #91. 2. | A spider bite is typical of the Community-associated MRSA; Health care-associated MRSA tends to cause more invasive infections, such as surgical or catheter insertion sites which may have redness, swelling, or tenderness. | Im | Sa/2 | Ap | 1 |
| #92. 4. | Studies show that respiratory distress syndrome is more common in babies born by cesarean section than those born vaginally. | As | He/3 | K | 4 |
| #93. 3. | Clients have a legal right to self-determination, even when it results in self-harm. The nurse must accept that clients are responsible for themselves and will do what they want. However, clients also have a right to have the consequences of their decisions explained to them in a language that they understand. | As | Sa/1 | Co | 1 |
| #94. 4. | Making the client physically comfortable and relaxed promotes sleep. A warm beverage is relaxing; the calcium in milk has a sedative effect. | An | Ph/5 | Ap | 1 |
| #95. 1. | Contact precautions are used for pathogens that may be spread by contact with wound drainage. Standard precautions are routinely used in addition to contact precautions. | As | Sa/2 | Co | 1 |
| #96. 3. | The PTT is an indicator of the effectivenss of anticoagulant therapy. | As | Ph/7 | Ap | 1 |
| #97. 1. | Ménière's disease is a disorder of the inner ear affecting balance and hearing, characterized by dizziness and loss of hearing. Fall precautions should be initiated. | An | Sa/1 | Ap | 1 |
| #98. 4. | A major preventable complication of chronic fibrillation is the develoment of atrial thrombus (clot), which can embolize to the brain and cause a stroke. Long-term anticoagulation using warfarin (Coumadin) decreases the risk of stroke. | Ev | Ph/8 | Ap | 1 |
| #99. 3. | Pyridium is a azo dye with local analgesic effect on the urinary tract mucosa. Wearing of contact lenses should be avoided during the treatment, as it may also stain them. | Im | Ph/6 | Ap | 5 |
| #100. 2. | Fibromyalgia is an idiopathic condition characterized by tender points, fatigue, morning stiffness, sleep problems, and depression. | An | Ph/8 | Ap | 1 |

# Practice Test 11

1. The client is receiving total parenteral nutrition (TPN) via a triple lumen catheter. The nurse knows which of the following actions is essential?
   1. Evaluate the peripheral intravenous (IV site).
   2. Confirm the tube is in the stomach.
   3. Obtain 10-mL syringes for flushes on the adjoining lines.
   4. Report WBC of 6000 cells/mm³ to the physician.

2. A client is in for a preoperative assessment. Which statement by the client would the nurse identify as the highest risk for developing postoperative complications?
   1. "I am 60 years old."
   2. "My blood pressure is 150/95."
   3. "My creatinine is 0.8 mg/dL."
   4. "My hemoglobin is 15 gm/dL."

3. The client on the oncology unit has developed stomatitis as a result of chemotherapy and radiation. Which of these nursing diagnoses is appropriate for this problem?
   1. Fatigue
   2. Disturbed body image
   3. Impaired tissue integrity: alopecia
   4. Impaired oral mucous membrane

4. A nurse is caring for four clients. After receiving report, which client should the nurse see first?
   1. A client who has a serum sodium of 144 mEq/L.
   2. A client who had a PICC line inserted yesterday.
   3. A client with a chest tube whose pulse ox shows 95%.
   4. A client with hypertension complaining of a headache.

5. The client is exhibiting Kussmaul's respirations. Which of these nursing measures would be most effective to assist this client to achieve a positive outcome?
   1. Hold all insulin injections.
   2. Provide client with food.
   3. Start 0.9% NS IVF.
   4. Instructions on incentive spirometer use.

6. Crohn's disease and ulcerative colitis have similarities and differences. Which of the following statements is accurate about these disorders?
   1. Crohn's disease generally causes pain in the distal ileum.
   2. Crohn's disease presents as a protrusion from its normal cavity in a weakened area.
   3. Ulcerative colitis presents with a hard, rigid abdomen.
   4. Ulcerative colitis can lead to fistula formation.

7. A client is diagnosed with diverticulitis. Which instruction would the nurse provide to the client?
   1. You need to decrease fiber in your diet.
   2. Check your stool for blood.
   3. An upper GI study will help to look at this problem.
   4. You need to increase your exercise activity.

8. The nurse is developing the care plan for a client after bariatric surgery. Which would be a priority nursing intervention?
   1. Keep skin around ostomy bag clean and dry.
   2. Prevent wound infection.
   3. Discuss with client an ideal weight loss goal.
   4. Serve liquids with meals.

9. The client has been using a patient-controlled analgesia after surgery. Which of these client findings would indicate that the desired outcome of this analgesia has been unsuccessful?
   1. The client states he has pushed his button several times the last hour.
   2. The client's heart rate has decreased from 90 to 75.
   3. The client rates his pain at 10 out of 10.
   4. The client is asking for more ice.

10. An elderly client calls for the nurse and states a pain level of "3 out of 10." What would be the nurse's best response?
    1. Administer a prescribed pain medication.
    2. Tell the client that a "3" is too low to receive medication.

3. Ask the client "Why do you think you need pain medication?"

4. Educate the client that pain medication can cause constipation.

11. A client who has a history of heart failure arrives in the emergency department. The assessment reveals severe dyspnea, blood-tinged frothy sputum, and anxiety. What will be an appropriate intervention for this client?

1. Provide instruction on the use of incentive spirometry.

2. Administer sublingual nitroglycerin.

3. Allow client to visit the bathroom as needed.

4. Position client in upright position with legs dangling.

12. The client is taught how to self-administer nitroglycerin. Which of the following statements by the client would require further teaching?

1. "If 3 tablets are ineffective, I will call 911."

2. I will obtain a new supply every 30 days."

3. "The pills should always be stored in a dark, glass bottle."

4. "A pill melts under my tongue."

13. For which client would the medication sumatriptan (Imitrex) be contraindicated?

1. A 75-year-old man with diabetes.

2. A 37-year-old with cluster headaches.

3. A 16-year-old who is taking birth control pills.

4. A 31-year-old who is 18 weeks pregnant.

14. A new nurse is describing diabetic ketoacidosis (DKA). Which component of the disorder would require further clarification?

1. Acidosis

2. Dehydration

3. Hyperglycemia

4. Insulin overdose

15. The client is diagnosed with cor pulmonale and asks for more explanation. What is the nurse's best response?

1. The right ventricle is enlarged to make up for the left ventricle's weakness.

2. It's enlarged because the right atria is putting more pressure on it.

3. It's enlarged as a result of a disease that affected the structure or function of the lungs.

4. It's been enlarged since birth due to a congenital condition.

16. What fetal development would be found at 13 weeks gestation?

1. Insulin in pancreas

2. Open eyelids

3. Tooth enamel

4. Gingivitis

17. A nurse discovers a positive Tinel's sign during the client assessment. Which condition would the nurse know this is associated with?

1. Orthopnea

2. Hypertension

3. Leukemia

4. Carpal tunnel syndrome

18. The nurse instructs a client who has congestive heart disease to avoid which item in the diet?

1. Decaffeinated coffee

2. Canned vegetables

3. Fresh fruit

4. Skim milk

19. The nurse is observing a nursing assistant (NA) providing care to a client with a fractured hip. Which action would require immediate intervention?

1. The client's bed is raised up all the way for the breakfast meal.

2. The NA places pillows between the client's legs.

3. The traction bar is placed so the client can reach it.

4. The NA assists the client onto the raised toilet seat.

20. What would be the most appropriate toy for a 6-year-old child in a hip spica cast?

1. Hand puppets

2. Tinkertoys

3. A board game

4. A small ball

21. What analgesic should the emergency department nurse prepare to administer IV to a client suffering myocardial infarction (MI)?

1. Demerol

2. Morphine

3. Nitroglycerin

4. Valium IV

22. A term infant born 30 minutes ago is assessed as having respirations of 70 per minute with acrocyanosis. What action must the nurse take?

1. Suction and keep warm; place the infant in the Trendelenburg position.
2. Administer O$_2$ via an oxyhood.
3. Alert the physician for an emergency.
4. Monitor vital signs every 30 minutes.

23. A client is scheduled for a total gastrectomy with jejunostomy. During preoperative instructing, what statement will indicate the client requires additional teaching about the postoperative period?
    1. "I hope I can eat, but if not I will have TPN."
    2. "My spouse will help fix the six small meals every day."
    3. "I will drink my fluids in between my meals instead of with them."
    4. "I'm glad that the B$_{12}$ shots will only be for a few weeks."

24. The client is prescribed aspirin 325-mg enteric coated every day. What essential teaching information should be performed by the nurse?
    1. "Expect to have a little dizziness while taking the aspirin."
    2. "Don't take this with alcohol."
    3. "Take on an empty stomach before meals."
    4. "It will keep your fever down."

25. After receiving report, which client needs the most urgent care?
    1. A 45-year-old male with intermittent left lower quadrant (LLQ) abdominal and back pain; his urine is positive for blood. VS: T 99°F, BP 130/78, HR 78, RR 18.
    2. An 80-year-old female with a history of diverticulitis; complaining of LLQ pain and has a board-like abdomen, left shoulder pain. VS: T 100.4°F, BP 120/80, HR 112, RR 22.
    3. A 17-year-old female with cramping periumbilical pain that has been moving toward the right lower quadrant (RLQ) the last 2 hours; has vomited once, rates pain as a "3". VS: T 99°F, BP 112/74, HR 100, RR 22.
    4. A 52-year-old male who complains of lower abdominal and scrotal pain and has a burning sensation when voiding. VS: T 100.4°F, BP 110/70, HR 80, RR 16.

26. Which nursing diagnosis is most appropriate for the AIDS client who has been admitted with pneumocystis carinii?
    1. Fluid volume deficit
    2. Body image disturbance
    3. Impaired gas exchange
    4. Ineffective individual coping

27. The client has returned from PACU after a modified radial mastectomy of the left side. Which of the following nursing actions would be contraindicated?
    1. Position the client on the right side.
    2. Elevate the left arm on a pillow.
    3. Place a sign in the room that states BP cannot be taken in the right arm.
    4. Instruct the client to flex and extend the left fingers and wrist.

28. Which of the following patients is at the highest risk for osteoarthritis?
    1. A 85-year-old female who has always run 5 miles per day and was anorexic.
    2. A 32-year-old male banker who exercises moderately 3–5 times per week.
    3. An African-American female who is 40 years old, is a normal weight for her height and has never broken a bone.
    4. A 60-year-old male who is retired from the Air Force and still maintains an active lifestyle and adequate nutrition.

29. What is the maternal response most common during the second stage of labor?
    1. Alopecia
    2. Active pushing
    3. Anger
    4. Loss of control

30. To combat the most common adverse effects of chemotherapy, what medication would the nurse administer?
    1. Antibiotic
    2. Antiemetic
    3. Anticoagulant
    4. Anti-inflammatory

31. The nurse knows that the plan of care for a client taking lithium would include which of the following considerations?
    1. Reduce caffeine intake.
    2. Stop the medication immediately if hand tremors appear.
    3. Adverse side effects include blurred vision.
    4. Hallucinations and delusions are considered positive symptoms in mental disorders.

32. The nurse teaches a client who has had a biological (xenograft) valve replacement for his damaged mitral valve. Which of the following

statements, if made by the client, would require immediate follow-up by the nurse?

1. "I will get enough anticoagulation to last me for 3 months."
2. "I will notify my dentist before visits."
3. "I have found a counseling service to help me through this event."
4. "I would like to know what happened to the person I got my valve from."

33. The client reports having the flu recently after a camping trip and now has a left-sided rash on the rib cage. What discharge teaching should be included concerning this event?

1. Watch out for snakes when camping.
2. Use tweezers to remove ticks.
3. Wear dark colored clothes so bugs will not be attracted to you.
4. Dogs and cats are a tick's transportation system.

34. A client was evaluated for orthostatic hypotension. Which of the following statements by the nurse is most accurate?

1. "Keep the head of your bed flat when you sleep."
2. "You will most likely need a higher dose of your diuretic."
3. "Dangle on the side of the bed before getting up."
4. "The blood is rushing to your head."

35. A client is brought into the emergency room following a fall off a ladder. What priority action would the nurse perform?

1. Insert a foley catheter.
2. Apply a Crutchfield traction tong.
3. Remove client from backboard to prevent pressure ulcers.
4. Ask client to describe the accident.

36. Which action demonstrates the nurse knows that it is a legal duty to cause no harm to clients?

1. The nurse did not take vital signs after surgery.
2. A client asks for food after surgery, but the nurse tells him he cannot have it.
3. The client complains all the time and the nurse states, "You are our worst patient."
4. The nurse does not put on the client's slippers before ambulation.

37. A man is admitted for treatment of benign prostatic hypertrophy (BPH). Which of the following questions should the nurse ask first?

1. "How many bowel movements do you have per day?"
2. "When did you have your prostate removed?"
3. "Do you have to push when you urinate?"
4. "Do you take vitamins every day?"

38. A client is admitted with influenza. What will be the nurse's best action to prevent it being passed to others?

1. Instruct the client to use tissues when sneezing.
2. Wash hands after touching the client.
3. Wear gloves when taking the client's tray out of the room.
4. Instruct all visitors to wear a gown in the room.

39. The nurse is teaching a community group about the causes of peptic ulcer disease. When asked what causes the problem, which answer would indicate teaching has been successful?

1. Stress
2. Smoking
3. Spicy foods
4. *H. pylori*

40. Which nursing diagnosis should receive priority for a patient experiencing pregnancy-induced hypertensive disorder (PIH)?

1. Ineffective tissue perfusion
2. Fear related to loss of fetus
3. Imbalanced nutrition, more than body requirements
4. Nausea

41. The nurse should be on alert for what condition in a child with cystic fibrosis?

1. Fibrosis of the lung
2. Respiratory infections
3. High surfactant levels
4. Hyperventilation

42. A client enters the emergency room with hemoptysis. Which of the following actions would be the most appropriate for the nurse to take?

1. Determine the cause of the problem.
2. Request an operating room.
3. Start a transfusion.
4. Ask the client to sign consent for catherization.

43. A client is admitted for a paracentesis after a 3-year history of cirrhosis. Which position

should the nurse place the client for the procedure?

1. Prone
2. Dorsal recumbent
3. Supine
4. Sitting in a chair

44. A school-age child weighing 55 pounds has been ordered meperidine (Demerol) 1.5 mg/kg IM for pain. What amount should the nurse administer to the child?

1. 1.5 mg
2. 8.25 mg
3. 41.25 mg
4. 55 mg

45. A client is to have a CT with contrast to evaluate a possible tumor. It would be most important for the nurse to ask which of the following questions?

1. "Do you have many headaches?"
2. "Are you a diabetic?"
3. "Do you have any metal parts in your body?"
4. "Are you claustrophobic?"

46. The client is ordered a D-Dimer assay, fibrinogen, FDP, PT, and aPTT. The nurse should be alert for which of the following problems?

1. Bleeding
2. Ketoacidosis
3. Pancreatitis
4. Coronary heart disease

47. The client's hemoglobin is low at 7.5 and the physician's orders state to infuse immunoglobulin IVIG. What would be the nurse's best action?

1. Tell the client it will take 2 to 4 hours for the infusion.
2. Inquire why the client is receiving this infusion.
3. Instruct the client to inform staff of any adverse effects occurring during infusion.
4. Obtain a consent.

48. The nurse is caring for a client with rheumatoid arthritis. The nurse would be most concerned if the client made which statement?

1. "I try to take a walk every day."
2. "I have lactose intolerance."
3. "I take aspirin and motrin every day for the pain."
4. "I feel the most stiff in the morning."

49. A client has returned from an arthroscopy of the left knee. Which assessment should be performed every hour?

1. Pain rating
2. Bowel sounds
3. Pedal pulses
4. Respiration rate

50. A client had her pituitary gland removed because of a tumor. Which observation should the nurse expect after this surgery?

1. The client will be voiding massive amounts.
2. The client's serum sodium will be elevated.
3. The client's potassium will be elevated.
4. The client's temperature will fluctuate.

51. The nurse is observing a newly hired nursing assistant (NA). Which behavior by the NA would cause the nurse to intervene?

1. The NA puts gloves on when emptying all urinals.
2. The NA closes the door to a negative-pressure room.
3. The NA puts on gloves to give a MRSA client a bath.
4. The NA gives tissues to a client coughing.

52. A client has been receiving an antibiotic for a urinary tract infection. The nurse would be most concerned if the client made which one of the following statements?

1. "I have a little itching with urination."
2. "I am drinking and voiding more."
3. "I don't hear as well as I used to."
4. "I can't eat as much as I used to."

53. The nurse explains to the family why the client is going to receive palliative surgery. Which statement by family member demonstrates successful teaching?

1. "This surgery will cure the illness."
2. "This surgery will restore the ability that was lost."
3. "It will be good that this may reduce the pain."
4. "It will be good to know exactly why this illness is present."

54. A child is placed in a spica cast. What action should the nurse plan to implement?

1. Keep upper arms restrained.
2. Hang toys above the crib.
3. Provide cheese and milk for protein.
4. Change position every 4 hours to prevent skin breakdown.

55. How many calories does a 7 lb 10 oz infant require per 24-hour period?
    1. 300–350
    2. 400–412
    3. 500–520
    4. 600–620

56. For a client suffering with abruptio placentae, which of these is the most important for a nurse to monitor?
    1. Vaginal bleeding that is bright red or dark
    2. Soft abdomen
    3. Symptoms of hypoglycemia
    4. Hypotension

57. The nurse is working with a client who often threatens suicide to get attention but does not verbalize a plan. How should the nurse interpret this behavior?
    1. Hopelessness
    2. Confrontation
    3. Manipulation
    4. Self-anger

58. Which question would be most important to ask a client before going to surgery?
    1. "Are you allergic to bees?"
    2. "Can you eat shellfish?"
    3. "Do foods with red dye bother you?"
    4. "Can you blow up balloons?"

59. The physician states the client will be monitored using capnography. What explanation will the nurse give the family about this term?
    1. "It measures the arterial blood pressure."
    2. "It will measure the oxygen saturation."
    3. "It will record brain activity."
    4. "It records the level of carbon dioxide exhaled."

60. The nurse starts an IV antibiotic piggybacked onto normal saline. Five minutes after it is started, the client begins to exhibit shortness of breath and wheezing. Which of the following actions should the nurse take first?
    1. Obtain vital signs.
    2. Stop the infusion.
    3. Administer IV Benadryl.
    4. Notify the physician.

61. What would be a priority nursing diagnosis for a client diagnosed with Kaposi's sarcoma?
    1. Social isolation
    2. Potential for injury
    3. Disturbed body image
    4. Self-care deficit

62. A client has had a stroke and now has left homonymous hemianopsia. What would be appropriate actions by the staff?
    1. Approach the client from the right side.
    2. Place objects on the left side of the client.
    3. Stand on the client's left side when assisting with meals.
    4. Instruct client to turn head to the right to be able to see better.

63. Which would be a priority nursing diagnosis for a client with post-polio syndrome?
    1. Imbalanced nutrition: Less than body requirements
    2. Impaired urinary elimination
    3. Risk for delayed development
    4. Impaired walking

64. A client has been prescribed corticosteroids daily for severe asthma and now has an elevated blood glucose. He asks the nurse if he is now diabetic. What would be the nurse's explanation?
    1. "Yes, the steroids alter the pancreas' ability to produce insulin."
    2. "Yes, any time blood glucose levels are high, it means diabetes is present."
    3. "No, the steroids increase the synthesis of glucose."
    4. "No, the insulin production is down due to the asthma condition."

65. The client is diagnosed with hyperpituitarism and acromegaly. Which nursing diagnosis is listed on the care plan?
    1. Risk for injury
    2. Disturbed body image
    3. Constipation
    4. Decreased cardiac output

66. The client is told that preventricular contractions (PVCs) are occurring. What should the nurse know about this condition?
    1. A PVC is a late depolarization that happens after the beat.
    2. PVCs are one of the most common dysrhythmias.
    3. A PVC occurs during the down stroke of an R wave.
    4. Three successive PVSs at a rate over 100/min is atria tachycardia.

67. A new graduate nurse obtains equipment and supplies needed for a sickle-cell client that has just been admitted. Which equipment will the new nurse need to return?
   1. A patient-controlled analgesia pump
   2. An IV pump
   3. Blood tubing
   4. A fan

68. At what age will the first outward signs of muscular weakness begin to appear in a child with muscular dystrophy?
   1. Infant to age 2
   2. Age 2 to 5
   3. Age 7 to 12
   4. Age 12 to 14

69. Teaching is provided for a client being discharged after being seen for herpes simplex Type 1 (HSV-1). What information should the nurse tell the client?
   1. Inform sexual partner of the infection.
   2. Use sunblock when out in the sun.
   3. Stay away from others who have not had chickenpox.
   4. Scrape blisters away as soon as they appear.

70. A client returns from PACU following a transsphenoidal hypophysectomy. What would be an appropriate nursing intervention?
   1. Encourage coughing and deep breathing.
   2. Measure the blood saturation on the dressing.
   3. Test the clear drainage for glucose.
   4. Expect a fever post-operatively.

71. A client has had an artificial pacemaker implanted. What should the nurse know about pacemakers?
   1. They can be used to pace the atria and/or ventricles.
   2. Pacemaker spikes will only appear if the battery is low.
   3. All pacemakers are located on the outside of the chest wall near the heart.
   4. A permanent pacemaker would treat a fast heart rate.

72. The Joint Commission on Accreditation of Healthcare Organizations (JCAHO) has developed four phases of emergency management. Which one would be absent from the list?
   1. Mitigation
   2. Preparedness
   3. Reaction
   4. Recovery

73. A client is desmopressin acetate (DDAVP) after having radiation for a brain tumor. The nurse recognizes the client's condition and has placed which nursing diagnosis on the care plan?
   1. Fluid volume deficit
   2. Excess fluid volume
   3. Impaired mobility
   4. Stress overload

74. Immunocompromised children are at risk of contracting illness spread by some animals. For this reason, which animal is the better choice of a companion for a child?
   1. A bird
   2. A dog
   3. A turtle
   4. An iguana

75. A new nursing assistant (NA) was assigned to particular rooms. An experienced nursing assistant found dirty linen in the bathroom in one of the assigned rooms and enters into the break room with 4 other staff present and states "You left dirty linen in the bathroom! The client's husband could have fallen on it!" As the charge nurse, what would be the first step in resolving this conflict?
   1. Ask the new NA to tell the experienced NA why she left the linen in the bathroom.
   2. Ask the two NAs to meet with the charge nurse privately and discuss the situation.
   3. Thank the experienced NA for picking up the dirty linen.
   4. Tell the new NA to ignore the verbal threats of the experienced NA.

76. Which of the following would be considered a delegation instead of an assignment to an unlicensed assistive personal (UAP)?
   1. Take vital signs in rooms 1–7.
   2. Give bed baths to room 8–12.
   3. Inspect patient's IV site for bleeding in room 13.
   4. Feed patients in room 14–18.

77. If a client states dizziness upon getting out of bed, the nurse would initiate which of the following actions?
   1. Instruct client to rise slowly when getting out of bed.
   2. Obtain order to discontinue blood pressure medication.

3. Take a standing blood pressure.

4. Encourage PO fluids.

78. The client is diagnosed with myasthenia gravis. What is one of the goals for the medication treatment?

1. Increase heart rate

2. Decreased GI motility

3. Decrease ptosis

4. Improve sensation

79. The client states he has been experiencing some angina symptoms several times a week. What would be an appropriate question to ask him?

1. "Have you changed your diet?"

2. "Are you still participating in your exercise program?"

3. "Are you still taking your Atenolol?"

4. "Have you notified your insurance company?"

80. The client is suspected of having a pheochromocytoma. What intervention would be included in the care plan?

1. Instruct client to touch chin to chest.

2. Take vital signs every hour.

3. Ask client to plantar and dorsiflex both feet.

4. Avoid abdomen palpation.

81. What would be an appropriate nursing diagnosis for a child who has been burned on a large body surface?

1. Ineffective health maintenance

2. Risk for injury

3. Hypothermia

4. Social isolation

82. A 75-year-old client who is receiving medications that suppresses the immune system says to a nurse, "My 23-year-old neighbor is also receiving treatment like me. He told me what to watch for." Which of these responses would be the most appropriate one for the nurse to make initially?

1. "You will have the same side effects as your neighbor."

2. "You may have different side effects to the medication than your neighbor."

3. "Report any side effects your neighbor experiences."

4. "What type of cancer does your neighbor have?"

83. The client presents the following complaints: weight loss, irritability, muscle weakness, palpitations. You suspect the patient is suffering from what condition?

1. Cirrhosis

2. Hyperthyroidism

3. Cushing's disease

4. Addison's disease

84. What is a reason that anti-infective drugs must be monitored in the older adult?

1. Older adults are not susceptible to infection complications.

2. Excretion of these agents is very quick.

3. Acute renal failure may occur.

4. They are taken TID.

85. Your co-worker asks you for your suggestions about a large dressing change. What style of leadership is the co-worker demonstrating?

1. Autocratic

2. Democratic

3. Laissez-faire

4. Recognition

86. Which statement reflects the nurse providing negative feedback to the nursing assistant (NA) in a professional manner?

1. "The I&O flow sheet needs to be charted before the second shift begins. Let me know if you need help with it."

2. "I see you emptied the foley by the end of shift. I appreciate that."

3. "Thank you for rechecking Mr. Jones', temperature."

4. "There was dirty linen on the floor in Mrs. Smith's room."

87. Why is it important to distribute the work among nursing assistants after the change of shift report?

1. The charge nurse will know how many patients are on the unit.

2. The charge nurse will distribute workload equally.

3. The charge nurse will distribute the patients equally.

4. The charge nurse will know how many nurses there are.

88. The nurse is aware that the action of anticholinergic agents will produce what physiological changes in a client?

1. Increasing intraocular pressure
2. Decrease mouth secretions
3. Increase GI secretions
4. Decrease heart rate

89. The client is complaining of shortness of breath, edema at lower extremities, and hunger. Which of the following actions would the nurse initiate first?
    1. Apply O$_2$
    2. Elevate legs
    3. Provide clear liquids
    4. Notify the physician

90. A pregnant client has been admitted due to persistent vomiting and has not eaten for 4 days. What condition will the nurse suspect?
    1. Anticipatory nausea
    2. Hyperemesis gravidarum
    3. Psychogenic vomiting
    4. Retching

91. The client who had a coronary artery bypass graft is receiving discharge teaching. Which of the following statements demonstrates successful teaching?
    1. "It will be good to get back to work next week."
    2. "I will limit exercise to avoid stress on my heart."
    3. "I'm glad I don't have to watch my diet as close, since the surgery fixed my heart disease."
    4. "I can lift objects less than 10 pounds."

92. The 16-year-old client is a diabetic who has been admitted with a blood sugar of 800. What will the nurse need to be aware of when discussing the diabetic condition with the client?
    1. The amount of carbohydrates the patient is eating.
    2. How often the patient is checking her blood sugar?
    3. Rebellion can be a factor in this age bracket.
    4. Does the patient wear her medical identification bracelet?

93. When assessing a wound area, the nurse notes the following information: Right foot – warm and dry, small amount of bloody drainage on dressing, foul odor, and no pain reported. Which of the previous assessments would warrant further investigation?
    1. Foot warm and dry
    2. Small amount of bloody drainage on dressing
    3. Foul odor
    4. No pain reported

94. The first assignment of a licensed registered nurse is on a unit that has a reputation for having a very "tough" charge nurse. What should be the attitude of the new employee upon taking this position?
    1. Be prepared to face a challenge with the charge nurse.
    2. Plan to carry out job responsibilities as taught.
    3. Ask the co-workers for advice.
    4. Speak with the supervisor about this position.

95. Which would be included in the statements given to a care giver of an older adult living in the home?
    1. "Caring for your mom will bring you closer."
    2. "Caring for your mom will get easier as time goes on."
    3. "It's normal to feel some anxiety and anger. It will pass."
    4. "You need to set time frames for the other family members to help."

96. What is the most important reason to control vomiting?
    1. Inhibit impulses from the brain
    2. To prevent motion sickness
    3. Relieve distress
    4. To prevent aspiration

97. If Ativan is available in 2 mg/mL, how much would be given if the order states 0.75 mg?
    1. 0.25 mL
    2. 0.37 mL
    3. 0.55 mL
    4. 0.75 mL

98. The client is having nausea and vomiting 3 hours before a chemotherapy treatment. What condition does the nurse suspect?
    1. Anticipatory nausea and vomiting
    2. Hyperemesis gravidarum
    3. Postoperative nausea and vomiting
    4. Psychogenic vomiting

**99.** Cannabinoids are used as antiemetics in what type of client?
1. Chemotherapy clients
2. Pregnant clients
3. Postoperative clients
4. Clients with ascites

**100.** The client with diabetes calls out and states he is sweating and shaky. What would be your first action?
1. Take his blood sugar.
2. Give him some orange juice.
3. Give him his scheduled insulin.
4. Notify the physician.

# Answers and Rationales for Practice Test 11

| ANSWER | RATIONALE | NP | CN | CL | SA |
|---|---|---|---|---|---|
| **#1. 3.** | The TPN is infused in the central line, not a peripheral one; there is no tube associated with TPN and the WBC count is within normal limits. It is recommended by most facilities to use 10-mL syringes when administering medication through central or PICC lines to prevent a greater pressure than from a small-size syringe. | Pl | Ph/6 | An | 5 |
| **#2. 3.** | Having high blood pressure is a risk factor, and surgery may be postponed because of it. The other choices are within normal limits (WNL) and are not considered risk factors. | An | Ph/7 | An | 1 |
| **#3. 4.** | Stomatitis is an inflammation of the mouth that can develop after oncology treatment. | An | Ph/8 | An | 1 |
| **#4. 4.** | All clients except "4" have no abnormalities cited. A headache with hypertension could be a forewarning of a serious problem. | An | Ph/7 | An | 1 |
| **#5. 3.** | Kussmaul's respirations are seen in diabetic ketoacidosis. Respirations increase in rate and depth in an attempt to blow off the carbon dioxide accumulating with the acidosis state. Dehydration from hyperglycemia is present and IVF is needed quickly. The event may have occurred from either lack of insulin or noncompliance with the therapeutic regimen. | Pl | Ph/8 | An | 1 |
| **#6. 1.** | The other choices describe a hernia, peritonitis, and fistulas that are more associated with Crohn's disease. | As | Ph/8 | Ap | 1 |
| **#7. 2.** | Diverticulitis is an inflammation of the diverticula and may present with alternating constipation and diarrhea with blood and mucus. Diagnostics would include barium enema or a lower GI study (colonoscopy). The client is put on a clear liquid diet during the inflamed period, then a high or low residue diet depending on the findings. | Im | Ph/8 | An | 1 |
| **#8. 2.** | Infection is a common complication after bariatric surgery and the client's vital signs and lab work should be monitored carefully. | Im | Ph/7 | An | 1 |
| **#9. 3.** | An unsuccessful report would be the pain is still rated high. The other choices are normal occurrences. | An | Ph/7 | An | 1 |

| ANSWER | | RATIONALE | NP | CN | CL | SA |
|---|---|---|---|---|---|---|
| #10. | 1. | If the client called out with a complaint of pain, the nurse must accept the client's pain for what the client says it is. The client may not understand the rating scale or may not want to complain. The nurse should ask further assessment questions. | Im | Ph/8 | Ap | 1 |
| #11. | 4. | The client's dyspneic condition warrants a sitting position to facilitate breathing. Nitroglycerin would be used if chest pain, angina, or a heart attack was suspected. The client would be given a urinal in order not to expend energy walking to the bathroom. | An | Ph/8 | An | 1 |
| #12. | 2. | A new supply should be obtained every 6 months. The other choices are all true of the medication. | Ev | Ph/8 | An | 5 |
| #13. | 4. | Sumatriptan is indicated for cluster headaches. Pregnant clients should not take 5-HT agonists such as this medication. | Ev | Ph/6 | An | 5 |
| #14. | 4. | In DKA, there is little or no insulin. The client will be hyperglycemic, in a state of acidosis and dehydrated. | An | Ph/8 | An | 1 |
| #15. | 3. | The right ventricle is enlarged due to increased pressure in the pulmonary circulatory system and pulmonary hypertension. | Im | Ph/8 | Ap | 1 |
| #16. | 1. | The pancreas secretes insulin around 12–13 weeks gestation. | As | He/3 | Ap | 3 |
| #17. | 4. | This is a tingling sensation produced by pressing on or tapping the median nerve. | As | Ph/7 | Ap | 1 |
| #18. | 2. | Clients with congestive heart disease are usually already on diuretics to control excess fluid, therefore a diet low in sodium should be followed. Canned vegetables are usually high in sodium content and should be avoided, whereas fresh vegetables and fruits should be encouraged. | Im | Ph/5 | An | 1 |
| #19. | 1. | The leg and hip must be maintained in an abducted position to prevent dislocating the head of the femur. The head of bed should not be elevated more than 60 degrees to prevent hip flexion of greater than 90 degrees. | Im | Sa/1 | Ap | 1 |
| #20. | 1. | Because children may stuff food or toys in the cast, a hand puppet should keep the child active and entertained and should be difficult to stuff in the cast. A ball might roll off the bed. | An | Sa/2 | Ap | 4 |
| #21. | 2. | Severe MI pain demands a powerful drug. Control of pain is essential in preventing cardiogenic shock. It is also suspected that unrelieved pain may cause a cascade of infarctions. | As | Ph/6 | Ap | 5 |
| #22. | 4. | The respiratory rate of 60–70 per minute for 2 hours after delivery is normal. Acrocyanosis is normal until 24 hours postdelivery. Routine vital signs should be monitored every 30 minutes for 2 hours postdelivery. | Im | He/3 | Ap | 3 |
| #23. | 4. | Dietary B$_{12}$ is absorbed in the stomach and because the stomach is removed, injections will be required for life. | Ev | He/3 | An | 1 |
| #24. | 2. | Aspirin can cause gastric irritation or bleeding, especially when taking with alcohol ingestion. Clients should report ringing in the ears, dizziness, abdominal pain, and the | Im | Ps/6 | An | 5 |

| ANSWER | RATIONALE | NP | CN | CL | SA |
|--------|-----------|-----|-----|-----|-----|
| | medication should be taken with meals or milk to prevent lodging in the esophagus. | | | | |
| #25. 2. | This client has the classic signs of peritonitis, probably secondary to perforation and needs care right away. Her temperature may be low due to her age, but her pulse is an indicator of fluid volume deficit. | An | Sa/1 | An | 1 |
| #26. 3. | Pneumocystis carinii pneumonia is seen in immunodeficient adults with AIDS and impedes the respiratory system. | An | Ph/8 | An | 1 |
| #27. 3. | The sign should state no blood pressures or venipunctures in the left arm to avoid the occurrence of lymphedema. | Im | Ph/7 | An | 1 |
| #28. 1. | This patient's age, intense and prolonged exercise as well as nutritional deficiencies from anorexia put her at the highest risk for developing osteoarthritis. | An | Ph/7 | An | 1 |
| #29. 2. | Maternal behavior changes from coping with contractions to actively pushing during the second stage of labor. | An | He/3 | Ap | 3 |
| #30. 2. | Nausea and vomiting are the most common side effects, and antiemetics should be given before chemotherapy treatment. | Im | Ph/6 | Ap | 5 |
| #31. 1. | Caffeinated beverages/foods may aggravate mania, especially in bipolar disorder. The most common side effects are fine hand tremors, polyuria, thirst, and mild nausea. Blurred vision is a sign of toxicity and immediate emergency treatment initiated. Negative symptoms would include social withdrawal, lack of initiative, apathy, and decreased energy, as in schizophrenia. | Pl | Ps/4 | An | 5 |
| #32. 4. | A xenograft is harvested from an animal, usually a pig, not from a human donor. Some clients have difficulty adjusting to the lifestyle changes with valvular disorders and may experience some fear or anxiety, and may benefit from counseling. | Im | Ph/7 | An | 1 |
| #33. 2. | The symptoms described are indicative of Lyme disease from a tick bite. Ticks should be removed by grasping close to the skin with tweezers and slowly pulling the tick from the skin, washing the affected area and hands, and disinfecting the tweezers. Deer are responsible for transporting ticks. | Im | He/3 | An | 1 |
| #34. 3. | This condition presents as dizziness or syncope when there is a decreased blood flow to the brain. Treatment options will depend on the underlying cause, but clients should be taught to sit and stand up slowly, sleep with head of bed raised, drink plenty of fluids, and exercise if appropriate. | Im | Sa/2 | An | 1 |
| #35. 1. | The client may experience a spinal cord injury (SCI) in which a backboard and neck brace remain in place until a CT rules out the injury. If the client does have SCI, the bladder becomes atonic due to a disruption of the spinal cord and bladder retention or incontinence may occur. | Im | Ph/8 | An | 1 |
| #36. 2. | Nonmaleficence is demonstrated here, as taking in food before the physician orders may cause harm to the client's physical state. The other choices are: 1-malpractice; 3-abuse; 4-negligence. | As | Sa/1 | An | 1 |

| ANSWER | RATIONALE | NP | CN | CL | SA |
|--------|-----------|----|----|----|----|

**#37. 3.** BPH is a non-cancerous enlargement of the prostate gland and will affect urination. — As — Sa/1 — An — 1

**#38. 1.** It is recommended the affected client use tissues or a mask if coughing or sneezing. Individuals who enter the room should also wear a mask. The other choices are standard precautions for anyone with symptoms of respiratory infection. — Im — Sa/2 — An — 1

**#39. 4.** The majority of gastric ulcers and duodental ulcers are caused by the bacterium *Helicobacter pylori*. — Ev — He/3 — Ap — 1

**#40. 1.** PIH, or pre-eclampsia is characterized by generalized vasospasm, a significant decrease in circulating blood volume. — An — He/3 — An — 3

**#41. 2.** Secretions usually harbor bacteria. Because the client is unable to expectorate, the child is predisposed to infections. — An — Ph/8 — Ap — 4

**#42. 1.** The first priority is to try and determine the cause of bleeding, by auscultation, labs, and/or bronchoscopy. If the amount is less than 200 mL in less than a 24-hour period, then a watch-and-wait approach is initiated with close monitoring. — Im — Ph/8 — An — 1

**#43. 4.** The client's abdomen will be assessed through a small incision below the umbilicus, as fluid then drains via gravity from the peritoneal cavity into a clear container. If the client is bed-bound, the Fowler's position would be appropriate. — Pl — Ph/8 — Ap — 1

**#44. 3.** First, calculate the weight in kg: 27.5 kg. Set up the proportion with the ordered dosage in one fraction and the unknown dosage and the client's weight in the other fraction: — Im — Ph/8 — An — 5

$$\frac{1.5 \text{ mg}}{1 \text{ kg/dose}} = \frac{X}{27.5 \text{ kg}}$$

Cross multiply the fractions:

$$X \times 1 \text{ kg/dose} = 1.5 \text{ mg} \times 27.5 \text{ kg}$$

Solve for X by dividing each side of the equation by 1 kg and cancel units:

$$X = 41.25 \text{ mg}$$

**#45. 2.** If a client has diabetes, he may be taking metformin (Glucophage). The client would be advised he cannot take the drug for 48 hours after the scan to prevent lactic acidosis and he should check with his physician how to manage blood glucose during that time. — As — Ph/7 — An — 1

**#46. 1.** These tests together are indicative of evaluating the client for disseminated intravascular coagulation (DIC) which is a bleeding problem. — As — Ph/8 — An — 1

**#47. 2.** IVIG is usually given for T-cell and B-cell deficiencies. Double-check to make sure the right order is for the right client. — Pl — Sa/2 — An — 1

**#48. 3.** Next to *H. pylori* infection, the use of aspirin and NSAIDs is the most common cause of gastric and duodenal ulcers, and this occurs in many individuals with arthritis. The nurse will need to assess for this possible complication. — An — Ph/8 — An — 1

| ANSWER | RATIONALE | NP | CN | CL | SA |
|---|---|---|---|---|---|
| **#49. 3.** | An hourly assessment would be performed on the pedal pulses as part of the neurovascular system. Pain assessment is important, but it is done as pain medicine is given and an hour after, and PRNs are usually only allowed every 3–6 hours. | An | Ph/8 | Ap | 1 |
| **#50. 1.** | The posterior pituitary gland houses the antidiuretic hormone, which acts to reduce the volume of urine produced. The hormone will be absent and large amounts of water will be excreted in the urine. | An | Ph/8 | An | 1 |
| **#51. 3.** | An MRSA client would be on contact precautions and the closeness of the NA to the client would also require a gown. | Im | Sa/2 | An | 1 |
| **#52. 3.** | This client's statement may be the signal that ototoxicity is occurring and needs immediate attention. The medication may need to be stopped and changed. | An | Ph/6 | An | 1 |
| **#53. 3.** | Palliative surgery is done only for the purpose of improving the quality of a person's life. It is not intended to cure the person or even prolong life. | Ev | Ps/4 | Ap | 1 |
| **#54. 2.** | Hanging toys would encourage use of upper extremities. Restriction of arms would be frustrating; diet should include bulk and bran to prevent constipation; position changes should occur every 2 hours. | Pl | Ph/7 | Ap | 4 |
| **#55. 2.** | An infant requires approximately 50–55 calories per pound in a 24-hour period. | An | Ph/5 | Ap | 4 |
| **#56. 2.** | Abruptio placentae is a separation of the placenta from its implantation site before delivery of the fetus. The most common presenting symptoms are abdominal pain and vaginal bleeding. | As | He/3 | Ap | 3 |
| **#57. 3.** | All threats of suicide should be explored. However, the client who repeatedly uses threats of suicide to get attention is manipulative, and this behavior should be confronted. If the client verbalizes a plan, this indicates a serious threat of suicide. | An | Ps/4 | An | 2 |
| **#58. 4.** | Individuals who have been exposed to latex on a frequent basis, such as health care workers, food handlers, or spina bifida patients, are more prone to latex allergy. If this occurs, precautions will be taken in the OR to use non-latex items. | An | Sa/2 | An | 1 |
| **#59. 4.** | Capnography is the continuous reading of carbon dioxide in expired air in mechanically ventilated patients, whereas pulse oximetry only monitors oxygenation. | Im | Ph/7 | An | 1 |
| **#60. 2.** | The client's condition is indicative of an anaphylactic reaction and the infusion should be stopped immediately. Vital signs would be taken, the physician called, and possibly Benadryl may be ordered. | Im | Ph/6 | An | 1 |
| **#61. 3.** | Kaposi's sarcoma is a rare skin cancer that occurs more in HIV clients, which manifests as maculopapular lesions that range in color from pink to bluish-purple. | An | Ph/8 | An | 1 |
| **#62. 2.** | This condition is the loss of half of the visual field. The client can see more on the right and should be encouraged to turn the head left to compensate for the part that is lost. | Im | Ph/8 | An | 1 |

| ANSWER | | RATIONALE | NP | CN | CL | SA |
|---|---|---|---|---|---|---|
| #63. | 4. | This is a neurological disorder of unknown etiology that presents with signs and symptoms of poliomyelitis, which the client had survived from the 1950s. | An | Ph/8 | An | 1 |
| #64. | 3. | Corticosteroids cause blood sugar to rise by stimulating liver synthesis of glucose. The pancreas is unaffected. | An | Ph/8 | An | 1 |
| #65. | 2. | The skeletal changes and organ enlargements are visible and not reversible. | An | Ph/8 | An | 1 |
| #66. | 2. | PVCs are associated with cardiac as well as non-cardiac conditions. | An | Ph/8 | An | 1 |
| #67. | 4. | A fan will not be needed as a vaso-occlusive crisis may have arisen from an extreme temperature change, and the client will most likely request the room to be warm. The client may require a blood transfusion, IVF, and need pain medication. | Pl | Ph/8 | An | 1 |
| #68. | 2. | At this age, the child may have difficulty puckering his lips or be unable to change his facial expression when he laughs or cries. Other classic signs are clumsiness, falling, and difficulty climbing stairs. | As | Ph/8 | Ap | 4 |
| #69. | 2. | For Type 1, the client should use sunscreen to avoid sun-related outbreaks, avoid sharing eating utensils, towels, or razors. It can be passed via skin-to-skin contact. There is also a Type 2 (genital herpes) and Herpes Zoster (shingles). | Im | He/3 | Ap | 1 |
| #70. | 3. | Clear or yellow-tinged drainage could be cerebrospinal fluid (CSF) which contains glucose. Activities that increase intracranial pressure should be avoided. | An | Ph/8 | An | 1 |
| #71. | 1. | This is the only true statement. Spikes will appear on the ECG strips; they can be implanted internally or externally; a slow heart rate would be the reason for a permanent pacemaker. | An | Ph/8 | An | 1 |
| #72. | 3. | The third phase is Response—a phase that encompasses the actions all staff must take in the event of an attack. Mitigation—assessment and analysis to identify kinds of emergency situations that could occur; Preparedness—taking steps to manage the effects of an attack; Recovery—steps taken to restore normal operations. | Pl | Ph/8 | An | 1 |
| #73. | 1. | The condition is diabetes insipidus, in which the radiation has damaged the pituitary gland. The antidiuretic hormone (ADH) will not be produced and the client will complain of thirst, yet void very large amounts of urine. The DDAVP is a replacement agent to help correct this problem. | An | Ph/8 | An | 1 |
| #74. | 2. | Other animals such as birds and reptiles should be avoided, as they are associated with arboviruses and salmonellosis, have few vaccines, and are most likely to transmit disease. Precautions must be taken and taught to a child and family to limit the exposure to harmful bacteria, viruses, and fungi. | As | Sa/2 | An | 4 |
| #75. | 2. | A therapeutic relationship, such as explained by Peplau, consists of working together to allow growth and resolve problems. | Im | Sa/1 | Ap | 2 |

| ANSWER | RATIONALE | NP | CN | CL | SA |
|---|---|---|---|---|---|
| #76. 3. | A delegation is a transfer of authority to a competent individual, however it does not require the unlicensed assistive personal (UAP) to make clinical judgment. The nurse will then need to determine the appropriate plan of care. | An | Sa/1 | Co | 1 |
| #77. 1. | The client may be experiencing orthostatic hypotension or the cause may be from medications. Whatever the cause, the client needs to adjust positions to prevent a fall. | Im | Sa/2 | Ap | 1 |
| #78. 3. | Myasthenia gravis is characterized by weakness of the voluntary muscles. Initial manifestations usually involve the ocular muscles, causing diplopia (double vision) and ptosis (drooping of the eyelids). | Ev | Ph/8 | An | 1 |
| #79. 3. | Atenolol is a beta-adrenergic blocking agent, which reduces myocardial oxygen consumption; thereby controlling chest pain and delaying the onset of ischemia during activity. | As | Ph/8 | An | 5 |
| #80. 4. | Pheochromocytomas are found in the abdomen or on adrenal glands. Palpation should be avoided as it may stimulate a hypertensive crisis. | Im | Ph/8 | An | 1 |
| #81. 3. | It is imperative that hypothermia is avoided, as it may intensify a shock condition, which will cause further ischemic injury to the burned area. | An | Ph/8 | An | 4 |
| #82. 2. | Side effects can vary with individuals, as the medications are given based on a variety of factors, such as the route of administration, the dosage, and how often given. | Im | Ph/8 | An | 1 |
| #83. 2. | Hyperthyroidism is caused by excessive circulating thyroid hormones which produces these symptoms. | An | Ph/8 | An | 1 |
| #84. 3. | Aminoglycosides are antibiotics that are capable of producing nephrotoxicity and ototoxicity even in conventionally used doses, so peak and trough plasma concentrations are also ordered with the drug. The client is also encouraged to maintain good hydration. Examples are amikacin and gentamicin. | Pl | Ph/6 | An | 5 |
| #85. 2. | This action would display a democratic action, in which the task and employee is the focus. Policies are enforced, but a sharing of responsibility is achieved. | As | Sa/2 | Ap | 1 |
| #86. 1. | It is important to provide feedback to other co-workers, and negative feedback provides information about what behaviors need modification. In this example, the NA either forgot to chart the I&O information or did not finish it by the required time. | Pl | Sa/1 | An | 1 |
| #87. 2. | Each day the client census and workload may change. | An | Ph/8 | An | 1 |
| #88. 2. | Anticholinergic drugs have long been used to treat Parkinson's disease, which act by reducing excessive cholinergic activity. Adverse effects include dry mouth, urinary retention, and blurred vision. | As | Ph/6 | Ap | 5 |
| #89. 1. | The ABCs (airway, breathing, circulation) is the first priority. | Im | Sa/1 | An | 1 |
| #90. 2. | The cause of hyperemesis gravidarum is unknown, but is a serious complication of pregnancy which would perpetuate into weight loss, dehydration, and electrolyte imbalance. | As | He/3 | Ap | 3 |

| ANSWER | RATIONALE | NP | CN | CL | SA |
|---|---|---|---|---|---|
| #91. 4. | The client may lift up to 15 pounds on week 3, and a cardiac rehabilitation program will most likely be devised. | Ev | He/3 | An | 1 |
| #92. 3 | G. Stanley Hall, known as the "Father of Adolescence," stated that this period of growth is filled with storm and stress. Adolescents may be angry with the medical conditions they have, family problems at home, or other causes that may precipitate this elevated blood sugar. | An | Ps/4 | An | 4 |
| #93. 3. | The foul odor will signal an infection is occurring and will need a culture performed and possible antibiotics. | As | Sa/2 | Ap | 1 |
| #94. 2. | A professional attitude should be maintained while on the job. Any conflicts should be discussed with the charge nurse. The nurse should remember the priority responsibility is to take care of the clients. | An | Sa/1 | Ap | 1 |
| #95. 4. | The care giver can become overwhelmed in taking care of an older adult, which can affect physical, emotional, and socioeconomic health status. Either other family members need to help or elicit respite care. | An | He/3 | An | 1 |
| #96. 4. | Aspiration is the passage of food or solid particles into the lungs. It tends to occur in individuals who have impaired swallowing, those with a decreased level of consciousness, or those with a central nervous system abnormality. Suction should be immediately available at all times. | An | Ph/8 | An | 1 |
| #97. 2. | Ordered dose over dose available: 0.75 mg ÷ 2 mg = 0.37 mL | Im | Ph/6 | An | 5 |
| #98. 1. | The nausea and vomiting appear earlier than these symptoms would normally be expected. | An | Ph/8 | Co | 1 |
| #99. 1. | Cannabis derivatives (a derivative of the hemp plant, i.e., marijuana) has been used medically to reduce nausea in clients undergoing cancer chemotherapy and to reduce intraocular pressure in clients with glaucoma. | An | Ph/6 | An | 5 |
| #100. 2. | These are typical symptoms for a client with diabetes whose blood sugar is low. The first priority is to treat the client by giving a simple sugar to raise the blood sugar, then take a blood glucose reading, and follow up by giving a complex carbohydrate with protein. | Im | Ph/8 | Ap | 1 |

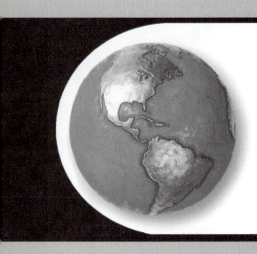

# INDEX

Male infertility, 608
Male reproductive system, 342–343
  age-related changes, 175
  chemotherapy and, 193
  cystic fibrosis and, 488
Male reproductive system disorders, 353–355
  benign prostatic hypertrophy, 354
  epididymitis, 353
  prostate cancer, 354
  prostatic surgery, 354–355
  prostatitis, 353
Malignancies, 277–278
  Hodgkins and non-Hodgkin's lymphoma, 528–529
  leukemia, 192, 525
  multiple myeloma, 277–278
  polycythemia vera, 278
Malignant cells
  differentiation, 191
  rate of growth, 191
  spead (metastasis), 191
Malignant hypertension, 250
Malignant melanoma, 409
Malpractice, 117
Management of care, 2
Mandelamine (methenamine mandelate), 92, 348
Mandibulectomy, 316
Mandol (cefamandole naftate), 88
Mania, 650
Mania with delirium, 650
Mannitol (Osmitrol), 71–72, 209, 226, 452
MAOIs. *See* Monoamine oxidase inhibitors (MAOIs)
Marasmus, 147
Marcaine (bupivacaine), 24, 574
Marezine (cyclizine), 315
Marijuana, 644
Marplan (isocarboxazid), 651, 652
Maslow, Abraham, 118–119, 625
Maslow's hierarchy of needs, 118–119
Massage, 413
Mastectomy, 613–614
Mastitis, 587
Maternal adjustment, 583
Maternal assessment, during labor, 565
Matulane (procarbazine), 103, 297, 529
Maturation, 422
Maxaquin (lomefloxacin), 93
Maxipine (cefepine), 88
MDI. *See* Metered dose inhaler (MDI)
Measles, mumps, rubella vaccine, 109
Measles (rubeola), 435
Measurement tools, for development, 423–424
Meat exchanges, 688–689, 693
Mebendazole (Vermox), 96
Mechanical ventilation, 289–290
Mechlorethamine HCl (Mustargen), 98
Meclizine (Antivert), 82, 228, 315
Medical asepsis, 127
Medical-biologic model, 623
Medication calculations, 18–23
  approximate equivalents, 19
  conversions, 18–19
  dosage calculations, 19–21
Medroxyprogesterone (Provera), 51
Medulloblastoma, 525
Mefenamic acid (Ponstel), 367
Mefoxin (cefoxitin sodium), 88

Megesterolacetate (Megace), 51
Meiosis, 441, 538
Melanocytes, 406
Melanocyte-stimulating hormone (MSH), 382, 383
Melanoma, malignant, 409
Mellaril (thioridazine), 33
Melphalan (Alkeran), 277
Menarche, 430, 536, 610
Mendel's law, 441
Ménière's disease, 228
Meninges, 201
Meningioma, 212
Meningitis, 211
Meningomyelocele, 454
Menopause (climateric), 536, 610, 614–615
  complications, 615
Menorrhagia, 611
Menotropins (Pergonal), 51
Men's health agents, 52
Menstrual cycle, 536, 537
Menstrual disorders, 610–611
Menstruation, 536
  postpartum, 582
Mental age, 423
Mental health. *See* Psychiatric-mental health nursing
Mental retardation, 639
  Down syndrome, 443
  seizures and, 458
Mental status assessment, 204, 626–627
Meperidine (Demerol), 28, 331, 573, 643
Mepivacaine (Carbocaine), 24, 574
Mercaptopurine (Purinethol), 99
Mescaline, 643
Mesoderm, 540
Mesoridazine (Serentil), 33
Mestinon (pyridostigmine), 42, 217
Metabolic acidosis, 161
Metabolic alkalosis, 161
Metabolic effects of immobility, 126
Metabolic rate, in children, 444
Metabolism
  basal, 147
  drug, 9
  energy, 147
  skin and, 406
Metamucil (psyllium hydrophilic muciloid), 80
Metaproterenol (Alupent), 39, 292
Metaraminol (Aramine), 40
Metastasis, 191
Metered dose inhaler (MDI), 487
Metformin (Glucophage), 396
Methadone (Dolophine), 28, 643
Methamphetamine, 643
Methenamine mandelate (Hiprex, Mandelamine), 92, 348
Methergine (methylergonovine), 53
Methimazole (Tapazole), 50, 391
Methohexital (Brevital), 185
Methotrexate, 297, 348, 367
Methotrexate with leucovorin rescue, 98
Methoxamine (Vasoxyl), 38
Methoxyflurane (Penthrane), 574
Methylcellulose (Citrucel, Cologel), 80
Methyldopa (Aldomet), 66, 68, 215
Methylergonovine (Methergine), 53
Methylprednisolone sodium succinate (Solu-Medrol), 49, 352

Methylsergide maleate (Sansert), 211
Methytestosterone (Android), 52
Metoclopramide (Reglan), 82, 315
Metolazone (Zaroxolyn), 67, 70
Metric system, 18–19
  approximate equivalents to household system, 19
  conversions within, 19
  conversion to household system, 19
  prefixes, 18
Metronidazole (Flagyl, Protostat), 318, 320, 499, 612, 613
Metrorrhagia, 611
Mevacor (lovastatin), 65, 251
Mexiletine (Mexitel), 60
MI. *See* Myocardial infarction (MI)
Microdrop, 21–22
Micronase Diabeta (glyburide), 396
Midamor (amiloride), 71
Midazolam (Versed), 30, 185
Middle ear, 203
Midrin, 211
Miglitol (Glyset), 396
Migraine, 210, 211
Milia, 595
Milieu therapy, 629
Milk exchanges, 687, 692
Milk of magnesia (magnesium hydroxide), 78, 80, 319
Milwaukee brace, 508, 511
Mineralocorticoids, 382, 383, 388
Mineral oil, 80
Minerals, 104–105, 147, 148–149
Minipress (prazosin), 66
Minocycline (Minocin), 90
Minoxidil (Loniten), 67
Mintezol (thiabendazole), 96
Miochol (acetylcholine), 42, 54
Miotics, 54–55
Mirtazapine (Remeron), 652
Misoprostol (Cytotec), 82, 320
Mist tent, 483
Mithramycin (plicamycin), 100, 277
Mitomycin-C, 348
Mitomycin (Mutamycin), 100
Mitosis, 441
Mitotic inhibitors, 102
Mitral valve, 236
Mixed-acting adrenergics, 39–41
MMR (measles, mumps, rubella) vaccine, 109
M'Naghten rule, 118
Moban (molindone), 33
Modified Trendelenburg, 124
Moist heat, 127
Moles (nevi), 409
Molindone (Moban), 33
Mongolian spots, 595
Monoamine oxidase inhibitors (MAOIs), 35–36, 651, 652, 653
Monocid (cefonicid), 88
Monocytes (macrophages), 145, 266
Mononuclear cells, 266
Monopril (fosinopril), 67
Mons veneris, 534
Montelukast (Singulair), 73
Mood, 626
Mood disorders, 649–653
  analysis, 649
  assessment, 649

bipolar disorders, 649, 650, 651
dysthymic disorder, 649, 650, 653
evaluation, 651
major depression, 650, 651–653
patterns of mood disturbances, 651
planning and implementation, 649–651
Morals, 116
Moricizine (Ethmozine), 60
Morning sickness, 548
Moro reflex, 424, 592
Morphine, 185, 218, 478, 573, 643
Morphine sulfate, 27, 247, 331
Mosaicism, 442
Motor neurons, 200
Motor pathways, 201
Motor skills, parenthood and, 582
Motrin (ibuprofen), 26, 156, 367
Mourning, 679–680
Mouth, 307–308
  cancer of, 316
Moxifloxacin (Avelox), 93
MRI. *See* Magnetic resonance imaging (MRI)
MS. *See* Multiple sclerosis (MS)
MSH. *See* Melanocyte-stimulating hormone (MSH)
Mucolytics, 74–75
Mucomyst (acetylcysteine), 74–75, 447
Multigravida, 543
Multilumen catheters, 163
Multipara, 543
Multiple myeloma, 192, 277–278
Multiple sclerosis (MS), 216–217
Multiple trauma, 166
Multisystem stressors (adult), 144–173
  acid-base balance, 161–162
  fluids and electrolytes, 158–161
  immune response, 144–145
  infection, 155
  inflammatory response, 144
  intravenous therapy, 162–164
  multiple trauma, 166
  nutrition, 146–155
  pain, 155–158
  sample questions, 166–172
  shock, 164–165
  stress and adaptation, 144
Multisystem stressors (pediatric), 441–450
  accidents, poisonings, and ingestion, 446–448
  fluid and electrolyte, acid-base balances, 443–446
  genetic disorders, 441–443
  sample questions, 448–450
Mumps (parotitis), 435
Muscle relaxants, 32
Muscles, 362
  childhood development, 507
Muscular dystrophy, 512
Musculoskeletal effects of immobility, 126
Musculoskeletal injuries, 166
Musculoskeletal system (adult), 361–381
  age-related changes, 174
  analysis, 363
  assessment, 362–363
  bones, 361
  cartilage, 362
  evaluation, 366
  joints, 362
  muscles, 362

# S

Saccular aneurysm, 252
Saddle block, 185
Safe, effective care environment, 2
Safety, 121–129
  asepsis, 127–128
  body mechanics, 122
  client positioning, 123–125
  cold application, 125
  equipment, 122
  external heat application, 127
  fire safety/preparedness practices, 121–122
  immobility, 125, 126–127
  pressure ulcer, 128–129
  principles and interventions for specific aspects of care, 122–128
  restraints, 122
  transfer and movement principles and techniques, 122–123
  universal/clinical issues, 128–129
Safety and infection control, 2
Salicylate poisoning, 447
Salicylates, 25, 156, 250, 472
Saline abortion, 610
Salivary glands, 307
  autonomic nervous system effect on, 203
Sandimmune (cyclosporine), 104, 352
SA node. See Sinoatrial (SA) node
Sansert (methylsergide maleate), 211
Saquinavir (Fortovase), 275
Sarcoma, 192
  Ewing's, 530
  osteogenic, 530
Sarfak (docusate calcium), 316
SASH method, 17
Saw palmetto, 108
Scarf sign, 593
Schilling test, 272
Schizophrenia, 647–649
School-age children
  developmental stage, 429–430
  response to death, 437
Sclera, 202
Scleral buckling, 226
Scoliosis, 510–511
  surgery for, 511
Scopolamine (Hyoscine, Transderm-Scop), 43, 82, 184
Scoring, 3
Scrotum, 342, 343
Sebaceous glands, 407
Secobarbital (Seconal), 30, 184, 573
Secondary hypertension, 250
Second stage of labor, 567–568
Second trimester bleeding complications, 549
Secretory phase, of menstrual cycle, 536
Sedatives, 29–31
  for labor analgesia, 573
  preoperative, 184
Seizure disorders, 456–457
Selective alpha agonists, 38
Selective beta-1 agonists, 39
Selective beta-2 agonists, 39
Selective estrogen receptor modulators (SERMs), 52
Selective serotonin reputake inhibitors (SSRIs), 36, 640, 652, 654
Selegilene (eldepryl), 216

Self-mutilation, 633
Self-needs analysis, 3–4
Semi-Fowler's position, 123
Semilunar vales, 236–237
Seminal vesicles, 343
Sengstaken-Blakemore tube, 329
Senile dementia, 178–179
Senile keratoses, 409
Senna (Senokot), 80, 316
Sensorineural hearing loss, 205
Sensory neurons, 200
Sensory pathways, 201
Sensory perception, 406
Sensory system, newborn, 591–592
Separation anxiety, 428, 639
Sepsis, neonatal, 602–603
Septic shock, 164
Septra (trimethoprim-sulfamethoxazole), 275, 348
Serax (oxazepam), 654
Serentil (mesoridazine), 33
SERMs. See Selective estrogen receptor modulators (SERMs)
Seroquel (quetapine), 648
Serotonin-blocking agents, 81, 82
Serpalan (reserpine), 66, 215
Sertraline (Zoloft), 36, 651, 652
Serum globulins, 265
Serzone (nefazodone), 37, 652
Seventh-Day Adventists, 130
Sex hormones, 382, 383
  as chemotherapeutic drugs, 192
Sex-linked (X-linked) inheritance, 442
Sexual abuse, 434, 675
Sexual development
  boys, 430
  girls, 430
Sexually transmitted disease (STD), 612
Sexual response, in female, 536
SGA. See Dysmature infant (SGA)
Shingles, 410
Shock, 164–165, 166
  anaphylactic, 164
  assessment findings, 165
  body's response to, 164–165
  cardiogenic, 164
  classification of, 164
  drugs used to treat, 165
  hypovolemic, 164
  neurogenic, 164
  nursing interventions, 165
  postoperative, 187
  septic, 164
  spinal, 220
Shock lung (adult respiratory distress syndrome), 165
Shoulder presentation, 560, 561
Shunts, 453–454
SIADH. See Syndrome of inappropriate antidiuretic hormone secretion (SIADH)
Sickle-cell anemia, 476, 477–478
Sickle cell crisis, 477
Sickling tests, 477–478
Side effects, cancer treatment, 524
SIDS. See Sudden infant death syndrome (SIDS)
Sigmoidoscopy, 312
Sildenafil (Viagra), 52
Silvadene (silver sulfadiazine), 410, 412
Silver nitrate, 410, 412

Venules, 237
VePesid (etoposide), 102
Verapamil (Calan, Isoptin), 56, 58–59, 249
Vermox (mebendazole), 96
Vernix, 595
Versed (midazolam), 30, 185
Vertex presentation, 562, 563
Vesicle, 408
Vesicoureteral reflux, 502
Vestibular apparatus, 203
Vestibule, 534
Viagra (sildenafil), 52
Vibramycin (doxycycline), 90
Victims of abuse, 674
Videx (didanosine), 275
Villi, 308
Vinblastine (Velban), 102
Vincristine (Oncovin), 102, 297, 528
Viokase, 488
Viracept (nelfinavir), 275
Viral theory of cancer, 191
Viramune (nevirapine), 95, 275
Virazole (ribavirin), 95, 486
Vision, 202–203
    age-related changes in, 174
    care of client with diminished, 209–210
    eye, 202
    newborn, 592
    pediatric, 451
    visual pathways, 203
Vision tests, 451
Vistaril (hydroxyzine), 156, 315, 573
Vital signs, in neuro check, 205
Vitamins, 104–105, 147, 149–150
    A, 149
    $B_1$, 149
    $B_2$, 149
    B3, 65
    $B_6$, 150
    $B_{12}$, 150, 272
    C, 150
    D, 149, 393
    deficiency syndromes, 148–150
    E, 149, 615
    fat-soluble, 147, 149
    K, 149, 594
    need during pregnancy, 545
    water-soluble, 147, 149–150
Vitreous humor, 202
Voluntary commitment, 118
Vomiting, 314–315, 446
VP-16 (etoposide), 102
VSD. See Ventricular septal defect (VSD)
Vulva, cancer of, 614

## W

Walker, 363
Walking, assistive devices, 363–364
Wallaby blanket, 601
Warfarin (Coumadin), 62, 63, 213, 254, 255
"Watchful waiting," 354
Water, 147, 150
Water deficit syndromes, 159, 161
Water excess syndromes, 159, 161
Water-seal drainage systems, 287, 288
Water-soluble vitamins, 147, 149–150

WBCs. See White blood cells (WBCs)
Weber's test, 205
Weight
    height and weight charts, 150
    newborn, 594
Weight control diets, 152
Weight gain, during pregnancy, 545
Wellbutrin (bupropion), 37, 652
West nomogram, 21
Wet suction, 287
Wharton's jelly, 539
Wheal, 408
Wheelchair transfers, 122
Wheezing, 482
Whipple's procedure, 333
White blood cells (WBCs), 145
    disorders of, 479
White matter, 201
Whole blood, 270
Whooping cough, 435
Wilms' tumor (nephroblastoma), 529
Withdrawal, 633
Women's health agents, 51–52
Worms, parasitic, 498
Wound care treatments, 129
Wound complications, 187–188

## X

Xanax (alprazolam), 30, 654
Xanthine-derivatives, 487
X-linked inheritance, 442
X-rays, 207, 362, 546
Xylocaine (lidocaine), 23–24, 56, 60, 244, 249, 574
Xylometazoline, 38

## Y

Yellow marrow, 264
Yutopar (ritodrine), 39, 569–570

## Z

Zafirlukast (Accolate), 73
Zagam (sparfloxacin), 93
Zantac (ranitidine), 76, 319
Zarontin (ethosuximide), 31
Zaroxolyn (metolazone), 67, 70
ZDV (zidovudine), 95, 275
Zefazone (cefmetazole), 88
Zerit (stavudine), 275
Zestril (lisinopril), 67
Ziagen (abacavir), 275
Zidovudine (AZT, Retrovir), 95, 275
Zileuton (Zyflo), 73
Zinecard
Ziprasidone (Geodon), 648
Zithromax (azithromycin), 89
Zocor (simvastatin), 65
Zofran (ondansetron HCl), 82
Zoloft (sertraline), 36, 651, 652
Zolpidem (Ambien), 30
Zovirax (acyclovir), 95, 410
Z-track injection, 16
Zyflo (zileuton), 73
Zygote, 538
Zyloprim (allopurinal), 84, 368
Zyprexa (olanzapine), 37, 648
Zyrtec (cetirizine), 74
Zyvox (linezolid), 86

## SYSTEM REQUIREMENTS FOR NCLEX-RN

Operating Systems: Microsoft® WindowsTM XP, Microsoft Vista

- RAM: Minimum required by operating system
- Hard disk space: 100MB
- Display: SVGA-compatible
- Graphics adapter: SVGA or higher: 800 × 600, true color (24-bit or 32-bit), or high color (16-bit) modes
- CD-ROM drive: 8x or faster

### Setup Instructions

1. Insert disc into CD-ROM drive. The setup routine should automatically start. You will be prompted by install instructions. Follow through to end. If it does not automatically start, go to step 2.
2. From "My Computer," double click the icon for the CD-drive.
3. Double click on "setup.exe"

CENGAGE LEARNING HAS PROVIDED YOU WITH THIS PRODUCT FOR YOUR REVIEW AND, TO THE EXTENT THAT YOU ADOPT THE ASSOCIATED TEXTBOOK FOR USE IN CONNECTION WITH YOUR COURSE, YOU AND YOUR STUDENTS WHO PURCHASE THE TEXTBOOK MAY USE THE MATERIALS AS DESCRIBED BELOW.

**IMPORTANT! READ CAREFULLY**: This End User License Agreement ("Agreement") sets forth the conditions by which Cengage Learning will make electronic access to the Cengage Learning-owned licensed content and associated media, software, documentation, printed materials, and electronic documentation contained in this package and/or made available to you via this product (the "Licensed Content"), available to you (the "End User"). BY CLICKING THE "I ACCEPT" BUTTON AND/OR OPENING THIS PACKAGE, YOU ACKNOWLEDGE THAT YOU HAVE READ ALL OF THE TERMS AND CONDITIONS, AND THAT YOU AGREE TO BE BOUND BY ITS TERMS, CONDITIONS, AND ALL APPLICABLE LAWS AND REGULATIONS GOVERNING THE USE OF THE LICENSED CONTENT.

### 1.0 SCOPE OF LICENSE

1.1 <u>Licensed Content.</u> The Licensed Content may contain portions of modifiable content ("Modifiable Content") and content which may not be modified or otherwise altered by the End User ("Non-Modifiable Content"). For purposes of this Agreement, Modifiable Content and Non-Modifiable Content may be collectively referred to herein as the "Licensed Content." All Licensed Content shall be considered Non-Modifiable Content, unless such Licensed Content is presented to the End User in a modifiable format and it is clearly indicated that modification of the Licensed Content is permitted.

1.2 Subject to the End User's compliance with the terms and conditions of this Agreement, Cengage Learning hereby grants the End User, a nontransferable, nonexclusive, limited right to access and view a single copy of the Licensed Content on a single personal computer system for noncommercial, internal, personal use only, and, to the extent that End User adopts the associated textbook for use in connection with a course, the limited right to provide, distribute, and display the Modifiable Content to course students who purchase the textbook, for use in connection with the course only. The End User shall not (i) reproduce, copy, modify (except in the case of Modifiable Content), distribute, display, transfer, sublicense, prepare derivative work(s) based on, sell, exchange, barter or transfer, rent, lease, loan, resell, or in any other manner exploit the Licensed Content; (ii) remove, obscure, or alter any notice of Cengage Learning's intellectual property rights present on or in the Licensed Content, including, but not limited to, copyright, trademark, and/or patent notices; or (iii) disassemble, decompile, translate, reverse engineer, or otherwise reduce the Licensed Content. Cengage reserves the right to use a hardware lock device, license administration software, and/or a license authorization key to control access or password protection technology to the Licensed Content. The End User may not take any steps to avoid or defeat the purpose of such measures. Use of the Licensed Content without the relevant required lock device or authorization key is prohibited. UNDER NO CIRCUMSTANCES MAY NON-SALEABLE ITEMS PROVIDED TO YOU BY CENGAGE (INCLUDING, WITHOUT LIMITATION, ANNOTATED INSTRUCTOR'S EDITIONS, SOLUTIONS MANUALS, INSTRUCTOR'S RESOURCE MATERIALS AND/OR TEST MATERIALS) BE SOLD, AUCTIONED, LICENSED OR OTHERWISE REDISTRIBUTED BY THE END USER.

### 2.0 TERMINATION

2.1 Cengage Learning may at any time (without prejudice to its other rights or remedies) immediately terminate this Agreement and/or suspend access to some or all of the Licensed Content, in the event that the End User does not comply with any of the terms and conditions of this Agreement. In the event of such termination by Cengage Learning, the End User shall immediately return any and all copies of the Licensed Content to Cengage Learning.

### 3.0 PROPRIETARY RIGHTS

3.1 The End User acknowledges that Cengage Learning owns all rights, title and interest, including, but not limited to all copyright rights therein, in and to the Licensed Content, and that the End User shall not take any action inconsistent with such ownership. The Licensed Content is protected by U.S., Canadian and other applicable copyright laws and by international treaties, including the Berne Convention and the Universal Copyright Convention. Nothing contained in this Agreement shall be construed as granting the End User any ownership rights in or to the Licensed Content.

3.2 Cengage Learning reserves the right at any time to withdraw from the Licensed Content any item or part of an item for which it no longer retains the right to publish, or which it has reasonable grounds to believe infringes copyright or is defamatory, unlawful, or otherwise objectionable.

## 4.0 PROTECTION AND SECURITY

4.1 The End User shall use its best efforts and take all reasonable steps to safeguard its copy of the Licensed Content to ensure that no unauthorized reproduction, publication, disclosure, modification, or distribution of the Licensed Content, in whole or in part, is made. To the extent that the End User becomes aware of any such unauthorized use of the Licensed Content, the End User shall immediately notify Cengage Learning. Notification of such violations may be made by sending an e-mail to infringement@cengage.com.

## 5.0 MISUSE OF THE LICENSED PRODUCT

5.1 In the event that the End User uses the Licensed Content in violation of this Agreement, Cengage Learning shall have the option of electing liquidated damages, which shall include all profits generated by the End User's use of the Licensed Content plus interest computed at the maximum rate permitted by law and all legal fees and other expenses incurred by Cengage Learning in enforcing its rights, plus penalties.

## 6.0 FEDERAL GOVERNMENT CLIENTS

6.1 Except as expressly authorized by Cengage Learning, Federal Government clients obtain only the rights specified in this Agreement and no other rights. The Government acknowledges that (i) all software and related documentation incorporated in the Licensed Content is existing commercial computer software within the meaning of FAR 27.405(b)(2); and (2) all other data delivered in whatever form, is limited rights data within the meaning of FAR 27.401. The restrictions in this section are acceptable as consistent with the Government's need for software and other data under this Agreement.

## 7.0 DISCLAIMER OF WARRANTIES AND LIABILITIES

7.1 Although Cengage Learning believes the Licensed Content to be reliable, Cengage Learning does not guarantee or warrant (i) any information or materials contained in or produced by the Licensed Content, (ii) the accuracy, completeness or reliability of the Licensed Content, or (iii) that the Licensed Content is free from errors or other material defects. THE LICENSED PRODUCT IS PROVIDED "AS IS," WITHOUT ANY WARRANTY OF ANY KIND AND CENGAGE LEARNING DISCLAIMS ANY AND ALL WARRANTIES, EXPRESSED OR IMPLIED, INCLUDING, WITHOUT LIMITATION, WARRANTIES OF MERCHANTABILITY OR FITNESS FOR A PARTICULAR PURPOSE. IN NO EVENT SHALL CENGAGE LEARNING BE LIABLE FOR: INDIRECT, SPECIAL, PUNITIVE OR CONSEQUENTIAL DAMAGES INCLUDING FOR LOST PROFITS, LOST DATA, OR OTHERWISE. IN NO EVENT SHALL CENGAGE LEARNING'S AGGREGATE LIABILITY HEREUNDER, WHETHER ARISING IN CONTRACT, TORT, STRICT LIABILITY OR OTHERWISE, EXCEED THE AMOUNT OF FEES PAID BY THE END USER HEREUNDER FOR THE LICENSE OF THE LICENSED CONTENT.

## 8.0 GENERAL

8.1 Entire Agreement. This Agreement shall constitute the entire Agreement between the Parties and supercedes all prior Agreements and understandings oral or written relating to the subject matter hereof.

8.2 Enhancements/Modifications of Licensed Content. From time to time, and in Cengage Learning's sole discretion, Cengage Learning may advise the End User of updates, upgrades, enhancements and/or improvements to the Licensed Content, and may permit the End User to access and use, subject to the terms and conditions of this Agreement, such modifications, upon payment of prices as may be established by Cengage Learning.

8.3 No Export. The End User shall use the Licensed Content solely in the United States and shall not transfer or export, directly or indirectly, the Licensed Content outside the United States.

8.4 Severability. If any provision of this Agreement is invalid, illegal, or unenforceable under any applicable statute or rule of law, the provision shall be deemed omitted to the extent that it is invalid, illegal, or unenforceable. In such a case, the remainder of the Agreement shall be construed in a manner as to give greatest effect to the original intention of the parties hereto.

8.5 Waiver. The waiver of any right or failure of either party to exercise in any respect any right provided in this Agreement in any instance shall not be deemed to be a waiver of such right in the future or a waiver of any other right under this Agreement.

8.6 Choice of Law/Venue. This Agreement shall be interpreted, construed, and governed by and in accordance with the laws of the State of New York, applicable to contracts executed and to be wholly preformed therein, without regard to its principles governing conflicts of law. Each party agrees that any proceeding arising out of or relating to this Agreement or the breach or threatened breach of this Agreement may be commenced and prosecuted in a court in the State and County of New York. Each party consents and submits to the nonexclusive personal jurisdiction of any court in the State and County of New York in respect of any such proceeding.

8.7 Acknowledgment. By opening this package and/or by accessing the Licensed Content on this Web site, THE END USER ACKNOWLEDGES THAT IT HAS READ THIS AGREEMENT, UNDERSTANDS IT, AND AGREES TO BE BOUND BY ITS TERMS AND CONDITIONS. IF YOU DO NOT ACCEPT THESE TERMS AND CONDITIONS, YOU MUST NOT ACCESS THE LICENSED CONTENT AND RETURN THE LICENSED PRODUCT TO CENGAGE LEARNING (WITHIN 30 CALENDAR DAYS OF THE END USER'S PURCHASE) WITH PROOF OF PAYMENT ACCEPTABLE TO CENGAGE LEARNING, FOR A CREDIT OR A REFUND. Should the End User have any questions/comments regarding this Agreement, please contact Cengage Learning at delmar.help@cengage.com.